Community and Public Health Nursing | 3rd edition

EVIDENCE FOR PRACTICE

Rosanna F. DeMarco, PhD, RN, FAAN
Chair and Professor
Department of Nursing
College of Nursing and Health Sciences
University of Massachusetts Boston
Boston, Massachusetts

Judith Healey-Walsh, PhD, RN
Clinical Associate Professor
Director of the Undergraduate Program
Department of Nursing
College of Nursing and Health Sciences
University of Massachusetts Boston
Boston, Massachusetts

Wolters Kluwer

Philadelphia • Baltimore • New York • London
Buenos Aires • Hong Kong • Sydney • Tokyo

Vice President and Publisher: Julie K. Stegman
Senior Acquisitions Editor: Christina Burns
Director of Product Development: Jennifer K. Forestieri
Supervisory Development Editor: Greg Nicholl and Staci Wolfson
Editorial Coordinator: John Larkin
Editorial Assistant: Kate Campbell
Production Project Manager: Linda Van Pelt
Design Coordinator: Terry Mallon
Marketing Manager: Brittany Clements
Manufacturing Coordinator: Karin Duffield
Prepress Vendor: Aptara, Inc.

3rd Edition

Library of Congress Cataloging-in-Publication Data

Names: DeMarco, Rosanna F., author. | Healey-Walsh, Judith, author. |
    Preceded by (work): Harkness, Gail A. Community and public health
nursing.
Title: Community and public health nursing : evidence for practice / Rosanna
    F. DeMarco, Judith Healey-Walsh.
Description: 3. | Philadelphia : Wolters Kluwer, [2020] | Preceded by
    Community and public health nursing / Gail A. Harkness, Rosanna F.
    DeMarco. Second edition. [2016]. | Includes bibliographical references
and index.
Identifiers: LCCN 2018058862 | ISBN 9781975111694 (paperback)
Subjects: | MESH: Community Health Nursing | Public Health Nursing |
    Evidence-Based Nursing | Nursing Theory | United States
Classification: LCC RT98 | NLM WY 108 | DDC 610.73/43—dc23
LC record available at https://lccn.loc.gov/2018058862

Care has been taken to confirm the accuracy of the information presented and to describe generally accepted practices. However, the author(s), editors, and publisher are not responsible for errors or omissions or for any consequences from application of the information in this book and make no warranty, expressed or implied, with respect to the currency, completeness, or accuracy of the contents of the publication. Application of this information in a particular situation remains the professional responsibility of the practitioner; the clinical treatments described and recommended may not be considered absolute and universal recommendations.

The author(s), editors, and publisher have exerted every effort to ensure that drug selection and dosage set forth in this text are in accordance with the current recommendations and practice at the time of publication. However, in view of ongoing research, changes in government regulations, and the constant flow of information relating to drug therapy and drug reactions, the reader is urged to check the package insert for each drug for any change in indications and dosage and for added warnings and precautions. This is particularly important when the recommended agent is a new or infrequently employed drug.

Some drugs and medical devices presented in this publication have Food and Drug Administration (FDA) clearance for limited use in restricted research settings. It is the responsibility of the health care provider to ascertain the FDA status of each drug or device planned for use in his or her clinical practice.

CCS0319

Contributors

Stephanie M. Chalupka, EdD, RN, PHCNS-BC, FAAOHN, FNAP
Associate Dean for Nursing
Department of Nursing
Worcester State University
Worcester
Visiting Scientist
Environmental and Occupational Medicine and
Epidemiology Program
Department of Environmental Health
Harvard T. H. Chan School of Public Health
Boston, Massachusetts
(Chapter 9, Planning for Community Change)

Susan K. Chase, EdD, RN, FNAP
Professor
College of Nursing
University of Central Florida
Orlando, Florida
(Chapter 23, Faith-Oriented Communities and Health Ministries in Faith Communities)

Sabreen A. Darwish, RN, BScN, MScN
Second Year PhD Student/Research Assistant
College of Nursing and Health Sciences
University of Massachusetts
Boston, Massachusetts
(Chapter 3, Health Policy, Politics, and Reform)

Karen Dawn, RN, DNP, PHCNS, CDE
Assistant Professor
School of Nursing
George Washington University
Ashburn, Virginia
(Chapter 4, Global Health: A Community Perspective)

Pamela Pershing DiNapoli, PhD, RN, CNL
Associate Professor of Nursing and Graduate Programs
College of Health and Human Services
University of New Hampshire
Durham, New Hampshire
(Chapter 22, School Health)

Merrily Evdokimoff, PhD, RN
Consultant
Clinical Associate Lecturer
Department of Nursing
University of Massachusetts
Boston, Massachusetts
(Chapter 20, Community Preparedness: Disaster and Terrorism)

Barbara A. Goldrick, MPH, PhD, RN
Epidemiology Consultant
Chatham, Massachusetts
(Chapter 8, Gathering Evidence for Public Health Practice; Chapter 14, Risk of Infectious and Communicable Diseases; Chapter 15, Emerging Infectious Diseases)

Patricia Goyette, DNP-PHNL, RN
Educational Consultant
Everett, Massachusetts
(Chapter 25, Occupational Health Nursing)

Cheryl L. Hersperger, MS, RN, PHNA-BC, PhD Student
Assistant Professor
Department of Nursing
Worcester State University
Worcester, Massachusetts
(Chapter 9, Planning for Community Change)

Anahid Kulwicki, PhD, RN, FAAN
Dean and Professor
School of Nursing
Lebanese American University
Beirut, Lebanon
(Chapter 3, Health Policy, Politics, and Reform)

Annie Lewis-O'Connor, PhD, NP-BC, MPH, FAAN
Senior Nurse Scientist and Founder and Director of C.A.R.E Clinic
Brigham and Women's Hospital
Boston, Massachusetts
(Chapter 16, Violence and Abuse)

Patricia Lussier-Duynstee, PhD, RN
Assistant Dean
Assistant Professor
School of Nursing
MGH Institute of Health Professions
Boston, Massachusetts
(Chapter 6, Epidemiology: The Science of Prevention;
Chapter 7, Describing Health Conditions: Understanding
and Using Rates)

Kiara Manosalvas, MA
Reseach Assistant II The Following & Mental Health
Counselor
Teachers College
Columbia University
Chestnut Hill, Massachusetts
(Chapter 16, Violence and Abuse)

Patrice Nicholas, DNSc, DHL (Hon.), MPH, MS, RN, NP-C,
FAAN
Professor
School of Nursing
MGH Institute of Health Professions
Director, Global Health and Academic Partnerships
Brigham and Women's Hospital
Boston, Massachusetts
(Chapter 6, Epidemiology: The Science of Prevention;
Chapter 7, Describing Health Conditions: Understanding
and Using Rates)

Christine Pontus, RN, MS, BSN, COHN-S/CCM
Associate Director in Nursing and Occupational Health
Massachusetts Nurses Association (MNA)
Canton, Massachusetts
(Chapter 25, Occupational Health Nursing)

Joyce Pulcini, PhD, RN, PNP-BC, FAAN, FAANP
Professor
Director of Community and Global Initiatives
Chair, Acute and Chronic Care Community
School of Nursing
George Washington University
Washington, DC
(Chapter 4, Global Health: A Community Perspective)

Teresa Eliot Roberts, PhD, RN, ANP
Clinical Assistant Professor
College of Nursing and Health Sciences
University of Massachusetts Boston
Boston, Massachusetts
(Chapter 10, Cultural Competence: Awareness, Sensitivity,
and Respect)

Judith Shindul-Rothschild, PhD, MSN, RN
Associate Professor
Connell School of Nursing
Boston College
Chestnut Hill, Massachusetts
(Chapter 17, Substance Use;
Chapter 21, Community Mental Health)

Joy Spellman, MSN, RN
Director, Center for Public Health Preparedness
Mt. Laurel, New Jersey
(Chapter 20, Community Preparedness: Disaster and
Terrorism)

Tarah S. Somers, RN, MSN/MPH
Senior Regional Director
Agency for Toxic Substances and Disease Registry,
New England Office
US Public Health Service Commissioned Corps
Boston, Massachusetts
(Chapter 19, Environmental Health)

Patricia Tabloski, PhD, GNP-BC, FGSA, FAAN
Associate Professor
Connell School of Nursing
Boston College
Chestnut Hill, Massachusetts
(Chapter 24, Palliative and End-of-Life Care)

Aitana Zermeno, BS
Research Assistant
Connors Center for Women's Health and Gender Biology
Division of Women's Health
Brigham and Women's Hospital
Boston, Massachusetts
(Chapter 16, Violence and Abuse)

Reviewers

Elizabeth Armstrong, DNP, MSN, RN, CNE
Assistant Professor
School of Nursing
University of Bridgeport
Bridgeport, Connecticut

Karen Cooper, MS, RN
Clinical Assistant Professor
Department of Nursing
Towson University
Towson, Maryland

Teresa E. Darnall, PhD, MSN, RN, CNE
Assistant Dean
Assistant Professor
May School of Nursing and Health Sciences
Lees-McRae College
Banner Elk, North Carolina

Florence Viveen Dood, DNP, MSN, BSN, RN
RN-BSN Program Coordinator
Assistant Professor
School of Nursing
Ferris State University
Big Rapids, Michigan

Aimee McDonald, PhD, RN
Assistant Professor
Department of Nursing
William Jewell College
Liberty, Missouri

Rita M. Million, PhD, RN, PHNA-BC, COI
Nursing Faculty
School of Nursing
College of Saint Mary
Omaha, Nebraska

Deanna R. Pope, DNP, RN, CNE
Professor
School of Nursing
Marshall University
Huntington, West Virginia

Kendra Schmitz, RN, MSN
Assistant Professor
School of Nursing
D'Youville College
Buffalo, New York

Kathleen F. Tate, MSN, MBA, CNE, RN
Assistant Professor
School of Nursing
Northwestern State University
Natchitoches, Louisiana

Preface

"If you want to go quickly, go alone. If you want to go far, go together."
African Proverb

"The idea that some lives matter less is the root of all that is wrong in the world."
Paul Farmer

"No matter what people tell you, words and ideas can change the world."
Robin Williams

We are experiencing extraordinary changes in healthcare in this new century; changes that call upon the most creative, analytical, and innovative skills available. While the world has the resources to reduce healthcare disparities and eliminate the differences in healthcare and health outcomes that exist between various population groups across the globe, accomplishing this is a long-term and complicated task. Improvement in the social structure within which people live, and a redistribution of resources so that all people have access to the basic necessities of life, require an unprecedented global consciousness and political commitment.

Ultimately, reducing health disparities and promoting health equity occur within the local community where people reside. Nurses are by far the largest group of healthcare providers worldwide and, as such, have the ability and responsibility to be change agents and leaders in implementing change in their communities. They can be the primary participants in the development of health policy that specifically addresses the unique needs of their communities. Through implementation and evaluation of culturally appropriate, community-based programs, nurses can use their expertise to remedy the conditions that contribute to health disparities. People need to be assured that their healthcare needs will be assessed and that healthcare is available and accessible.

In the United States, public health has resurged as a national priority. Through *Healthy People 2020*, national goals have been set to promote a healthy population and address the issue of health disparities. The process of implementing the *Healthy People 2020* objectives rests with regional and local practitioners, with nurses having a direct responsibility in the implementation process. The nurse practicing in the community has a central role in providing direct care for the ill as well as promoting and maintaining the health of groups of people, regardless of the circumstances that exist. Today, there are unparalleled challenges to the nurse's problem-solving skills in carrying out this mission.

Whether caring for the individual or the members of a community, it is essential that nurses incorporate evidence from multiple sources in the analysis and solution of public health issues. *Community and Public Health Nursing: Evidence for Practice* focuses on evidence-based practice, presenting multiple formats designed to develop the abstract critical thinking skills and complex reasoning abilities necessary for nurses becoming generalists in community and public health nursing. The unique blend of both the nursing process and the epidemiologic process provides a framework for gathering evidence about health problems, analyzing the information, generating diagnoses or hypotheses, planning for resolution, implementing plans of action, and evaluating the results.

"To every complex question there is a simple answer ... and it is wrong." **H. L. Mencken (writer and wit, 1880–1956)**

CONTENT ORGANIZATION

It is the intention of *Community and Public Health Nursing: Evidence for Practice* to present the core content of community and public health nursing in a succinct, logically organized, but comprehensive manner. The evidence for practice focus not only includes chapters on epidemiology, biostatistics, and research but also integrates these topics throughout the text. Concrete examples assist students in interpreting and applying statistical data. *Healthy People* goals and measurable objectives serve as an illustration of the use of rates throughout the text. Additionally, we have added brief learning activities and questions throughout the text to allow students to apply the *Healthy People* goals to real-life scenarios. Groups with special needs, such as refugees and the homeless, have been addressed in several chapters; however, tangential topics that can be found in adult health and maternal-child health textbooks have been omitted. A chapter on environmental health concerns has been included, along with a chapter on community preparedness for emergencies and disasters. Also, a global perspective has been incorporated into many chapters.

Challenges to critical thinking are presented in multiple places throughout each chapter. Case studies are integrated into the content of each chapter and contain critical thinking questions imbedded in the case study content. Also, a series of critical thinking questions can be found at the end of each chapter. (Please see the description of features below.) Considering the onus presented by Mark Twain: *"Be careful about reading health books. You may die of a misprint,"* every attempt has been made to present correct, meaningful, and current evidence for practice.

Part One presents the context within which the community or public health nurse practices. An overview of the major drivers of healthcare change leads to a discussion of evolving trends, such as the emphasis on patient/client-centered care, the effects of new technology upon the delivery of care, and the need for people to assume more responsibility for maintaining their health. Community and public health nursing as it presently exists is analyzed and reviewed from a historical base, and issues foreseen for both the present and immediate future are discussed. The nursing competencies necessary for competent community and public health practice are also presented.

A more in-depth discussion of the complex structure, function, and outcomes of public health and healthcare systems follows. National and international perspectives regarding philosophical and political attitudes, social structures, economics, resources, financing mechanisms, and historical contexts are presented, highlighting healthcare organizations and issues in several developed countries. The World Health Organization's commitment to improving the public's health in developing countries follows, with an emphasis on refugees and disaster relief. With the burden of disease growing disproportionately in the world, largely due to climate, public policy, socioeconomic conditions, age, and an imbalance in distribution of risk factors, the countries burdened by disease often have the least capacity to institute change. Part One concludes with examination of the indicators of health, health and human rights, factors that affect health globally, and a framework for improving world health.

Part Two provides the frameworks and tools necessary to engage in evidence-based practice focused on the population's health. Concepts of health literacy, health promotion, disease prevention, and risk reduction are explored, and a variety of conceptual frameworks are presented with a focus on both the epidemiologic and ecologic models. Epidemiology is presented as the science of prevention, and nurses are shown how epidemiologic principles are applied in practice, including the use of rates and other statistics as community health indicators. Specific research designs are also explored, including the application of epidemiologic research to practice settings.

Part Three is designed to develop the skills necessary to implement nursing practice effectively in community settings. Since healthcare is in a unique state of transformation, planning for community change is paramount. The health planning process is described, with specific attention given to the social and environmental determinants of change. Lewin's change theory, force-field analysis, and the effective use of leverage points identified in the force-field analysis demonstrate the change process in action.

Changes directed at decreasing health disparities must be culturally sensitive, client-centered, and community-oriented. A chapter on cultural diversity and values fosters the development of culturally competent practitioners, and the process of cultural health assessment is highlighted. Frameworks of community assessment are presented and various approaches are explored. Management of care and the case management process follows. The role and scope of home care nursing practice and the provision of services is presented along with the challenges inherent with interdisciplinary roles, advances in telehealth, and other home care services.

Although content on family assessment can be found in other texts, it is an integral component of community and public health practice. Therefore, theoretical perspectives of family, and contemporary family configurations and life cycles are explored. Family Systems Nursing and the Calgary Family Assessment and Intervention Model are provided as guides to implementing family nursing practice in the community. Evidence-based maternal-child health home visiting programs and prominent issues related to family caregiving are also highlighted.

Part Four presents the common challenges in community and public health nursing. The chapter addressing the risk of infectious and communicable diseases explores outbreak investigation with analysis of data experience provided by the case studies. Public health surveillance, the risk of common foodborne and waterborne illnesses, and sexually transmitted diseases are followed by a discussion of factors that influence the emergence/reemergence of infectious diseases, examples of recent outbreaks, and means of prevention and control.

The challenge presented by violence in the community is presented with an emphasis on intimate partner violence and the role of the healthcare provider. Because of the cultural variations in substance use disorder, multifaceted approaches to the problem are discussed with the recommendation that evidence-based prevention and treatment protocols for substance use disorder are incorporated by community health nurses in all practice settings. Meeting the healthcare needs of vulnerable and underserved populations is another challenge. Health priorities for people who live in rural areas; are gay, lesbian, bisexual, or transgender; are homeless; or live in correctional institutions are reviewed.

The issues of access to quality care, chronic disease management, interaction with health personnel, and health promotion in hard-to-reach populations among these populations are also presented.

The environmental chapter demonstrates how to assess contaminants in the community by creation of an exposure pathway. The health effects of the exposure pathway can then be ascertained. Individual assessment of contaminant exposures, interventions, and evaluations are also explored, ending with a focus on maintaining healthy communities. The final chapter in Part Four presents the issue of community preparedness. The types of disasters along with classification of agents are described, disaster management outlined, and the public health response explained. The role and responsibility of nurses in disasters and characteristics of the field response complete the content.

Part Five describes five common specialty practices within community and public health nursing. All have frameworks that define practice and reflect the competencies necessary for competent practice in a variety of community settings. These include application of the principles of practice to community mental health, school health, faith-oriented communities, palliative care, and occupational health nursing.

Features Found in Each Chapter

CHAPTER HIGHLIGHTS

Brief outline of the content and direction of the chapter

OBJECTIVES

Observable changes expected following completion of the chapter

KEY TERMS

Essential concepts and terminology required for comprehension of chapter content

CASE STUDIES

Vignettes presented throughout the content of each chapter, designed to stimulate critical thinking and analytic skills

Evidence for Practice

Examples of objective evidence obtained from research studies that provide direction for practice

Practice Point

Highlighting of essential facts relevant to practice

Student Reflection

Student stories of their own experience and reflections

KEY CONCEPTS

Summary of important concepts presented in the chapter

CRITICAL THINKING QUESTIONS

Problems requiring critical analysis that combines research, context, and judgment

COMMUNITY RESOURCES

List of resources that support the content of selected chapters

I didn't fail the test, I just found 100 ways to do it wrong.
Benjamin Franklin

Acknowledgments

It is difficult to embark on the development of a new textbook without the support of colleagues, family, and friends. A special thanks belongs to our contributors, both returning and new, who were willing to share their expertise by writing chapters filled with the passion and commitment to community and public health. In addition, we are thankful for the invaluable experiences we obtained from our community and public health work that interfaced and informed the production of this book. Those experiences ranged from developing interventions with and for women living with HIV/AIDS in Boston, to implementing community-based programs that addressed the health needs of diverse populations, to teaching students about the social determinants of health, and to assuming leadership roles on local boards that are responsible for the health of our local communities. Our editorial coordinator, John Larkin, was very helpful in answering questions, calming frustrations, and solving problems. Greg Nicholl, our development editor, provided the consistency found throughout the chapters. Thank you all for helping us create this unique approach to community and public health nursing!

Rosanna F. DeMarco
Judith Healey-Walsh

A Special Thanks in Memoriam to Dr. Gail A. Harkness, DPH, FAAN

The first and second editions of this textbook were led by the efforts of Dr. Gail Harkness. Gail was a mentor and friend. While she is no longer with us to help support, guide, and enliven this newest edition, we wanted to take time to honor her memory and produce this edition in her honor.

Gail was such an intelligent, warm, and wise public health expert who was most passionate about population health and epidemiology, and particularly infectious diseases past, present, and evolving. She was a prolific writer and teacher. When I met her, she reached out to me, asking if I could help her with her vision of a community health and public health textbook for nursing students that was affordable and succinct and did not just "rattle on" with facts but situated public health ideas in the context of evidence, student stories, and current disease prevention and health promotion innovations. She brought to my mentorship opportunity her global experiences from the UK (University of Leeds) to Japan (Osaka), as well as her own local work on a town Board of Health in Massachusetts. Gail loved public health research and the evidence it yielded to inform policy decisions toward all our health. She was a graduate of the University of Rochester (undergraduate and graduate programs) in Nursing and received her Doctorate in Public Health from the University of Illinois, School of Public Health in Epidemiology and Biometry (the application of statistical analysis to biologic data).

More than being an epidemiologist, she loved the opportunity as an academician to teach nursing students at all levels to be as passionate about public health as she was. She was a professor emerita from University of Connecticut. We know her family and friends miss Gail very much, but her energy and spirit will always be in this textbook.

Rosanna F. DeMarco

Contents

Part 1

The Context of Community and Public Health Nursing

Public Health Nursing: Present, Past, and Future

Judith Healey-Walsh

Nursing is based on society's needs and therefore exists only because of society's need for such a service. It is difficult for nursing to rise above society's expectations, limitations, resources, and culture of the current age.
Patricia Donahue, *Nursing, the Finest Art: An Illustrated History*

I believe the history of public health might be written as a record of successive redefinings of the unacceptable.
George Vicker

Some people think that doctors and nurses can put scrambled eggs back into the shell.
Dorothy Canfield Fisher, social activist and author

The only way to keep your health is to eat what you don't want, drink what you don't like, and do what you'd rather not.
Mark Twain

CHAPTER HIGHLIGHTS

- Healthcare changes in the 21st century
- Characteristics of public health nursing
- Public health nursing roots
- Challenges for practice in the 21st century

OBJECTIVES

- Outline three major changes in healthcare in the 21st century.
- Identify the eight principles of public health nursing practice.
- Explain the significance of the standards and their related competencies of professional public health nursing practice.
- Discuss historical events and relate them to the principles that underlie public health nursing today.
- Consider the challenges for public health nurses in the 21st century.

KEY TERMS

Aggregate: Population group with common characteristics.
Competencies: Unique capabilities required for the practice of public health nursing.
District nurses: Public health nurses in England who provide visiting nurse services; historically, they cared for the people in the poorest parish districts.
Electronic health records: Digital computerized versions of patients' paper medical records.
Epidemiology: Study of the distribution and determinants of states of health and illness in

KEY TERMS *(continued)*

human populations; used both as a research methodology to study states of health and illness, and as a body of knowledge that results from the study of a specific state of health or illness.

Evidence-based nursing: Integration of the best evidence available with clinical expertise and the values of the client to increase the quality of care.

Evidence-based public health: A public health endeavor wherein there is judicious use of evidence derived from a variety of science and social science research.

Health disparities: Differences in healthcare and health outcomes experienced by one

population compared with another, frequently associated with race/ethnicity and socioeconomic status

Health information technology: Comprehensive management of health information and its secure exchange between consumers, providers, government and quality entities, and insurers.

Public health: What society does collectively to ensure that conditions exist in which people can be healthy.

Public health interventions: Actions taken on behalf of individuals, families, communities, and systems to protect or improve health status.

Public health nursing: Focuses on population health through

continuous surveillance and assessment of the multiple determinants of health with the intent to promote health and wellness; prevent disease, disability, and premature death; and improve neighborhood quality of life (American Nurses Association [ANA], 2013).

Telehealth: Use of electronic information and tele-communications technologies to support long-distance clinical healthcare, patient and professional health-related education, public health, and health administration.

Social determinants of health: Social conditions in which people live and work.

CASE STUDY   *References to the case study are found throughout this chapter (look for the case study icon). Readers should keep the case study in mind as they read the chapter.*

The Department of Health and Human Services (HHS) in a southeastern state has begun implementing the recommendations from both the U.S. Institute of Medicine's publication *The Future of the Public's Health in the 21st Century* and the 10-year national objectives for promoting health and preventing disease in the United States established by *Healthy People 2020*. A task force is developing a new vision

for **public health** in the state. Sandy is a program developer in the state's Department of Public Health, with the primary responsibility of assisting local public health departments in developing, implementing, and evaluating public health nursing initiatives. Sandy represents public health nursing on the task force. (Adapted from Jakeway, Cantrell, Cason, & Talley, 2006).

HEALTHCARE CHANGES IN THE 21ST CENTURY

A worldwide phenomenon of unprecedented change is occurring in healthcare. There are new innovations to test, ethical dilemmas to confront, puzzles to solve, and rewards to be gained as healthcare systems develop, refocus, and become more complex within a multiplicity of settings. Nurses, the largest segment of healthcare providers in the world, are on the frontline of that change.

Demographic characteristics indicate that people in high-income countries are living longer and healthier lives, yet tremendous health and social disparities exist. The social conditions in which people live, their incomes, their social statuses, their educations, their literacy levels, their homes and work environments, their support networks, their genders, their cultures, and the availability of health services are

the **social determinants of health**. These conditions have an impact on the extent to which a person or community possesses the physical, social, and personal resources necessary to attain and maintain health. Some population groups, having fewer resources to offset these effects, are affected disproportionately. The results are **health disparities**, or differences in healthcare and health outcomes experienced by one population compared with another.

For example, the World Health Organization (WHO) estimates that almost half of all countries surveyed have access to less than half the essential medicines they need for basic healthcare in the public sector. These essential medicines include vaccines, antibiotics, and painkillers. Children in low-income countries are 16 times more likely to die before reaching the age of 5 years, often because of malnourishment, than children in high-income countries. The double burden of both undernutrition and overweight conditions causes serious health problems and affects survival (WHO, 2017). Globally, resources exist to remedy these circumstances, but does the political commitment exist?

> The development of society, rich or poor, can be judged by the quality of its population health, how fairly health is distributed across the social spectrum, and the degree of protection provided from disadvantage as a result of ill health. **World Health Organization**

Role of the Government in Healthcare

A government has three core functions in addressing the health of its citizens: (1) it assesses healthcare problems; (2) it intervenes by developing relevant healthcare policy that provides access to services; and (3) it ensures that services are delivered and outcomes achieved. The United States, the United Kingdom, the European community, and some newly industrialized countries have embraced these principles. However, governments in other countries struggle to build any semblance of a health system. Unstable governments struggle with mobilizing the concern, motivation, or resources to address healthcare issues.

There were unprecedented public health achievements in the United States during the 20th century. The Centers for Disease Control and Prevention (CDC) has listed the Ten Great *Public Health* Achievements as the legislature amends the law based on supportive epidemiologic analyses and comparisons of health factors over 30 years (Box 1.1). However, healthcare expenditures are now more than $3.2 trillion per year (CDC, 2016). Infant mortality, longevity, and other health indicators still fall behind those of many other industrialized nations. The current U.S. healthcare system faces serious challenges on multiple fronts. Although the United States is considered the best place for people to obtain accurate diagnoses and high-quality treatment, until

1.1	Ten Great Public Health Achievements in the United States, 1900 to 1999

Vaccination
Motor vehicle safety
Safer workplaces
Control of infectious diseases
Decline in coronary heart disease and stroke deaths
Safer and healthier foods
Healthier mothers and babies
Family planning
Fluoridation of drinking water
Recognition of tobacco as a health hazard

Source: Centers for Disease Control and Prevention. (1999). Ten great public health achievements—United States, 1900–1999. *Morbidity Mortality Weekly Report, 48*(12), 241–243.

2014 nearly 45 million Americans lacked health insurance and therefore access to care. These uninsured Americans were primarily young people, low-income single adults, small-business owners, self-employed adults, and others who did not have access to employer-sponsored health insurance.

The Patient Protection and Affordable Care Act (PPACA) was signed into law by President Barack Obama in 2010. The goal of the PPACA is to help provide affordable health insurance coverage to most Americans, lower costs, improve access to primary care, add to preventive care and prescription benefits, offer coverage to those with pre-existing conditions, and extend young adults' coverage under their parents' insurance policies. It is estimated that 95% of legal U.S. residents will ultimately be covered by health insurance, although implementation will evolve over time (Doherty, 2010). The passage of the PPACA was the first step in providing Americans with the security of affordable and lifelong access to high-quality healthcare. More information about the Affordable Care Act is found in Chapter 3.

> It is cheaper to promote health than to maintain people in sickness. **Florence Nightingale**

Practice Point

Making healthcare a right rather than a privilege has global implications.

The United States assesses and monitors people's health through an intricate system of surveillance surveys conducted by the HHS, the CDC, and the state and local governments. Health policy development focuses on cost, access to care, and quality of care. *Access* is defined as the ability to get into the healthcare system, and *quality care* is defined as receiving appropriate healthcare in time for the services to be effective. Outcomes are ensured by a continual evaluation system linked in part with the CDC surveys. Despite this elaborate healthcare system, health disparities related to race, ethnicity, and socioeconomic status still pervade the healthcare system. Health disparities vary in magnitude by condition and population, but they are observed in almost all aspects of healthcare, in quality, access, healthcare utilization, preventive care, management of chronic diseases, clinical conditions, and settings, and within many subpopulations.

The *National Healthcare Quality and Disparities Report* (NHQDR) measures trends in the effectiveness of care, patient safety, timeliness of care, patient centeredness, and efficiency of care. The report presents, in chart form, the latest available findings on quality of and access to healthcare (Agency for Healthcare Research and Quality [AHRQ], 2018). For example, Figure 1.1 indicates that quality of healthcare improved overall from 2000 to 2014, although the pace of improvement varied

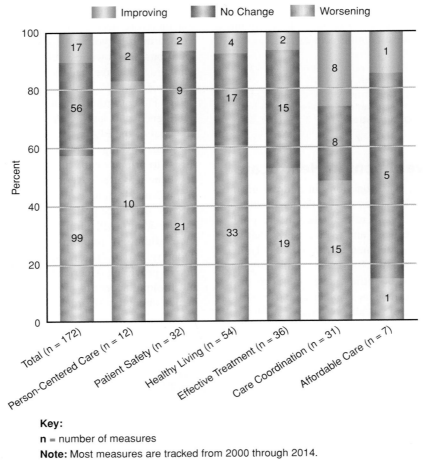

Key:

n = number of measures

Note: Most measures are tracked from 2000 through 2014.

FIGURE 1.1 Number and percentage of all quality measures that were improving, not changing, or worsening, total and by priority area, from 2000 through 2014.

based on priority area. In addition, as Figure 1.2 demonstrates, that although some gaps in measures by race/ethnicity are improving, health disparities in quality healthcare remain.

The challenge for the United States in the 21st century is to create a dynamic, streamlined healthcare system that produces not only the finest technology and research, but also the most accessible, efficient, low-cost, and high-quality healthcare in the world. The current healthcare system also must be transformed to become one of the most competitive and successful systems in the world. Innovative and creative changes will be needed to create a patient/client-centered, provider-friendly healthcare system that is consumer-driven. The political will does exist to create a better future: patient/client-centered care is evolving, new technology is shaping delivery of care, and people are assuming more responsibility for maintaining their health.

Patient/Client-Centered Care

Healthcare has been evolving toward a multifaceted system that empowers patients and clients rather than providers, as was common in the past. This transformation is considered the best way to ensure that patients have access to high-quality care, regardless of their income, where they live, the color of their skin, or how old or ill they are.

Patient/client-centered care considers cultural traditions, personal preferences, values, families, and lifestyles. People requiring healthcare, along with their families or significant others, become an integral part of the healthcare team, and clinical decisions are made collaboratively with professionals. Clients become active participants in their own care, and monitoring health becomes the client's responsibility. Support, advice, and counsel from health professionals are available, along with the tools that are needed to carry out that responsibility.

The shift toward patient/client-centered care means that a broader range of outcomes needs to be measured from the patient's perspective to understand the true benefits and risks of healthcare interventions.

Practice Point

The AHRQ has developed a series of tools to assist clients in making healthcare decisions.

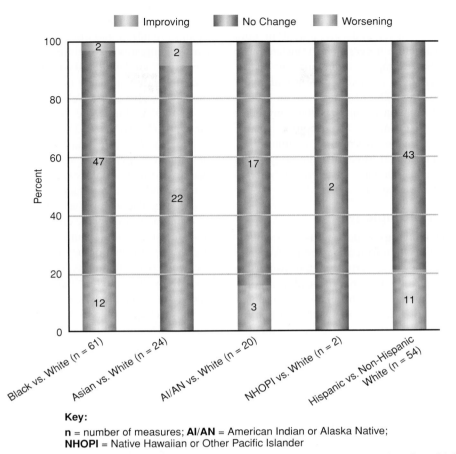

Key:

n = number of measures; **AI/AN** = American Indian or Alaska Native;
NHOPI = Native Hawaiian or Other Pacific Islander

FIGURE 1.2 Number and percentage of quality measures with disparity at baseline for which disparities related to race and ethnicity were improving, not changing, or worsening (2000 through 2014 to 2015).

To help clients and their healthcare providers make better decisions, the AHRQ has developed a series of tools that empower clients and assist providers in achieving desired outcomes. Tools include questionnaires to help determine important treatment preferences and decisions, symptom severity indexes, client fact sheets, client-reported functional status indicators, and other helpful decision-making guidelines. AHRQ (2016) developed the SHARE Approach, a model to promote shared decision-making between a healthcare provider and patient/client. The model has five steps that encourage a conversation between the provider and patient in order to gain a clear understanding of the benefits, harms, and risks of the care options and to identify the patient's values and preferences. The steps include:

1. **S**eek the patient's participation
2. **H**elp the patient to review and compare care options
3. **A**ssess the patient's values and preferences
4. **R**each a consensus decision with the patient
5. **E**valuate the decision

These tools are available to both consumers and healthcare providers at the AHRQ website.

For the system to work effectively, transitions between providers, departments, various healthcare settings, and the home must be coordinated and efficient so that unneeded or unwanted services can be reduced. Americans are sophisticated, empowered consumers in almost every aspect of their lives and will make the best decisions both for themselves and collectively for the healthcare economy and society itself.

Technology

Rapidly advancing forms of technology are dramatically improving lives. Thousands of new ideas are investigated each year, with hundreds of new medical devices submitted to the U.S. Food and Drug Administration annually. Medical devices vary considerably, such as computer-assisted robotic surgical techniques, artificial cervical disks, new diagnostic techniques, implantable microchip-containing devices that control dosing from drug reservoirs, continuous glucose-monitoring systems for detecting trends and tracking patterns in people with diabetes, and many more.

The benefits of biomedical progress are obvious, clear, and powerful. The hazards are much less well appreciated. **Leon Kass, physician**

Although massive investments in medical research have been made, there has been an underinvestment in both research and the infrastructure necessary to translate basic research into results. For example, studies indicate that it takes physicians an average of 17 years to adopt widely the findings from basic research. The healthcare sector invests nearly 50% less in information technology than any other major sector of the U.S. economy. More comprehensive knowledge bases of healthcare information, computerized decision support, and a health information technology (HIT) infrastructure with national standards of interoperability to promote data exchange are necessary.

Health Information Technology

Health information technology is defined as the comprehensive management of health information and its exchange between consumers, providers, government, and insurers in a secure manner. HIT makes it possible for healthcare providers to better manage patient care through secure use and sharing of health information. It is viewed as the most promising tool for improving the overall quality, safety, and efficiency of the health delivery system.

> Health information technology and electronic health information exchange have emerged as a primary means of shaping a healthcare system that is effective, safe, transparent, and affordable. When linked with other health system reforms, technology can support better quality healthcare, reduce errors, and improve population health. **State Alliance for e-Health**

Health information technology includes the use of **electronic health records** (EHRs), digital computerized versions of patients' paper medical records, to maintain people's health information. EHRs and other HIT systems are powerful tools that are having a significant impact on healthcare. Consumers are empowered with more information, choices, and control, and providers have reliable access to complete personal health information that can help them make the right decisions. All necessary health information, from medical histories to billing information, will be accessible from the internet and readily available to all appropriate healthcare facilities and providers of care (with permission of the client). With faster diffusion of medical knowledge through the internet, decision-making will be expedited, medical errors reduced, and duplication of tests and misdiagnosis decreased. However, to protect these records from unauthorized, inappropriate, or unethical use, national privacy laws must be in place.

In the United States, the Office of the National Coordinator for Health Information Technology (ONC) is the principal federal entity responsible for the coordination and safety of information technology issues. It is a resource to the entire health system to support the adoption of HIT and to promote nationwide health information exchange to improve healthcare. ONC is organizationally located within the Office of the Secretary for the U.S. HHS. The ONC has developed SAFER guides for EHRs, consisting of nine guides organized into three broad groups that enable healthcare organizations to address EHR safety in a variety of areas. The guides identify recommended practices to optimize the safety and safe use of EHRs and can be found on the ONC website (see web Resources on thePoint®).

The ONC funds the Nationwide Health Information Network (NwHIN, 2013), a collaborative organization of federal, local, regional, and state agencies. Its mission is to develop the envisioned secure, nationwide, interoperable health information infrastructure to connect providers, consumers, and organizations involved in supporting health and healthcare. The major goals of NwHIN are to enable health information to follow the consumer, to be available for clinical decision-making, and to support appropriate use of healthcare information beyond direct client care to improve the health of communities. The conceptual model that guides NwHIN is illustrated in Figure 1.3. The NwHIN has developed a set of standards, services, and policies that enable the secure exchange of health information nationwide over the internet. Health information will follow the patient and be available for clinical decision-making as well as for uses beyond direct patient care, such as measuring quality of care. It is proposed that the NwHIN will be the vehicle through which health information will be exchanged.

Telehealth

Telehealth is the use of electronic information and telecommunications technologies to support long-distance clinical healthcare, patient and professional health-related education,

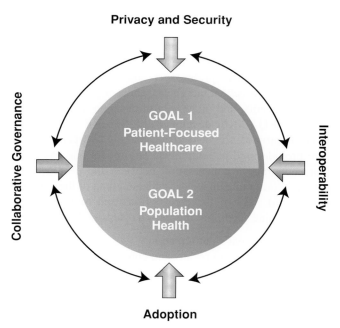

FIGURE 1.3 The nationwide health information network conceptual model. (From Nationwide Health Information Network [NwHIN]. Retrieved from http://www.ahrq.gov/research/findings/nhqrdr/nhdr12/highlights.html.)

public health, and health administration (Health Resources and Services Administration, 2014). Telehealth is becoming a necessity, due in part to the aging population, the rising number of people with chronic conditions, and the need to increase healthcare delivery to medically underserved populations. Findings from the 2015 National Nursing Workforce Survey indicated that nearly half of the registered nurses surveyed had provided nursing services through the use of telehealth products (Budden, Moulton, Harper, Brunell, & Smiley, 2016).

Advances in technology, specifically those involving video-conferencing, medical devices, sensors, high-speed telecommunication networks, store-and-forward imaging, streaming media, and terrestrial and wireless communications have made it possible to assess clients' conditions remotely in their homes. Information can be stored for later access or assessments can be performed in real time using internet video systems. It is also possible to obtain the advice of expert specialty consultants without meeting in person. The increasing complexity of telehealth requires ongoing communication, training, cultural sensitivity, and customization for individual clients. However, access, availability, and cost issues can be barriers to use of this technology (Standing, Standing, McDermott, Gururajan, & Mavi, 2016; Tuckson, Edmunds, & Hodgkins, 2017).

Evidence for Practice

The use of home telehealth devices as an alternative for chronic disease management by nurses has the potential to assist many older people in their homes with the goal of decreasing hospital readmission, and improving the quality of life through early detection and prompt treatment of symptoms. However, long-term outcomes and sustainability have been a concern and challenge. Radhakrishnan, Xie, and Jacelon (2015) studied a telehealth program at a home health agency (HHA) in Texas that ended the program after 10 years of service. The researchers designed a descriptive qualitative study using semistructured interviews to explore the reasons for starting the program, the progressive decline, and the barriers to and facilitators for sustainability of home telehealth programs. The sample included 13 home health staff, including six visiting nurses, two telehealth nurses, four nursing administrators, and nine adult patients, all of whom were over 55 years of age.

Of them, 77% were over 60, and all had Medicare benefits. The service was provided on average for 60 days to patients who were dealing with self-management of chronic diseases, such as cardiovascular disease, respiratory conditions, and diabetes. The telehealth system used at the agency transmitted the patient's biometric and symptom status data to the HHA, but it did not have audio or video capacity. A technician and LVN trained the patient on the use of the device. The telehealth nurse would review the data, and if they were above or below the pre-determined parameters, the nurse would call the patient and the visiting nurse, who would call or visit the patient or contact the MD.

Data on telehealth utilization and patient outcomes were tracked by the HHA. The researchers used conventional content analysis (reading and coding) of the interview transcripts, from which five themes emerged. Subthemes and the barriers and facilitators toward program sustainability were identified. The five themes and aligned subthemes included (a) impact on patient-centered outcomes (self-management, quality of life, and patient characteristics); (b) impact on cost-effectiveness (return on investment), impact on healthcare utilization, and telehealth update and maintenance costs; (c) patient–clinician and interprofessional communication (nurse–patient, nurse–physician, and patient–physician communication); (d) technology usability (cumbersome installation process, device usability); and (e) home health management culture (top-down decision-making, support for supplementary telehealth resources.)

The major barriers were lack of reimbursement, fewer than expected referrals from MDs, minimal impact on re-hospitalization rate, nurses' caseloads usability of the device, high maintenance time and costs, poor interoperability with MD offices, frustration with the amount and delays in communication, lack of administrative and technical support, and patient preference for in-person interaction. Positive features and outcomes that could support sustainability included early identification of a problem and ability to intervene quickly, at-home convenience and ability to remain at home, family caregiver support, feeling of security and support for the patient and family, cost-sharing with other institutions, understanding and buy-in at all levels of management, ease of use and communication to the nurse, and MD involving end users in decision-making in all aspects of program development.

The study's findings support the complexity of a telehealth program, as having potentially positive and negative features. Program design and implementation needs to be intentionally addressed with involvement of the end users nurses, patients, and MDs. The program also must have an ongoing assessment and quality improvement approach, so that barriers are identified early and solutions found to maximize the benefits and sustainability of the program.

Personal Responsibility for Health

Increased personal responsibility for preventing disease and disability is a vital component of healthcare change. The underlying premise holds that if people have a vested interest in their health, they will do more to maintain it. However, if a person is healthy, he or she may not focus on maintaining individual health, yet no one is more seriously affected when illness or disability occurs. Preventing or modifying unhealthy behaviors can save both lives and money, but can

1. Attain high-quality, longer lives free of preventable disease, disability, injury, and premature death.
2. Achieve health equity, eliminate disparities, and improve the health of all groups.
3. Create social and physical environments that promote good health for all.
4. Promote quality of life, healthy development, and healthy behaviors across all life stages.

personal responsibility regarding one's health be truly mandated and regulated?

Personal responsibility for health involves active participation in one's own health through education and lifestyle changes. It includes responsibility for reviewing one's own medical records, including laboratory test results, and monitoring both the positive and negative effects of prescription and over-the-counter medications. It means showing up for scheduled tests and procedures, following dietary recommendations, losing weight if needed, avoiding tobacco and recreational drug use, engaging in exercise programs, and educating oneself about one's own conditions. Ultimately, people must take the responsibility for making their own choices and healthcare decisions.

The patient should be made to understand that he or she must take charge of his own life. Don't take your body to the doctor as if he were a repair shop. **Quentin Regestein, psychiatrist, Harvard University**

U.S. government initiatives have been implemented to encourage personal responsibility for health. *Healthy People 2020* is a national, science-based plan designed to reduce certain illnesses and disabilities by reducing disparities in healthcare services in people of different economic groups. Since 1979, *Healthy People* programs have measured and tracked national health objectives to encourage collaboration, guided people toward making informed health decisions, and assessed the impact of prevention activity. Specific objectives with baseline values for measurement are developed, setting specific targets to be achieved by 2020. The four major overarching goals that incorporate these objectives are listed in Box 1.2 (*Healthy People 2020,* n.d.).

PUBLIC HEALTH NURSING TODAY

The shorter length of stay in acute care facilities, as well as the increase in ambulatory surgery and outpatient clinics, has resulted in more acute and chronically ill people residing in the community who need professional nursing care. Fortunately, these people can have their care needs met cost-effectively outside of expensive acute care settings. As a

result, demand has increased for nurses in ambulatory clinics, home care, and care management.

Hospitals remain the most common workplace for RNs in the United States (54%) (Budden et al., 2016). However, the number of RNs working in home health service units or agencies is increasing (13%) (U.S. Department of Labor, 2017). Public health, ambulatory care, and other noninstitutional settings have historically had the largest increases in RN employment. These statistics indicate a shift in the roles of nurses, particularly for those working in public health settings.

Nursing is the protection, promotion, and optimization of health and abilities, prevention of illness and injury, alleviation of suffering through the diagnosis and treatment of human response, and advocacy in the care of individuals, families, communities, and populations. **American Nurses Association**

Public Health Nursing

A decades-long debate about terminology has fostered confusion regarding the roles of nurses who serve the community. However, public health professionals nationwide have come together to define the principles of public health (Box 1.3). Embracing these fundamental principles for all public health professionals, the Quad Council of Public Health Nursing Organizations established eight principles of public health nursing practice (Box 1.4). The Quad Council of Public Health Nursing Organizations is an alliance of four national nursing organizations that address **public health nursing** issues in the United States, comprising the following:

- Association of Community Health Nurse Educators (ACHNE)
- ANA's Congress on Nursing Practice and Economics (CNPE)
- American Public Health Association (APHA)—Public Health Nursing Section
- Association of State and Territorial Directors of Nursing (ASTDN)

Public health is what we, as a society, do collectively to assure the conditions in which people can be healthy. **Institute of Medicine, 1988**

1.4 | Principles of Public Health Nursing: The Public Health Nurse Is Guided by Adherence to All of the Following Principles

The client or unit of care is the population.

The primary obligation is to achieve the greatest good for the greatest number of people or number of people as a whole.

Public health nurses collaborate with the client as an equal partner.

Primary prevention is the priority in selecting appropriate activities.

Public health nursing focuses on strategies that create healthy environmental, social, and economic conditions in which populations may thrive.

A public health nurse is obligated to actively identify and reach out to all who might benefit from a specific activity or service.

Optimal use of available resources and creation of new evidence-based strategies is necessary to assure the best overall improvement in the health of populations.

Collaboration with other professions, populations, organizations, and stakeholder groups is the most effective way to promote and protect the health of the people.

Source: American Nurses Association (ANA). (2013). *Public health nursing: Scope and standards of practice*. Silver Spring, MD: Nursesbooks.

Scope and Standards of Practice

The ANA sets the scope and standards for all professional nursing practice. The publication *Public Health Nursing: Scope and Standards of Practice* establishes the characteristics of competent public health nursing practice and is the legal standard of practice. It defines the essentials of public health nursing, the activities, and the accountabilities that are characteristics of practice at all levels and settings. An important component of this document is the designation of **competencies** required to meet each standard of practice. This scope and standards document can be used by PHNs from entry-level to senior management in a variety of practice settings and is an indispensable publication reference for every practicing PHN (ANA, 2013).

Competencies for Public Health Nursing Practice

The core competencies for public health nurses (CCPHN) defined in the ANA (2013) publication are aligned with core competencies developed by other public health organizations. The CCPHN reflect the unique capabilities required for the practice of public health nursing. Three tiers of practice are defined, along with competencies associated with that level of practice. Tier 1 core competencies apply to entry-level public health professionals at the basic or generalist level. For example, individuals who have limited experience working in the public health field and are not in management positions would be considered practicing at Tier 1. Tier 2 core competencies apply to individuals with management and/or supervisory responsibilities and are considered specialists or mid-level practitioners. Tier 3 core competencies apply to senior managers and leaders at the executive level who deal with multisystems. Essentially, these competencies underlie the wide variety of roles and responsibilities that PHNs accept in the workplace.

The CCPHN are integrated into the *Standards of Practice for Public Health Nursing* (ANA, 2013). Each standard of practice is followed by the essential competencies required to meet that standard. Following each standard of practice, additional competencies are presented for practice as an advanced PHN.

Public Health Nursing Interventions

The **public health intervention** (wheel) model illustrated in Figure 1.4 is (1) a population-based model that (2) is applied to individuals, families, communities, or within systems and (3) defines 17 public health interventions focusing upon prevention. It is a way of defining public health nursing by the type of actions taken on behalf of clients to protect or improve health status. The interventions in the wheel model complement the competencies that each PHN must demonstrate for safe practice. The competencies define what should be done while the interventions provide a means to accomplish those actions. Table 1.1 describes the 17 interventions illustrated in the wheel. Other interventions have been suggested, such as that of change agent, culture broker, and researcher. The wheel creates a structure for identifying and documenting interventions, thereby capturing the nature of public health nursing practice.

Two years ago, Sandy participated in a statewide survey of both the public health nurses in the state as well as their employers. The purpose of the survey was to determine the characteristics of public health nursing practice, especially the use of principles of population health. Results indicated that the majority of the public health nurse's time is spent in the provision of primary care and clinical services to individual clients. The major factors that contribute to this finding include the number of uninsured people (16%) and a large population of medically underserved people.

Define the type of practice (tier) that the public health nurses were performing.

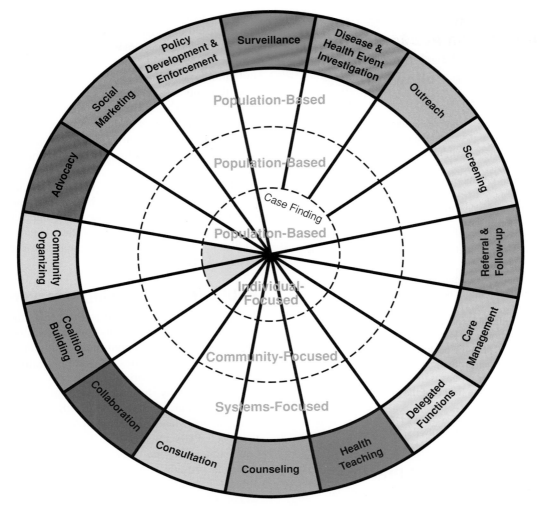

FIGURE 1.4 Public health intervention wheel.

The new vision for public health being designed by the task force promotes a shift from a predominantly individual and clinic-based care model to a population health practice model. The public health nurses in the state were unprepared for this transition and lacked a strong understanding of population health concepts and competencies. Using the standards of practice and associated competencies outlined in *Public Health Nursing: Scope and Standards of Practice*, and with assistance from faculty members at the state university, the task force is helping to develop an online population-based health course to meet the needs of the public health nurses in the state. The priorities of the online course are as follows:

- Community assessment and diagnosis
- Interpreting and presenting health information
- Using computer technology in health planning and policy development
- Building community coalitions

Using *Public Health Nursing: Scope and Standards of Practice*, choose the appropriate standards and competencies

that the public health nurses should demonstrate to meet these priorities.

Education for Public Health Nursing Practice

The educational credential for entry into public health nursing practice is the baccalaureate degree in nursing. This can be a baccalaureate in nursing (BS or BSN) or a generalist master's degree as a clinical nurse leader (CNL). Public health nursing specialists in population health may have a master of science in nursing (MSN), master of public health (MPH), a joint MSN/MPH, or a doctoral degree. Doctoral degrees may be doctor of philosophy (PhD), doctor of nursing practice (DNP), or doctor of public health (DrPH). Diploma- and associate degree-prepared RNs and licensed practical nurses may practice in some public health settings. In these positions, nurses provide care for individuals or families but not for populations (ANA, 2013).

TABLE 1.1 Public Health Nursing Interventions

Intervention	Definition
Surveillance	Monitors health events through ongoing, systematic collection, analysis and interpretation of health data for planning, implementing, and evaluating public health interventions
Investigation of disease and other health events	Systematically gathers and analyzes data about threats to population health, determines the source, identifies cases and those at risk, and determines control measures
Outreach	Locates populations at risk, provides information, identifies possible actions, and identifies access to services
Screening	Identifies individuals with unrecognized risk factors or asymptomatic conditions
Case-finding	Locates individuals and families with identified risk factors and connects them with resources
Referral and follow-up	Assists in identifying and accessing necessary resources to prevent or resolve concerns
Case management	Coordination of a plan or process to bring health services and the self-care capabilities of the client together as a common whole in a cost-effective way
Delegation	Direct care tasks an RN entrusts to other appropriate personnel
Teaching	Develops a health education plan and teach clients and other caregivers leading to behavior change
Counseling	Develops an interpersonal relationship with the client to increase his or her capabilities to address or solve issues
Consultation	Seeks information and generates solutions to health problems or issues through interactive problem-solving
Collaboration	Works with people or representatives of organizations to achieve a common goal
Coalition-building	Fosters, mobilizes, and participates in community-wide alliances to achieve a specific goal
Community organizing	Helps community groups to identify common problems or goals, mobilizes resources, and develops and implements strategies for reaching those goals
Advocacy	Acts on behalf of clients who have lost control of factors that affect their health and a need is unmet; strengthens clients' capacity to act
Social marketing	Uses marketing principles and technology to design programs to address needs of the client
Policy development	Promotes beneficial social changes that influence the health of groups and populations
Policy enforcement	Compels others to comply with the laws, rules, regulations, and ordinances created in conjunction with policy development

Source: Adapted from *Public Health Interventions: Application for Nursing Practice.* Retrieved from www.health.state.mn.us/divs/opi/cd/phn/wheel.html.

ROOTS OF PUBLIC HEALTH NURSING

Exploring the roots of the healing professions provides the background for understanding the characteristics of nursing practice today (Table 1.2). Since the beginning of civilization, people in all cultures have focused on birth, health, illness, and death. Historical records indicate that early societies engaged in public health measures by burying wastes away from water supplies, developing sewage systems, and draining marshes to control communicable disease. In these times, people spent their lives with their family and community, especially when they were ill and needed care. Early caregivers, usually women, cultivated healing herbs, applied poultices, applied heat and cold, immobilized fractures, delivered babies, and attended the dead.

In the Middle Ages, care of ill people was based in the household. Care was haphazard. The few hospitals that existed were run by monks and nuns, primarily for residents of monasteries, and only the wealthy could afford assistance with their care. Changes in social structures encouraged the development of cities, but overcrowding, lack of sanitation, and an ever-increasing susceptible population contributed to recurring epidemics. During the 14th century, the Black Plague alone killed approximately one fourth of the population of Europe. From the 1500s through the 1700s, the Renaissance in Europe stimulated the rise of scientific thought and inspired social consciousness.

The English Poor Law of 1601 marked the beginning of state-provided relief for the poor, placing a legal responsibility on each district to care for people within its boundaries who, either because of age or infirmity, were unable to work.

TABLE 1.2 Milestones in Public Health and Public Health Nursing

1601	Poor Law instituted in England; beginning of state-supported assistance for the poor
1617	Sisters (or Daughters) of Charity founded in France
1789	First local permanent health department in the United States founded in Baltimore, MD
1798	Marine Hospital Service established in the United States; later became the Public Health Service
1809	Sisters of Charity founded by Elizabeth Ann Seton in Maryland
1813	Ladies' Benevolent Society of Charleston, SC, established to provide home care to the sick
1825	154 hospitals had been established in England
1836	Training school for deaconesses established by Theodore Fliedner, a German Lutheran pastor
1840/1841	Dorothea Dix began her lifelong campaign to improve the life of the mentally ill
1850	Shattuck Report published by the Massachusetts Sanitary Commission; recommended the establishment of a state health department and local health boards in every town, collection of vital statistics, sanitation, disease control, health education, town planning, and teaching of prevention in medical schools
1851	Florence Nightingale attended Fliedner's school for deaconesses
1859	William Rathbone established district nursing in England
1860	Florence Nightingale established the first school for nurses at St. Thomas Hospital in London
1861	Soldiers in the American Civil War attended by visiting nurses
1870s	First nursing schools opened in the United States based on the Nightingale model
1872	American Public Health Association established
1882	Clara Barton convinced the U.S. Congress to establish the American Red Cross with an extended mission to provide aid for natural disasters
1885/1886	Visiting nurse associations established in Boston, Philadelphia, and Buffalo
1893	Lillian Wald established the Henry Street Settlement in New York City for the sick poor
1895	Ada Steward employed by Vermont Marble Works as the first occupational health nurse
1898	Significant use of trained nurses in military hospitals
1901	U.S. Army Nurse Corps established
1908	U.S. Navy Nurse Corps established
1912	National Organization for Public Health Nursing established, with Lillian Wald the first President; U.S. Children's Bureau established; Marine Hospital Service changed to U.S. Public Health Service
1914	First postgraduate program in public health nursing at Teachers College in New York City, affiliated with the Henry Street Settlement, established by Mary Adelaide Nutting
1920	90% of the ill were cared for at home with assistance from the community
1925	Frontier Nursing Service in the United States established by Mary Breckinridge to provide access to healthcare in remote Appalachian regions of southeastern Kentucky
1933	Pearl McIver became the first nurse employed by the U.S. Public Health Service
1935	U.S. Social Security Act passed
1943	Frances Payne Bolton was instrumental in founding the Cadet Nurse Corps as a part of the Public Health Service to train nurses during World War II
1953	U.S. Department of Health, Education, and Welfare established
1957	Nationalized Canadian healthcare system established
1965	Public health pediatric nurse practitioner program established at University of Colorado
1966	Medicare for the elderly established in the United States
1967	Medicaid for the medically indigent established in the United States
1970	Occupational Safety and Health Administration established
1974	National Health Planning and Resources Development Act passed
1975	Certification for community health nurses established by the American Nurses Association (ANA)

1979	Smallpox eradication worldwide certified by the WHO[a]
1980	First national health objectives for the United States established: *Promoting Health/Preventing Disease: Objectives for the Nation*
1980	Direct reimbursement through Medicaid for nurse practitioner in rural health clinics, United States
1984	Behavioral Risk Factor Surveillance System (BRFSS) established
1989	*Guide to Clinical Preventive Services* (standardizing screening and prevention strategies) published by the U.S. Public Health Services Task Force
1990	*Healthy People 2000: National Health Objectives for Health Promotion and Illness Prevention* published
1991	*Nursing's Agenda for Health Care Reform* published by a coalition of more than 60 nursing organizations
1998	*The Public Health Workforce: An Agenda for the 21st Century* published by U.S. Public Health Service
2000	*Healthy People 2010* published
2002	European region of WHO declared free of polio
2002	U.S. Office of Homeland Security established
2003	U.S. Institute of Medicine recommends that undergraduate nursing students understand the ecological model of health and core competencies of population-based practice
2010	Patient Protection and Affordable Care Act (PPACA) passed

[a]WHO, World Health Organization.

The Sisters (or Daughters) of Charity, known as the "Grey Sisters," was founded in 1617 in France, with members taking vows to provide care to the sick poor. The organization was so successful that it spread from the rural districts to Paris, and a training program was established in 1633 for young women who were devoted to serving people in need. From that time through the 19th century, this nursing community spread throughout the world. Today, the mother house is located in Paris.

In the 1800s, a variety of reforms were initiated to care for the sick poor throughout Europe that interacted and built on one another. Hospitals were established. By 1825, there were 154 in England alone. However, the fatality rates in these institutions were high, particularly for newborns and people with open wounds; the hospitals were called "death houses." So-called "ward maids," equivalent to housekeepers, provided care.

In Holland, Mennonites recruited women of the church to form deaconess groups to care for the poor. In 1836, Theodore Fliedner, a German Lutheran pastor, established a three-year training school for deaconesses, which was associated with a new hospital. Fliedner also founded parish districts by dividing towns geographically into smaller areas to provide care to residents.

In Victorian times, poorhouses or workhouses existed for chronically ill poor people who were often elderly, without families. The primary reason for poverty was illness, and tuberculosis was rampant. Each parish had its own poorhouse. "Pauper nurses" were poor residents themselves, given the responsibility to care for the destitute. Conditions in many of these poor houses were deliberately harsh and often abysmal. Unfortunately, some pauper nurses were illiterate, irresponsible drunks who were vicious to residents, prolonging their illness (The Public Health [Scotland] Act, 1897). One of the most famous comical, fictional characters in Charles Dickens's works is Nurse Sairey Gamp in *The Life and Adventures of Martin Chuzzlewit*. She was a nurse of sorts who dealt with the "lying in and the laying out" extremities of life, representing some of the more questionable characteristics of the so-called nurses at the time (Fig. 1.5).

During the latter part of the 19th century, when district nursing was established, meeting the needs of the ill became more organized in England. At that time, William Rathbone, a Quaker merchant and philanthropist in Liverpool, England, organized help for the poor. In 1859, he hired Mary Robinson, a nurse who previously had cared for his terminally ill wife, to provide care for the people in one of the poorest parish districts in Liverpool. Mary became the first **district nurse** in England. Box 1.5 lists the duties of district nurses in Liverpool. District nursing soon sprang up in other towns, cities, and rural areas in England, funded by local philanthropists.

Rathbone devoted the rest of his life to expanding services for the sick poor, with assistance from his friend Florence Nightingale and others. Nightingale, the daughter of a wealthy English landowner, devoted her life to the prevention of needless illness and death. In 1851, she attended Theodore Fliedner's program for deaconesses—for nurse training—in Kaiserswerth, Germany. She formed a team of nurses that assisted soldiers during the Crimean War (1854 to 1856) and statistically documented her successes saving lives through

FIGURE 1.5 Dickens's character, Sairey Gamp. (From Kalisch, P. A. & Kalisch, B. J. [2004]. *American nursing: A history*. Philadelphia, PA: Lippincott Williams & Wilkins.)

1.5	Duties of District Nurses in Liverpool, England: 1865

Investigate new referrals as soon as possible.

Report to the superintendent situations in which additional food or relief would improve recovery.

Report neglect of patients by family or friends to the superintendent.

Assist physicians with surgery in the home.

Maintain a clean, uncluttered home environment and tend fires for heat.

Teach the patient and family about cleanliness, ventilation, giving of food and medications, and obedience to the physician's orders.

Set an example for "neatness, order, sobriety, and obedience."

Hold family matters in confidence.

Avoid interference with the religious opinions and beliefs of patients and others.

Report facts to and ask questions of physicians.

Refer the acutely ill to hospitals and the chronically ill, poor without family to infirmaries.

Source: Brainard, M. (1985). *The evolution of public health nursing* (pp. 120–121). New York: Garland. (Original work published in 1922. Philadelphia, PA: W.B. Saunders.)

prevention of infections and improving environmental conditions (Fig. 1.6). In 1860, following the war, Nightingale opened the first school of nursing, and Rathbone hired several graduates as district nurses. Two years later, with Nightingale's assistance, he established a nursing school in Liverpool.

Public Health Initiatives in Early America

American social values were strongly influenced by British traditions, including care for the sick poor. Care of destitute and infirm residents was the responsibility of the town or county, similar to the English Poor Law of 1601. In the 1700s, early public health efforts in the colonies were focused on sanitation, collection of vital statistics, and control of infectious diseases. People with contagious diseases were isolated in "pesthouses," and home quarantines were instituted. Women of the house were responsible for care of the ill, and treatments consisted of home remedies that were often passed down through generations.

Occasionally, a board of health would be established to address a specific problem, but it was then disbanded. In 1789, the first local health department with a permanent board of health was formed in Baltimore, MD. In 1798, the Marine Hospital Service was established by Congress to provide for the temporary relief and maintenance of sick and disabled seamen, as a means to protect the public from contagious diseases brought into port by the sailors. This was the first prepaid medical care program in the United States, financed through compulsory employer tax and federally administered.

At the beginning of the 1800s, people recognized that they needed a more organized public health system. In 1809, Elizabeth Ann Seton founded the Sisters of Charity in Maryland. The Sisters of Charity (also called Daughters of Charity) established and operated many hospitals, orphanages, and educational institutions over the years. In 1813, the Ladies' Benevolent Society of Charleston, SC, was established to provide organized home care to the sick. Knowing the threats that sick merchant seamen posed to the general population, Congress passed the Act for the Relief of Sick and Disabled Seamen in 1798 (amended in 1802) to establish hospitals for merchant seamen. However, conditions in many cities remained nearly intolerable.

The Industrial Revolution resulted in the transformation of primarily agricultural economies to large industrial centers. Large numbers of people migrated into cities, living in crowded tenement houses. Working conditions were poor, people were overworked and underpaid, and child labor was prevalent. Poor nutrition and overcrowded living conditions led to the rapid spread of communicable diseases. For example, New York City's streets were piled with garbage and sewage, and tenements were filthy and crowded, providing breeding grounds for tuberculosis, smallpox, and typhus. Although initial attempts were made to protect residents from infectious diseases by providing healthcare to merchant seamen, diseases became epidemic and quarantine

FIGURE 1.6 Florence Nightingale, the "Lady with the Lamp." (From Kalisch, P. A. & Kalisch, B. J. [2004]. *American nursing: A history*. Philadelphia, PA: Lippincott Williams & Wilkins.)

became inadequate. Few advances in public health were made other than scattered smallpox regulations until the Shattuck Report was published.

Lemuel Shattuck

Lemuel Shattuck prepared a report for the Massachusetts Sanitary Commission that pointed out that much of the ill health and disability in American cities in 1850 could be traced to unsanitary conditions. The report is now considered one of the fundamental documents in public health in the United States. It provided for the first systematic use of birth and death records and demographic data to describe the health of a population. The recommendations became the foundation of the sanitation movement in the United States, which laid the framework for the dramatic increase in life expectancy that occurred in the next 150 years. In 1850, the average lifespan was 25 years, and by 2000, it was more than 75 years. The Shattuck Report recommended the establishment of a state health department and local health boards in every town, and resulted in the first attempt to write a comprehensive public health code. Following the Civil War, many states and localities adopted these recommendations, ultimately resulting in the public health system that exists today.

Perhaps the most significant single document in the history of public health—I know of no single document in the history of that science quite so remarkable in its clarity and completeness and in its vision of the future. **C. E. A. Winslow, bacteriologist and public health expert, on the Shattuck Report**

Dorothea Dix

Dorothea Dix was also an American political activist in the 19th century who became aware of the dreadful conditions in prisons and mental hospitals, and she vigorously lobbied state and federal officials to remedy the situation. She had traveled to England in 1836, and during her time there, she met William Rathbone, who was spending a year as a guest at the family estate in Liverpool. In addition, she met political activists who believed that government should take an active role in social welfare. The lunacy reform movement was underway in England at the time, and the detailed investigations of the madhouses were published, resulting in legislative changes. After returning from England in 1840, Dix traveled the state of Massachusetts, visiting jails and insane asylums. She was appalled by conditions there and compiled a report that she presented to the Massachusetts Legislature. Considered the most progressive state in the union, Massachusetts quickly allocated funds to establish the first hospitals for the mentally ill. After making changes in Massachusetts, Dorothea moved on to other states and other countries, establishing hospitals and improving life for the mentally ill.

I proceed, Gentlemen, briefly to call your attention to the present state of Insane Persons confined within this Commonwealth, in cages, stalls, pens! Chained, naked, beaten with rods, and lashed into obedience. **Dorothea Lynde Dix**

Clara Barton

Clara Barton achieved widespread recognition during the Civil War, distributing supplies to wounded soldiers and caring for the casualties with the help of her team of nurses. As a result of these experiences, she recognized the need for a neutral relief society in the United States that could be activated in times of war, similar to the International Committee of the Red Cross that was founded in 1863 in Geneva, Switzerland, by Henry Dunant. Barton lobbied tirelessly, and in 1882, she convinced Congress to ratify the Treaty of Geneva, and the American Red Cross was established with an extended mission—to provide aid for natural disasters.

Lillian Wald

In the 1880s, 20 years following the establishment of district nursing in England, a similar movement began in the United States. Urban tenement houses in the large American cities across the country were crowded and unsanitary, and infectious diseases such as tuberculosis, typhoid fever, smallpox, and scarlet fever were prevalent. A number of initiatives were undertaken in the major cities to improve the life of residents. An increased understanding of communicable disease indicated that education about prevention of infections would reduce these illnesses. Teaching methods to prevent infectious disease, implementing sanitary reforms, and fostering better nutrition became the foundations of community nursing practice in the United States.

Lillian Wald, the founder of public health nursing, was born into a life of privilege (as was Florence Nightingale) (Fig. 1.7). At the age of 22, Wald attended the New York Hospital School of Nursing. While taking classes at the Women's Medical College, she became involved in organizing a class in home nursing for poor immigrants on New York's Lower East Side. Distressed by the living conditions in the dingy multistorey flats, Wald moved to the neighborhood, and she and her classmate Mary Brewster volunteered their services. With the aid of several patrons, they founded the Henry Street Settlement in 1893; fees were based on the patient's ability to pay. In addition to providing acute and long-term care for the sick, Wald and Brewster taught health and hygiene to the immigrant women, stressing the importance of preventive care. Wald called her services "public health nursing." Similar settlement houses in other American cities developed rapidly.

> The vermin in these old houses are terribly active at night . . . there is nothing harder to endure than to watch by a night sickbed in these old worn houses and see the crawling creatures, and the babes so accustomed to them that their sleep is scarcely disturbed. **Lillian Wald, *The House on Henry Street***

Wald devoted herself full time to the Lower East Side community, ultimately becoming one of the most influential and respected social reformers and humanitarians of the 20th century. Within a decade, the Henry Street Settlement included a team of 20 nurses, and it offered an astonishing array of innovative and effective social, recreational, and educational services. Eventually, the organization incorporated housing, employment, educational assistance, and recreational programs. It also placed nurses in public schools and businesses. Later, the Henry Street Settlement became the Visiting Nurse Association of New York City (Henry Street Settlement, 2004).

> Nursing is love in action, and there is no finer manifestation of it than the care of the poor and disabled in their own homes. **Lillian Wald**

In 1912, Wald helped found the National Organization for Public Health Nursing, which set the first professional standards for the practice of public health nursing. These standards were a precursor to ANA's *Public Health Nursing: Scope and Standards of Practice*, which guides the practice of public health nursing today. As a founder of Columbia University's School of Nursing, she persuaded the administration to appoint the first professor of nursing in the country, laying the foundation for nursing education in institutions of higher learning. Wald also was an advocate for children and women's rights, helping with the establishment of the United States Children's Bureau, National Child Labor Committee, and the National Women's Trade Union League (Ruel, 2014).

Public Health Initiatives in the 20th Century

Public Health in the First Half of the Century

Public health and nursing initiatives grew exponentially in the 1900s, a century dominated by two world wars and an

FIGURE 1.7 Lillian Wald (center, second row) and nurses of the Henry Street Settlement. (From Kalisch, P. A. & Kalisch, B. J. [2004]. *American nursing: A history*. Philadelphia, PA: Lippincott Williams & Wilkins.)

astounding increase in scientific knowledge. Recognition of public health nursing as a necessary function of government came about gradually in the early part of the 20th century. Local health departments, charged with control of communicable diseases, sanitation, maintaining a safe water supply, food inspection, health education, and other functions, began hiring more nurses. Although there was a rapid growth in the number of hospitals, few resources were available to people who had to be cared for in their homes. The first PHNs focused on care at the bedside, but they soon realized that their efforts had little effect if conditions were unsanitary and if there was no food in the house. PHNs effectively served as sanitary inspectors, tenement house inspectors, probation officers, and social welfare service workers. Before long, it was clear that nursing practice demanded psychosocial and political skills, along with a broad understanding of the community.

As demand for services grew, the role of PHNs became more focused on teaching and counseling, showing others how to care for the sick, instructing them on how to prevent illness, and promoting maternal and child health (Kalisch & Kalisch, 1978). Health promotion and disease prevention began with the need for health education during home visits to the poor living in large cities and expanded over time to schools, employees, and the rural population.

Mary Breckinridge

An innovation in the provision of health services occurred when Mary Breckinridge founded the Frontier Nursing Service in 1925 (Fig. 1.8). Following the death of her two children, she decided to devote her life to improving the health of children and developing a system of rural healthcare in the remote regions of Kentucky and throughout the world.

Traveling on horseback, Breckinridge studied the health needs of the mountain people. She found that women lacked prenatal care, gave birth to an average of nine children, and primarily had self-taught midwives in attendance at their delivery. Maternal and infant mortality were high. Breckinridge realized that children's healthcare must begin before birth with care of the mother and continue throughout childhood, while including care for the entire family (Schminkey & Keeling, 2015). She founded the Frontier Nursing Service, which continues to provide family-oriented healthcare to rural and underserved populations today. In 1939, she helped establish the Frontier Graduate School of Midwifery, one of the first midwifery programs in the country (Frontier Nursing Service Inc., n.d.)

Our aim is to see ourselves surpassed. **Mary Breckinridge**

Early 20th Century Federal Healthcare Initiatives

The Spanish–American War of 1898 led to a significant use of trained nurses in military hospitals. For the first time, the graduates of nearly 200 nurse training schools throughout the country were incorporated into a single nursing corps. These nurses were the forerunners of women in the armed services. A permanent Army Nurse Corps was established in February, 1901, followed by creation of a Navy Nurse Corps in 1908 (Kalisch & Kalisch, 1978).

Prior to the 20th century, government involvement in healthcare was left to the states. By 1900, health departments had been established in the majority of states, but their function was limited. By 1912, there was a growing acceptance that the U.S. government should take an active

FIGURE 1.8 Mary Breckinridge and a frontier nursing visit. (From Kalisch, P. A. & Kalisch, B. J. [2004]. *American nursing: A history*. Philadelphia, PA: Lippincott Williams & Wilkins.)

role in the health and welfare of the people. The need for a permanent federal agency that was responsible for the health of citizens was recognized, and the Marine Hospital Service, originally established in 1798 for seamen, was reorganized to form the U.S. Public Health Service (USPHS). The office of the U.S. Surgeon General was also founded that year. Federal programs focused on the health of mothers and children, the poor, the mentally ill, and those with sexually transmitted diseases were implemented. For example, the Maternal and Infancy Act (Sheppard–Towner Act), passed in 1921, provided matching funds to states that developed maternal and child divisions in their health departments. Home visits by PHNs encouraged prenatal care and health promotion for mother and child, and maternity centers and child health clinics were established (Kalisch & Kalisch, 2004).

World War I (1914 to 1918) was a military conflict centered in Europe that involved most of the world's great powers. Although the Army Nurse Corps and the Navy Nurse Corps had expanded, care of the wounded was still insufficient, and civilian nurses were in short supply. The types of wounds from modern weapons and the use of poisonous gases required new nursing skills, and wound infections were rampant. Then, in late 1918, when the armistice occurred, an influenza pandemic spread throughout the world, with soldiers becoming vectors of the viral infection.

By 1920, there was a significant shortage of nurses, and patient care suffered. It was estimated that 90% of ill people were cared for at home with assistance from the community (Kalisch & Kalisch, 1978). The Great Depression began in 1929, resulting in widespread unemployment, including nurses. At the same time, the need for health services expanded, especially for charity cases. The federal government became even more active in health and social welfare programs, employing nurses through the Federal Emergency Relief Act, the Civil Works Administration, and other agencies. In 1933, Pearl McIver became the first nurse to be employed by the USPHS. Her primary role was to provide consultation services to state public health departments, resulting in an increase in local PHN employment.

The Social Security Act of 1935 was passed to help prevent a recurrence of the problems associated with the Depression, especially for poor elderly people. It provided a system of federal old-age benefits and enabled states to make more adequate provision for elderly people, the blind, dependent and crippled children, maternal and child welfare, public health, and the administration of state unemployment compensation laws. Financial support was provided to increase public health programs, particularly for mothers and children in rural areas. Local health departments designed their programs on the basis of the funding that was available, rather than directing their efforts toward a comprehensive community health program. A component of the federal approach to health policy today still directs funding to special population groups or to the prevention and control of specific diseases.

With the onset of the United States' involvement in World War II, it became clear that the United States would soon face a critical shortage of nurses nationwide. Through the work of Congresswoman Frances Payne Bolton, the Cadet Nurse Corps was founded as a part of the USPHS to train nurses during World War II. Applicants were granted subsidization of nursing school tuition and associated expenses, and schools were funded to provide expedited training. In exchange, applicants agreed to provide nursing services to the military or other essential civilian industries for the duration of the war. The number of PHNs employed by industry almost doubled during this time. Public health nursing also expanded in rural areas during World War II, and some official agencies began to offer bedside care.

Public Health in the Second Half of the Century

After the war, the increased demand for healthcare services led to increased opportunities for PHNs, changes in healthcare delivery and financing, and the growth of health insurance. Local health departments faced increases in demand for services related to community problems such as alcoholism and mental illness. Their services increased to include screening for tuberculosis and sexually transmitted diseases as well as treatment of infectious diseases, and services were extended to rural areas.

By mid-century, a number of social improvements resulted in an increased lifespan. Public health measures such as improved sanitation, provision of potable water, better nutrition, and better housing contributed to this phenomenon, along with medical developments such as immunizations and antibiotics. Childhood mortality decreased, and more Americans lived into middle and old age. Infectious diseases were the leading causes of mortality in 1900; by 1950, the leading causes of death were heart disease, cancer, and cerebrovascular disease, as they remain today. With the increased lifespan, new challenges related to chronic diseases emerged.

In 1966, the Social Security Act was amended and Medicare was created to provide healthcare funding to the elderly. The next year, Medicaid was established to provide funding for the indigent (see Chapter 2). These programs contributed to the continued increase in demand for services, and costs of healthcare escalated. Some people perceived these programs to be the first step toward universal healthcare coverage in the United States. To address increased demands, the federal government passed health planning legislation to meet differing needs throughout the country. Although this legislation had merit, it failed to produce expected results. Federal efforts to reform healthcare continued to focus on organization of services and financing, rather than implementing changes in the social conditions that led to health disparities.

The roles and responsibilities of PHNs continued to expand during the 1970s, and they contributed significantly to the improvement of the health of communities. A wide variety of programs were implemented according to need. Hospice services, day care centers for the disabled, alcohol and drug abuse programs, halfway houses, and rehabilitation centers are just a few of the public health initiatives that nurses helped create. Home nursing visits increased following Medicare's implementation of diagnosis-related groups (DRGs) that were designed to lower costs through reduced hospital stays. Medicaid also reimbursed some home care services, as did the Veterans Administration and private medical insurance. More and more acutely ill people were cared for in the home, creating an ongoing demand for PHNs.

Despite the increased need for nursing services, public health as a whole declined in the 1980s. The economic recession resulted in decreased funding for social programs. The Institute of Medicine (IOM) published *The Future of Public Health* in 1988, finding that public health services varied considerably across the United States. The system was in disarray, controlled more by the political system than by public health professionals. This study set the stage for the development of the *Healthy People* initiative that designed a national strategy to improve the health of Americans. *Healthy People 2020*, discussed earlier in this chapter, is the most recent vision for the next decade. Many of these measurable objectives (see Box 1.2) are discussed throughout this text.

The task force decides that a written and pictorial presentation on the historical roots of public health nursing practice will be a component of the online course.

Describe three characteristics of population-based nursing practice that have been present since the first district nurse was appointed in England.

The First Decade of the 21st Century

The Department of Homeland Security (DHS) was created by the Department of Homeland Security Act of 2002 and is an outgrowth of the Office of Homeland Security established by President George W. Bush shortly after the terrorist attacks of September 11, 2001. The primary mission of DHS is to lead the unified national effort to secure the United States, reducing the vulnerability of the United States to terrorism and protecting against and responding to threats and hazards to the United States.

The DHS fosters an all-hazards, all-disciplines approach to emergency management that allows effective response to all emergencies, whether natural or human-made, or caused by terrorists. To meet this mission, the DHS builds collaboration and partnerships with all levels of government, the private sector, academia, and the general public. Because all disaster response begins at the local level, all cities and towns in the United States are now required to have all-hazards

local emergency preparedness plans (see Chapter 20). The National Response Framework, established by DHS, guides the overall conduct and coordination of all-hazards incident responses when the scope of a disaster extends beyond the capability of local and state governments to respond.

Through education and outreach, homeland security expertise is fostered across multiple disciplines to serve as an indispensable resource for the United States. The Federal Emergency Management Agency, as the lead agency for emergency management, offers courses for first responders. The CDC also offers many online training sessions, and many states and localities have developed their own training programs.

The aftermath of the destruction of the World Trade Center in 2001 also identified a lack of trained leaders and workers in all areas of public health service. In an era in which public health threats range from pandemics of emerging infectious diseases to obesity epidemics to the opioid epidemic to bioterrorism, the need for an effective public health workforce is paramount. PHNs constitute the single largest group of professionals practicing public health; however, all nurses, to some degree, are involved in public health. Therefore, the IOM (2003) has recommended that undergraduate nursing students have an understanding of the ecological model of health (see Chapter 5) and the core competencies of population-based practice discussed earlier in this chapter.

Some of the issues that were characteristic of public health nursing in the past are still prevalent today, and a multitude of new challenges exists. To provide the most comprehensive care to clients, whether individual people, families, or groups, PHNs must be flexible, be politically active, embrace change, and refresh their knowledge of public health issues on a continual basis.

CHALLENGES FOR PUBLIC HEALTH NURSING IN THE 21st CENTURY

Many yet-unknown challenges will develop during the 21st century. Communities will evolve and change, cultures will merge, environments worldwide will undergo transformation, and advances in technology and therapeutic techniques will result in dramatic changes to healthcare. The following are some of the challenges for PHNs foreseen at present.

Engaging in Evidence-Based Practice

Nurses have always used the knowledge gained through education and experience in making decisions about the care of clients—accentuated by a dose of intuition. The challenge today and for the future is to document and use the best evidence available in making decisions with clients about their care. **Evidence-based nursing** is the integration of the best evidence available with clinical expertise and the values of the client to increase the quality of care. Similarly,

evidence-based public health is a public health endeavor in which there is judicious use of evidence derived from a broad variety of science and social science research. In addition to published research, PHNs can gather information from interviews and through observation of specific population groups and gather pertinent information about the geographic locale.

Epidemiology is the science of prevention. Epidemiologic research has provided knowledge of the natural history of diseases and identified the (risk) factors that increase a person's susceptibility to illness. Nurses use the evidence that epidemiologic research has established when assessing clients and using data for planning and implementing interventions. Using the epidemiologic body of knowledge that has been developed for specific conditions, nurses can determine the stage of the illness in question and decide with the client what type of interventions are most appropriate for preventive or therapeutic purposes (see Chapters 5 and 6 for discussions of primary, secondary, and tertiary prevention strategies). Nurses engaging in community assessment also use epidemiologic methods to determine the assets and health needs of populations, and the evidence is used to create a variety of intervention programs. The public health approach to problem-solving is illustrated in Figure 1.9.

> Sandy and other members of the task force think that evidence-based practice should be part of the online population-based health course.
>
> What activities could be assigned that would foster evidence-based practice?

Practice Point

Systematic reviews of research evidence, such as those included in the Cochrane Database of Systematic Reviews, are instrumental in implementing evidence-based practice.

Helping Eliminate Health Disparities in Underserved Populations

Eliminating health disparities is a combined effort of health professionals in all settings, but PHNs deal directly with these issues, often on a personal basis. Ultimately, the most important changes occur at the local level. By participating in the development, implementation, and evaluation of culturally appropriate, community-based programs, nurses use their expertise to remedy the conditions that contribute to health disparities.

Demonstrating Cultural Competence

Countless cultures in the world are constantly changing. The shared cultural symbols and meanings that are a part of people's daily social interactions have an impact on their acceptance or rejection of actions taken to promote their health. Therefore, nursing strategies that are focused on people with little attention as to how they think, feel, and interact with their world are not sufficient.

Cultural competency is an expected component of nursing practice, but it will become even more essential as interaction and integration among cultures increases. The characteristics of the major cultural groups that make up a community must be understood, along with those aspects of the community that give it its own unique subculture. It is

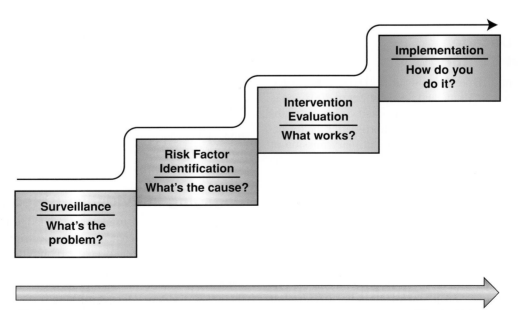

FIGURE 1.9 The public health approach to problem-solving.

necessary for nurses to be aware of cultural interpretations of healthcare activities so that they know what questions to ask and interventions to suggest. To achieve cultural competence, nurses should respect differences, understand their own beliefs, and not let personal beliefs have an undue influence on others. Nurses need to communicate curiosity and openness to others' ideas and ways of life, respect their decisions, and demonstrate patience and humility (see Chapter 10).

> Misunderstanding a culture's symbols is a common root of prejudice. **Dan Brown, *The Lost Symbol***

Evidence for Practice

The delivery of culturally competent public health nursing that can address health disparities depends on competent nursing practice. Understanding the nurse characteristics, care situations, and training associated with culturally competent awareness and behavior provides a basis for planning and developing interventions to ensure competent nursing care. To meet this objective, a cross-sectional, descriptive, and exploratory study was conducted among 31 PHNs in a southeastern U.S. public health department using a cultural competence assessment tool with an internal consistency reliability of 0.90.

The self-reported study findings showed moderate competence in awareness and sensitivity. Although nursing care was consistent with guidelines and mandates found in the National Standards for Culturally and Linguistically Appropriate Services in Healthcare (U.S. Office of Minority Health), the nurses did not assess their behaviors at comparable levels. While providing care, the nurses encountered multiple racial/ethnic and special population groups, including many that are at risk for or experiencing health disparities and poor outcomes. Therefore, being culturally competent in both thought and actions is necessary and important for these nurses. These nurses felt frustrated in their attempts to provide care that was consistent with their perceptions of culturally competent care. Lack of human or financial resources, interpreters, gender-specific providers, and time were the most common barriers. In addition, the nurses expressed a desire for additional diversity training. To meet the goals of a culturally competent workforce, formal courses, continuing education programs, and practical experiences should focus on awareness, sensitivity, and behaviors consistent with culturally competent care. To develop additional evidence-based knowledge for practice, additional studies of clients' perceptions and evidence of culturally competent care are needed. This information is necessary for the development of practice interventions with measurable outcomes that can be evaluated for effectiveness in addressing health disparities (Starr & Wallace, 2009).

Planning for Community Change

Change in healthcare at all levels can occur through behavior change, or through modifications in the environment, public policy, social or cultural norms, or healthcare delivery. Often, interventions at institutional or societal levels may lead to significant changes in public health without the need for behavior change on the part of individual people; fluoridation of water is an example. Even small changes in health behavior at the community or population level have the potential to significantly affect health status. The use of gel alcohol in hospitals and the availability of disinfectant wipes in grocery stores and other public places are examples.

Change should be planned and should meet specific needs to be the most effective. The impetus for change varies considerably. For example, installation of home monitoring devices may require new responsibilities, an influx of immigrants may increase the healthcare needs of a community, data may indicate that substance use disorder and violence are increasing in specific groups, or new state regulations may require the establishment of new programs. On a community basis, health planning occurs on both an ongoing and an episodic basis depending on the need and usually is a collaborative effort between multiple groups and organizations. A good example is the development of emergency preparedness plans in cities and towns (see Chapter 20).

Monitoring and evaluating the health status of individual people, families, and community groups are primary components of nursing practice in the community, as is the investigation of emerging health and environmental problems. Therefore, accepting responsibility for contributing to community health change as a policy advocate and political activist is essential. Few practitioners are as well prepared to address community health issues as PHNs. See Chapter 9 for more information on planning for community change.

The state department of public health recognizes that increasing the knowledge base of PHNs in population-based practice is just one step in implementing the new vision of public healthcare delivery. Knowledge alone cannot change practice from a clinical focus to a population-based focus if the work environment does not support the transition. Sandy is preparing another survey to determine current practices that need to be discontinued, strengthened, or developed within the next five years. Although the new vision for PHNs will include primary care, the majority of skills in the new model of practice will focus on population-based competencies.

Design a simple public health nursing model that incorporates the basic principles of population-based nursing.

Evidence for Practice

Intimate partner violence (IPV) is a serious and prevalent public health issue. Given the complexity of IPV, there have been efforts to integrate social and healthcare services. Public health nurses are well positioned to work collaboratively with social service agencies to provide health education and assistance in accessing healthcare services. Providing health education at social service agencies gives public health nurses access to IPV survivors and is also convenient for the IPV survivors, who typically spend significant amounts of time at the agencies. Prior to developing any educational offering it is imperative that the nurse assess the perceived needs of the survivors. Ferranti, Lorenzo, Munoz-Rojas, and Gonzalez-Guarda (2017) studied the health education needs and learning preferences of female IPV survivors who were receiving assistance at a social service agency in South Florida. Using an exploratory two-phase sequential mixed method, the researchers first conducted semistructured interviews with 10 service providers to gain their perspective on the health needs of women they served. The interviews were analyzed to extract themes, and the themes guided the development of a survey that contained 10 close-ended questions. Three themes were identified: (a) multidimensional health needs of families (primary care, mental health, reproductive/sexual health, chronic disease management); (b) complexities of navigating the health system, including structural barriers (insurance, transportation, finances, and immigration status) and health literacy (finding a doctor); and (c) self-improvement specific to IPV survivors (empowerment and vocational skills).

There were 122 female IPV survivors who completed the survey. The sample was primarily Hispanic, ranging in age from 19 to 65, with a mean age of 34.8 and the majority having a high school education or higher (81%). Of them, 57% were born outside of the United States. Physical health proved to be a lower priority for the participants, as almost 70% of them identified depression as the top health education need. Over 50% of the women chose abuse and mental health as the next greatest concerns, with anxiety selected by 45%. For health topics, over half of the women selected self-esteem, nutrition, and women's health, with 45% identifying children's health as an important health topic. With respect to learning preference, hands-on activities and talking to an expert were the top two choices, with 50% of the participants selecting them. The relationships between most learning preferences and demographic factors, as analyzed using chi-square and t-tests, were nonsignificant. However, age was significantly related to learning preference of brochures/books. Those who selected brochures/books were significantly older (mean = 37.6) compared to those who did not. Also, language preference (English vs. another language, Spanish or Creole) was significantly associated with presentation preference and group discussion. The women who preferred English were more apt to select both presentation and group discussion when compared with those who preferred another language.

The study highlights the importance of health education in the continued recovery of IPV survivors. The differences that were found between the service providers and recipients supports the critical importance of public health nurses including the IPV survivors prior to planning any health education program so that it targets the participants' priorities and learning preferences. The strong emphasis on mental health acknowledges the psychological toll that IPV has on the survivors.

Contributing to a Safe and Healthy Environment

Where people live, work, and spend their time can have direct consequences on their health. In every community in the world, clients are part of the environment, which has a direct impact on their health and well-being. The WHO (2016) reports that 23% of the global burden of disease is attributable to the environment. There are two ways to examine the effects of the environment on human health. The first focuses on how contaminants in the environment, such as asbestos, lead, or radon, influence human health. The second focuses on how the entire environment surrounding the community, such as the climate, neighborhood safety, access to grocery stores, and the physical layout of the community, affects health. Often, the two types of environmental effects interact.

The challenge for environmental health nurses is to use the best science available to assess how the local environment affects human health, to formulate evidence-based or best-practice interventions, and to evaluate the effectiveness of those interventions. Nurses are in a strong position to advocate for healthier environments in both the workplace and community (see Chapter 19).

Responding to Emergencies, Disasters, and Terrorism

All disaster response begins at the local level, and PHNs have always responded to community emergencies and disasters. They play an important role in all phases of the disaster management continuum, whether anticipating potential emergencies, developing appropriate community preparedness plans, building system-wide partnerships, practicing implementation of disaster management plans and skills on a regular basis, or evaluating outcomes (see Chapter 20).

Disaster preparedness plans are proactive planning efforts that are developed in anticipation of disaster scenarios, providing structure to a response before the disaster occurs. In an all-hazards event plan, the response must be a coordinated community effort in which members of the community are engaged in ongoing preparedness activities focused on a variety of disaster situations. The capacity to respond to threats depends in part on the ability of healthcare professionals and public health officials to rapidly and effectively detect, manage, and communicate during an event. The terrorist attacks in 2001 identified a lack of workers in all areas of public health, as well as a growing appreciation of the first responders, primarily firemen, police, and healthcare personnel. Increased competency in disaster response added a new dimension to nursing practice. The public health workforce continues to be mobilized to ensure the training and education of communities across the nation regarding biological, chemical, and radiological attacks. It is necessary to learn how to prepare for events that are difficult to imagine, and it is even more challenging to mount a response.

Responding to the Global Environment

The burden of disease is growing disproportionately in the world and is largely affected by climate, public policy, age of the population, socioeconomic conditions, and factors that place people at risk for illness. Most of the countries burdened by disease have the least amount of human and economic capacity to effect change. Extreme poverty is the driving force behind increased mortality, and women are disproportionately affected.

Although maternal deaths have dropped worldwide by almost 50% in the last decade, maternal mortality is still unacceptably high. On any given day, approximately 800 women die from preventable causes related to pregnancy and childbirth, nearly all (99%) occurring in low-income countries. Many of the complications resulting from childbirth can be prevented by skilled care before, during, and after childbirth by midwives and nurses. When a mother dies or is disabled, her children may be forced to live in poverty. Presently, about 6.6 million children younger than 5 die each year; poor nutrition is the underlying cause of death (WHO, 2017).

The leading causes of mortality and global burden of disease worldwide have shifted from communicable to noncommunicable chronic diseases as a result of population aging and better control of infectious diseases. Cardiovascular disease is already the leading cause of death in the world, followed by stroke. Figure 1.10 shows the 10 leading causes of death worldwide. Only lower respiratory infections, diarrheal diseases, and tuberculosis are infectious diseases remaining in the top 10. Chronic diseases such as COPD; Alzheimer disease; tracheal, broncial, and lung cancers; and diabetes mellitus are causing increased numbers of deaths

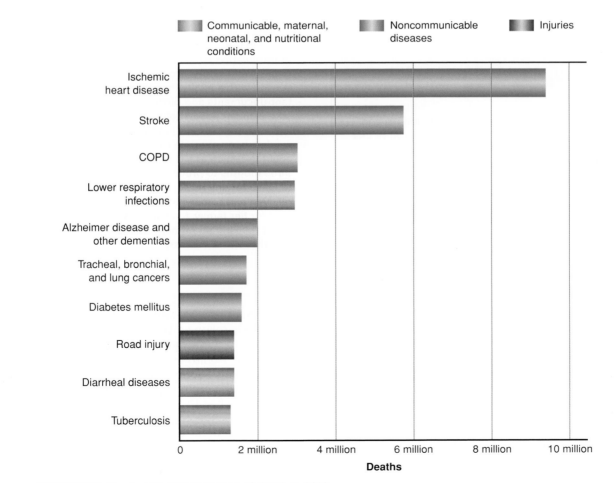

FIGURE 1.10 The top 10 global causes of death in 2016.

worldwide. Traffic injuries worldwide are expected to grow from the eighth leading cause of death in 2016 to the fifth in 2030. The global burden of disease and methods to improve global quality of care are discussed in Chapter 4.

With the world becoming a global village, problems that affect people in other countries also affect people in their own countries. Nurses and community healthcare providers need to be knowledgeable about the needs of all people, as well as their patients, in the global society. Opportunities have expanded for nurses to work internationally in a wide variety of roles: working side by side with local people in healthcare, initiating health education programs, establishing local primary healthcare programs, and participating in countless other activities. Advanced technology and knowledge transfer techniques will allow rapid transfer of information from electronic monitoring equipment, presenting exciting opportunities to improve health in remote locations. New cooperative healthcare ventures will occur throughout the world in the 21st century.

Practice Point

In this dynamic time, care will be transformed as needs rapidly evolve. Newly prepared nurses will experience events never before thought possible.

Student Reflection

Over the spring vacation, a group of eight undergraduate nursing students, three graduate students, and three faculty members flew to Nicaragua to work in a clinic for the week. There was one person who stands out in my mind. She was a 25-year-old woman who came to the clinic complaining of diarrhea, accompanied by her 6-year-old son and 3-year-old daughter. One of our nurse practitioners (NPs) cared for her while I observed. After the NP determined that the woman had a gastrointestinal parasite that was common in Nicaragua and prescribed treatment, the nurse asked the client about her wishes to have more children. The woman responded quietly that she did not want more children, but that her husband was adamant that she did not use birth control. When the NP asked if birth control was a sensitive subject between them, the woman began to cry. She told us that after the birth of her daughter, she began birth control without consulting her husband, and when he found out, he became verbally and physically abusive. Since that point, their relationship had become increasingly violent and the woman said she feared for her life, along with the lives of her children. Her husband felt that if she used birth control she was cheating. He told her that he was not going to use a condom, and if she did not want to have his children, she didn't love him.

This situation made me realize just how dismal it can be for women in violent relationships. Because of lack of resources, it is very difficult for abused women to find help, and many lose hope, believing that nothing can be done. Their situation is complicated since the majority of women are financially dependent on their partners. Our client was in a similar situation. She was afraid of her husband, vulnerable financially, and had two children to protect. Her situation would be further complicated if she continued without birth control. During the visit, the NP and I listened and provided the emotional support that she so desperately needed. We began to discuss some options and actions that she might be able to take. Just as we would in the United States, we discussed the necessity of formulating a plan before acting, helping to ensure success and safety. We talked about the possibility of staying with a family member and reviewed the important documents and birth certificates that she should take with her. Also, I told her about a domestic violence support group that the clinic provided. Finally, we discussed multiple forms of birth control that she could use, such as the hormone injection that lasts for three months to prevent pregnancy, if she were unable to leave for any reason. I think the woman left feeling relieved and somewhat hopeful for what the future held for her family. Even if I was only able to get my client thinking about her options, I feel that our time together was a success.

KEY CONCEPTS

- Three major changes in healthcare in the 21st century include the development of patient/client-centered care, increased use of technology, and increased personal responsibility for health.
- The practice of public health nursing is defined in the ANA (2013) publication *Public Health Nursing: Scope and Standards of Practice*. It defines the essentials of public health nursing, the activities, and the accountabilities that are characteristic of practice at all levels and settings. It is the legal standard of practice set by the profession.

- In the ANA (2013) publication, each standard of practice is followed by the essential competencies required to meet that standard.
- The Public Health Intervention Wheel defines 17 interventions—actions taken on behalf of individuals, families, communities, and systems to protect or improve health status.
- Entry into public health nursing practice requires a baccalaureate degree.
- The historical roots of public health nursing have set the framework for current nursing practice in the community.

- Multiple challenges face PHNs in the 21st century:
  - Engaging in evidence-based practice
  - Helping eliminate health disparities in under-served populations
  - Demonstrating cultural competence
- Planning for community change
- Contributing to a safe and healthy environment
- Responding to emergencies, disasters, and terrorism
- Responding to the global environment

CRITICAL THINKING QUESTIONS

1. Review the public health milestones presented in Box 1.1. What potential health successes might be cited in the next decade?
2. Identify a new role for nursing that will most likely evolve in the first half of the 21st century.
3. Analyze the roots of public health nursing and its influence on practice today.

HEALTHY PEOPLE 2020 LEARNING ACTIVITY

Social Determinants of Health

Healthy People 2020 provides a blueprint which identifies nationwide health improvement priorities. This national consensus plan includes 42 topics, with a subset of 12 leading health indicators (LHI) and over 1,200 objectives. It offers a framework for strategic planning to promote health improvement and achieve health equity through measurable objectives and deliberate actions. The *Healthy People 2020* website is dense with important information on the development, implementation, and progress of this national plan. Learning to navigate the website, to access the rich materials offered is vital to gain a deep understanding of the national health improvement priorities, specific objectives, and initiatives seeking to achieve the national goals and objectives.

Social Determinants of Health is a new topical area identified as a priority in *Healthy People 2020*. To learn more about this topic go to: https://www. healthypeople.gov.

Click on Topics & Objectives: Topics are listed alphabetically, scroll down to "S" and click on **Social Determinants of Health.**

Click on "Overview" and find the answers to the following questions:

- What is the goal for this topic?
- What are some examples of social and physical determinants of health?
- What are the five determinants selected for *Healthy People 2020*?

Click on "Objectives" and select one objective from each of the five determinants: Analyze the data, looking specifically at any disparities, progress made, and thinking about continued barriers to achievement.

Click on "Resources and Interventions" and select one resource from the national, state, and local groupings: Review the resource to explore how community and public health groups are working to address and improve the social determinants of health across the nation.

REFERENCES

Agency for Healthcare Research and Quality (AHRQ). (2016). The SHARE approach: A model for shared decision-making. Retrieved from https://www.ahrq.gov/professionals/education/curriculum-tools/shareddecisionmaking/index.html

Agency for Healthcare Research and Quality (AHRQ). (2018). National health care quality and disparities report, 2016. U.S. Department of Health and Human Services. Retrieved from https://nhqrnet.ahrq.gov/inhqrdr/reports/qdr

American Nurses Association (ANA). (2013). *Public health nursing: Scope and standards of practice.* Silver Spring, MD: Nursesbooks.

Budden, J.S., Moulton, P., Harper, K. J., Brunell, M. L., & Smiley, R. (2016). The 2015 national nursing workforce survey. *Journal of Nursing Regulation, 7*(1), S1–S90.

Centers for Disease Control and Prevention. (1999). 10 great public health achievements—United States, 1900–1999. *Morbidity Mortality Weekly Report, 48*(12), 241–243.

Centers for Disease Control and Prevention (CDC). (2016). FastStats: Health expenditures. Retrieved from https://www.cdc.gov/nchs/fastats/health-expenditures.htm

Doherty, R. B. (2010). The certitudes and uncertainties of health care reform. *Annals of Internal Medicine, 152*(10), 679–682.

Ferranti, D., Lorenzo, D., Munoz-Rojas, D., & Gonzalez-Guarda RM, (2017). Health education needs of intimate partner violence survivors: Perspectives from female survivors and social service providers. *Public Health Nursing, 35,* 118–125.

Frontier Nursing Service Inc. (n.d.). A brief history of the Frontier Nursing Service. Retrieved from http://www.frontiernursing.org

Health Resources and Services Administration. (2014). Retrieved from http://www.hrsa.gov/ruralhealth/about/telehealth/

Healthy People 2020. (n.d.). Retrieved from http://www.healthypeople.gov/2020/about/default.aspx

REFERENCES *(Continued)*

Henry Street Settlement. (2004). About our founder, Lillian Wald. Retrieved from http://www.henrystreet.org/about/history/.org/

Institute of Medicine (IOM). (2003). Who will keep the public healthy? Educating public health professionals for the 21st century. Retrieved from http://books.nap.edu/openbook.php?record_id= 10542&page =R2

Jakeway, C. C., Cantrell, E. E., Cason, J. B., & Talley, B. S. (2006). Developing population health competencies among public health nurses in Georgia. *Public Health Nursing, 23*(2), 161–167.

Kalisch, P. A., & Kalisch, B. J. (1978). *The advance of American nursing.* Boston, MA: Little Brown.

Kalisch, P. A., & Kalisch, B. J. (2004) *American nursing: A history.* Philadelphia, PA: Lippincott, Williams & Wilkins.

Nationwide Health Information Network (NwHIN). (2013). Retrieved from https://www.healthit.gov/sites/default/files/hie-interoperability/nationwide-health-information-network-exchange-data-sheet.pdf

The Public Health (Scotland) Act. (1897). Pauper nurses. *The British Medical Journal, 2,* 104. Retrieved from http://www.ncbi.nlm.nih.gov/pmc/articles/PMC2407239/pdf/brmedj08725–0040a.pdf

Radhakrishnan, K., Xie, B., & Jacelon, C. S. (2015). Unsustainable home telehealth: A Texas qualitative study. *Gerontologist, 58*(5), 830–840.

Ruel, S. R. (2014). Lillian Wald. Home Healthcare Nurse. *Home Health Nurse, 32*(7), 597–600.

Standing, C., Standing, S., McDermott. M. L., Gururajan, R., & Mavi, R. K. (2016). The paradoxes of telehealth: A review of the literature 2000–2015. *Systems Research and Behavioral Science. 35,* 90–101.

Schminkey, D. L., & Keeling, A. W. (2015). Frontier nurse-midwives and antepartum emergencies, 1925 to 1939. *Journal of Midwifery & Women's Health, 60*(1), 48–55.

Starr, S. & Wallace, D. C. (2009). Self-reported cultural competence of public health nurses in a southeastern U.S. public health department. *Public Health Nursing, 26*(1), 48–57.

Tuckson, R. V., Edmunds, M., & Hodgkins, M. L. (2017). Telehealth. *New England Journal of Medicine. 377*(16), 1585–1592.

U.S. Department of Labor. (2017). Bureau of labor statistics: Occupational employment and wages registered nurses. Retrieved from https://www.bls.gov/oes/current/oes291141.htm

World Health Organization. (2016). Preventing disease through healthy environments: A global assessment of the burden of disease from environmental risks. Retrieved from http://www.who.int/quantifying_ehimpacts/publications/preventing-disease/en/

World Health Organization. (2017). World health statistics *2017.* Retrieved from http://www.who.int/gho/publications/world_health_statistics/2017/en/

WEB RESOURCES

- Please visit thePoint® for up-to-date web resources on this topic.

Chapter 2

Public Health Systems

Rosanna F. DeMarco

> It is no measure of health to be well adjusted to a profoundly sick society.
> **Jiddu Krishnamurti**
>
> Without health, life is not life; it is only a state of languor and suffering—an image of death.
> **Buddha**
>
> America's healthcare system is neither healthy, caring, nor a system.
> **Walter Cronkite**
>
> Everyone should have health insurance? I say everyone should have healthcare.
> I'm not selling insurance.
> **Dennis Kucinich**

CHAPTER HIGHLIGHTS

- Public health and healthcare systems as a complex organization of institutions and structures
- National and international perspectives on public health structure, function, and outcomes differ by fiscal support and philosophical attitudes concerning health
- Public health administration as a reflection of health, politics, economics, and social structures
- Influences of history, resources, financing mechanisms, interest groups, and environmental conditions on public health
- Governmental and nongovernmental organizations and public health

OBJECTIVES

- Understand and describe the challenges in reducing the gap between healthcare expenditures and healthcare disparities.
- Compare and contrast differences across international public health systems.
- Explain the different contributions of governmental and nongovernmental structures in public health systems in different countries.

KEY TERMS

Bilateral agency: Refers to two agencies that conduct business within one country.
Department of Health and Human Services: U.S. branch of government responsible for health and welfare of citizens.
Health disparities: Difference in the quality of healthcare delivered or obtainable, often tied to race or ethnicity or socioeconomic status.

Healthy People 2020: A U.S. national consensus plan with specific health goals.
International Council of Nurses (ICN): A federation of more than 130 national nurses associations (NNAs), representing the more than 16 million nurses worldwide.

KEY TERMS *(continued)*

Millennium Development Goals (United Nations): Eight goals that all 191 UN member states have agreed to try to achieve by the year 2015 to combat poverty, hunger, disease, illiteracy, environmental degradation, and discrimination against women.

Multilateral agencies: Agencies that use both governmental and nongovernmental resources.

National Health Expenditure Accounts (NHEA): Comprised of measures of costs of healthcare goods and services in the United States.

Nongovernmental organization (NGO): Agency that acquires resources to help others from private (vs. public) sources.

Organization for Economic Cooperation and Development (OECD): A group that collects data related to healthcare use across a variety of professional and service parameters.

Philanthropic organization: An organization that uses endowments or private funding to address the needs of individuals, families, and populations.

Refugee: Person who leaves his or her place of origin and cannot return because of a well-founded fear of being persecuted for reasons that include race, religion, nationality, membership of a particular social group, or political opinion.

United Nations Educational, Scientific, and Cultural Organization (UNESCO) Sustainable Development Goals: A global framework of 17 goals to coordinate efforts from 193 nations represented by the United Nations around ending poverty and hunger, combating inequality and disease, and building a just and stable world.

World Bank: International organization that uses funds from developed countries to help initiatives of developing countries.

World Health Organization (WHO): International center that collects data, advances initiatives, and offers support related to public health.

CASE STUDY   *References to the case study are found throughout this chapter (look for the case study icon). Readers should keep the case study in mind as they read the chapter.*

When Clara arrived in the United States as a refugee* after surviving many years of violence and brutality in her native Sudan, she was barely 20 years of age (an estimate). Many girls like Clara do not know their age; they often do not know the year in which they were born. Clara represents a community or population of women who have experienced hard realities related to the genocide in Sudan. War between the North and the South, which still continues, results from different religious views and ethnicity, and it puts all people, particularly some young women, in a vulnerable position. In their commitment to ethnic cleansing, men in the army have raped young girls without hesitation, leaving them to face pregnancy with no women's healthcare and with very little support to change their future circumstances in a patriarchal society.

Clara has found asylum in the United States through the generosity of a nongovernmental health organization. She now enters a healthcare system that offers screening, care, follow-up, and support as she learns that she and her child are human immunodeficiency virus (HIV)-seropositive. Although Clara and her young child face the prospect of a life-threatening illness, she is supported by a system that seems to care about her progress and future health, as well as the health of the entire population.

_____

*The United States provides refuge to persons who have been persecuted or have well-founded fear of persecution through two programs: one for refugees (persons outside the United States and their immediate relatives) and one for asylees (persons in the United States and their immediate relatives) (https://www.dhs.gov/sites/default/files/publications/Refugees_Asylees_2015.pdf).

Comparing healthcare systems allows for an examination of how these systems, which help ensure the health or wellness of populations, are organized and financed; cost control is important. Comparing helps develop standards and initiatives directed by organizations discussed in this chapter, such as the **World Health Organization (WHO)**, the **World Bank**, and the **Organization for Economic Cooperation and Development (OECD)**.

In addition, such comparisons aid researchers who study specific healthcare interventions and outcomes internationally. The fundamental challenge in making comparisons is the difficulty in finding universal measures of health which can be compared fairly. In the final analysis, what should be of most interest is learning which healthcare system yields the highest quality of care and universal access at a reasonable cost.

IMPORTANCE OF UNDERSTANDING HOW PUBLIC HEALTH SYSTEMS ARE ORGANIZED

Public health involves organized efforts to improve the health of communities rather than individual people. Thus, the central goal of public health is the reduction of disease through prevention and the improvement of health in the community, both nationally and internationally (Schnieder, 2017). As shown in Chapter 1, it has been the characteristics of population health and illness over time that have directed how public health is defined, organized, delivered, and evaluated. But it would be naive to believe that these characteristics are the only things that contribute to the ways in which public health initiatives and the structure behind them have developed. So, to understand how public health systems are organized in a city, state, or country, it seems logical and necessary to explore a variety of components to fully realize why public health systems exist and how they function. To that end, the following section explores a variety of general health and public health systems ranging from those in industrialized countries to those in developing countries. The text discusses the role of public health personnel in the context of how local and global communities organize their efforts to keep the population disease- and injury-free. For people who are committed to the ideals of prevention and access to care for all, public health is not without challenges.

STRUCTURE OF PUBLIC HEALTHCARE IN THE UNITED STATES

In the midst of many successes and challenges related to health and illness, the public health delivery system in the United States supports efforts to address significant healthcare concerns that affect both citizens and refugees/asylees through government agencies, **nongovernmental organizations** (NGOs), and **philanthropic organizations** (Office for Refugees and Immigrants [ORI], 2017). The following section describes the complexity of relationships among the agencies devoted to public health delivery at the local and state levels. The activities of these agencies vary widely because local priorities and values influence availability and operations.

Government Agencies and Public Health

Through public efforts, the U.S. government becomes involved with providing services that benefit the social welfare of citizens in terms of health at national, state, and local levels. The federal government creates policy, financing, and regulatory enforcement when a service that would benefit citizens is identified and available (Shi & Johnson, 2014). Good examples of government efforts to improve public health include providing free drug information on government published databases, establishing disaster preparedness plans, and creating quality indicators for child health (Agency for HealthCare Research and Quality [AHRQ], 2017a; American Red Cross, 2017; National Library of Medicine, 2017).

The federal government plays an important role in regulation. Public health entities of regulation are often related to (1) food, (2) drugs, (3) devices, (4) occupation health, and (5) the environment through the Centers for Disease Control and Prevention (CDC) Public Health Law Program (2017) and **Department of Health and Human Services**, National Prevention Strategy created by the National Prevention Council (2011). However, out of concern related to the quality of healthcare, the government can "step in" to assist private citizens on different occasions. Two examples are federal regulations related to women delivering children who need at least 48 hours of inpatient care and making sure that mental healthcare is in parity with medical care (Harwood et al., 2017).

The federal government allocates tax funds to state governments in support of specific public health programs. For example, block grants give money to specific programs and providers based on state health needs (Urban Institute, 2013). Some examples of block grants include Maternal and Child Health Services and Prevention and Treatment of Substance Abuse Block Grants. Entitlement programs to support the healthcare needs of low-income families come from the federal government. Three important examples of entitlement programs are Medicare, Medicaid, and the Special Supplemental Food Program for Women, Infants, and Children (WIC) (Jackson & Mayne, 2016). The Medicaid program requires matching funds from the states to provide for the healthcare needs of citizens (Fig. 2.1) (Centers for Medicare and Medicaid Services [CMS], 2018).

State governments also play a large role in public health regulatory activities, program responsibility, and resource allocation—to varying extents. Local governments implement the public health activities within communities.

Generally, from either an economic or theoretical perspective, the private sector often does not provide services that would improve social welfare, although in many ways, private organizations often directly assist the common good of populations through their endowment funds (endowed with monies often directly assists the common good of populations); they direct their efforts to key initiatives that are altruistic and very helpful to community dwellers. Examples include philanthropies such as the Kellogg Foundation and the Robert Wood Johnson Foundation (Kellogg Foundation, 2017; Robert Wood Johnson Foundation, 2017).

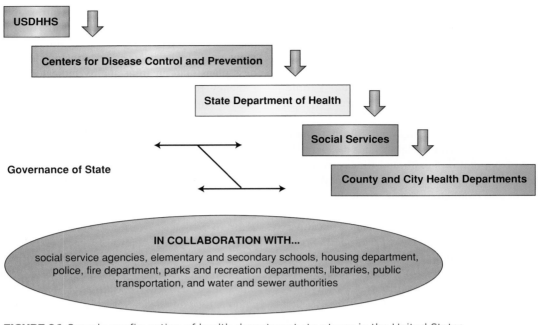

FIGURE 2.1 Sample configuration of health department structures in the United States. USDHHS, U.S. Department of Health and Human Services. (From http://www.hhs.gov/about/orgchart.)

Clara is a good example of a person who came to the United States with no resources. She has no income and is trying to find a way to sustain herself and her child while dealing with the trauma of her past life, and her future life with a chronic life-threatening illness. She is receiving Medicaid from the state in which she now lives in the United States, WIC for her child, and support from the Ryan White HIV/AIDS Program. Since 1991, this program has provided supplemental support for medical care, medications, housing, and public health services for those living with HIV.

Evidence for Practice

The Ryan White Program funds networks of care, which include medical care providers and support services, for people living with HIV or acquired immunodeficiency syndrome (AIDS) (PLWHA) in 51 eligible metropolitan areas (EMAs). Researchers created a survey to measure characteristics of care networks and the quality, accessibility, and coordination of services from the perspective of case management and medical providers, administrators, and consumers (Hirschhorn et al., 2009), and they administered the surveys in 42 EMAs.

The investigators then rated the care networks highly on access, quality, and coordination between case management and primary care providers.

However, there were frequent differences in ratings of quality and barriers by the type of respondents (consumer representatives, grantees, and providers). There were also substantial variations across EMAs in network characteristics, perceived effectiveness, performance measurement, and quality improvement activities. The results indicated that the Ryan White Program has been somewhat successful in developing networks of care. However, support is needed to strengthen the comprehensiveness and coordination of care.

Specific Agencies

United States Department of Health and Human Services

The U.S. Department of Health and Human Services or USDHHS (USDHHS, 2017a) is the federal agency that is directly involved with the health and healthcare of U.S. citizens or refugees/asylees. The Office of the Secretary of Health and Human Services oversees the work of 11 agencies (Fig. 2.2). These agencies work in collaboration with state and local governments in the United States to provide (1) assessment information regarding the level of health or illness in the nation; (2) assurance that the infrastructure, including trained personnel, is available to all citizens and refugees/asylees; and (3) legislation and implementation of health policy. The federal government makes public health policy. By producing information gathered through research,

FIGURE 2.2 Federal agencies with public health responsibilities. (Redrawn from U.S. Department of Health and Human Services organizational chart.) *Designates components of the Public Health Service. (From http://www.hhs.gov/about/orgchart.)

it provides evidence that can effectively change public health practice (Bekemeier, Zahner, Kulbok, Merrill, & Kub, 2016). Thus, the federal government supports research efforts that can help citizens improve their health significantly, and promotes ways to implement the evidence from a culturally relevant and sensitive perspective. For example, the National Institutes of Health (NIH, 2017), Agency for Healthcare Research and Quality (AHRQ, 2017b), and the Centers for Disease Control and Prevention (CDC, 2017a) are three important organizations in which research is undertaken and used effectively to address healthcare concerns

such as HIV screening and care, adverse events in hospital settings, and measures to decrease the rates of emerging infectious diseases (USDHHS, 2017a).

State and Local Health Departments

State agencies, which administer specific federal public health activities throughout a particular state, are influenced from a structural and functional perspective by the federal government. However, state departments of health can be diverse for political and environmental reasons (CDC, 2017a), and they influence NGOs as well as local health departments.

According to Schneider (2017), there are several types of models of health department structure. Most commonly, a state health department is an independent organization that is in communication with the head of the executive branch of the state government (governor). (Within the health department are core public health areas, such as infectious disease control, preventive health, health institution licensing, and epidemiology, but they may relate to a political agenda or worldview of the state leadership.) The head of the state health department can be, but is not necessarily, a physician, although in some states, this is a statutory requirement. The state governor may choose the head of the department of health, or members of a state board of health may make the appointment. These boards of health are representative of the state demographics and may include residents who may be health professionals or may simply be healthcare consumers.

Another model is the state department of health and human services. This model focuses on public health, social service, and medical assistance programs. This relationship between public health and social services often helps bring together related expertise to address complex problems that frequently require coalition building with the public (Janosky et al., 2013).

Although local health departments (city or county) can be governed by state health departments, the local departments often create their own structure based on the needs of the local community, and these local health departments implement programs that serve local citizens. In a county health department, it would not be unusual to see a functioning tuberculosis clinic and tuberculosis surveillance program that works in collaboration with the state health department to care for patients exposed to or infected with the tuberculosis bacillus.

Finally, many other contributors to public health initiatives have strong relationships and interagency affiliations with state and local health departments. They include social service agencies, elementary and secondary schools, housing departments, police and fire departments, parks and recreation departments, libraries, public transportation systems, and water and sewer authorities. Government authorities are often involved in these areas within the context of public health. Generally, localities create relationships and lines of authority that make sense for the particular needs of their citizens (see Fig. 2.1).

FUNCTIONS OF PUBLIC HEALTH IN THE UNITED STATES

In the chapters that follow, there are specific explanations with examples of the functions that public health offers to people in the United States. However, it is important to review several key components of the function public health serves, including a national consensus on goals (USDHHS, 2017b); provision of systems of health insurance based on risk, not necessarily on health; and the role of nongovernmental

entities in disease prevention and health promotion. In the United States, public healthcare includes disease prevention and health promotion based on science and cultural relevance. It is not focused on the health of the individual person, but on the population as a whole. The goal of public healthcare is to keep populations healthy through a broader "reach" than connection at the individual level.

One way to develop a system that advises people with backgrounds similar to Clara's involves strategically putting language-sensitive notices in places where these people live, congregate, or travel. They need to (1) go to their local healthcare centers to get tested for the HIV virus and (2) receive appropriate care. This "reach" may help more at-risk members of a community than discussing the HIV-testing program with people at healthcare facilities. This approach uses broad strategic planning, including the voices of community members, multidisciplinary teams, and nongovernmental not-for-profit sectors of health organizations, which focuses on key target objectives.

Public health goals and focused target objectives are identified and promulgated by a national publication called **Healthy People 2020**. *Healthy People 2020* is a national consensus plan identifying focal areas which need active and specific plans and implementations, based on levels of illness (morbidity) and death (mortality) that account for the physical, psychosocial, and financial suffering of citizens (USDHHS, 2017a). *Healthy People 2020* is mentioned throughout this book as a source of goals and indicators that should direct community healthcare at the local, state, and federal level. However, the United States and its system of healthcare have historically given, and continue to give, stronger support to (1) individual rather than community care and (2) cure rather than prevention. It involves highly specialized healthcare providers who have little contribution to community outreach.

Funding for the healthcare system in the United States comes primarily from privately owned health insurance companies. Exceptions include programs that are publicly funded, such as Medicare, Medicaid, TRICARE (civilian health benefits for military personnel, retirees, and dependents), Children's Health and Insurance Program (CHIP), and Veterans Health Administration (Centers for Medicare and Medicaid Services, 2017; Children's Health Insurance Program, 2017; U. S. Department of Veterans Affairs Health Benefits, 2017). At least 15.7% of the U.S. population is completely uninsured (Kaiser Foundation, 2013), and a substantial portion of the population (35%) is underinsured. More is spent on healthcare in the United States than in any other nation in the world. Even though not all citizens have health insurance, according to the OECD, the United States has the third highest public healthcare expenditure per capita,

TABLE 2.1 Measures of Healthcare in Selected Developed Countries

Country	Life Expectancy (years)	Infant Mortality	No. of Physicians/ 1,000 People	No. of Nurses/ 1,000 People	Per Capita Spending on Healthcare (U.S.$)	Healthcare Costs (GDP)^a	Percentage of Government Revenue Spent on Health/ Percentage of Healthcare Costs Paid by the Government
Australia	81.4	4.2	2.8	9.7	3,137	8.7	17.7/67.0
Canada	80.7	5	2.2	9	3,895	10.1	16.7/69.8
France	81	4	3.4	7.7	3,601	11	14.2/79.0
Germany	79.8	3.8	3.5	9.9	3,588	10.4	17.6/76.9
Japan	82.6	2.6	2.1	9.4	2,581	8.1	16.8/81.3
Sweden	81	2.5	3.6	10.8	3,323	9.1	13.6/81.7
United Kingdom	79.1	4.8	2.5	10	2,992	8.4	15.8/81.7
United States	78.1	6.7	2.4	10.6	7,290	16	18.5/45.4

^{a}GDP, gross domestic product.
Source: Organization of Economic Cooperation and Development. Retrieved from http://www.oecd.org/els/health-systems/49105858.pdf.

and still lags behind in measures to decrease infant mortality and raise life expectancy, as compared with other nations in the world (Table 2.1) (OECD, 2017a). Active debate about healthcare in the United States includes serious ethical questions about whether health is a right or a privilege, and whether all people should have equal access to quality healthcare. In 2010, controversial federal legislation took positive steps to give access to healthcare to all citizens through private and public funding through health insurance. This effort evolved into a federal program called Obamacare after then President Barack Obama and has since been evolving into a new health coverage program that seems to hold a difficult political road ahead. Taking into account the expense and the assurance of efficiency, effectiveness, access, and quality for all to be insured will be the challenge of the current White House administration (The White House, 2017).

Beyond the system of public and private control and ownership of healthcare services in the United States, a vast array of NGOs helps keep people healthy through voluntary and philanthropic services. For example, private community hospitals are sometimes supported by community groups which ensure that vulnerable populations have access to healthcare. The care may be free. In addition, the community facility may sponsor community health education programs and prevention/screening clinics for underserved populations. Although many states provide communities with (community) municipal or neighborhood health centers and ambulatory/outpatient services through local or federal funding, health services can be offered through private groups who are interested in supporting specific areas of need, such as migrant or school-based health programs (McGuire, 2014). These programs are often run by altruistic, nonprofit organizations. Examples of some NGOs in the

United States include the American Diabetes Association, Citizens for Global Solutions, AmeriCorps, and the U.S. Fund for UNICEF (United Nations Children's Fund, 2017).

TRENDS IN PUBLIC HEALTH IN THE UNITED STATES

In the United States, the federal government expends time and effort every year to create a report of the trends in the following areas: (1) health status and what determines health (determinants), (2) how communities use healthcare services (health utilization) and healthcare resources to help communities stay healthy, (3) how much money is spent on healthcare (expenditures), and (4) which citizens are the most vulnerable. The following sections explain these four areas more specifically.

Health Status and Its Determinants

Measuring the health status of citizens in communities helps the U.S. public health system determine how to direct resources (money and services) to keep people healthy. Despite the fact that life expectancy is higher for both men and women in countries such as Japan, the overall health of people in the United States has improved over the years. However, in the United States, current data show a downward shift related to malignancies, obesity, and dental care (Organization of Economic Cooperation and Development [OECD], 2017a). It is believed that the health successes found in the United States result from money spent on health education programs, public health programs, health research, and healthcare itself. The trend has been toward using larger sums of money to help Americans keep healthy. Much of the funding currently spent on healthcare is spent on prescription drugs and care of chronic conditions, which often affect the elderly or disabled. A good example of how increases in funding have improved health is the significant improvement in mortality (numbers of deaths) and morbidity (numbers of recorded illnesses) statistics in a variety of health-related actions, such as the use of corticosteroids in acute lung injury or disease (Tang, Craig, Eslick, Seppelt, & McLean, 2009).

Mortality (death rates) and morbidity (illness rates) have improved for many reasons, but a primary reason is that an organized effort on the part of the American public health system has injected resources to study certain prominent problems in the United States. A good example is the provision of services to prevent progression of cardiac illness. Thus, the death rate from heart disease has decreased, primarily because health education has emphasized a healthier lifestyle and cholesterol screening (Speroni, Williams, Seibert, Gibbons & Early, 2013). Another example is the decrease in mortality and morbidity rates of individuals living with HIV/AIDS. The use of highly active antiretroviral therapy, including protease inhibitors, has dramatically changed patterns of survival; these patterns now assume the trajectory of a chronic illness. Regardless of inequalities in gender, race, and socioeconomic status, people who once lived for five years after being diagnosed with HIV now live for 15 years, and children born with HIV infection from perinatal transmission are now teens who deal with HIV, safe sex behaviors, and disclosure issues with sexual partners (Regidor et al., 2009).

> ### ✎ Practice Point
>
> It is easy to receive morbidity and mortality information in the United States by going to the CDC website and electronically subscribing to the *Morbidity and Mortality Weekly Report (MMWR)* for free. The *MMWR* reports are very informative about trends in assessing the public health status of the United States. More specifically, the *MMWR* reports publicly, in a systematic way, the frequencies of diseases, disabilities, or health-related events, and it supplies information about trends provided by the CDC and other health officials.

Despite these successes, key social and behavioral determinants of health still need to be addressed. For example, obesity, diabetes, and cigarette smoking are significant risk factors for diseases that may interfere with healthy brain functioning (Lal, Strange, & Bachman, 2012). Although much effort has been given to preventive education in these areas, a high percentage of adults and adolescents continue to make no effort to change their exercise, smoking, or eating patterns. In addition, rates of reportable childhood infectious diseases have decreased and cancer has declined in men, but there has been no significant change in the rates for women's cancers. In fact, many believe that there has been

an epidemic of breast cancer in non-Hispanic white women in recent years (Sexton et al., 2011).

Utilization of Healthcare Resources

Changes in payment policies, which are intended to decrease direct and indirect costs, as well as losses from billing fraud/abuse, continue to change healthcare delivery in the United States. There is less use of institutions (i.e., hospitals). Highly complex diagnostic procedures and surgical interventions like cardiac surgery are more likely to take place in hospitals. However, emergency departments and office-based physician and physician-group visits, as well as ambulatory surgical procedures, have increased. In particular, emergency department admissions have increased for those citizens who are asthmatic, especially children (Banda et al., 2013). At the same time, there has been a significant decrease in Medicare-certified home health agencies. In 1997, there were 10,800 agencies, and in 2002, there were 6,800 agencies, primarily because the Balanced Budget Act of that year forced either consolidations or closing of existing services (Center of Budget and Policy Priorities, 2017).

Prevention-oriented approaches and services decrease morbidity and mortality rates (Friis & Sellers, 2014). For example, distribution of flu or pneumonia vaccines as a form of prevention and a common public health campaign demonstrates a commitment of public health to decreasing morbidity and mortality. However, the funding for such programs is often slashed when fiscal constraints cause fiscal intermediaries to (address) pay for treatment of well-known illnesses and disabilities, rather than provide funding for prevention programs which have the potential to impact large populations. Despite decreases in financial support for vaccination programs, there have been increases in the number of children 19 to 35 months of age who have received combined vaccinations (Chidiac & Ader, 2009). In addition, the number of women older than 18 obtaining a Papanicolaou (Pap) smear screen has also increased. However, there is a link between this preventive intervention, some college training, and the vaccine that counters certain strains of human papillomavirus (HPV) (CDC, 2017b).

> ### ✎ Practice Point
>
> *Assurance* is a word used in public health to identify an important concept: that individual people, families, and populations have the healthcare personnel and systems needed to address their respective healthcare needs. Assurance as a goal is highly related to the goal of maintaining healthcare professionals in the work force who are competent and stay in the work force. It is possible to think about schools of nursing as a way in which nursing programs are supporting assurance. To understand the level of commitment to healthcare education for nursing professionals in the state in which you live, determine the number of

schools of nursing in the state, which ones specifically offer advanced practice specialties in community/ public health, the number of schools of public health, and the number of medical schools. In addition, check labor statistics related to trends in the retirement of health professionals. Each of these efforts can help make it possible to understand trends in the preparation of healthcare providers and also help assess needs for the future from the local perspective. Comparison among states gives a larger perspective and can be obtained by accessing the Health Resources and Services Administration (HRSA) website, which is the federal organization specifically responsible for health professional resources in the United States.

Clara is a good example of someone who has been courageous in coming to the United States but is compromised in terms of literacy and socioeconomic needs. She also is unfamiliar, at a basic level, with how healthcare systems work, and how to access them effectively. She needs someone to advocate for her. Even if there are services available to help her, she may not know how to gain access to these services.

Expenditures and Health: Trying to Improve Public Health Economically

Access to healthcare is critical for prevention and treatment of illness and injury. Health insurance and appropriate coverage often determine access. Lack of health insurance is related to poverty, and puts residents in a position of vulnerability. The United States spends more on healthcare than any industrialized country. Although hospital care accounts for the largest share of healthcare spending, prescription drugs are the fastest growing healthcare expenditure. Medicare pays for only a little of this expense, even though citizens aged 65 and older, who are the primary recipients of Medicare, have the greatest need for therapeutic drugs. Thus, people whose income is reduced through retirement, or death of a family member, may have a substantial out-of-pocket expense (Baird, 2016).

National Health Expenditure Accounts (NHEAs) are a measure of expenditures on healthcare goods and services in the United States. These accounts are prepared by the National Health Statistics Group. Government public health activity constitutes an important service category in NHEAs. In the most recent set of estimates, expenditures totaled $56.1 billion in 2004, or 3.0% of total U.S. health spending (CMS, 2017). What becomes challenging is specifically identifying what is considered "public health" in an expenditure.

Vulnerable Populations and Healthcare

Key indicators in the United States reveal a healthcare gap between the overall American population and people of different genders and ethnicities. There is also a healthcare gap for those who have less education, lower socioeconomic status, and live in certain geographic areas in the United States. These disparities are characteristic of people who have been marginalized and oppressed. Marginalization often occurs in people who live below the poverty level in the United States, and these people frequently are poorly educated. In the chapters that follow, higher rates of morbidity, mortality, difficulty in accessing care, and negative outcomes when receiving care will be seen as key issues in such populations.

Historically, in 2002, the Institute of Medicine released a document called *Unequal Treatment: Confronting Racial and Ethnic Disparities in Healthcare* (Institute of Medicine, 2002). The report defines **health disparities** as "racial or ethnic difference in the quality of healthcare which is not due to access-related factors or clinical needs, preferences, and appropriateness of intervention" (Institute of Medicine, 2002, p. 3). Disparities are found in certain types of illness, such as cardiovascular disease, cancer, HIV, diabetes, end-stage renal disease, and certain surgical procedures. Surgical procedures such as amputations have been found to be more common within minority groups.

The Department of Health and Human Services has identified six areas for which it has oversight. These areas are (1) infant mortality, (2) cancer screening, (3) cardiovascular disease, (4) diabetes, (5) HIV/AIDS, and (6) immunizations. In addition, there are also several areas that need special emphasis, including mental health, hepatitis, syphilis, and tuberculosis.

HEALTHCARE SYSTEMS IN SELECTED DEVELOPED NATIONS

Overall, the commitment to prevention and the cost savings, whether a personal commitment or an economic commitment, is yet to become effective in the United States across a variety of parameters. However, other countries have been able to achieve success with their healthcare system structure, function, and outcomes. Figure 2.3 provides an overview of selected healthcare indicators of 17 countries including the United States. For purposes of comparison and contrast, the following section discusses how Canada, France, Germany, the Netherlands, and the United Kingdom keep their citizens healthy and well. These countries were chosen because they historically have had healthcare philosophies that are based on inclusivity of all citizens, lower cost, quality, and a perspective that healthcare is a right. No country is perfect, and many face the same escalating costs as the United States. However, a key international source, the OECD (OECD, 2017a), presents comparative data that demonstrate that these countries have better morbidity and mortality rates, as well as other health-related factors, than the United States. The approaches of these countries to the healthcare of their citizens can serve as important examples of goals which other countries may want to pursue. Key components to advancing

	AUSTRALIA	CANADA	GERMANY	NEW ZEALAND	UNITED KINGDOM	UNITED STATES
OVERALL RANKING (2007)	3.5	5	2	3.5	1	6
Quality Care	4	6	2.5	2.5	1	5
Right Care	5	6	3	4	2	1
Safe Care	4	5	1	3	2	6
Coordinated Care	3	6	4	2	1	5
Patient-Centered Care	3	6	2	1	4	5
Access	3	5	1	2	4	6
Efficiency	4	5	3	2	1	6
Equity	2	5	4	3	1	6
Long, Healthy, and Productive Lives	1	3	2	4.5	4.5	6
Health Expenditures per Capita, 2004	$2,876*	$3,165	$3,005*	$2,083	$2,548	$8,102

Country Rankings: ☐ 1.0–2.66   ☐ 2.67–4.33   ☐ 4.34–6   * 2003 data

FIGURE 2.3 Overall ranking of countries according to various healthcare indicators (2007). *2003 data. (From The Commonwealth Fund. [2013]. International Health Policy Survey, the Commonwealth Fund 2005; International Health Policy Survey of Sicker Adults; the 2006 Commonwealth Fund International Health Policy Survey of Primary Care Physicians; and the Commonwealth Fund Commission on a High-Performance Health System National Scorecard.)

public health and public health systems are (1) identifying indicators of health, (2) being committed to providing healthcare professionals and the public with a system that works, and (3) generating policy that allows for the production of positive outcomes. The following countries have been selected because of unique positive contributions they have made in healthcare outcomes, through creative funding and infrastructure adjustments to meet the unique needs of their respective populations. In many cases, comparisons have been made to these countries because of the positive experiences that have been reported from health outcome data as it relates to costs.

Canada

According to Health Canada (2017) and the OECD Canada (2017b), Canada is the second largest country in the world, with 10 provinces and two territories. Its 31.5 million people have a life expectancy of 78 years (men) and 82 years (women). Seventeen percent of the population is older than 60 years of age. Cancer is the leading cause of mortality, followed by congestive heart failure.

Canada's healthcare system is a national health program; it is considered a single-payer system with universal coverage. This means that all Canadian citizens are covered for healthcare by one government-run system. Canadian Medicare, the healthcare insurance coverage for all, began

in 1968 to eliminate financial barriers to care and to allow citizens to have choice in what physician they chose for their care (Health Canada, 2017). Culturally, Canada is made up of multicultural and multilingual populations because of high immigration rates over the years. Canadians view healthcare as a right, not a privilege, and more specifically, as a social responsibility.

Funding for the Canadian healthcare system comes from personal, sales, and corporate taxes, and federal transfer payments (<25%). The federal government provides healthcare only for special populations (military personnel, native Canadians, and federal prisoners [<2% of the population]). The government of Canada has the responsibility for what are considered the public health arms of the National Institutes of Health, occupational and environmental health, health promotion, Indian Health Service, and health protection.

Despite a single-payer reimbursement system, the 12 provinces determine the management, delivery, and financial arrangements for the Canadian Medicare services. Private insurance exists to cover services not covered under Medicare, such as vision needs, dental services, and pharmaceuticals for nonelderly people. This type of private insurance is acquired through employment contributions, and represents a small portion of total health expenditures (15%). Provinces raise money specifically for Medicare through taxes, corporate contributions, personal income, fuel taxes, and lottery profits.

The money allocated through these approaches supports the individual health costs of citizens in each unique province or territory, hospital payments, and physician salaries which are capped and negotiated, drugs, long-term care and mental health institutions, and provincial healthcare planning. At the national level, there is oversight of the development and safety of pharmaceuticals and reviews that survey physician production, practice, and quality.

The most powerful individuals in the healthcare system are health administrators, not physicians. These health administrators put an emphasis on cost, efficiency, and social responsibility. Unlike in the United States, most of the physicians are generalists who are reimbursed by provincial health plans (99%) through fee-for-service, capitation (maximal amount of money based on patient caseload), or salaries in health centers. Nevertheless, the majority of care occurs in the private physician's office. Nurses have little autonomy and often migrate to the United States to practice in order to gain higher salaries (Health Canada, 2017).

Capital expenditures are separate from operating expenditures, which gives provinces control over facility development and renovation. There is a trend toward delivering healthcare and performing medical and surgical procedures outside of hospital settings, with an increasing focus on health promotion and disease prevention. Most procedures are scheduled in advance and take place in outpatient or ambulatory areas. Although there may be long waits for care, it is important to remember that the wait time is not for emergency or life-threatening conditions. It is a way to distribute care more evenly and to control costs.

Individual provinces closely monitor quality of care, with strong emphasis on decreasing duplication of services across all levels of care. Hospitals, in particular, are used not just for acute care, but for long-term care of patients (23% of hospital beds). There have been reports of inequities between provinces (Health Canada, 2017) and fear that cost containment may limit the use of newer and developing technologies. The balanced benefit of this approach is that Canada has better health outcomes than the United States (30th vs. 37th) in OECD rankings (OECD Canada, 2017b) while spending less money per person on healthcare. Many people believe that it is far better to wait for nonemergent care than to be uninsured (see Table 2.1).

Evidence for Practice

Brehaut and colleagues (2009) used population-based data to evaluate whether caring for a child with health problems had implications for caregiver health after controlling for relevant covariants. They used data on 9,401 children and their caregivers from a population-based Canadian study to analyze and compare 3,633 healthy children with 2,485 children with health problems. Caregiver health outcomes included chronic conditions, activity limitations, self-reported general health, depressive symptoms, social support, family functioning, and marital satisfaction. Covariants included family (single-parent status, number of children, income adequacy), caregiver (gender, age, education, smoking status, biologic relationship with child), and child (age, gender) characteristics. Their findings showed that caregivers of children with health problems had more than twice the odds of reporting chronic conditions, activity limitations, and elevated depressive symptoms, and had greater odds of reporting poorer general health than did caregivers of healthy children. This study points out that caregivers of children with health problems had substantially greater odds of also having health problems than did caregivers of healthy children. From a public health assurance perspective, this indicates that healthcare initiatives need be directed not only to individual children who are chronically ill but also to families. There is an important link between those with chronic illness and those who care for them.

 ## Student Reflection

We were asked in clinical seminar to think about and discuss the prejudices we may have heard about other healthcare systems in the world, and I immediately thought of Canada because it is our next-door neighbor. Everybody says that healthcare is rationed, there aren't enough doctors, the quality of care is poor, and that it is "socialized medicine." I have realized that although there may be a wait for specialist care, there is no wait for the most common need for care . . . primary care. There is rationing related to immediate need versus needs that can be delayed. The most important thing is that everybody has insurance, and nobody is denied care because they can't pay for it. Although there are some shortages of physicians, there is more of a sense of balance in having more physicians available to take care of the common illnesses of the population (primary care). From what I have read, the quality of care is acceptable, especially in light of the fact that in our own country some have no ability to obtain care. I guess the bottom line is, as I prepare to practice nursing, I am keenly aware of the need to ensure all populations of having access to get help for common problems and to have, most importantly, equal access to quality care.

France

Despite the French people's dissatisfaction with their healthcare system, many consider their system one of the best in the world (Bourdelais, 2010). According to the OECD

(OECD, 2017c), France, a republic with a population of 61,000,000, is a healthy country in terms of infant mortality, life expectancy, and healthcare-related costs (see Table 2.1).

The Ministry of Health runs two large organizations that cover the funding and provision of health services in 22 regional services agencies: (1) General Health Management and (2) Hospital and Healthcare Management. The structure of the healthcare system in France includes the National Institute of Health, established in 1998; the French Agency of Health Safety of Health Products, which functions similarly to the Food and Drug Administration (FDA) of the United States, also established in 1998; the Agency of Environmental Health Safety (established in 2000); French Institute of Blood, established in 1992; French Institute of Transplants (established in 1994); and the Ministry for Health, Family and the Disabled.

The government presents a law to the parliament every year as a way to use public policy to finance a social security fund, which includes the national expenditure on health insurance. This public policy effort also specifies goals for the healthcare system, similar to the *Healthy People 2020* effort in the United States. The Ministry of Health delegates the planning and implementation of health initiatives to regions that make up the country in order to decentralize and make care plans specific to each region. A national health insurance guarantees universal access to 80% of the French people by offering health coverage to wage earners through what is called the CNAMTS (Caisse Nationale de l'Assurance Maladie des Travailleurs Salariés or French National Health Insurance Agency for Wage Earners). The rest of the national funding is divided among other funds that are occupationally specific (physicians, agricultural workers, and students). Therefore, the French population is 100% covered by a public mandatory health insurance. Funds are financed by payroll taxes (60%) and since 1990, by a proportional income tax (40%) called the CSG ("contribution sociale généralisée"). The funds are governed by boards with representatives of the government, the main workers unions, and the association of French manufacturers. France has an essential single-payer system. More than 80% of French people carry a supplemental form of private insurance often linked to employment. Public payment covers 76% of French health expenditure. Patients pay physicians directly and apply for reimbursement, and 21% of expenditures are on pharmaceuticals. For 96% of the population, healthcare is entirely free; it is reimbursed up to 100%. Users of this system can select any physician—even a specialist and hospital (public or private)—with the belief that choice leads to successfully managed competition and quality care.

In France, there are more than 1.2 million employees in the health service sector. Physicians consider public hospital jobs undesirable, and often foreign physicians fill these positions. The majority of physicians in private practice participate in a government-fixed fee-for-service scheme, and the remainder charge what they wish. Physicians accept

2.1 Characteristics of Physicians in France

- Physicians are unevenly distributed between rural and urban areas.
- About 50% of physicians are women.
- Physician visits can take 15 to 30 minutes.
- Physicians see about 10 patients per day.
- Medical education for physicians is publicly funded.
- Ratio of generalists to specialists is 1:1.
- Ranking system of hospital practitioners is nationwide.
- Physicians, biologists, and dentists are all salaried hospital practitioners.
- Advancement is based on seniority.

Source: Organization of Economic Cooperation and Development. (2006). *The supply of physician services in OECD countries* (OECD health working papers No. 21). Retrieved from http://www.oecd.org/els/health-systems/35987490.pdf.

what the government pays, and the patient pays the difference. French general practitioners earn the equivalent of about $55,000 per year. Other characteristics of physicians working in France are presented in Box 2.1.

The French healthcare system is made up of public, private, and not-for-profit sectors, which avoids the long waiting lists characteristic of other socialized medicine systems. Health insurance supplies a large majority (91%) of the funds for the 1,032 (85% of total) public hospitals, which account for 65% of all hospital beds in France. Private, not-for-profit hospitals account for 15% of all hospital beds, and specialize in medium- to long-term care. Private, for-profit hospitals account for 20% of all hospital beds. The private hospitals conduct 50% of surgeries and 60% of cancer care.

A key ethic of this system is individual choice of physician and place of service, including a tradition of long-term care in the private home. France maintains strict boundaries between health and social services, and outcomes and performance are benchmarks for both home healthcare and nursing homes. Financial aid is given to people in the form of *allocation personnalisée d'autonomie*, or allocation for loss of autonomy, to purchase care—even from family members or other unskilled labor—as a way to promote employment.

Evidence for Practice

The following two survey studies are examples of this commitment to the health of the French population.

1. Constant, Salmi, Lafont, Chiron, and Lagarde (2009) investigated behavioral changes in a cohort of car drivers to understand why there was a decrease in motor vehicle road casualties in France. Researchers offered self-report survey questions to more than 11,000 people between 2001 and 2004 to explore attitudes related to road safety and driving

behaviors. Investigators found that adequate sleep was related to positive outcomes in road safety. Decreases in cell phone use and speeding over this time period demonstrated decreases in road mortality in France.

2. Nayaradou, Berchi, Dejardin, and Launoy (2010) elicited preferences of the population for willingness to participate in a mass colorectal cancer screening initiative in northwest France. (The implementation of a mass colorectal cancer screening program is a public health priority.) They interpreted the results of a survey conducted by mail from June 2006 to October 2006 on a representative random sample of 2,000 inhabitants, aged 50 to 74 years. On the questionnaire, each person made three or four discrete choices between hypothetical tests that differed in eight ways: how screening is offered, process, test sensitivity, rate of unnecessary colonoscopy, expected mortality reduction, method of screening, test result transmission, and cost. Results from the 32.8% of respondents indicated that expected mortality reduction, sensitivity, cost, and process were among the population preferences. Researchers found that the sensitivity of the test was most important in respondents with higher financial resources. Key implications included how adherence to screening could be accomplished in light of these data.

Clients in nursing homes pay for their room and board separately from nursing/healthcare, and these costs come from pension funds or welfare funds. The residents of nursing homes are legally entitled to be involved in the governance of their home, and in France, this system is highly respected and well run with little inefficiency. Finally, there is a strong emphasis on prevention as a priority.

Germany

Germany, the largest country in Europe, is made up of 82.4 million people divided into 16 states. From a vital statistics perspective, life expectancy varies between men and women (76 and 82 years, respectively), and 19% of the population is older than 65 years of age. The leading causes of death include heart disease and lung cancer (OECD, 2017d).

Germany has a universal healthcare system (OECD, 2017d). Historically, health insurance was a requirement and directed at low-income workers and certain government employees. Eventually, all people were able to obtain insurance. Currently, physicians in private practice provide ambulatory care, and centralized nonprofit hospitals offer the majority of inpatient care. Most of the population has health insurance; individuals can obtain coverage from a variety of "sickness funds" financed by public and private sources. Funds for standard insurance come from a combination of employee/employer contributions and government subsidies, which are scaled on the basis of need. An option exists for individuals to choose to pay a tax and opt out of the standard plan in favor of "private" insurance. Many people with higher salaries choose this option, but their premiums are linked to health status, not to income level.

Regional physicians' associations negotiate provider reimbursement for specific services. A commission composed of representatives of business, labor, physicians, hospitals, and insurance and pharmaceutical industries meets annually. The commission takes into account government policies and makes recommendations on overall expenditure targets to regional associations. Although reimbursement of providers is on a fee-for-service basis, including co-payments, the amount to be reimbursed for each service is determined retrospectively to ensure that spending targets are not exceeded. The average length of hospital stay in Germany has decreased in recent years from 14 to nine days, still considerably longer than the five- to six-day average in the United States (OECD, Health Statistics, Definitions, Sources, and Methods, 2016). Drug costs have increased substantially each year, despite attempts to contain costs. Overall healthcare expenditures have risen, but costs are substantially less than those in the United States (OECD, 2017d).

The reunification of East and West Germany, which occurred in 1990, did increase variation in health statistics by lowering infant mortality and increasing life expectancy. However, differences continue to exist between the two parts of the country because of differences in philosophy and distribution of care in the past. Philosophically, the idea that all people should have health insurance and that the nation is responsible to provide systems of healthcare to its citizens is common to both regions. Health insurance coverage is maintained by all citizens sharing in the effort to have an insurance pool, and payment is based on income, not risk. The healthcare benefits are extremely comprehensive and include medications, dental, vision, medical treatments, and even health spas. Decentralization of healthcare administration includes a federal institute for communicable and noncommunicable disease similar to the CDC in the United States. The organizations of a variety of institutes are grouped across a regional healthcare system which is managed by the sickness funds and physician associations.

Prevention has an important role in the German system, not only as an effort toward cost saving but also in increasing the quality of life of citizens. Public health efforts include not only primary prevention but also health screening with a special emphasis on youth development.

Evidence for Practice

Stolle, Sack, and Thomasius (2009) have expressed concern about episodic excessive alcohol consumption (binge drinking) in children and adolescents as a serious public health problem in Germany because of its associated risks with further morbidities and mortality. An extensive literature search for evidence related to binge drinking from 1998 to 2008 revealed that episodic excessive alcohol consumption is associated not only with somatic complications, but also with traffic accidents and other types of accidents, violent behavior, and suicide. The more frequently a child or adolescent drinks to excess, and the younger he or she is, the greater is the risk of developing an alcohol-related disorder (alcohol misuse or dependence syndrome). Although in the United States, brief motivational interventions have been shown to have a small to medium-sized beneficial effect in reducing further binge drinking and its complications, the Germans use an intervention called HaLT ("stop," also an acronym for hart am limit—"near the limit"). Further types of brief motivating intervention could be integrated in this approach as another variable to decrease binge drinking behavior and prevent the development of alcohol-related disorders.

Nurses in the German healthcare system are mostly diploma-educated individuals working with a physician. There has been a protracted history of shortages of nurses in the 831 public hospitals, 835 independent nonprofit hospitals, and 374 private hospitals. As a final comparison, Germany's healthcare system is sixth in financial fairness, 14th in overall goal attainment, and 14th in terms of overall performance. America's system is 54th in financial fairness, 15th in goal attainment, and 37th in overall performance.

 Student Reflection

It is stunning to me that when you explore different healthcare systems in the United States, the systems seem so wasteful or greedy or just not inclusive enough to allow everyone to have the same healthcare opportunities. One of the things I was thinking about is that, in the United States, we have accepted for a long time the necessity of education. Whether the quality of the education is there or not...the idea is that education is a significant predictor of success and gainful employment in life. Well, if that is the case why would we not have the same perspective for health? Isn't good health a predictor of future good health? Recently, some people in the United States were very worried about the effort to create opportunities for all people to have access to healthcare...not necessarily effective or efficient healthcare but healthcare, period. My sense was that people were divided about using tax money for healthcare. Some felt that the United States was becoming "socialized." I guess it made me sad to think about so many people I have met in poor, run-down neighborhoods who could use the benefits of a philosophy that does not forget them, that cares for them, and wants them to have an equal share of a quality life.

The Netherlands

According to the OECD (2017e), total health spending in the Netherlands accounted for 9.8% of the GDP, slightly more than the average of other OECD countries. The Netherlands also ranks above the OECD average in terms of health spending per capita, with current spending of U.S.\$3,52 (adjusted for purchasing power parity), compared with an OECD average of U.S.\$2,964. Health spending per capita in the Netherlands remains much lower than in the United States, Norway, Switzerland, and Luxembourg.

The Netherlands has a dual-level healthcare payment system. All primary and acute care is financed from private mandatory insurance. Long-term care for the elderly, dying, long-term mentally ill, and so on is covered by money acquired from taxation and is considered a "social insurance." Insurance companies must offer a core universal insurance package for universal primary, curative care, which includes the cost of all prescription medicines at a fixed price without discrimination by age or levels of health or illness. Otherwise, they are considered to be operating illegally.

According to OECD health data (2017e), for people whose health expenses are higher because of illness, insurance companies receive more compensation if they have to pay out more than might be expected. This allows them to accept all patients in an ethically sound way and take care of their needs, rather than strategizing savings by not insuring those who have expensive, long trajectories of needed care. Insurance companies compete with each other on price for insurance premiums and negotiate deals with hospitals to keep costs low and quality high. There is formal regulation that includes checking for abuse and for acts that are against consumer interests. An insurance regulator ensures that all basic policies have identical coverage rules so that no person is medically disadvantaged by his or her choice of insurer.

Payroll taxes paid by employers and a fund controlled by the health regulator, or the "regulator's fund," finance the healthcare system. The government contributes 5% to the regulator's fund. The remaining money needed to cover the country's health expenses is collected as premiums paid by those insured. Insurance companies, many of which are private, can offer additional services, such as dental care, at extra cost over and above the universal system. The standard monthly premium for healthcare paid by individual adults is about €100 (currently about U.S.\$129) per month, and people with low incomes can get help from the government to pay for the premiums. The regulator's fund pays for all children's healthcare in the country.

Hospitals in the Netherlands, which have been advancing in quality over time, are regulated and inspected regularly. They are privately run and for-profit. People can choose where they want to be treated; on the internet, they can obtain access to information about the performance and waiting times at each hospital. Those who are dissatisfied with their insurer and choice of hospital can cancel at any time, but they must make a new agreement with another insurer.

The Netherlands primarily funds what is considered one of the best long-term care systems through non–means-tested social insurance programs financed by national premiums. The programs cover a broad range of institutional and noninstitutional services (OECD, 2017e). This system includes mental health and substance abuse care. Prescriptions are covered by insurers who use specific cost formularies. Generally, co-payments, with options to pay more for certain drugs, are available.

Evidence for Practice

Investigators in the Netherlands examined the association between dairy product intake and the risk of bladder cancer in 120,852 men and women 55 to 69 years of age (Keszei, Schouten, Goldbohm, & Van Den Brandt, 2009). By using a 150-item food frequency questionnaire, several researchers studied a cohort for 16 years and identified and examined 1,549 people. The findings suggested a positive correlation in women between butter intake and bladder risk.

United Kingdom

The National Health Service (NHS), which provides healthcare in the United Kingdom, began in 1948 (U.K. Department of Health, 2017). The system operates across the four countries that make up the United Kingdom (England, Scotland, Wales, and Northern Ireland). Although there are differences in how the health system is implemented, its basic organization and functions are detailed in a constitution which includes specific rights and governance.

The NHS constitution states that healthcare will be provided for all permanent residents of the United Kingdom, regardless of age, gender, disability, race, sexual orientation, religion, or belief, and access to healthcare is based only on need. People are able to choose their own physician; if necessary, this may involve traveling outside the United Kingdom to see other medical professionals for healthcare. About 36% of clients wait for hospital admission for treatment of non-acute conditions, and emergencies are addressed immediately. Two-thirds of patients are treated in less than 12 weeks (OECD, 2017f).

The NHS system is decentralized, with access to care and prevention provided by the Strategic Health Authorities. The primary treatment centers are structured like departments of health in the United States and are responsible for (1) assessing healthcare needs of communities, (2) commissioning health services needed by these communities based on this assessment, (3) identifying goals for improving the health of communities, (4) ensuring access to care, (5) assessing the interaction between healthcare organizations and social services organizations, and (6) assessing the quality of healthcare personnel.

Each of the foundation trusts, which are decentralized departments whose goal is the health of specific sectors of the population, acts as a department of health (U.K. Department of Health, 2017). There is also a central Department of Health which is not involved in day-to-day decision-making and implementation of care. This department makes policy decisions on a large scale, and local governments can define how they will uniquely carry out those policies for their citizens. The NHS provides primary, inpatient, long-term, psychiatric, and eye care free to many people, including children, the elderly, the unemployed, and low-income residents. Private healthcare does exist in the United Kingdom, but only a small percentage of the population use it, generally for specialty care. Private insurance does not cover the cost of pre-existing conditions, chronic conditions, or pregnancy.

Access to medications and healthcare personnel and facilities include prescriptions which are paid by either a flat rate or through annual capped charges. Physicians contract with the NHS to provide services and receive a salary. The majority of the hospitals are owned and run by the NHS trusts. Of the 2.1 physicians per 1,000 population, most are general practitioners. They can have both a public and private practice. They are paid by a mix of capitation, salary, and fees. Those physicians who are specialists are called "consultants," and they are based in hospitals. Nurses make up the largest group of NHS staff and are paid from 40% of the NHS budget. As in most parts of the world, there is a nursing shortage. Although most nurses work in hospital systems, they are educated as specialists, and focus on particular specialty areas such as maternal health.

Revenues for all NHS health services come from taxes (83%), employer–employee contributions (13%), and user fees or co-payments (4%). Expenditures come from the NHS (88%) and private insurance (12%). All people in the United Kingdom have health insurance; in comparison, 44 million in the United States are uninsured, with no access to healthcare. Although there are questions about the level of quality of care in the NHS when compared to the United States, there is much better cost control, and access to care for all people, which translates into better health for the U.K. population.

Evidence for Practice

The Royal College of Paediatrics and Child Health (RCPCH) in the United Kingdom introduced guidelines for re-immunization of children after completion of standard-dose chemotherapy and after hematopoietic stem cell transplantation (HSCT) (Patel, Chisholm, & Health, 2008). To understand if the guidelines were properly applied and whether they created a positive standard, researchers offered an online anonymous survey to pediatric principal treatment center (PTC) consultants and shared care (SC) consultants. Results from 55 PTC consultants and 54 SC consultants demonstrated that most PTC and SC consultants recommend initiating re-immunization at six months after completion of standard-dose chemotherapy. Between 93% and 100% of respondents reported re-immunization at the recommended time after HSCT for each transplant type. (Physicians recommended pneumococcal conjugate vaccine after chemotherapy by 58.3% (35/60) of respondents and by 51.7% (30/58) after HSCT.) There were distinct differences between PTC and SC consultants in their choice of varicella postexposure prophylaxis.

PUBLIC HEALTH COMMITMENTS TO THE WORLD: INTERNATIONAL PUBLIC HEALTH AND DEVELOPING COUNTRIES

The following section addresses public health commitment from an organizational perspective. The WHO will be discussed, especially in relation to its current health goals, and the structures and processes which are intended to yield positive outcomes. Initiatives to address refugees internationally through the United Nations and other organizations across the globe (bilateral, multilateral, NGOs) will also be considered. In addition, the international face of nursing will be discussed with its focus on offering nursing science and evidence-based practice internationally.

FIGURE 2.4 World Health Organization Director General Adhanom Ghebreyesus (Image courtesy of the World Health Organization).

World Health Organization

When the United Nations was established in 1945, a key directive and commitment was to protect human rights, security, and the social development of all countries. The WHO was established in 1946 as part of the United Nations to maximize health and wellness for all (World Health Organization [WHO], 2017a). The WHO is located in Geneva, Switzerland, and has six regional offices, including a U.S. branch located in Washington, DC (Pan American Health Organization, PAHO). The relationship of the United Nations to the WHO is similar to that of the USD-HHS and the NIH to the CDC. For example, there is a keen focus on supplying current information about disease and disability and establishing standards of care on the basis of evidence found in health research. In the WHO, efforts are directed primarily to safely conquer disease and to help advance professionals and healthcare systems which allow this to occur with efficiency and effectiveness. In addition, the WHO, led by Director General Adhanom Ghebreyesus (Fig. 2.4), focuses on policy development through a process of supporting annual commissions and assemblies (e.g., World Health Assembly) as a means of advancing policies and guidelines to countries with common, or uniquely specific, healthcare problems (WHO, 2013b). The development of the WHO's Child Growth Standards used data collected in the WHO Multicentre Growth Reference Study. The WHO provides international access to

documentation on how physical growth curves and motor-skill milestones of achievement were developed, as well as application tools to support implementation of the standards (WHO, 2013c).

The 63rd session of the World Health Assembly in Geneva in May 2010 (WHO, 2017d) discussed a number of public health issues, including (1) implementation of the International Health Regulations (IHR), (2) monitoring of the achievement of the health-related **Millennium Development Goals (MDGs)**, (3) strategies to reduce the harmful use of alcohol, and (4) counterfeit medical products.

The IHR document is a legal brief that addresses transnational control of infectious diseases and was developed as a response to the increase in international travel and trade. On June 15, 2007, the IHRs became international law; 194 countries have agreed to implement the regulations. The IHR requires nations to strengthen core surveillance and response capacities to infection control at the primary, intermediate, and national level, as well as at designated international ports, airports, and ground crossings. The regulations further introduce a series of health documents, including ship sanitation certificates and an international certificate of vaccination or prophylaxis for travelers. The document is available at the WHO website.

Historically, the United Nations MDGs were eight goals that all 189 UN member states at the time agreed to try to achieve by the year 2015 (WHO, 2017d). The United Nations Millennium Declaration, signed in September 2000, committed world leaders to combat poverty, hunger, disease, illiteracy, environmental degradation, and discrimination against women. The MDGs were derived from this Declaration, and all have specific targets and indicators. The following are the specific goals:

1. To eradicate extreme poverty and hunger
2. To achieve universal primary education
3. To promote gender equality and empowering women
4. To reduce child mortality rates
5. To improve maternal health
6. To combat HIV/AIDS, malaria, and other diseases
7. To ensure environmental sustainability
8. To develop a global partnership for development

The UN MDGs have, overall, been remarkably successful in focusing attention and mobilizing resources to address the major gaps in human development. Some of the MDGs' key targets, such as halving the poverty rate were met; however, achieving the health goals continues to look very challenging (Center for International Governance Innovation, 2017).

These goals are now further empowered with the **United Nations Educational, Scientific, and Cultural Organization (UNESCO) Sustainable Development Goals**. The Sustainable Development Goals, or SDGs, are a global framework to coordinate efforts around ending poverty and hunger, combating inequality and disease, and building a just and stable world. There are 17 goals in all, and all 193 nations represented at the United Nations agreed to them (UNESCO, 2017).

The World Bank, the International Monetary Fund, and the African Development Bank agreed to cancel debt of the poorest countries so that resources could be used to improve health. Key criticisms about this monetary support has been related to the fact that much of the money (at least 50%) was diverted to disaster relief and military aid, areas for which it was not intended (World Bank Annual Report, 2010).

Refugee and Disaster-Relief Assistance

A **refugee** is defined as "any person who is outside his or her country of origin and who is unwilling or unable to return there or to avail him or herself of its protection because of a well-founded fear of being persecuted for reasons of race, religion, nationality, membership in a particular social group, or political opinion or a threat to life or security as a result of armed conflict and other forms of widespread violence which seriously disturb the public order" (Office of the United Nations High Commissioner for Human Rights [UNHCR], 2017). The United Nations High Commissioner for Refugees (UNHCR) was established by the International Refugee Organization, an organization that was founded on April 20, 1946, to deal with the massive refugee problem created by World War II.

Internally displaced persons are people who have been forced to flee their homes suddenly or unexpectedly in large numbers because of armed conflict, internal strife, systematic violations of human rights, or natural disasters, and who are *within* the territory of their own country (Office of the United Nations High Commissioner for Human Rights [OHCHR], 2017).

Most conflicts occur within rather than between countries. Compared with other continents, Africa and Asia have consistently registered high numbers of civil armed conflicts (Relief Web, 2013). Some of the countries that have experienced violent conflicts and prominent humanitarian interventions in the past two decades include Liberia, Angola, Sierra Leone, Rwanda, Sudan, Chechnya, Bosnia and Herzegovina (formerly Yugoslavia), Somalia, Sri Lanka, Azerbaijan, Armenia, Democratic Republic of Congo (DRC), Kosovo, East Timor, Afghanistan, and Iraq (Relief Web, 2017).

The health consequences experienced by populations affected by armed conflict are generally similar in nature. War-induced displacement is psychologically and physically traumatizing to everyone affected. People are rarely prepared for flight and have no time to gather clothes, food, or anything that can sustain their lives during displacement. Their search for safety can last for long periods, depending on the nature of war, prevailing geographical conditions, and the willingness of host communities to welcome them. Relatives and family members are often separated. Some are lost to capture, displacement, and/or death (Brown, deGraaf, Annan, & Betancourt, 2016).

The health effects of armed conflict may be direct or indirect. The direct effects include injuries (e.g., due to land mines, weapons), sexual violence, human rights violations, psychological trauma, and death. Indirect effects include food scarcity, population displacement, high levels of morbidity and mortality, infectious disease, complications of chronic disease, reproductive health morbidities, malnutrition, and disruption of health services (Levy & Sidel, 2016). It is significant that the United Nations, in its human rights activities, works with bilateral and multilateral agencies, NGOs, and the World Bank to offer health assistance in addition to the many other competing direct and indirect needs related to refugees.

Multilateral, Bilateral, and Nongovernmental Organizations as International Organizations for Health

International health organizations are classified on the basis of their relationships with other distinguished organizations which match their commitment to specific aspects of population-based health, the specific implementation of health goals both directly and indirectly, and their particular resources, including financial contributions. **Multilateral agencies** and organizations receive funding from both governmental and nongovernmental sources. Examples of these multilateral agencies include the United Nations and the WHO, which were discussed previously. The World Bank is another multilateral organization. Its major goal is to lend money to countries in need of developing their infrastructure on a variety of fronts. Some of the projects undertaken by the World Bank and related to health include addressing access to safe drinking water, soil development so that healthy foods can be grown and eaten, building sanitation systems so that water drainage is not connected directly to sewage, and promotion of vaccination programs, as well as promoting primary healthcare, which includes screening programs. Specific programs include Roll Back Malaria, the Joint United Nations Programme on HIV/AIDS, the Global Alliance for Vaccines and Immunizations, Onchocerciasis Control Program (river blindness control), and the Global Water Project (World Bank, 2017). (See the earlier discussion of WHO, United Nations, and MDGs for a critique of the use of promised monies to assist with health goals by World Bank and other funding organizations.)

Bilateral agencies and organizations conduct their services within one specific country. The U.S. Agency for International Development (USAID) is a good example in the United States. It is a committed initiative which works with developing countries to enhance systems to fortify the health and welfare of international populations. USAID focuses specifically on support directed to sub-Saharan Africa, Asia, Latin America, the Caribbean, Eurasia, and the Middle East. Key health prevention initiatives focus on larger areas of child, maternal, and reproductive health, and have specific interests in HIV/AIDS, malaria, and tuberculosis care (USAID, 2017). Many of the healthcare systems in countries described earlier in this chapter have parallel organizations to USAID.

NGOs, discussed earlier in this chapter, are private agencies that voluntarily use their resources to address a variety of healthcare initiatives in the United States. Some of these organizations have specific goals or roles in global health. For example, the International Committee of the Red Cross (2017) is known most for its role in disaster relief. Some groups, such as Catholic Relief Services, (2017), have a particular religious affiliation, and others, such as Oxfam International (2017), are directed specifically to issues related to hunger and nutritional health. Philanthropies are organizations that are similar to NGOs, but they receive funding through personal endowments. For example, the Bill and Melinda Gates Foundation (2017) focuses on health, poverty, and development in Africa, South America, Asia, and Australia. Specifically, The Living Proof Project supports vaccine and nutrition programs, as well as decreasing the incidence of diseases such as polio, HIV/AIDS, and tropical illnesses. In all cases, NGOs and philanthropies view human rights as a fundamental (motivation) basis for addressing the unseen and unfelt pain of many people in the world who suffer needlessly.

Practice Point

The United States offers a process of applying for tax-exempt status for not-for-profit NGOs, which are focused on national or international public health. This process requires filing specific forms with the Internal Revenue Service (IRS) and a fee, and there must be no involvement with or by any political campaigns. The organizational status acquired through this process is a tax-exempt, nonprofit corporation or association (a 501c3). It requires a board of directors be formed, with a stipulation in its by-laws which states the work intended to be done by the organization. In return, the IRS gives the organization tax exemption for purchases aligned with the mission of the organization, as well as other benefits and protections. Donations and contributions made to nonprofit organizations may be claimed as tax deductions on individual or corporate tax returns. Check out your local rules and regulations, or discuss this idea with any legal consultant you may know (perhaps a law student at your university or town).

International Council of Nurses

The International Council of Nurses (ICN) is a federation of more than 130 national nurses associations (NNAs), representing more than 13 million nurses worldwide. Founded in 1899, ICN is the world's first and widest-reaching international organization for health professionals. Operated by internationally prominent nurses, ICN works to ensure quality nursing care for all, sound health policies globally, the advancement of nursing knowledge, and the presence worldwide of a respected nursing profession and a competent and satisfied nursing work force (International Council of Nurses [ICN], 2017).

ICN advances nursing, nurses, and health through its policies, partnerships, advocacy, leadership development, networks, congresses, and special projects, and by its work in the arenas of professional practice, regulation, and socioeconomic welfare. ICN is particularly active in the following:

- International classification of nursing practice
- Advanced nursing practice
- Entrepreneurship
- HIV/AIDS, tuberculosis, and malaria
- Women's health
- Primary healthcare
- Family health
- Safe water

Despite the variation in healthcare structures between countries, and the varying degrees of both fiscal and health outcomes, nurses continue to advance the health of the public. Through (1) assessment of health across a variety of specialties and patient groups, (2) education of other nurses in health promotion and disease prevention, and (3) contributions to health policy development, nurses represent the voice of patients and clients worldwide.

KEY CONCEPTS

- Healthcare systems are organized based on philosophies of care and are culturally influenced.
- The United States healthcare system includes structure and functions to support assessment, assurance, and health policy related to the health of populations.
- Despite the economic strength of the United States and other industrialized nations, many countries have found more efficient and effective ways to care for all by decreasing health disparities and giving equal access to care.
- Public, philanthropic, and nongovernmental agencies all contribute to the health of populations through diverse structures, financing, and personnel approaches to the health needs of citizens.

CRITICAL THINKING QUESTIONS

1. Give three reasons why you think that comparing healthcare systems between countries is an important approach to serving the healthcare needs of people.
2. In thinking about multilateral, bilateral, and nongovernmental organizations, where would you see the role of a community/public health nurse? Give some examples, and explain why public health nurses provide a unique contribution.
3. How do cultural and philosophical factors play an important role in how healthcare systems are developed and supported? Give explicit examples.

COMMUNITY RESOURCES

- Local philanthropies and foundations with goals focused on healthcare
- State Department of Health
- Organizational chart of the (state house) legislative governance in your state (look for Health and Human Services)
- Insurance companies (private, HMOs)
- Departments of Social Services (Medicaid Division)

REFERENCES

Agency for Health Care Research and Quality (AHRQ). (2017a). *Child health quality toolbox*. Retrieved on June 23, 2017, from https://www.ahrq.gov/research/findings/factsheets/children/toolbox/index.html.

Agency for Health Care Research and Quality (AHRQ). (2017b). Retrieved on June 24, 2017, from https://www.ahrq.gov/.

American Red Cross. (2017). *Make a plan*. Retrieved on June 23, 2017, from http://www.redcross.org/get-help/how-to-prepare-for-emergencies/make-a-plan

Baird, K. E. (2016). Recent trends in the probability of high-out-of-the-pocket medical expenses in the United States. *Sage Open Medicine*, 9, 2050312116660329. *Date of Electronic Publication*: 20160909 (*Print Publication*: 2016).

Banda, E., Persky, V., Chisum, G., Damitz, M., Williams, R., & Turyk, M. (2013). Exposure to home and school environmental triggers and asthma morbidity in Chicago inner city children. *Pediatric Allergy and Immunology: Official Publication of the European Society of Pediatric Allergy and Immunology*, 24(8), 734–741.

Bekemeier, B., Zahner, S. J., Kulbok, P., Merrill, J. & Kub, J. (2016). Assuring a strong foundation for our nation's public health systems. *Nursing Outlook*, 64(6), 557–565.

Bourdelais, P. (2010). *Improving public health in France. The local political mobilization in the nineteenth century*. Retrieved on June 7, 2010, from http://www.ep.liu.se/ej/hygiea/ra/026/paper.pdf

Brehaut, J. C., Kohen, D. E., Garner, R. E., Miller A. R., Lach, L. M., Klassen, A. F., & Rosenbaum, P. L. (2009). Health among caregivers of children with health problems: Findings from a Canadian population-based study. *American Journal of Public Health*, 99, 1254–1262, doi: 10.2105.

Brown, F. L., deGraaf, A. M., Annan, J, & Betancourt, T. S. (2016). Annual research review: Breaking cycles of violence-a systematic review and common practice elements analysis of psychosocial interventions for children and youth affected by armed conflict. *Journal of Child Psychology and Psychiatry and Allied Disciplines*, Date of Electronic Publication: December 10, 2016, doi: 10.1111/jcpp.12671.

Catholic Relief Services. (2017). Retrieved on June 7, 2017, from http://crs.org/

Center for International Governance Innovation. (2017). Retrieved on June 25, 2017, from https://www.cigionline.org/publications/post-2015-development-agenda-goals-targets-and-indicators?gclid=CjwKEAjwvr3KBRD_i_Lz6cihrDASJADUkGCah44hcsQZEDWWf-NZT1e19P72Hif7TKLlb8gS4Ez3uihoCihnw_wcB

Center on Budget and Policy Priorities. (2017). Retrieved on June 24, 2017, from http://www.cbpp.org/

Centers for Disease Control and Prevention (CDC). (2017a). Retrieved on June 8, 2017, from http://cdc.gov

Centers for Disease Control and Prevention (CDC). (2017b). Pap Smears. Retrieved on June 24, 2017, from https://www.cdc.gov/nchs/fastats/pap-tests.htm

Centers for Medicare and Medicaid Services (CMS). (2017). Retrieved on June 8, 2017, from http://www.cms.gov/

Centers for Medicare and Medicaid Services [CMS]. (2018). Retrieved on November 2, 2018 from https://www.cms.gov/

Chidiac, C., & Ader, F. (2009). Pneumococcal vaccine in the elderly: A useful but forgotten vaccine. *Aging Clinical & Experimental Research*, 21(3), 222–228.

Children's Health Insurance Program. (2017). CHIP. Retrieved on June 24, 2017, from https://www.medicaid.gov/chip/index.html

REFERENCES *(Continued)*

Constant, A., Rachid Salmi, L., Lafont, S., Chiron, M., & Lagarde, E. (2009). Road casualties and changes in risky driving behavior in France between 2001 and 2004 among participants in the GAZEL Cohort. *American Journal of Public Health*, 99, 1247–1253, doi: 10.2105.

Friis, R. H., & Sellers, T. A. (2014). *Epidemiology for public health practice* (5th ed.). Sudbury, MA: Jones & Bartlett.

Gates Foundation. (2017). Retrieved on June 8, 2017, from http://www.gatesfoundation.org/Pages/home.aspx

Harwood, J. M., Azocar, F., Thalmayer, A., Xu, H., Ong, M. K., Tseng, C. H., … Ettner, S. L. (2017) The Mental Health Parity and Addiction Equity Act Evaluation Study. *Medical Care*, 55(2), 164–172.

Health Canada. (2017). Retrieved on June 8, 2017, from https://www.canada.ca/en/health-canada.html

Hirschhorn, L. R., Landers, S., McInnes, D. K., Malitz, F., Ding, L., Joyce, R., & Cleary, P. D. (2009). Reported care quality in federal Ryan White HIV/AIDS Program supported networks of HIV/AIDS care. *AIDS Care*, 21(6), 799–807.

Institute of Medicine. (2002). Unequal Treatment: Confronting Racial and Ethnic Disparities in Healthcare. *National Academies of Sciences, Engineering and Medicine.* Retrieved on November 2, 2018 from http://www.nationalacademies.org/hmd/Reports/2002/Unequal-Treatment-Confronting-Racial-and-Ethnic-Disparities-in-Health-Care.aspx

Internal Displacement Monitoring Center (IDMC). (2010). *Internal Displacement: Global Overview of Trends and Developments in 2008.* Retrieved on February 26, 2010, from http://www.internald-isplacement.org/8025708F004BE3B1/%28httpInfoFiles%29/82D A6A2DE4C7BA41C12575A90041E6A8/$file/IDMC_Internal_ Displacement_Global_Overview_2008.pdf

International Committee of the Red Cross. (2017). Retrieved on June 8, 2017, from http://www.icrc.org/

International Council of Nurses (ICN). (2017). Retrieved on June 8, 2017, from http://www.icn.ch/

Jackson, M. I. & Mayne, P. (2016). Child access to nutritional safety net during and after the great recession: The case of WIC. *Social Science & Medicine*, 170, 197–207.

Janosky, J. E., Armoutliev, E. M., Benipal, A, Kingsbury, D., Teller, J., Snyder, K. L. & Penny, R. (2013). Coalitions for impacting the health of a community: The Summit County, Ohio, Experience. *Population Health Management*, 16(4), 246–254.

Johnson, T. V., Schnatz, P. F., Johnson, A. M., & Sorosky, J. I. (2007). Update on cervical cancer screening. *Hospital Physician*, 4(5), 15–24.

Kaiser Foundation. (2010). *Health Coverage & the Uninsured: Profile of the Uninsured.* Retrieved on June 8, 2010, from http://www.kff.org/uninsured/profile.cfm

Kellogg Foundation. (2017). Retrieved on June 8, 2017, from http://www.wkkf.org/Default.aspx?LanguageID = 0

Keszei, A. P., Schouten, L. J., Goldbohm, R. A., & Van Den Brandt, P. A. (2009). Dairy intake and the risk of bladder cancer in the Netherlands cohort study on diet and cancer. *American Journal of Epidemiology*, 171(4), 436–446.

Lal, C., Strange, C., & Bachman, D. (2012). Neurocognitive impairment in obstructive sleep apnea. *Chest*. 141(6), 1601–1610.

Lassey, M., Lassey, W., & Jinks, M. (1997). *Health care systems around the world: Characteristics, issues and reforms.* Upper Saddle River, NJ: Prentice-Hall.

Levy, B. S. & Sidel, V. W. (2016). Documenting the effects of armed conflict on population health. *Annual Review of Public Health*, 37, 205–218.

McGuire, S. (2014). Borders, centers, and margins: Critical landscapes for migrant health. *Advances in Nursing Science*, 37(3), 197–212.

National Conference of State Legislatures. (2009). *Final maternity length-of-stay rules published*. Retrieved on June 24, 2017, from http://www.ncsl.org/research/health/final-maternity-length-of-stay-rules-published.aspx

National Institutes of Health (NIH). (2017). Retrieved on June 8, 2017, from http://nih.gov

National Library of Medicine. (2017). Drug information portal. Retrieved on June 23, 2017, from https://druginfo.nlm.nih.gov/drugportal/drugportal.jsp

National Prevention Council, National Prevention Strategy. (2011). Retrieved on November 2, 2018 from https://www.surgeonge-neral.gov/priorities/prevention/strategy/report.pdf

Nayaradou, M., Berchi, C., Dejardin, O., & Launoy, G. (2010). Eliciting population preferences for mass colorectal cancer screening organization. *Medical Decision Making*, 30(2), 224–233.

Office for Refugees and Immigrants (ORI). (2017). Retrieved on June 23, 2017, from http://www.mass.gov/eohhs/gov/departments/ori/

Office of the United Nations High Commissioner for Human Rights (OHCHR). (2017). *Questions and answers about IDP*. Retrieved on June 14, 2017, from http://www.ohchr.org/EN/pages/home.aspx

Organization of Economic Cooperation and Development, Health Statistics, Definitions, Sources, and Methods. (2016). Retrieved on June 14, 2017, from http://stats.oecd.org/fileview2.aspx?IDFile = efc0d5e1-1350-4d26-a1ff-7d17533dede5

Organization of Economic Cooperation and Development (OECD). (2017a). *United States Health Data.* Retrieved on June 9, 2017, from https://data.oecd.org/healthres/health-spending.htm

Organization of Economic Cooperation and Development (OECD). (2017b). Canada. Retrieved on June 25, 2017, from http://www.oecd.org/canada/

Organization of Economic Cooperation and Development (OECD). (2017c). France. Retrieved on June 25, 2017, from http://www.oecd.org/france/

Organization of Economic Cooperation and Development (OECD). (2017d). Germany. Retrieved on June 25, 2017, from http://www.oecd.org/germany/

Organization of Economic Cooperation and Development (OECD). (2017e). Netherlands. Retrieved on June 25, 2017, from http://www.oecd.org/netherlands/

Organization of Economic Cooperation and Development (OECD). (2017f). United Kingdom. Retrieved on June 25, 2017, from http://www.oecd.org/united kingdom/

Organization of Economic Cooperation and Development (OECD). (2017g). Health Data 2009. Retrieved on June 10, 2010, from http://www.oecd.org/dataoecd/46/8/38980162.pdf

Overview of Uninsured in the United States. (2011).*Office of the Assistant Secretary for Planning and Evaluation.* Retrieved on November 2, 2018 from https://aspe.hhs.gov/basic-report/overview-uninsured-united-states-summary-2011-current-population-survey

Oxfam International. (2017). Retrieved on June 11, 2017, from http://www.oxfam.org/

Patel, S. R., Chisholm, J. C., & Health, P. T. (2008). Vaccinations in children treated with standard-dose cancer therapy or hematopoietic stem cell transplantation. *Pediatric Clinics of North American*, 55(1), 169–186.

Regidor, E., Sánchez, E., de la Fuente, L., Luquero, F. J., de Mateo, S., & Domínguez, V. (2009). Major reduction in AIDS-mortality inequalities after HAART: The importance of absolute differences in evaluating interventions. *Social Science & Medicine*, 68(3), 419–426.

Relief Web. (2013). Retrieved on November 2, 2018 from https://reliefweb.int/report/world/reliefweb-highlights-2013

Relief Web. (2017). Retrieved on June 11, 2017, from http://relief-web.int/

Robert Wood Johnson Foundation. (2017). Retrieved on June 8, 2017, from http://www.rwjf.org/

Schnieder, M. J. (2017). *Introduction to public health.* (5th ed.). Burlington, MA: Jones and Barlett.

Sexton, K. R., Franzini, L., Day, R. S., Brewster, A., &Vernon S. W. (2011). A review of body size and breast cancer risk in Hispanic and African American women. *Cancer, 117*(23), 5271–5281.

Shi, L. & Johnson, J. A. (2014). *Novick and Morrow's Public health administration: Principles for population-based management.* 3rd ed. Boston, MA: Jones and Bartlett Learning LLC.

Speroni, K. G., Williams, D. A., Siebert, D. J., Gibbons, M. G., & Earley, C. (2013). Helping nurses care for self, family, and patients through the nurses living fit intervention. *Nursing Administration Quarterly, 37*(4), 286–294.

Stolle, M., Sack, P., & Thomasius, R. (2009). Binge drinking in childhood and adolescence: Epidemiology, consequences, and interventions. *Deutsches Ärzteblatt International, 106*(19), 323–328.

Tang, B. M., Craig, J. C., Eslick, G. D., Seppelt, I., & McLean, A. S. (2009). Use of corticosteroids in acute lung injury and acute respiratory distress syndrome: A systematic review and meta-analysis. *Critical Care Medicine, 37*(5), 1594–1603.

The White House. (2017). Retrieved on May 25, 2017, from https://www.whitehouse.gov/repeal-and-replace-obamacare.

U.K. Department of Health. (2017). Retrieved on June 8, 2017, from http://www.dh.gov.uk/en/index.htm

UNESCO. (2017). *Sustainable development goals.* Retrieved on June 25, 2017, from http://en.unesco.org/sdgs

United Nations Children Fund. (2017). Retrieved on June 10, 2017, from https://www.unicef.org/

Urban Institute. (2013). Retrieved on November 2, 2018 from https://www.urban.org/search?search_api_views_fulltext=block%20grants

U.S. Agency for International Development (USAID). (2017). Retrieved on June 8, 2017, from https://www.usaid.gov/

U.S. Department of Health and Human Services (USDHHS). (2017a). Retrieved on June 8, 2017, from https://www.hhs.gov/

U.S. Department of Health and Human Services. (2017b). *Healthy People 2020.* Retrieved on June 8, 2010, from https://www.healthypeople.gov/2020/topics-objectives

U.S. Department of Veterans Affairs. (2017). Retrieved on June 8, 2017, fromhttps://www.va.gov/healthbenefits/

World Bank. (2017). Retrieved on June 8, 2017, from http://www.worldbank.org/

World Bank Annual Report. (2010). Retrieved on November 2, 2018 from http://siteresources.worldbank.org/EXTANNREP2010/Resources/WorldBank-AnnualReport2010.pdf

World Health Organization (WHO). (2017a). Retrieved on June 8, 2017, from http://www.who.int/about/en/

World Health Organization (WHO). (2010b). *Governance.* Retrieved on June 8, 2017, from http://www.who.int/mediacentre/events/governance/wha/en/

World Health Organization (WHO). (2017c). *Child growth standards.* Retrieved on June 8, 2017, from http://www.who.int/childgrowth/en/

World Health Organization (WHO). (2017d). *Millennium development goals.* Retrieved on June 8, 2017, from http://www.who.int/topics/millennium_development_goals/en/

Chapter 3

Health Policy, Politics, and Reform

Anahid Kulwicki and Sabreen A. Darwish

Healing is a matter of time, but it is sometimes also a matter of opportunity.

Hippocrates

Disruptive innovation is not about pushing out the incumbent, it's about giving the consumer a choice.

Dr. Jason Hwang, co-author of *The Innovator's Prescription: A Disruptive Solution for Healthcare*

CHAPTER HIGHLIGHTS

- Healthcare policy and the political process
- Healthcare finance and cost–benefit in relation to health policy
- Access to healthcare and insurance facts in the United States
- Healthcare workforce diversity and its effects on the quality of healthcare
- Nursing's role in shaping healthcare policy
- Quality of care and evaluation
- Information management facts
- Equity in healthcare access
- Ethical consideration in health policy
- Political advocacy, how to be politically active and advocate
- Health advocacy and healthcare reform
- Affordable Care Act (ACA) overview and updates
- Community-based services and healthcare reform
- Health services research application to healthcare policy

OBJECTIVES

- Define public health, policy, and politics while identifying the relationships between concepts.
- Explain the effect of politics in healthcare policy.
- Identify the steps of policymaking and understand them comprehensively.
- Apply the process of policymaking to explain daily decisions regarding health and health choices.
- Understand facts regarding the healthcare system, access to care, and insurance issues.
- Identify the basic economic and financial concepts in relation to healthcare services.
- Identify the definition and determinants of quality of care.
- Understand the critical role of nurses in healthcare reforms through political advocacy.
- Explain the importance of workforce diversity, and the concept of cultural competency.
- Understand the information management involved in the healthcare system.
- Explain the ethical and legal considerations in the policymaking process.
- Explain the major reforms in the healthcare system in the United States.
- Understand the main foundations and premises of the Affordable Care Act (ACA), community health services, and the role of the ACA
- Understand the value of health services research in the healthcare system.

KEY TERMS

Affordable Care Act (ACA): The comprehensive healthcare reform law enacted in March 2010 (sometimes known as the Patient Protection and Affordable Care Act [PPACA], the Health Care and Education Reconciliation Act, or "Obamacare") designed to improve the quality and accessibility of healthcare while reducing its cost.

Centers for Medicare and Medicaid Services (CMS): Federal agency that runs the Medicare, Medicaid, and Children's Health Insurance Programs, and the federally facilitated marketplace that was designed to enact and achieve the goals of the ACA, which were first articulated by the Institute for Healthcare Improvement.

Cost–benefit: An economic approach or analysis tool used to evaluate the effectiveness of a treatment or intervention. Mathematically speaking, the net economic benefit can be calculated by subtracting the costs for a service from the benefits of this service. If this value is positive, it implies that the benefit from a specific intervention exceeds its cost. An intervention is judged to be unworthy if its cost exceeds the benefits gained from carrying it out.

Cost sharing: The arrangement that defines how you and an insurer pay for insured services or items. Coinsurance, copayment, and deductibles are all forms of cost sharing. Premiums, payments for uncovered healthcare supplies or services, or fees paid to out-of-network providers are not shared costs.

Cultural competency: The knowledge, skills, attitudes, and behaviors that are learned in order to provide the optimal health service to individuals from a variety of ethnic, racial, and cultural backgrounds.

Deductibles: The amount you pay in a calendar year before your health plan begins to pay. For instance, if your deductible is $2,000, you must pay that amount out-of-pocket for covered health services before your insurer begins paying your healthcare costs.

Economics: The study of how individuals, groups, organizations, and society allocate and utilize finances, personnel, time, and physical space as components of resources. Economic tools and other quantitative financial measures are used as a method of evaluating the existing governmental, private programs or public, and private policy alternatives.

Equity: As applied to healthcare, the notion that healthcare does not vary in quality because of gender, race, age, ethnicity, geographic location, or socioeconomic status.

Gross domestic product (GDP): The main economic indicator used to evaluate the degree of economic growth in the United States. It is defined as the final and total output of goods and services produced in 1 year by labor input within the United States. The figure of GDP is reported quarterly.

Health policy: Policy that has an impact on the health of an individual, a family, a population, or a community and is created by the government, institution(s), or professional association(s).

National health expenditure: The total spending in dollars for the costs of healthcare goods and services in a 1-year period. National health spending is one of the many parts that constitute the GDP, and the growth in health expenditure is usually compared to the GDP growth.

Out-of-pocket costs: The costs that aren't covered by your health plan. Deductibles,

coinsurance, copayments, and some supplies or services are examples.

Patient advocacy: A vital nursing professional duty of supporting actions that are in the best interest of patients' health and that defend patient rights via speaking on patients' behalf. Such support is targeted toward the overall well-being and the contribution to the healing process.

Policy: Principles that govern an action to achieve a given outcome. Policies are guidelines that direct individuals' behavior toward a specific goal. They are deliberate courses of action chosen by an individual or group to confront problems.

Politics: Process of influencing the allocation of resources (financial, human, time, or physical space). Additionally, politics represents how conflicts are expressed and resolved in a society. Politics also may be a factor in deciding who participates or who influences governmental decision-making.

Public health policy: A set of policies (governing principles) that has a health-related mission and has an impact on the health and well-being of the population.

Political advocacy: Being involved in the legislative process and influencing decision-making in relation to healthcare to best serve the public interest as well as the profession by enacting the advocacy role to influence a change in policies, laws, or regulations that govern the larger healthcare system.

Quality of care: A concept used to evaluate the extent of how efficiently and effectively healthcare systems provide safe patient care at a reasonable cost to people in

KEY TERMS *(continued)*

need. It is the degree to which health services for individuals and populations increase the likelihood of a desired health outcome.

Reform: Form again; improvement of what is wrong or

unsatisfactory. It is for the better, especially as a result of improvement of legal or political abuses or malpractices.

Workforce diversity: The presence of a variety of ethnic,

religious, age, gender, sexual orientation, socioeconomic status, nationality, disability, geographic location, racial, and cultural backgrounds of the workers in a specific area such as the health sector.

CASE STUDY   *References to the case study are found throughout this chapter (look for the case study icon). Readers should keep the case study in mind as they read the chapter.*

You are caring for an 8-year-old African American female patient on the general pediatrics floor. She was transferred from the PICU, where she was admitted for respiratory failure and status asthmaticus. She has a history of "wheezing" but has never been diagnosed with asthma. She receives the majority of her care in the emergency department (ED) and urgent care centers. She has never been on asthma medications. She lives at home with her mother and two siblings. Her mother is employed as a clerk at a hospital and earns $29,942 per year. Her mother's employer provides health insurance. However, she cannot afford to add all three of her children to her health insurance plan. As you read through the chapter, consider the following questions.

Lack of health insurance limits this patient's access to quality asthma care. Barriers to quality care exist even for those who are insured. What are some of those barriers? Are there differences in asthma prevalence by race and income? Are there differences in how children in minority groups access medical care? How do these differences affect asthma care? How are most children in the United States insured? Do you think it is common for a person to have a job yet not have health insurance coverage for their children? What are other health insurance options available to this family? How can you advocate for this child? How can you help ensure improved asthma care for all?

Being engaged in the healthcare system as a healthcare professional providing care, as an administrator, or even as a client, it is important to have a general understanding of how the healthcare system works. What are the guiding principles that affect individuals' daily decisions regarding their health and health choices? Who is involved in the process of decision-making? What are the steps that are followed during this process? How can nurses be an active part in the process of developing or changing healthcare policies? Do patients have input into these policies? How does a healthcare policy affect an individual's access to healthcare? Are politics different from healthcare policies? Are politics isolated from any ethical or legal considerations? As healthcare providers, how can nurses be involved in reforming the healthcare system? How can they do so by using research or evidence in reforming healthcare?

This chapter will answer these questions. Moreover, it will give the reader the opportunity to start thinking about the challenges and problems in the healthcare system in a broad and comprehensive manner, to analyze these problems critically, and to find solutions by considering the political process and policy actions. In other words, the reader will be able to better understand challenges addressed

by health policies and understand researcher input that may improve the U.S. healthcare system.

HEALTHCARE POLICY AND THE POLITICAL PROCESS

Policy can be created in the form of a law or a guideline of public and private institutions (Centers for Disease Control and Prevention [CDC], 2015). Health policy refers to decision-making to reach health goals and these decisions are made to direct future health planning and outcomes within a framework of time (World Health Organization [WHO], 2017).

Porche (2012) defines policies as a set of principles that govern an action to achieve a given outcome, or guidelines that direct individuals' behavior toward a specific goal. Kraft and Furlong (2013) define policy as decisions characterized by behavioral consistency, which reflect the values and beliefs of two parties, namely, policymakers and policy followers. Moreover, they claim that policy refers to the goals, plans, and specific strategies or programs used in achieving a given outcome. Public policies address community problems and are developed by public or government officials (Kraft & Furlong, 2013). Health policy broadly describes the actions taken by governments—national, state, and local—to advance the public's health (Acuff, 2017).

Health policies are those policies that have an impact on the health of an individual, a family, and a population or community and are created within the government, institution, or professional association (Porche, 2012). Health policies are crafted to alleviate issues of health or healthcare (Mason, Leavitt, & Chaffee, 2012). "States use health policies to specify requirements for licensure in the health professions, to set criteria for eligibility for Medicaid, and to mandate immunization requirements for public university students" (Mason et al., 2012, p. 3). Furthermore, U.S. states are involved with healthcare policy in many ways; some directly operate public hospitals and mental health facilities, while others administer public health departments that operate public health clinics (Acuff, 2017). In addition to the state level, policies can be separated into local or national. An example of a state-level policy would be a school board crafting a policy in regard to contraceptive care, whereas an example of national policies would include laws and regulations in regard to access to care and reimbursement for advanced practice nurses (Leavitt, 2009). In times of emergency at the local, state, or national levels there is concentration of effort through the Federal Emergency Management Administration (FEMA). The FEMA addresses through organized coordination of a variety of key services assistance when natural and man-made disasters occur but they also do this work successfully by being responsible in getting all of these levels of services prepared in light of a disaster or any kind (Acuff, 2017).

Moreover, three main components of **public health policy** are reported consistently in the literature, namely, (1) health-related decisions guided by the stated laws written by legislators, (2) rules and regulations designed to operate the health-related activities and programs, and (3) the judicial decisions related to health, which involve both federal and state governments (Porche, 2012).

Practice Point

As was previously discussed, politics cannot be separated from the process of policymaking. There are many different ways to describe the impact of politics. First, politics are concerned with the exercising of power and decision-making in a society (Kraft & Furlong, 2013). Second, politics are usually studied as the process of formulating and adopting policies along with focusing on the role of both governmental institutions and the public.

Involving Politics

Politics are the process of influencing the allocation of resources needed to enable policies, and involves the strategies needed to achieve the desired goals (Mason et al., 2012). Politics also reflects how conflicts and problems are expressed and resolved in the context of society, and involves choices and influences based on power dynamics (Leavitt, 2009). Additionally, politics helps in answering questions regarding who participates or who influences governmental decision-making, and who benefits or who does not. Therefore, it is impossible to understand health policy or any type of public policy without considering political factors, which affect every level of policy formulation.

Kraft and Furlong (2013) discussed many reasons to involve the government in the policymaking process. These reasons usually reflect political, moral, ethical, and economical responsibilities. The two latter reasons will be discussed later in this chapter. In reference to a political issue, the government should be interested in problems that affect a specific group or a whole population. This interest usually takes the form of legislations that provide substantial solutions for the health problems that threaten the safety of the citizens and/or their environment. There are many examples of the positive role that governments play through policies and legislations—to name a few: providing equal opportunity through universal provision of education, healthcare, and often, housing and nutrition programs (Grogan, 2012).

Solutions can be achieved by working at either the federal or the state level. However, Rice and team (2013) explain that there is little agreement between the two major U.S. political parties (Democrats and Republicans) when it comes to how, when, to whom, and what kind of healthcare should be provided, and who should pay for it. Rice and colleagues (2013) concluded that in attempting to answer healthcare-related critical questions, disagreement between the two major political parties can create difficulty in finding solutions to the problems of the society, and hence to policies, including those of healthcare. Consequently, this can influence access to healthcare and the possibility of improving the **quality of care** provided (Rice et al., 2013).

Additionally, politics interacts with every aspect of healthcare in the United States (Morone, Litman, & Robins, 2008). Accordingly, U.S. politicians are interested in making decisions for the society that can be enforced by rules, laws, and regulations. Politics is sometimes perceived as a negative and unfavorable way to deal with social issues. However, politics provides the power needed to influence critical decisions regarding the allocation and distribution of resources in a society. Moreover, political actions are the tools used by politicians and the official representatives of the citizenry to shape decisions.

In summary, Mason and colleagues (2012) identified three common themes, which can be extracted from the different definitions of politics. First, the power of influence implies there is room for shaping desired outcomes by having an impact on the decisions made by governments, communities, or associations. Second, the most critical process for politics is to make decisions regarding the distribution and allocation of resources. Third, resources vary and include financial, human (personnel), time, and physical space. These resources are often found to be scarce. It is argued by Brownson, Fielding, and Maylahn (2009) that the availability of adequate resources can strongly affect the decision-making process. Accordingly, resources are believed to affect the desired outcome and outputs from a given policy.

While the previous themes of governmental power, decision-making, and resources are vital in understanding the political role in decision-making, it is crucial to acknowledge the fact that healthcare professionals, namely nurses, have political skills and active roles in healthcare leadership. As highlighted by Mason and colleagues (2012), those skills are as follows:

1. Having social skills and the ability to understand, interpret, and represent one's own and others' behaviors
2. Having the ability, qualifications, and power to influence others and make changes
3. Networking ability to develop, connect, and use different social networks
4. Having a high level of integrity, sincerity, and genuineness

Des Jardin (2001) notes that nurses, in the role of negotiating and finding moderating points of agreement in political charged areas of concern, are very skilled in negotiating, communicating clearly, solving problems and creating consensus (Boswell, Cannon, & Miller, 2005). Nurses are trusted nationally and internationally and trust is a significant ingredient to assisting with agendas focused on change and consequently to help in making improvements in healthcare and the healthcare system (Boswell et al., 2005; Williams, 1993). Because nurses are active at the point of care with many patients and families it brings them to see their role and act in the capacity to influence changes in policies, laws, or regulations that govern the larger healthcare system (Oestberg, 2013).

Politics are interconnected with policymaking because politicians can control and determine the allocation of resources. To put health policies in place, politicians must agree on the most prevalent health issues and on how to address these issues, as they greatly impact the nation's health (Porche, 2012). To best serve their patients and best understand their field, nurses and other healthcare professionals are encouraged to be involved in the political process and in the development of health policies.

For the previously mentioned reasons, it is important for healthcare professionals to understand some of the important terms and concepts that are related to healthcare politics and policy. Putting policies in place is a process. Policymaking takes a great deal of effort, time, and commitment. Porche (2012) laid out a dynamic series of events that take place in the policymaking process (Fig. 3.1).

- Setting an agenda: the crucial basic phase when the problem of common interest is identified for a specific community or a group. Three factors were found to play a role in this stage and were identified by Porche (2012): (1) the significance of the problem, (2) the political support for

FIGURE 3.1 Policy cycle.

addressing the problem, and (3) the ability to perceive the viability of proposed alternative solutions for the problem. For example, tobacco use is a major contributor to morbidity and mortality, which threaten populations globally. Consequently, governments play a critical role in encouraging or discouraging smoking behavior through different policies along with the role of nurses as political advocates for achieving health improvements.

- Policy formulation: the stage in which the possible and available alternative policies are identified and a specific policy is selected. Continuing the discussion on tobacco use, all possible and effective policy measures, such as smoke-free indoor air laws, tobacco industry–regulating policies at all levels—state, local, and national—should be addressed and discussed to select the most effective policy in reducing the prevalence of smoking.

- Policy adoption: the process of selecting the policy that should gain support, power, and directions for the legislators. In order to proceed in the process of fighting tobacco use, all proposed policies need to gain support from stakeholders at the different levels starting from state level and ending at the local level, along with nursing's role in reflecting and directing the selection of policies.

- Policy implementation: the stage in which the actual carrying out of the policy takes place by using the available human and financial resources. In terms of tobacco use, in this stage, real application of the anti-tobacco policies takes place when representatives at different political levels, including nurses, start to enhance and reinforce the application of smoke-free environments using all possible resources. Law enforcement is critical in this stage.

- Policy assessment: evaluation of the implemented policy in terms of being compliant or congruent with the statutory requirements, and whether it really serves the goal of solving the problem. Because the goal of anti-tobacco policies and regulations is to prevent tobacco-related diseases through reducing smoking prevalence, the success of these policies can be evaluated mainly by assessing the extent of achieving these goals, along with consideration for cost containment and effectiveness of policy-based interventions.

- Policy modification: depending on the prior step, the policy can be maintained, changed, or eliminated, according to its level of appropriateness. In this step, a decision takes place either to maintain working according to the anti-tobacco policies or to modify them and replace them, considering other alternative policies, and the process of policymaking repeats itself.

Evidence for Practice

Tobacco use is a major global contributor to illness and is projected to kill more than 1 billion people during this century if present trends continue (WHO, 2008). Nurses are increasingly engaged in community- and policy-level activities to improve health and prevent disease and disability by conducting research that focuses on the tobacco industry and related policies. Malone (2009) conducted a literature review on research studies conducted by nurses on the tobacco industry. The epidemic of tobacco and its health consequences result primarily from the industry's promotion through marketing to groups who already struggle with health challenges and may have literacy challenges. These approaches undermine public health interventions to address smoking behavior. The notion that smoking is a behavioral choice of individuals creates further barriers to understanding the larger social and political context within which individuals use and attempt to quit tobacco.

Nurses have been among the researchers worldwide who are studying tobacco industry activities and their role in policy and public health. Much of the nursing research to date focuses on four broad areas: (1) the tobacco industry's influence on policy, (2) its strategic responses to public health efforts, (3) its targeting of marginalized groups, and (4) its influence on research processes and outcomes.

Recommendations:

1. Traditional tobacco prevention and cessation efforts must accompany understanding of the role of the tobacco industry in shaping and contextualizing counseling programs.
2. Nurses need to be prepared to intervene as clinicians, community health proponents, policy advocates, researchers, and educators.
3. Nurses have the political power to influence perceptions about tobacco and the tobacco industry because they are highly trusted by the public and respected by policymakers for their numbers and political savvy.
4. Innovative archival research on the tobacco industry can help nurses reframe tobacco as a nursing issue, and link practices and government policies to their clinical practice.
5. Finally, nurses working in public health and policy arenas can help educate the public about the tobacco industry's ongoing efforts to encourage tobacco use, with major health consequences.

In the United States, both state legislatures and the U.S. Congress are responsible for determining appropriate healthcare policies. These state and national government representatives work on creating policies to solve problems affecting a specific group, a geographic area, or the entire population (Kraft & Furlong, 2013). These policies usually take the form of legislation, which provides substantial solutions for the health problems that threaten the health and safety of the citizens. This legislation can be achieved by working at either the federal or the state level. Health policy is not a single action but needs a range of legislative and regulatory efforts from ensuring air and water quality to supporting health-related research (Acuff, 2017). Although state legislatures and members of Congress can work collaboratively to solve problems and distribute resources, there is often much delay and disagreement between major political parties such as the Democratic and Republican parties (Rice et al., 2013). Because of such disagreements, it is difficult to build an effective collaboration in healthcare policymaking, and this can influence the individual's access to care and the possibility of improving the quality of care (Rice et al., 2013).

HEALTHCARE FINANCES AND COST–BENEFIT

Economics is the study of how individuals, groups, organizations, and society allocate and utilize resources (Porche, 2012). Consequently, it is critical to apply economic tools and various quantitative measures as a method of evaluating the existing governmental programs or public policy alternatives (Kraft & Furlong, 2013). Politics and economics interact at either the microeconomic level, which concerns the allocation of resources at the individual decision-making level, or the macroeconomic level (Porche, 2012). Economically speaking, any process of allocating fiscal resources is usually directed to best meet the human need and to improve their well-being (Kraft & Furlong, 2013). In the health context, for example, if the government spends more on medical visits than is needed to benefit its populations, this will lead to a decrease in resources available for other services such as education. Hence, the role of economics is extremely vital to enforce appropriate, effective, and efficient allocation of resources on the different areas of services provided for populations, and to achieve balance and justice reinforced by policies, laws, and regulation.

In studying health finance, it is critical to understand key terms. In the United States, the **gross domestic product** (GDP) is the main economic indicator used in the processes of evaluating policies in terms of their contribution to the economic growth. GDP is defined as the final and total output of goods and services produced by labor input within the United States in 1 year as determined by the Bureau of Economic Analysis (USBEA, 2013) in the U.S. Department of Commerce. The GDP figure is reported and released quarterly each year by the BEA. **National health expenditure** is one of the many components of the GDP, and the growth in health expenditure is usually compared to the GDP. As highlighted by Hartman, Martin, Benson, and Catlin (2013), the total U.S. healthcare spending reached $2.7 trillion in 2011, representing a 3.9% increase from 2010.

There is a set of economic analysis processes used to evaluate economic policy outcomes. The **cost–benefit** approach has been considered pivotal in evaluating the effectiveness of a treatment or intervention (Sorbello, 2008). It is the most frequently used approach because it serves to illustrate both the strengths and weaknesses of a given policy (Kraft & Furlong, 2013). Consequently, economists were found to be continuously interested in finding answers for the questions such as *who gets the benefit and who bears the burden of a policy? How should we measure the values, costs, and benefits of a specific policy?* In this type of analysis, economists are concerned with measuring the relative costs (in actual monetary value) against the benefits (both monetary and quality-of-life value) of a given program or any aspect of healthcare (Sorbello, 2008).

Practice Point

Mathematically speaking, the net economic benefit can be calculated by subtracting the costs from the benefits. If this value is positive, this implies that the benefit from a specific intervention exceeds its cost, so a decision is made to adopt such intervention. In contrast, an intervention is judged to be ineffective in terms of its costs if its cost exceeds the benefits gained from carrying it out. Although this process seems to be easily accomplished, it is a complicated process when it involves the healthcare system.

As described by Sorbello (2008), cost can be direct, in which the patient as a consumer is supposed to pay these costs at the time of service. For example, direct costs can be supplies or medications. Indirect costs are costs that are not assigned directly to the patient, but are related to the provision of services at the organizational level. Similarly, health benefits or outcomes can vary from simple, direct benefits to more complicated benefits. Outcomes should be objective, measurable, and representative of the treatment interventions, which is not an easy task to calculate, especially if the outcomes need to be expressed in dollars (Kraft & Furlong, 2013). However, less tangible outcomes, such as prevention of long-term suffering or disability, and quality of life, are more difficult to quantify. On the other hand, hospital days or dollars spent in a specific health service, for example, can be easily measured and evaluated.

There is one important process, which should not be ignored in cost–benefit analysis. Economists in their analysis of the costs and benefits must involve the perspectives of the different healthcare components that are participants in providing or receiving this service. Morone and colleagues (2008) explain there are many perspectives that should be considered and satisfied when providing a specific healthcare service. In other words, it is crucial for economists to consider the costs of the people who are counted, the type of costs involved, and the type of outcome that is desired. From the patients' perspectives, patients usually are more interested in their own costs and benefits. In other words, they are interested in their own expenses and **out-of-pocket** (OOP) expenses. Patients are also concerned about other types of costs, such as their psychological costs, suffering, and pain, which are difficult to quantify yet have long-lasting negative effects. Regarding the payer's perspective, the actual payment for the service is usually what matters. The providers are usually concerned with the actual and direct cost of providing a service.

Finally, it is critical to consider the societal concern, which usually includes all direct and indirect costs and benefits at the broader community level regardless of who benefits from or pays for the services. However, using the cost–benefit analysis as the only criterion in evaluating the efficiency and effectiveness of a policy is restricted by the fact that cost and benefits are not distributed evenly among individuals, consumers, or providers (Kraft & Furlong, 2013). In other words, the economic analysis should involve the distribution of costs and accessibility of the benefits in their analysis. Equity will be discussed in the following sections.

In summary, health spending is a product of services and the cost associated with those services. When a policy is evaluated for its effectiveness, there is an interest in keeping the cost of a specific health program within reason. Moreover, there is consideration for the overall costs and benefits of the existing program, in the event a more efficient and effective service is identified.

ACCESS TO CARE AND HEALTH INSURANCE

Before discussing access to care and health insurance, it is important first to understand the nature of the U.S. healthcare system, which is a unique system of independent and collaborative powers of both federal and state governments (Morone et al., 2008).

Evidence for Practice

In a large exploratory study comparing the U.S. healthcare system with that of other countries, Rice and colleagues (2013) highlighted the following facts about the U.S. system:

1. Private sector stakeholders play a stronger role in the U.S. healthcare system than in other high-income countries.
2. The major federal government health insurance programs Medicare and Medicaid were established in the mid-1960s.
3. Medicare provides coverage for seniors and the disabled, while Medicaid covers healthcare services for qualified low-income individuals (also covering limited care needs for qualifying seniors).
4. Public sources constitute 48% of healthcare expenditures in the United States.
5. Private third-party payers pay 40%, with the remaining 12% being paid OOP by individuals.
6. Only a minority (30%) of the U.S. population is covered by the public financing system, mainly through Medicare and Medicaid. Currently, 54% of Americans receive their coverage from private health insurance, with most (36%) privately insured individuals obtaining coverage through an employer.
7. One in six Americans is uninsured and over 17% of the population are without health. Because of the Affordable Care Act, the number of nonelderly who was at 10.3% in 2016.
8. Even among those with coverage, high OOP costs can be a barrier to receiving timely care and medications. Many others face high OOP expenses due to underinsurance.
9. The underinsured include elderly individuals who receive Medicare but cannot afford supplemental insurance or the OOP expenses associated with Medicare.
10. Those covered by Medicaid have insurance, but may experience problems accessing primary care due to their inability to find a private physician who accepts Medicaid patients. OOP expenses may also be a factor in inability to access care.
11. Patients in rural areas may find it impossible to get to primary care facilities. Medical costs are responsible for over 60% of personal bankruptcies in the country.

Concerns regarding racial/ethnic minorities, low-income groups, and uninsured groups overlap because of similar barriers these populations experience in accessing healthcare and obtaining quality services. Many low-income and uninsured populations are from diverse racial and ethnic minorities. National programs for improvement of access to quality healthcare for low-income and ethnic and racial minorities in United States are often addressed simultaneously. There are, of course, special issues within each population that need to be taken into consideration. Frequently, community health agencies play an important role in providing access to healthcare for underserved groups, especially those who are uninsured and with low income.

HEALTHCARE WORKFORCE DIVERSITY

The United States is a home for individuals from different ethnic backgrounds. Although the numbers are not growing as rapidly as the immigration of ethnically diverse populations, the United States has had an increase in the number of healthcare professionals immigrating to the United States from other countries (Hohn, Lowry, Witte, & Fernadez-Pena, 2016). Workforce diversity can address two important areas of outreach and support to communities affected by health disparities by **reducing health** disparities themselves and encouraging minority health professionals to work in these areas of underrepresented racial and ethnic minority groups (White, Zangaro, Kepley, & Camacho, 2014). However, the shortage of healthcare providers in the United States and the higher pay of health professionals in high-income countries have led to the migration of healthcare professionals from developing countries. In addition to the higher wages in United States, the opportunities for advancement are an incentive for health professionals' migration to the United States. Although healthcare professionals emigrating from other countries have filled critical vacancies, helped improve culturally competent care, and played important roles in innovations to substantially improve healthcare for hard to reach populations, they have created global challenges to low-resource countries. When nurses' education was publicly funded or subsidized and then those nurses moved to work in wealthier countries, their countries of origin suffer the loss of intellectual and practice evolution (Li, Nie, & Li, 2014).

Evidence for Practice

The 2016 American Association of Colleges of Nursing policy brief and the 2015 National Council of State Board of Nursing (NCSBN) survey reported that minority nurses represent 19% to 19.5%, respectively, of the total of all registered nurses (RNs) in the United States. The Office of Health Resource Service Administration's (HRSA) brief on gender and racial/ethnic diversity in U.S. health occupations for 2010 to 2012 describes a rate of ethnic minorities of 21.4% (HRSA, 2015). These estimates are below the almost 40% of ethnic minorities in the U.S. population (U.S. Census Bureau, 2015). According to the 2016 National Healthcare Quality and Disparities Report, released by the Agency for Health Quality and Research (AHQR, 2016), it was reported that in 2015, there were also 2.7 million RNs. In terms of nursing workforce, current estimates show that men are approximately 9% to 11% of the nursing workforce (Budden, Shong, Moulton, & Cimiotti, 2013; HRSA,

2013), while racial and ethnic minorities compose 33% of the U.S. workforce. However, only 25% of the nursing workforce shows a modest increase in racial and ethnic minority nurses (HRSA, 2013). RNs in a recent national workforce survey by the NCSBN were 83% white/Caucasian, 6% black/African American, 6% Asian, 3% Hispanic/Latino, 1% Native Hawaiian or Pacific Islander ethnicity, and 1% other (Budden et al., 2013). The difference in the proportion of white RNs in this study and the 75% proportion reported by HRSA in a recent report (HRSA, 2013) was attributed to the different sampling method, in which the NCSBN drew its sample from RN licensing data and represents all RNs licensed in the United States. Meanwhile, the HRSA sample included currently employed RNs and those seeking employment as RNs (National Advisory Council on Nurse Education and Practice [NACNEP], 2013).

Reports indicate that while 6.7% of the RN workforce was made up of foreign-educated nurses, some states like California, Hawaii, Nevada, New Jersey, New York, and Washington, D.C., were found to have an amount greater than 10% of foreign-educated nurses who are currently practicing (NCSBN, 2015). There has been an incremental increase in nursing workforce diversity for RNs. HRSA reported in a survey that the number of RNs from minority or ethnic backgrounds has grown from 119,512 in 1980 to 513,860 in 2008 (HRSA, 2010). The survey also revealed that while only 65.6% of the U.S. population is white and non-Hispanic, 83.3% of RNs were white and non-Hispanic. RNs from Asian backgrounds were overrepresented at 5.8%, compared to 4.5% of the U.S. population. This imbalance of RNs from Asian ethnicity in the United States can be explained by the U.S. recruitment efforts directed toward RNs primarily from the Philippines and/or India as shown in Figure 3.2. In this survey, in terms of languages spoken, most RNs spoke only English. Only 5.1% spoke Spanish, 3.6% spoke Filipino languages, 1.1% spoke French, and less than 1% spoke Chinese, German, or other languages. There are 165,539 RNs living in the United States who were educated in other countries. This number accounts for 5.6% of the entire licensed RNs workforce in the United States.

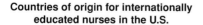

Countries of origin for internationally educated nurses in the U.S.

- Phillipines
- Canada
- India
- Korea/South Korea
- Nigeria
- United Kingdom
- Other

FIGURE 3.2 National Sample Survey of Registered Nurses (HRSA, 2010). (From U.S. Department of Health and Human Services, Office of Health Resources and Services Administration. [2010]. *Findings From the 2008 National Survey of Registered Nurses* [Chap 8, p. 192]. Retrieved from http://www.hrsa.gov/About/News/Pressreleases/2010/100922nursingworkforce.html.)

Practice Point

In the NCSBN survey, an examination of RNs by job title showed that "nurse executive" and "nurse faculty" roles had the least diversity, while "staff nurse" had the most diversity (Budden et al., 2013). Additionally, newly licensed nurses had a more diverse racial/ethnic composition (NCSBN, 2015). These data illustrate the need for diversity programs that focus on educational and career advancement for underrepresented minority RNs.

As minority populations increase at rapid rates, there is an increasing need for a diverse workforce of healthcare providers who can provide culturally competent care.

Transcultural and **cultural competency** is very important when addressing needs of diverse multicultural populations. Leininger (1999) defined transcultural nursing as a formal area of study, research, and practice focused on culturally based care beliefs, values, and practices to help achieving the goal of well-being, and prevention of disability in a culturally congruent and beneficial ways. Culture encompasses human beings, religion, kinship, education, technology, language, environmental context, and worldviews, and needs to be integrated into nursing care (Leininger, 1999). As defined by Bearskin (2011), cultural competence refers to the skills, knowledge, and attitudes required to provide care with consideration for various cultural differences. HRSA acknowledged that the most dominant determinant in RN cultural competency is the language used to communicate with the population being served by the RN. Similarly, a number of critical cultural competency interventions were proposed by Betancourt, Green, Carrillo, and Ananeh-Firempong (2003), which included minority recruitment into health professions, development of interpreter services and language-appropriate health educational materials, and education of healthcare providers on cross-cultural issues in order to best address health and healthcare disparities.

Consistently, Purnell has emphasized that healthcare providers must recognize, respect, and integrate clients' cultural beliefs and practices into health prescriptions allowing for the provider to be culturally aware, culturally sensitive, and have some degree of cultural competence to be effective in integrating health beliefs and practices into plans and interventions (Purnell, 2002; 2012). Purnell added that while cultural awareness has more to do with an appreciation of the external signs of diversity (e.g., arts, music, dress, etc.), cultural sensitivity has more to do with personal attitudes and not saying things that might be offensive to someone from a cultural or ethnic background different from what is considered normal.

FIGURE 3.3 A, B: Surrounded by registered nurses and legislators, on July 2, 2010, Gov. Deval Patrick signed into law a bill. **C:** Nurses testifying for one of the bills. (Adopted from the Massachusetts Nurse Newsletter July/August 2010.)

Practice Point

Purnell (2002) has identified cultural competence as having several characteristics that include knowledge and skills as well as the following:

- Exploring one's culture in a context of not trying to change others' cultures
- Making the effort to learn about others' cultures and cultural meanings
- Tolerating and embracing different ways of knowing and experiencing life by others
- Making no assumptions about what others believe
- Avoiding judgements around differences
- Opting to be available and being comfortable to experience other cultural interactions in persons or events
- Being versatile with other cultures
- Cultural competence is an individualized plan of care that begins with performing an assessment through a cultural lens.

It is also clear that cultural competency is required for achieving the aims of public health in the context of the client, individual, family, or community. Because healthcare professionals are involved in the process of policy formation, it is logical that the less diverse the workforce is, the less appropriate and effective the healthcare policies will be for disadvantaged populations. Healthcare professionals continue to report that marginalized (minority) populations experience greater healthcare needs and receive lower quality of care (Bearskin, 2011). As a result, the U.S. Health and Human Services and the Office of HRSA have taken bold steps to increase workforce diversity by providing funds for programs that address this important issue.

Despite all national efforts to improve the diversity of the healthcare workforce, Hunt (2007) reported that managing a racially and culturally diverse workforce is complex and challenging for nurses. He stated, "There are no ready-made tools to show them how to do so ... Achieving effective management of a culturally diverse workforce comes from an intrinsic motivation to develop the cultural competence to engage with them" (Hunt, 2007, p. 2252).

NURSING'S ROLE IN SHAPING HEALTHCARE POLICY

Historical Highlights on Nursing Political Involvement

Nurses have long been recognized as patient advocates. Today, more than ever, nurses need to be politically involved personally and professionally in the complex healthcare arena (Fig. 3.3). The process of gaining a position of influence in the legislative arena takes time.

William (1993) argues that the history for nurses being involved in political endeavors started in the mid-'70s and early '80s when nursing scholars and leaders advocated for political involvement of nurses. Furthermore, debate about nursing involvement in political issues within the profession and in societal issues occurred during 1976 (Powell, 1976). Nursing education efforts focused on legislative involvement at all government levels in this important year of advocacy (Williams, 1977). While Leininger (1978) described the need for political activism within the instruction of nursing students, Cowart and Allen (1981) described the rationale for curricular inclusion of politics and health policy content. Successful legislative lobbying toward healthcare policy formation included the voices of nurses in the 1990s (Milstead, 2013). Since then, organized nursing is included in the debates about healthcare reform. Nursing's presence in these debates was credited to the many years of public involvement by selected leaders in the nursing profession (Magnussen, Itano, & McGuckin, 2005.) There are many examples of the tremendous influence of nurses on healthcare. Nursing has a rich history of political activists in Florence Nightingale, Lillian Wald, and many others (Selanders, Louise, Crane, & Patrick, 2012).

Evidence for Practice

In a historical literature review of political activism in nursing conducted by Rubotzky (2000), it has been stressed that the years 1992 to 1994 were very influential.

1. Nursing in the United States started 1992 as an assertive, organized professional discipline with the intention of influencing national public policy. Such organized movement resolve was a clear break from the traditional, historical role of this traditionally women's profession.
2. The subsequent events of 1992 to 1994 illustrate a pivotal story of a discipline becoming an advocate of political significance, overcoming the barriers of traditional views, organizing as an identifiable political interest group, and speaking out with clarity as an advocate for the health of all Americans.
3. In 1993, the newly elected President of the United States, William Clinton, directed the formation of a national Task Force for Health Care Reform, including professional nurses in its membership.

In the modern era, there have been outstanding examples of individual nurses as well as associations throughout the history of the profession who have demonstrated their capacity to shape healthcare by being active in directing healthcare through legislation. Nurses have done this through initiating/revising healthcare goal policy proposals and influencing the implementation of health policy. For example, nurses who wanted to secure state registration for Michigan nurses created the Michigan Nurse Association. It took them over 5 years of lobbying to accomplish their goal and that was before women could even vote (Nault & Sincox, 2014).

What Does It Mean to Be Politically Active and Involved?

It's been argued that being personally involved in politics means being active in the political process as a citizen of the country. A good example of personal involvement is voting (Boswell et al., 2005). Nurses have long been recognized as patient advocates. Today, more than ever, nurses need to be politically involved personally as well as professionally in the complex healthcare arena. However, being politically involved means being knowledgeable about issues, laws, and health policy. Nurses need to be both personally and professionally involved but they need to be involved in an informed way more than ever today.

Oestberg (2013) highlighted many important reasons why nurse-informed political involvement is necessary: (1) nurses are direct caregivers, who spend more time with patients than other healthcare providers; (2) nurses come face to face with issues associated with patient safety and

satisfaction, access to services, clinical outcomes, and health disparities and (3) nurses are positioned on a daily basis to see not only the impact of health policy on individual patients but also the need for more comprehensive changes in the policies that address many health-related issues. Nursing exists to serve the public. It is a duty to be active politically and work to influence public policy especially when nurses are in a position to be aware of injustices in the healthcare system and the political arena. Nurses have a duty to set an example and become involved (Des Jardin, 2001; King, 2015).

In addition to their clinical expertise, nurses are being sought out to serve in a variety of leadership positions and develop policy recommendations related to a wide range of healthcare policy issues (Dean, 2011). Accordingly, policymakers need to hear nurses articulate their perceptions of needed change in policy or the need to create policy anew because they are in the best position to communicate citizens' problems and be advocates for individual, family, and community rights and healthcare needs.

As highlighted by Porche (2012), nurses and other healthcare professionals have a rich preparation in knowledge and personal and professional experiences within the healthcare system that enable them to influence the development of health policy. Nurses are experts as clinicians, educators, researchers, and administrators and need to acknowledge and use the power they have in numbers in public policy. Nurses are experts and should use their expertise to translate new worldviews into the policy arena. In the policy arena, they can utilize their knowledge, perspective, experiences, and skills to be change agents for public policy at all levels of government (Leavitt, 2009). Nurses also represent communities and speak as trusted and respected professionals, evidenced by annual surveys, which indicate that the public continues to rate RNs as the most trusted profession on the basis of their professional honesty and ethical standards (Norman, 2016; Williamson, 2017).

Nursing Advocacy and Policy Participation

"Nurses are natural advocates, but this advocacy does not stop at the patient and family level. Every nurse has a voice and can lead change locally and globally" (Carol Ann King, 2015, p. 13). Nurses consistently play the role of advocate as they support each patient's emotional well-being, contribute to the healing process and speak on their patients' behalf. On the other hand, nurses can use their **patient advocacy** and **political advocacy** skills to work in supporting each other and for the nursing profession as a whole (Krischke, 2011). Fulfilling the role of patient and public advocate, requires nurses to support actions that are in the best interest of public health and also that defend patient as well community rights. Therefore, nurses have a professional duty to protect many interests (Des Jardin, 2001; King, 2015). As indicated by Milstead (2008, 2013), nurses are experts who can address both the rational shaping of the policy, and the emotional

aspects of the process, and should feel morally obligated to advocate for their patients.

"As nursing advocates, we start with the foundation that we are servants to others and stewards of our profession. We choose to lead from that servant position, making sure peoples' needs are being met through wise and thoughtful interactions." (Noel, in Krischke, 2011). When nurses act as patient advocates, many of them are referencing to what happens at the point of care. It is often not the case to see oneself as a nurse equipped of able to discuss concerns related to health and healthcare with legislators (Nault & Sincox, 2014). Many nurses today are inspired to take on some form of advocacy to bring about change in the current policies, laws, or regulations that govern the larger healthcare system (Abood, 2007).

How to Be Politically Involved?

Nursing as an organized labor force makes up the largest group of healthcare professionals. Because of the extent of their knowledge of health principles and their ability to shape healthcare policy, nurses have a valuable part to play. According to Catalano (2015), political involvement comprises activities, methods, tactics, and behaviors that shape or have the possibility to affect governmental and/or legislative strategies and outcomes. Dealing with numerous concerns daily and other workplace issues, nurses have the choice to motivate themselves to act and find opportunities to bring about change in the healthcare system itself (Abood, 2007). Additionally, nurses can play a leading role in influencing their elected representatives to enact needed changes in healthcare and nursing policy and electing pro-nursing politicians to make sure that nurses and patients have partners at the state level and federal levels in gaining quality, affordable, and accessible healthcare (Artz, 2006).

Practice Point

Oestberg (2013) indicates that nursing and nurses can only be effective if they not only have deep knowledge about how the health system functions (structure and process) but also understand who are the decision-makers in the context of structure and process that can impact policy. In being knowledgeable in these areas, nurses can strategize effectively to impact policy development and change at the local, state, and federal level.

Nurses continuously demonstrate evidence-based care, and they share decision-making with patients and families, resulting in improved quality and reduced cost. Nurses have also been active in the development of public policies as members of the legislative and executive branches at national and state levels (Dean, 2011; Leavitt, 2009). Furthermore, elected officials are selected as representatives and they make decisions based on the information that is shared with them. Therefore, it is critical for nurses to become one of the key sources of information to legislators when the issues with which they deliberate on impact healthcare and the well-being of our population (King, 2015).

Oliver (2012) argued that legislators must make decisions about a large number of issues in a short time frame as they cannot be experts in every field, so they rely heavily on their staffers to research issues and on the experts in those fields with whom they have developed. In the research arena, all nurses engaged in research usually consider the policy implications of their work, and even if the researcher is not the advocate, those who are engaged in workplace, organizational policy, or public policy can use research studies to propose policy alternatives and enhance policy modification accordingly (Leavitt, 2009). Evidence-based practice is the gold standard for the interventions used in individual, family and community care efforts. Evidence-based practice examples are needed in nursing advocacy efforts because through research evidence can be gathered to be presented to decision makers about the changes nurses want to see and strive to accomplish (Oestberg, 2013). Nurses have many milestones in policy development as addressed by Leavitt (2009) through their practice and research, which have contributed to (1) quality outcomes, (2) decreases in cost, (3) expanded access, and (4) major differences to the health of the nation. To name a few:

1. The magnet process, which was originated by the American Academy of Nursing (AAN), has been integrated into The Joint Commission's standards.
2. School-based health centers, as demonstrated by advanced practice and public health nurses, can improve access for underinsured and uninsured children and can reduce some of the disparities in healthcare access.
3. Linda Aiken and colleagues' groundbreaking research on nurse staffing and the effect on patient outcomes has resulted in laws and regulations that created guidelines for staffing criteria of hospital units in many states (Aiken, Xue, Clarke, & Sloane, 2006).

In terms of policymaking, nurses have the basic vital evidence either supporting or opposing a policy. Nurses can also serve on a personal and professional level in the process of political election to be instrumental in serving the nation's health (Porche, 2012). They can be members of an organization or a group, which enables them to be involved in agenda setting and the introduction of a specific problem into the national agenda, identifying the goals and tools, and advocating and disseminating health issues through the media (Milstead, 2008).

ADVOCACY ACTIVITIES OF PROFESSIONAL NURSING ORGANIZATIONS

Central to all nursing practice is the role of nurses as advocates. Advocacy allows nurses to use their voice of experience to represent patients, families, causes, and professional issues. Nurses who are advocates in these areas often use their moral and ethical decision-making based on principles of fairness and equity and use them to influence political process that can lead to decisions in resource allocation (Matthews, 2012).

The Role of Professional Nursing Organizations

The American Nurses Association (ANA) is the only full-service professional organization representing the interests of the nation's 3.1 million registered nurses through its constituent member nursing associations and its organizational affiliates (Mathews, 2012). The ANA has issued *Nursing's Agenda for Health Care Reform*, endorsed by over 60 other nursing groups (ANA, 2010a). Myers (2010) pointed out that the ANA which serves as the strongest nursing organization in the United States, has been engaged in helping its members play a significant role in advocating for their patients by closing the gaps in the healthcare access for patients and their families through testifying at congressional hearings, healthcare summits, and regional forums. For example, nurses who are members of the ANA and their state nurses' association can apply to participate in the American Nurses Advocacy Institute (ANAI) which focuses on advocacy initiatives and political strategies (Vencill & Lemmons, 2015). Furthermore, ANA works with other health coalitions and advocates for nurses to serve as members of governing boards in each state, to advance the role of and recognition of nurses, to prevent potential declines in quality, and to communicate with the Congress in the prevention of harmful changes in Medicare actions (Dean, 2011; Spring, 2013). However, Myers (2010) stated there is a concern that too many nurses have been absent from policy deliberations despite ANA's calls for advocacy, minimizing the collective power of nurses in the legislative process.

Nursing organizations with legislative departments provide analysis on current issues in health policy and tips on how to communicate with legislators. Many also offer workshops on nursing advocacy, or legislative days at the state house, both excellent opportunities to begin an advocacy career (Oestberg, 2013). For example, the National League for Nursing (NLN) advocates a curriculum revolution and incorporates political activism in their strategic plan (Williams, 1993). The International Council of Nurses (ICN) is a federation of more than 130 national nursing associations where the ANA is the U.S. representative, along with other nursing associations, representing more than 13 million nurses worldwide. The ICN was founded in 1899 as an international center for nurses and other health professionals. The goal of the organization is to assure that quality nursing care is rooted in reasonable and effective health policies through the generation of nursing knowledge (research). The primary focus of this work is to benefit patients, families, communities, and the professional nurse workplace on the global stage (ICN, 2011).

CURRENT SITUATION OF NURSING POLITICAL INVOLVEMENT: CHALLENGES AND BARRIERS

Among the challenges that have been identified as negatively affecting nursing's political involvement include (1) living a fast-paced stressful life in today's world with not enough time to get involved; (2) heavy workloads with understaffing; (3) a perception of powerlessness; (4) gender issues that often support not being direct but indirect with upset and concerns; (5) fear that political action will create a breach of family time; (6) anxiety with public speaking; (7) complex public policy coupled with lack of knowledge in the legislative process; and (8) fear of retaliation for raising controversial positions related to justice and parity (Des Jardin, 2001). Furthermore, Boswell and colleagues (2005) added that time constraints, lack of resources, political awareness, role modeling, peer support, frustration, and burnout may also lead to minimal political involvement. Last, political involvement is further weakened by role ambiguity, role issues, and role incongruity (Des Jardin, 2001; Oliver, 2012).

Strategies for Nursing Involvement in Policy and Politics

There have been many co-authors in the policy arena who have developed strategies to guide nurses to find the best opportunity for policy involvement. Oestberg (2013) highlighted that nurses can make phone calls to elected representatives about bills under consideration, testify before committees, become involved in practice councils or boards at the workplace, and even run for elected office. Oestberg (2013) added that other strategies can include (1) establishing a mentor relationship with an experienced nurse advocate; (2) seeking formal education on health policy or public health, (3) searching for an internship with one's local or state representative to work on health-related legislation to understand how the system works and gain networking contacts; (4) using local and state resources or national nursing advocacy groups to gain an understanding of current issues and learn about involvement; (5) networking with other nurses to create a unified voice in addition to the elected representatives and their staff by first building credibility with them; and (6) avoiding underestimating personal experiences because legislators like to hear how legislative issues would affect their constituents. An example of nursing involvement in policy and passing laws that had a direct impact on the nursing profession is when Governor Patrick signed the Assault Bill announcing a zero tolerance for violence against healthcare professionals, namely nurses.

Practice Point

Nurses as educators have a particular responsibility to teach students how to translate issues into health policy. They can serve as both role models and teachers when there is a need to include political competence and citizenship in the education system (Carnegie & Kiger, 2009). Because nursing roles are interrelated, educators can work with researchers, and administrators can work with clinicians to share their perspectives and diverse knowledge to make tremendous contributions to policy development (Hewlett et al., 2009). Whitehead (2003) highlighted the vital role of the nursing education curriculum as an integral part in achieving many goals for nurses early on in their careers. These goals are: (1) reinforcing and ensuring nursing's active role in initiating and developing health policy; (2) creating politically involved nurses; and (3) developing nurses who are health policy experts and entrepreneurs. However, he observed that the available literature suggests that the majority of nursing curricula are yet to fulfil this role.

In summary, the nursing profession is one of the largest sectors of the healthcare industry in the United States and has a rich history as a unique profession with its own values, ethics, respect, integrity, and responsibility. Nurses' opportunities for contributions to healthcare policies are unlimited. As Fyffe (2009) pointed out, there is a need for greater coordination of action to ensure that nursing is represented and actively supported in influencing and shaping health and healthcare policy.

QUALITY OF CARE

The healthcare system in the United States is very complex, made up of diverse patients, healthcare providers, and healthcare payers. With patients, providers, and payers constantly interacting for varying reasons and in a variety of environments, it is extremely difficult to evaluate the complexities of the quality of care for the U.S. population. Despite the difficulties in evaluating the quality of healthcare, much is being done by the federal government, U.S. Department of Health and Human Services, the **Centers for Medicaid and Medicare Services** (CMS), and private institutions and organizations to examine the healthcare system in terms of quality, access, and cost. Mason and colleagues (2012) report several examples as to how efficiently and effectively healthcare systems provide safe patient care to people in need at a reasonable price and with equal distribution. Mason and colleagues (2012) reference the Institute of Medicine report (2001), which lists the following dimensions of healthcare systems that should be considered when quality, cost, and access are examined:

1. Safety: avoiding injury and harm from care that is meant to aid patients

2. Effectiveness: assuring that "evidence-based" care is actually delivered by avoiding overuse of medically unproven care and underuse of medically sound care
3. Patient-centeredness: involving patients thoroughly in the decision-making process about their care, thereby respecting their cultures, social circumstances, and needs
4. Timeliness: avoiding unwanted delays in treatment
5. Equality: closing racial, ethnic, gender, and socioeconomic gaps in care and outcomes

Quality of care is defined by the Institute of Medicine (2001) as the degree to which health services for individuals and populations increase the likelihood of desired outcomes and are consistent with current knowledge. Additionally, the U.S. Department of Health and Human Services (HHS) defines quality improvement efforts as "systematic and continuous actions that lead to measurable improvement in healthcare services and the health status of targeted patient groups" (AHRQ, 2016).

In demonstrating quality care, patients receive correct assessment and diagnosis, are given appropriate and effective treatment, and are monitored closely.

The Commonwealth Fund Commission on a High Performance Health System (Mongan, 2006) states the following six drivers of high performance in healthcare systems: (1) patient information is available to patients and all providers through health record systems; (2) patient care is coordinated among multiple providers and managed accurately; (3) all providers have accountability to each other and to the patient and collaborate to reliably deliver high-quality care; (4) patients have access to appropriate and culturally competent care and information; (5) accountability is present for the care of patients; and (6) the system is working to improve the quality of healthcare.

In an update on U.S. healthcare quality improvement efforts cited by Harvard School of Public Health, it has been reported that "Healthcare quality in the United States is improving, but there is still a lot that needs to be done. The National Healthcare Quality and Disparities Report (NHQDR) gives one benchmark we can use to assess the impact of current improvement efforts on healthcare outcomes" (Berger, 2015). The report added that the ACA mandated that the *National Strategy for Quality Improvement in Health Care* established in March 2011 by the Agency for Healthcare Research and Quality (AHRQ) to guide quality improvement efforts at the local, state, and national levels through three key aims (below) and six priorities:

1. Improving overall quality by making healthcare more patient-centered, reliable, accessible, and safe
2. Improving the health of the population by supporting proven interventions to address behavioral, social, and environmental determinants of health
3. Reducing the cost of quality care for individuals, families, employers, and government

Priority 1: Making care safer by reducing harm caused in the delivery of care

Priority 2: Ensuring that each person and family are engaged in care

Priority 3: Promoting effective communication and care coordination

Priority 4: Promoting the most effective prevention and treatment practices for the leading causes of mortality, starting with cardiovascular disease

Priority 5: Working with communities to promote wide use of best practices to enable healthy living

Priority 6: Making quality care more affordable for individuals, families, employers, and governments by developing new healthcare delivery models

Evidence for Practice

On the global level, quality of care is tracked based on attainment, equity of health outcomes across populations, and fairness of financial contributions. Additional measures include how investments in public health impact social objectives like reducing health disparities, improving health, and providing responsive services that best assist patients (Murray & Frenk, 2010). On the basis of these measures, the World Health Organization (WHO) public health leaders (2010) explained that governments including the Americas on average allocate more to health than the other regions. Americans spend a significant amount for health insurance but receive little in terms of quality of care. As described in Chapter 2, comparative evidence has shown that the U.S. healthcare system is gradually slipping behind less-industrialized countries each year, and improvements in healthcare have been slower when compared to other industrialized or developed countries (Murray & Frenk, 2010). Furthermore, the U.S. healthcare system has been deemed broken by many people, with skyrocketing costs and plummeting coverage for middle-class and low-income families (Jacobs & Skocpol, 2012).

In evaluating the extent that the goals and priorities addressed by the AHRQ have been achieved, in 2013 (Berger, 2015), the NHQD found the following:

- Half of all patient safety measures improved, with a median improvement of 3.6% per year.
- There was a 17% reduction in hospital-acquired conditions (including pressure ulcers, falls, and infections), resulting in approximately 50,000 fewer patient deaths and $12 billion in healthcare cost savings.
- A significant reduction in adverse drug reactions
- Patient–provider communication improved from 2005 to 2012, with the percentage of adults who reported poor communication with health providers decreasing.

- Parents also reported a significantly lower degree of poor communication with their children's health providers.
- Healthcare facilities saw improved discharge processes and care coordination, facilitated by the adoption of health information technologies such as electronic medical records.
- A significant increase in the percentage of patients with serious conditions who received complete written discharge instructions. For example, the percentage of heart failure patients who received full discharge instructions increased by 35%.
- Half of effective treatment measures improved for life-threatening conditions. For instance, from 2005 to 2012, the percentage of heart attack sufferers treated within 90 minutes of their arrival to a hospital increased.
- The overall performance of 10 other treatment measures improved, leading to better outcomes in cancer, pneumonia, and HIV care.
- Half of measures of healthy living improved. Adolescent vaccines were among notable improvements from 2008 to 2012—including increases in the percentage of adolescents receiving the meningococcal and tetanus-diphtheria-acellular pertussis vaccines. The recent anti-vaccination movement seems to be reversing this trend.
- Access and cost barriers to health insurance are being targeted through tax credits, more coverage options within the Health Insurance Marketplace, and cost-sharing reductions. According to the Kaiser Family Foundation, the average U.S. insurance premium increased by 3% in 2014, which is the smallest increase since 1999.

However, the NHQD reported several areas where disparities and gaps were evident in quality: (1) the development of special efforts is under way to address disparities; for instance, only 70% of people with high blood pressure are receiving the recommended level of care; (2) disparities in two areas—hospice care and chronic disease management—increased; (3) healthcare affordability is not yet decreasing; and (4) across all six priorities, disparities still exist according to income, race, and ethnicity.

To overcome this downward spiraling of quality and access to healthcare, it is essential that the United States better evaluate performance of healthcare and compare results with other countries (refer to Chapter 2 comparisons for data supporting this key point) (Murray & Frenk, 2010).

INFORMATION MANAGEMENT

As highlighted earlier in this chapter, information management of the U.S. healthcare system must be improved to advance the overall delivery of healthcare. Healthcare experts and the U.S. Congress overwhelmingly agree that implementing electronic information systems could greatly improve the efficiency of the healthcare system and the health of Americans (Blumenthal, 2009). In such efforts, U.S. policymakers have adopted the health information technology (HIT), labeled HITECH in law, a high priority through the American Recovery and Reinvestment Act (ARRA) (Jha, DesRoches, Kralovec, & Joshi, 2010). The ARRA offers significant incentives through Medicare and Medicaid funding to physicians and hospitals if they adopt effective HIT and electronic health records (EHRs). Through ARRA, $17 billion in financial aid was used as incentive for doctors and hospitals to utilize EHRs. Physicians who adopt and use EHRs meaningfully can be reimbursed for their services up to $44,000 over 5 years. Similarly, hospitals that effectively utilize EHRs earn an incentive of $2 million through a one-time bonus. Furthermore, HITECH provides $2 billion in assistance to put systems in place and offers grants that assist providers' installation of EHRs. Physicians and hospitals refusing to implement EHRs face penalties, such as losing a percentage of their Medicare fees (Blumenthal, 2009; Fonkych & Taylor, 2005). HITECH "provisions created an essential foundation for restructuring healthcare delivery and for achieving the key goals of improving healthcare quality; reducing costs; and increasing access through better methods of storing, analyzing, and sharing health information" (Buntin, Jain, & Blumenthal, 2010, p. 1).

The Office of the National Coordinator for Information Technology (Charles, Gabriel, & Searcy, 2015, OCN Data Brief) reported that in 2014, three out of four (76%) of hospitals had adopted at least a basic EHR system which represents an increase of 27% from 2013 and an eightfold increase since 2008 (Charles, Gabriel, & Searcy, 2015, OCN Data Brief). Nearly all reported hospitals (97%) possessed a certified EHR technology in 2014, increasing by 35% since 2011. Fewer hospitals are using basic EHRs without clinical notes, while the systems with more advanced functionality have increased significantly. Additionally, hospital adoption of comprehensive EHR systems has increased 11-fold since 2009, rising to a third (34.4%) of hospitals in 2014 (Charles et al., 2015, OCN Data Brief). Barriers to adopting systems include, but are not limited to, high costs, technical challenges in implementing and maintaining the system, and concerns of privacy (Blumenthal, 2009; Fonkych & Taylor, 2005). Providers who have not implemented an EHR system have difficulty in coordinating care, evaluating quality of care, and avoiding medical errors.

EQUITY IN HEALTHCARE ACCESS AND QUALITY

Equity is defined by the Institute of Medicine (2001) as healthcare that does not vary in quality because of gender, race, ethnicity, geographic location, or socioeconomic status. The U.S. Department of Research and Quality (USDHHS, AHRQ, 2007) indicates that significant healthcare disparities exist and the progress in eliminating health disparities is limited. Eliminating health disparities has became a priority of the

Barack Obama administration as the U.S. population became increasingly diverse (Mason et al., 2012). Furthermore, insurance rates are rising more rapidly than wages, and middle- and low-income families and employers are having great difficulty affording insurance (Institute of Medicine, 2003).

Schoen, Davis, How, and Schoenbaum (2006) developed a scoring system of equity in the U.S. healthcare system and concluded that there were major inequities in health, quality, access, and efficiency. More researchers have reported that individuals living in low-income communities are associated with significant disparities. For example, researchers found that whites, blacks, and Hispanics with cancer who lived in high-poverty geographic areas, experienced a systematically lower 5-year survival rate. In addition to disparities due to poverty, there were disparities found in terms of race and ethnicity as well. In terms of getting effective and appropriate care, white patients were more likely to receive timely, patient-centered care than African Americans and Hispanics. Additionally, African Americans and Hispanics had higher mortality rates than were whites. Researchers went further to explain, "black, Hispanic, low-income and uninsured patients are less likely to have primary care providers to coordinate care, are more likely to experience test results/records delays and duplication, are more likely to go to the emergency departments when other care was not available, and more likely to be admitted to the hospital for potentially preventable conditions, than white, higher-income, and insured patients" (Schoen et al., 2006, p. 472). In summary, because there is an abundance of evidence indicating increased disparities in healthcare delivery when assessed by income, insurance, and race, it is imperative that appropriate efforts continue in reducing health disparities in the United States.

Because of such vast disparities in healthcare access and quality, President Obama made healthcare a priority issue. In March of 2010, President Obama signed the Patient Protection and **Affordable Care Act** (ACA) into law (Jacobs & Skocpol, 2010). As of late 2018, different measures of the law had been diminished and were being challenged by the Trump administration and a majority-Republican Congress.

COMMUNITY-BASED SERVICES ASSOCIATED WITH HEALTHCARE REFORM

Efforts put forth through the ACA, such as the Community Transformation Grant (CTG) program, provide funds to organizations, health centers, and initiatives with goals of creating healthy communities and assisting vulnerable populations (Hennrikus, 2013). The CTG grants fund programs that promote tobacco-free living, physical activity, healthy eating, services to prevent and control high blood pressure and high cholesterol, social and emotional wellness, and healthy and safe environments. It is estimated the CTG program will affect 40% of the U.S. population with health promotion and disease prevention efforts with vast opportunities for nurses to get involved.

Achieving health equity is and must continue to be a priority for this country to move forward. It is critical that nurses stay involved and offer their expertise. Nurses' involvement with research, advocacy, community outreach, and policy efforts will help underserved populations receive the care that they need and deserve (Mason et al., 2012). Community-based prevention commonly refers to a range of prevention strategies including upstream interventions that address underlying social and economic factors; public policies, including regulations and legislation, that support healthy behaviors; and interventions directed at high-need, low-income neighborhoods (Goodman, 2009).

There is also a critical need to increase the prevention resources available in impoverished communities to achieve the breadth and depth of influence necessary to shift the distribution of risk factors, exposures, and chronic diseases to healthier patterns. Finally, there needs to be better alignment with and support for community programs that have been traditionally viewed as outside of the public health sector but which nonetheless exert a fundamental influence on population health (e.g., early childhood development, income support for families living in poverty, and access to quality schools and educational opportunities). Such interventions create an infrastructure in public health departments to support and implement community-based prevention programs aimed at improving population health (Goodman, 2009).

The website, Healthcare.gov referred to home and community-based services (HCBS) as the services and support provided by most state Medicaid programs in a home or community that give help with such daily tasks as bathing or dressing where such care is covered when provided by care workers or by a family member if permitted. Calman, Golub, and Shuman (2012) have highlighted four vital models that are congruent with the ACA Triple Aim that includes: (1) better healthcare for individuals; (2) better health outcomes in the community; and (3) lower healthcare costs. Healthcare reform was designed to address both the quality and accessibility of healthcare while reducing its cost. This article by Calman and colleagues (2012) provides an overview of models that are considered as foundations for healthcare reform and are supported by the ACA and its core principles of primary care: comprehensive, coordinated and continuous primary care; preventive care; and the sophisticated implementation of HIT designed to promote communication between healthcare providers, enhance coordination of care, minimize duplication of services, and permit reporting on quality. These models included:

1. Federally qualified health centers: also, known as community health centers, have been a key component of the primary care safety net in the United States since 1965 and became a focus of the Obama administration's health-reform plan.
2. Patient-centered medical home (PCMH): describes the model of care in the most advanced primary care centers, focus is on the provision of primary and preventive care by qualified primary care providers, supported by an interdisciplinary team of health professionals. Care must be accessible, high-quality, safe, and efficient, as well as continuous, comprehensive, and coordinated with other healthcare providers as needed. The basic requirements to achieve PCMH recognition include measures in the following areas: (1) access and communication, (2) patient tracking and registry functions, (3) care management, (4) patient self-management and support, (5) electronic prescribing, (6) test tracking, (7) referral tracking, (8) performance reporting and improvement, and (9) advanced electronic communication.
3. Accountable care organizations (ACOs): an initiative supported by the ACA. ACOs are based in part on the models developed between 2005 and 2010 by the CMS demonstration project, the Physician Group Practice Demonstration. Like PCMHs and health homes, ACOs provide a structure for reforms in the way that healthcare is financed in order to incentivize collaborating organizations to provide better care at lower costs, with the goal of generating both overall savings and greater earnings for the provider organization.
4. Meaningful use: The goals of the meaningful use (MU) initiative are to (1) improve the quality, safety, and efficiency of care and to reduce health disparities; (2) engage patients and their families; (3) improve care coordination; (4) improve population and public health; and (5) ensure adequate privacy and security protection for personal health information.

Evidence for Practice

A program designed and implemented in collaboration with a Certified Home Healthcare Agency and regional hospital addresses the serious issue of increasing hospital readmission rates by focusing on transitional care needs of patients and families. The researchers who designed this experiment to see how re-hospitalization could be affected compared the odds of re-hospitalization among patients who received the transitional care services ($n = 223$) and a similar group of patients who received usual home care services ($n = 224$). Findings indicate that patients who received the transitional care services were significantly less likely to be readmitted to the hospital than the patients in the control group who received usual care (Russell, Rosati, Sobolewski, Marren, & Rosenfeld, 2011).

ETHICAL CONSIDERATION

Nursing has an ethical obligation to society to improve quality of life by maximizing the potential of the individual patient according to his or her needs (Des Jardin, 2001). In that capacity, nurses have a duty to support professional nursing goals that relate to healthcare for consumers; yet, each distinct group of healthcare professionals has its own priorities that might not be congruent with the institutional values (Indiana State Nurse Association, 2013). This section will explain how the Nursing Code of Ethics strengthens nursing's position as an advocate and will describe how professional associations advocate for the nursing profession, nurses, and healthcare for the citizens of the United States.

Practice Point

Des Jardin (2006) states clearly that differences in stakeholder interests puts parties such as nurses, patients, and institutions into a political-ethical clash at times. Guidelines are available to help nurses know how they can be involved in the political process.

By using these guidelines and an ethical framework for political decision-making, nurses can evaluate issues while assessing problems, planning for action, and evaluate the effectiveness and benefits of those strategies effectively.

Individuals have their own moral lens through which they view the world, and where they can judge what is right and wrong. No matter what a nurse's personal moral views may be, employers establish policies regarding appropriate behavior in the workplace and these expectations are known as organizational ethics, which are defined as expectations about the "right" behaviors for healthcare professionals in the work setting (Indiana State Nurse Association, 2013). An example of such ethics are the standards provided in the *Code of Ethics for Nurses* (ANA, 2010a). Advocacy by the profession of nursing developed within the United States as visionaries, leaders, and nurses from across the nation formulated the first (and subsequent) revisions of the *Code of Ethics for Nurses with Interpretive Statements*, often referred to as the *Code of Ethics* (ANA, 2001). The concluding statement of the *Code of Ethics* preface states: "…the Code of Ethics is the ethical standard for all members of the profession. No one outside of nursing can alter it" (Mathews, 2012). The ANA *Code of Ethics with Interpretive Statements* has been updated in later versions (ANA, 2015a, 2015b) and have addressed nine main nursing ethical principles or known as provisions:

1. Provision 1: The nurse practices with compassion and respect for the inherent dignity, worth, and unique attributes of every person.
2. Provision 2: The nurse's primary commitment is to the patient, whether an individual, family, group, community, or population.
3. Provision 3: The nurse promotes, advocates for, and protects the rights, health, and safety of the patient.
4. Provision 4: The nurse has authority, accountability, and responsibility for nursing practice; makes decisions; and

takes action consistent with the obligation to promote health and to provide optimal care.
5. Provision 5: The nurse owes the same duties to self as to others, including the responsibility to promote health and safety, preserve wholeness of character and integrity, maintain competence, and continue personal and professional growth.
6. Provision 6: The nurse, through individual and collective effort, establishes, maintains, and improves the ethical environment of the work setting and conditions of employment that are conducive to safe, quality healthcare.
7. Provision 7: The nurse, in all roles and settings, advances the profession through research and scholarly inquiry, professional standards development, and the generation of both nursing and health policy.
8. Provision 8: The nurse collaborates with other health professionals and the public to protect human rights, promote health diplomacy, and reduce health disparities.
9. Provision 9: The profession of nursing, collectively through its professional organizations, must articulate nursing values, maintain integrity of the profession, and integrate principles of social justice into nursing and health policy.

It's noteworthy to address the role of the ANA in the following:

1. The *Code of Ethics for Nurses*—asserts the values and commitment to excellence for patients, society, and nurses individually and collectively as a profession (ANA, 2015a, 2015b);
2. The *Social Policy Statement*—details the authority based on the social responsibility of the profession to society. It serves as nursing's contract between the profession of nursing and society to uphold the highest values and standards in delivering its service of nursing care (ANA, 2010a); and
3. The *Scope and Standards of Practice in Nursing*—delineates the scope of nursing practice and then defines the standards of professional nursing practice and accompanying competencies (ANA, 2010b).

Healthcare workers encounter complicated ethical issues in their practice, however, and nursing particularly is involved in infinite judgments regarding the morality and immorality of their actions or interventions toward their patient. This has resulted mainly from the radical progress in biomedical sciences and the technological piece of the healthcare, which affects the lives of billions of people throughout the world. Consequently, nurses are required to hold the responsibility of both safeguarding the values of their society and developing their own moral framework for dealing with the moral dilemmas. The role of the nurse as a member of the interprofessional care team is to identify potentially ethics-related situations, work with others to address these issues, and provide holistic support for patients, families, and colleagues. Thus, in order to guide the process of moral decision-making, for example, the Ohio Nurses Association (2013) developed a process to guide RNs in the process of working through ethical ambiguity or dilemmas, which includes the following:

1. Identifying the existence of the ethical dilemma (conflict in values)
2. Gathering and analyzing relevant information—including identification of stakeholders, interdisciplinary team members, and other sources of relevant information
3. Clarifying personal values and moral position, including the moral perspectives of other "players" in the scenario
4. Determining options, based on careful consideration of alternatives' benefits and risks
5. Making responsible decisions about actions or recommendations, in collaboration with other interested parties
6. Evaluating the impact of the action and outcomes

Evidence for Practice

Technological and societal changes have created both ethical issues and new requirements for nursing education in the context of ethics (Ramos et al., 2013). However, a lack of ethical confidence is reported among newly graduated nurses (Park, 2009). In a qualitative case study conducted by Ramos and colleagues (2013), the participants, who were nursing teachers, expressed that reflection on nurses' ethics education should take place and that this reflection should not be limited to discussing content or instructional methods but should be extended to engage the student in critical analysis of moral scenarios. Students should actively pursue the building of their professional values (Ramos et al., 2013).

As concluded by Park (2009), nursing students have not been prepared to encounter ethical dilemmas in their nursing practice. The author also proposes the need for pragmatic teaching methods as a solution. In other words, planned ethics content in the nursing curriculum is necessary to improve moral sensitivity and moral reasoning of students (Park et al., 2012). Students must also be prepared to adopt different ways of thinking, to be open to the ethical issues by utilizing their absolute professional values and their professional code of ethics, and to apply them by using the lenses of their clients in order to achieve moral sensitivity.

HEALTH ADVOCACY AND HEALTHCARE REFORM

The concept of advocacy is both a morally and professionally important duty in nursing practice. This implies that nurses are required to help the patient make decisions according to their personal beliefs and values and to protect the patient's right through communicating with other healthcare providers (Leavitt, 2009; Park, 2009). Advocacy is a requirement for nurses. Advocacy is collaborating with colleagues or other healthcare professionals and engaging in conversations with decision-makers (Carnegie & Kiger, 2009). Because nurses have the position of communicating, interacting with, and caring for individuals and communities, it is extremely important that they listen to the experiences of individuals, and offer them the opportunity to address, and contribute to policies that affect their health (Carnegie & Kiger, 2009).

Healthcare systems are dynamic. Overall, they have been changing worldwide for decades, particularly in the United States. O'Grady (2009) made it clear that as communities are engaging in complex and dynamic health **reforms**, nurses are required to develop the language for a healthcare delivery system that is patient-centered, longitudinal and sustainable, relationship-based, and evidence-based. RNs are increasingly being recognized as leaders in transforming the healthcare system to meet the demand for illness prevention, wellness, and primary care services, with special attention to improving quality and managing costs (Dean, 2011).

Prior to the signing of the ACA in 2010, efforts were made for universal health insurance coverage dating back to the 1910s during the presidential campaign of Theodore Roosevelt. Even though such coverage has been established in all other industrial or industrializing nations, healthcare reformers have faced daunting political opposition in attempts at universal coverage in the United States (Jacobs & Skocpol, 2010). Although halted on universal coverage in the 1960s, reformers were able to establish Medicare to help cover costs for the elderly and Medicaid to help cover costs for low-income individuals. After incredible efforts that lasted over a decade, the ACA of 2010 became a monumental milestone but currently may be in jeopardy of being repealed under a new presidential administration and worldview as mentioned previously.

OVERVIEW OF THE ACA PRIOR TO THE END OF OBAMA PRESIDENCY

Generally speaking, health insurance is a contract that requires the health insurer to pay some or all of one's healthcare costs in exchange for a premium (Centers for Medicare and Medicaid Services [CMS], 2017; Healthcare.gov, 2017). The comprehensive healthcare reform law enacted in March 2010 (sometimes known as ACA, PPACA, or Obamacare), has two parts: (1) the Patient Protection and Affordable Care Act and (2) the Health Care and Education Reconciliation Act. The ACA is designed to address these concerns by improving the quality and accessibility of healthcare while reducing its cost. First articulated by the Institute for Health-care Improvement as the Triple Aim and later by the CMS as the Three-Part Aim, the goal of the ACA is to achieve better healthcare for individuals, better health outcomes in the community, and lower healthcare costs.

In May 2017, among the 48 states reporting both total Medicaid and CHIP enrollment and child enrollment data for the current period, total enrollment was comprised of 50.3% enrolled in the Medicaid child and CHIP, while 49.7% of adults were enrolled in Medicaid. Medicaid provides health coverage to millions of Americans, including eligible low-income adults, children, pregnant women, elderly adults and people with disabilities. Medicaid is administered by states according to federal requirements. The program is funded jointly by states and the federal government. Sixty-nine million people are covered. On the other hand, Medicare is a health insurance program for people age 65 or older, people under age 65 with certain disabilities, and people of all ages with end-stage renal disease (permanent kidney failure requiring dialysis or a kidney transplant). Medicare has three parts:

1. Part A hospital insurance—Most people don't pay a premium for Part A because they or a spouse already paid for it through their payroll taxes while working. Medicare Part A (hospital insurance) helps cover inpatient care in hospitals, including critical access hospitals, and skilled nursing facilities (not custodial or long-term care). It also helps cover hospice care and some home healthcare. Beneficiaries must meet certain conditions to get these benefits.
2. Part B medical insurance—Most people pay a monthly premium for Part B. Medicare Part B (medical insurance) helps cover doctors' services and outpatient care and some other medical services that Part A doesn't cover (e.g., services of physical and occupational therapists) while Part B helps pay for these covered services and supplies when they are medically necessary.
3. Prescription drug coverage—Most people will pay a monthly premium for this coverage while everyone with Medicare can get this coverage that may help lower prescription drug costs and help protect against higher costs in the future. Medicare prescription drug coverage is insurance that is provided by private companies. Beneficiaries choose the drug plan and pay a monthly premium.

Through the Patient Protection and ACA, the Obama administration's goals in improving the overall healthcare system and the quality of care included expanding health insurance coverage, shifting the focus of the healthcare delivery system from treatment to prevention, and reducing the costs and improving the efficiency of healthcare (Hellerstedt, 2013). The ACA was put in place to improve the quality, access, and affordability of healthcare. "The American College of Physicians hopes that the legislation will advance key priorities on coverage, workforce, and payment and delivery system reform" (Doherty, 2010, p. 679).

Additionally, the ACA expanded healthcare access to children (Oberg, 2013). Through the ACA, youth are allowed to remain on their parents' healthcare plan to the age of 26, insurers are no longer allowed to exclude children from coverage because of preexisting conditions, and access had been expanded through state-based health insurance exchanges for uninsured families (Oberg, 2013). Medicaid and Children's Health Insurance Program (CHIP) provisions have been administered through the ACA with goals of enrolling uninsured children. Such reforms will work to insure vulnerable childhood populations like children aging out of the foster care system (Oberg, 2013). Furthermore, reforms in healthcare for children will help reduce the cost of healthcare for families so that more children will be covered.

The U.S. Department of Health and Human Services, AHRQ (2012) reported that although indicators have shown that quality of healthcare for the general population is improving, quality of care is still not up to par for minorities and low-income communities. Furthermore, although the ACA has made strides for healthcare for all, an estimated 49 million Americans are still without health insurance (Hellerstedt, 2013).

Evidence for Practice

There has been considerable debate on repealing, replacing, or updating the ACA by President Donald Trump and his administration as well as members of the Congress. The proposed revised version of the ACA was reviewed by the Congressional Budget Office (CBO) and concluded that the new proposed version of the ACA would reduce the deficit by $337 billion in the next 10 years due to removal of premium tax credits and cuts in Medicaid. However, if the revised bill is enacted, it is estimated that 24 million people will lose health coverage by 2026. On March 24, 2017, the Speaker of the House of Representatives withdrew the ACA repeal-and-replace bill and stated that the ACA will be left intact for the time being. On March 6, 2017, House Republicans announced a bill to partially repeal and replace the ACA. There remains disagreement among members of Congress as to the details of the bill.

Next Steps

1. Elimination of additional Medicare taxes
There has been considerable discussion about repealing the additional Medicare tax, which imposes additional tax to individuals with high incomes. The repeal of the current bill will have

considerable payroll implications. Effective January 2018, the bill would repeal the additional Medicare tax that imposes an additional tax on income of $200,000 or more for individuals, $250,000 or more for joint returns, and $125,000 or more for married taxpayers filing separate returns. This would have payroll implications as employers have been required to withhold an additional 0.9% of Medicare subject wages over $200,000 to support the additional tax.

2. Premium tax credits and subsidies repealed
The proposed bill would eliminate premium tax credits for individuals who obtain health insurance through a federal or state health insurance market-place (exchange) as of January 1, 2020. It would also repeal cost-sharing reductions (and payments to issuers for such reductions) for plan years beginning after December 31, 2019.
More changes have included the following areas as well:

3. Health insurance tax credit
4. Continuous coverage
5. Elimination of other ACA taxes
For more information on the ACA updates, please visit https://www.paychex.com/articles/health-reform/aca-update-march-2017.

Evidence for Practice

In measuring the equity of healthcare and in working on reform, it is also important to review the effects of social determinants of health, which include early childhood education, employment opportunities, treatment of women, the effects of poverty, and individual empowerment on humans' health status and life expectancy (Wilensky & Satcher, 2009). The WHO's Commission on the Social Determinants of Health was created in 2005 to focus on the social determinants as a means of reducing health disparities (Wilensky & Satcher, 2009). This group explains that healthcare reform must focus on nutrition, education, reducing substance abuse, and access to care. In the United States, the following four components have been, or need to be, addressed in the following ways:

1. Nutrition: Over the years, the federal government has put in place systems that work to improve nutrition for low-income communities such as the federal food stamp program and the Special Supplemental Nutrition Program for Women, Infants, and Children (WIC and SNAP, respectively).
2. Education: Programs like the No Child Left Behind Act and the Action for Healthy Kids Program work to help low-income students by providing additional academic support and proper nutrition and physical activity.

3. Reducing substance use: Because many children are born with medical challenges due to their mother's substance abuse, more aggressive intervention must be put in place to help pregnant women deal with substance abuse. Programs for mothers should be free to those who cannot afford them.
4. Access to care: Medicaid and the State Children's Health Insurance Program (SCHIP) were put in place to ensure low-income children were provided with appropriate care. Although such systems were put in place, many children who are eligible are not enrolled. More aggressive outreach campaigns must be established to educate families on the care they are eligible to receive.

HEALTH SERVICES RESEARCH

Although the ACA has been passed and efforts to improve healthcare are increasing, the quality of healthcare and services has not improved significantly. Researchers, healthcare professionals, and other advocacy groups continue to push for an improved healthcare system in the United States with appropriate health services for all, and to do this, the healthcare system needs an accelerated transformation, which brings about quality care, proper information management, insurance for all, and equity to access (Dougherty & Conway, 2008). Dougherty and Conway (2008) proposed a model to transform the U.S. healthcare system, explaining how to deliver high-quality healthcare. Their plan outlines the activities, participants, investments, and fundamental shifts required to create and sustain a high-quality, patient-focused, healthcare system. Porter (2009) lists the following steps that must take place to improve the U.S. healthcare system:

1. Measurement and dissemination of health outcomes must be shared.
2. The delivery of prevention, wellness, screening, and routine health maintenance services must be fundamentally restructured.
3. Care delivery must be reorganized around medical conditions.
4. A reimbursement program for healthcare professionals as incentives to achieve better outcomes for patients should be introduced.
5. Providers must compete for patients based on the quality of the care provided.
6. All providers must establish electronic medical records.
7. Patients' involvement in their health must improve and incentives for patient involvement should be considered.

Porter explains that all items must happen simultaneously to build an effective healthcare system. Conway and Clancy (2009), in speaking of improving the healthcare system on the front line, emphasize the importance of improving measurements, adopting information technology, accelerating the production and use of requisite research, improving collaborations and networks, and increasing clinical training. Taking such action, Conway and Clancy claim, may significantly improve clinician engagement and patient care.

CONCLUSION

At this moment in history, healthcare is at the forefront of the public's attention. As an item on the President's platform, as the most popular topic on the news and radio, and as an issue greatly impacting individuals and employers, healthcare is an important topic, which is receiving attention from everyone. During this significant moment in the history of healthcare, nurses play an important role in providing quality healthcare, tracking patient progress, and being active members in healthcare reform. It is important that nurses are knowledgeable about health policy, politics, and healthcare reform because it will improve their understanding about where they work, the patients they care for, and government efforts that will impact both.

KEY CONCEPTS

- Because policy development and formulation is concerned with providing population-based interventions which will greatly impact the nation's health, the political process has a close relationship with health policies.
- Making health policy takes great time, effort, and commitment. This process is presented as a dynamic and cyclic series of six events, namely, agenda-setting, policy formulation, policy adoption, policy implementation, policy assessment, and finally policy modification.
- When a policy is evaluated for its effectiveness, there is an interest in keeping the cost of a specific health program within reason, and it is critical to consider the overall costs and benefits of an existing program when a more efficient and effective service is identified and adopted.
- The U.S. healthcare system is a unique system of both independent and collaborative power and action by both federal and state governments.
- Healthcare issues of racial and ethnic minorities, low-income individuals, and the uninsured overlap. Community health agencies play an important role in providing access to healthcare for those who are underserved, whether from uninsured or low-income communities.
- The United States has an increasing healthcare professional immigration from other countries.
- There is an increasing need for a diverse workforce of healthcare providers who can provide culturally competent care for the growing minority population. The less diverse the workforce, the less representative and influential will be the impact of the healthcare providers on healthcare policies.
- Nursing has a rich history as a unique profession, with its own values, ethics, respect, integrity and responsibility. Nurses' contributions to the policies are unlimited; there is a need for greater coordination of action to ensure that nursing is actively supported and involved in influencing and shaping health and healthcare policy.
- It is extremely difficult to evaluate the complexities of the quality of care for the U.S. population.
- U.S. policymakers have made the adoption of HIT a priority so that health records can be kept electronically, assisting patients, providers, and insurers.
- Because of the vast disparities in healthcare access and quality, President Obama made healthcare his top priority, promising affordable and adequate healthcare insurance for all Americans.
- Healthcare is closely linked with ethical issues and decisions and has implications for patients, providers, and healthcare leaders.
- Although most politicians agree a reform must take place, many cannot agree on what the change should look like. Consequently, healthcare reform in the United States has been a long political battle for quite some time.
- Research continues to be an influencing power by documenting the need for an accelerated reform in order to achieve quality care, proper information management, and insurance for all, and equity to access.

CRITICAL THINKING QUESTIONS

1. Consider that you are a nurse working with a patient who is from a different cultural and ethnic background from your own. Explain how you could translate the concept of cultural competency into practice. Do not forget ethical considerations.
2. After reading this chapter, you have learned about the six stages of the process of policy. Give at least one example showing how nurses can be engaged in each stage of the process.
3. You have read a lot about President Obama's Patient Protection and Affordable Care Act:
   a. What are the major milestones of this act that represent the healthcare reform?
   b. Explain how this act helps in delivering better healthcare services.
   c. Explain why this act has been considered a long political battle for a period of time.

CRITICAL THINKING QUESTIONS *(Continued)*

4. You have learned about health information technology (HIT) in this chapter:
   a. Give a few examples for the application of HIT in the clinical practice.
   b. Explain the main barriers of using HIT in the healthcare system.
   c. How has the American Recovery and Reinvestment Act (ARRA) reinforced the use of HIT in different healthcare settings?
5. How can research help in improving the U.S. healthcare system?
6. After carefully reading about Rice's exploratory study regarding the U.S. healthcare system, summarize in a short paragraph the major problems in this system.
7. Please visit this website https://www.healthy-people.gov/2020/topics-objectives and answer the following questions:
   a. What is the role that the *Healthy People 2020* initiative plays in healthcare reforms?
   b. What are the objectives that include professional nursing activities?
   c. How do you relate this to healthcare reforms and quality improvement?

REFERENCES

Abood, S. (2007). Influencing healthcare in the legislative arena. *Online Journal of Issues in Nursing, 12*(1), 2.

Acuff, K. (2017). Definition of Health care Policy. Last Updated August 14, 2017. Retrieved from http://www.livestrong.com/article/259661-definition-of-health-care-policy/

Agency for Healthcare Research and Quality. (2016). National Healthcare Quality and Disparities Report and 5th Anniversary Update on the National Quality Strategy. AHRQ Publication No. 16-0015. Updated May 21, 2016. Retrieved from http://www.ahrq.gov/research/findings/nhqrdr/nhqdr15/index.html

Aiken, L. H., Xue, Y., Clarke, S. P., & Sloane, D. M. (2006). Supplemental nurse staffing in hospitals and quality of care. *The Journal of Nursing Administration, 37*(7–8), 335–342.

American Nurse Association. (2010a). *Nursing social policy statement: The essence of the profession* (3rd ed.). Silver Spring, MD: Nursingbook.org.

American Nurse Association. (2010b). *Nursing: Scope and standards of practice* (2nd ed.). Silver Spring, MD: Nursebooks.org.

American Nurses Association (ANA); Winland-Brown, J., Lachman, V. D., & Swanson, E. O. C. (2015a). The new "code of ethics for nurses with interpretive statements": Practical clinical application, part I. *Medsurg Nurs, 24*(4), 268. Retrieved from http://web.b.ebscohost.com.ezproxy.lib.umb.edu/ehost/pdfviewer/pdfviewer?vid=2&sid=5 67b6248-a412-42d7-b804-56e9f2067741%40sessionmgr103

American Nurses Association (ANA); Lachman, V. D., Swanson, E. O. C., & Winland-Brown, J. (2015b). The New 'Code of Ethics for Nurses with Interpretive Statements' (2015): Practical clinical application, Part II. *Medsurg Nursing, 24*(5), 363. Retrieved from http:// www.nursingworld.org/code of ethics

American Nurses Association (ANA). (2001). The code of ethics for nurses with interpretive statements. Washington, DC: Nurses-books.org.

Artz, M. (2006). Ask not what nursing can do for you…. Nurses have a lot of power. *American Journal of Nursing, 106*(9), 91.

Bearskin, R. (2011). A critical lens on culture in nursing practice. *Nursing Ethics, 18*(4), 548–559.

Berger K, (2015). An Update on United States Healthcare Quality Improvement Efforts. Retrieved from https://www.hsph.harvard.edu/ecpe/an-update-on-united-states-healthcare-quality-improve-ment-efforts/. Accessed December 22, 2015.

Betancourt, J. R., Green, A. R., Carrillo, J. E., & Ananeh-Firempong, II, O. (2003). Defining cultural competence: A practical framework for addressing racial/ethnic disparities in health and healthcare. *Public Health Reports, 118*(4), 293.

Blumenthal, D. (2009). Stimulating the adoption of health information technology. *New England Journal of Medicine, 360*(15), 1477–1479.

Boswell, C., Cannon, S., & Miller, J. (2005). Nurses' political involvement: Responsibility versus privilege. *Journal of Professional Nursing, 21*(1), 5–8.

Brownson, R., Fielding, F., & Maylahn, C. (2009). Evidence-based public health: A fundamental concept for public health. *Annual Review of Public Health, 30*(1), 313–315.

Budden, J. S., Zhong, E. H., Moulton, P., & Cimiotti, J. P. (2013). Highlights of the national workforce survey of registered nurses. *Journal of Nursing Regulation, 4*(2), 5–14.

Buntin, M. B., Jain, S. H., & Blumenthal, D. (2010). Health information technology: Laying the infrastructure for national health reform. *Health Affairs, 29*(6), 1214–1219.

Calman, N. S, Golub, M., & Shuman, S. (2012). Primary care and health reform. *Mount Sinai Journal of Medicine, 79*, 527–534.

Carnegie, E., & Kiger, A. (2009). Being and doing politics: An outdated model or 21st century reality? *Journal of Advanced Nursing, 65*(9), 1976–1984. doi:10.1111/j.1365-2648.2009.05084.x

Catalano, J. T. (2015). *Nursing now! Today's issues, tomorrow's trends.* Philadelphia, PA: F.A. Davis. Retrieved from http://scholar.google.com/scholar?hl=en&as_sdt=0,5&q=Catalano+Nursing+now%3A+Today%27s+issues,+tomorrow%27s+trends

Centers for Disease Control and Prevention, Office of the Associate Director for Policy. (2015). Definition of Policy. Last updated May 29, 2015. Retrieved from https://www.cdc.gov/policy/analysis/process/definition.html

Centers for Medicare and Medicaid Services (CMS). (2017). Retrieved from Healthcare.gov.

Charles, D., Gabriel, M., & Searcy T. (2015). *Adoption of Electronic Health Record Systems among U.S. Non-Federal Acute Care Hospitals: 2008–2014.* ONC Data Brief, no. 23. Washington DC: Office of the National Coordinator for Health Information Technology (ONC).

Conway, P., & Clancy, C. (2009). Transformation of healthcare at the front line. *Journal of the American Medical Association, 301*(7), 763–765.

Cowart, M. E., & Allen, R. F. (1981). *Changing conceptions of healthcare: Public policy and ethical issues for nurses.* Thorofare, NJ: Charles B. Slack.

Dean, E. (2011). Reforms forum fails to insist on nurse role in commissioning. *Nursing Standard, 25*(41), 9–9. Retrieved from http://ezproxy.lib.umb.edu/login?url = http://search.ebscohost.com/login.aspx?direct = true&db = ccm&AN = 2011184887&site = ehost-live

Des Jardin, K. E. (2001). Political involvement in nursing—politics, ethics, and strategic action. *AORN journal, 74*(5), 613–622.

Des Jardin, K. E. (2006). Political involvement in nursing-Education and empowerment. *AORN Journal.* doi: org/10.1016/S0001-2092(06)61679-7.

Doherty, R. B. (2010). The certitudes and uncertainties of healthcare reform. *Annals of Internal Medicine, 152*(10), 679–682.

Dougherty, D., & Conway, P. (2008). The "3T's" road map to transform US healthcare: The "How" of high-quality care. *Journal of the American Medical Association, 299*(19), 2319–2321.

Fonkych, K., & Taylor, R. (2005). *The State and Pattern of Health Information Technology Adoption.* Santa Monica, CA: Rand Corporation.

Fyffe, T. (2009). Nursing shaping and influencing health and social care policy. *Journal of Nursing Management, 17*(6), 698–706.

Goodman, A. (2009). President Obama's health planned community-based prevention. Editorial. *American Journal of Public Health, 99*(10), 1736–1738.

Grogan, C. M. (2012). The murky relationship between ideology and the role of government in health policy. *Journal of Health Politics, Policy & Law, 37*(3), 361–364. doi:10.1215/03616878-1573058.

Hartman, M., Martin, A., Benson, J., & Catlin, A. (2013). National health spending in 2011: Overall growth remains low, but some payers and services show signs of acceleration. *Health Affairs, 32*(1), 87–99.

Health Resources and Services Administration (HRSA). (2013). The U.S. nursing workforce: Trends in supply and education. National Center for Health Workforce Analysis. Available from http://bhpr.hrsa.gov/healthworkforce/supplydemand/nursing/nursingworkforce/nursingworkforce fullreport.pdf. Accessed October 30, 2013.

Health Resources and Services Administration (HRSA). (2015). The U.S. nursing workforce: Trends in supply and education. National Center for Health Workforce Analysis. Retrieved from http://bhpr.hrsa.gov/healthworkforce/supplydemand/nursing/nursingworkforce/nursingworkforce fullreport.pdf.

Healthcare.gov. (2017). Centers for Medicare and Medicaid Services (CMS), 2017. ACA

Hellerstedt, W. L. (2013). The Affordable Care Act: What are its goals and do we need it? Retrieved from http://www.epi.umn.edu/mch/wp-content/uploads/2013/09/ACA-Overview.pdf.

Hennrikus, D. (2013). The Community Transformation Grant Program. *Healthy Generations, 16.* Retrieved from http://www.epi.umn.edu/mch/wpcontent/uploads/2012/05/HG_Fall20132.pdf"; \l "page = 18

Hewlett, P. O., Bleich, M., Cox, M. F., & Hoover, K. W. (2009). Changing times: The role of academe in health reform. *Journal of Professional Nursing, 25*(6), 322–328. doi:10.1016/j.profnurs.2009.10.008

Hohn, M. D., Lowry, J. P., Witte, J. C., & Fernández-Pena, J. R. (2016). Immigrants in healthcare keeping Americans healthy through care and innovation. Executive Summary. Retrieved from http://www.immigrationresearch-info.org/system/files/health_care_report_FINAL_20160607.pdf. Accessed June 2016.

Hunt, B. (2007). Managing equality and cultural diversity in the health workforce. *Journal of Clincial Nursing, 16*(12), 2252–2259.

Indiana State Nurse Association. (2013). *Public Policy Platform 2013.* Retrieved from http://www.IndianaNurses.org.

Institute of Medicine. (2001). *Crossing the Quality Chasm: A New Health System for the 21st Century.* Washington, DC: National Academies Press.

International Council of Nursing (ICN) (2011). About ICN. Updated November 1,2011. Retrieved from http://www.icn.ch/"; \t "_blank.

Jacobs, L. R., & Skocpol, T. (2012). *Health Care Reform and American Politics: What Everyone Needs to Know.* New York, NY: Oxford University Press.

Jha, A., DesRoches, C., Kralovec, P., & Joshi, M. (2010). A progress report on electronic health records in US hospitals. *Health Affairs, 29*(10), 1951–1957.

King, C. A. (2015). Nursing advocacy 101: Start where you are to do what you can. *Tar Heel Nurse, 77*(2 Spec No), 12–15.

Kraft, M., & Furlong, S. (Ed.). (2013). *Public Policy, Politics, Analysis and Alternatives.* California: Sage Publication.

Krischke, M. (2011). Nursing Advocacy: Standing Up for Patients and the Profession. *Travel Nursing.* Retrieved from http://www.travelnursing.com/news/nurse-news/nursing-advocacy-standing-up-for-patients-and-the-profession.

Leavitt, J. K. (2009). Leaders in health policy: A critical role for nursing. *Nursing Outlook, 57*(2), 73–77. doi: 10.1016/j.outlook.2009.01.007.

Leininger, M. M. (1978). *Caring: An essential human need.* Detroit, MI: Wayne State University Press.

Leininger, M. M. (1999). What is transcultural nursing and culturally competent care? *Journal of Transcultural Nursing, 10*(1), 9.

Li, H., Nie, W., & Li, J. (2014). The benefits and caveats of international nurse migration. *International Journal of Nursing Sciences, 1*(3), 314–317.

Magnussen, L., Itano, J., &McGuckin, N. (2005). Legislative advocacy skills for baccalaureate nursing students. *Nurse Educator, 30*(3), 109–112.

Malone, R. E. (2009). The social and political context of the tobacco epidemic: Nursing research and scholarship on the tobacco industry. *Annual Review of Nursing Research, 27*, 63–90. doi:10.1891/0739-6686.27.63.

Mason, D., Leavitt, J., & Chaffee, M. (2012). *Policy and politics in nursing and healthcare* (6th ed.). Missouri, MO: Elsevier Sauders.

Massachusetts Nurse Newsletter July/August. (2010). In Press Release on Assault Bill from the Governor's Office. Retrieved from https://www.massnurses.org/files/file/News/newsletter/2010/Jul_Aug.pdf

Matthews, J. (2012). Role of professional organizations in advocating for the nursing profession. *Online Journal of Issues in Nursing, 17*(3). Retrieved from nursingworld.org.

Milstead, J. (Ed.). (2008). *Health policy and politics: A nurse's guide.* Boston, MA: Jones and Bartlett Publishers.

Milstead, J. A. (2013). Advanced practice nurses and public policy, naturally. *Health policy and politics: A nurse's guide,* 1–27.

Mongan, J. (2006). Commonwealth Fund Commission Framework for a High Performance Health System for the United States. Retrieved from http://www.commonwealthfund.org/publications/fund-reports.

Morone, J., Litman, T., & Robins, L. (Eds.). (2008). *Health Politics and Policy.* New York, NY: Delmar.

Murray, C., & Frenk, J. (2010). Ranking 37th—measuring the performance of the US healthcare system. *New England Journal of Medicine, 362*(2), 98–99.

Myers, C. (2010). Being there: Policy making and nurses. *Tennessee Nurse, 73*(3), 9–10.

National Advisory Council on Nurse Education and Practice (NACNEP). (2013) The Eleventh Report to the Secretary of the Department of Health and Human Services and the Congress of the NACNEP 123rd and 124th Meetings. Health Resources and Services Administration (HRSA). Retrieved from https://www.hrsa.gov/advisorycommittees/bhpradvisory/nacnep/Reports/eleventhreport.pdf

National Council of State Board of Nursing (NSCBN). (2015). National Nursing Workforce Study. Retrieved from https://www.ncsbn.org/workforce.htm.

Nault, D. S., & Sincox, A. K. (2014). Nursing voice in politics: The ongoing relationship with nurses and legislators. Independent Study 1.0 contact hour. July 2014 Expires. July 2016. Retrieved from Minurses.org.

REFERENCES *(Continued)*

Norman, J. (2016). *Americans rate healthcare providers high on honesty, ethics*. Washington, DC: Gallup Inc. Social Issues. Updated December 19, 2016. Retrieved from https://news.gallup.com/poll/200057/americans-ratehealthcare-providers-high-honesty-ethics.aspx

O'Grady, E. (2009). Health policy and politics. Acknowledge the paradoxes and advance the profession. *Nursing Economics, 27*(5), 337. Retrieved from http://web.a.ebscohost.com.ezproxy.lib.umb.edu/ehost/pdfviewer/pdfviewer?sid = 32b50468-22d0-47c3-ab5e-26cb8e67064b%40sessionmgr4001&vid = 1&hid = 4214

Oberg, C. N. (2013). The Affordable Care Act and children. *Healthy Generations*, 26. Retrieved from http://www.epi.umn.edu/mch/wp-content/uploads/2013/09/ACA-Children.pdf.

Oestberg, F. (2013). Getting involved in policy and politics. *Nursing Critical Care, 8*(3), 48.

Ohio Nurses Association. (2013). What do I do now? Ethical dilemmas in nursing and healthcare. *ISNA Bulletin, 39*(2), 5–12. Retrieved from http://ezproxy.lib.umb.edu/login?url = http://search.ebscohost.com/login.aspx?direct = true&db = ccm&AN = 2012007375&site = ehost-live

Oliver, J. D. (2012). Communicating with your legislator. *Perioperative Nursing Clinics, 7*(4), 393–396.

Park, M. (2009). The legal basis of nursing ethics education. *Journal of Nursing Law, 13*(4), 106–113. doi:10.1891/1073-7472.13.4.106.

Park, M., Kjervik, D., Crandell, J., & Oermann, M. (2012). The relationship of ethics education to moral sensitivity and moral reasoning skills of nursing student. *Nursing Ethics, 19*(4), 568–580.

Porche, D. (2012). *Health policy, application for nurses and other healthcare professionals*. Canada: Jones and Bartlett Learning.

Porter, M. (2009). A strategy for healthcare reform—toward a value-based system. *New England Journal of Medicine, 361*(2), 109–112.

Powell, D. J. (1976). Nursing and politics: The struggles outside nursing's body politic. *Nursing Forum, 15*(4), 341–336.

Purnell, L. (2002). The Purnell model for cultural competence. *Journal of Transcultural Nursing, 13*(3), 193–196.

Purnell, L. D. (2012). *Transcultural healthcare: A culturally competent approach*. Philadelphia, PA: F.A. Davis.

Ramos, F., de Pires, D., Brehmer, L., Gelbcke, F., Schmoeller, S., & Lorenzetti, J. (2013). The discourse of ethics in nursing education: Experience and reflection of Brazilian teachers-case study. *Nurse Education Today, 33*, 1124–1129.

Rice, T., Rosenau, P., Unruh, L. Y., Barnes, A. J., Saltman, R. B., & van Ginneken, E. (2013). United States of American: Health system review. *Health Systems in Transition, 15*(3), 1–431.

Rubotzky, A. M. (2000). Nursing participation in healthcare reform efforts of 1993 to 1994: Advocating for the national community. *Advances in Nursing Science, 23*(2), 12–33.

Russell, D., Rosati, R. J., Sobolewski, S., Marren, J., & Rosenfeld, P. (2011). Implementing a transitional care program for high-risk heart failure patients: Findings from a community-based partnership between a certified home healthcare agency and regional hospital. *Journal for Healthcare Quality, 33*(6), 17–24.

Schoen, C., Davis, K., How, S., & Schoenbaum, S. C. (2006). US health system performance: A national scorecard. *Health Affairs, 25*(6), w457–w475.

Selanders, L. C., & Crane P. C. (2012). The voice of Florence Nightingale on advocacy. *Online Journal of Issues in Nursing. 17*(1), 1.

Sorbello, B. (2008). Finance: It's not a dirty word. *American Nurse Today, 3*(8), 32–35.

Spring, S. (2013). Nurses earn highest ranking ever, remain most ethical of professions in poll: ANA urges policymakers to listen to nurses on healthcare policy, funding. *New Mexico Nurse, 58*(1), 13–13. Retrieved from http://web.b.ebscohost.com/ehost/pdfviewer/pdfviewer.

U.S. Bureau of Economic Analysis (USBEA). (2013). GDP and the economy: Survey of current business. Retrieved from http://www.bea.gov.

U.S. Census Bureau. (2015). Quick Facts. Retrieved from https://census.gov/quickfacts/.

U.S. Department of Health and Human Services, Agency for Healthcare Research and Quality. (2012). *2012 National healthcare disparities report*. Retrieved from http://www.ahrq.gov/research/findings/nhqrdr/nhdr12/.

U.S. Department of Health and Human Services, Office of Health Resources and Services Administration (HRSA). (2010). Findings from the 2008 national survey of registered nurses (chap 8, p. 192). Retrieved from http://www.hrsa.gov/about/news/pressreleases/2010/100922nursingworkforce.html.

Vencill, B. P., & Lemmons, K. Doing your part professional advocacy. *Or Nurse, 9*(3), 48. doi: 10.1097/01.ORN.0000464758.25224.fc.

Vencill, B. P., & Lemmons, K. (2015). Doing your part for professional advocacy. Retrieved from http://www.resolver.ebscohost.com.ezproxy.lib.umb.edu/openurl?sid=EBSCO%3accm&genre=article&issn=19333145&ISBN=&volume=9&issue=3&date=20150501&spage=48&pages=48-48&title=OR+Nurse&atitle=Doing+your+part+for+professional+advocacy.&aulast=Vencill%2c+Bonnie+R.&id=DOI%3a10.1097%2f01.ORN.0000464758.25224.fc&site=ftf-live.

White, K. M., Zangaro, G., Kepley, H. O., & Camacho, A. (2014). The Health Resources and Services Administration Diversity Data Collection. *Public Health Reports, 129*(Suppl 2), 51–56.

Whitehead, D. (2003). The health-promoting nurse as a health policy career expert and entrepreneur. *Nurse Education Today, 23*(8), 585–592.

Wilensky, G., & Satcher, D. (2009). Don't forget about the social determinants of health. *Health Affairs, 28*(2), w194–w198.

Williams, A. (1993). Community health learning experiences and political activism: A model for baccalaureate curriculum revolution content. *Journal of Nursing Education, 32*(8), 352–356.

Williams, C. A. (1977). Making things happen: Community health nursing and the policy arena. *Nursing Outlook, 25*(4), 250–254.

Williamson, E. (2017). Nurses rank # 1 once again in Gallup Poll for ethics and honesty. Retrieved from https://www.nurse.com/blog/2016/12/21/nurses-rank-1-once-again-in-gallup-poll-for-ethics-and-honesty/

World Health Organization (WHO). (2008). *World Health Report 2008*. Geneva, Switzerland.

World Health Organization. (2017). *Heath Policy*. Retrieved from http://www.who.int/topics/health_policy/en/.

WEB RESOURCES

Please visit thePoint® for up-to-date web resources on this topic.

Please watch the following YouTube video titled as: Governor Patrick Signs Assault Bill. https://www.youtube.com/watch?v=bdsgDoS8amY. Massnurses Published on Jul 8, 2010.

Chapter 4

Global Health: A Community Perspective

Joyce Pulcini and Karen Dawn

> It is health that is real wealth and not pieces of gold and silver.
> **Mahatma Gandhi**
>
> Of all the forms of inequality, injustice in healthcare is the most shocking and inhumane.
> **Martin Luther King Jr.**

CHAPTER HIGHLIGHTS

- Definitions of global health and global burden of disease
- Indicators of health
- Health and human rights
- Factors that affect health globally
- Framework for improving world health
- Sustainable Development Goals

OBJECTIVES

- Identify critical determinants of global health and the intersection between health and the environment.
- Describe the approaches to achieving maximum health outcomes in poor countries and affluent countries.
- Define the concept of burden of disease, how it is measured, and the ultimate effect on a population's health.
- Identify and explain the effects of political, economic, and sociodemographic factors on health.
- Describe the purpose of the Sustainable Development Goals and their future impact on improving global health.
- Describe key indicators of health that can be measured or used as benchmarks to examine the health outcomes of a population.

KEY TERMS

Communicable disease: An illness caused by an infectious agent or its toxins that occurs through the direct or indirect transmission of the infectious agent or its products from an infected individual or by an animal, vector, or the inanimate environment to a susceptible animal or human host (Centers for Disease Control and Prevention, 2010).

Demographic and epidemiologic transitions: Progressive improvement in health from a global perspective.

Determinants of health: Factors that affect outcomes of health status, such as physical environment, social environment, health behaviors, and individual health, as well as broader factors such as access to health services and overall health policies and interventions.

Global burden of disease: The importance of risks to health and their outcomes in different demographic populations and social settings.

Global health: "An area for study, research, or practice that places a priority on improving health and achieving equity for all people worldwide. Global

KEY TERMS *(continued)*

health emphasizes transnational health issues, determinants, and solutions, involves many disciplines within and beyond the health sciences, and promotes interdisciplinary collaboration, and is a synthesis of population-based prevention with individual-level clinic care" (Koplan et al., 2009).

Health: A state of complete physical, mental, and social well-being, not merely the absence of disease or infirmity.

Health indicators: Descriptors of the general health of a nation

that are grouped into four categories: morbidity and mortality, risk factors, health service coverage, and health system resources.

Noncommunicable disease: Diseases that afflict a population which are chronic in nature and may be due to lifestyle changes, sometimes as a result of modernization of societies. Examples include cardiovascular diseases, cancers, diabetes, obesity, and chronic respiratory diseases.

Risk factors: Personal habits and behaviors, social, and

environmental conditions, or inborn or inherited characteristics that are known to affect a health-related condition which could be alleviated or managed.

Public health: Ensuring that every person in the community has a standard of living adequate for the maintenance of health. This involves the science and art of preventing disease, prolonging life, and promoting physical health and efficiency through organized community efforts.

CASE STUDIES

References to case studies are found throughout this chapter (look for the case study icon). Readers should keep the case studies in mind as they read the chapter.

CASE 1

Haweeyo is a 30-year-old woman living in extreme poverty just outside Mogadishu. She is pregnant by a man who sexually assaulted her several months ago. She reported the incident to the police but they did nothing. In her culture, pregnancy without marriage carries great stigma and shame. She and her family have become social outcasts in their community and are having difficulty finding work and paying for food. Haweeyo received threats of violence repeatedly by people in her community and was taken from her home and severely beaten 2 days ago. Haweeyo has received no prenatal care and did not seek treatment for her injuries because she feared she would be treated poorly by the health providers. A few hours after being attacked by her neighbors she went into early labor and her sister called the birth attendant. As her labor continued, the community health worker (CHW) birth attendant recognized the labor was complicated and needed to get Haweeyo to the hospital to deliver her baby. Her family did not have funds or transportation to get her to the city hospital. Haweeyo died in her own home a few hours later.

CASE 2

Vikram is a 68-year-old father of seven children, who shares a small home with his wife, three of his adult children and their families, his mother, and older brother in India. He is recently recovering from a third episode of diarrheal illness in the past 3 months. He experienced weight loss of almost 20 lb in 4 weeks, complained of feeling fatigued most of the time, shortness of breath, persistent cough, night sweats, and low-grade fever. Two years ago, he was diagnosed with tuberculosis. He took medications for a short time, but due to lack of finances and availability of the medications he stopped. Vikram visited the small health clinic where he was seen by the only medical practitioner in the village. With no x-ray facilities available, a TB skin test (TST) was performed and he was sent home. Three days later he returned to the clinic. The skin test was positive and TB was confirmed by a sputum smear test. While at the health clinic he was also tested for HIV, which was negative. He was started again on TB medications, but developed multidrug-resistant tuberculosis (MDR-TB) and subsequently his condition deteriorated.

We live in a global environment. Recent examples of how health in one region of the world affects other regions include both the Ebola epidemic and Zika infections. News of both of these infections have spread rapidly through world news and are exacerbated by widespread global migration.

What does it mean to be healthy in a global context? A person's health status is highly dependent on his or her living environment, social norms, gender, and age, specifically in low-resourced settings. Access to and utilization of healthcare is highly dependent on where you live in the world and the community definition of health. In addition, the health of individuals depends on the social and economic conditions in which they live. Many factors affect the health and well-being of individuals. This chapter explores an array of factors that affect health and the global environment.

DEFINITIONS OF HEALTH

The World Health Organization (WHO) in 1947 defined **health** as "a state of complete physical, mental, and social well-being and not merely the absence of disease or infirmity" (WHO, 1947, p. 1). The WHO definition of health encompasses the highest level of health, involving self-actualization or reaching one's true potential. The more specific concepts of public health or global health may be important when the concept of an individual's health is considered. All are interrelated in a global context.

Winslow (1920), often called the father of public health, defined **public health** as "the science and art of preventing disease, prolonging life, and promoting physical health and efficiency through organized community efforts for the sanitation of the environment, the control of community infections, the education of the individual in principles of personal hygiene, the organization of medical and nursing service for the early diagnosis and preventive treatment of disease, and the development of the social machinery which will ensure to every individual in the community a standard of living adequate for the maintenance of health" (p. 23). The identification of nursing in 1923 as a key participant in the social construct of health recognized the contribution that nurses could make to promote health and well-being of all humankind.

Dunn (1959) placed health on a continuum, ranging from premature death to wellness to high-level wellness, which can be equated to self-actualization. In this model, the environment (i.e., factors outside of the person) plays a major role in health (Fig. 4.1)

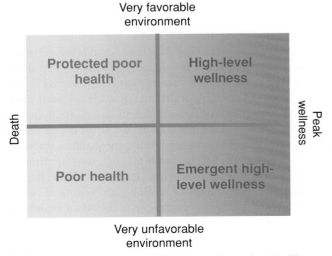

FIGURE 4.1 The health grid, its axes and quadrants. (From Dunn, H. [1959]. High-level wellness for man and society. *American Journal of Public Health, 49*[6], 788.)

In her classic work, Smith (1981) identified four models of health:

1. *Clinical model:* elimination of disease or symptoms. Some people feel that they are well when they have no symptoms or diagnosed diseases and would not classify themselves as sick otherwise.
2. *Role-performance model:* health that involves a match between people and social roles. For example, some people, even if they have symptoms of disease, would classify themselves as unhealthy only if they could not fulfill their roles in life, such as parent or worker.
3. *Adaptive model:* health that involves adaptation to the environment. For example, some people consider health to be determined by their ability to adapt in the face of adversity or disease.
4. *Eudaimonistic model:* health that is the actualization or realization of human potential. In this model, for example, people would consider themselves to be healthy if they are functioning not only physically but also emotionally and socially. The WHO (1947) definition of health actually strives for this level of health.

Global health was defined by the Institute of Medicine (IOM, 1997) as "health problems, issues, and concerns that transcend national boundaries and may best be addressed by cooperative actions and solutions" (p. 2). Each of Smith's four models can be viewed within the definition of the IOM and includes people's definition of health based on their culture, role in life, and environmental resources. A person's definition of health determines how and when he or she seeks assistance from the health-care system and may ultimately affect the outcome of long-term health.

The evolution of the definition of health clearly shows an increased appreciation of the biophysical, sociodemographic, and environmental influences on individual, family, and community health. Health is a complex concept that can be conceptualized in many ways, from a broad to narrow disease-specific view. Further, complexity comes into play when the social, political, and economic conditions are factored into the equation.

In each of these case studies, internal factors—the way a person views health—and external factors outside of the individual such as the environment, affect whether a person is viewed as healthy, unhealthy, or at risk. The way women view health, in particular pregnancy, can affect birth outcomes. Environment is key and ultimately changes the context in which health or illness conditions are experienced or played out. When dimensions of poverty, education, culture, lifestyle, norms, beliefs, and political and economic instability are added to the equation, it is possible to further understand the complexity of the concept of health and its determinants.

GLOBAL HEALTH CONCEPTS

Determinants of Health

Global health is a dynamic concept with many components. In examining this concept, several factors need to be considered. Skolnik (2016) identifies the key **determinants of health**, which encompass the following domains: (1) physical environment; (2) social environment; (3) health behaviors and coping skills; (4) access to health services; (5) healthy child development; and (6) employment and working conditions, in the context of the broader factors of access to health services, as well as health policies and interventions (p. 21).

Demographic and Epidemiologic Transitions

When it comes to global health, there is no "them"…only "us." **Global Health Council**

Demographic and epidemiologic transitions refer to the improvement in global health indicators (WHO, 2013a). Changes in these demographic indicators signify improvement in health over time. In addition, specific indicators provide a unique picture of community health: life expectancy and morbidity and mortality, selected infectious diseases, health service coverage, health systems expenditure and inequities, and demographic and socioeconomic statistics (WHO, 2014a). They include many factors, such as age, gender, socioeconomic status, and disease prevalence, and taken together, they can portray the health of a community and identify areas in need of intervention.

In addition, these indicators are tracked by the demographic and health survey (DHS) program, which is conducted at the household level to evaluate the health of a nation (United States Agency for International Development, 2014). Every 3 to 4 years, a DHS is conducted to describe the health of a country and define specific demographics that can be compared to each other. These transitions are used as a measure of health improvement of a nation.

Demographic transitions may progress from low to high levels:

1. High fertility and high mortality, resulting in slow population growth
2. Improvement in hygiene and nutrition, leading to less infectious disease
3. Mortality declines, and later fertility declines
4. Elderly population increases

Epidemiologic transitions include the following:

1. High and fluctuating mortality, due to poor health, epidemics, and famine
2. Progressive declines in mortality, as epidemics become less frequent
3. Further decline in mortality, increasing life expectancy, and predominance of noncommunicable diseases (NCDs)

As a country becomes more developed, levels of demographic or epidemiologic transitions shift upward. For example, as mortality rates decrease, more attention can be paid to increase the quality of life of all citizens, including the elderly. As the number of children involved in agrarian functions decreases and as the need for formal education increases, fertility rates tend to decrease. As more members of a population are educated, indicators of health, such as higher life expectancy and lower mortality rates, improve.

Global Burden of Disease

Every observer of human misery among the poor reports that disease plays the leading role. **Fisher** (1909, p. 124)

Global burden of disease (GBD) is the risks to health and health outcomes in different demographic populations and social settings related to a set of diseases and injuries. There are 18 components of GBD that are interrelated and create the changing picture of burden related to specific communities (Institute for Health Metrics and Evaluation, 2014). The largest study of these indicators was published in 2012, revealing that women and men are living longer but spending more time living with illness and injury (Horton, 2013). The collection of specific data related to risk factors, health indicators, and health outcomes of 291 diseases and injuries in 20 regions of the world determines the GBD (Murray et al., 2012). Indicators include lower respiratory tract infection, diarrheal disease, malaria, and protein malnutrition as well as road injuries and pollution (Institute of Health Metrics and Evaluation, 2014). Changes in these factors can identify areas of improvement or the need for intervention. The goal of analyzing these data is to summarize measures of a population's health and to identify risk factors that affect health. The concept of disease burden first occurred in the early 1980s, when the World Bank signaled the need for a better understanding of disease control and mortality to set priorities for resource-limited countries. In an era of unmet needs, economic divisions, and health inequalities, the need for rigorous data for decision-making despite limited resources was, and still is, vital (Lopez, Mathers, Ezzati, Jamison, & Murray, 2006). Examining the effects of health indicators and risk factors on the overall health of a community can guide healthcare planners and providers in choosing those services and interventions that can improve health.

As health policymakers and governments better understood the impact of disease, the need for an analysis of the circumstances grew. In 1990, the World Bank commissioned the first study on disease burden (World Bank, 1993). In 1994, Jamison and Jardel (1994) incorporated the concept of cost–benefit analysis related to disease burden to assist countries in decision-making about health interventions. Murray and Lopez (1996) edited a publication called *The Global Burden of Disease*. All of these reports later influenced the ongoing analysis by the World Bank, as well as work by the Fogarty International Center at the U.S. National Institutes of Health and the Bill and Melinda Gates Foundation, to form the Disease Control Priorities Project (DCPP). The project's purpose has been "to review, generate, and disseminate information that contributes to the scientific evidence base for improving population health in developing countries" (DCPP, 2008, p. 1). Murray and colleagues (2012) compared data on disease and injury from 1990 through 2010, providing a longitudinal assessment of effects of disease and injury on specific populations. Integrating collected health data, using evidence that supports the data, and applying to disease outcomes is paramount to improving global health.

Noncommunicable Diseases

In 2012, the World Health Assembly endorsed an important new health goal: to reduce avoidable mortality from **noncommunicable diseases** (NCDs) by 25% by 2025 (the 25 × 25 goal) (Alleyne et al., 2013). The *Global Burden of Disease and Risk Factors* study built upon earlier versions, providing a comprehensive analysis of the health of the world's population, including health indicators for disease outcomes, as well as risk factors and monitoring strategies that can be used for program planning to improve health outcomes (Murray et al., 2012).

While **communicable disease** is still prevalent, 70% of all deaths globally are caused by NCDs. Four common behavioral risk factors that occur globally—tobacco use, excessive alcohol consumption, poor diet, and lack of physical activity—are associated with four health diseases—cardiovascular disease, cancer, chronic pulmonary disease, and diabetes that account for 80% of deaths from NCDs (Hunter & Reddy, 2013, WHO 2017a). Clearly, the leading causes of mortality and burden of disease worldwide have shifted from communicable to NCDs. This change represents an opportunity for communities to address behaviors that can affect overall health (Fig. 4.2). When examining the GBD chart, many diseases can be ameliorated through health promotion, education, and the provision of skilled healthcare (Box 4.1).

According to the *WHO Global Status Report on Noncommunicable Diseases* (2014b), of the 56 million global deaths in 2012, 38 million, or 68%, were due to NCDs, the most prominent of which were cardiovascular diseases, diabetes, cancers, and chronic respiratory diseases. Nearly 15 million of all deaths attributed to NCDs occur between the ages of 30 and 69 years and 80% of these deaths from NCDs occur in low- and middle-income countries (Lozano et al., 2012). The report states that, "almost three quarters of all NCD deaths (28 million), and 82% of the 16 million premature deaths, occur in low- and middle-income countries"

(WHO, 2015, p 1). Low-income countries are mostly situated in middle Africa, but middle-income countries include most of Central and South America, Eastern Europe, and Asia. While NCDs are still not the most frequent causes of death in African nations, these diseases are rising rapidly and are projected to exceed communicable, maternal, perinatal, and nutritional diseases as the most common causes of death by 2030 (Southern African Development Community, 2012).

More than half of all cancer deaths occur in developing nations (Cancer Research U.K., 2014). NCDs also cause death at younger ages in low- and middle-income countries. For example, 29% of deaths due to NCDs in low- and middle-income countries occur among people under the age of 60, compared to 13% in high-income countries. A WHO report (2011) stated that the estimated percentage increase in cancer incidence by 2030, compared with 2008, will be greater in low-income (82%) and lower–middle-income countries (70%) compared with the upper–middle-income (58%) and high-income countries (40%).

Key factors in the rise of NCDs are similar in all countries, and the diseases are often preventable (Box 4.2). In low- and middle-income countries that are now seeing increases in the rate of NCDs, the process is accelerated by urbanization, culture change especially among the young, increasing sedentary lifestyles, and corporate marketing that targets these populations. One might see older populations still eating more healthy traditional foods, and younger populations lured in by fast food marketing, for example. Recommendations are being made, especially in low-resource settings, for increased surveillance and reporting of these diseases as well as increased efforts to educate the public on this important health area. NCDs play an important role not only on their effect on individuals but also on social, economic, and environmental factors that affect human development (Alleyne et al., 2013; WHO, 2017a).

An important factor in the increase in NCDs is also the aging of the global population. As we look to the future, the combination of aging and increased NCDs is likely to cause a higher disease burden.

The Impact of Disease Burden

The burden of disease is growing disproportionately in the world and is largely affected by climate, public policy, aging of the population, socioeconomic conditions, and risk factors (Fig. 4.3). Most of the countries burdened by disease have the least amount of human and economic capacity to effect change (Farmer, Furin, & Katz, 2004). Sub-Saharan Africa is unique in having an overwhelming share of the disease burden related to poverty and people living with HIV/AIDS (United Nations, 2012).

Women are disproportionately affected by the disease burden related to reproductive health and HIV infection (Hawkes & Buse, 2013). Globally, an estimated 830 women die daily from complications of childbirth (WHO, 2016a). Many of the complications resulting from childbirth can be prevented with the use of skilled midwives and nurses at birth. When a

1990 **2016**

Disease or injury	Rank	Rank	Disease or injury
Diarrhea/LRI/other	1	1	Cardiovascular diseases
Cardiovascular diseases	2	2	Diarrhea/LRI/other
Neonatal disorders	3	3	Neoplasms
Other noncommunicable	4	4	Other noncommunicable
Neoplasms	5	5	Neonatal disorders
Unintentional injuries	6	6	Mental and substance use
Mental and substance use	7	7	Musculoskeletal disorders
NTDs and malaria	8	8	Diabetes/urog/blood/endo
Chronic respiratory	9	9	Unintentional injuries
Musculoskeletal disorders	10	10	Neurologic disorders
HIV/AIDS and tuberculosis	11	11	HIV/AIDS and tuberculosis
Diabetes/urog/blood/endo	12	12	Chronic respiratory
Transport injuries	13	13	Transport injuries
Nutritional deficiencies	14	14	NTDs and malaria
Neurologic disorders	15	15	Nutritional deficiencies
Self-harm and violence	16	16	Self-harm and violence
Other group I	17	17	Cirrhosis
Digestive diseases	18	18	Digestive diseases
Cirrhosis	19	19	Other group I
Maternal disorders	20	20	Maternal disorders
War and disaster	21	21	War and disaster

DALYs = Disability Adjusted Life Years
The sum of years of potential life lost due to premature mortality and the years of productive life lost due to disability.
This category also includes other noninfectious causes arising in the perinatal period apart from prematurity, low birth weight, birth trauma, and asphyxia. These noninfectious causes are responsible for about 20% of DALYs shown in this category.

Communicable, maternal, neonatal, and nutritional diseases

Noncommunicable diseases

Injuries

FIGURE 4.2 The leading causes of death worldwide. (Institute for Health Metrics and Evaluation. [2017]. University of Washington. Retrieved from https://vizhub.healthdata.org/gbd-compare.)

4.1 Top 10 Facts According to the Global Burden of Disease

Fact 1: Global average life expectancy increased by 5 years between 2000 and 2015, the fastest increase since the 1960s.

Fact 2: Globally, healthy life expectancy (HLE) at birth in 2015 was estimated at 63.1 years.

Fact 3: In 2015, more than 16 000 children under age 5 died every day.

Fact 4: 45% of deaths among children under age 5 occur during the first 4 weeks of life.

Fact 5: In 2015, an estimated 2.6 million babies were stillborn.

Fact 6: 1.3 million deaths in 2015 were attributable to hepatitis.

Fact 7: Noncommunicable diseases (NCDs) caused 37% of deaths in low-income.

Fact 8: Ischemic heart disease and stroke killed 15 million people in 2015.

Fact 9: Diabetes is among the 10 leading causes of deaths and disability worldwide.

Fact 10: Injuries claimed nearly 5 million lives in 2015.

Source: World Health Organization. (2017c). *10 Facts on the State of Global Disease*. Retrieved from http://www.who.int/features/factfiles/global_burden/en.

4.2 Key Factors in the Rise of Noncommunicable Diseases

- Noncommunicable diseases (NCDs) kill 40 million people each year, equivalent to 70% of all deaths globally.
- Each year, 15 million people die from a NCD between the ages of 30 and 69 years; over 80% of these "premature" deaths occur in low- and middle-income countries.
- Cardiovascular diseases account for most NCD deaths, or 17.7 million people annually, followed by cancers (8.8 million), respiratory diseases (3.9 million), and diabetes (1.6 million).
- These four groups of diseases account for over 80% of all premature NCD deaths.
- Tobacco use, physical inactivity, the harmful use of alcohol, and unhealthy diets all increase the risk of dying from a NCD.
- Detection, screening, and treatment of NCDs, as well as palliative care, are key components of the response to NCDs.

Source: World Health Organization. (2017b). Global status report on noncommunicable diseases. Retrieved from http://www.who.int/mediacentre/factsheets/fs355/en.

mother dies or is disabled, her children may be forced to live in poverty. Addressing the causes of these health discrepancies with education, specifically education for girls, and creating integrated health programs, such as HIV treatment and prenatal care, will improve the quality of care and thus decrease the disease burden (Potter et al., 2008; UNAIDs, 2017). Girls and young women aged 15 to 24 years are twice as likely to become infected with HIV and account for 22% of new HIV infections (United Nations AIDS, 2013). Women now comprise 51% of individuals infected with HIV worldwide (amfAR, 2016). Of adults living with HIV in sub-Saharan Africa, 58% are women, compared with 26% in North America. HIV/AIDS is the leading cause of death among women of reproductive age (aged 15 to 44) (amfAR, 2016).

Children younger than 5 years who may be malnourished shoulder a significant portion of the disease burden. Nutrition is related to access to a food source and the quality of the food. In many countries, staple food such as rice, nshima, or millet, and other grain-based substances is abundant but lacks basic nutrients. Undernutrition and a diet of foods with poor nutritional content contribute to 45% of deaths in children younger than 5 years in developing countries (WHO, 2014c). Optimal breast-feeding could save more than 800,000 lives of children younger than 5 years each year. This primarily results from the lack of national infrastructure to adequately measure the effects of ill health on the entire country. Women are often essentially "invisible" to the healthcare system after childbirth. Compound this with poverty and lack of access, and women and children will remain in a state of poor health.

 The community response to outcast Haweeyo and her family because of her pregnancy and unmarried status represents discrimination. As a woman, she suffers the triple

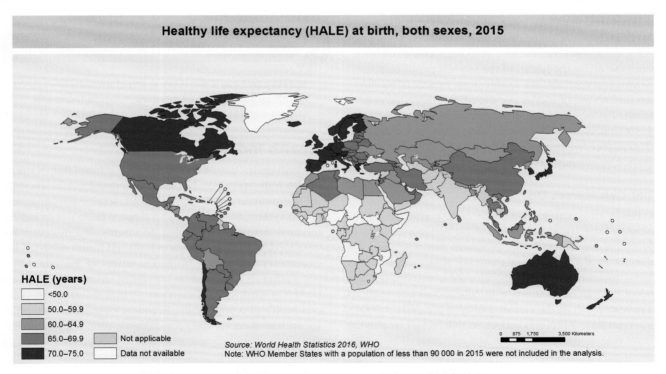

Healthy life expectancy (HALE) at birth, both sexes, 2015

HALE (years)
- <50.0
- 50.0–59.9
- 60.0–64.9
- 65.0–69.9
- 70.0–75.0
- Not applicable
- Data not available

Source: *World Health Statistics 2016, WHO*
Note: WHO Member States with a population of less than 90 000 in 2015 were not included in the analysis.

The boundaries and names shown and the designations used on this map do not imply the expression of any opinion whatsoever on the part of the World Health Organization concerning the legal status of any country, territory, city or area or of its authorities, or concerning the delimitation of its frontiers or boundaries. Dotted and dashed lines on maps represent approximate border lines for which there may not yet be full agreement.

Data Source: World Health Organization
Map Production: Information Evidence and Research (IER)
World Health Organization

FIGURE 4.3 Global healthy life expectancy at birth. (World Health Organization [2016e]).

stigma of being "immoral," pregnant, and poor because the cultural norm in her country is to marry before conceiving a child. Why do you think stigma, shame, and social outcasting continue to be a challenge for women and their families in this region of the world? How might you explain the relationship between culture and perceived women's role and behavior? As a nurse working in this community, what might be the best practice for intervening and preventing violence and death toward young girls and women who find themselves in a situation such as Haweeyo's?

What Risk Factors Affect the Disease Burden?

In a health context, **risk factors** are defined as personal habits and behaviors, environmental conditions, or inborn or inherited characteristics that are known to affect a health-related condition. Many of these can be reduced or prevented. Addressing risk factors and how they relate to the population can improve the health status of a nation. Risk factors occur in combination and change with age, creating different risks over a lifetime. Risk factor categories found to be associated with overall health include the following:

- *Childhood and maternal undernutrition:* Underweight children and conditions related to iron, vitamin A, and zinc deficiencies contribute to poor health outcomes.
- *Other nutrition-related risk factors and inactivity:* Obesity and physical inactivity, coupled with hypertension and hyperlipidemia, affect adults as well as children worldwide.
- *Addictive substances:* Tobacco smoking, alcohol and illicit drug use affect the health of the world's population.
- *Sexual and reproductive health:* Risk factors of unsafe sex and no use or ineffective use of contraception contribute to decreased health of women and children.
- *Environmental risks:* Unsafe drinking water, unsanitary conditions, poor hygiene, urban air pollution, and indoor smoke created by burning solid fuels, contribute to poor health.

What Can Nurses Do?

The health of a nation is overwhelmingly affected by the presence of specific risk factors and the nation's capacity to support and implement health programs that will affect the major causes of morbidity and mortality. Risk factors such as tobacco use, nutritional status, alcohol consumption, and condom use can be modified with educational interventions and have an effect on the overall quality of life (WHO, 2004). Nurses can have a profound effect on risk factors by playing a major role in health promotion and education. The quality of health service coverage, even in settings with few resources or ones where an extreme nursing shortage exists, can be improved by nurses who target health promotion issues within their community. One example is educating families on the daily use of insecticide-treated bed nets (ITNs) in

regions where malaria is highly endemic, and use of artemisinin-based combination therapies (ACTs) in high-prevalence regions (WHO, 2013b). Artemisinin is a drug known for its ability to swiftly reduce the number of *Plasmodium* parasites in the blood of patients with malaria. The 2016 WHO Malaria Report (2016b) states that between 2010 and 2015, malaria incidence rates fell by 21% globally and in the WHO African Region. During this same period, malaria mortality rates fell by an estimated 29% globally and by 31% in the Region. During this same period, malaria mortality rates fell by an estimated 29% globally and by 31% in the African region. However, as cases of malaria have diminished, the use of ITNs has decreased. The public health sector needs to advocate that the ITNs are essential for all areas, and that they be retreated annually for efficacy. The Roll Back Malaria project of the WHO focuses on the community commitment to fight malaria (WHO, 2013b), and ITNs are one method of prevention. Promoting the proper use of ITNs would be an example of a program based on a specific demographic risk factor that nurses, as trustees of health, could promote.

Risk factors can be addressed both at the individual and the societal level. Often, the way in which various risk factors interact with one another, and the best approach to addressing each one, is not well understood or defined. If demographics and geographic patterns are applied to each of the risk categories, different patterns of need emerge. Using risk factors as a guide to which interventions will work (i.e., the package of interventions) greatly improves outcomes in specific communities. Removal of major risk factors, could improve healthy life expectancy worldwide.

Practice Point

Nurses can have a substantial effect on people's health by focusing their teaching on modifiable risk factors such as changing lifestyle behaviors.

Health Indicators

According to the WHO statistical information system, **health indicators** may be placed in four categories: morbidity and mortality, risk factors, health service coverage, and health system resources. Each category has a list of indicators and universal definitions. Morbidity and mortality are measured by life expectancy at birth and health-adjusted life expectancy (HALE) at birth. The effect of mortality on a population is reported as disability-adjusted life years (DALYs) (Box 4.3). These three indicators reflect the general health of a population. Secondary measures of mortality, such as maternal and neonatal rates, reflect at-risk groups that affect overall mortality. Risk factor reduction focuses on healthy nutrition, improving health behaviors, and ameliorating environmental factors such as clean water and burning solid fuels. Health service coverage data identify uptake of specific services known to improve or promote health and well-being, such as reproductive health services, infant and

4.3 Health Indicator Descriptions

Life expectancy at birth (years): average number of years a newborn is expected to live if the current mortality rates continue to apply

HALE (health-adjusted life expectancy at birth [years]): average number of years that a person can expect to live in "full health" by taking into account years lived in less than full health due to disease and/or injury

DALYs (disability-adjusted life years): quantifying the burden of disease to a healthy life. The loss of years related to burden of disease. The gap in years reflects the current state of health versus an optimum state of health of a nation.

Source: World Health Organization. (2014). *Health statistics and health information systems.* Retrieved from http://www.who.int/healthinfo/en.

child health and immunization, HIV, and tuberculosis (TB) care. Health system resources focus on the capacity and supply of healthcare providers. These indicators in the aggregate provide valuable data that are used by health ministries and nongovernmental organizations (NGOs) as benchmarks for measuring target interventions.

Box 4.4 reflects the 10 highlights of the WHO Health Statistics Report for 2016 (WHO, 2016d). These highlights indicate that health discrepancies continue, and that interventions and benchmarks targeted at health indicators need to be based on the community-specific risk factors. In addition, these highlights suggest that global health continues to have an immense disease burden that is filled with opportunities for nurses to make a difference. Programs should focus on areas that have high impact on the overall health

4.4 Ten Highlights of the 2016 WHO World Health Statistics Report

Every year:
- 303,000 women die due to complications of pregnancy and childbirth
- 5.9 million children die before their fifth birthday
- 2 million people are newly infected with HIV, and there are 9.6 million new TB cases and 214 million malaria cases
- 1.7 billion people need treatment for neglected tropical diseases
- more than 10 million people die before the age of 70 due to cardiovascular diseases and cancer
- 800,000 people commit suicide
- 1.25 million people die from road traffic injuries
- 4.3 million people die due to air pollution caused by cooking fuels
- 3 million people die due to outdoor pollution
- 475,000 people are murdered, 80% of them men

Source: World Health Organization (2016d). *World Health Statistics 2016.* Retrieved from http://www.who.int/mediacentre/news/releases/2016/health-inequalities-persist/en.

4.5 Six Lines of Action to Promote Health in the 2030 Agenda for Sustainable Development

1. Monitoring the health-related Sustainable Development Goals (SDGs)
2. Health system strengthening for universal health coverage
3. Health equity—leave no one behind
4. Sustainable health financing
5. Innovation, research and development
6. Intersectoral action for health

Source: World Health Statistics Report. (2017c). *World Health Statistics Report 2017.* Retrieved from http://apps.who.int/iris/bitstream/10665/255336/1/9789241565486-eng.pdf?ua=1.

and well-being of the population they are intended to serve. The six lines of action (Box 4.5) of the WHO Health Statistics Report for 2017 (WHO, 2017b) provide guidance in promoting health equity and sustainable development through 2030.

Practice Point

Culturally appropriate, community-driven, and community-based programs are critical for eliminating disparities; strategies directed at individuals are not sufficient.

From what you know about global risk factors that affect burden of disease, in reviewing the highlights of the WHO report (2017c) what nursing interventions should be implemented to address improved health outcomes? What risk factors could be targeted that would address some of the issues highlighted within the report? For example, we know that unsafe sex practices is a major risk factor affecting reproductive health—maternal mortality is declining too slowly and cases of HIV infection are still on the rise in young women. What other factors would we need to know within a global setting before we could conduct a community needs assessment about unsafe sex practices? For example, how should we address unsafe sex practices for both men and women?

Statistics on population health indicators are used by governments and donor agencies. Health statistics will become vital to cost–benefit analysis for program development, with the shift in the developing world toward implementing a sector-wide approach program for health planning (WHO, 2008).

A sector-wide approach promotes the collective agreement of the government entity (e.g., a ministry of health), donor countries, and other key stakeholders in the community such as physician and nurse organizations, NGOs, and researchers. The process ensures that the government assumes leadership in developing a common policy and program for health, including monitoring arrangements and instituting more coordinated procedures for funding and procurement (WHO, 2013c). The challenge for ministries of health will be to administer, implement, and evaluate their annual healthcare goals and to work to identify ways and means to address the shortcomings that most affect the communities.

Evidence for Practice

Deaths from injuries and car accidents are about as prevalent as HIV/AIDS in the world. Bus accidents also cause many injuries in countries where safety laws are not well enforced. More than 90% of injury deaths occur in low- and middle-income countries, where preventive efforts are often nonexistent and healthcare systems are least prepared to meet the challenge, according to the WHO (2009b). What interventions can nurses implement that can reduce this problem?

Addressing the burden of highly infectious diseases such as TB is an urgent global health priority. TB is one of the 10 leading causes of death worldwide. In 2015 alone, an estimated 1.8 million people died from the disease, including 0.4 million with a dual diagnosis of TB and HIV. Despite a decrease in the incidence of the disease, approximately 10.4 million new cases were diagnosed in 2015 alone with most infections occurring among people living in crowded conditions in low-income countries. Treatment of TB involves following a strict drug regimen for several months, and completing the full course of treatment is critical. Unfortunately, failure to complete the drug regimen is very common, often attributed to cost and availability of medications. One of the consequences when patients stop taking their medications is the emergence of multidrug-resistant disease (MDR-TB). An estimated 480,000 people who started treatment developed multidrug-resistant TB (MDR-TB) in 2015. Ending the TB epidemic by 2030 is a key health target among the Sustainable Development Goals (SDGs) (WHO, 2017c).

As you reflect upon Vikram, what are some of the important preventive measures Vikram could have taken to reduce the risk of TB for himself and his family? What may have put Vikram at risk for MDR-TB? As a nurse, what are some of the important teaching points you should emphasize about taking TB medications? Why do you think Vikram was tested for HIV when he presented to the clinic with symptoms of TB?

Poverty and Risk Factors

Only when (and if) the "haves" develop genuine empathy for the "have-nots," and come to acknowledge their own long-term interdependence with all other humans, will the global economy be improved to any significant advantage for the desperately poor. **SR Benatar in PLOS Medicine** (2005)

Low- and middle-income countries have an increased burden of the risk factor of poverty. Extreme poverty—the inability to meet the basic needs of adequate nutrition, safe drinking water, basic education, and primary health services, and a livelihood that can generate the means to secure these basic needs—is the driving force behind increased mortality. Unlike those who are moderately and relatively poor, those who are extremely poor cannot access healthcare and are chronically hungry (Sachs, 2010, 2015). With a substantial segment of the world population existing on less than a dollar a day, the choices within the environment for sustenance create health risks. Nearly half the world's population and about 81% of sub-Saharan African households rely on wood-based biomass energy (fuel wood and charcoal) for cooking (World Bank, 2011). Continuous smoke from burning air-polluting solid fuels affects the population's health, and negatively impacts the economy. Attention to achieving sustainable energy sources, particularly in Africa, will help to alleviate poverty, improve healthcare status, and address ever-expanding greenhouse gas emissions (Venro, 2009). This continued reliance on air-polluting fuels, such as in China, affects the population's health (which, in turn, affects their economic prospects).

Unclean water remains a major problem in reducing diarrheal illness and waterborne and water-related illnesses and their health consequences. Between 1990 and 2011, 1.9 million people gained access to improved sanitation facilities (United Nations, 2013a) and the proportion of people using an improved water source rose from 76% to 89%. Developing basic sanitation expectations for communities and decreasing reliance on traveling great distances to acquire water will improve health overall.

WOMEN, POVERTY, AND HEALTH

"There are two powers in the world; one is the sword and the other is the pen. There is a third power stronger than both, that of women." **Malala Yousafzai** author of *I Am Malala: The Girl Who Stood Up for Education and was Shot by the Taliban*

Gender impacts health, both biologically and socially. The health of women and girls is affected by many social issues, particularly education. A lack of basic education worsens a female's risk of poverty, which impacts childhood marriage, early childbirth, lack of birth control, and increased vulnerability to HIV/AIDS (Jackson, 2009; WHO, 2017b).

Some of the sociocultural factors that prevent women and girls from benefiting from quality health services and attaining the best possible level of health include:

- unequal power relationships between men and women;
- social norms that decrease education and paid employment opportunities;
- an exclusive focus on women's reproductive roles; and
- potential or actual experience of physical, sexual and emotional violence (WHO, 2017b).

Poverty is a barrier to health for both men and women, but it yields a higher burden on women and girls' health.

The burden of disease associated with reproductive health affects the health indicators of a nation. Thompson (2007) described the deadly combination of poverty, the right to economic development, and the poor health of women as barriers to improving the health of the world's families. If maternal and child healthcare is left unattended, the rates of maternal and neonatal mortality will rise and national development in those nations with the fewest resources will be limited. The continued low status of women, despite years of policy development, increases the risk of disease and disability. The power imbalances within households around the world affect the health of women and young girls.

Maternal, newborn, and child health affect population mortality and health in profound ways. An estimated 3 million unsafe abortions occur annually among girls and young women age 15 to 19 years (WHO, 2014d). Despite evidence of low-cost interventions that would improve reproductive health outcomes, scale-up for these interventions is lacking (Bhutta et al., 2008). The known interventions are focused on recognizing maternal and neonatal complications; procedures to prevent postpartum hemorrhage (PPH), such as active management of the third stage of labor; neonatal care at birth, such as drying the infant off and wrapping the infant immediately; and having a skilled provider examine the infant within 2 days of birth. Each of these interventions relies heavily on education of the mother and community and should be a primary focus of community-based programs to improve maternal and child health. As education increases in the community, evaluating the use of such interventions still remains low. Such low-cost, low-tech interventions can address the imbalances in maternal and child health, if used for every pregnancy and birth, and evaluated for quality of delivery and effectiveness. Refocusing efforts on the full cycle of quality improvement will greatly affect overall global health (Houweling et al., 2014).

In Case 1, Haweeyo benefited from the presence of an experienced CHW birth attendant and her ability to recognize the necessity for moving her to the hospital for advanced level of care for both mother and baby.

As the nurse, you recognize gender differences and acceptable roles and behaviors for women are evident in this community. How might you intervene to reduce gender discrimination and violence based on culturally specific restrictive beliefs and taboo regarding women, moral behaviors, and role of women in a community? How might you help women like Haweeyo allay their fear of stigma and shame and become more aware of available services, transportation, and sensitive, caring providers who will care for her emotional and physical well-being?

SUSTAINABLE DEVELOPMENT GOALS

"Two years ago, world leaders adopted the ambitious 2030 Agenda for Sustainable Development, with 17 Sustainable Development Goals at its heart. The Agenda is our shared plan to transform the world in 15 years and, crucially, to build lives of dignity for all." **UN Secretary-General António Guterres**

The Sustainable Development Goals (SDGs) were adopted by the United Nations in 2015 to replace the Millennium Development Goals (MDGs) (Fig. 4.4). The SDGs are a universal set of goals, targets, and indicators that the United Nations 191 member states are using to frame their agendas and political policies through 2030 (United Nations, 2017). The SDGs aim to address inequalities between nations, but also within nations. The SDGs contain 17 goals covering a broad range of sustainable development issues for the world. In addition to the overarching goals, there are targets within each goal for a total of 161 targets. Goal number 3: Good health and well-being for all, specifically addresses health.

The 17 SDGs:

1. End poverty in all its forms everywhere
2. End hunger, achieve food security and improved nutrition, and promote sustainable agriculture
3. Ensure healthy lives and promote well-being for all at all ages
4. Ensure inclusive and equitable quality education and promote lifelong learning opportunities for all
5. Achieve gender equality and empower all women and girls
6. Ensure availability and sustainable management of water and sanitation for all
7. Ensure access to affordable, reliable, sustainable, and modern energy for all
8. Promote sustained, inclusive, and sustainable economic growth, full and productive employment, and decent work for all
9. Build resilient infrastructure, promote inclusive and sustainable industrialization, and foster innovation

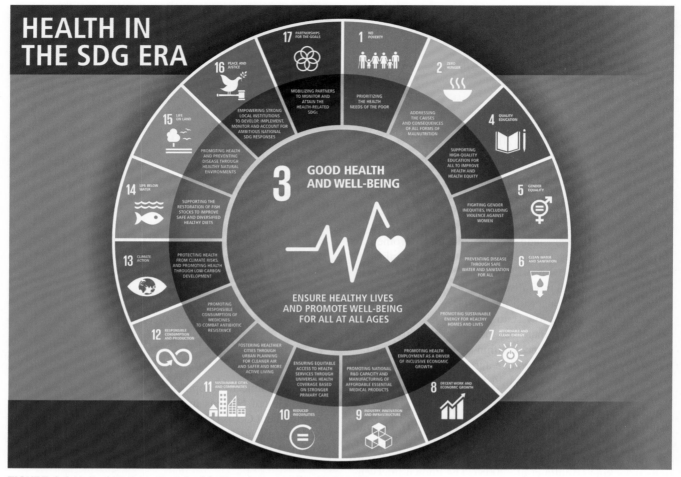

FIGURE 4.4 United Nations Sustainable Development Goals. (WHO).

10. Reduce inequality within and among countries
11. Make cities and human settlements inclusive, safe, resilient, and sustainable
12. Ensure sustainable consumption and production patterns
13. Take urgent action to combat climate change and its impacts
14. Conserve and sustainably use the oceans, seas, and marine resources for sustainable development
15. Protect, restore, and promote sustainable use of terrestrial ecosystems, sustainably manage forests, combat desertification and halt and reverse land degradation, and halt biodiversity loss
16. Promote peaceful and inclusive societies for sustainable development, provide access to justice for all and build effective, accountable, and inclusive institutions at all levels
17. Strengthen the means of implementation and revitalize the global partnership for sustainable development

Over the past decade, significant improvements have occurred in global health outcomes, but it is important to note that health inequalities are prevalent throughout the globe. According to the International Counsel of Nurses

(2017), the social determinants of health (SDH) are the conditions and systems that shape health throughout the life cycle. The SDH are the conditions in which people are born, grow, live, work, and age (Marmot, 2016). These circumstances are shaped by the distribution of money, power, and resources at the local, national, and global levels. Social factors, including education, employment status, income level, gender, and ethnicity have a direct influence on a person's health. The SDH are mostly responsible for health inequities—the unfair and avoidable differences in health status seen within and between countries. Health equity and social determinants are acknowledged as an important component of the SDGs agenda and of the achievement of universal health coverage (UHC). To reduce health inequities, both SDH and UHC need to be addressed in an integrated and systematic manner (WHO, 2016c).

Evaluating the SDGs

The United Nations has extensive and continuous targets for evaluating all 17 goals. The High-Level Political Forum (HLPF) has a central role in the follow-up and review of the 2030 Agenda and the 17 SDGs at the global level. The HLPF facilitates sharing successes, challenges, and lessons learned, and provides political leadership, guidance, and recommendations for follow-up. The HLPF also coordinates sustainable development policies, ensures that the 2030 Agenda remains relevant and ambitious, assesses progress, achievements, and challenges faced by developed and developing countries, and addresses emerging issues. A central feature of the HLPF is the voluntary national reviews (VNRs) that it receives from member states on their implementation of the 2030 Agenda and the SDGs. Regularly undertaken by both developed and developing countries, the VNRs provide a platform for partnerships between groups and stakeholders (United Nations, 2017). Global progress on meeting each SDG is summarized in Table 4.1. Progress on SDG #3 (health), is summarized in Box 4.6.

How Can Nurses Help Implement the STGs?

Global health is encompassed in all the SDGs, and most prominently in SDG #3: Ensure healthy lives and promote well-being for all and all ages. Our nursing role directly impacts this SDG. While nurses seek to help people achieve their optimal health, our work frequently includes addressing the SDH and nurses understand the links between wider conditions on individual and population health. As nurses, we have a responsibility to care for our patients, communities, country, and the globe, by staying informed and continually educating ourselves on how to improve health for all. Suggestions on how to implement the SDGs from the International Council of Nursing (2017) include (1) becoming a leader and (2) raising your voice at the policy table. Becoming a leader involves working with groups within the healthcare system and larger community. Leadership includes both social responsibility and good citizenship, which connects to nurses' professional and ethical responsibilities to improve health for all. According to the Institute of Medicine (2011), "a shift must take place in how nurses view their responsibility to those they care for; they must see themselves as full partners with other health professionals" to be effectively involved in improving overall health.

Evidence for Practice

The 2015 countdown report for maternal, newborn, and child survival outlines the progress that has been made in improving the lives of families. Yet more can be done with basic, low-cost interventions (United Nations, 2013b; WHO, 2012b). Sustaining focused interventions on early detection and treatment of diarrhea and pneumonia will decrease mortality (Walker et al., 2013). Four interventions known to affect both diarrhea and pneumonia include the following (Bhutta et al., 2013):

- Breast-feeding. Not breast-feeding resulted in a 165% increased risk of acquiring diarrhea from 0 to 5 months of age (Lamberti, Walker, Noiman, Victora, & Black, 2011). Education on exclusive breast-feeding. Significant results, as high as 90%, were attributed to promotional interventions for children from 0 to 6 months of age (Bhutta et al., 2013).
- WASH interventions. Water, sanitation, and hygiene (WASH) interventions demonstrated a risk reduction of 17% with proper excreta disposal, and risk reductions of up to 48% with water and soap handwashing (Cairncross et al., 2010).
- Zinc supplementation. Supplementation resulted in a reduction in diarrhea and acute lower respiratory tract infection mortality (Yakoob et al., 2011).
- Postpartum hemorrhage. PPH is the leading cause of maternal death, claiming an estimated 140,000 lives in low-resource settings, with an additional 2 million women left to recover from anemia (Prata, Passano, Sreenivas, & Gerdts, 2010; Smith, Gubin, Holston, Fullerton, & Prata, 2013). The use of uterotonics such as oxytocin or misoprostol can have a profound effect on preventing and treating PPH. Several large randomized controlled trials (RCTs) have shown that the use of such medications will improve delivery of the placenta, decrease blood loss, and avert death and disability. Implementation of such treatments as a standard of care requires a reliable supply chain for medications and the support of nurse leaders to implement the procedures for every delivery, since we know that long labors and multiple gestations increase the risk for PPH, but many women with no risk factors suffer hemorrhage.
- Creating political will is important to improving health. Countries that improved care by strengthening their health system with education and deployment of midwives reduced their maternal mortality rate by 2% to 5% and will have a median drop of maternal mortality ratio by 63% over 20 years (Van Lerberghe et al., 2014). Countries with sustainable changes focused on improving access as close to the family as possible, scaling up birth care in line with the population, decreasing fees and financial barriers to care, and making quality care a priority. In countries where these four elements have been most successful, nurse midwifery has become more visible and accepted.
- Preterm birth and stillbirth have been neglected in improving child mortality (WHO, 2012a). Investing in low-cost interventions, such as universal kangaroo care, and high-cost interventions, such as corticosteroid injections, could save up to 950,000 infants per year. Education of skilled health personnel, specifically nurses and midwives, on tools to support preterm care and access to essential equipment and education can have a profound effect on neonatal survival. The global action report by WHO *Born Too Soon* (WHO, 2012a) outlines steps that can improve preterm birth and prevent causes of stillbirth, such as maternal malnutrition.

TABLE 4.1 Progress to Date: Sustainable Development Goals, 2017

Sustainable Development Goals	Progress at Meeting Goal
1. End poverty in all its forms everywhere	An estimated 767 million people lived below the extreme poverty line in 2013, down from 1.7 billion people in 1999. This represents a reduction in the global rate of extreme poverty from 28% in 1999 to 11% in 2013.
2. End hunger, achieve food security and improved nutrition, and promote sustainable agriculture	The proportion of undernourished people worldwide declined from 15% in 2000–2002 to 11% in 2014–2016. Globally, approximately 793 million people were undernourished in 2014–2016, down from 930 million in 2000–2002.
3. Ensure healthy lives and promote well-being for all at all ages	See Box 4.6 for extensive progress at meeting this health goal.
4. Ensure inclusive and equitable quality education and promote lifelong learning opportunities for all	Despite gains in primary school enrollment between 2000 and 2014, 9% of primary school–aged children worldwide were out of school in 2014, with little progress since 2008.
5. Achieve gender equality and empower all women and girls	Women's participation in national parliaments worldwide were 23% in 2017. In the majority of the 67 countries with data from 2009 to 2015, fewer than a third of senior- and middle-management positions were held by women.
6. Ensure availability and sustainable management of water and sanitation for all	In 2015, 5.2 billion people (71% of the global population) used a safely managed drinking water source located on premises, available when needed and free from contamination.
7. Ensure access to affordable, reliable, sustainable and modern energy for all	In 2014, 85% of the global population had access to electricity, up from 78% in 2000. However, 1.06 billion people still lived without this basic service
8. Promote sustained, inclusive and sustainable economic growth, full and productive employment, and decent work for all	The average annual growth rate of real gross domestic product (GDP) per capita expanded from 0.9% in 2005–2009 to 1.6% in 2010–2015. Real GDP growth in the least developed countries (LDCs) averaged 4.9% in 2010–2015, short of the target of at least 7% annually.
9. Build resilient infrastructure, promote inclusive and sustainable industrialization, and foster innovation	Global investment in research and development increased at an average annual rate of 4.5% between 2000 and 2014.
10. Reduce inequality within and among countries	In 49 of 83 countries with data from 2011–2015, the per capita incomes of the poorest 40% of the population grew more rapidly than the national average, leading to a reduction in income inequality.
11. Make cities and human settlements inclusive, safe, resilient, and sustainable	In 2014, nine in 10 people living in urban areas breathed air that did not meet the World Health Organization's air quality guidelines value for particulate matter.
12. Ensure sustainable consumption and production patterns	Globally, the material footprint of human beings increased from 48.5 billion metric tons in 2000 to 69.3 billion metric tons in 2010. The material footprint per capita increased from 8 metric tons per person in 2000 to 10 metric tons per person in 2010.
13. Take urgent action to combat climate change and its impacts	As of 2017, 148 parties ratified the Paris Agreement.
14. Conserve and sustainably use the oceans, seas, and marine resources for sustainable development	Of the 63 large marine ecosystems, 16% are in the "high" or "highest" risk categories for coastal eutrophication (oxygen depletion leading to animal death). By 2050, it is estimated that coastal eutrophication will increase in 21% of large ecosystems.
15. Protect, restore and promote sustainable use of terrestrial ecosystems, sustainably manage forests, combat desertification and halt and reverse land degradation, and halt biodiversity loss	From 2010 to 2015, the annual net loss of forest area globally was less than half that of the 1990s. The proportion of land area covered by forest decreased from 32% in 1990 to 32% in 2010 and 31% in 2015.

Sustainable Development Goals	Progress at Meeting Goal
16. Promote peaceful and inclusive societies for sustainable development, provide access to justice for all, and build effective, accountable, and inclusive institutions at all levels	Globally, the proportion of people held in detention without being tried or sentenced for a crime was 31% in 2013–2015.
17. Strengthen the means of implementation and revitalize the global partnership for sustainable development	In 2016, approximately 80% of the population in developed regions had internet access, compared to 40% in developing regions and 15% in LDCs.

Source: United Nations. (2017). *Sustainable Development Goals Report 2017*. Retrieved from https://unstats.un.org/sdgs/files/report/2017/TheSustainableDevelopmentGoalsReport2017.pdf.

4.6 Progress on SDG 3—Health

Goal 3 addresses all major health priorities and calls for improving reproductive, maternal and child health; ending communicable diseases; reducing noncommunicable diseases and other health hazards; and ensuring universal access to safe, effective, quality, and affordable medicines and vaccines as well as health coverage. Between 2000 and 2015, global health indicator changes included:

- Maternal mortality ratio declined by 37%, and the under 5 mortality rate fell by 44%. However, 303,000 women died during pregnancy or childbirth and 5.9 million children under age 5 died worldwide in 2015; most from preventable causes.
- 46% reduction in HIV incidence
- 17% decline in the incidence of tuberculosis
- 41% decrease in the incidence of malaria
- 21% drop in people requiring mass or individual treatment and care for neglected tropical diseases.
- The risk of dying between the ages of 30 and 70 from one of four main NCDs—cardiovascular disease, cancer, diabetes, or chronic respiratory disease—fell from 23% to 19% between 2000 and 2015, but not rapidly enough to meet the 2030 target.
- Nearly 800,000 suicides occurred worldwide in 2015, with men twice as likely to die by suicide as women.
- In 2013, approximately 1.25 million people died from road traffic injuries, an increase of 13% since 2000.
- Globally in 2012, household air pollution from cooking with unclean fuels and inefficient technologies led to an estimated 4.3 million deaths; another 3 million deaths were attributed to ambient air pollution from traffic, industrial sources, waste burning, and residential fuel combustion.

OTHER FACTORS THAT AFFECT GLOBAL HEALTH

Economics and Politics

The global environment is intricately intertwined with the economic and political status of a nation. As one area improves, so do others, and vice versa. It is known that health and education are clearly linked, in that the better educated the population is, the better the health of the population (Ross & Wu, 1995). Political and economic instability, which leads to poverty, is a major barrier to achieving health for a population. When economies and political systems are stable, the health of a population generally improves.

Over the past 60 years, the world economy has increased, and yet has spawned greater disparities. For example, the global economy increased sevenfold since 1950, whereas the disparity in gross domestic product between the 20 richest and 20 poorest nations more than doubled between 1960 and 1997 (British Medical Journal, 1999). Extreme poverty is decreasing in every region of the world, according to the 2017 Sustainable Development Goals Report of the United Nations. The proportion of people living on less than $1.25 a day fell from 43% in 1990 to 21% in 2010 (World Bank, 2014). An estimated 767 million people, or 10.7% of the population lived on less than $1.90 a day in 2013, with decreasing numbers of people living in conditions of extreme poverty. Yet living in poverty remains the driving economic condition that significantly affects health and well-being in sub-Saharan Africa and in southern Asia (United Nations, 2013a; World Bank, 2016).

The current economic and political instability of many parts of the world only exacerbates the difficulties for the world's poor. The effects of a slowdown of the world economy on the incomes of other less wealthy nations have become evident. This ripple effect is felt by the poorest people of the world.

The first wealth is health. **Ralph Waldo Emerson**

Even with these enormous disparities in health, poor countries can learn to become more economically self-sufficient by producing enough basic commodities and foods for their population to survive, and also by producing specific goods for export that are not readily available in wealthier countries. Poor countries must grow staple foods that lead to nutritionally balanced diets for the local people. It is possible to achieve high levels of health even without high levels of income. Disparities between the wealthiest and poorest nations must be reduced; in the end, each individual is inextricably linked as the world quickly becomes a global community. Maintaining communities and honoring cultural norms and traditions can only help populations become more self-sufficient. It is inherently necessary for health planners to understand this basic fact.

In Case 2, consider some of the social and economic factors that may influence the health of Vikram and his family. How might access to healthcare services, education about prevention, and treatment of communicable diseases prevent transmission of TB from occurring in Vikram's community and other rural, poorly resourced areas? How do diagnoses and treatments of communicable and infectious diseases differ both globally and culturally within different regions of the world?

Factors Associated With Healthcare Systems

Healthcare systems differ in terms of the degree to which they can adequately serve the population and the degree to which they are centralized in the government. They range from national healthcare systems, such as those in the United Kingdom or Spain, to pluralistic free-market systems, such as those in the United States. National healthcare systems are highly regulated, tend to have salaried physicians and other providers, are funded by governments, and involve relatively high taxes. Free-market healthcare systems depend more on individual or employer and employee contributions than on taxes. In between these two extremes are the systems of various countries whose citizens have access to universal health insurance and pay higher taxes for these services, such as the Scandinavian countries of Denmark, Norway, and Sweden. Other health insurance funding methods include national health insurance programs with single-payer systems, such as those in Canada, and programs with multipayer health insurance systems that offer universal health insurance via sickness funds, such as those in Germany and France.

The U.S. system, which is often characterized as highly fragmented and segmented, depending on the individual's insurance status or level of wealth, spends far more per capita on health than any other country in the world. Although the United States spends the most on healthcare per capita, it has the worst rating in preventable deaths (treatable cancer, diabetes, childhood infections/disease, and complications from surgery); it ranked last among 16 industrialized nations. From 1997–1998 to 2006–2007, the United States lowered its preventable mortality rate by only 20% compared to an average decrease of 31% in other nations (Nolte & McKee, 2011). The United States ranked last among 11 industrialized countries in access, administrative efficiency, equity, and healthcare outcomes in 2017 (Schneider et al., 2017). Figure 4.5 compares countries of the world on these measures (Schneider et al., 2017)

The United States passed the Patient Protection and Affordable Care Act in March 2010, a landmark national healthcare reform law that was expected to allow 94% of all Americans to obtain health insurance, reduce the growth in healthcare costs, and decrease the federal budget deficit by $143 billion over the next 10 years (Congressional Budget Office, 2010). This legislation has had many hurdles and had gradually increased the number of insured individuals in spite of opposition by many Americans and various states until 2017 when significant challenges occurred. So how does this translate to poorer countries with less wealth than the United States or Europe? Lessons learned from decades of work focusing on a specific disease of a population have provided data to suggest that focusing on the system may garner better health indexes for global health delivery (Kim, Farmer, & Porter, 2013). Care delivery value chains (CDVCs) targeted at a specific problem can create a system that engages all aspects of care toward one outcome. Creating a value-based delivery system which is focused on the value it achieves for the patient and society, and which emphasizes best practice and includes the need to understand the combined effect of interventions over a cycle of care, is an important aspect of CDVCs (Kim et al., 2013). The elements of the value chain include the following:

- Monitoring and prevention
- Diagnosing
- Preparing
- Intervening
- Recovering and rehabilitation
- Monitoring and managing overall outcomes

Integrating this model into health systems may move health indexes to the next level.

Strong healthcare systems are vital, yet they also need sustainable financial support. Some countries are turning to insurance mechanisms. Smith and Sulzbach (2008) describe voluntary, nonprofit health insurance schemes, organized and managed at the community levels, that they call "community-based health insurance" (p. 2461). This concept is based on the principle of risk pooling and involves regular payments of a small premium in exchange for reducing direct payments at the point of service. These types of financing are also referred to as prepayment schemes, private prepaid programs, microinsurance, and mutual health organizations (Dror et al., 2016; Smith & Sulzbach, 2008). Although care in these poorer countries involves a completely different paradigm than in developed countries, lack of the greatest resource—healthcare providers—is one of the most compelling problems. Lack of financing either

Exhibit ES-1. Overall Ranking

COUNTRY RANKINGS

| | Top 2 |
| Middle |
| Bottom 2 |

	AUS	CAN	FRA	GER	NETH	NZ	NOR	SWE	SWIZ	U.K.	USA
OVERALL RANKING (2013)	4	10	9	5	5	7	7	3	2	1	11
Quality care	2	9	8	7	5	4	11	10	3	1	5
Effective care	4	7	9	6	5	2	11	10	8	1	3
Safe care	3	10	2	6	7	9	11	5	4	1	7
Coordinated care	4	8	9	10	5	2	7	11	3	1	6
Patient-centered care	5	8	10	7	3	6	11	9	2	1	4
Access	8	9	11	2	4	7	6	4	2	1	9
Cost-related problem	9	5	10	4	8	6	3	1	7	1	11
Timeliness of care	6	11	10	4	2	7	8	9	1	3	5
Efficiency	4	10	8	9	7	3	4	2	6	1	11
Equity	5	9	7	4	8	10	6	1	2	2	11
Healthy lives	4	8	1	7	5	9	6	2	3	10	11
Health expenditures/capita, 2011	$3,800	$4,522	$4,118	$4,495	$5,099	$3,182	$5,669	$3,925	$5,643	$3,405	$8,508

FIGURE 4.5 Healthcare System Performance Rankings. (Schneider, E., Sarnak, D., Squires, D., Shah, A., Doty, M. [2017]. *Mirror, Mirror 2017: International comparison reflects flaws and opportunities for better U.S. healthcare*. The Commonwealth Fund. Retrieved from http://www.commonwealthfund.org/~/media/files/publications/fund-report/2017/jul/schneider_mirror_mirror_2017.pdf.)

from the government or from the population further exacerbates this problem.

Extreme shortages of healthcare workers are an endemic problem in developing countries, and yet again, these countries share the greatest burden of disease, spend the least on healthcare expenditures, and have the lowest number of healthcare workers. Fifty-seven countries, most of them in Africa and Asia, face a severe health workforce crisis. With most recent data available, the WHO (2006) estimated that at least 2,360,000 health service providers and 1,890,000 management support workers, or a total of 4,250,000 health workers, are needed to fill the gap. Without prompt action, the shortage will worsen, especially in the poorest countries. Sub-Saharan Africa, for example, had 11% of the world's population and 24% of the GBD, and it manages with only 3% of the world's health workers (WHO, 2006). The number of health workers is directly related to the health of global populations. Further, country-specific data can be found at the website of Global Atlas of the Health Workforce, WHO, Geneva: http://www.who.int/hrh/statistics/hwfstats/.

To add to this problem, many factors that affect the health of global populations are often beyond the control of individual people. Wars, political instability, famine, ecologic factors such as climate change and subsequent environmental disasters, and economic trends may lead members of the local health workforce (such as nurses and physicians) to move to highly developed countries where they can work in more favorable conditions.

What has occurred is a global shortage of nurses and physicians in areas of need, and workforce migration leading to a "brain drain" of workers moving from lesser-developed countries to more developed countries. In 2010, the WHO introduced the *Global Code of Practice of the Recruitment of Health Personnel* (WHO, 2010). The code promotes the ethical recruitment of personnel and provides a focus on health work force development and health systems sustainability, and strengthening local health systems. Table 4.2 lists the key facts related to health worker migration. The WHO (2011) assembly on strengthening nursing and midwifery supported a continued focus on including nursing

TABLE 4.2 Background on Health Workforce Shortage

- Globally, health workforce shortages are highest in sub-Saharan Africa, which bears 24% of the world's disease burden but has only 3% of health workers and less than 1% of the world's financial resources to respond to this burden (WHO, 2006).

- Adding to the shortage and inequitable distribution of the health workforce, the past 20 years have seen an increase in international health worker migration, with patterns of migration becoming increasingly complex (Nair & Webster, 2013; Taylor & Dhillon, 2011). In this period, developed nations have become more and more reliant on international migrants to fill health workforce positions—including nursing assistants, nurses, physicians, and medical specialists.

- With rising life expectancy and expanding elderly populations, this reliance is expected to continue.

- Migration, undeveloped health systems, and poor wages and working conditions are some of the factors that impact limited health workers in countries with the poorest health indicators.

- WHO estimates that the basic healthcare system of 57 countries is affected by shortage of human resources and about 1/3 of these countries are the emerging market economies (Nair & Webster, 2013).

and midwifery in health system planning and employment, and transforming education systems to meet the needs of each country. Gostin (2008) states that the factors contributing to a shortage of healthcare workers are globalization, which has increased over the past 20 to 30 years, and a decreased supply of healthcare workers along with an increased demand for well-trained workers. He says that this leads to a "push–pull" situation, in which healthcare workers are "pushed" from developing countries and "pulled" to developed countries with the promise of a brighter future. Factors leading to this problem include low wages, unsafe environments, the need for better living conditions and facilities, lack of opportunity to be promoted, and unusually heavy workloads and long working hours (Gostin, 2008). The WHO (2010) suggests that in-source countries need to consider better health workforce retention by focusing on maldistribution of nurses and quality of life. Health systems need to provide protection and better treatment of workers in general, as often there are poor working conditions and poor pay. Finally, in accordance with the WHO goal of improving nursing education, countries need to invest in improving the initial education and training of midwives so that they are better prepared as professional healthcare workers (WHO, 2009a). Because migration is a human right, the WHO supports destination or receiving countries to act as responsible global citizens in recruiting migrant workers. This includes building capacity in their own countries as well as treating expatriate workers with the same dignity and respect as all healthcare workers.

Gostin (2008) does suggest an upside to migration for the worker and the community: workers who migrate also gain new skills in the receiving countries and can return to their native countries revitalized with education and new outlooks on solving the problems—in other words, "brain gain." Those who leave may also come back with the skills to educate other workers. For example, nurses may return with advanced practice nursing skills and become educators in their respective countries.

When a country invests in its healthcare workers through improved training, improved working conditions, career ladders, and allocation of financial resources toward improving salaries and systems, workers are more likely to remain in that country. HIV protection and treatment, as well as plans for emergency preparedness, are paramount if workers are to feel safe in their environments. The "pull" to other countries is great, and healthcare workers must feel that their contribution is valued and that their future will be improved if they resist the perceived benefits of moving to more developed countries to live out their lives and careers.

ROLE OF NURSES

The world is now a global village. Problems that affect people in other countries also affect people in their own countries. Nurses and community healthcare providers need to be knowledgeable about the needs of all people, as well as of their patients, in the global society. Knowledge of the goals for worldwide health can lead to new cooperative ventures and unique solutions using technology and knowledge transfer techniques. Do all citizens of the world deserve access to good health and a sense of well-being? It is expected that the answer to this question will be "yes," but such a goal can be accomplished only through international cooperation, regardless of national boundaries. Larger questions of inequalities in wealth and resources must be addressed, and as a new generation of providers emerge, they may have the answers that have eluded societies before them.

Nurses are a major part of the solution to world health problems. The ability of nurses to assess patients and communities, set realistic goals, develop interventions partnered with local community resources, and continually evaluate progress toward meeting goals will move the global environment on a path toward improved health. Nurses' enlightenment about global health issues will enable our valuable profession to be part of the solution toward a healthier global population.

KEY CONCEPTS

- Global health encompasses the behavioral and environmental risk factors of a community, which are influenced by politics, economics, and culture.
- Monitoring health indicators and ensuring the inclusion of vulnerable and invisible populations will improve packaged interventions to affect health outcomes.
- Global burden of disease is a term that reflects the health of a nation and the level of opportunity to improve health.
- The Sustainable Development Goals are a framework for achieving improved global health and outcomes. Nurses should participate in both policy and leadership working toward meeting the SDGs.
- The road map to achieving health relies on the participation of all individuals and nations to address the basic needs of clean drinking water, sanitation, and alleviating poverty.
- Education is the key to improving the community environment, which, in turn, will improve health.
- Health worker migration increases the burden of care for a society and results in the need to shift tasks primarily to nurses and community health workers.

CRITICAL THINKING QUESTIONS

1. Imagine the role that nurses can play in a more egalitarian world where all healthcare providers can contribute equally to the pressing global problems presented here. What are some of your proposed solutions?
2. How can nurses work within communities of interest to determine how the burden of disease is affected by poverty?
3. How can nurses influence the major risk factors related to maternal mortality and HIV?
4. What health factors can nurses address to work with young males of a community to improve overall health?

COMMUNITY RESOURCES

- World Health Organization
- International Council of Nurses
- United Nations

REFERENCES

Alleyne, G., Binagwaho, A., Haines, A., Jahan, S., Nugent, R., Rojhani, A., & Stuckler, D.; Lancet NCD Action Group. (2013). Embedding non-communicable diseases in the post-2015 development agenda. *The Lancet, 381*(9866), 566–574.

Foundation for AIDS Research (amfAR). (2016). Statistics: Women and HIV/AIDS. Retrieved from http://www.amfar.org/about-hiv-and-aids/facts-and-stats/statistics–women-and-hiv-aids/.

Benatar, S. (2005). Moral imagination: The missing component in global health. *PLoS Medicine, 2*(12), e400.

Bhutta, Z. A., Das, J. K., Walker, N., Rizvi, A., Campbell, H., Rudan, I., & Black, R. E.; Lancet Diarrhoea and Pneumonia Interventions Study Group. (2013). Interventions to address deaths from childhood pneumonia and diarrhoea equitably: What works and at what cost? *The Lancet, 381*(9875), 1417–1429.

Bhutta, Z., Ali, S., Cousens, S., Ali, T. M., Haider, B. A., Rizvi, A., ... Black, R. E. (2008). Alma-Ata: Rebirth and Revision 6 Interventions to address maternal, newborn, and child survival: What difference can integrated primary health care strategies make. *The Lancet, 372*(9642), 972–989.

British Medical Journal. (1999). The champagne glass of world poverty. *British Medical Journal, 318*, 7189.

Cairncross, S., Hunt, C., Boisson, S., Bostoen, K., Curtis, V., Fung, I. C., Schmidt, W. P. (2010). Water, sanitation and hygiene for the prevention of diarrhoea. *International Journal of Epidemiology, 39*(Suppl 1), i193–i205.

Cancer Research UK. (2014). Cancer stats: Cancer statistics for the UK. Retrieved from http://www.cruk.org/cancerstats.

Center for Disease Control and Prevention. (2010). Retrieved from https://www.cdc.gov/tb/programs/laws/menu/definitions.htm.

Congressional Budget Office. (2010). Retrieved from http://www.cbo.gov/ftpdocs/113xx/doc11379/Manager'sAmendmenttoReconciliationProposal.pdf

Disease Control Priorities Project. (2008). Retrieved from http://www.dcp2.org/main/Home.html.

Dror, D. M., Hossain, S. A. S., Majumdar, A., Pérez Koehlmoos, T. L., John, D., & Panda, P. K. (2016). What factors affect voluntary uptake of community-based health insurance schemes in low- and middle-income countries? A systematic review and meta-analysis. *PLoS ONE, 11*(8), e0160479. http://doi.org/10.1371/journal.pone.0160479.

Dunn, H. (1959). High-level wellness for man and society. *American Journal of Public Health, 49*(6), 786–792.

Farmer, P., Furin, J., & Katz, J. (2004). Global health equity. *The Lancet, 363*, 182.

Fisher, I. (1909). *Report on national vitality, its wastes and conservation. Prepared for the National Conservation Commission.* Washington, DC: Government Printing Office.

Gostin, L. (2008). The international migration and recruitment of nurses: Human rights and global justice. *JAMA, 299*(15), 1827–1829.

Hawkes, S., & Buse, K. (2013). Gender and global health: Evidence, policy, and inconvenient truths. *The Lancet, 381*(9879), 1783–1787.

REFERENCES *(Continued)*

Horton, R. (2013). Non-communicable diseases: 2015 to 2025. *The Lancet, 381*(9866), 509–510.

Houweling, T. A. J., Morrison, J., Azad, K., Manandhar, D. S., Alcock, G., Shende, S., … Costello, A. (2014). How to reach every newborn: Three key messages. *The Lancet Global Health, 2*(8), e436–e437.

Hunter, D. J., & Reddy, K. S. (2013). Noncommunicable diseases. *New England Journal of Medicine, 369*(14), 1336–1343.

Institute of Health Metrics and Evaluation. (2014). Global burden of disease. Retrieved from http://www.healthmetricsandevaluation.org/gbd.

Institute of Medicine. (1997). *America's vital interest in global health: Protecting our people, enhancing our economy, and advancing our international interests.* Washington, DC: National Academies Press. Retrieved from http://books.nap.edu/openbook.php?record_id=5717&page=11.

Institute of Medicine. (2011). *The future of nursing: Focus on scope of practice.* Retrieved from http://nationalacademies.org/hmd/reports/2010/the-future-of-nursing-leading-change-advancing-health/report-brief-scope-of-practice.aspx?_ga=2.178996644.1245131437.1508119332-661089218.1508119332.

International Council of Nursing. (2017). *Nurses a voice to lead: Achieving the SDGs.* Geneva, Switzerland. Retrieved from https://www.icnvoicetolead.com/wp-content/uploads/2017/04/ICN_AVoiceToLead_guidancePack-9.pdf.

Jackson, L. W. (2009). Educate the women and you change the world: Investing in the education of women is the best investment in a country's growth and development. *Forum on Public Policy Online.* Retrieved from http://forumonpublicpolicy.com/summer09/womenandleadership.html.

Jamison, D. T., & Jardel, J. P. (1994). Comparative health data and analyses. In C. J. L. Murray & A. D. Lopez (Eds.), *Global comparative assessments in the health sector: Disease burden, expenditures, and intervention packages (pp. v–vii).* Geneva: World Health Organization.

Kim, J. Y., Farmer, P., & Porter, M. E. (2013). Redefining global health-care delivery. *The Lancet, 382*(9897), 1060–1069.

Koplan, J. P., Bond, T. C., Merson, M. H., et al. (2009). Towards a common definition of global health. *The Lancet, 373*(9679), 193–195.

Lamberti, L., Walker, C. F., Noiman, A., Victora, C., & Black, R. E. (2011). Breastfeeding and the risk for diarrhea morbidity and mortality. *BMC Public Health, 11*(Suppl 3), S15.

Lopez, A., Mathers, C., Ezzati, M., Jamison, D., & Murray, C. (Eds.). (2006). *Global burden of disease and risk factors* (2nd ed.). New York: Oxford University Press. Retrieved from http://www.dcp2.org/pubs/GBD/1/Section/27.

Lozano, R., Naghavi, M., Foreman. K., Lim, S., Shibuya, K., Aboyans, V., … Memish, Z. A. (2012). Global and regional mortality from 235 causes of death for 20 age groups in 1990 and 2010: A systematic analysis for the Global Burden of Disease Study 2010. *The Lancet, 380*(9859), 2095–2128.

Marmot, M. B. (2016). Lectures: Sir Michael Marmot highlights health inequalities and 'causes of the causes'. Retrieved from http://www.abc.net.au/news/2016-09-03/boyer-lecture-sir-michael-marmot-highlightshealth-inequalities/7810382.

Murray, C., & Lopez, A. (Eds.). (1996). *The global burden of disease.* New York: Oxford University Press.

Murray, C. J., Vos, T., Lozano, R., Naghavi, M., Flaxman, A. D., Michaud, C., … Memish, Z. A. (2012). Disability-adjusted life years (DALYs) for 291 diseases and injuries in 21 regions, 1990–2010: A systematic analysis for the Global Burden of Disease Study 2010. *The Lancet, 380*(9859), 2197–2223.

Nair M., & Webster P. (2013). Health professionals' migration in emerging market economies: patterns, causes and possible solutions. *Public Health, 35*(1), 157–163. Retrieved from http://www.ncbi.nlm.nih.gov/pubmed/23097260.

Nolte, E., & McKee, M. (2011). Variations in amenable mortality—Trends in 16 high-income nations. *Health Policy, 103*(1), 47–52.

Potter, D., Goldenberg, R., Chao, A., Sinkala, M., Degroot, A., Stringer, J. S. A. … Vermund, S. H. (2008). Do targeted HIV programs improve overall care for pregnant women? Antenatal syphilis management in Zambia before and after implementation of prevention of mother-to-child HIV transmission programs. *Journal of AIDS, 47*(1), 79–85.

Prata, N., Passano, P., Sreenivas, A., & Gerdts, C. E. (2010). Maternal mortality in developing countries: Challenges in scaling-up priority interventions. *Women's Health, 6*(2), 311–327.

Ross, C., & Wu, C. (1995). Links between education and health. *American Sociological Review, 60,* 719–745.

Sachs, J. (2015). *The end of poverty.* London: Penguin.

Sachs, J. (2010). The MDG decade: Looking and conditional optimism for 2015. *The Lancet, 376,* 950–951.

Schneider, E., Sarnak, D., Squires, D., Shah, A., Doty, M. (2017). Mirror, Mirror 2017: International comparison reflects flaws and opportunities for better U.S. health care. The Commonwealth Fund. Available at: http://www.commonwealthfund.org/~/media/files/publications/fund-report/2017/jul/schneider_mirror_mirror_2017.pdf.

Skolnik, R. (2016). *Essentials of global health.* Boston, MA: Jones and Bartlett.

Smith, J. A. (1981). The idea of health: A philosophical inquiry. *Advances in Nursing Science, 3*(3), 43.

Smith, K. V., & Sulzbach, S. (2008). Community-based health insurance and access to maternal health services: Evidence from three West African countries. *Social Science and Medicine, 66,* 2460–2473.

Smith, J. M., Gubin, R., Holston, M., Fullerton, J., & Prata, N. (2013). Misoprostol for postpartum hemorrhage prevention at home birth: An integrative review of global implementation experience to date. *BMC Pregnancy and Childbirth, 13*(1), 44.

Southern African Development Community. (2012). Towards a common future: Non-communicable diseases. Retrieved from http://www.sadc.int/themes/health/non-communicable-diseases/.

Taylor A. L., Dhillon, I. S. (2011). The WHO Global Code of Practice on the International Recruitment of Health Personnel: The Evolution of Global Health Diplomacy. *Global Health Governance, 5*(1). Retrieved from http://papers.ssrn.com/sol3/papers.cfm?abstract_id=1970315.

Thompson, J. (2007). Poverty, development and women: Why should we care? *Journal of Obstetrics, Gynecology and Neonatal Nursing, 36,* 523–530.

United Nations AIDS. (2013). *Women, girls, gender equality and HIV.* New York: United Nations. Retrieved from http://www.unaids.org/en/media/unaids/contentassets/documents/factsheet/2012/20120217_FS_WomenGirls_en.pdf.

United Nations. (2012). *The Millennium Development Goals Report 2012.* New York: United Nations. Retrieved from http://www.undp.org/content/dam/undp/library/MDG/english/The_MDG_Report_2012.pdf.

United Nations. (2013a). *The Millennium Development Goals 2013 Report.* New York: United Nations. Retrieved from http://www.un.org/millenniumgoals/pdf/report-2013/mdg-report-2013-english.pdf.

United Nations. (2013b). *Countdown to 2015. Maternal, newborn, and child health survival.* New York: United Nations. Retrieved from http://www.countdown2015mnch.org/documents/2013Report/Countdown_2013-Update_noprofiles.pdf.

United Nations AIDS. (2017). When women lead change happens. Available at: http://www.unaids.org/sites/default/files/media_asset/when-women-lead-change-happens_en.pdf.

United Nations. (2017). *Sustainable Development Goals Report 2017.* Retrieved from https://unstats.un.org/sdgs/files/report/2017/TheSustainableDevelopmentGoalsReport2017.pdf.

United States Agency for International Development. (2014). Demographic and Health Survey Program. Retrieved from http://www.dhsprogram.com/.

Van Lerberghe, W., Matthews, Z., Achadi, E., Ancona, C., Campbell, J., Channon, A., … Turkmani, S. (2014). Country experience with strengthening of health systems and deployment of midwives in countries with high maternal mortality. *The Lancet, 384*(9949):1215–1225.

Venro. (2009). Re-thinking biomass energy for sub-Saharan Africa. Retrieved from http://www.venro.org/fileadmin/redaktion_afrikas_perspektive/publikationen/Projekt-Publikationen/091124_Arfikas-Perspektive_Bioenergiestudie_Final.pdf.

Walker, C. L. F., Rudan, I., Liu, L., Nair, H., Theodoratou, E., Bhutta, Z. A., … Black, R. E. (2013). Global burden of childhood pneumonia and diarrhoea. *The Lancet, 381*(9875), 1405–1416.

Winslow, C. E. A. (1920). The untilled fields of public health. *Science, 51*(1306), 23–33.

World Bank. (1993). *Investing in health: World development report*. New York: Oxford University Press.

World Bank. (2011). Wood-based biomass energy development for Sub-Saharan Africa: Issues and approaches. Energy Sector Management Assistance Program (ESMAP). Retrieved from https://openknowledge.worldbank.org/handle/10986/26149.

World Bank. (2014). Poverty overview. Retrieved from http://www.worldbank.org/en/topic/poverty/overview.

World Bank. (2016). Poverty and Prosperity: 2016. Available at: http://www.worldbank.org/en/publication/poverty-and-shared-prosperity.

World Health Organization. (1947). Constitution of the World Health Organization (p. 1). Retrieved from http://whqlibdoc.who.int/hist/official_records/constitution.pdf.

World Health Organization. (2004). *World development report 2004: Making services work for poor people*. Washington, DC: The World Bank.

WHO (2006). Health workers: a global profile. In: *The World Health Report 2006 – Working together for health*. Geneva: World Health Organization. http://www.who.int/whr/2006/whr06_en.pdf.

World Health Organization. (2008). Definition of the sector wide approach in glossary of globalization trade and health terms. Retrieved from http://www.who.int/trade/glossary/story081/en/.

World Health Organization. (2009a). *Global standards for the initial education of professional nurses and midwives (WHO/HRH/HPN/08.6) (pp. 40)*. Geneva, Switzerland: World Health Organization. Retrieved from http://www.who.int/hrh/nursing_midwifery/hrh_global_standards_education.pdf.

World Health Organization. (2009b). Injuries: The neglected burden in developing countries. *Bulletin of the World Health Organization, 87*, 246–246.

World Health Organization. (2010). Global code of practice on the International Recruitment of Health Personnel. Retrieved from http://www.who.int/hrh/migration/code/code_en.pdf.

World Health Organization. (2011). *Global status report on non-communicable diseases*. Geneva, Switzerland: World Health Organization.

World Health Organization. (2012a). Born too soon: The global action report on preterm birth. Retrieved from http://www.who.int/pmnch/media/news/2012/preterm_birth_report/en/index2.html.

World Health Organization. (2012b). Countdown 2015. Partnership for maternal child health. Geneva, Switzerland: World Health Organization. Retrieved from http://www.countdown2015mnch.org/documents/2012Report/2012-part-2.pdf.

World Health Organization. (2013a). Achieving health-related MDGs. Retrieved from http://www.who.int/hrh/workforce_mdgs/en/index.html.

World Health Organization. (2013b). Roll back malaria program. Retrieved from http://www.rollbackmalaria.org/keyfacts.html.

World Health Organization. (2013c). World Health Report 2013, Research for universal health coverage. Retrieved from http://www.who.int/whr/2013/report/en/.

World Health Organization. (2014a). Global health observatory. Retrieved from http://www.who.int/gho/en/.

World Health Organization. (2014b). Global status report on noncommunicable diseases. Geneva, Switzerland: World Health Organization.

World Health Organization. (2014c). Infant and young children: Fact sheet. Retrieved from http://www.who.int/mediacentre/factsheets/fs342/en/.

World Health Organization. (2014d). Maternal mortality: Fact sheet. Retrieved from http://www.who.int/mediacentre/factsheets/fs348/en/.

World Health Organization. (2015). Noncommunicable diseases prematurely take 16 million lives annually, WHO urges more action. News release. Retrieved from http://www.who.int/mediacentre/news/releases/2015/noncommunicable-diseases/en/.

World Health Organization. (2016a). Maternal Mortality Fact sheet. Available at: http://www.who.int/mediacentre/factsheets/fs348/en/.

World Health Organization. (2016b). Fact Sheet: World Malaria Report 2016. Available at: http://www.who.int/malaria/media/world-malaria-report-2016/en/.

World Health Organization. (2016c). *What are the social determinants of health?* Retrieved from http://www. who.int/social_determinants/sdh_definition/en/.

World Health Organization. (2016d). *World Health Statistics 2016*. Retrieved from http://www.who.int/mediacentre/news/releases/2016/health-inequalities-persist/en/.

World Health Organization. (2016e) http://gamapserver.who.int/mapLibrary/Files/Maps/Global_HALE_2015.png.

World Health Organization. (2017a). *Non-communicable diseases Fact Sheet*. Available at: http://www.who.int/mediacentre/factsheets/fs355/en/.

World Health Organization. (2017b) *World Health Statistics Report 2017*. Retrieved from http://apps.who.int/iris/bitstream/10665/255336/1/9789241565486-eng.pdf?ua=1.

World Health Organization (WHO). (2017c). *Tuberculosis*. Retrieved from http://www.who.int/mediacentre/factsheets/fs104/en.

Yakoob, M. Y., Theodoratou, E., Jabeen, A., Imdad, A., Eisele, T., Ferguson, J., … Bhutta, Z. A. (2011). Preventive zinc supplementation in developing countries: Impact on mortality and morbidity due to diarrhea, pneumonia and malaria. *BMC Public Health, 11*(Suppl 3), S23.

WEB RESOURCES

Please visit thePoint® for up-to-date web resources on this topic.

Part | 2

Evidence-Based Practice and Population Health

Chapter 5

Frameworks for Health Promotion, Disease Prevention, and Risk Reduction

Rosanna F. DeMarco and Judith Healey-Walsh

Perplexity is the beginning of knowledge.
Khalil Gibran

In theory there's no difference between theory and practice. In practice there is.
Yogi Berra

If the facts don't fit the theory, change the facts.
Albert Einstein

CHAPTER HIGHLIGHTS

- Influences on health and well-being
- Role of the nurse as an interdisciplinary team member in health promotion and prevention
- Health promotion programs
- Epidemiologic models of health promotion and public health science
- Levels of prevention and pathogenesis

- Immunizations
- Screening
- Behavior change theories
- Ecologic model and women living with HIV/AIDS
- Health literacy
- Interactive health literacy and health education
- Critical health literacy and health promotion

OBJECTIVES

- Discuss the contribution of the Centers for Disease Control and Prevention to the health and well-being of people in the United States.
- Explain three levels of prevention in relation to levels of pathogenesis.
- Identify and define health behavior change models and their practical use in altering behavior to enhance health and well-being.
- Identify a multisystem prevention approach to people, families, and communities.

- Describe epidemiologic models of health promotion and modifiable risk reduction.
- Describe the relationship among health literacy, health education, and health promotion.
- Compare the three levels of health literacy: functional, interactive, and critical.
- Identify requisite health literacy knowledge and skills for self-management of health.
- Describe essential health literacy practices for community health nurses.

KEY TERMS

Behavior change models: Models that assist clients, groups, and communities to redirect activities toward health and wellness.

Ecologic model: Model that considers intrapersonal attributes, interpersonal dynamics, person/environment interactions, cultural beliefs, and attitudes.

Health: A quality, an ability to adapt to change, or a resource

KEY TERMS (continued)

to help cope with challenges and processes of daily living.

Health belief model: A behavior change model that considers the severity of the potential illness or physical challenge, the level of conceivable susceptibility, the benefits of taking preventive action, and the challenges that may be faced in taking action toward the goal of health promotion.

Health literacy: The degree to which individuals have the capacity to obtain, process, and understand basic health information and services needed to make appropriate decisions.

Health literacy universal precautions: Practices that healthcare providers use to make all health information easier to understand, to confirm client–provider comprehension, and to reduce the difficulty of health-related tasks.

Health promotion: The process of enabling people to increase control over all modifiable determinants of health to improve their health and well-being.

Learning model: A behavior change model emphasizing reinforcement of social competence, problem solving, autonomy, and sense of purpose.

Modifiable risk: Susceptibility to disease or injury that can be controlled by individual people, families, or communities.

Motivational interviewing: Client-centered communication style for eliciting behavior change by helping clients and groups explore and resolve ambivalence to change.

Primary prevention: Maximizing health and wellness through strategies that are set in place before illness or injury is present.

Relapse prevention model: A change model that is used primarily to assist people struggling with relapse and recovery from substance use.

Risk reduction: Decreasing the chance of developing an illness, experiencing an injury, or being faced with chronic consequences of both.

Secondary prevention: Maximizing health and wellness through strategies set in place at the early and active chronic stages of illness and injury.

Social learning: A behavior change model that considers environmental influences, personal factors, and behavior as key components to change.

Social support: A component of change in which community members, friends, neighbors, and adjacent communities influence change by offering instrumental assistance, informational support, emotional support, and appraising support.

Tertiary prevention: Maximizing health and wellness through strategies that are set in place at the palliation and end stage of disease and injury trajectories.

Theory of reasoned action: A behavior model emphasizing that individual performance of a given behavior is primarily determined by a person's intention to perform that behavior.

Transtheoretical model: Sequential approach to behavior change on the basis of process across stages and timely readiness of the learner.

Well-being: A subjective perception of full functional ability as a human being.

CASE STUDIES

References to case studies are found throughout this chapter (look for the case study icon). Readers should keep the case studies in mind as they read the chapter.

The following three case studies are examples of prevention research by the Centers for Disease Control and Prevention (CDC) to address community health **risk reduction** and health promotion initiatives in people of various ages. They illustrate how healthy behaviors and risk reduction can be addressed through culturally relevant avenues using both epidemiologic evidence and the behavior change models presented in this chapter. The key to success in promoting health and reducing risk in these cases is the thoughtful, planned building of coalitions among individuals, communities, and health professionals. For example, nurses who address a particular healthcare concern need to involve members of communities in identifying goals, objectives, and solutions that can affect lifelong health promotion. It is critical that the risk be modifiable (sometimes referred to as a "modifiable risk"), which means that individual people or groups can actually do something about the problem using social competence, problem solving, autonomy, and purpose.

CASE 1

At the CDC Prevention Research Centers' (PRCs) annual program meeting, 300 participants received a bag that was a product of community prevention research. The PRC program purchased the bags from Threads of Hope, a small business developed by community partners and the Center for Health Promotion and Disease Prevention of the University of North Carolina at Chapel Hill, one of 33 CDC-funded PRCs. Threads of Hope is a spin-off of the center's core research project, HOPE Works, which trains community facilitators to run support groups enabling women to help each other make health and lifestyle changes. The women, who are African American, Native American (Coharie tribe), Latina, or white, live in Sampson and Duplin Counties in eastern North Carolina, where unemployment has been high since the mid-1990s, when tobacco and textile production ceased in the area. At the time, the poverty rate was close to 20%.

Fifteen years of researcher–community collaboration in the area has indicated that income, education, occupation, and community factors are playing a greater role in health than individual health behaviors or access to healthcare. The economic depression contributed to a sense of hopelessness that made some women less motivated to address health behaviors. The women who participate in this community-owned business receive a living wage, training in textile production and business management, health insurance, a chance to pursue higher education, and access to health promotion interventions primarily concerning nutrition and physical activity (CDC, 2017a; HOPE (Health Opportunity, Partnerships, Empowerment) WORKS, 2017).

CASE 2

An organization known as Program to Encourage Active, Rewarding Lives for Seniors (PEARLS) was developed at the Health Promotion Research Center of the University of Washington to help combat depression in seniors. The CDC provided funding for this program, which lasts for six months and consists of eight in-home visits by a counselor.

Minor depression is characterized by loss of interest or pleasure in activities, and feelings of sadness or hopelessness. It strikes about 14% of seniors, many of whom are dealing with isolation, loss of friends and family, and debilitating chronic diseases. For example, seniors who have diabetes are more than twice as likely as other people of the same age to have depression. One client who had limited vision said, "I just can't contribute anymore." Another woman spent weeks lying hopelessly in bed after recovering from pneumonia. Counselors help clients identify and write down the factors contributing to their depression as well as develop and evaluate solutions. One counselor said, ". . . just like the cold or the flu has symptoms, so does depression. … There is a close connection between depression and unsolved problems. If the problem is, 'I can't do anything worthwhile,' the goal can be, 'Find something I can do on a small scale that will be beneficial to other people.'" Both the client with limited vision and the one recovering from pneumonia found help in PEARLS, which uses structured behavioral therapy and positive events to resolve depression. A counselor helped the woman with limited sight find ways to help others, such as knitting baby blankets and calling isolated people, which were activities suited to her skills, interests, and personality. Other components of PEARLS include scheduling social and physical activities and planning simple pleasures, such as taking a walk, calling a friend, or soaking in a hot bath.

In its 3-year study phase, PEARLS eliminated depression completely for more than a third of participants. Of seniors in a comparison group who received usual care, only 12% reportedly eliminated depression completely. PEARLS also reduced depressive symptoms by half for 43% of participants—with almost three times as many people achieving that result as in the comparison group.

Investigators have also found that PEARLS reduces hospitalizations, for any reason, among participants. Researchers attribute the success of PEARLS to the behavioral therapy, which affects the same parts of the brain as some antidepressant drugs. Behavioral therapy can be more permanent than drugs, is less expensive, and can be used outside a clinical setting. Because the clients come up with solutions of their own, they feel capable of following through on them (CDC, 2015e).

CASE 3

A project called Planet Health, developed by the Prevention Resource Center on Nutrition and Physical Activity at Harvard University, combines important messages on nutrition and physical activity with four academic subjects in public schools: social studies, math, science, and language arts. Even though obesity affects many American children, officials still find they must eliminate health classes, nurses, and physical education from public schools because of tight budgets.

The Planet Health curriculum meets Massachusetts academic standards and includes lessons designed to fit into a teacher's busy schedule. The program consists of 24 lessons a year, six in each of the four main subjects—language arts, math, science, and social studies—plus special activities for physical education classes. Planet Health also challenges students to turn off televisions. Harvard researchers have shown that television viewing is directly related to obesity. The curriculum encourages children to spend less time watching television, playing video games, or using the computer—to reduce their "screen time" to two hours or less per day. The curriculum also includes innovative exercises to learn more about food and the properties of food and styles of eating that make kids healthy.

In a two-year study at 10 middle schools, Planet Health reduced the amount of time boys and girls watched television and also lowered the prevalence of obesity among girls. According to another study, the program will save money for children later in life; for every dollar spent on the program in middle school, $1.20 in medical costs and lost wages will be saved by the time the children reach middle age. Blue Cross Blue Shield of Massachusetts picked up Planet Health as part of an overall school wellness program, and it is now used in more than 120 schools across the state. The YMCA has also started offering a version of Planet Health during after-school programs in Massachusetts. Since 2001, when the curriculum was put into book form, more than 4,000 copies have been sold. Researchers are working on a new edition that will add and update information about sugar-sweetened beverages, the different types of fats, and whole grains.

Researchers and administrators say Planet Health's greatest success can be seen in the lifestyle changes it inspires—not just in the classroom, but in the community. Schools that use Planet Health have begun to hold fitness days for families, and teachers have started yoga classes for themselves (CDC, 2017f).

INTRODUCTION

According to Glanz, Rimer, and Viswanath (2015), health is a quality, an ability to adapt to change, or a resource to cope with challenges and processes of daily living. Whether **health** is defined as an attribute that helps individuals, families, and communities navigate the stormy sea of life, or as an ideal state of physical, social, and mental **well-being**, the notion of health being the absence of disease is superseded by a complex relationship between health and a person's sense of wellness. For example, it is true that people who make up neighborhoods, communities, and populations can die from lack of health, but they can die well (i.e., with a sense of well-being and at a high level of human functioning). This chapter explores models of health promotion through public health science, with specific emphasis on models of risk prevention and behavior change as vehicles to well-being. In this chapter, "disease" refers to illness or injury not just at the individual level, but also from the perspective of the larger community of people in neighborhoods, cities, states, countries, and the world. An important underpinning to every effort described in this chapter is the ethical imperative to address health as a proactive approach to wellness. The chapter ends with the discussion of an inclusive and integrative behavior change model that describes the need to consider multiple influences on positive health outcomes. This is in contrast to single-focused measures that have been used in the past to develop health promotion interventions and healthcare policy. The issue of African American women living with human immunodeficiency virus/acquired immunodeficiency syndrome (HIV/AIDS) in the United States is used as an example of how a formidable infectious and communicable disease can be addressed using this model to identify key components that influence behavior change. It also illustrates how interdisciplinary teams that include nurses identify and foster health promotion and policy change.

> Every human being is the author of his own health or disease. **Buddha**

HEALTH PROMOTION, DISEASE PREVENTION, AND RISK REDUCTION AS CORE ACTIVITIES OF PUBLIC HEALTH

Health has different meanings to individuals, families, and communities. Nurses working with clients in communities with a focus on population-based health gain knowledge about subjective well-being by observing individuals, families, and communities who are directly participating in improving their health. Individuals and groups interact in partnership with public health professionals to enhance their well-being and maximize their progress toward health, rather than just avoid illness, such as in the case studies at the beginning of this chapter.

Improving health is a journey of discovery among health professionals, the science of public health (epidemiology), and people who are motivated to effect change across varied and complex influences on well-being. Ten key components of public health practice are central to keeping populations healthy and safe. Nurses promote health through prevention efforts by belonging to interdisciplinary teams that address the following core activities (American Public Health Association, 2017):

1. Providing essential input to interdisciplinary programs that monitor, anticipate, and respond to public health problems in population groups, regardless of which disease or public health threat is identified
2. Evaluating health trends and risk factors of population groups and helping to determine priorities for targeted interventions
3. Working with communities or specific population groups within the community to develop public policy and targeted health promotion and disease prevention activities
4. Participating in assessing and evaluating healthcare services to ensure that people are informed of available programs and services and are assisted in the utilization of available services

It is important to understand that promoting health and wellness behaviors in individuals as members of a group or population depends on addressing all 10 core activities of public health simultaneously as an integrated whole. Each of these areas is addressed throughout this chapter in more detail. In this chapter, health promotion is presented through frameworks or models that can direct nursing practice to (1) focus on how to approach this complex and almost overwhelming concept of health at the population level; (2) become knowledgeable about how and why behavior change needs to be addressed, related to disease prevention and health promotion, depending on levels of control over an outcome; and (3) devise creative, cost-effective interventions and policy changes related to levels of prevention.

HEALTHY PEOPLE INITIATIVES

The *Healthy People* initiatives and *Healthy People 2000, 2010,* and *2020* (HP 2000, HP 2010, and HP 2020) are a set of health objectives established nationally to address keeping individuals, families, and populations safe and healthy (Koh, Blakey, & Roper, 2014). Chapter 4 discusses international approaches to public health issues on the global scale. In the United States, the CDC promotes health at the global level by promoting the sharing of knowledge, tools, and other resources as a global responsibility, as well as creating partnerships throughout the world through health promotion, health protection, and health diplomacy (CDC, 2017b). From a national perspective, HP 2020 is a guidepost for nurses and interdisciplinary teams in community and public health. HP 2020 has historic roots in efforts by the U.S. Surgeon General to establish a definitive plan for state and community organizations to address the health of citizens. The effort to establish measurable objectives was developed through a planned process that involves consulting healthcare experts locally and nationally, collecting data obtained from studies of population illness (morbidity, natural progression of disease and injury, and mortality patterns over time), engaging businesses in the process, and listening to the needs and barriers identified by citizens in the United States. HP 2020 is designed to achieve two primary goals: (1) to increase quality and years of healthy life and (2) to eliminate any barriers to accessing care, specifically through health disparities. Currently, 42 topic areas with congruent objectives and data are available for consideration. Of this current grouping, new seminal areas have been identified that include genomics, global health, healthcare-associated infections, LGBT (lesbian, gay, bisexual, and transgender) health, preparedness, and social determinants of health (HP 2020, 2017a). Box 5.1 lists all the new areas of interest in HP 2020. Please note that HP 2030 is on the way (HP 2020, Development of the National Health Promotion and Disease Prevention Objectives for 2030, 2017b).

> Where would the first case study, about Threads of Hope, fit in terms of addressing HP 2020 indicators and focal areas? Identifying specific indicators and focal areas that support health promotion means very little unless professionals in community or public health practice, such as nurses, consider partnerships to be necessary in the promotion of community health. Do you think that Threads of Hope addresses a particular focal point that is missing from the HP 2020 project?

Knowing how to address the need for change and the actual change at a personal, family, and community level must be based on science—evidence based on rigorous

5.1 *Healthy People 2020* New Areas

1. Adolescent health
2. Blood disorders and blood safety
3. Dementias, including Alzheimer disease
4. Early and middle childhood
5. Genomics
6. Global health
7. Healthcare-associated infections
8. Health-related quality of life and well-being
9. Lesbian, gay, bisexual, and transgender health
10. Older adults
11. Preparedness
12. Sleep health
13. Social determinants of health

Source: http://www.healthypeople.gov/2020/about/new2020.aspx.

understanding of a problem. Specific actions that can best achieve positive health outcomes can then be determined. Consideration must be given to realistic availability of solutions, cost and benefits, and the degree to which individual people will accept these approaches. It seems too simple to assume that promoting identified HP 2020 goals and objectives in tandem with known scientific methods will promote the health of the nation. Many complicated factors affect the process of educating the public about health, such as people's knowledge of their risk of disease, subsequent health outcomes, and the personal or communal choice to be healthy. It is necessary to consider individual and family perspectives about health and wellness, as well as community definitions of these concepts.

Student Reflection

I will never forget giving a presentation to a group of men and women in a senior center as my first effort in trying to convince them that cholesterol was a silent killer. After sharing age- and education-specific information from the American Heart Association and the CDC demonstrating dietary and exercise choices to promote health, one man got up and said, "What difference does it make; we all are going to die from something and I would rather eat fried foods than not eat them." Many people around him nodded their heads, and I realized that until people are convinced that scientific evidence applies to them and that their choices affect their personal well-being, family, and increasing costs in healthcare, we are stuck with lofty goals by tradition rather than through transformation into something new.

The role of the community and the public health nurse in promoting health encompasses advocacy, community organizing, health education, and political and social reform in collaboration with agencies and community members (Kulbok, Thatcher, Park, & Meszaros, 2012).

Thus, it is critical to seek out health promotion and behavior change models to provide direction in making health promotion, disease prevention, and risk reduction efforts meet the realities of communities and the agencies serving communities.

ROAD MAPS TO HEALTH PROMOTION

Epidemiologic Model and Prevention

Although illness care is a primary component of the art and science of nursing, health promotion and disease prevention are important, closely related public health efforts in achieving the goals of nursing care. "Health Promotion is the art and science of helping people discover the synergies between their core passions and optimal health, enhancing their motivation to strive for optimal health, and supporting them in changing their lifestyle to move toward a state of optimal health.

Optimal health is a dynamic balance of physical, emotional, social, spiritual, and intellectual health. Lifestyle change can be facilitated through a combination of learning experiences that enhance awareness, increase motivation, and build skills and, most important, through the creation of opportunities that open access to environments that make positive health practices the easiest choice" (O'Donnell, 2009, p. 4).

In this chapter, the word "disability" is replaced with the words "physically challenged" or "differently abled" to emphasize that there is always "ability" to deal with structural and functional problems (Smeltzer, Robinson-Smith, Dolen, Duffin, & Al Maqbali, 2010).

Community health nurses are focused specifically on **modifiable risks** of acquiring disease. This requires nurses to analyze trends in risk surveillance data and consider the physical, emotional, and psychosocial challenges people face when confronting disease, physical stressors, and the possibility of premature death. Public health science uses in-depth processes of data collection across the natural history of disease to define trends, and in this way assists nurses and other public health officials in prioritizing the steps they need to take to minimize risk and improve the quality of care in populations.

Keeping in mind the subjectivity of wellness, how would you develop outreach in the PEARLS program to elderly members of the community who are isolated and may want to preserve their privacy?

What would be a convincing argument to make to women who are not involved in making bags with Threads of Hope? How could you convince them that doing so would actually be an act of health promotion and would have a positive effect on their well-being?

Practice Point

The *Morbidity and Mortality Weekly Report* (MMWR), published weekly by the CDC and available online, contains useful public health information and guidelines that address trends in illness and disease. MMWR readership predominantly consists of physicians, nurses, public health practitioners, epidemiologists and other scientists, researchers, educators, and laboratory-oriented professionals. The data provided in the MMWR come from state health departments and compare morbidity and mortality rates annually. These records are very helpful to public health clinicians because they supply information that promotes a proactive approach to resource planning when the rates are increasing (CDC, 2017c).

Although the morbidity and mortality data reports are quantitative, it is important to understand that in most cases, perceptions of health or well-being on the part of individuals, families, and communities are subjective. The science of diagnosis and healthcare follow-up may be present, but it is the subjective perceptions of others that often determine a person's willingness to participate in health promotion initiatives. For example, if people perceive that health or "low risk" means the absence of acute symptoms or the absence of disease, many of them may consider themselves healthy and in no need of making an effort toward health promotion. In fact, they could actually be living with real, chronic morbid or comorbid conditions such as diabetes, hypertension, congestive heart failure, or hepatitis C, or they may be at risk for acquiring these conditions.

Health promotion is a strategy that is used in partnership with health professionals, individuals, and communities. It includes all three levels of disease prevention and has the potential to or can directly change health and well-being. Healthcare professionals or people in communities can institute these strategies. In reality, disease and physical challenges can occur at any time. In many cases, predictions made from statistical conclusions (probabilities) through the science of epidemiology are the basis for determining the possibility of getting a disease or becoming physically or emotionally challenged (see Chapters 6 and 7). Analysis of epidemiologic data occurs while health professionals consider what happens at the prepathogenic, early pathogenic, and late pathogenic phases of diseases and physical or emotional disorders. The basis of this scientific approach is the study of causal relationships that yield pathology. Epidemiologists make conclusions about the direction of further study by considering (1) relative risk of an agent causing a problem (e.g., smoking and lung cancer); (2) consistency (i.e., similar results across other studies); (3) exposure (i.e., correlation with a certain distinct pathologic condition, such as for asbestos and mesothelioma); (4) timing (i.e., cause and resulting condition both occurring within a short period of time, such as inhaled fumes and an asthma attack); and (5) plausibility (i.e., existence of a biologic process) (Wakeford, 2015).

The central idea here is to prevent illness and physical or emotional challenges from occurring. Or, if they do occur, the goal is to lessen their effects and enhance clients' quality of life. The science of epidemiology helps health professionals such as nurses, and coalitions of interested citizens, develop interventions for the stages of illness or physical or emotional challenges, which enhance the quality of life of individuals and communities. In Figure 5.1, health and wellness change along a developmental timeline. After a disease or physical challenge is identified, it progresses and eventually becomes life threatening. Although this pattern appears to be linear, in reality the linearity is theoretical. Illness occurs erratically; there are times of stability and times of acute and stressful exacerbation (Yohannes et al., 2017). At each pathogenic level, health promotion is intimately linked to prevention.

Health & Wellness	Disease Identified	Chronic Illness	Physical/Emotional Challenges
Prepathogenic Period	Early Pathogenic Period	Pathogenic Period	Late Pathogenic Period

FIGURE 5.1 Natural history of disease and levels of wellness/illness continuum.

Levels of Prevention

Activities classified as "preventive" are directed at eradicating, eliminating, or reducing the impact of disease and injury on individuals and populations, thus promoting health instead of disease (Gasink & Lautenbach, 2008). *Disease* in this context refers to communicable and noncommunicable conditions. Examples of noncommunicable diseases (noninfectious diseases or physical or emotional challenges) are substance abuse, obesity, depression, or workplace injuries. Physical or emotional challenges, as well as genetic disorders, are conditions that are generally noncommunicable in nature but cause structural and functional changes that are not statistically normal in the general population. Some examples include glaucoma, scoliosis, Down syndrome, neurofibromatosis, hearing loss, and learning disabilities. Communicable diseases are caused by pathogens (e.g., viruses and bacteria) that multiply and enter hosts through a variety of mechanisms and influences. These diseases have the capacity to cause infections across living organisms, with life-threatening and potentially chronic effects. Examples include HIV, malaria, swine flu, and smallpox (Webber, 2016).

What type of diseases (communicable or noncommunicable) do the programs in each case study address? Could addressing noncommunicable diseases or physical or emotional challenges through these programs influence vulnerability or resistance to communicable diseases in these populations?

To understand specific health promotion approaches, nurses should think in terms of three levels: primary, secondary, and tertiary prevention. The individual person's or the community's state of health and well-being, as studied within the science of identification, description, and prediction of illness, serve as the basis for the levels.

Primary Prevention

When an individual or a group is considered in good health and shows no signs or symptoms of disease or physical challenges, nurses in interdisciplinary teams and community partnerships are involved in **primary prevention**. They seek to maximize health and wellness, using a variety of strategies, at a time when they or the clients have some level of control over the trajectory of health and wellness. Examples of primary prevention include the use of seat belts, hand washing, proper preparation of food, exercise, and balanced nutrition (Box 5.2).

Surveillance of healthy populations is a continual, dynamic method of gathering data about the health of the general public for the purpose of primary prevention of illness. The CDC and individual states monitor emerging and endemic health hazards that occur in community settings on an ongoing basis. Data are systematically collected, analyzed, interpreted, and disseminated so that they can be used to develop activities and programs that will reduce morbidity and mortality and improve health. The functions of public health surveillance are described in Box 5.3. In addition, local surveillance of community populations can be obtained by using various records—from clinics, community health and visiting nurses, worker's compensation settlements, personnel files, and the like.

5.2 Examples of Primary Prevention

Immunizations
Driver's safety classes
Healthy water quality
Healthy air quality
Health education classes
Improving safety designs of equipment
Fire safety
Decreasing exposure to sun
Use of environmentally safe products
Using seat belts
Using earplugs and safety glasses

5.3 Functions of Public Health Surveillance

Estimating the impact of a disease or injury
Portraying the natural history of a health condition
Determining the distribution and spread of illness
Generating hypotheses and stimulating research
Evaluating prevention and control measures
Facilitating planning for program activities
Detecting outbreaks

Source: Centers for Disease Control and Prevention. (2004). Framework for evaluating public health surveillance systems for early detection of outbreaks. *Morbidity and Mortality Weekly Report, 53*(RR-05), 1–11.

It is critical to understand that there are situations in which primary prevention is difficult to achieve at the individual or community level. Sometimes, even with professional support and healthcare information, clients are unable to avoid experiencing disease or physical challenges because the causative agents are "not modifiable," for example, genetic conditions, unexpected tragedies (natural disasters such as floods or tornados), and situations in which there is no developmental control, such as the effect of secondhand smoke. These would be considered conditions for which primary prevention strategies are difficult to implement and not modifiable.

> Great things are done by a series of small things brought together. **Vincent Van Gogh**

An important example of primary prevention is the availability and dispensing of vaccines developed to enhance the body's ability to create antibodies to either live or attenuated antigens. This approach protects individuals and populations from getting communicable diseases or lessens the severity of the disease. Immunization with vaccines is an effective way to promote primary prevention. Nurses who actively participate in the immunization of children in well-child clinics, young adults in university health clinics, and adults in international travel clinics are promoting primary prevention of measles, human papillomavirus (American Cancer Society, 2017), and yellow fever, respectively. See Box 5.4 for a list of vaccine-preventable diseases (CDC, 2017g).

According to the CDC (2017g), immunity to a disease results from the presence of antibodies to that disease. Antibodies are proteins produced by the body to neutralize or destroy toxins or disease-carrying organisms, and they are disease-specific. For example, antibodies to measles protect a person who is exposed to measles but have no effect if the person is exposed to mumps. There are two types of immunity: active and passive.

Active immunity results when exposure to a disease organism triggers the immune system to produce antibodies to that disease. Exposure to the disease organism can occur through infection with the actual live organism (resulting in natural immunity) or introduction of a dead or weakened form of the disease organism through vaccination (vaccine-induced immunity). Either way, if an immune person comes into contact with a disease, his or her immune system will recognize it and immediately produce the antibodies needed to fight it. Active immunity is long-lasting, sometimes lifelong.

Practice Point

It may be important for nurses working with clients older than 60 or in communities where chronic illnesses abound to consider the use of the vaccine against shingles. Shingles is a painful localized skin rash, often accompanied by blisters, caused by the varicella zoster virus (VZV), the same virus that causes chickenpox. Any person who has had chickenpox can develop shingles because VZV remains in the nerve cells of the body after the chickenpox infection clears and can reappear many years later. Shingles most commonly occurs in people 50 years of age or older, in those who have medical conditions that keep the immune system from working properly, or in those who receive immunosuppressive drugs. The vaccine against shingles is recommended by the Advisory Committee on Immunization Practices (ACIP) to reduce the risk of this condition and its associated pain in people 60 years of age or older. See http://www.cdc.gov/vaccines/vpd-vac/shingles/default.htm for further information.

Passive immunity results when a person is given antibodies to a disease rather than producing them through his or her own immune system. A newborn infant acquires passive immunity from its mother through the placenta. This type of immunity can also occur with the use of antibody-containing blood products such as immune globulin, which may be given when immediate protection from a specific disease is needed. This is the major advantage to passive immunity; protection is immediate, whereas active immunity takes time (usually several weeks) to develop. However, passive immunity lasts only for a few weeks or months. Only active immunity is long lasting. *Herd immunity* is a type of passive immunity; the presence of a large proportion of immune individuals in a community decreases the chances of contact between any infected people and susceptible individuals. An entire population need not be immune to prevent an epidemic of a disease. Herd immunity is often attributed to either antibody formation, which occurs when populations acquire an illness in a non–life-threatening form as a result of medical care interventions or reduced virulence, or to vaccination programs.

5.4 Vaccine-Preventable Diseases

Anthrax	Mumps
Cervical cancer	Pertussis (whooping cough)
Diphtheria	Pneumococcal pneumonia
Hepatitis A	Poliomyelitis (polio)
Hepatitis B	Rabies
Haemophilus influenzae type b (Hib)	Rotavirus
Human papillomavirus (HPV)	Rubella (German measles)
Influenza (flu)	Shingles (herpes zoster)
Japanese encephalitis	Smallpox
Lyme disease	Tetanus (lockjaw)
Measles	Tuberculosis
Meningococcal disease	Typhoid fever
Monkeypox	Varicella (chickenpox)
	Yellow fever

Secondary Prevention

Secondary prevention is a planned effort to minimize the impact of a disease or injury once it is in effect. Secondary prevention is used at an early stage of pathogenesis or physical or emotional challenges. It includes, through the science of screening, initial recognition of the stage of an illness or physical challenge, which can progress to greater or lesser severity over time. The types of screening procedures and examples are found in Box 5.5.

Women diagnosed with HIV/AIDS and children who are identified as having scoliosis are examples of the need for secondary prevention. To screen effectively for the presence of these conditions, a test should be (1) cost-effective, meaning that the cost of producing and distributing the screening tool is justified by the positive effect on protecting the public; (2) easy to use; (3) available to large sectors of the population at risk; (4) sensitive and specific enough to identify true positives and true negatives; (5) backed by a healthcare infrastructure that can implement programs of care for people who have a verified risk of disease or physical challenge; and (6) acceptable to clients. Sensitivity and specificity are criteria used to measure how valid and reliable a screening test can be. Sensitivity measures the strength of a screening test's ability to correctly identify people who have a disease or physical challenge. Specificity measures the strength of a screening test's ability to correctly identify people who do not have a disease or physical challenge. In an ideal world, all screen tests should have both high sensitivity (100%) and high specificity (100%). The 100% level is approached but

5.5	**Types and Examples of Screening Procedures**

Mass screening: applied to entire populations
- Blood lead level screening
- Papanicolaou (Pap) smears
- Phenylketonuria of newborns

Selective screening: performed for specific high-risk populations
- Mammographies for young women at high risk for cancer
- Tuberculin tests for hospital employees
- Occupational diseases
- Exposure to radiation

Multiphasic screening: a variety of screening tests applied to the same population on the same occasion. Data can be used for establishing baseline data in a healthcare facility and for risk factor appraisal
- Series of tests performed on a single blood sample
- Periodic surveillance of drug therapy
- Monitoring the stage of an illness
- Case finding: clinician's search for illness as a part of a client's periodic health examination
- Monitoring the health of individuals in a case load

Source: U.S. Preventive Services Task Force. (2002). *Guide to clinical preventive services* (3rd ed.). McLean, VA: International Medical Publishing.

5.6	**Sensitivity and Specificity**

Sensitivity = testing correctly to identify persons who have the disease/physical challenge
High sensitivity: True positive (people who have the disease and test positive)
Low sensitivity: False negative (people who have the disease but test negative [normal])
Specificity = testing to identify persons who do not have the disease
High specificity: True negative (people who do not have the disease and test negative)
Low specificity: False positive (people who do not have the disease but test positive [abnormal])

not met. Thus, confirmatory studies need to be undertaken to verify the presence of the disease. In the case of diseases that could be fatal, sensitivity is crucial (Box 5.6). For nurses participating in screening and delivering results of screening, it is most important to be aware of the test's limitations of validity and reliability and to remember that serious economic costs to communities and health systems can be incurred when testing is not accurate. Nurses should also be aware of the psychological costs when a false-positive result occurs, which can create debilitating fear and anxiety. Calculation of sensitivity and specificity is discussed in Chapter 7.

Student Reflection

I recently participated in an immersion trip to Central America as a nursing student. I kept asking questions to our guides about disease screening and secondary prevention related to breast cancer, HIV, human papillomavirus, cholesterol, and high blood pressure. In several instances, it was clear that no screening was being performed in some of the areas. I was upset that screening, which has been established as reputable and accurate, was not occurring—especially in population groups that suffered from poverty and suboptimal living situations (lack of running water, outdoor ditches for latrines, garbage dumps as housing, unavailable barrier protection with sexual intimacy). After discussions with local health officials, it was clear that the lack of health personnel to offer the screening, the cost of the necessary materials, and the severe lack of infrastructure to follow up if people tested "positive" meant that there could be no screening at all. This stunned me and allowed me to understand the economic and ethical considerations related to screening and secondary prevention.

For example, when a client is tested initially for HIV with the OraQuick HIV test for oral fluid, a test supported by the CDC based on many years of serum testing (CDC, 2017d), the healthcare team has a responsibility to verify these findings despite the high sensitivity and specificity of this test (99.3% and 99.8%, respectively). If a person tests positive for HIV, the initial result is confirmed by using an HIV antibody test known as the enzyme-linked immunosorbent assay (ELISA), which was developed in the 1980s (Homsy, Thomson-Honnebier, Cheng-Mayer, & Levy, 1988). After all confirmatory HIV testing has been completed and infectious disease experts, including physicians and nurses specializing in infectious disease, have reviewed the findings, these professionals may consider the client to be at the stage of illness early in the trajectory of pathogenesis. For example, the client may have a low viral load or absent viral load with a CD4 count greater than 200 cells/µL. This would mean that the client has the ability to fight infection and that replication of the virus is not high. Involving this client in medical care, with the support of infectious disease services such as housing, nutrition services, counseling, addiction recovery, financial support, and primary care services, offers him or her the potential to maintain health and wellness.

Some may question the use of the word "prevention" here, when indeed the person already has a confirmed diagnosis of HIV. In this context, secondary prevention means that efforts are being made to minimize (1) any further extension of the HIV illness to "full-blown" AIDS (CD4 count less than 200 cells/µL, with detectable viral loads); (2) the need to use antiretroviral medications, which have severe and debilitating side effects; (3) any exacerbation of other comorbidities that could affect HIV status, such as intravenous drug use; and (4) any possibility of communicating the virus to others. People living with HIV/AIDS need to have support to counter perceptions of stigma and discrimination that can lead to depression. Depression can be linked with decreased healthcare adherence, which can cause HIV to worsen and AIDS to develop. If these clients are sexually active and not using safe sex practices, which include not maintaining recovery from substance abuse and not using barrier protection, the virus will be spread to others and they, in turn, may become infected with another strain of the virus.

Is it possible to screen for the problems identified in the three case studies (depression, nutrition, and physical activity)? How would this screening occur? What resources would be used?

In a school screening program for idiopathic scoliosis, a school nurse may find that a child has an anatomical abnormality. Depending on the stage of the abnormality, the school nurse makes appropriate referrals on the basis of orthopedic and neurologic screening standards (Scoliosis Screening, 2017). Generally, scoliosis screening is conducted because of evidence-based predictions of development at a cross-section of time when identification of the problem is critical to timely interventions.

Sometimes, when screening is completed, the client's level of disease or injury is found to be at a more advanced stage and is not considered to have been "caught early." This is true for many women of color who are tested for HIV. History of

intimate partner violence may inhibit personal motivation to receive care or may create situations in which the client may not be free to get care. Lack of healthcare insurance, mental health challenges, and active substance addictions can also cause women to delay testing for HIV. Subsequently, when they are diagnosed, they may be very ill, experiencing the life-threatening chronic and/or end stage of the illness called AIDS (Earnshaw, Smith, Chaudoir, Lee, & Copenhaver, 2012).

The U.S. government requires screenings for some conditions and not others. Some screenings are mandatory because of the physical and economic costs that may result if they are not performed (e.g., newborn screenings). On the other hand, some people see screenings as stigmatizing and may experience feeling of vulnerability or discrimination in a variety of ways (interpersonally, with regard to health insurance, and at work).

Tertiary Prevention

Tertiary prevention is the long-term management and treatment of clients with chronic conditions, such as HIV/AIDS and cancer, so that quality of life is maintained, despite the fact that the condition will not improve and will most likely worsen. Tertiary prevention includes rehabilitation and palliative care. AIDS-related cancers such as lymphoma are not uncommon. In general, cancer is a life-threatening illness that may occur along with other conditions. Cardiovascular disease, diabetes, and pulmonary disease may be present as well and require clinicians such as nurses to plan clients' cancer treatment, continue to assess HIV/AIDS disease progression, watch for opportunistic infections, and control pain or other side effects of the treatment. Care also includes supporting life choices that bring emotional comfort to clients such as family involvement, decreased isolation, supportive spiritual development, and organized help from communities.

Practice Point

Public health nurses should become familiar with those resources available to communities that can help address prevention at all levels. Local and state health departments have directories of both publicly and privately funded prevention support programs and services, and many hospital systems provide directories for clients to consider in their time of need. Finally, internet-based directories are being created to help citizens find a network of services in their community or region.

For example, nurses involved in cardiac care might do the following: Rather than envisioning end-stage cardiac rehabilitation as the focus of prevention after a cardiovascular event, or when cardiovascular disease is prominent in a community, they could think about approaches to prevention that are inclusive of all stages of health promotion and prevention. Many cardiovascular centers provide unique,

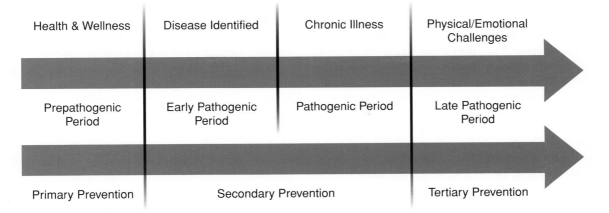

FIGURE 5.2 Natural history of disease, levels of wellness/illness, and levels of prevention continuum.

prevention-as-treatment approaches for communities with high incidence and prevalence rates for heart disease or an unusual number of people who are at risk for developing heart disease. Interdisciplinary teams of clinicians, including nurses, offer clients and communities the strategies and tools necessary to reduce their risks. For example:

- Primary prevention programs: Clients and families who are at risk for heart disease because of family history are treated. This level of prevention focuses on evaluation of personal risks in light of family history to help clients reach their heart health goals.
- Rehabilitation: Cardiac rehabilitation programs assist clients and families in recovery from heart attacks, angioplasty, and cardiac surgery and provide them with important information to make lifestyle changes to prevent recurrence.
- Associated comorbidities programs: Clients and families at risk for, or who already have, diabetes are assisted in weight loss and in managing other cardiac risk factors such as hypertension and high cholesterol. In addition, they are assisted in managing the combination of effects the illnesses have on daily life.

Therapies can include monitored exercise, stress management, yoga and meditation, nutrition counseling, smoking cessation, weight management, and stress testing.

In summary, prevention efforts are intended to decrease the physical, psychological, and economic costs of chronic, serious illness as well as physical and emotional challenges. Efforts to address these potential costs use an epidemiologic model of levels of prevention throughout the natural history of disease (prepathogenesis, early pathogenesis, and pathogenesis across time). These efforts include the use of immunizations, screening, and rehabilitation (see Figs. 5.1 and 5.2). Health promotion using this model is based on public health science and surveillance of trends related to diagnoses that are identified through sensitive and specific screening tests and the natural history of particular diseases. Nurses in public and community health practice, being advocates of

decreasing risk in populations, use this model to care for individuals, groups, and communities through instrumental care or through health policy.

BEHAVIOR MODELS

The focus of prevention efforts is the development of culturally relevant and gender-sensitive interventions that demonstrate positive outcomes in health and well-being. To promote health and well-being, one of the key approaches of primary, secondary, and tertiary prevention is a focused effort to change behaviors that have a negative impact on the natural history of disease and to promote behaviors that have a positive impact on the natural history of disease. Approaching individuals and groups about behavior change must incorporate knowledge of diverse client perspectives and include the use of counseling skills and motivational interviewing.

Motivational interviewing, which was developed by Rollnick and Miller (1995), is defined as a "directive, client-centered communication style for eliciting behavior change by helping clients/[groups] to explore and resolve ambivalence" (Motivational Interviewing, 2017). It is a focused, goal-directed approach (Box 5.7). It originated with problem drinkers who presented themselves to clinicians; the drinkers

---

5.7 Actions Involved in Motivational Interviewing Behaviors for Clinicians

Seek to understand the person's frame of reference through reflective listening.

Express acceptance and affirmation.

Elicit and select reinforcing motivational statements of problem recognition, concern, desire, intention, and ability to change.

Monitor the degree of readiness to change and ensure that resistance is not generated by clinician control.

Affirm freedom of choice and direction.

Source: www.motivationalinterview.org/clinical/whatismi.html.

needed help to change a behavior, although they wanted to continue it (ambivalence). To address behavior change using this method, the motivation comes from the client and is not imposed by a clinician. The client needs to resolve ambivalence to change a behavior with autonomy. Persuasion on the part of the clinician only intensifies resistance. The communication style is therefore one of directing the client to examine and resolve ambivalence. This method does not (1) argue with a group or community by insisting it has a problem that needs to change, (2) offer advice without actively encouraging group-identified choices, (3) give advice while the group is put in a passive role, (4) impose diagnostic labels, or (5) use coercive tactics. Motivational interviewing teaches all clinicians that making efforts to change behavior is based on a clinician–client exchange. Whether individuals or groups represent specific interests in communities, participation in decision making, informed consent, advocacy, and health literacy must be considered in using models of behavior change.

The quality of health at the individual, family, and community level is influenced by many factors. As discussed earlier, decreasing health disparities was an objective of HP 2010 and was identified as a key component in addressing barriers for some community dwellers who may desire to keep healthy and are ready to do so. So, despite the desire to change a behavior, there may be social, economic, or biologic nonmodifiable influences that prevent change. Behavior health models describe, explain, or predict prevention health behaviors. The models discussed here are available to help nurses consider creative methods of implementing the preventive measures identified earlier in this chapter. Although they appear to stand alone as unique and unrelated frameworks of behavior change, consideration of multiple influences cannot help but foster health, as in a "perfect world" (i.e., one in which nurses understand this concept and use all these methods together). The following section describes the theoretical frameworks of behavior change and many of the **behavior change models** that have been used to address health promotion and risk reduction (Glanz et al., 2015). This section ends by describing the ecologic model. The ecologic model is a model that considers multiple influences as a way to address complex behaviors to promote health at the individual, environmental, and policy level.

Learning Theories

According to Skinner (1953), health behaviors are seen as incremental steps toward a final goal. In the so-called **learning model**, a goal is established and reinforced by the nurse, with rewards given for partial accomplishment, if necessary. Incremental increases are then made as the pattern of behavior is shaped toward a specific goal. Reinforcement is used as motivation to either continue or discontinue a behavior. This model uses extrinsic, or external, factors for reinforcement. Although extrinsic factors are successful in the adoption of initial behavior, intrinsic, or internal, factors are more effective in long-term adherence. Praise, encouragement, or prizes are examples of

extrinsic rewards for the initial adoption of healthy behaviors. Feelings of accomplishment and changes in personal health habits are examples of intrinsic rewards that are often used in the long-term adoption of healthy behaviors.

A good example of the use of a classic learning model is the syndicated weight reduction program called Weight Watchers. Through the use of group encouragement, incremental weight loss is rewarded with public recognition and even a presented "ribbon" or "star" to indicate success. Intrinsic rewards, including the ability to show successful weight loss, as well as leadership opportunities within the program, can be helpful to people just beginning Weight Watchers, and have been documented within the past 10 years (Mitchell, Ellison, Hill, & Tsai, 2013).

Nurses in home care situations who work with clients with chronic illnesses, such as diabetes, congestive heart failure, and hypertension, have used the learning approach successfully while being actively involved in teaching and surveillance of client care. The difficulty with this approach is that there is a high level of expectation that intrinsic rewards will last over time, despite the influence of social norms and economic conditions. For example, in inner city and rural area communities, it is not uncommon to find a dearth of grocery stores, fresh fruit and vegetable stands, and farmer's markets as options for purchasing low-calorie, low-fat, and low-cost healthy foods. Instead, small stores sell high-calorie, high-fat processed foods (Liu, Stephenson, Houlihan, & Gustafson, 2017). Thus, clients with diabetes may have received intrinsic and extrinsic rewards for glycemic control but have little opportunity for continuity given the economic and social choices available in their communities.

> Anything that changes your values changes your behavior. **George A. Sheehan**

Evidence for Practice

Barch and colleagues (2017) explored how an important aspect of motivation in behavior is reinforcement learning that is implicit (outside of conscious awareness) or explicit (direct examples of rewards), as well as direct positive reinforcement or punishment. Motivational impairments are core features of a variety of types of psychopathology. Positive reinforcement is an important aspect of motivational function (learning about actions that lead to reward) and punishment (learning to avoid actions that lead to loss). In examining performance on tasks among individuals with schizophrenia, schizoaffective disorder, and bipolar disorder with psychosis, individuals with schizophrenia and schizoaffective disorder performed significantly worse than controls, but the individuals with bipolar disorder did not. Worse performance on an explicit reinforcement learning task, but not the implicit reinforcement learning task, was related to worse motivation and pleasure symptoms across all diagnostic categories. Performance on explicit reinforcement learning, but not implicit reinforcement learning, was related to working memory, which accounted for some of the diagnostic group differences.

Positive reinforcement has been used successfully in research studies to increase social behavior, improve cognitive and language skills, increase functional skills, and improve play skills. The questions that should be asked in reference to practices related to clients, groups, and communities are as follows:

- How do I deal with challenging behaviors during an interaction?
- How do I structure care to facilitate appropriate behaviors?
- What strategies do I use to teach new behaviors?
- How am I currently using positive reinforcement in my practice?
- How can I use positive reinforcement more effectively in my practice?

Health Belief Model

The **health belief model**, developed by Hochbaum (1956) and Rosenstock (1974), specifies that individual, family, or community health–related behavior depends on (1) the severity of the potential illness or physical challenge, (2) the level of conceivable susceptibility, (3) the benefits of taking preventive action, and (4) what stands in the way of taking action toward the goal of health promotion. This model uses cues as an important way to remind people of healthy behaviors and to promote these actions. Examples of this model include posting a note stating, "Don't overdo it at dinner" (individual) or "Let's try to do one thing tonight that is not related to a television set" (family), and placing a "Got Milk?" billboard in the neighborhood (community/population). Critical to this approach is the belief that the cue messages can be accomplished. If a community group does not believe that they can sustain a "walking" club in a safe section of a neighborhood, cues will not successfully encourage community members to follow a walking program. At the individual level, age-specific considerations are important. If people think they are healthy, they will not adhere to a preventive health program. Older people, who more readily see chronic illness and death as imminent, may become frightened with the prospect of susceptibility, while younger people often believe that they are invincible and impervious to illness and physical challenges.

Evidence for Practice

VanDyke and Shell (2017) explored the role of the health belief model in predicting breast cancer screening among women in rural Appalachia. Health beliefs (perceived susceptibility to breast cancer, severity of breast cancer, and benefits and barriers to screening) were used to predict health behavior through frequency of mammograms in a total of 170 women aged 18 to 78. Demographic characteristics, mammogram frequency, and perceived susceptibility, severity, and benefits and barriers to mammography were assessed. Findings included that women with objectively elevated risks for breast cancer (history of abnormal mammograms or family history of breast cancer) perceived themselves to be at higher risk for breast cancer, and those with a history of abnormal mammograms were more likely to receive mammograms regularly. Consistent with the health belief model, fewer perceived barriers to mammography predicted greater mammogram frequency. However, the model was not fully supported because perceived susceptibility, severity, and benefits to mammography did not predict mammogram frequency.

Student Reflection

My instructor in community health asked us to use the health belief model in caring for clients who were receiving care in a sexually transmitted infection (STI) clinic. He suggested that I show the clients some of the consequences of syphilis in particular (graphic pictures), because there had been a large increase in the incidence of the disease in the section of town where the clinic was situated. After I interviewed 10 different clients and really tried to increase their fear about the consequences of their actions, more than 50% stated that they never thought they would get an STI despite not using any precautions to reduce the chances of becoming infected. In fact, 30% of the clients revealed during assessment that this was their second or third diagnosis of syphilis. So, despite the severity of the results of the disease, other factors affected choices of risk about acquiring an STI. Some of those factors were alcohol abuse; inability to practice safe sex effectively; and trading unprotected sex for money, housing, and food.

Transtheoretical Model

The **transtheoretical model**, developed by Prochaska and DiClemente (1983), is a sequential approach to behavior change that involves timely readiness of the learner. This model promotes change using a five-stage process; the stages are (1) precontemplation, (2) contemplation, (3) preparation, (4) action, and (5) maintenance. Experts believe that individuals, families, and communities progress through these stages in a back-and-forth manner, not in a linear fashion. For nurses, the key to this approach is developing interventions tailored to clients' levels of readiness. For example, using this model to establish a twice-yearly blood pressure screening program in a community setting would require the following stages:

1. Precontemplation (no screening programs scheduled and no intention to schedule screening)
2. Contemplation (no screening programs scheduled but intent to start a program soon)
3. Preparation (no definite screening program but have taken steps to develop a program)
4. Action (a developed screening program and intent to sustain the program)
5. Maintenance (have had the program for some time and intend to continue)
6. Relapse (had a program, does not have a program currently but intends to be active with a program soon)

Evidence for Practice

Owusu, Quinn, Wang, Aibangbee, and Mamudu (2017) analyzed data from 43,540 participants of the Global Adult Tobacco Survey in low- and middle-income countries because over 80% of active smokers live in these countries. Intentions to quit smoking were categorized into precontemplation (referent category), contemplation, and preparation stages based on the transtheoretical model. Approximately 82%, 14%, and 4% of the smokers were in precontemplation, contemplation, and preparation stages, respectively. Rural residents had increased odds of being in contemplation stage (OR = 1.41, 95% CI = 1.09–1.83) compared with urban residents. Compared to homes where smoking was allowed, smoke-free homes were associated with increased odds of contemplation (OR = 1.77, 95% CI = 1.41–2.23) and preparation (OR = 2.18, 95% CI = 1.78–2.66). Exposure to anti-smoking messages in more than one media channel was associated with increased odds of contemplation (OR = 1.60, 95% CI = 1.33–1.92) and preparation (OR = 1.73, 95% CI = 1.28–2.33) compared with no exposure to anti-smoking messages. The results suggest that anti-smoking media campaigns and smoke-free policies may promote intention to quit smoking. While these suggest the need for implementation of comprehensive anti-smoking campaigns and smoke-free policies, longitudinal studies are required to confirm these findings and to evaluate how intention to quit translates into quit attempts.

Theory of Reasoned Action

The **theory of reasoned action** states that a person's given behavior is primarily determined by his or her *intention* to perform that behavior (Fishbein & Ajzen, 1975). This intention is determined by the person's attitude toward the behavior (beliefs about the outcomes of the behavior and value of these outcomes), and the influence of the person's societal environment or subjective norm (beliefs about what others think the person should do). The ability to perform the behavior (a belief that it can be done) is the critical aspect of the change process. Social or subjective norms are significant, and the importance of abiding by these norms is reflected in what people expect of individuals, families, and communities. For example, healthcare practitioners may use this model in smoking cessation. If a client believes that he or she cannot give up the addiction, no social norm will influence the behavior change. Smokers may isolate themselves from others or from circumstances which might influence their belief in their ability to change. Thus, the notion of addictive behaviors being hidden to decrease social pressure is a formidable challenge when trying to encourage healthy behaviors. The theory of planned behavior (a theory that links attitudes with behavior) is aligned with the theory of reasoned action, which states that perceived control over skills is needed to perform a behavior. This is similar to Bandura's concept of self-efficacy (the belief that one is capable of achieving a certain goal which may be a behavior).

Evidence for Practice

Kim, Darwish, Lee, and DeMarco (2017) used self-efficacy theory to create a community-engaged research protocol to help women living with HIV infection to quit smoking. Video conferencing to strengthen the belief that one can quit smoking was delivered on smart phones and was compared with telephone counseling. The counseling (video or phone) with actual treatment to quit (nicotine patches) were intended to be intervention components to help the women quit and sustain smoking cessation over time. Preliminary findings indicate that age predicts preference for phone call delivery of the intervention, thought to be chosen because of stigma related to smoking behavior.

Social Learning (Social Cognitive) Theory

Social learning, or social cognitive, theory is a behavior change approach in which environmental influences, personal factors, and attributes of the behavior itself have an effect. Most importantly, a person must believe in his or her capability to perform the behavior (self-efficacy) as well as perceive an incentive to do so (positive expectations outweigh negative). The immediate or long-term benefits must be valued. Providing skill development by modeling desired behavior can increase self-efficacy (Bandura, 1986).

Evidence for Practice

Wieland and team (2016) studied U.S. immigrants with increasing cardiovascular risk because of barriers to physical activity and health diets. They developed a physical activity and nutrition intervention through a community-based participatory research approach where they developed and used a modular content manual based on social learning theory. Family health promoters from the participating communities (Hispanic, Somali, Sudanese) were trained to deliver the intervention using the modules through 12 home visits during the first six months and up to 12 phone calls during the second six months. Key measurements included accelerometer-based assessment of physical activity and 24-hour dietary recall. Secondary measures included biometrics and social learning theory–based instruments. Of 150 individuals that included adolescents and adults, moderate levels of self-efficacy and social support were reported for physical activity and nutrition. What is particularly relevant in this study is how the processes and products from this program may be relevant to other social learning communities aiming to reduce cardiovascular risk and negative health behaviors among immigrants and refugees.

Theories of Social Support

Family members, friends, neighbors, and adjacent communities can influence change by offering **social support**—instrumental assistance, informational support, emotional support, and/or appraising support. An example of instrumental assistance is providing transportation to buy groceries or building a safe place to walk in a community. An example of informational support would be providing a community board with information on how to obtain assistance to clean a polluted pond. An example of emotional support is calling an isolated family that has lost a child to assist them in their bereavement. An example of appraising support is giving positive feedback about a new health skill (Berkman & Krishna, 2014). Although the literature suggests that social support is not equivalent to professional support, professionals can assist interested community members in organizing and developing social support opportunities that promote health in the community.

 Evidence for Practice

Rackow, Sholz, and Hornung (2015) studied the concept of "enabling" in exercise where it was hypothesized that social support has an indirect association on exercise through self-regulation and self-efficacy. These researchers examined the effects of different kinds of social support (emotion and instrumental) on exercise not only through self-efficacy but also through self-monitoring and action planning. Using an eight-week online program, study participants were randomly assigned to an intervention or a control group. The intervention included exercising regularly with a new exercise companion (social support). The researchers found that received emotional social support predicted self-efficacy, self-monitoring, and action planning in the intervention group. No direct or indirect effect of received instrumental social support on exercise emerged. In the control group, neither emotional nor instrumental social support was associated with any of the selfevidence for the enabling hypothesis of received social support via self-efficacy on physical exercise in an intervention study. This study demonstrated the contribution of received emotional and instrumental social support in the context of the "enabling" hypothesis.

The Relapse Prevention Model

The **relapse prevention model** has been used specifically with issues that relate to adherence. Relapse often occurs because of (1) negative emotional states; (2) lack of or limited coping skills; (3) decreased motivation; (4) stress; and (5) high-risk experiences. Taylor (2013) supports the idea that there are differences between a relapse and short lapse from healthy behavior and suggests that planning a strategy related to high-risk situations is critical for success, especially in the realm of harm reduction efforts. For example, communities interested in crime prevention and harm reduction may be aware that in certain months of the year, there is an increase in violent crime. They would then create a community campaign to promote nonviolence by increasing law enforcement presence and improving faith-based, school system, elder health, and neighborhood watch supports.

Evidence for Practice

Luciano and colleagues (2014) studied strategies of people with co-occurring disorders such as severe mental and substance use disorders. Strategies for relapse prevention described by men with co-occurring disorders with one or more years of sobriety were identified by analyzing semi-structured interviews from a sample of 12 men with demographic and diagnostic clinical data. The men were receiving treatment in residential or outpatient care and were primarily Caucasian (91.7%) and unmarried (100%) with ages ranging from 23 to 42. The two most common psychiatric disorders were schizoaffective disorder ($n = 4$, 33.3%) and bipolar disorder ($n = 4$, 33.3%), while the two most commonly misused substances were alcohol and cannabis. Qualitative analyses showed that participants maintained sobriety for at least one year by building a supportive community, engaging in productive activities, and carefully monitoring their own attitudes toward substances, mental health, and responsibility. Alcoholics Anonymous might act as a catalyst for building skills. The researchers concluded that a variety of self-management strategies are used to prevent relapse—seeking support, activities, and a healthy lifestyle. The researchers identified a relapse prevention model from this work, in which social networks, role functioning, and self-monitoring and conceptualizing self-care are critical to extending periods of health and wellness.

The Ecologic Model

The **ecologic model** stems from the original work of Bronfenbrenner (1979, 2004). This model is based on the belief that all processes occurring within individuals and their environment should be viewed as interdependent. It suggests that behavior change in individuals needs to be considered in a broader social context, including developmental history, psychological characteristics, interpersonal relationships, physical environment, and culture.

According to this model, behavior is a result of the knowledge, values, and beliefs of people, as well as numerous social influences. These social influences include relationships, social support networks, and community structure. According to the ecologic model, there are four levels of reciprocal influence, and it is necessary to consider all of these levels in order to change behavior. The four levels of influence, which may either promote risk or support protective factors, are (1) ontogenetic, (2) microsystem, (3) exosystem, and (4) macrocultural (Fig. 5.3) (El-Bassel et al., 2003). The influences represent biologic, environmental, and social influences as a dynamic and collective group of variables that need to be considered as a whole.

This model has been successfully used in health promotion and prevention research as a way to decrease barriers to mammography screening and safer sex practices (Eddy, Donahue, Webster, & Bjournstad, 2002; McLeroy, Bibeau, Steckler, & Glanz, 1988; Richards, Viadro, & Earp, 1998; Schaalma, Abraham, Gillmore, & Kok, 2004). Burke (2003) used the ecologic model to provide a better understanding of intrapersonal, interpersonal, and environmental factors associated with intimate partner violence in low-income communities. Others have used this model to identify individual and community resources, such as trust and partnership, to develop effective interventions for health access (Bhattacharya, 2003). El-Bassel and team (2003) used the ecologic model to study communication strategies for preventing HIV infection in African American and Latino heterosexual couples ($n = 217$).

USE OF THE ECOLOGIC MODEL: EVIDENCE FOR HEALTH PROMOTION INTERVENTION

The ecologic model is an appropriate framework to help identify and measure complex processes at a variety of levels for women living with HIV/AIDS. It allows public health interdisciplinary teams to (1) emphasize the unique developmental nature of variables that influence behaviors; (2) use a multilayered understanding of influence on behaviors; and (3) test variables from each of the identified systems in the model to guide the assessment, development, implementation, and evaluation of targeted interventions. The following is an example of how public healthcare providers implement each of the systems in the model in order to develop appropriate health promotion interventions. The ecologic model is more inclusive than many of the theories of behavior change

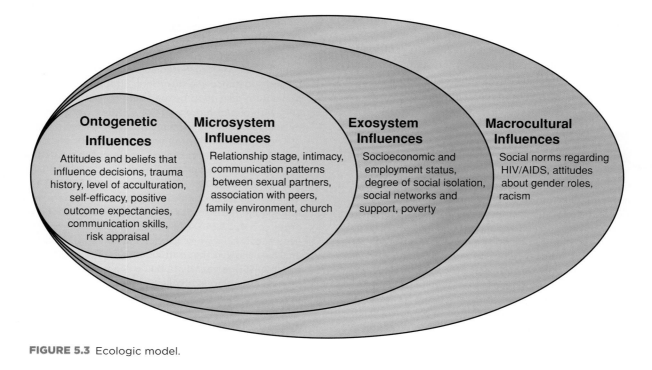

FIGURE 5.3 Ecologic model.

previously discussed. The references used include publications that are more than five years old, which indicates the historical development of evidence since the 1980s, when HIV was first identified in gay men in San Francisco, California.

Ontogenic System: Personal Factors

Characteristics such as race, marital status, and level of education are predictors of effective HIV prevention strategies (Hodder et al., 2013). Three trends emerging from these studies are as follows: (1) black women with lower levels of education are less likely to use HIV prevention measures than other groups surveyed; (2) older women and women of color are less likely to use condoms; and (3) strong correlations exist between education level and AIDS-related knowledge. In research which explores sexual risk factors, intimate partner violence, and selected psychosocial illnesses (injection drug use, alcohol abuse, anxiety, depression, psychosis, and dementia), HIV-positive menopausal women without childbearing issues have been overlooked (Stockman et al., 2013). Regardless of gender, identity, race, or ethnicity, traumatic events, mental illness, distrust, and stigma have all been linked to poor adherence to health promotion and prevention efforts, and behaviors associated with increased HIV risk (Kalichman, Katner, Banas, & Kalichman, 2017). These factors are barriers to HIV prevention for black women, and the lack of economic opportunity means they must focus on immediate survival, restricting their choices. In spite of the help of public funding and support services, lack of adequate and sustaining income is formidable (Chandler, Ansley, Ross, & Morrison-Beedy, 2016).

The relationship between trauma and HIV in African American–seropositive women and the contexts in which these risks occur are critical areas in need of understanding and successful intervention. Trauma, such as child sexual abuse, intimate partner violence, adult sexual abuse, and victimization from exposure to violent environments, contributes to behaviors associated with increased HIV risk and disease sequelae (Kalichman et al., 2017; Glover et al., 2010). "Research has shown that histories of physical and sexual trauma can affect the decisions women make with regard to risks for STIs and HIV, including the choice of partners and the ability to negotiate the use of barrier methods of protection" (Myers, Wyatt, Loeb, & Carmona, 2006, p. 401). In African American women, being a victim of violence increases depressive symptoms, decreases safe sex behaviors, increases the chance of becoming HIV-seropositive, and increases the chances of acquiring and being treated for an STI (Kalichman et al., 2017). Severe child sexual abuse is also associated with substance use and lower self-esteem (Willie, Overstreet, Sullivan, Sikkema, & Hansen, 2016).

In the health histories of aging African American women with no history of HIV, comorbid chronic conditions challenge self-care, especially when there is little or no social support (Willie et al., 2016). Risk-taking behaviors, such as having multiple sexual partners, unprotected sex, and drug and alcohol abuse greatly complicate HIV risk, HIV infection, and STIs when these behaviors are superimposed on chronic conditions such as hypertension, obesity, lupus, diabetes, and congestive heart failure. These behaviors continue to be major issues in prevention efforts (Buzi, Smith, Weinman, & Novello, 2013). Prevalence of hepatitis C virus is as high as 30% among those living with HIV and 90% if HIV was contracted through intravenous drug use. End-stage liver disease from hepatitis C virus is a major cause of death in people coinfected with HIV (HRSA, 2017). According to the CDC (2017c), the retrovirus responsible for HIV/AIDS targets the CD4$^+$ T lymphocyte as a primary target, thus crippling a number of important immunologic functions. Progressive impairment of the immune response leads to susceptibility in a variety of opportunistic infections and chronic life-threatening conditions. Measurements of CD4$^+$ T lymphocytes and the amount of HIV virus in the system (viral load in copies/mL), along with clinical manifestations of disease or infection, are used to guide clinical and therapeutic management of HIV-infected persons in the United States. Results of viral load assessments are used to make decisions regarding initiation of antiretroviral therapy and to determine whether current antiretroviral therapy is effective. These measures are critical in decreasing mortality and morbidity rates.

Microsystem: Relationship between Women and the Environment

Disclosing one's HIV status has been reported to increase feelings of shame and stigma, partner violence, rejection, depression, and high-risk sexual behavior (Herek, Gillis, & Cogan, 2009). Stigma is highly correlated with low self-image, depression, lack of social support, a lack of subjective social integration, and social conflict (Kalichman et al., 2017). Withdrawal from personal interaction as a way to reduce tension is part of stigmatization, and for persons living with HIV/AIDS who have strong histories of substance abuse, the temptation to fall out of recovery is profound (Logie & Gadalla, 2009). Poor self-image is linked to increased risk behaviors for HIV infection (Mahajan et al., 2008) and decreased disease adjustment, health promotion, self-advocacy, and self-efficacy for negotiating safe sex and safe sex practices (Herek et al., 2009). When women are empowered by HIV prevention efforts, they experience increased self-image, control over healthcare treatment decisions, self-efficacy, increased knowledge, and a positive sense of self as individuals and in relationships (Norris & DeMarco, 2005).

In non-HIV studies, such as breast cancer survivorship, self-image is related to relationship satisfaction and a positive feminine identity (Zimmermann, Scott, & Heinrichs, 2010). Self-image is a factor which affects risk behavior and perceptions of risk for unplanned pregnancies and is a predictor of the ability to negotiate safe sex behaviors

(Zimmermann et al., 2010). In women, there is a relationship between poor self-image, depression, and lack of self-advocacy in sexual relationships (DeMarco, Johnsen, Fukuda, & Deffenbaugh, 2001). From a treatment perspective, depressive symptoms are underdiagnosed and are associated with lower medication adherence, risky behaviors, and poor health outcomes (Lennon, Huedo-Medina, Gerwien, & Johnson, 2012). Lack of adherence to antiretroviral medication schedules has an effect on CD4 and viral load counts (i.e., adherence slows the progression of HIV, thereby maintaining health and survivorship). Substance abuse (drugs and alcohol) in HIV-infected persons decreases the use of appropriate and needed healthcare interventions, and in addition, it decreases HIV prevention by increasing the likelihood of risky sexual behavior (Liebschutz, Geier, Horton, Chuang, & Samet, 2005).

Exosystem: Formal and Informal Social Structures

Simoni, Walters, and Nero (2000) found that in women of African descent (black Hispanics, non-Hispanic blacks) living in New York City, disclosure of their HIV status to adult family members, friends, and coworkers was related to greater frequency of HIV-related social support but was not directly related to a decrease in depression or mood disturbance. During and after disclosure, social support was found to help with coping and improve psychological distress. Isolation, stigma, managing their medical care, and being a mother caused women to be unwilling to talk about their illness with their children, family, friends, and partners (DeMarco et al., 2001).

There is a strong connection between highly active antiretroviral therapy (HAART) and health. For poor women of color, adherence to medical protocols, which include HAART, and medical follow-up, as well as less high-risk behavior, is compromised by (1) believing that other people in their lives, specifically family and friends (children and sexual partners), come first; (2) subsisting on a low income, which affects resource allocation; (3) experiencing race discrimination, which magnifies the seropositive stigma; and (4) choosing to enter high-risk situations to obtain money (sex work) to change their circumstances. Many strategies are used to improve medication adherence, including counseling, support groups, educational information, telephone/computer-based feedback, improving motivation and self-efficacy, and directly observed therapy. Adherence may be improved with these strategies, but much needs to be understood within a particular group to determine their best use in a cost-effective manner (Haynes, Ackloo, & Sahota, 2008; Wolitski, Janssen, Onorato, Purcell, & Crepaz, 2005). However, despite the use of these methods, a proven method for implementing long-term behavior change remains unknown.

Social support includes relationships with family, friends, and community members. This is usually thought of as perceived social support; it represents the degree to which needs for relevant (or important) support are fulfilled by a person's social network. High levels of depressive symptoms are related to lack of HIV social support from friends, relatives, partners, groups, and organizations. In contrast, increased social support improves self-esteem and mastery. Thus, interventions that include group support can benefit psychological health (Simoni, Huang, Goodry, & Montoya, 2005).

Psychosocial factors contribute to disease progression, which can be measured by CD4 and viral load levels. These levels are indirect measures of adherence to HIV medications (Ironson et al., 2005). Factors that support adherence to HIV treatment protocols include supportive family members and other emotional support, whereas barriers to adherence include stigma, feeling unloved, and relationship turbulence (Edwards, 2006).

Macroculture: Values and Beliefs of Culture

To reduce the spread of HIV/AIDS, women who are seropositive must reduce the number of instances when reinfection by other HIV strains may occur, and protect partners from the virus by increasing safe sex behaviors. Safer sex strategies, from adolescence and onward in sexual development, include assertiveness, self-advocacy to negotiate protection during intercourse, verbal strategies, avoidance of drugs and/or alcohol consumption before or during sex, and avoidance of contact with potentially infected body fluids (Buzi et al., 2013). Negotiated safer sex in adults has almost exclusively been associated with condom use (Widman, Carol, & Noar, 2013). Because of the belief that partners are not sexually active with others, heterosexual adults use condoms less often with primary or regular partners than with casual sexual partners (Widman et al., 2013). In addition, as mentioned earlier, many social and situational factors contribute to decreases in behavior that may prevent HIV in women, such as feeling intense stigma, victimization, substance abuse, mental health problems, and contracting other STIs (Crepaz et al., 2007; Mize, Robinson, Bockting, & Scheltema, 2002).

Gender roles in women and, in particular, the need to maintain connection in relationships at the cost of one's own health are major issues for all women living with chronic diseases, but particularly for those who are HIV-positive (DeMarco & Johnsen, 2002, 2003; DeMarco, Lynch, & Board, 2002; DeMarco, Miller, Patsdaughter, Grindel, & Chisholm, 1998). Jack (1991, 1999) discussed the concept of silencing in the context of women's experiences with relationships. Jack's work is relevant today, since the experiences women have in relationships continue to be oriented toward understanding and defining themselves in the context of others. Jack supports the position that women's relationships are influenced not only by biologic factors but also by psychosocial factors (Bancroft, 2002) and asserts "women's orientation to relationships is the central component of female identity and emotional activity" (Jack, 1991, p. 3). This researcher's extensive exploratory and longitudinal studies with diverse groups of women resulted in the development of the concept of "silencing the self" and the Silencing the Self Scale. This concept of "silencing the self" has been used to explain how gender roles negatively influence self-advocacy behaviors in women. Women tend to silence their voice in relationships in order to maintain connections with others, even if that means they will subsequently suffer physically, psychologically, or socially. According to Jack (1991), women are reinforced culturally to (1) care for others' needs before their own, (2) abide by designated societal rules of behavior, (3) refrain from directly expressing their feelings and needs, and (4) outwardly maintain compliance, while feeling hostility inwardly because of their silencing behaviors. Silencing the self is relevant to the proposed study because it is a concept that is identified and understood in the context of relationships with others (i.e., a relational concept). The nature of intimate heterosexual relationships where seropositive safe sex occurs is an example of this relational context. Women living with HIV continue to be sexually active with men. Being quiet during times of sexual intimacy, rather than making direct requests and taking care of themselves, will not protect them against further strains of HIV and other STIs, and will infect others (DeMarco et al., 1998, 2001, 2002; DeMarco & Johnsen, 2002, 2003; DeMarco & Norris, 2004a, 2004b; Norris & DeMarco, 2004, 2005; Lanier & DeMarco, 2015).

HEALTH PROMOTION AND SECONDARY/TERTIARY PREVENTION FOR WOMEN LIVING WITH HIV/AIDS

Using the ecologic model, the aim of any intervention to promote health and minimize the spread of HIV/AIDS requires the creative inclusion of a prevention initiative that is community-based, peer-led, and interdisciplinary. Advancing the scientific understanding of secondary HIV prevention (what is called *positive prevention*) and exploring ways to reduce behavioral risk in African American women may prevent further transmission of HIV and the serious negative psychological consequences of living with HIV disease. African American women experience disproportionate levels of (1) interpersonal mistrust and fear of disclosure because of the fear of stigma, (2) poor adherence to treatment and other health promotion and disease prevention efforts, (3) delay in seeking care related to mental health comorbidities and addiction recovery issues, and (4) compromised self-advocacy in sexual relationships. An innovative, culturally relevant, and gender-sensitive intervention that would address these barriers for women who are already disproportionately saddled with HIV/AIDS, racism, ageism, and poverty would be beneficial not only to them but also to their families and the communities in which they live. Ultimately, public health nurses would be trying to improve health outcomes for this underserved population of women.

Within the context of HIV physical care and efforts to decrease communicability using the ecologic model, consideration should be given to mental health symptoms, severity/frequency of the effects from significant trauma (PTSD), substance use, abuse, and addiction. In Table 5.1, the sectors of the model and areas that need to be considered to address prevention are shown as a process of collaboration between interdisciplinary teams, evidence, and real, population-based needs.

The previous sections of this chapter provided a theoretical grounding in varied frameworks, which can guide the planning, implementation, and evaluation of health promotion and disease prevention interventions and programs. In addition, empirical evidence of the use and effectiveness of

TABLE 5.1 Ecologic Model with Health Promotion and Disease Prevention Considerations for African American Women Living with HIV

Ontogenetic System: *Personal Factors*	Microsystem: *Relationship between the Individual and the Environment*	Exosystem: *Formal and Informal Social Structures*	Macroculture: *Values and Beliefs of Culture*
Health history	Relationships and influences in interactions in relationships	Stressors or buffers that influence risky behaviors	Culture of women
Physiologic indicators	Stigma related to disclosure	Relationships with family, friends, community members	Culture of African American women
Comorbidities	Substance abuse/recovery		Self-advocacy in sexual relationships
Mental health	Healthcare adherence	Healthcare adherence, substance use, self-advocacy in sexual relationships	Stigma
Age, education, marital status, income, pregnancies, health history, sexual history, mental health symptoms	Self-advocacy in sexual relationships	Stigma	
Effect of trauma			
CD4 count/viral load			
Sexually transmitted infections			

the frameworks was discussed. The following sections explore the centrality of health literacy in its relationship with health education and health promotion.

Health literacy, health education, and health promotion are interrelated concepts, which individually and collectively have substantial effects on the health and well-being of individuals, families, and communities. Health literacy, health education, and health promotion seek to change knowledge, skills, attitudes, behavior, and social determinants to improve the health outcomes of individuals, families, and communities. Community and public health nurses are well-positioned to partner with individuals, families, and communities and to work collaboratively to initiate and maintain needed change. To be effective, nurses and their clients must understand health literacy and how the level impacts both access to healthcare and health outcomes. In addition, nurses must have skill in adapting health communication, health education, and health promotion strategies so that they can be clearly understood and acted upon by individuals, families, and communities at varied levels of health literacy.

The promise of health literacy is the promise of improved health. **Pleasant et al., 2016**

HEALTH LITERACY

Origins of Health Literacy

The concept of **health literacy** has evolved over the past two decades. Initial interest in health literacy stemmed from population studies of adult literacy. The 1992 National Adult Literacy Survey (NALS) conducted by the U.S. Department of Education revealed a surprisingly high prevalence of low literacy among the U.S. adult population (Weiss et al., 2005; Zarcadoolas, Pleasant, & Greer, 2009). This survey defined literacy as "the ability to use printed and written information to function in society, to achieve one's goals, and to develop one's knowledge and potential" (National Center for Education Statistics, 1993, p. 6). The survey categorized literacy into three general kinds of tasks: (1) prose tasks, which measure reading comprehension and ability to extract themes; (2) document tasks, which assess the ability of readers to interpret documents (consent forms, insurance forms); and (3) quantitative tasks, which assess the ability to work with numerical information embedded in written material (figure taxes, calculate calories on a nutrition checklist) (National Center for Education Statistics, 1993). As low literacy can negatively impact everyday functioning, questions were raised as to how low literacy might affect health and healthcare. Therefore, the concept of health literacy began getting attention in the 1990s.

The initial focus was on the content of health-related written materials, and the readability of that content. It was assumed at the time that most health consumers had the literacy skills to be able to read and understand materials disseminated by healthcare providers. However, multiple studies that examined the reading level and suitability of health materials across an array of health topics found repeatedly that the written materials exceeded the average reading ability of the public. For example, one out of five American adults read at the fifth grade level or below, and the average American adult reads at the eighth or ninth grade level, yet most healthcare materials are written at the 10th grade level (NPSF, 2018). This serious mismatch was found to contribute to inaccessibility of understandable health education and communication and to adverse events, compromising healthcare safety and quality.

In 2003 and most recently in 2016, the U.S. Department of Education, National Center for Education Statistics conducted the National Assessment of Adult Literacy (NAAL) and the Program for the International Assessment of Adult Competencies (PIAAC, 2016), which assessed the status of English adult literacy in the United States. For the first time, health literacy was included as a component of the larger assessment, providing the first nationally representative sample measuring the ability of the American public to read, understand, and apply health-related information (White, 2008). The results of this study provided insight into the levels of health literacy in the U.S. population. As community health nurses provide both individual and group health education and health promotion interventions, understanding the definitions and levels of health literacy is critical.

Definitions and Basic Level of Health Literacy

The definition of health literacy has and continues to evolve (Cutilli & Bennett, 2009; Nuttbeam, 2000). Initially health literacy was viewed primarily as an individual's ability to read health information. As the routes (verbal, written, media, internet) of health communication were viewed more broadly, the healthcare system became more complex, and the expectations for shared decision making (health consumer and health provider) and self-care increased, the definition of health literacy expanded (Cutilli & Bennett, 2009). Rather than just focusing on an individual's ability to read health information, the Institute of Medicine (now the National Academies of Science) (2004) expanded the definition of health literacy to include, "The degree to which individuals have the capacity to obtain, process, and understand basic health information and services needed to make appropriate decisions" (p. 32). This is one of the most widely used definitions and, like others, considers the individual's capacities, such as conceptual knowledge, and listening, speaking, numeracy, reading, and writing skills, along with abilities to access information and services, and uses all this information to make effective health-related decisions (*Healthy People 2020*, 2017a; IOM, 2004; Speros, 2006). Attention, although broadened beyond the written word, still was directed toward the abilities of the individual health consumer, and there was a widely held assumption that general literacy assured health literacy, and that most of the American public could understand basic health information as it was presented in health-related materials. This level of health literacy is referred to as functional health literacy, as it involves the basic level of reading and writing skills to obtain, understand, and apply information related to health risks, medication prescriptions, or access to health services (Nutbeam, 2000). The results of the NAAL were eye-opening, as it had a subsection specifically on health literacy, in demonstrating that health literacy was different than general literacy, and that proficiency in health literacy was very low in the U.S. population.

The 2003 NAAL study remains the only population-level study of health literacy and continues to be cited in the literature (National Center for Education Statistics, 2006). The health literacy tasks focused on the skills needed to address typical health-related materials, including insurance forms, medication labels, and pamphlets about specific diseases. The health-related tasks were divided among three principal healthcare domains: (a) clinical, (b) preventative, and (c) navigation of the healthcare system. The results showed that many U.S. adults struggle to understand healthcare information, with over one third (77 million people) at a basic or below basic health literacy level, who could therefore be confused about basic healthcare tasks such as how to take their medications by reading the label, how to follow a childhood immunization schedule by reading a standard chart, or how to understand critically important warnings on the label of an over-the-counter medication. Just over half demonstrated intermediate health literacy, whereby an individual could determine cause and effect, make simple inferences, and read instructions on a prescription label and determine what time to take the medication. Only 12% of Americans were proficient in health literacy, meaning that they could handle more complex health-related tasks, for example, using a table to calculate an employee's share of health insurance costs for the year, or understanding a risk–benefit ratio. The results of the study also provided insights about risk factors for low health literacy and preferences for sources of health information. Other studies have identified an array of knowledge and skills that are related to health literacy (Speros, 2011).

Increasing Interest in Health Literacy

Beyond the shocking prevalence of limited health literacy, three other factors fueled increasing interest in and study about health literacy: the risk factors contributing to low health literacy, the wide range of knowledge and skill required for proficient health literacy, and the relationship between health literacy and health outcomes. The increasing and ongoing study of health literacy revealed that limited health literacy can affect anyone and crosses gender, age, race, ethnicity, and socioeconomic status (IOM, 2004; Speros, 2011). However, beginning with the NAAL study and supported by subsequent studies, factors such as age, income, education, race, and linguistic ability were found to influence health literacy and contribute to health disparities

(Rikard, Thompson, McKinney, & Beauchamp, 2016). Box 5.8 identifies the populations that have been found to be at the highest risk for limited health literacy.

Health literacy has been described as a state, not a trait, as it can be variable within the same individual, based on context (Berkman, Davis, & McCormack, 2010). The complexity of the task and the condition of the individual influence health literacy. Even adults with strong literacy skills can face health literacy challenges and feel overwhelmed, typically in situations when they (a) are not familiar with medical terms or how their body works, (b) have to interpret numbers or risks to make a healthcare decision, (c) are diagnosed with a serious illness and are scared or confused, or (d) have complex conditions that require complicated self-care. Therefore, health literacy is not a fixed characteristic but able to change during an individual's lifespan, influenced by education, aging, culture, social interaction, life experiences, and specific context (IOM, 2004; Nutbeam, 2008).

Knowledge and Skills Related to Health Literacy

Adults at the below basic level for health literacy were the least likely to use any written material to obtain information on health topics with 43% indicating that they used written information infrequently, far less than those at the intermediate or proficient level. Nonprint sources, including broadcast media, such as radio or television, were rated higher than any type of print source. The lower the health literacy level, the less apt the individual would be to use the internet as a source of health information. Only 15% of adults with below basic health literacy used the internet "some" or " a lot" compared to 31% of adults with basic health literacy, 49% of adults with intermediate health literacy, and 62% of adults with proficient health literacy. This is an issue, as being computer-literate (able to operate and navigate a computer, portals with health information, and web-based health information) has been identified as one of the competencies for health literacy. Figure 5.4 illustrates the role of the community health nurse in educating an older adult in the use of computer technology to gain access to trustworthy health information. All adults, regardless of their

5.8	**Populations at Risk for Low Health Literacy**

Adults over 65
Individuals with limited education or low income
Non-native speakers of English
Racial and ethnic minorities
Recent refugees and immigrants
Adults with any type of disability, difficulty, or illness

Source: National Center for Education Statistics. (2006). *The health literacy of America's adults: Results from the 2003 national assessment of adult literacy.* Washington, DC: U.S. Department of Education.

health literacy skills, reported that they were more likely to get health information from nonprint sources, such as radio/television, friends/family, and most often health professionals (National Center for Education Statistics, 2006).

Further exploration of what constitutes health literacy has revealed that it requires broad knowledge and skills applied to a wide range of health topics, tasks, and situations. Beyond reading, health literacy involves a complex group of listening, computational, navigational, analytical, and decision-making skills, and the ability to apply these skills to varied health situations. Healthcare consumers need to be able to obtain, evaluate, and apply health-related information, which can require the use of technology. They need computational skills to calculate insurance premiums, deductibles, and copays, and analytical skills to make comparisons. For safe and accurate medication administration, the healthcare consumer must be able to read and interpret the prescription label or over-the-counter medication instructions and warnings, calculate or measure doses, understand the desired effect and potential side effects, obtain refills,

FIGURE 5.4 A community health nurse teaching an older adult how to navigate the web and find credible health information.

and determine insurance medication benefit. Table 5.2 identifies the varied health literacy skills and tasks required for self-health management.

TABLE 5.2 Skills and Tasks Required for Health Literacy

Aspects of Health Literacy	Examples of Skills and Tasks
Information-literate	Reading ability Comprehend complex health information Identify key information from dense text Understand directions for medication Understand nutrition labels Understand and follow directions for varied health-related procedures and treatments Understand information to give informed consent Read and follow appointment slips Apply written information to make effective health-related decisions Find credible health-related information independently
Visually literate	Understand and apply information from graphs, charts, diagrams, pictures, graphic instructions
Communication-literate	Provide a health history Describe symptoms Ask and respond to health-related questions Listen and understand verbal instructions and teaching
Computationally literate	Calculate doses Calculate calories within specialized diets Measure liquid medications Calculate deductibles, co-payments, and premium costs
Analytically literate	Compare and analyze insurance costs and covered benefits Understand risk–benefit ratio of treatment options and health promotion activities Interpret test results (blood glucose, peak flow results, etc.)
Computer-literate	Operate a computer Navigate the internet Obtain, evaluate, and apply web-based health-related information Access and use personal information from a health portal

Source: Agency for Healthcare Research and Quality. (2010). *Health literacy universal precautions tool-kit. AHRQ publication no. 10-0046-EF.* Rockville, MD: AHRQ. Retrieved from http://www.ahrq.gov/qual/literacy/index.html; Institute of Medicine. (2004). *Health literacy: A prescription to end confusion.* Washington, DC: The National Academies Press; and Speros, C. (2011). Promoting health literacy: A nursing imperative. *Nursing Clinics of North America, 46,* 321–333.

Health Outcomes Linked to Health Literacy

Studies have shown that limited health literacy is associated with multiple suboptimal health outcomes. Adults with low health literacy have a higher risk and rate of hospitalization, and higher use of emergency room service (Baker et al., 2002; Schillinger, 2002). However, they are less likely to access preventative care, and had lower use of mammography and receipt of flu shots (IOM, 2004; White, Chen, & Atchison, 2008). Other problematic areas revealed that adults with low health literacy had less ability to interpret labels and health messages, and demonstrated poor ability in accurate self-administration of medications (Bennett et al., 2009). Among older adults, those with low health literacy presented lower overall health status and higher mortality (Baker et al., 2007). Patients with low health literacy and chronic diseases such as diabetes, asthma, or hypertension have less knowledge of their disease and its treatment and fewer correct self-management skills than literate patients (AHRQ, 2010a). Among primary care patients with type 2 diabetes, inadequate health literacy is independently associated with worse glycemic control and higher rates of retinopathy. Inadequate health literacy may contribute to the disproportionate burden of diabetes-related problems among disadvantaged populations (Schillinger, 2002).

In addition to the effects of low health literacy on the individual, there are economic consequences of low health literacy to society. Low health literacy is an enormous cost burden on the U.S. healthcare system. According to the report *Low Health Literacy: Implications for National Health Policy*, "low health literacy is a major source of economic inefficiency in the U.S. healthcare system" (Vernon, Trujillo, Rosenbaum, & DeBuono, 2007). Annual costs for individuals with low health literacy are four times higher than those with higher literacy skills. The annual cost of low health literacy to the U.S. economy was $106 billion to $238 billion (Vernon et al., 2007). This represents between 7% and 17% of all personal healthcare expenditures. Medical errors and behaviors labeled as noncompliant may be based on poor understanding of the healthcare information. Inpatient spending increases by approximately $993 for patients with limited health literacy (Howard, Gazmararian, & Parker, 2005). Improving health communication reduces healthcare costs and increases the quality of healthcare.

Expanding Responsibility for Health Literacy

Low health literacy was initially viewed as an individual client's deficit, that is, a client's lack of knowledge and skills regarding health issues. The alarming prevalence of low health literacy and the concerning, varied, and serious negative health outcomes linked to limited health literacy drew increasing attention. It was evident that issues of health literacy went beyond reading written materials and individuals' abilities. Health literacy began to be viewed as a systems problem within healthcare, reflecting the complexity of both the presentation of health information and navigation of the healthcare system (Parker & Ratzan, 2010; Rudd, 2010). It

was becoming apparent that the healthcare consumer, healthcare provider, healthcare system, and government all have a role to play in addressing limited health literacy.

The Joint Commission (TJC), the major accrediting organization for healthcare organizations in the United States, recognizes the importance of health literacy and health communication as a critical component of patient safety and quality healthcare. TJC acknowledged the relationship among health literacy, health communication, and patient safety, stating in a 2007 report, "Health literacy issues and ineffective communications place patients at greater risk of preventable adverse events. If a patient does not understand the implications of her or his diagnosis and the importance of prevention and treatment plans, or cannot access healthcare services because of communications problems, an untoward event may occur" (TJC, 2007, p. 7). In addition, TJC's accreditation standards "underscore the fundamental right and need for patients to receive information—both orally and written—about their care in a way in which they can understand this information" (TJC, 2007, p. 7). TJC called for more attention to the structure and function of the healthcare system and the manner in which it can be changed to "permit patients to receive more time, attention, education and understanding of their conditions and their care" (TJC, 2007, p. 49).

Three federal policy initiatives also addressed health literacy. The Affordable Care Act of 2010 addressed efforts to improve health literacy in two areas: (a) incorporating health literacy into professional training; and (b) requiring that the health plans and insurers provide consumers with clear, consistent, and comparable health information in a standardized summary of benefits and coverage template. The National Action Plan to Improve Health Literacy provided seven coordinated health literacy goals (Box 5.9) for the United States, based on the following two principles: (a) all people have the right to health information that helps them make informed decisions, and (b) health services should be delivered in ways that are understandable and lead to health longevity, and good quality of life (USDHHS, 2010). The Plain Writing Act of 2010 requires all new publications, forms, and publicly distributed documents from the federal government to be written in a clear, concise, and well-organized manner so that the public can understand and use them.

These notable reports and regulations have moved health literacy from a limited focus on an individual's capacity to read and comprehend health information to a healthcare system's issue related to the responsibilities of provider communication, and the challenges of navigating the complex system, and further to an issue of health policy and reform.

Practice Point

Health literacy influences the ability to understand, interpret, and act on health information.

5.9 The National Action Plan to Improve Health Literacy's Seven Health Literacy Goals

1. Develop and disseminate health and safety information that is accurate, accessible, and actionable.
2. Promote changes in the healthcare system that improve health information, communication, informed decision making, and access to health services.
3. Incorporate accurate, standards-based, and developmentally appropriate health and science information and curricula in childcare and education through the university level.
4. Support and expand local efforts to provide adult education, English language instruction, and culturally and linguistically appropriate health information services in the community.
5. Build partnerships, develop guidance, and change policies.
6. Increase basic research and development, implementation, and evaluation practices and interventions to improve health literacy.
7. Increase the dissemination and use of evidence-based health literacy practices and interventions.

Source: U.S. Department of Health and Human Services, Office of Disease Prevention and Health Promotion. (2010). *National action plan to improve health literacy.* Washington, DC: Author. Retrieved from https://health.gov/communication/hlactionplan/pdf/Health_Literacy_Action_Plan.pdf.

HEALTH LITERACY AND HEALTH EDUCATION

As further understanding of the impact of low health literacy emerged, efforts were directed at communication between healthcare providers and their clients, and clients' ability to navigate the healthcare delivery system and more actively participate in self-care. Expectations in healthcare are changing and moving away from the healthcare provider as the expert and in charge of care. Health promotion and disease management are becoming more of a shared responsibility of the individual and the healthcare provider. In actuality, more and more is being expected of individuals and their informal family caregivers. If individuals are unable to understand what is taught or prescribed, then follow-through will be poor in relation to health behavior changes and the many tasks needed to manage chronic disease and to promote health. Consequently, another level of healthcare literacy, beyond functional health literacy, was proposed. Interactive health literacy refers to more advanced cognitive and social skills that empower an individual's active participation in healthcare, promotes more shared decision making between the healthcare provider and their clients, and increased responsibility for self-care management of both disease and health promotion (Fernandez-Gutierrez, Bas-Sarmiento, Albar-Marin, Paloma-Castro, & Romero-Sanches, 2017; Nutbeam, 2000). Community health nurses provide health education and care coordination, and promote the client's self- management of chronic conditions and health maintenance in many settings,

including homes, schools, and ambulatory clinics. Therefore, nurses must have the knowledge and skill to assess and understand the health literacy levels of their clients in order to improve the safety and quality of the care they provide.

Health Literacy Competencies and Practices Useful in Health Education

Health communication and health education seek to change knowledge, skill, and behavior, and ultimately to improve health and well-being. For change to occur, nurses and other healthcare providers must ensure that their oral and written health communication is presented in a manner that clients can comprehend and utilize. Addressing health literacy requires the use of clear and effective communication practices. Coleman, Hudson, and Pederson (2017) had 25 health literacy experts examine 32 previously identified health literacy and clear communication practices and competencies (knowledge, skills, and attitudes) (Coleman, Hudson, & Maine, 2013; Toronto, 2016; Toronto & Weatherford, 2015), and rank them in order from high to low importance. Consensus among the experts revealed a cluster of eight top-rated practices. Box 5.10 describes these practices, which provide guidance for healthcare providers in improving their health communication and health education strategies and outcomes. Toronto's (2016) study of health literacy competencies for nurses examined knowledge, skills, and attitudes. The highest-rated knowledge competency focused on the

5.10 Eight Top-Rated Health Literacy Practices (Consensus From Experts)

1. In written and oral communication avoids using medical terminology, and when avoidable, clearly defines using lay terms
2. To assess understanding (knowledge) and ability (skill) and correct any misunderstandings of material taught/shared, uses a "teach-back" or "show-me" method
3. Invites questions from patients using a patient-centered approach (e.g., "what questions do you have" rather than "do you have any questions")
4. Uses health literacy universal precautions method in written and oral communication with all patients
5. Uses a professional medical interpreter when communicating with a patient whose preferred language is other than English
6. Partners with the patient from the outset of the encounter negotiating a mutual agenda
7. Prioritizes health messages/teaching with emphasis on one to three "need to know" or "need to do" concepts during a clinical encounter
8. At the beginning of the clinical encounter asks the patient to share all of his or her concerns

Source: Coleman, C. A., Hudson, S., & Maine, L. L. (2013). Health literacy practices and educational competencies for health professionals: a consensus study. *Journal of Health Communication, 18*(Suppl 1), 82–102.

importance of knowing that all individuals, regardless of their literacy level, prefer and benefit from clear, plain language communication. The most frequently identified skill related to the nurse's ability to speak slowly and clearly. Regarding attitude, the findings emphasized the nurse's understanding that you cannot tell who is at risk for low literacy by looking or even interacting with them. Therefore, nurses need to approach all health communication and education using health literacy universal precautions.

Health Literacy Universal Precautions

As limited health literacy is so prevalent in the United States, is difficult to determine, and can vary based on the client's current condition and the complexity of the health-related information or task, experts recommend that healthcare providers adopt the use of health literacy universal precautions, meaning that "healthcare providers make all health information easier to understand, confirm everyone's comprehension, and reduce the difficulty of health-related tasks" (Liang & Brach, 2017, p. e216). Through the use of health literacy universal precautions, community health nurses can structure health communication and education to improve client understanding, informed decision-making, and ability to follow-through on a mutually established plan of care. **Health literacy universal precautions** promote specific strategies and practices that should be used with all clients to reduce the common mismatch that occurs between a clinician's level of communication and a client's level of comprehension. In fact, evidence shows that clients often misinterpret or do not understand much of the health information given to them by healthcare providers. This lack of understanding can lead to medication errors, poor self-management of chronic conditions, limited participation in health promotion activities, and adverse health outcomes (AHRQ, 2010a; Bennett et al., 2009).

ESTABLISHING A SUPPORTIVE LEARNING ENVIRONMENT

No matter what the setting in which the community health nurse is providing health teaching, a supportive, shame-free learning environment in which clear communication is intentionally used must be established. The learning environment should foster clients as active partners in their healthcare, specifically by encouraging clients to ask questions. Clients may be embarrassed to ask questions, or not know how to express their question, particularly when the nurse appears pressed for time or unsupportive. Asking "What questions do you have?" communicates to the client an expectation that they should have questions and will more likely encourage questions, rather than saying "Do you have any questions?" which typically leads to a "no" answer by clients even if they do have questions. In addition, the nurse can support client questioning by (a) making it clear that the nurse has time and wants to address questions; (b) sitting at the same level as the client (not standing); (c) looking at the client, listening attentively, and not interrupting;

(d) helping the client to prioritize his or her questions; and (e) encouraging the client to write down questions before interactions with any healthcare provider (primary care provider, specialist, pharmacist) (AHRQ, 2010b).

EFFECTIVE QUESTIONING

An effective tool for community health nurses to teach clients is the Ask Me 3 Good Questions for Good Health developed by the National Patient Safety Foundation (now available through the Institute for Healthcare Improvement). Community health nurses should teach these three questions to their clients, and encourage them to ask these questions every time they meet with a healthcare provider. The questions are:

- What is my main problem?
- What do I need to do?
- Why is it important for me to do this?

Ask Me 3 can provide a useful guide for clients, encouraging them to speak up and ask questions. These three questions are useful in focusing important conversations; making all clinical encounters and health education sessions interactive can increase understanding for both the provider and the client. Clients are more apt to follow a plan of care if they understand what the problem is, specifically what they need to do, and the rationale for the actions advised. However, community health nurses can also use it to structure how they share information with clients to ensure that the answers to the three questions are provided in the course of the conversation.

EVIDENCE-BASED HEALTH LITERACY UNIVERSAL PRECAUTIONS

The Agency for Healthcare Research and Quality has developed a Health Literacy Universal Precautions Toolkit (https://www.ahrq.gov/professionals/quality-patient-safety/quality-resources/tools/literacy-toolkit/index.html) that provides evidence-based guidance to improve health communication between healthcare providers and clients at all levels of health literacy. The toolkit includes 21 tools and 30 resources addressing four domains that are essential for the promotion of health literacy: (a) spoken communication, (b) written communication, (c) self-management and empowerment, and (d) supportive services.

Research has demonstrated that for spoken language, the healthcare provider should avoid medical jargon; use simple, clear, lay terms; speak clearly and slowly; and listen attentively. The amount of information should be limited with no more than four main messages all focusing on the desired behaviors and actions, which are repeated and reinforced during the session. Most people prefer clear communication using simple words and short sentences, covering the essential, need-to-know information. Using pictures or other visuals and everyday examples to supplement the teaching is effective (Speros, 2011).

Written health education materials should also use simple terms, active voice, and short sentences. They should be easy to read, using bulleted lists, beginning with the most important information first and limiting the amount of information. Headings and subheadings are useful in separating and introducing new information. Pictures and graphic illustrations are helpful in improving understanding and retaining information (Speros, 2011).

The focus of health communication and education should be on moving the client to well-informed, self-care management of all aspects of their health, including management of illnesses and preventative and health promoting activities. Promoting clients as active partners in their healthcare decisions and management supports client empowerment.

Table 5.3 summarizes health literacy universal precautions evidence-based practices.

Studies have shown that 40% to 80% of the medical information patients receive is forgotten immediately and nearly half of the information retained is incorrect (Kessels, 2003). It cannot be assumed that what the nurse has taught has been understood by the client and that the client can act on it. Therefore, another important health literacy–health education related tool is using the teach-back method every time the nurse shares health-related information with a client. The purpose of this teach-back technique is to ensure that the nurse has explained the information clearly and that the client has accurately understood the information. The nurse asks clients to explain in their own words what they have been taught, what they need to know, and what they need to do. If a client is unable to teach back the information, the nurse would explain the information again, reassess, and repeat the process until the client can demonstrate understanding. A variation of the teach-back method is the show-me method, wherein the nurse has the client demonstrate a skill, such as blood glucose monitoring or medication administration, so that the nurse and client are confident in the client's ability to perform the skill at home. Effectiveness of the teach-back technique has been shown to improve client–provider communication, client follow-through on plans of care, and client health outcomes (Sudore & Schillinger, 2009). Clients who understand their personal health information make fewer mistakes and demonstrate greater follow-through with instructions. Health literacy can be improved through intentional provision of information, effective communication, and structured education.

TABLE 5.3 Health Literacy Universal Precautions Practices in Health Communication and Education

Health Literacy Domain	Practices
Written communication	Use plain, simple words
	Avoid medical jargon
	Write at the fifth grade level
	Use short sentences
	Use bulleted lists
	Use active voice
	Focus on no more than four key points
	Begin with most important point
	Use headings and subheadings to separate information
	Chunk similar information
	Use white space and reasonable font size
	Add pictures graphic illustrations to illustrate information
	Summarize key points at the beginning and the end
Spoken communication	Establish a shame-free learning environment
	Show respect and a helpful, caring attitude
	Face the client
	Speak slowly, clearly
	Use simple, everyday language, avoiding medical jargon
	Encourage questions
	Teach clients to use Ask Me 3
	Repeat and review key points
	Use written information, pictures, videos, and other visual aids to reinforce spoken communication
	Use teach-back and show-me methods to verify comprehension
	Summarize at the end

Source: Agency for Healthcare Research and Quality (AHRQ). (2010). *Health literacy universal precautions tool-kit.* AHRQ publication no. 10-0046-EF. Rockville, MD: AHRQ. Retrieved from http://www.ahrq.gov/qual/literacy/index.html; Speros, C. (2011). Promoting health literacy: A nursing imperative. *Nursing Clinics of North America, 46,* 321–333.

Evidence for Practice

Bailey and team (2016) completed a mixed-methods study to determine if a health literacy universal precautions approach resulted in similar or different satisfaction levels among low and high health literacy participants. This study was part of a larger research project that tested the effectiveness of SIP*smart*ER, a six-month behavioral intervention designed using a health literacy universal precaution approach. The intervention was directed at reducing the sugar-sweetened beverage (SSB) intake in a population of rural-dwelling, low socioeconomic adults. The intervention was comprised of several health education components including 3 small group classes, one live teach-back call, 11 interactive voice response (IVR) calls, personal action planning, and self-monitoring (SSB) logs. The researchers analyzed the program's interview-administered summative evaluation, which was completed by 105 participants (68 identified as high and 37 low health-literate).

Overall results demonstrated no significant differences in the satisfaction of each of the interventions components and that participants with low and high health literacy benefitted from and were satisfied with an intervention designed using health literacy universal precautions. Quantitative data revealed that each component was positively evaluated. The small group classes received the highest rating and were chosen as the most motivating by both groups. A higher number of low health literacy participants liked the content and length of the IVR system as compared to the high health literacy participants. The IVR calls reviewed and reinforced information from the small group sessions and may have been more beneficial to the low health literacy participants; however, the completion rate of the IVR calls was the same for both groups. Qualitative findings indicated more likes than dislikes in both groups.

HEALTHY PEOPLE 2020 AND HEALTH LITERACY

Healthy People 2020 acknowledges the relationship among health literacy, health communication, and health outcomes. Health communication objectives were identified to improve population health outcomes and healthcare quality and to achieve health equity. The objectives proposed that improvements in health communication will provide accurate, understandable, actionable, tailored health information that will contribute to improved health literacy, which should support better health outcomes.

Two overarching health communication objectives identified in HP 2020 are:

(a) Improve the health literacy of the population
(b) Increased proportion of persons who report that their healthcare providers have satisfactory communication skills

5.11 *Healthy People 2020:* Health Communication Objectives

- Increase the proportion of persons who report that their healthcare providers always explained things so they could understand them.
- Increase the proportion of persons who report that their healthcare provideres always gave them easy-to-understand instructions about what to do to take care of their illness or health conditions.
- Increase the proportion of persons who report that their healthcare provider always asked them to describe how they will follow the instructions.
- Increase the proportion of persons who report that their healthcare providers always involved them in decisions about their healthcare as much as they wanted.

Source: Healthy People 2020. (2017a). *2020 Topics and objectives.* Retrieved from https://www.healthypeople.gov/2020/topics-objectives.

Improved health literacy can empower individuals to assume more responsibility for their health and actively participate in better informed, shared decision making with their healthcare providers. The health communication sub-objectives measure an increase in the evidence-based practices outlined in health literacy universal precautions (Box 5.11).

Evidence for Practice

Improving health literacy is a goal included in the U.S. Department Health and Human Services' national health promotion and disease prevention initiative, *Healthy People 2020* (USDHHS, 2010). To track progress in the adoption of health literacy universal precautions, *Healthy People 2020* selected measures of three health literacy strategies: (1) providing easy-to-understand instructions about what to do for self-management of an illness or health condition; (2) asking patients to describe in their own words, how they will follow the instructions (teach-back method); and (3) offering assistance in completing a form. Liang and Brach (2017) used data from the Agency for Healthcare Research and Quality's Medical Expenditure Panel Survey (MEPS)— Household Component, which tracks progress in *Healthy People 2020* healthy literacy measures to examine the extent of health providers' use of recommended health literacy universal precautions. The findings, which analyzed changes from 2011 to 2014, did reveal an improvement in each measure. Seventy percent of adults reported always receiving easy-to-understand instructions (increased from 64% in 2011), 29% (up from 24% in 2011) reported that their providers always asked them to explain how they will follow the instructions, and 17% (up from 14% in 2011) were offered assistance in completing a form.

Health communication, health literacy, and health education can be more than the sum of their parts. By working together we can progress farther to improve individual and community health. **Allen et al., 2017**

HEALTH LITERACY AND HEALTH PROMOTION

Both in practice and research, the focus of health literacy has been on individual abilities in basic functional literacy and interactive literacy, and health communication between clients and healthcare providers. Attention has been on the effect of low health literacy and the implementation of practices to alleviate the potential negative outcomes. Health literacy researchers and experts have suggested an additional perspective that views health literacy as an asset, which can increase through health education and health promotion (Pleasant et al., 2015). Low health literacy is linked to poor health outcomes and health disparities, while strong health literacy is connected to improved health outcomes. It has been suggested that improving health literacy could contribute to decreasing health disparities. To improve health literacy, health providers and consumers need to look beyond individual health literacy capacities and health providers' health literacy competencies, to necessary system's level changes in the social, economic, and environmental context (Allen, Auld, Logan, Henry Montes, & Rosen, 2017; Chinn, 2011; Rudd, 2015). In its landmark report, *Health Literacy: A Prescription to End Confusion* (IOM, 2004), the Institute of Medicine noted "improving individual health literacy requires great effort from the public health and healthcare systems, the education system, and society overall" (IOM, 2004, p. xiv). To realize the broader goal of improving health literacy across populations requires a larger effort, one that addresses health literacy at the community and population levels. This requires broadening definitions and another level of health literacy that are closely related to health promotion and public health, which address the social determinants of health and health disparities.

The following three expanded definitions of health literacy recognize the relationships among health literacy, health promotion, and public health. According to the World Health Organization's (WHO) definition, health literacy "represents the cognitive and social skills which determine the motivation and ability of individuals to gain access to, understand and use information in ways which promote and maintain good health. By improving people's access to

health information and their capacity to use it effectively, health literacy is critical to empowerment" (WHO, 2018b). Sørensen and colleagues (2012) also included health promotion in their enhanced definition, "Health literacy is linked to literacy and entails people's knowledge, motivation, and competences to access, understand, appraise, and apply health information in order to make judgments and take decisions in everyday life concerning healthcare, disease prevention and health promotion to maintain or improve quality of life during the life course" (p. 3). In these expanded definitions, health literacy is viewed as an asset, an outcome of health promotion efforts, and as having both personal and social benefits. Advanced cognitive skills include critical thinking, analysis, decision making, and problem solving in a health-related context. These cognitive skills are combined with social skills of communication and questioning to empower individuals to improve their personal health status and the health of the communities in which they live (Crondahl & Karlsson, 2016).

Freedman and colleagues (2009) broadened the definition of health literacy to include a focus on public health and the community, "The degree to which individuals and groups can obtain, process, understand, evaluate and act upon information needed to make public health decisions that benefit the community" (p. 448). The authors propose that in addition to individual-level health literacy efforts, equal attention should be given to literacy about public health with more emphasis on primary prevention and population health. Health literacy is not just a personal resource; higher levels of health literacy within populations, such as public health literacy, yield social benefits, for example, by mobilizing communities to address the social, economic, and environmental determinants of health, which can be the root causes of health illiteracy. An emphasis on community recognizes that individuals and families are embedded in environmental and sociocultural contexts. This understanding supports the perspective that health literacy is a collaborative responsibility among individuals, communities, the healthcare system, the government, and other related societal institutions, to promote health and reduce health disparities among individuals, families, communities, and societies (Rudd, 2015).

Critical Health Literacy

Critical health literacy reflects elements of the above definitions. This level of health literacy requires more advanced cognitive skills, coupled with social skills that can "be applied to critically analyse (sic) information, and to use information to exert greater control over life events and situations" (Nutbeam, 2000, p. 264). Chinn's (2011) concept analysis of critical health literacy revealed three domains, including (a) critical appraisal of information, (b) understanding the social determinants of health, and (c) collective action. Similarly, Nutbeam (2000, 2008) asserts that critical literacy requires individual and collective action to understand and address the social, economic, and environmental determinants of health. People with critical health literacy can change general and organizational practices related to health, and communicate with leaders and politicians to realize changes they consider important. The author suggests a strong relationship between health promotion and health literacy. Nutbeam (2000) references the WHO's (1986) *Ottawa Charter for Health Promotion*'s influence on defining health promotion, "as public health action directed toward improving people's control over all modifiable determinants of health" (p. 261). Concern is not only for personal behaviors and lifestyle, but also for living and working conditions and public policy, all of which influence public health.

International Health Promotion Efforts Supporting Critical Health Literacy

The United Nations ECOSOC Ministerial Declaration of 2009 provided a clear mandate for action: "We stress that health literacy is an important factor in ensuring significant health outcomes and in this regard, call for the development of appropriate action plans to promote health literacy. Indeed, knowledge and understanding remain powerful tools in health promotion" (WHO, 2016). Improving health literacy in populations provides the foundation for self and community empowerment, whereby individuals are enabled to assume an active role in improving their own health, and coalitions form to promote community action for health, and to move local, state, and national governments to meet their obligations in addressing public health issues.

Health Promotion and the Social Determinants of Health

The *Ottawa Charter for Health Promotion* is an international agreement signed at the First International Conference on Health Promotion, organized by the WHO and held in Ottawa, Canada, in November 1986. The charter defines **health promotion** as "the process of enabling people to increase control over, and to improve, their health. It moves beyond a focus on individual behaviour (sic) and toward a wide range of social and environmental interventions" (WHO/Ottawa Charter for Health Promotion, 1986; WHO/Health Promotion, 2018). Health promotion seeks to both support individuals to assume responsibility for their own health and to work to create an environment in which they can be successful. It involves motivation and self-efficacy, community empowerment, and health-promoting political and social activism. Good health is a major resource for personal, family, community, social, and economic development and has an essential impact on the quality of life. Political, economic, social, cultural, environmental, behavioral, and biologic factors can either foster or limit health. Most communication and health education interventions remain focused on personal health and lifestyles. There is a real need to develop, implement, and evaluate interventions to improve knowledge, understanding and capacity to act on social, economic, and environmental determinants of health, thus developing individual and community empowerment. Public health literacy is as much citizen-based as it is expert-driven, and it can take multiple forms from voting to organizing grassroots initiatives to establishing healthy policies and structures.

The Ottawa charter identified five action areas for health promotion, which remain relevant today:

- Build healthy public policies: Health promotion goes beyond healthcare. Health and health consequences should be considered in all public policies, including non-health sectors.
- Create supportive environments: Health is strongly affected by environmental factors. The environments in which people live, work, learn, and play must be structured to promote health and well-being.
- Strengthen community action: Community empowerment in health promotion activities must be emphasized. Community stakeholders need to be involved in all areas of community action including setting priorities, making decisions, and planning, implementing, and evaluation strategies to improve health.
- Develop personal skills: Health education is a component of health promotion that supports the acquisition of knowledge and skills required for self-management of health, informed decision-making, and participation in community action.
- Reorient health services: Responsibility for health is shared among individuals, community groups, health professionals and service institutions, and governments. Healthcare needs to move beyond its focus on illness and clinical interventions and services, toward a health promotion direction that embraces broader social, economic, cultural, political, and physical environmental factors that exert a strong influence on health.

As community health nurses focus on the multiple determinants of health, stressing the crucial social factors, and emphasize health promotion and disease prevention, they are well positioned to support the development of critical health literacy and community empowerment. The five action areas emphasized by the *Ottawa Charter* provide guidance for community health nurses as they develop individual and community-based health promotion activities, form community health action coalitions, and support efforts to address health in all public policies and create environments where healthy choices are accessible by all.

Health literacy at the community level has many implications regarding daily decisions about health promotion and disease prevention, not only for individuals, but decisions for and by the family and community units. Community-based health literacy interventions have been defined as "Any purposeful, organized activity to help a group of people find, understand, use, or communicate about health information, services, or issues for themselves or their communities" (National Academies of Sciences, Engineering and Medicine, 2018, p. 8). Health literacy in the community setting has profound influence on an individual's and community's ability to engage in negotiations, decision making, activism, and community level empowerment and development focused on health (Batterham, Hawkins, Collins, Buchbinder, & Osborne, 2016).

Practice Point

Health literacy, including all three levels (functional, interactive, and critical), is an asset that improves individual, family, and community health, and has the potential to reduce health inequities.

Evidence for Practice

Low health literacy among Korean American women has been identified as a significant barrier to their participation in breast and cervical cancer screening. Han and colleagues (2017) tested a community health worker (CHW)–led health literacy intervention on mammogram and Papanicolaou test screening among Korean American women. The authors used a cluster randomized control design to compare a CHW-led health literacy intervention with an educational control group. Participants had to be Korean American women aged 21 to 65, who were able to read and write in either English or Korean, and had not had a mammogram or Pap test in the past 24 months. Trained CHWs from 23 ethnic churches recruited the study sample of 560 women (intervention *n* = 278 and control *n* = 282). The control group received publicly available educational breast and cervical cancer brochures. The intervention group received an educational brochure tailored specifically to their risk factors. After receiving this, they received a two-hour health literacy training facilitated by the trained CHW, within a small group community-based setting. The training introduced key medical terms, and allowed practice of phrases in English and role play of a typical screening process. In addition, participants received practice reading and interpreting appointment slips and instructions, and guidance on how to effectively navigate the healthcare system screening process.

At the end of the small group meeting, participants received a DVD and guidebook that reinforced all aspects of the class. For six months, the CHWs initiated monthly calls to reinforce the knowledge and skill gained in the health literacy session, and assist with any navigational barriers. The researchers assessed self-report of mammogram and Pap test utilization at baseline, and medical record review at three- and six-month intervals. At six months, 56.1% and 54.5%, respectively, of those in the intervention group had received a mammogram and Pap test compared with 10.0% and 9.2%, respectively, of women in the control group. Having read all of the intervention materials was an important factor, as completing a screening test doubled for both cancers when a participant had read all materials compared to a participant who read only some or none. The CHW-led health literacy intervention was successful in promoting mammogram and Pap test screening among Korean American women, which could contribute to decreasing existing cancer health disparities among this population. In addition, the findings support the importance of transforming the design of health literacy training from a knowledge-based to a skills-building and empowerment focus.

ROLE OF NURSES

This chapter addresses real examples of how nurses, as part of an interdisciplinary team, can be involved in fundamental prevention and health promotion efforts. After using public health science and evidence to identify risk, the focus of prevention and health promotion can proceed using culturally relevant, sensitive, ethical, and creative ways to motivate others to consider health and wellness as individuals, groups, and communities. Historical behavior change theories are examples of how health science has developed in using psychology, sociology, anthropology, and ethical perspectives to advance efforts at the national level and beyond. Although primary prevention in particular is often overlooked as a critical component to health and wellness when it comes to resource allocation in the U.S. health system, in truth it is one of the most influential areas where nurses as teachers can make a difference in people's lives.

In addition, the chapter explores the relationship among health literacy, health education, and health promotion, areas of healthcare in which community health nurses have a central role and responsibility. Understanding the complexities of health literacy is a core responsibility. Community health nurses need to integrate health literacy universal precautions best practices into their health education and health promotion interventions to improve health outcomes. Knowledge of the three levels of health literacy—functional, interactive, and critical—allows the community health nurse to intervene at the individual, provider, and community level.

KEY CONCEPTS

- National goals and directives to maintain the health of individuals, families, and communities are important road maps for healthcare professionals.
- Three levels of prevention assist health professionals to advance quality of life and health through the natural history of disease and disability.
- Identifying modifiable risk and using health promotion models to address change in behaviors, beliefs, attitudes, and intentions can significantly increase the health of individuals, families, and communities.

- Health literacy involves three levels: functional, interactive, and critical, all of which must be addressed to improve individual and public health.
- Health literacy, health education, and health promotion are interrelated and collectively work to support health self-management, effective provider–client communication and collaboration, and community engagement and activism to address the social determinants of health.

CRITICAL THINKING QUESTIONS

1. What does it mean to be healthy and well when diagnosed with multiple sclerosis?
2. Name community indicators that would demonstrate health and wellness for a particular geographic area.
3. What are the responsibilities of community and public health nurses in promoting health and decreasing illness and injury in populations, families, and individuals?
4. Identify five key influences on health and wellness in the United States.
5. If national health policies are identified but cannot be funded because of national fiscal deficits, how would community/public health nurses initiate support for these policies?
6. Choose a data-based publication that represents each level of prevention and take a position about which level is the most complex to put into action for advancing health and wellness.

7. Critique behavior change from the perspective of measuring the change after a health promotion intervention has been implemented (e.g., teaching communities to decrease saturated fat in their diet and to exercise more).
8. Evaluate the written teaching materials used at your clinical placement. Do they reflect the use of health literacy universal precautions? If not, take one and revise it using the universal precautions practices.
9. Reflect on your spoken communication with clients. Do you consider health literacy issues? List five ways that you can use health literacy universal precautions in your spoken communication and then practice them at clinical and evaluate your competence.

COMMUNITY RESOURCES

- State and local departments of health (divisions of maternal and child health, communicable disease, occupational health, addictions, gerontology)
- YMCA/YWCA programs
- Gyms/athletic complexes
- State and local police departments
- Parks and recreation departments
- Places where blood pressure equipment is sold or screenings are available (local retail stores)

- School systems (school nurse associations)
- Local restaurants
- Air and water control areas
- Primary care physician and advanced nurse practices
- Dentists
- Elder services

REFERENCES

Agency for Healthcare Research and Quality (AHRQ). (2010a). *Health literacy interventions and outcomes: An update of the literacy and health outcomes systematic review of the literature.* Retrieved from https://effectivehealthcare.ahrq.gov/sites/default/files/pdf/health-literacy_research-protocol.pdf

Agency for Healthcare Research and Quality (AHRQ). (2010b). *Health literacy universal precautions toolkit.* AHRQ publication no. 10-0046-EF. Rockville, MD: AHRQ. Retrieved from https://www.ahrq.gov/professionals/quality-patient-safety/quality-resources/tools/literacy-toolkit/index.html

Allen, M. P., Auld, E., Logan, R., Henry Montes, J., & Rosen, S. (2017). *Improving collaboration among health communication, health education, and health literacy. NAM Perspectives, Discussion Paper.* Washington, DC: National Academy of Medicine. Retrieved from https://nam.edu/improving-collaboration-among-health-communication-health-education-and-health-literacy

American Cancer Society. (2017). Retrieved from https://www.cancer.org/cancer/cancer-causes/infectious-agents/hpv/acs-recommendations-for-hpv-vaccine-use.html

REFERENCES *(Continued)*

American Public Health Association. (2017). *The role of public health nurses.* Retrieved from https://www.apha.org/apha-communities/member-sections/public-health-nursing

Bailey, A. N., Porter, K. J., Hill, J. L., Chen, Y., Estabrooks, P. A., & Zoellner, J. M. (2016). The impact of health literacy on rural adults' satisfaction with a multi-component intervention to reduce sugar-sweetened beverage intake. *Health Education Research, 31*(4), 492–508.

Baker, D. W., Gazmararian, J. A., Williams, M. V., Scott, T., Parker, R. M., Green, D., … Peel J. (2002). Functional health literacy and the risk of hospital admission among medicare managed care enrollees. *American Journal of Public Health, 92*(8), 1278–1283.

Baker, D. W., Wolf, M. S., Feinglass, J., Thompson, J. A., Gazmararian, J. A., & Huang, J. (2007). Health literacy and mortality among elderly persons. *Archives of Internal Medicine, 167*(14), 1503–1509.

Bancroft, J. (2002). Biological factors in human sexuality. *The Journal of Sex Research, 39*(1), 15–21.

Bandura, A. (1986). *Social foundations of thought and action: A social cognitive theory.* Englewood Cliffs, NJ: Prentice-Hall.

Barch, D. M., Carter, C. S., Gold, J. M., Johnson, S. L., Kring, A. M., MacDonald, A. W., … Strauss, M. E. (2017). Explicit and implicit reinforcement learning across the psychosis spectrum. *Journal of Abnormal Psychology, 126*(5), 694–711.

Batterham, R. W., Hawkins, M., Collins, P. A., Buchbinder, R., & Osborne, R. H. (2016). Health literacy: applying current concepts to improve health services and reduce health inequalities. *Public Health, 132*, 3–12.

Bennett, I. M., Chen, J., Soroui, J. S., & White, S. (2009). The contribution of health literacy to disparities in self-rated health status and preventive health behaviors in older adults. *Annals of Family Medicine, 7*(3), 204–211.

Berkman, N. D., Davis, T. C., & McCormack, L. (2010). Health literacy: what is it?. *Journal of Health Communication, 15*(S2), 9–19.

Berkman, L. F., & Krishna, A. (2014). Social network epidemiology. In L. F. Berman & I. Kawachi (Eds.). *Social epidemiology* (2nd ed.). New York: Oxford University Press.

Bhattacharya, G. (2003). Social-environmental influences on HIV risks: Implications for HIV prevention. *Journal of HIV/AIDS & Social Services, 2*(3), 11–31.

Bronfenbrenner, U. (1979). *The ecology of human development: Experiments by nature and design.* Cambridge, MA: Harvard University.

Bronfenbrenner, U. (2004). *Making human beings human: Bioecological perspectives on human development.* Thousand Oaks, CA: Sage Publications.

Burke, J. G. (2003). Intimate partner violence among low income women: Associated individual and contextual risk factors (Doctoral dissertation, Johns Hopkins University). *Dissertation Abstracts International, 64*(O2), 659B University Microfilms No. 3080630.

Buzi, R. S., Smith, P. B., Weinman, M. L., & Novello, G. (2013). HIV risk perceptions among adolescents attending family planning clinics: An integrated perspective. *AIDS Care, 25*(1), 20–27.

Centers for Disease Control and Prevention (2017a). *Prevention research centers: Building a healthy world.* Retrieved from https://www.cdc.gov/prc/pdf/PRC-Building-A-Healthly-World.pdf

Centers for Disease Control and Prevention. (2017b). *Global health.* Retrieved from https://www.cdc.gov/globalhealth/index.html

Centers for Disease Control and Prevention. (2017c). *Morbidity mortality weekly report.* Retrieved from https://www.cdc.gov/mmwr/mmwr_wk.html

Centers for Disease Control and Prevention. (2017d). *Supplemental testing for confirmation of reactive oral fluid rapid HIV antibody tests.* Retrieved from https://www.cdc.gov/mmwr/preview/mmwrhtml/mm5450a5.htm

Centers for Disease Control and Prevention. (2017e). PE*ARLS—A Depression Management Program for Elderly Adults.* Retrieved from https://www.cdc.gov/prc/prevention-strategies/program-encourage-active-rewarding-lives-seniors-depression-management.htm

Centers for Disease Control and Prevention. (2017f). *Reading writing and reducing obesity.* Retrieved from https://www.cdc.gov/prc/pdf/prc_planethealth_story.pdf

Centers for Disease Control and Prevention. (2017g). *Vaccines and preventable diseases.* Retrieved from https://www.cdc.gov/vaccines/vpd/index.html

Chandler, R., Ansley, E. H., Ross, H., & Morrison-Beedy, D. (2016). Perceptions of Black college women on barriers to HIV-risk reduction and their HIV prevention intervention needs. *The Journal of the Association of Nurses in AIDS Care : JANAC, 27*(4), 392–403.

Chinn, D. (2011). Critical health literacy: A review and critical analysis. *Social Science and Medicine, 73*, 60–67.

Coleman, C. A., Hudson, S., & Maine, L. L. (2013). Health literacy practices and educational competencies for health professionals: a consensus study. *Journal of Health Communication, 18*(Suppl 1), 82–102.

Coleman, C., Hudson, S., & Pederson, B. (2017). Prioritized health literacy and clear communication practices for health care professionals. *HLRP: Health Literacy Research and Practice, 1*(3), e91–e99.

Crepaz, N., Horn, A. K., Rama, S. M., Griffin, T., DeLuca, J. B., Mullins, M. M., & Aral, S. O. (2007). The efficacy of behavioral interventions in reducing HIV risk sex behaviors and incident sexually transmitted disease in Black and Hispanic sexually transmitted disease clinic patients in the United States: A meta-analytic review. *Sexually Transmitted Diseases, 34*, 319–332.

Crondahl, K., & Eklund Karlsson, L. (2016). The nexus between health literacy and empowerment: A scoping review. Sage Open, April-June 2016, 1–7. doi: 10.1177/2158244016646410

Cutilli, C. C., & Bennett, I. M. (2009). Understanding the health literacy of America: Results of the National Association of Adult Literacy. *Orthopaedic Nursing, 28*(1), 27–32.

DeMarco, R., & Johnsen, C. (2002). Vulnerable populations: Women living with HIV/AIDS. In E. A. Mahoney & J. K. Shaw (Eds.). *HIV/AIDS nursing secrets* (pp. 135–142). Philadelphia, PA: Hanley & Belfus, Inc.

DeMarco, R., & Johnsen, C. (2003). Taking action in communities: Women living with HIV lead the way. *Journal of Community Health Nursing, 20*(1), 51–62.

DeMarco, R., Johnsen, C., Fukuda, D., & Deffenbaugh, O. (2001). Content validity of a scale to measure silencing and affectivity among women living with HIV/AIDs. *Journal of Association of Nurses in AIDS Care, 12*(4), 49–60.

DeMarco, R., Lynch, M. M., & Board, R. (2002). Mothers who silence themselves: Clinical implications for women living with HIV/AIDS and their children. *Journal of Pediatric Nursing, 17*(2), 89–95.

DeMarco, R. F., Miller, K., Patsdaughter, C., Grindel, C., & Chisholm, M. (1998). From silencing the self to action: Experiences of women living with HIV/AIDS. *Women's Health Care International, 19*(6), 539–552.

DeMarco, R., & Norris, A. E. (2004a). Women's voices women's lives: A Web-based HIV prevention film project. In J. V. M. Welie & J. Lee (Eds.). *Jesuit health sciences and the promotion of justice: An invitation to a discussion* (pp. 203–209). Milwaukee, WI: Marquette University Press.

DeMarco, R., & Norris, A. E. (2004b). Culturally relevant HIV interventions: Transcending ethnicity. *Journal of Cultural Diversity, 11*(2), 65–68.

Earnshaw, V. A., Smith, L., Chaudoir, S. R., Lee, I., & Copenhaver, M. M. (2012). Stereotypes about people living with HIV: Implications for perceptions of HIV risk and testing frequency among at-risk populations. *AIDS Education & Prevention, 24*(6), 574–581.

Eddy, J. M., Donahue, R. E., Webster, R. D., & Bjournstad, E. D. (2002). Application of an ecological perspective in worksite health promotion: A review. *American Journal of Health Studies, 17*(4), 197–202.

Edwards, L. V. (2006). Perceived social support and HIV/AIDS medication adherence among African American women. *Qualitative Health Research, 16*(5), 679–691.

El-Bassel, N., Witte, S. S., Gilbert, L., Wu, E., Chang, M., Hill, J., & Steinglass, P. (2003). The efficacy of a relationship-based HIV/STD prevention program for heterosexual couples. *American Journal of Public Health, 93*(6), 963–969.

Fernandez-Gutierrez, M., Bas-Sarmiento, P., Albar-Marin, M. J., Paloma-Castro, O., & Romero-Sanches, J. M. (2017). Health literacy interventions for immigrant populations: A systematic review. *International Nursing Review, 65*, 54–64.

Fishbein, M., & Ajzen, I. (1975). *Belief, attitude, intention, and behavior: An introduction to theory and research.* Reading, MA: Addison-Wesley.

Freedman, D. A., Bess, K. D., Tucker, H. A., Boyd, D. L., Tuchman, A. M., & Wallston, K. A. (2009). Public health literacy defined. *American Journal of Preventative Medicine, 36*(5), 446–451.

Gasink, L. B., & Lautenbach, E. (2008). Prevention and treatment of health care-acquired infections. *Medical Clinics of North America, 92*(2), 295–313.

Glanz, K., Rimer, B. K., & Viswanath, K. (2015). *Health behavior, theory, research, and practice* (5th ed.). San Francisco, CA: Jossey-Bass.

Glover, D. A., Loeb, T. B., Carmona, J. V., Sciolla, A., Zhang, M., Myer, H. F., & Wyatt, G. E. (2010). Childhood sexual abuse severity and disclosure predict posttraumatic stress symptoms and biomarkers in ethnic minority women. *Journal of Trauma & Dissociation, 11*(2), 152–173.

Han, H. R., Song, Y., Kim, M., Hedlin, H. K., Kim, K., Ben Lee, H., & Roter, D.. (2017). Breast and cervical cancer screening literacy among Korean American women: A community health worker-led intervention. *American Journal of Public Health, 107*(1), 159–165.

Haynes, R. B., Ackloo, E., & Sahota, N. (2008). Interventions for enhancing medication adherence. *Cochrane Database of Systematic Reviews, 2*, CD000011.

Healthy People 2020. (2017a). *2020 Topics and objectives.* Retrieved from https://www.healthypeople.gov/2020/topics-objectives

Healthy People 2020. (2017b). *Development of the national health promotion and disease prevention objectives for 2030.* Retrieved from https://www.healthypeople.gov/2020/About-Healthy-People/Development-Healthy-People-2030.

Herek, G., Gillis, J. R., & Cogan, J. C. (2009). Internalized stigma among sexual minority adults: Insights from a social psychological perspective. *Journal of Counseling Psychology, 56*, 32–43.

Hochbaum, G. (1956). Why people seek diagnostic x-rays. *Public Health Reports, 71*, 377–380.

Hodder, S. L., Justman, J., Hughes, J. P., Wang, J., Haley, D. F., Adimora, A. A., … El-Sadr, W. M. (2013). HIV acquisition among women from selected areas of the United States: A cohort study. *Annals of Internal Medicine, 158*(1), 10–18.

Homsy, J., Thomson-Honnebier, G. A., Cheng-Mayer, C., & Levy, J. A. (1988). Detection of human immunodeficiency virus (HIV) in serum and body fluids by sequential competition ELISA. *Journal of Virological Methods, 19*(1), 43–56.

HOPE (Health, Opportunities, Partnerships, Empowerment) WORKS. (2017). Retrieved from http://hpdp.unc.edu/research/projects/hope-works/. Accessed November 18, 2017.

Howard, D. H., Gazmararian, D. H., & Parker, J. (2005). The impact of low health literacy on the medical costs of medicar managed care enrollees. *The American Journal of Medicine, 118*, 371–377.

HRSA. (2017). *A guide for evaluation and treatment of Hepatitis C in adult co-infected with HIV.* Retrieved from https://hab.hrsa.gov/sites/default/files/hab/clinical-quality-management/hepccoinfectguide2011.pdf.

Institute of Medicine. (2004). *Health literacy: A prescription to end confusion.* Washington, DC: The National Academies Press.

Ironson, G., O'Cleirigh, C., Fletcher, M. A., Laurenceau, J. P., Balbin, E., Klimas, N., & Solomon, G. (2005). Psychosocial factors predict CD4 and viral load change in men and women with human immunodeficiency virus in the era of highly active antiretroviral treatment. *Psychosomatic Medicine, 67*(6), 1013–1021.

Jack, D. C. (1991). *Silencing the self.* Cambridge, MA: Harvard University Press.

Jack, D. C. (1999). *Behind the mask.* Cambridge, MA: Harvard University Press.

The Joint Commission. (2007). *What did the doctor say?: Improving health literacy to protect patient safety.* Retrieved from https://www.jointcommission.org/assets/1/18/improving_health_literacy.pdf

Kalichman, S., Katner, H., Banas, E., & Kalichman, M. (2017). Population density and AIDS-related stigma in large-urban, small-urban, and rural communities of the Southeastern USA. *Prevention Science, 18*(5), 517–525.

Kessels, R. P. (2003). Patients' memory for medical information. *Journal of the Royal Society of Medicine, 96*(5), 219–222.

Kim, S., Darwish, S., Lee, S., & DeMarco, R. (2017). A Pilot Smoking Cessation Intervention Study for Women Living with HIV: Study Protocol. *Open Access Journal of Clinical Trials, 9*, 11–20.

Koh, H. K., Blakey, C. R., & Roper, A. Y. (2014). Health People 2020: A report card on the health of the nation. *Journal of the American Medical Association, 311*(24), 2475–2476.

Kulbok, P. A., Thatcher, E., Park, E., & Meszaros, P. S. (2012). Evolving public health nursing roles: Focus on community participatory health promotion and prevention. *The Online Journal of Nursing Issues, 17*(2). doi: 10.3912/OJIN.Vol17No02Man01

Lanier, L. R., & DeMarco, R. F. (2015). A Synthesis of the Theory of Silencing the Self and the Social Ecological Model: Understanding Gender, Race, and Depression in African American Women Living with HIV Infection. *AIDS Patient Care and STDs, 29*(3), 142–149. doi: 10.1089/apc.2014.0116.

Lennon, C. A., Huedo-Medina, T. B., Gerwien, D. P., & Johnson, B. T. (2012). A role for depression in sexual risk reduction for women? A meta-analysis of HIV prevention trials with depression outcomes. *Social Science & Medicine, 75*(4), 688–698.

Liang, L., & Brach, C. (2017). Health literacy universal precautions are still a distant dream: Analysis of US data on health literate practices. *HLRP: Health Literacy Research and Practice, 1*(4), e216–e230.

Liebschutz, J. M., Geier, J. L., Horton, N. J., Chuang, C. H., & Samet, J. H. (2005). Physical and sexual violence and health care utilization in HIV-infected persons with alcohol problems. *AIDS Care, 17*(5), 566–578.

Liu, E., Stephenson, T., Houlihan, J., & Gustafson, A. (2017). Marketing strategies to encourage rural residents of high obesity counties to buy fruits and vegetables in grocery stores. *Preventing Chronic Disease, (14),* E94.

Logie, C., & Gadalla, T. M. (2009). Meta-analysis of health and demographic correlates of stigma towards people living with HIV. *AIDS Care, 21*(6), 742–753.

Luciano, A., Bryan, E. L., Carpenter-Song, E. A, Woods, M., Armstrong, K., & Drake, R. E. (2014). Long-term sobriety strategies for men with co-occurring disorders. *Journal of Dual Diagnosis, 10*(4), 212–219.

Mahajan, A. P., Sayles, J. N., Patel, V. A., Remien, R. H., Sawires, S. R., Ortiz, D. J., & Coates, T. J. (2008). Stigma in the HIV/AIDS

REFERENCES *(Continued)*

epidemic: A review of the literature and recommendations for the way forward. *AIDS, 22*(Suppl 2), S67–S79.

McLeroy, K. R., Bibeau, D., Steckler, A., & Glanz, K. (1988). An ecological perspective on health promotion programs. *Health Education Quarterly, 15*(4), 351–374.

Mitchell, N. S., Ellison, M. C., Hill, J. O., & Tsai, A. G. (2013). Evaluation of the effectiveness of making weight watchers available to Tennessee Medicaid (TennCare) recipients. *Journal of General Internal Medicine, 28*(1), 12–17.

Mize, S. J., Robinson, B. E., Bockting, W. O., & Scheltema, K. E. (2002). Meta-analysis of the effectiveness of HIV prevention interventions for women. *AIDS Care, 14*(2), 163–180.

Motivational Interviewing. (2017). Retrieved from https://www.umass.edu/studentlife/sites/default/files/documents/pdf/Motivational_Interviewing_Definition_Principles_Approach.pdf

Myers, H. F., Wyatt, G. E., Loeb, T. B., & Carmona, J. (2006). Severity of child sexual abuse, post-traumatic stress and risky sexual behaviors among HIV-positive women. *AIDS and Behavior, 10*(2), 191–199.

National Academies of Sciences, Engineering and Medicine. (2018). *Community-based health literacy interventions: Proceedings of a workshop.* Washington, DC: National Academy Press.

National Center for Education Statistics. (1993). *Adult literacy in America: National Adult Literacy Survey.* Washington, DC: US Department of Education.

National Center for Education Statistics. (2006). *The health literacy of America's adults: Results from the 2003 national assessment of adult literacy.* Washington, DC: US Department of Education.

National Patient Safety Foundation [NPSF]. (2018). *Health literacy.* Retrieved from https://www.npsf.org/page/healthliteracy?&hhsearchterms=%22health+and+literacy%22

Norris, A. E., & DeMarco, R. (2004). The mechanics of conducting culturally relevant HIV prevention research with Haitian American adolescents: Lessons learned. *Journal of Multicultural Nursing and Health, 11*(1), 69–76.

Norris, A. E., & DeMarco, R. (2005). The experience of African American women living with HIV creating a prevention film for teens. *Journal of the Association of Nurses in AIDS Care, 16*(2), 32–39.

Nutbeam, D. (2000). Health literacy as a public health goal: A challenge for contemporary health education and communication strategies into the 21st century. *Health Promotion International, 15*(3), 259–267.

Nutbeam, D. (2008). The evolving concept of health literacy. *Social Science and Medicine, 67*, 2072–2078.

O'Donnell, M. P. (2009). Definition of Health Promotion 2.0: Embracing Passion, Enhancing Motivation, Recognizing Dynamic Balance, and Creating Opportunities. *American Journal of Health Promotion, 24*(1), 4–5.

Owusu, D., Quinn, M., Wang, K. S., Aibangbee, J., & Mamudu, H. M. (2017). Intentions to quit smoking in 14 low and middle income countries based on the transtheoretical model. *Drug and Alcohol Dependence, 178*, 425–429.

Parker, R., & Ratzan, S. C. (2010). Health literacy: A second decade of distinction for Americans. *Journal of Health Communication, 2*(15), S20–S33.

Plain Writing Act of 2010 (the Act). (2010). *Public Law 111–274. 111th Congress.* Washington, DC: Congress of the United States. October 13, 2010. Retrieved from http://www.gpo.gov/fdsys/pkg/PLAW-111publ274/pdf/PLAW-111publ274.pdf

Pleasant, A., Cabe, J., Patel, K., Cosenza, J., & Carmona, R. (2015). Health literacy research and practice: A needed paradigm shift. *Health Communication, 30*, 1176–1180.

Pleasant, A., Rudd, R. E., O'Leary, C., Paasche-Orlow, M. K., Allen, M. P., Alvarado-Little, W., … Rosen, S. (2016). *Considerations for a new definition of health literacy.* Discussion Paper, Washington, DC: National Academy of Medicine. Retrieved from http://nam.edu/wp-content/uploads/2016/04/Considerations-for-a-New-Definition-ofHealth-Literacy.pdf.

Prochaska, J. O., & DiClemente, R. (1983). Stages and processes of self-change of smoking: Toward an integrative model of change. *Journal of Consulting and Clinical Psychology, 5*(3), 390–395.

Program for the International Assessment of Adult Competencies. (2016). Retrieved from https://nces.ed.gov/surveys/piaac/.

Rackow, P., Scholz, U., & Hornung, R. (2015). Received social support and exercising: An intervention study to test the enabling hypothesis. *British Journal of Health Psychology, 20*(4), 763–776.

Richards, C. L., Viadro, C. I., & Earp, J. A. (1998). Bringing down the barriers to mammography: A review of current research and interventions. *Breast Disease, 10*(4), 33–44.

Rikard, R. V., Thompson, M. S., McKinney, J., & Beauchamp, A. (2016). Examining health literacy disparities in the United States: A third look at the national assessment of adult literacy (NAAL). *BMC Public Health, 16*, 975–985.

Rollnick, S., & Miller, W. R. (1995). What is motivational interviewing? *Behavioral and Cognitive Psychotherapy, 23*, 325–334.

Rosenstock, I. (1974). The health belief model and preventive health behavior. *Health Education Monographs, 2*, 354–385.

Rudd, R. (2010). Improving Americans' health literacy. *New England Journal of Medicine, 363*(24), 2283–2285.

Rudd, R. E. (2015). The evolving concept of Health literacy: New directions for health literacy studies. *Journal of Communication in Healthcare, 8*(1), 7–9.

Schaalma, H. P., Abraham, C., Gillmore, M. R., & Kok, G. (2004). Sex education as health promotion: What does it take? *Archives of Sexual Behavior, 33*(3), 259–269.

Schillinger, D., Grumbach, K., Piette, J., Wang, F., Osmond, D., Daher, C., … Bindman, A. B. (2002). Association of health literacy with diabetes outcomes. *Journal of the American Medical Association, 288*(4), 475–482.

Scoliosis Screening. (2017). Retrieved from http://iscoliosis.com/symptoms-screening.html

Simoni, J. M., Huang, B., Goodry, E. J., & Montoya, H. D. (2005). Social support and depressive symptomatology among HIV-Positive women: The mediating role of self-esteem and mastery. *Women and Health, 42*(4), 1–15.

Simoni, J. M., Walters, K. L., & Nero, D. K. (2000). Safer sex among HIV-positive women: The role of relationships. *Sex Roles, 42*, 691–708.

Skinner, B. F. (1953). *Science and human behavior.* New York: Macmillan.

Smeltzer, S. C., Robinson-Smith, G., Dolen, M. A., Duffin, J. M., & Al Maqbali, M. (2010). Disability-related content in nursing textbooks. *Nursing Education Perspectives,31*(3), 148–155.

Sørensen, K., Van Den Broucke, S., Fullam, J., Doyle, G., Pelikan, J., Slonska, Z., & Brand, H. (2012). Health literacy and public health: A systematic review and integration of definitions and models. *BMC Public Health, 12*, Article 80.

Speros, C. (2006). Health literacy: Concept analysis. *Journal of Advanced Nursing, 50*, 633–640.

Speros, C. (2011). Promoting health literacy: A nursing imperative. *Nursing Clinics of North America, 46*, 321–333.

Stockman, J. K., Lucea, M. B, Draughon, J. E., Sabri, B., Anderson, J. C., Bertrand, D., … Campbell, J. C. (2013). Intimate partner violence and HIV risk factors among African-American and African-Caribbean women in clinic-based settings. *AIDS Care, 25*(4), 472–480.

Sudore, R. L., & Schillinger, D. (2009). Interventions to improve care of patients with limited health literacy. *Journal of Clinical Outcomes Management, 16*(1), 20–29.

Taylor, M. (2013). Exploring practices of harm reduction. *Alberta Association of Registered Nurses, 68*(4), 17–19.

Toronto, C. E. (2016). Health literacy competencies for registered nurses: an e-Delphi study. *The Journal of Continuing Education in Nursing, 47*(12), 558–565.

Toronto, C. E., & Weatherford, B. (2015). Health literacy education in health professions schools: an integrative review. *Journal of Nursing Education, 54*(12), 669–676.

U.S. Department of Health and Human Services, Office of Disease Prevention and Health Promotion. (2010). *National action plan to improve health literacy.* Washington, DC: Author. Retrieved from https://health.gov/communication/hlactionplan/pdf/Health_Literacy_Action_Plan.pdf

VanDyke, S. D., & Shell, M. D. (2017). Health beliefs and breast cancer screening in rural Appalachia: An evaluation of the Health Belief Model. *The Journal of Rural Health, 33*(4), 350–360.

Vernon, J. A., Trujillo, A., Rosenbaum, S. J., & DeBuono, B. (2007). *Low health literacy: Implications for national health policy.* Washington, DC: Department of Health Policy, School of Public Health and Health Services, The George Washington University. Retrieved from https://hsrc.himmelfarb.gwu.edu/sphhs_policy_facpubs/172/

Wakeford, R. (2015). Association and causation in epidemiology-Half a century since the publication of Bradford Hill's interpretational guidance. *Journal of the Royal Society of Medicine, 108*(1), 4–6.

Webber, R. (2016). *Communicable diseases: A global perspective* (5th ed.). Boston, MA: CABI.

Weiss, B. D., Mays, M. Z., Martz, W., Castro, K. M., DeWalt, D. A., Pignone, M. P., … Hale, F. A. (2005). Quick assessment of literacy in primary care: the newest vital sign. *The Annals of Family Medicine, 3*(6), 514–522.

White, S. (2008). *Assessing the nation's health literacy: Key concepts and findings of the national assessment of adult literacy (NAAL).* Chicago, IL: American Medical Association Foundation.

White, S., Chen, J., & Atchison, R. (2008). Relationship of preventive health practices and health literacy: a national study. *American Journal of Health Behavior, 32*(3), 227–242.

Widman, L., Golin, C. E., & Noar, S. M. (2013). When do condom use intentions lead to actions? Examining the role of sexual communication on safer sexual behavior among people living with HIV. *Journal of health psychology, 18*(4), 507–517.

Wieland, M. L., Weis, J. A., Hanza, M. M., Meiers, S. J., Patten, C. A., Clark, M. M., … Sia, I. G. (2016). Healthy immigrant families: Participatory development and baseline characteristics of a community-based physical activity and nutrition intervention. *Contemporary Clinical Trials, 47*, 22–31.

Willie, T. C., Overstreet, N. M., Sullivan, T. P., Sikkema, K. J., & Hansen, N. B. (2016). Barriers to HIV medication adherence: Examining distinct anxiety and depression symptoms among women living with HIV who experienced childhood sexual abuse. *Behavioral Medicine,42*(2), 120–127.

Wolitski, R. J., Janssen, R. S., Onorato, I. M., Purcell, D. W., & Crepaz, N. (2005). An overview of prevention with people living with HIV. In S. C. Kalichman (Ed.), *Positive prevention: reducing HIV transmission among people living with HIV/AIDS* (pp. 1–28). New York: Kluwer.

World Health Organization. (1986). *The Ottawa Charter for Health Promotion … 21 November 1986.* Geneva: World Health Organization. Retrieved from http://www.euro.who.int/__data/assets/pdf_file/0004/129532/Ottawa_Charter.pdf

World Health Organization. (2016). United Nations Development Program. Policy brief 4: Health literacy. In: 9th Global Conference on Health Promotion. Retrieved from file:///C:/Users/judith.walsh/Downloads/Policy%20brief%204%20-%20Health%20literacy%20-%20FINAL%20-%20CORR3.pdf

World Health Organization. (2018). *Health Promotion-promoting healthier populations.* Retrieved from http://www.who.int/topics/health_promotion/en/

World Health Organization (WHO). (2018b). *Health Promotion Track 2: Health literacy and health behavior. 7th Global Conference on Health Promotion: track themes.* Retrieved from https://www.who.int/healthpromotion/conferences/7gchp/track2/en/

Yohannes, A. M., Mulerova, H., Vestbo, J., Rennard, S. I., Wouters, E., & Hanania, N. A. (2017). The association of depressive symptoms with rates of acute exacerbations in patients with COPD: Results from a 3-year longitudinal follow-up of the ECLIPSE cohort. *Journal of the American Medical Directors Association, 18*(11), 955–959.

Zarcadoolas, C., Pleasant, A., & Greer, D. S. (2009). *Advancing health literacy: A framework for understanding and action* (Vol. 45). San Francisco, CA: John Wiley & Sons.

Zimmermann, T., Scott, J. L., & Heinrichs, N. (2010). Individual and dyadic predictors of body image in women with breast cancer. *Psycho-oncology, 19*(10), 1061–1068.

6

Epidemiology: The Science of Prevention

Patrice Nicholas and Patricia Lussier-Duynstee

There are in fact two things, science and opinion, the former begets knowledge, the latter ignorance.

Hippocrates

Science is organized common sense, where many a beautiful theory was killed by an ugly fact.

Thomas Huxley

Get your facts first, then you can distort them as you please.

Mark Twain

CHAPTER HIGHLIGHTS

- Defining epidemiology
- Development of epidemiology as a science
- Epidemiologic conceptual frameworks
- Applying epidemiologic principles in practice
- Assessment of health needs and assets
- Using assessment data for planning and implementing interventions
- Promoting healthy lifestyles
- Preventing and controlling outbreaks
- Contributing to a safe and healthy environment
- Evaluating the effectiveness of health services

OBJECTIVES

- Trace the origins of epidemiology.
- Comprehend the basic principles and scope of epidemiology.
- Contrast three epidemiologic conceptual models.
- Apply principles of epidemiology to *Healthy People 2020*.
- Relate the problem-solving process to both the epidemiologic process and the nursing process.
- Apply epidemiologic principles to the practice of public health nursing.

KEY TERMS

Epidemic: An outbreak that occurs when there is an increased incidence of a disease beyond that which is normally found in the population.

Epidemiologic triad: Model based on the belief that health status is determined by the interaction of the characteristics of the host, agent, and environment.

Epidemiology: Study of the distribution and determinants of states of health and illness in human populations; used both as a research methodology to study states of health and illness, and as a body of knowledge that results from the study of a specific state of health or illness.

Natural history: Course of a disease or condition from the onset to resolution.

Outbreak: Epidemic usually limited to a localized increase in the incidence of the illness.

Rate: Primary measurement used to describe either the occurrence or the existence of a specific state of health or illness.

Risk: Probability or likelihood that a disease or illness will occur in a group of people who presently do not have the problem.

Risk factor: Characteristics or events that have been shown to increase the probability that a specific disease or illness will develop.

Web of causation: Epidemiologic model that strongly emphasizes the concept of multiple causation while

de-emphasizing the role of agents in explaining illness.

Wheel of causation: Epidemiologic model that de-emphasizes the agent as the sole cause of disease while emphasizing the interplay of physical, biologic, and social environments.

CASE STUDY

References to the case study are found throughout this chapter (look for the case study icon). Readers should keep the case study in mind as they read the chapter.

In 2011, there were an estimated 782,500 gang members in the United States. In 2012, an increase brought the known total to 850,000, with an estimated 30,700 gangs, up from 29,900 in 2011. Gang members often come from socially and economically disadvantaged communities. In 2012, cities with populations of 50,000 or more had a prevalence of 85.6 as compared to suburban counties at 49.5, smaller cities at 25.4, and rural counties at 16.0. Gang members commit a disproportionate amount of violence and crime compared with youths not involved in gangs. Gang members are also more likely to use drugs and alcohol, as well as engage in unsafe sex. As a result, youths who belong to gangs can be considered a vulnerable population at increased risk for negative health outcomes. Public health nurses in large cities have developed programs that target youths in gangs. These nurses represent local healthcare facilities, community service agencies, churches, schools, businesses, and other neighborhood groups focusing on increasing access to expanded community health services, promoting healthy living behaviors and fostering a positive community environment. *Healthy People 2020* (Centers for Disease Control and Prevention [CDC], 2010a) objectives

include decreasing the proportion of secondary school students who report the presence of youth gangs at school during the school year with a baseline of 12.4% and a target of 10.4%.

(2012 National Youth Gang Survey; Healthy People 2020)

Katie, a public health nurse in Los Angeles, has developed a partnership with a local police department juvenile diversion program that offers a delinquency prevention program to young people from 13 to 18 years of age. These young people have been arrested for nonviolent offenses, such as possession of drugs, burglary, theft, joy riding, and vandalism. Some of these young people are gang members, and others are at risk for joining gangs because they come from neighborhoods with long histories of gang activity. Katie's responsibilities are to lead interactive three-hour sessions that primarily focus on health-related issues for the youths. She identifies three topics for discussion: (1) major causes of morbidity and mortality in youth, (2) major health issues common in a particular age group, and (3) risk prevention and health promotion (adapted from Sanders, Schneiderman, Loken, Lankenau, & Bloom, 2009).

L ike other types of modern science, epidemiology arose from building blocks constructed by ancient civilizations. Humans have experienced disease for as long as they have existed, and in the early days, attempts that people made to understand the onset of disease and to prevent its occurrence were crude. People perceived health as something holy, and healers looked to the spiritual world to protect health and prolong life. People often considered disease and disability as a great curse and a divine punishment, and they believed that amulets, totems, charms, and rituals prevented all sorts of evils. However, early cave dwellers experimented with medicinal plants and became adept at treating some illnesses. These discoveries were

primarily a direct result of trial-and-error observations, enhanced by doses of curiosity, common sense, and chance.

For thousands of years, the practice of healing slowly developed as humans observed that more and more herbal remedies and therapeutic treatments had beneficial results. Some cultures, such as in Egypt, had an extensive repertoire of treatments. More than 700 remedies existed for ailments resulting from crocodile bites to infections following childbirth. Practitioners at that time reduced dislocations, aligned and immobilized fractures, and applied hot and cold treatments to reduce inflammation. People recognized and understood differences in individual constitutions and observed that many diseases were contagious in nature.

Interestingly, they conceptualized the influence of the environment on the occurrence of disease. However, priests and religious healers kept most of this knowledge secret.

Hippocrates of Cos (460 to 370 BC), considered the father of modern medicine, was the first person to record these secrets in writing. In a textbook of medicine that was used for centuries, he recorded the belief that external factors in the environment were a cause of illness in humans. He wrote of the effects of seasons, winds, and water, as well as the characteristics of the ground. He encouraged healers to observe what are known today as lifestyle patterns: "what are their pursuits, whether they are fond of drinking and eating to excess, and given to indolence, or are fond of exercise and labor" (Hippocrates, 1938). Hippocrates also wrote *On Air, Waters and Places*, a book that provided details on the relationship between humans and the environment. Experts now consider this book as a milestone in the development of the science of epidemiology, illustrating the connection between human life and the environment. However, people overlooked this concept for centuries, and it was not seriously considered again until investigators in the late 19th century developed the science of bacteriology.

Men and women today still search for reasons for their illnesses, and many still perceive illness as a punishment for sins. However, the wealth of scientific knowledge developed within the last 160 years has permitted the understanding of the complexities of the human body and the effects of internal and external stressors. This knowledge has provided the means for preventing and modifying illness and repairing disabilities. Much of this knowledge has been gained through the extension of the observations of the past to the rigorous study of specific illnesses or disabilities in large groups of people.

DEFINING EPIDEMIOLOGY

Early attempts to understand illness and disease focused on studying the experiences of individual people. Today, clinicians consider these case reports or case studies. Studying individual experiences is invaluable for forming ideas, or hypotheses, about possible causes of specific diseases. However, studying individual people may not provide accurate information about the characteristics of the disease being investigated, because individual experiences with a disease may vary. Also, examining the experiences of individual persons does not provide evidence of causality (see Chapter 8). To gather more accurate information about disease, studying groups of people is essential.

An example is the relationship between smoking and lung cancer that experts statistically determined in the 20th century. Without studying the experiences of groups of people, they may never have identified this relationship. Some smokers never develop lung cancer, and some nonsmokers do develop lung cancer. However, epidemiologists Doll and Hill, in the 1950s, demonstrated the relationship between lung cancer and smoking by comparing a group of people with lung cancer to a group of people without lung cancer. They discovered that the people with lung cancer had smoked significantly more cigarettes than those without lung cancer (Doll & Hill, 1950). Further epidemiologic research studies provided more evidence of a causal link between smoking cigarettes and lung cancer.

Unfortunately, after 50 years, smoking is still a cause of significant illness and death throughout the world. In the United States alone, in 2015, 15.1% of all adults were identified as smokers, as defined by smoking every day. The percentage is even greater in American Indians/Alaska Natives, multiple race individuals, and non-Hispanic Blacks (CDC, 2016).

Epidemiology as the science of prevention emerged from the rigorous study of disease and illness in groups of people. **Epidemiology** is defined as the study of the distribution and determinants of states of health and illness in human populations. States of health and illness include health, disease, morbidity, injuries, disability, and mortality. The goals of epidemiology are to prevent or limit the consequences of illness and disability in humans, as well as to maximize their state of health (Harkness, 1995). The word *epidemiology* is derived from the word **epidemic** in the Greek language: *epi*—upon, *demo*—people, and *logos*—thought. In epidemiology, the community replaces the individual client as the primary focus of concern (Mausner & Kramer, 1985).

The science of epidemiology has been traditionally associated with infectious disease. Many of the techniques used in epidemiologic investigations were developed when cholera was killing much of the population of Europe. Therefore, early epidemiologic attempts to control and prevent infectious disease involved altering the characteristics of the agent, the host, and the environment (see Chapter 14).

The scope of epidemiology has expanded and shifted substantially. Primarily as a result of improved public health practices in the early 20th century, life expectancy in the United States, the United Kingdom, and European countries, as well as in other developed countries, rose. With it, a change in the patterns of disease occurred. No longer are infectious diseases the leading causes of death; the morbidity and mortality from noninfectious diseases and chronic degenerative conditions have increased (Table 6.1). Advancing technology in the 20th century made everyday life increasingly complex. There were unparalleled changes in diagnostic practices and therapeutic methods, resulting in expanded strategies for the prevention and control of disease. A focus on maintenance of wellness evolved.

> All truths are easy to understand once they are discovered—the point is to discover them. **Galileo Galilei**

Investigators now use epidemiologic techniques to study all aspects of health, including factors that keep people well. Chronic disease, psychosocial problems, occupational injuries, environmental effects, and the planning and evaluation of health services are but a few of the disciplines that have

TABLE 6.1 Comparison of the Leading Causes of Death in the United States, 1900 and 2010

1900[a]	2010[b]
1. Major cardiovascular–renal disease	1. Heart disease
2. Influenza and pneumonia	2. Malignant neoplasms (cancer)
3. Tuberculosis	3. Chronic lower respiratory diseases
4. Gastritis, duodenitis, enteritis, and colitis	4. Cerebrovascular diseases (stroke)
5. Accidents	5. Unintentional injuries
6. Malignant neoplasms	6. Alzheimer disease
7. Diphtheria	7. Diabetes mellitus
8. Typhoid and paratyphoid fever	8. Nephritis, nephritic syndrome, and nephrosis
9. Measles	9. Influenza and pneumonia
10. Cirrhosis of the liver	10. Suicide

[a]United States Census Bureau. (1975). *Historical statistics of the United States, colonial times to 1970,* bicentennial edition, Part 2. Washington, DC.
[b]Centers for Disease Control and Prevention. *Health, United States, 2013.* Retrieved from http://www.cdc.gov/nchs/hus.htm.

been enhanced by using principles of epidemiology. Today, epidemiology is both a *research methodology* used to study states of health and illness and a *body of knowledge* that results from the study of a specific state of health or illness. When using epidemiology as a research methodology, the calculation of **rates** is the primary measurement used to describe either the occurrence or the existence of a specific state of health or illness (see Chapter 7).

How can Katie use these principles of epidemiology, both as a research method and as a body of knowledge, in her preparation for the three-hour sessions? How does her knowledge interface with *Healthy People 2020* (CDC, 2010a) data?

DEVELOPMENT OF EPIDEMIOLOGY AS A SCIENCE

John Graunt and the Bills of Mortality

The study of illness in groups of people developed gradually. One of the first people to study patterns of disease in populations was a London haberdasher, John Graunt. In 1662, he analyzed the weekly reports of births and deaths in London; his analyses were the precursor of modern vital statistics. Graunt found that more male infants were born than female infants and that more men died than women. He also observed that infant mortality was high, and he noted that seasonal variations occurred in deaths.

Through his analysis of the Bills of Mortality, Graunt developed a better understanding of diseases and conditions that led to death. He published his observations and findings in *Natural and Political Observations Made Upon the Bills of Mortality.* Graunt added an essential step in the development of epidemiology as a science. He developed a new logic of statistical inference, demonstrating that examining routinely collected data from groups of people would yield clues to human illness. His publication can be found online.

Two centuries passed before William Farr expanded Graunt's work. In the meantime, James Lind instituted the precursor of the clinical trial when he compared responses to dietary treatments for scurvy, and Percivall Pott observed cancer of the scrotum in English chimney sweeps, hypothesizing that soot was the cause. Edward Jenner performed the first successful vaccination against smallpox with the liquid from a cowpox pustule, resulting in the vaccination of more than 100,000 people in England within three years. These accomplishments in the 18th century linked specific diseases with the characteristics of groups of people and documented the effects of various treatments. Table 6.2 summarizes the milestones in the evolution of epidemiology from 460 BC through the 20th century.

William Farr, Registrar General

In 1839, William Farr was appointed to the new Office of the Registrar General for England and Wales. Farr set up a system for the consistent collection of the numbers and causes of deaths. With these data, he was able to compare the death rates of workers in various occupations, the differences in mortality according to gender, and the effect of imprisonment on mortality. He also discovered an inverse relationship: deaths from cholera decreased with an increase in elevation above sea level (Farr, 1852).

Farr and his predecessors contributed significantly to the understanding of the distribution of illness and death. As one of the first epidemiologists, he recognized (1) the value of a precise definition of both the illness and the population at risk for the illness, (2) the importance of using appropriate comparison groups, and (3) that factors such as age, health status, and environmental exposure can confound statistical results.

TABLE 6.2 Selected Milestones in the Evolution of Epidemiology

Time	Person	Accomplishment or Event
460–377 BC	Hippocrates of Cos	First to record the relationship of the external environment to the health of individuals. Considered the first epidemiologist.
ca. 81 AD	Aretaeus, the Cappadocian	Described pulmonary tuberculosis in detail.
129	Claudius Galen	Described the four humors and introduced many drugs derived from plants. First to describe smallpox.
500	Susruta	Brahmin physician who associated malaria with the mosquito.
850	Rhazes	Arab physician who wrote *al-Hawi*, papers that incorporated all known medical, anatomical, and pharmacologic knowledge of the time. Differentiated smallpox from measles.
1347		Italian 40-day ban on travel and trade was established to control bubonic plague. Quarantine comes from the Italian word *quarentina*, meaning 40 days.
1589	Thomas Moffet	First description of living organisms causing disease: lice, fleas, and scabies mites.
1662	John Graunt	London haberdasher who analyzed weekly reports of births and deaths. Found infant mortality was high and deaths varied according to seasons.
1683	Anton van Leeuwenhoek	Used a microscope to observe and describe "animalcules" from pond water and human saliva.
1701	Nicolas Andry	French surgeon who proposed that infection by germs was a cause of disease.
1747	James Lind	Observed and compared responses to dietary treatments for scurvy—the first evidence of a clinical trial. Recommended preventive techniques for typhus.
1760	Daniel Bernoulli	Demonstrated that smallpox conferred lifelong immunity through the use of the first life table techniques.
1775	Percivall Pott	Observed that many English chimney sweeps developed cancer of the scrotum; hypothesized that exposure to soot was the cause.
1779	Johann Peter Frank	German who wrote *A System of a Complete Medical Policy*, the first book about public health.
1798	Edward Jenner	Discovered the first vaccination against smallpox with cowpox pustule liquid. Within three years, 100,000 people in England were vaccinated.
1800	William Cruikshank	Scottish surgeon who used chlorine to purify water.
1836	Pierre-Charles-Alexandre Louis	Conducted observational studies demonstrating the ineffectiveness of bloodletting. Emphasized statistics.
1840–1860s	William Farr	First Registrar General in England. Considered father of modern statistics. Developed mortality surveillance systems and addressed basic epidemiologic concepts. Pioneered public health reforms.
1846	Peter Ludvig Panum	Danish physician who described the epidemiology of measles and the mechanism for spread of disease.
1847	Ignaz Semmelweis	Hungarian obstetrician who demonstrated that mortality from puerperal fever could be dramatically reduced if doctors washed their hands.
ca. 1850	Jean Baptiste Emile Vidal	French dermatologist responsible for the introduction of an efficient sewage system in Paris.
ca. 1854	John Snow	Performed epidemiologic research on transmission of cholera using natural experiments, mapping, and rates. Removed London's Broad Street drinking water pump handle to stop the spread of cholera.
1854	Florence Nightingale	Initiated sanitary reforms in the Crimean War and demonstrated that preventable or contagious diseases were the primary cause of mortality. Later used statistics to improve public health in England. Considered the founder of the nursing profession.

Time	Person	Accomplishment or Event
ca. 1860	John Parkin	English surgeon who used charcoal filters to purify water in an attempt to prevent the spread of cholera.
1860–1880s	Louis Pasteur	Developed pasteurization. Suggested that living organisms called "germs" caused infectious diseases.
1864		Contagious Diseases Act passed in England to combat the spread of venereal disease.
1865–1880s	Robert Koch	German who discovered the causal agents for anthrax, cholera, and tuberculosis. Developed criteria for identifying cause. Won Nobel Prize for bacteriology in 1905.
1866	Joseph Lister	Developed a carbolic acid spray for surgical disinfections.
1921		Johns Hopkins University established the first academic program in epidemiology.
1927	Wade Hampton Frost	Developed cohort analysis of mortality data and developed life tables. Credited for moving epidemiology from a descriptive to an analytical discipline.
1930		National Institutes of Health established in the United States.
1946		U.S. Communicable Disease Center was established. Now Centers for Disease Control and Prevention (CDC).
1948		Framingham cohort study of cardiovascular disease initiated.
1950s	Richard Doll and A. Bradford Hill	English researchers who conducted the landmark studies on the relationship between smoking and lung cancer.
Second half of the 20th century		Chronic degenerative diseases replaced infectious diseases as leading causes of death worldwide.

Sources: Lee, H. S. J. (2002). *Dates in infectious diseases: A chronological record of progress in infectious diseases over the last millennium.* New York: Parthenon Publishing Group.; Timmreck, T. C. (2002). *An introduction to epidemiology.* Boston, MA: Jones and Bartlett; and Lilienfeld, D. E., & Stolley, P. D. (1994). *Foundations of epidemiology.* New York: Oxford University Press.

John Snow and the Broad Street Pump

Perhaps the best known epidemiologist of the 19th century was John Snow, a contemporary of William Farr. He was a British physician who used population data and his own observations to investigate the epidemic of cholera that occurred from 1848 through 1854. He observed that deaths from cholera were particularly high in the parts of London supplied by two water companies the Lambeth Company and the Southward and Vauxhall Company.

Sewage heavily polluted a section of the Thames River, and interwoven water mains piped untreated water into the homes of two thirds of London's residents. Houses on the same street received water from different companies.

Sometime between 1849 and 1854, the Lambeth Company changed its water source to a less contaminated location upstream. During a particularly bad cholera outbreak from 1853 to 1854, Snow demonstrated through calculation of death rates from cholera that the disease decreased in those areas supplied by the Lambeth Company but remained the same in those areas supplied by the Southward and Vauxhall Company (Table 6.3).

The most severe outbreak during this time was in the area of Broad Street, Golden Square, where people obtained their water from a local pump. More than 500 people died from cholera within 10 days. Believing that the water delivered by the pump was responsible for the cases of cholera, Snow

TABLE 6.3 Death Rates From Cholera by Water Company, London, 1853–1854

Water Company	Population, 1851	Cholera Deaths	Deaths/100,000
Southwark and Vauxhall	167,654	192	114
Both companies	301,149	182	60
Lambeth	14,632	0	0

Source: Snow, J. (1855). *On the mode of communication of cholera.* London: John Churchill. Retrieved from http://www.ph.ucla.edu/epi/snow/snowbook.html.

removed the handle, and the number of cases immediately declined. However, there also were a number of other factors that contributed to this event, for example, an exodus of the population to other locations. Nonetheless, he is credited for "staying the epidemic," and a pump now has been erected in his honor on the corner of Broad Street in Soho.

Snow, during his investigations, mapped the areas where cholera occurred, developed rates as an objective measure to compare populations, made use of the natural experiment provided by the unusual pattern of water mains, and found evidence for the cause of cholera. These were outstanding accomplishments in an era that preceded bacteriology. He published his findings in *On the Mode of Communication of Cholera* (Snow, 1855). The entire document is available online.

Florence Nightingale, Nurse and Epidemiologist

Florence Nightingale, the daughter of a wealthy Englishman, was also a contemporary of William Farr and John Snow. She devoted her life to the prevention of needless illness and death. She used compelling statistics to bring about healthcare reforms, both during the Crimean War and later in her English homeland. Also, she is credited with founding the profession of nursing.

Prior to leading a group of nurses to aid the British soldiers in the Crimean War, Nightingale was superintendent of a London hospital. There she supervised nurses, the operation of the physical plant, and the purity of the medicines. In 1854, she and a group of carefully chosen nurses and servants joined the troops in Scutari, in the Crimea. She was appalled by the conditions of the hospital barracks. Rats and fleas infested buildings, facilities were overcrowded, linen was filthy, essential supplies were missing, and an open sewer ran underneath the barracks. The soldiers suffered not only from wounds, but also from dysentery, malnutrition, frostbite, cholera, typhus, and scurvy. The mortality rate for the soldiers was 42.7% (Cohen, 1984).

Using carefully gathered data that were unique at the time, Nightingale documented the results of her sanitary reforms. The polar area diagram she designed (Fig. 6.1) illustrates the needless deaths in the military hospitals during the Crimean War. Deaths peaked in January 1855. During that month, 83 soldiers died from wounds, but 2,700 died from infectious diseases. If the dead soldiers had not been replaced, infectious diseases would have wiped out the entire army. By the end of the war, the death rate in British soldiers in the Crimea was less than that of the troops at home (Cohen, 1984).

With the help of William Farr, Nightingale continued documenting events after the war that were associated with poor sanitary conditions. She compared mortality in civilians with that in soldiers and found that in peacetime, the soldiers in England had a mortality rate nearly twice that of civilian males. Nightingale asked for and received a formal investigation of military healthcare, and eventually, the

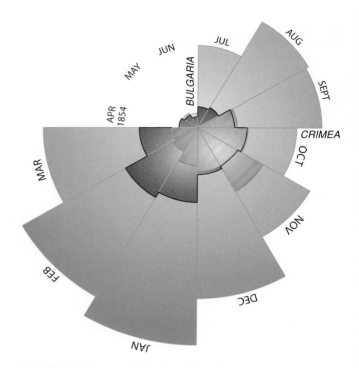

FIGURE 6.1 Florence Nightingale's polar area diagram illustrating the extent of needless deaths in British military hospitals during the Crimean War, April 1854 to March 1855. The *blue wedges* measured from the center of the circle represent area for area the deaths from preventable zymotic diseases, the *red wedges* measured from the center the deaths from wounds, and the *black wedges* measured from the center the deaths from all other causes. The *black lines* across the *red triangles* in September and November 1854 mark the boundaries of the deaths from all other causes during those months. In October 1854, the *black area* coincides with the *red*. The entire areas may be compared by following the *blue*, the *red*, and the *black lines* enclosing them. (From Aiken, L. [1988]. *Assuring the delivery of quality patient care. State of the Science Invitational Conference, Nursing resources and the delivery of patient care [NIH Publication No. 89–3008, pp. 3–10]*. Washington, DC: U.S. Department of Health and Human Services, Public Health Service; Cohen, I. B. [1984]. Florence Nightingale. *Scientific American*, 250[3], 129.)

government implemented her sanitary reforms. She studied the health of soldiers in India, the mortality in British hospitals, and the mortality following surgery. Throughout her career, she experimented with graphs and diagrams that everyone could understand and tried to introduce statistics into higher education. As a pioneering epidemiologist, she effectively demonstrated that statistics provide an organized way of learning from experience.

EPIDEMIOLOGIC MODELS

Epidemiologic Triad

The **epidemiologic triad** is the classic model based on the belief that health status is determined by the interaction of the characteristics of the host, agent, and environment, not by any single factor. The host is the client whose health status is the concern, whether it is a person, a family, a group of high-risk people, or the community as a whole. Agents are an element or force that under proper conditions can initiate or perpetuate a health problem. Environment refers to the context within which the agent and host interact (Fig. 6.2).

Host factors, sometimes called intrinsic factors, include both variable (modifiable) and absolute (nonmodifiable) factors. Age, race, and genetic makeup are examples of absolute, or nonmodifiable, factors. Lifestyle, exercise level, nutrition, health knowledge, and motivation for achieving optimal wellness are examples of host factors that are variable, or modifiable.

Agents can be classified into five groups. These agents may be *physical*, such as heat and trauma; *chemical*, such as pollutants, medications, and drugs; *nutritional*, such as the absence or excess of water, vitamins, fats, proteins, and carbohydrates; *psychosocial*, such as stress, social isolation, and social support; and *biologic*, such as bacteria, viruses, arthropods, toxins, and conditions that interfere with the normal function of the body.

Environmental factors are frequently divided into three categories: biologic, physical, and social. The biologic environment is composed of plants, animals, and the toxins they produce; this includes pathogenic microorganisms, vectors that carry the infectious agents, and the reservoirs where infectious agents are normally found. The physical environment includes light, heat, air, atmospheric pressure, radiation, geologic factors, and the structures in the environment. The social environment includes culture, technology, educational opportunities, political systems, demographic characteristics, sociologic factors, and economic and legal systems.

The Wheel of Causation

Many diseases, illnesses, and conditions have multiple or no discernible agents, or the agent may be a part of the environment. An alternate model is conceptualized as a

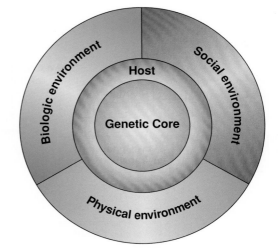

FIGURE 6.3 The wheel of causation.

wheel, with a circle as the genetic core of the host, surrounded by a larger, segmented wheel representing the biologic, physical, and social environments (Fig. 6.3). The **wheel of causation** de-emphasizes the agent as the sole cause of disease, whereas it emphasizes the interplay of physical, biologic, and social environments. Interaction between the host and environment, with or without an identifiable agent, remains the major determinant of health status in all epidemiologic models.

The Web of Causation

The **web of causation** is an epidemiologic model that strongly emphasizes the concept of multiple causation while de-emphasizing the role of agents in explaining illness. At the time of development, there was a need to create a model that would help describe the multiple factors underlying chronic illnesses. These causal webs are more focused and realistic, and they may be as intricate and complex as needed. In this model, it is necessary to identify all possible antecedent factors that could influence the development or prevention of a particular health condition. Each factor is perceived as a link in multiple interrelated chains. By making the pathways explicit in a web of causation, a diagram deepens understanding and provides a framework for statistical analysis. It also serves as a valuable practical guide. Direct and indirect factors can be identified that can be changed or modified to improve health. Not only does it provide multiple entry points for intervention, but it also has the capacity to demonstrate the interrelationship of different factors. These can include both unpredicted and possibly undesirable side effects. Public health professionals use web of causation models such as this to design methods that interrupt the chain of events that lead to adverse states of health. Figure 6.4 exemplifies a classic web of causation that identifies multiple ways to reduce health problems, in this case drug use and abuse in adolescents.

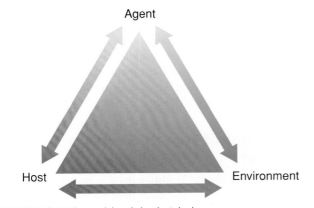

FIGURE 6.2 The epidemiologic triad.

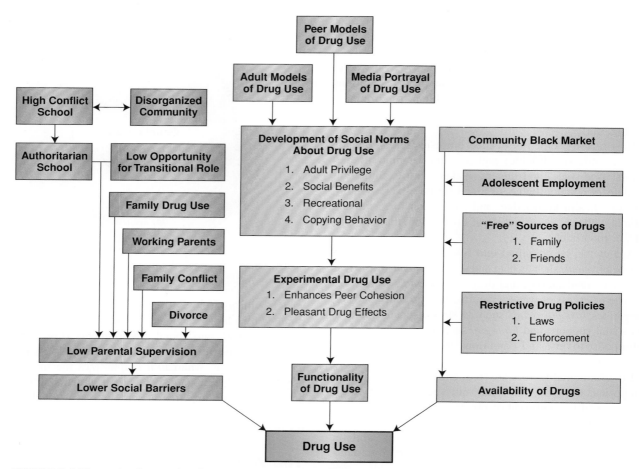

FIGURE 6.4 The web of causation for drug use. (Used with permission from Duncan, D. F., & Petrosa, R. [1999]. Social and community factors associated with drug use and abuse among adolescents. In T. P. Gullotta, G. R. Adams, & R. Montemayor (Eds.). *Substance misuse in adolescence (pp. 56–91)*. Thousand Oaks, CA: Sage Publications.)

Natural History of Disease

In 1958, Leavell and Clark developed a conceptual model for the **natural history** of any disease affecting humans (Leavell & Clark, 1965). This groundbreaking model integrated the pathogenesis of an illness with primary, secondary, and tertiary prevention measures (Fig. 6.5). The initial interactions between the agent, host, and environment occur during the prepathogenesis period. Primary prevention measures specific to the disease can be implemented at this stage to prevent its onset in a population of well people. The period of pathogenesis begins when there are biologic, psychological, or other responses within the host. Secondary prevention measures focus on early diagnosis and prompt treatment. This can limit resulting disabilities when implemented during the early stages of the disease. Tertiary prevention follows with rehabilitation measures that enable the individual to function at his or her maximum capability. This model, used widely in practice, is discussed in more detail in Chapter 5 (see Fig. 5.2).

Every human being is the author of his own health or disease. **Buddha**

APPLYING EPIDEMIOLOGIC PRINCIPLES IN PRACTICE

The epidemiologic process and the nursing process are both derived from the problem-solving process that provides a framework for gathering data about health problems, analyzing the information, generating diagnoses or hypotheses, planning for resolution, implementing plans of action, and evaluating results (Table 6.4). The focus of the nursing process is on caring for the client within his or her family, whereas the focus of the epidemiologic process is on caring for the population of the community as a whole. Whether caring for the individual or the members of a community, nurses need access to data, abstract critical thinking skills, and complex reasoning abilities.

Assessment of Health Needs and Assets

Community and public health nurses assess both health needs and health assets for individual people within their environment and for the population within the community as

FIGURE 6.5 Leavell and Clark's natural history of any disease affecting humans. (From Leavell, H. R. & Clark, E. G. (1979). *Preventive medicine for the doctor in his community: An epidemiological approach.* Malabar, FL: Krieger Publishing Company.)

a whole. Both the individual and the community are considered clients.

Individual Assessment

Providing personal healthcare services to individual persons is a cornerstone of nursing practice. Community health and public health nurses often provide direct health services, including preventive services, to high-risk, displaced, and vulnerable populations. The nurse is usually the first person to systematically observe the individual person, either in the home, clinic, parish, or healthcare facility. The public health nurse takes a nursing history, performs a physical assessment, and makes both objective and subjective observations about the condition of the person. He or she establishes where the person is in relation to the full spectrum of health and identifies the person's assets as well as needs. Assets include strengths and resources of the client such as general state of health, prior use of healthcare services, health behaviors, lifestyle, motivation, and other factors. This information establishes the database about the client. The planning process and the interventions that are subsequently implemented are based on this assessment. Also, the database becomes a baseline for measuring the outcomes of care.

TABLE 6.4 Similarities Between the Nursing Process and the Epidemiologic Process

Nursing Process, Client Based	Epidemiologic Process, Population Based
Assessment	
• An individual client database is established	• Data are gathered from reliable sources
• Data are interpreted	• Nature, extent, and scope of problem are defined
	• Problem described by person, place, and time
Diagnosis	
• Healthcare needs and assets are identified	• Tentative hypothesis is formulated
• Goals and objectives for care are established	• Data analyzed to test the hypothesis
Planning	
• Processes for achieving goals are selected	• Plans are made for control and prevention of the condition or event
Implementation	
• Actions initiated to achieve goals	• Actions are initiated to implement the plan
Evaluation	
• Extent of goal achievement is determined	• Actions are evaluated and report is prepared
	• Further research is conducted if necessary

Considering the goals of the delinquency prevention program, what information does Katie need to gather from her group of young people? How could she access this information?

What factors increase the risk of negative health outcomes for youths in gangs?

Practice Point

You have to ask the right questions to gather the information (data) you need.

Nurses use the information that epidemiologic research has established when performing most client assessments, although they may not be aware that they are doing so. For example, a common process is to assess individuals for risk factors that have been associated with a disease or illness through epidemiologic research. **Risk** refers to the probability or likelihood that a disease or illness will occur in a group of people who presently do not have the problem. **Risk factors** are those characteristics or events that have been shown to increase the probability that a specific disease or illness will develop. Some risk factors are modifiable, and others such as age are not. For example, epidemiologic research has established that certain risk factors, such as a sedentary lifestyle, obesity, increased cholesterol, hypertension, and smoking, are associated with cardiovascular disease. These risk factors are now a part of the epidemiologic body of knowledge, or the epidemiology, of heart disease. As a result, several health appraisal approaches are now commonly used to profile client risk.

Epidemiologic research has also established the natural history of most illnesses. This refers to the course of a disease or condition from onset to resolution. It includes (1) pathologic onset stage, (2) the presymptomatic stage, and (3) the manifestation of clinical disease (Leavell & Clark, 1965). Through the individual assessment process, the nurse can begin to determine the stage of the illness in question. Cues identified at the initial assessment may indicate whether primary, secondary, or tertiary prevention interventions would be most appropriate.

Evidence for Practice

Decline in the physical functioning of the elderly is of concern worldwide. Chen, Chang, and Lan (2015) conducted a study that evaluated the association between changes in physical functioning and a variety of other factors in an older population in Taiwan. The data of 907 participants were derived from the *Functioning and Aging Study* conducted in Taipei between 2005 and 2009.

Functional status was assessed using activities of daily living, instrumental activities of daily living and mobility tasks, and classification as being normal, with mild disability, moderate disability, and severe disability.

The proportion of elderly participants with normal function decreased with time throughout the study period. Risk factors, both modifiable and nonmodifiable, that were associated with changes in physical functioning included the following:

- Age
- Living arrangements, social support
- Self-rated health
- Stroke
- Diabetes
- Parkinson disease
- Osteoporosis
- Depression
- Cognition
- Vision
- History of fracture and falls
- Incontinence of urine and feces
- Physical activity
- Body mass index (BMI), short physical performance

Researchers conclude that older persons with stroke, Parkinson disease, diabetes, osteoporosis, geriatric conditions, and poor short physical performance would benefit the most from prevention measures for functional decline. Older people not living with spouses, with poor self-rated health, with low social support, who are malnourished and live a sedentary lifestyle might also benefit from interventions protecting against functional decline. All public health nurses can assess their elderly clients and plan interventions that will protect them from excessive decline in the ability to function well in their daily lives.

Community Assessment

Conceptualizing the community as a client is difficult for the individual-oriented nurse. Assessing the health needs and assets of a community involves creating a comprehensive community profile or database. The individual nurse may be solely responsible for the assessment, but usually he or she contributes to the assessment as a member of a team. Epidemiologic statistical methods, such as calculation of rates, are used in this process (see Chapter 7). A detailed discussion of community assessment is found in Chapter 11.

Epidemiologists gather available demographic data that provide information about the age and sex distribution, socioeconomic characteristics, and cultural and ethnic distributions. They access vital statistics, including applicable epidemiologic morbidity and mortality rates. Additional data can be obtained from community members or community groups. Information about the accessibility and availability of healthcare services, such as health manpower, may or may not be community assets. To obtain information about health beliefs, norms, values, goals, perceived needs, and health practices, healthcare workers may use focus groups, interviews or observation, or surveys. Nurses may participate in field-testing new tools for data collection.

After epidemiologists collect the data, they synthesize and analyze the information and generate a list of community health needs and assets. Identifying patterns of disease, illness,

and injuries detects trends that form the rationale for program development. Critical thinking skills are essential for the appropriate analysis of this information. Finally, it is necessary to set goals and objectives to address high-priority problems.

Practice Point

A thorough and accurate client database, whether that of individuals, groups, or the community, provides the evidence and rationale for your interventions.

To understand the scope of the health problems facing the young people who were enrolled in the delinquency prevention program, a community assessment should be considered. What information does Katie need to gather, and where would she find that information?

Student Reflection

Although my nursing program focused a lot on research findings, particularly in writing assignments, I did not fully understand the impact that statistics can make in nursing until I had my community practicum in a local women's health center. When I arrived there, the staff was talking about a violent episode that had occurred the previous week. Everyone seemed to think that there was more violence in the community than there should be, and that we needed to know more about it.

My preceptor was a program developer, and the women at the center asked her if they needed a violence prevention program. One of my first assignments was to find out just how much and what types of violence had occurred in the last year. The first thing my preceptor suggested was to go online and look at websites for various states and towns. I was amazed at how much information was available. For example, I found out that the rates of homicide, assaults, and rapes in our town were greater than the average for both the state and the nation. Also, I found out that 45% of the poor, young males from minority groups were in jail for crimes of violence! I learned that most violence occurs between people who know each other, and that violence is related to substance abuse. I presented my information to the staff, and they all decided to have my preceptor contact other community agencies and the local college to form a coalition to address violence. I attended the first meeting, and people tossed around lots of ideas. They decided to look into a 24/7 free telephone line to give people support in a crisis, increase housing for women suffering from domestic violence, and consider a number of initiatives for youth in the town.

This experience taught me several things.

- Lots of information is available about health problems in a community.
- New ideas require presentation of supportive data.
- Involving other interested communities can enhance whatever is planned to reduce health problems.
- One person's efforts can really make a difference.

Using Assessment Data for Planning and Implementing Interventions

The individual or community client database, much of which has been gathered using epidemiologic methods, provides the rationale for planning and implementing interventions. It is possible to use the epidemiologic body of knowledge that describes the natural progression of specific diseases or illnesses to target ways to break the problem cycle once it has been identified. An intervention plan outlines the goals, objectives, and strategies for achieving the interventions and provides completion dates for their accomplishment. The type of health problem, the readiness of the individual or community to address the problem, the availability of health services, the nurse's role, the characteristics of social change, and other related factors influence successful implementation.

Three goals for the delinquency prevention program are presented at the beginning of this chapter.
Write an objective for each goal.

Promoting Healthy Lifestyles

Every phase of public health nursing involves the provision of health education whenever the opportunity arises. Lifestyle patterns are modifiable, and nurses can help make the public aware of the benefits of preventive health through use of the media and meeting with individuals and community groups.

Following the landmark epidemiologic studies of smoking and lung cancer in the 1950s, the general public gradually recognized that personal behaviors such as smoking were risk factors for the leading conditions causing morbidity and mortality in the United States and other countries. In 1984, the CDC and the U.S. state health departments collaboratively established the Behavioral Risk Factor Surveillance System (BRFSS). The goal of this surveillance system is to collect, analyze, and interpret specific behavioral risk factor data that can be used to plan, implement, and monitor health promotion and disease prevention programs.

The BRFSS gathers information about health behaviors, such as lack of physical activity, obesity, and safety belt use, primarily by telephone calls. It also gathers data about preventive health services, such as screening for breast and cervical cancer and elevated blood cholesterol. The BRFSS used these epidemiologic statistics when national objectives were established for *Healthy People 2000*, *Healthy People 2010*, and *Healthy People 2020*. *Healthy People 2020*, developed by the U.S. Department of Health and Human Services, sets behavioral objectives to be achieved over the second decade of the 21st century. Experts developed these objectives through a broad consultation process, built on the best scientific knowledge and designed to measure programs over time. Along with the BRFSS data, *Healthy People 2020* serves as the basis for the development of state and community plans to improve the health of their populations. Each state collects statistics for the BRFSS, and thus these data are available for nurses to access when planning educational programs for primary prevention.

Dietary factors are associated with 4 out of the 10 leading causes of death: heart disease, some types of cancer, stroke, and type 2 diabetes. Obesity rates have doubled in adults and tripled in children and adolescents over the last two decades. The data are alarming (CDC, 2015).

The prevalence in the United States between 2011 and 2014 is as follows:

- 36.5% of adults aged 20 years and older were obese
- 20.5% of adolescents aged 12 to 19 years were obese
- 17.5% of children aged 6 to 11 years were obese
- 8.9% of children aged 2 to 5 years were obese

These are significant increases in obesity as compared to the period of 1999–2000.

The estimated cost of these diet-related conditions is more than $123 billion annually in medical expenses. Including lost productivity in these statistics adds billions more (CDC, 2010b). The BRFSS data dramatically demonstrate the significant increase in the prevalence of overweight people in the United States (Fig. 6.6). Using these data, *Healthy People 2020* identified overweight and obesity as a major health issue in the United States. Sex and ethnicity are also important factors in the development of obesity (Fig. 6.7). Overweight is most prevalent in African American and Hispanic females. If nurses find that such statistics apply to the members of their own community, they can initiate programs to address the problem.

The burden of food-related ill health measured in terms of mortality and morbidity is similar to that attributable to smoking. The cost is twice the amount attributable to car, train, and other accidents, and more than twice that attributable to smoking. The vast majority of the burden is attributable to unhealthy diets rather than to food-borne diseases (Rayner & Scarborough, 2005).

Practice Point

Use statistics to demonstrate the need for program development and community interventions.

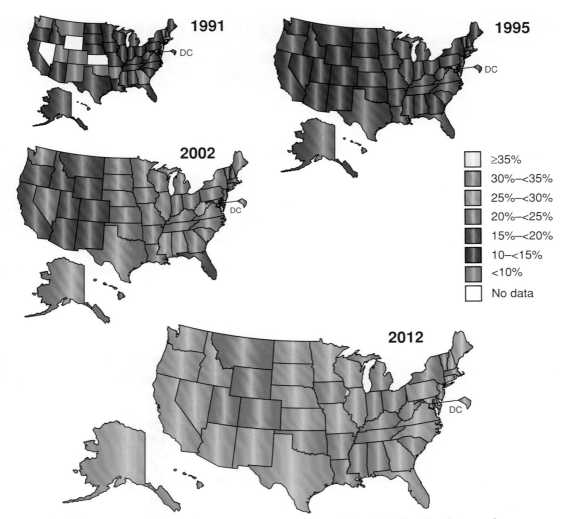

FIGURE 6.6 Changes in prevalence of obesity among U.S. adults. Note that the data are for ages 18 years and over, based on self-reported weight and height via telephone interview. Obesity is defined as body mass index ≥30. (From National Health and Nutrition Examination Survey, NCHS, CDC; BRFSS, 2012.)

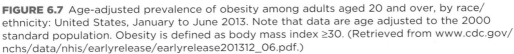

FIGURE 6.7 Age-adjusted prevalence of obesity among adults aged 20 and over, by race/ethnicity: United States, January to June 2013. Note that data are age adjusted to the 2000 standard population. Obesity is defined as body mass index ≥30. (Retrieved from www.cdc.gov/nchs/data/nhis/earlyrelease/earlyrelease201312_06.pdf.)

Evidence for Practice

Healthier food access in schools is a major objective of *Healthy People 2020*. To accomplish this goal, the United States has invested heavily in actions to prevent youth obesity by promoting healthy eating and physical activity. With support from the CDC, the Communities Putting Prevention to Work (CPPW) obesity prevention program was initiated in King County, Washington, during 2010 and 2012 (CDC, 2014). Components of the robust obesity prevention program included the following:

- Implementation of nutrition standards for school meals
- Student-led healthy eating and active living promotional campaigns
- Farm to school initiatives
- High-quality physical education
- Nutrition and culinary training for school cafeteria staff
- Participation in community health coalitions

The CPPW focused on low-income school districts and communities, since community health assessment data indicated that the prevalence of obesity, poor nutrition, and physical inactivity was disproportionately high relative to higher-income communities. Data were obtained from a school-based survey analogous to the national Youth Risk Behavior Survey. The Washington State Department of Health used self-reported height and weight from the survey to calculate BMI. The survey response rates ranged from 63% to 71%, resulting in approximately 34,000 respondents per survey year, for the project group, and 61% to 67% for the rest of the population of Kings County and the state of Washington resulting in approximately 18,500 respondents per survey year.

Results indicated a statistically significant 17% decline in youth obesity after implementation of CPPW school districts, but not in non-CPPW districts. Also, there was a statistically significant reduction in youth obesity in Kings County when compared with the rest of the state of Washington.

These findings suggest that focused, multifaceted, and comprehensive policy, systems, and environmental change interventions located in each community can reduce obesity in youth. Continued community level interventions such as these have the potential to meet the CDC's obesity prevention priority as one of its 10 "winnable battles."

Preventing and Controlling Outbreaks

The investigation of an epidemic or **outbreak** is an example of the epidemiologic process in action. Epidemics occur when there is an increased incidence of a disease or event beyond that which is normally found in the population. Although the term *outbreak* is often used synonymously with epidemic, outbreaks are usually limited to a localized increase

6.1 How to Investigate an Outbreak

- Establish the existence of the outbreak.
- Describe the outbreak according to person, place, and time.
- Formulate and test hypotheses as to the most probable causative factors.
- Implement a plan for control of the outbreak and prevention of further outbreaks.
- Evaluate results, prepare reports, and conduct further research if necessary.

in the incidence of the illness. The steps of investigating an outbreak are presented in Box 6.1. A detailed description of outbreak investigations is found in Chapter 14.

Public health nurses may be involved in any of the steps of the outbreak investigation. The nurse's role varies with the workplace. Generally, nurses are involved in education of the public, mobilization of community resources, and implementing regulatory and control measures.

Practice Point

When you are investigating unusual events, determine whether the incidence is greater than what normally would occur at that time and place.

 What types of outbreaks may occur during the delinquency prevention program?

Contributing to a Safe and Healthy Environment

Individual and community risk assessments should include detection of real or potential threats from the environment. Environment includes physical, biologic, social, cultural, or any other external factors that can influence the health status of individuals or populations. The principles of epidemiology, normally used in investigating disease and illness, can be applied to the human effects of natural disasters such as hurricanes and earthquakes, as well as to industrial disasters such as injuries, air pollution, nuclear accidents, and release of toxic chemicals.

Practice Point

Evaluate your community, and subsets of the community, for potential environmental hazards.

When healthcare professionals gather demographic data, vital statistics, and epidemiologic morbidity and mortality statistics, they should also consult environmental health sources. Using detailed individual or community client databases, nurses then have the potential to link environmental exposure to illness and disease. Nurses often provide case management for both communicable and chronic illnesses that result from environmental exposure. Nurses also may be risk consultants, communicators, and educators, working with community groups, agencies, and industry to protect the health of their workers.

 What are the environmental risks for the group of delinquent youth? How would Katie address these in her sessions with the youth?

The World Health Organization (WHO), the National Institute for Occupational Safety and Health (NIOSH) in the United States, and other international and national agencies review existing knowledge about chemicals, radiation, and other environmental hazards that have immediate and long-term effects on health, and issue reports concerning environmental health criteria. See Chapter 19 for detailed information regarding environmental assessment.

Evaluating the Effectiveness of Health Services

Public health professionals who collect epidemiologic data during assessments and use them for establishing the need for health programs can also use them to evaluate those services. Evaluation requires a systematic and objective process that determines the relevance, effectiveness, and impact of the health service. Creating objectives that are measurable assists in this process. Nurses should continuously monitor the health status indicators in the community, especially for vulnerable populations. Age-specific mortality rates, low birth rates, infant mortality rates, health services utilization, and other indexes specific to the characteristics of the community are examples (see Chapter 7). This information assists in identifying gaps and detecting emerging problems early so that appropriate responses can be facilitated. In addition, nurses and other healthcare professionals can also use epidemiologic principles to develop surveys to gather specific information from targeted populations such as child care centers or the population of census tracts that may be at high risk.

The primary way to demonstrate prevention or control of a health problem is to compare epidemiologic statistics before and after the implementation of the health service. Planning and evaluation are continuous processes. As new data become available, modification in health services may be necessary, and those modifications require evaluation.

Practice Point

Use your program objectives to evaluate your interventions.

 Outline an evaluation program for the delinquent youth prevention program discussed in the case at the beginning of this chapter.

KEY CONCEPTS

- Early attempts at understanding the reasons for disease were primarily a direct result of trial-and-error observations of individual people.
- Study of illness and causes of death in groups of people began in the 17th century. Founders of epidemiology as the science of preventive medicine included John Graunt, William Farr, John Snow, and Florence Nightingale.
- Epidemiology is defined as the study of the distribution and determinants of the states of health and illness in human populations, with the goal of preventing or limiting consequences and maximizing states of health.

- Individual and community assessments, using epidemiologic principles, form the database that provides the evidence and rationale for interventions.
- Promoting healthy lifestyles uses epidemiologic data such as that found in the BRFSS. The U.S. publication *Healthy People 2020* defines measurable objectives to be achieved over the second decade of the 21st century.
- Nurses, in their care of individual and community clients, have the potential to link environmental exposure to illness and disease.
- Epidemiologic data, collected during assessments that establish the need for health programs, are also used to evaluate those services.

CRITICAL THINKING QUESTIONS

1. Jeff is 11 years old and slightly overweight. His father is a truck driver who was recently diagnosed with type 2 diabetes. His mother is a licensed practical nurse at the local hospital. At a recent health science fair at his school, a student-led screening clinic documented Jeff's blood pressure at 140/92 mm Hg.
   a. Is Jeff at risk? If so, for what?
   b. Utilizing the *Guidelines for High Blood Pressure in Adults* (American College of Cardiology, 2017), what is Jeff's future risk from adolescence through adulthood?
   c. What other data do you need?
   d. How does epidemiologic data define hypertension in a child of Jeff's age?
   e. What recommendations would you make?
   f. Are there health promotion activities that you would recommend?

2. Look through several major newspapers for articles containing health statistics.
   a. What are the implications of these statistics for your community?
   b. What further data would you obtain to document the problem in your community?

3. Go to the CDC website www.cdc.gov. Pick a topic to explore. Show how epidemiologic information has been used to describe the topic.

4. Explore the website "Violence Prevention" (http://www.cdc.gov/ViolencePrevention/pub/PreventingYV.html). Identify at least one activity that Katie could use to meet each of the goals of her program.

REFERENCES

American College of Cardiology. (2017). *2017 Guideline for high blood pressure in adults*. Retrieved from http://www.acc.org/latest-in-cardiology/ten-points-to-remember/2017/11/09/11/41/2017-guideline-for-high-blood-pressure-in-adults

Centers for Disease Control and Prevention. (2010a). *Healthy people 2020*. Retrieved from https://www.healthypeople.gov/2020/About-Healthy-People

Centers for Disease Control and Prevention. (2010b). *National health priorities, reducing obesity, heart disease, cancer, diabetes and other diet and inactivity related diseases, costs, and disabilities*. Retrieved from http://www.cdc.gov/nccdphp/dnpao/index.html

Centers for Disease Control and Prevention. (2014). Declines in student obesity prevalence associated with a prevention initiative—King County, Washington, 2012. *Morbidity and Mortality Weekly Reports*, 63(07), 155–157.

Centers for Disease Control and Prevention. (2015). *Prevalence of obesity among adults and youth: United States, 2011–2014*. Retrieved from https://www.cdc.gov/nchs/data/databriefs/db219.pdf

Centers for Disease Control and Prevention. (2016). Current cigarette smoking among adults—United States, 2005–2015. *Morbidity and Mortality Weekly Report*, 65(44), 1205–1211. Retrieved from https://www.cdc.gov/mmwr/volumes/65/wr/mm6544a2.htm

Chen, C. M., Chang, W. C., & Lan, T. Y. (2015). Identifying factors associated with changes in physical functioning in an older population. *Geriatrics and Gerontology International*, 15(2), 156–164.

Cohen, I. B. (1984). Florence Nightingale. *Scientific American*, 250(3), 128–137.

Doll, R., & Hill, A. B. (1950). Smoking and carcinoma of the lung; preliminary report. *British Medical Journal*, 2(4682), 739–748.

Farr, W. (1852). Influence of elevation on the fatality of cholera. *Journal of the Statistical Society of London*, 15(2), 155–183.

Harkness, G. A. (1995). *Epidemiology in nursing practice*. St. Louis, MO: Mosby.

Hippocrates. (1938). On airs, waters, and places [400 BC]: Translated and republished. *Medical Classics*, 3, 19–42.

Leavell, H. R., & Clark, E. G. (1965). *Preventive medicine for the doctor in his community: An epidemiologic approach (p. 21)*. New York: McGraw-Hill.

Mausner, J. S., & Kramer, S. (1985). *Epidemiology—An introductory text* (2nd ed.). Philadelphia, PA: W. B. Saunders.

Rayner, M., & Scarborough, P. (2005). The burden of food related ill health in the UK. *Journal of Epidemiology and Community Health*, 59(12), 1054–1057.

Sanders, B., Schneiderman, J. U., Loken, A., Lankenau, S. E., & Bloom, J. J. (2009). Gang youth as a vulnerable population for nursing intervention. *Public Health Nursing*, 26(4), 346–352.

Snow, J. (1855). *On the mode of communication of cholera*. London: John Churchill. Retrieved from http://www.ph.ucla.edu/epi/snow/snowbook.html

WEB RESOURCES

Please visit thePoint® for up-to-date web resources on this topic.

Describing Health Conditions: Understanding and Using Rates

Patrice Nicholas and Patricia Lussier-Duynstee

Perplexity is the beginning of knowledge.
Khalil Gibran

There are three kinds of epidemiologists: those who can count and those who can't.
Anonymous

Prejudice is a great time saver. You can form opinions without having to get the facts.
E.B. White, author

CHAPTER HIGHLIGHTS

- Concept and calculation of rates
- Crude, specific, and adjusted rates
- Incidence and prevalence rates
- Sensitivity and specificity calculations

OBJECTIVES

- Describe the primary method used to measure the existence of states of health or illness in a population during a given time period.
- Explain the formula and rules for calculation of a rate.
- Differentiate between crude and adjusted rates.
- Contrast incidence rates and prevalence rates.
- Discuss the use of specific rates when describing characteristics of person, place, and time.
- Differentiate between incidence density, incidence rates, and relative risk ratio.
- Discuss differences between the sensitivity and specificity of tests.
- Using examples, interpret the relevance of the use of rates in nursing practice.

KEY TERMS

Adjusted rate: Statistical procedure that removes the effects of differences in the composition of a population, such as age, when comparing one to another.

Attack rate: An incidence or occurrence rate.

Attributable risk: The difference between the incidence rates in an exposed and an unexposed group of people.

Case fatality rate: Calculated by dividing the number of deaths from a specific disease by the number of people living with that disease during the year, and multiplying by 100.

Cause-specific mortality rate: The probability of death from a specific cause.

Crude rate: Measurement of the occurrence of the health problem or condition being investigated in the entire population.

Demographic data: The study of the size, distribution, and characteristics of human populations.

Epidemic curve: A graph that plots the distribution of cases by the time of onset of the disease.

Epidemiologic descriptive studies: Research studies designed to acquire more information about

KEY TERMS *(continued)*

the occurrence and distribution of states of health, such as characteristics of person, place, and time.

Incidence density: Use of a person-time denominator in the calculation of rates; a person-day reflects one person at risk for 1 day, and a person-year represents one person at risk for 1 year.

Incidence rate: Measure of the probability that people without a certain condition will develop that condition over a period of time.

Long-term change: Fluctuations in time surrounding health problems that extend over decades, reflecting gradual changes.

Morbidity: A departure from a state of physiologic or psychological well-being.

Mortality rate: The probability of death from any cause among the entire population within a given time frame.

Period prevalence: A prevalence rate that indicates the existence of a condition during an interval of time, often a year.

Periodic change: Seasonal or cyclic fluctuations in time surrounding health problems.

Point prevalence: A prevalence rate that indicates the existence of a condition at a specific point in time.

Populations at risk: Groups of people who have specific characteristics, or risk factors, that increase the probability of developing health problems.

Prevalence rate: Measures the number of people in a given population who have an existing condition at a given point in time.

Proportion: A type of ratio that includes the quantity in the numerator as a part of the denominator.

Proportional mortality ratio: A ratio that compares deaths from a specific illness with deaths from all other causes.

Rate: The primary measurement used to describe the occurrence (quantity) of a state of health in a specific group of people in a given time period.

Ratio: A fraction that represents the relationship between two numbers.

Relative risk ratio: The ratio of the incidence rate in the exposed group and the incidence rate in the nonexposed group.

Sensitivity: Ability of a test to correctly identify people who have a health problem; the probability of testing positive if the health problem is truly present.

Short-term change: Variations measured in hours, days, weeks, or months; commonly found in outbreaks of infectious disease.

Specific rates: Detailed rates that are calculated using the number of people in the smaller subgroups of the population in the denominator. Often, people are divided into subgroups by age and sex, although any characteristic can be used.

Specificity: Ability of a test to correctly identify people who do not have a health problem; the probability of testing negative if the health problem is truly absent.

CASE STUDY

References to the case study are found throughout this chapter (look for the case study icon). Readers should keep the case study in mind as they read the chapter.

The Visiting Nurse Association serving two rural counties in Florida has received a grant from the United States Office of Minority Health for a human immunodeficiency virus/acquired immunodeficiency syndrome (HIV/AIDS) prevention outreach program targeted toward the two counties' large African American population. The counties are adjacent to each other and have a combined population of 312,838 people. The number of African American people in the two counties is 57,875, or 18.5% of the population.

Lindsay is on the team that developed the program grant, and she is now the program director. She and the team members develop a HIV/AIDS outreach survey, a yes-or-no checklist that serves as a data collection form. Demographic information will be collected at the end of the interview. Outreach workers from the African American community are hired to interview people on the street and in their homes following a week-long training session on HIV/AIDS and methods of establishing rapport (adapted and updated from [Brown & Brown, 2003])

Data from a recent survey in seven African countries found that in 2016, an estimated 1.5 million females aged 15 to 24 years were living with HIV infection in Eastern and Southern Africa, where the prevalence of HIV infection among adolescent girls and young women (3.4%) is more than double that for males in the same age range (1.6%) (Brown et al., 2018). Consider the questions on the HIV/AIDS Outreach Survey below for both of these HIV surveys.

HIV/AIDS OUTREACH SURVEY FORM

1. Do you know about HIV/AIDS?
2. Are you doing anything to protect yourself from HIV?
3. Have you used drugs?
4. Have you been tested for HIV?
5. Modes of HIV transmission reviewed?
6. Risk factors reviewed?

7. Discussed HIV risk reduction?
   a. Correct condom use
   b. Monogamous partners
   c. Reduce number of partners
   d. Cleanliness of equipment
8. Literature given?
9. Condoms given?
10. Is subject male or female?
    Comments: _____

To understand the extent of a state of health, whether it is a disease, disability, or factors that keep people well, it is necessary to describe the magnitude or frequency of the condition. Since people differ in terms of health, it is important to know how they differ. By looking at the frequency of the condition in groups of people who either have or do not have the problem under investigation, it can be determined who is at risk or not at risk for that condition. Using this technique, descriptive epidemiology can demonstrate the seriousness of the problem, determine the characteristics of the people it affects, and identify where and when it occurs. It can also provide data, or clues, that suggest how the condition evolves and why the condition exists. This information can indicate which people are likely to develop certain health problems; what diseases, disabilities, or needs they have; how these health problems are distributed within the community; and what kind of health services are needed. The use of existing resources in a community can then be determined and programs planned to address the needs.

Using the information about the frequency and distribution of a condition, nurses and other healthcare professionals can examine the characteristics of groups of people in the community, or within institutions, who are most likely to develop health problems. These groups are considered to be **populations at risk**. Knowledge about the population at risk and risk factors can be also used to set priorities for the development of strategies to meet emerging health needs and for expansion or change in programs or services that are directed toward secondary or tertiary prevention.

The process of using epidemiologic techniques to generate a knowledge base about a specific health problem and plan for its control and prevention is best illustrated by cardiovascular disease. The knowledge gained from the study of populations at risk and identification of predisposing risk factors has been the foundation for the primary, secondary, and tertiary prevention strategies used widely today. Since the initial development of objectives in the earlier reports on *Healthy People 2000* and *2010*, *Healthy People 2020* (CDC, 2010a) has strengthened the focus on health promotion activities in the United States. With a vision based on developing a society in which all people live long, healthy lives, its mission is to identify nationwide health improvement priorities; increase public awareness and understanding of the determinants of health, disease, and disability and the oppor-

tunities for progress; provide measurable objectives and goals that are applicable at the national, state, and local levels; engage multiple sectors to take actions to strengthen policies and improve practices that are driven by the best available evidence and knowledge; and identify critical research, evaluation, and data collection needs.

The overarching goals of *Healthy People 2020* (CDC, 2010a) are:

- Attain high-quality, longer lives free of preventable disease, disability, injury, and premature death
- Achieve health equity, eliminate disparities, and improve the health of all groups
- Create social and physical environments that promote good health for all
- Promote quality of life, healthy development, and healthy behaviors across all life stages

Although most epidemiologic studies have focused on disease and disability, it should be emphasized that this process can also be used to study states of wellness. For example, studies of the factors that are associated with healthy, community-dwelling elderly people can lead to the implementation of strategies to enhance wellness in the elderly population.

To demonstrate that African American people are a population at risk, Lindsay examines Florida statistics. She finds that since the epidemic began, a cumulative total of 107,980 cases of HIV/AIDS have been diagnosed in Florida. Nearly half (48.7%) of these cases have occurred in African American people.

Make a list of other information that Lindsay needs to understand the scope of the HIV/AIDS problem in the two counties.

UNDERSTANDING AND USING RATES

Although the most basic measure of frequency involves counting the number of affected people, this may result in misleading impressions and usually is of limited use. A higher number of cases in one group of people versus another may mean that the number of susceptible people in that group is greater or that the counting took place over a longer period of time. To provide more valid descriptions of the frequency of various states of health, it is necessary to use ratios, proportions, and rates.

However, there are some statistics that are impressive even if they involve counting (or estimating) just the number of affected people. For example, Figure 7.1 illustrates the 10 leading causes of death in the world in 2015. The figure shows that ischemic heart disease and stroke caused 15 million deaths. Chronic obstructive pulmonary disease caused 3.2 million deaths, lung cancer 1.7 million deaths, and diabetes 1.6 million, an increase from 1 million in 2000 (World Health Organization [WHO], 2015).

A **ratio** is a fraction that represents the relationship between two numbers. It is the value obtained by dividing one quantity by another quantity. People (or things) counted in the numerator are not counted in the denominator. For example, the number of boys (160) in an elementary school could be contrasted with the number of girls (80) in that school using a ratio (160/80 = 2/1 = twice as many boys as girls).

A **proportion** is a type of ratio that includes the quantity in the numerator as a part of the denominator; it is the relationship of a part to the whole. Dividing the number of boys by the total number of children in the school results in a proportion (160 divided by 240 = 0.67; 67% of the students are boys).

The **rate** is the primary measurement used to describe the occurrence (frequency or quantity) of a state of health in a specific group of people in a given time period. It is a proportion that includes the factor of time. Therefore, rates are the best indicators of the risk (probability) that a specific disease, condition, or event will occur. The rules for calculation of rates are outlined in Box 7.1. Rates are used to quantify either the occurrence (incidence) or the existence (prevalence) of states of health or illness. Using rates rather than counting cases takes both the size of the population at risk and the time frame into account.

Not everything that counts can be counted, and not everything that can be counted counts. **Albert Einstein**

For example, suppose it is necessary to compare 2,250 cases of H1N1 influenza diagnosed in February in Lake County having a population of 104,000 with 10,500 cases of H1N1 influenza diagnosed in February in Barnes County having a population of 950,000. If only the frequency count is examined, Barnes County has the greatest number of people with the flu, and therefore, it could be concluded that Barnes County has the greater community problem. However, it is not appropriate to compare the raw numbers alone; more cases would be expected in a county with more residents. Indeed, the calculation of rates in Table 7.1 indicates that Lake County had the most severe outbreak of the illness in February.

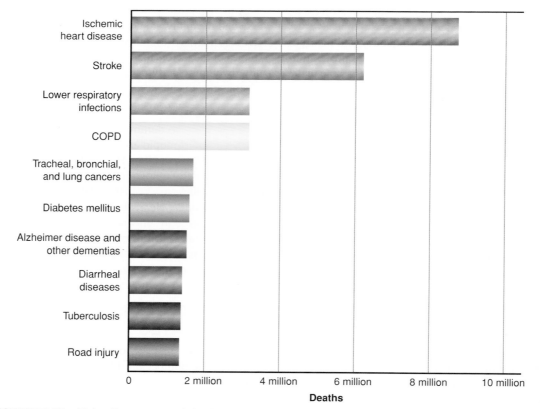

FIGURE 7.1 The 10 leading causes of death in the world (WHO, 2015). (Available from http://www.who.int/mediacentre/factsheets/fs310/en.)

7.1 How to Calculate Rates

1. All of the events being measured should be included in the numerator.
2. Everyone included in the denominator should be at risk for the event in the numerator. For example, it would be inappropriate to include males in the denominator when calculating a rate for ovarian cancer because no males are at risk for the illness.
3. A specific period of time for the observations must be clearly indicated. This can range from a single point in time to several years, depending on the type of rate that is being calculated.
4. A rate is a fraction or a proportion; therefore, it is necessary to multiply by a base, usually a multiple of 10, to make the rates understandable. This removes the decimal points and makes the comparison of rates easier to interpret. Any base multiple of 10 may be chosen that results in a rate above the value of 1. For large populations, 100,000 is often used. For smaller populations, 100 is often used, and the rate can then be expressed as a percentage.
5. Formula for calculation:

$$\text{Rate} = \frac{\text{Number of conditions or events within a designated period of time}}{\text{Population at risk during the same period of time}} \times \text{Base multiple of 10}$$

Practice Point

When assessing the extent of a health problem in a community at a given time, the number of cases should be counted, the number of people in the population should be obtained, and a rate should be calculated.

Crude Rates

Crude rates are general or summary rates that measure the occurrence of the condition being investigated in the entire population. Calculation of these rates usually involves averaging the population numbers at the beginning and end of the year, and that number is used in the denominator. However, smaller groups within the entire population (subgroups) may differ significantly with regard to their risk of developing the condition, and thus, calculating only crude rates may obscure important information. For example, the formula for a crude birth rate has the entire population in its denominator. Births can occur only to females who are of childbearing age; therefore, the total population may not be an ideal denominator.

 There are 2,150 people living with HIV/AIDS this year in two Florida counties. What is the crude rate of the HIV/AIDS burden in these two counties?

Adjusted Rates

There is often a need to remove the effects of differences in the composition of a population when comparing one with another. For example, an investigator may want to compare two or more groups knowing that they differ in terms of a characteristic, such as age, that may influence the results. The process of adjusting rates controls for these differences. Although age adjustment and other types of **adjusted rates** are artificial, they provide a valid way to compare two populations without the confounding variable (such as age) affecting the results.

As an example, Figure 7.2 illustrates age-adjusted death rates by race, Hispanic origin, state, and territory: United States and U.S.-dependent areas, average annual 1979 to 1981, 1989 to 1991, and 2013 to 2015 (Centers for Disease Control and Prevention [CDC], 2016).

Age-adjusted rates are meaningful only as a comparison and should not be used if an accurate description of a population is desired and not a comparison of populations. It is also possible to adjust rates to remove other variables, such as race or occupation, that are confounding an investigation.

Incidence Rates

An **incidence rate** (also an occurrence or **attack rate**) is a measure of the probability that people without a certain condition will develop the condition over a period of time, often a year. It measures the pace at which new illnesses, such as

---

TABLE 7.1 Calculation of Rates of H1N1 Influenza in Lake and Barnes Counties

Lake County	Barnes County
Influenza rate = $\frac{2,250}{104,000} \times 100,000$	Influenza rate = $\frac{10,500}{950,000} \times 100,000$
Influenza rate = 0.0216346 × 100,000	Influenza rate = 0.0110526 × 100,000
Influenza rate = 2,163.5 cases per 100,000 people	Influenza rate = 1,105.3 cases per 100,000 people

Note: A base multiplier of 10,000 would result in a rate of approximately 216 cases per 10,000 people in Lake County and 111 cases per 10,000 in Barnes County.

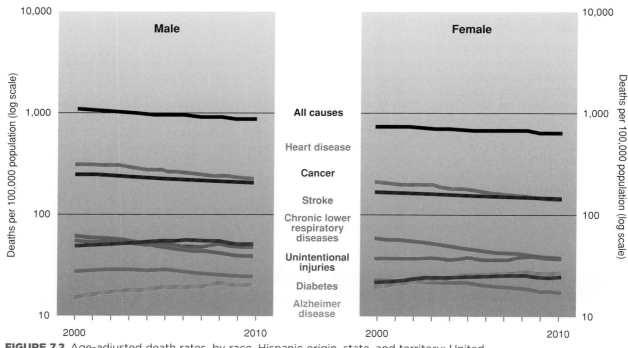

FIGURE 7.2 Age-adjusted death rates, by race, Hispanic origin, state, and territory: United States and U.S. dependent areas, average annual 1979–1981, 1989–1991, and 2013–2015 (CDC, 2016). (Available from https://www.cdc.gov/nchs/data/hus/2016/016.pdf.)

H1N1 influenza, occur in a previously disease-free group of people. The general rules that apply to rates also apply to calculation of incidence rates (see Box 7.1). However, only the *new* cases that have occurred in the designated time period are counted and placed in the numerator. Common incidence rates and ratios that provide indexes of the health of a community are presented in Table 7.2.

Determination of the date of onset is required for studies of incidence. For acute conditions, this can be quickly established. H1N1 influenza is an acute, time-limited condition; thus, the data in Table 7.1 result in incidence or occurrence rates. For other conditions such as cancer or depression, it may be difficult to determine the time of onset. In this case, an event that can be verified, such as the date of diagnosis, is considered as the time of onset.

Lindsay finds that 384 new cases of HIV infection were diagnosed in the two counties within the past year. What is the incidence rate? Contrast this incidence rate with: (1) the crude rate of the HIV/AIDS burden calculated above; and (2) the incidence rate in the United States of 83.7 new HIV infections per 100,000 in 1 year. Interpret the results.

Prevalence Rates

Both incidence rates and **prevalence rates** can be measures of **morbidity**—a departure from a state of physiologic or

psychological well-being. Prevalence rates measure the number of people in a given population who have a specific existing condition at a given point in time. The general rules that apply to rates also apply to calculation of prevalence rates (see Box 7.1). However, both new cases and existing cases (old and new cases) are counted in the designated time period and placed in the numerator.

There are two types of prevalence rates. **Period prevalence** indicates the existence of a condition during a period or an interval of time. **Point prevalence** refers to the existence of a condition at a specific point in time and provides a picture of an existing situation for a group of people. If the time frame is not given, point prevalence is inferred. Point prevalence does not have to be expressed in calendar time; it can refer to an event that happens to different people at different times. For example, it could refer to the day of discharge from an institution for a group of people or a specific day of attendance at a screening clinic.

Prevalence is influenced by two factors: the number of people who have developed the condition in the past and the duration of their illness. The longer the duration of a condition, the higher the prevalence rate. This is best illustrated with chronic diseases. Even if the incidence rate is low, the prevalence rate may be high. For instance, there are many more existing cases of cancer in a community than are indicated by examining the number of new cases of cancer.

Prevalence statistics are very important in identifying public health problems that exist in a community. They are particularly useful to health planning professionals because they measure the burden of a condition or illness in a community.

TABLE 7.2 Incidence Rates and Ratios That Provide Indexes of the Health of a Community

Indexes of Health	Calculation
General Mortality Rates	
Crude mortality rate	$\dfrac{\text{Number of deaths occurring in 1 year}}{\text{Mid-year population}} \times 100{,}000$
Cause-specific mortality rate	$\dfrac{\text{Number of deaths from a stated cause in 1 year}}{\text{Mid-year population}} \times 100{,}000$
Age-specific mortality rate	$\dfrac{\text{Number of people in a specific age group dying in 1 year}}{\text{Mid-year population of the specific age group}} \times 100{,}000$
Case fatality rate	$\dfrac{\text{Number of deaths from a specific disease}}{\text{Number of cases of the same disease}} \times 100$
Proportional mortality ratio	$\dfrac{\text{Number of deaths from a specific cause within a time period}}{\text{Total deaths in the same time period}} \times 100$
Maternal and Infant Rates	
Crude birth rate	$\dfrac{\text{Number of live births in 1 year}}{\text{Mid-year population}} \times 1{,}000$
General fertility rate	$\dfrac{\text{Number of live births in 1 year}}{\text{Number of females 15–44 years of age at mid-year}} \times 1{,}000$
Maternal mortality rate	$\dfrac{\text{Number of deaths from puerperal causes in 1 year}}{\text{Number of live births in the same year}} \times 1{,}000$
Infant mortality rate	$\dfrac{\text{Number of deaths of children 1 year of age in 1 year}}{\text{Number of live births in the same year}} \times 1{,}000$
Perinatal mortality rate	$\dfrac{\text{Number of fetal deaths plus infant deaths 7 days of age in 1 year}}{\text{Number of live births plus fetal deaths in same year}} \times 1{,}000$
Neonatal mortality rate	$\dfrac{\text{Number of deaths of children under 28 days of age in 1 year}}{\text{Number of live births in the same year}} \times 1{,}000$
Fetal mortality rate	$\dfrac{\text{Number of fetal deaths in 1 year}}{\text{Number of live births plus fetal deaths in the same year}} \times 1{,}000$

Note: A test with a high sensitivity has a low type II error rate. A test with a high specificity has a low type I error rate.

This information documents the need for developing programs such as the initiation of primary, secondary, or tertiary prevention strategies for people at risk. Also, these data provide the rationale for modification of facilities and hiring staff to meet the requirements of the community.

Evidence for Practice

Researchers at the Centers for Disease Control and Prevention (CDC, 2010b) used the results of the Oregon Healthy Teens Survey, which had questioned eighth-grade students to determine the demographic characteristics and risk factors for participation in the "choking game." This is an activity where youths become "high" by cutting off blood and oxygen to the brain with a belt, towel, rope, or other item. Evaluation of earlier studies had indicated that youths experiencing peer rejection or other disruptive factors are more likely to participate in strangulation activities.

This investigation (CDC, 2010b) reported prevalence rates as percentages because the base multiplier for calculation of the rates was 100. A total of 36.2% of the youths had heard of the choking game, 30.4% had heard of someone participating, and 5.7% had taken part themselves. Risk factors included substance use and mental health factors, such as depression. Youths with these factors had the highest participation rate (15.8%) and were approximately nine times more likely to participate. Of those who reported only substance use and no mental health factors, the participation rate was 7.9%, and of those who reported only mental health factors and no substance use, the participation rate was 4%. In students with no reported risk factors, the participation rate was 1.7%.

Public health surveillance of these strangulation activities in youths should be expanded to understand the frequency of the risk and the motives and circumstances surrounding participation. Along with parents and educators, nurses, counselors, and others who work with youths should be aware of strangulation activities and their serious health effects. They should watch for signs of participation in strangulation activities, especially in youths with suspected substance use or mental health risk factors. Three quarters of parents responding reported being familiar with the choking game, but considerably fewer (20%) reported having talked to their children about this activity. Ninety-six percent of parents reported knowing that unintentional death was a potential risk and 90% believe information about this activity should be included in school health curricula (Bernacki & Davies, 2012). In addition, this report indicated the importance parents' perspectives on the topic of the prevention of the choking. The association between participation in strangulation activities and other sensation-seeking behaviors or mental health risk factors suggests that effective methods for substance use prevention might serve as models for effective prevention strategies. However, prevention methods for this activity should be tested before being incorporated into general use. For example, an unintended consequence of prevention methods may be increased youth participation in the choking game. Effective prevention methods could be incorporated into existing substance use and mental health screening instruments, curricula, or related public health tools (CDC, 2010b).

SPECIFIC RATES: DESCRIBING BY PERSON, PLACE, AND TIME

Specific rates are more detailed rates and are calculated using the number of people in the smaller subgroups of the population in the denominator. Often, people are divided into subgroups by age and sex, although any characteristic can be used. The frequency and severity of most illnesses vary according to age more than any other personal characteristic.

When investigating the distribution and the determinants of a health condition, one of the first steps is to use statistics to find out who is experiencing the condition (person), where it is occurring (place), and when it appears (time). This information about the distribution of the condition is an essential step in the identification of high-risk groups and in the search for possible solutions.

There are three ways of examining descriptive information that can be helpful in developing plausible explanations (hypotheses) for the occurrence of the condition under study. First, look for *differences* in frequency of characteristics between groups; second, look for *areas of agreement* where factors are identified that are occurring frequently; and third, look for *variations* in the data that may present clues for

control and prevention of the condition. Rates are usually used in this process, and it is often helpful to use graphs or charts to depict the results.

> If you can't explain it simply, you don't understand it well enough. **Albert Einstein**

Person: Who

Within any general population, whether it consists of members of a neighborhood, the clients in a community clinic, or the residents in an assisted living facility, there are differences among the individual people. These differences are genetic, biologic, behavioral, and socioeconomic. Because of these variations, specific incidence and prevalence rates should be calculated according to these specific characteristics. Statistics of this type that are gathered to describe populations are referred to as **demographic data**, or the study of the size, distribution, and characteristics of human populations.

Two characteristics are considered routine descriptors of a person: age and sex. Most health problems vary in both frequency and severity by age, and many are sex-specific. Therefore, morbidity and mortality rates for almost all health conditions vary by age or sex. Because of this, age- and sex-specific incidence and prevalence rates should be calculated whenever describing a problem.

Practice Point

Age is the most important characteristic to address when describing the state of people's health; it is directly associated with risk for illness or disability.

The CDC has used specific incidence rates in its surveillance of injuries in the United States (CDC 2014a). Figure 7.3 shows the percentage distribution of injury episodes by place of occurrence in 2010. As can be expected, 47% of the nonfatal, medically attended injury episodes took place in or around the home. Nearly 40% of these injuries occurred while a person was engaged in leisure activities, including sports (CDC, 2012). Figure 7.3 shows percentages; however, these are also rates with a multiplier of 100. Knowing what an injured person was doing and where his or her injury occurred is very important for designing prevention programs.

Figure 7.4 presents an example of specific prevalence rates for adults aged more than 45 years who need help with routine activities, by age group and selected race or ethnicity. Again, this example shows rates expressed as percentages; examining this figure shows that needing help with routine activities increased steadily with age for all racial/ethnic groups. Non-Hispanic blacks were more likely to need help with routine activities compared with Hispanics and non-Hispanic whites for those aged 45 to 74 years. Among adults aged 45 to 54, Hispanics were least likely to

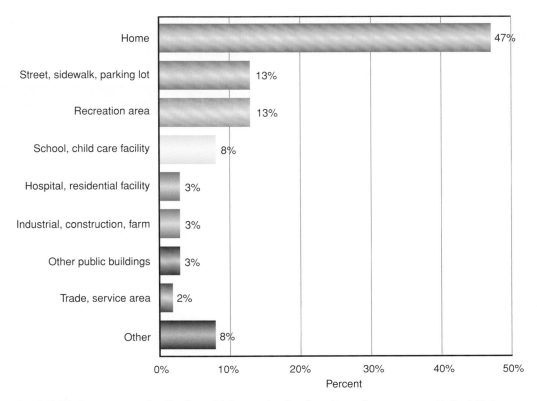

FIGURE 7.3 Percentage distribution of injury episodes, by place of occurrence: United States, 2010. (*Source:* National Health Interview Survey, 2010. Available from http://www.cdc.gov/nchs/data/factsheets/factsheet_injury.htm.)

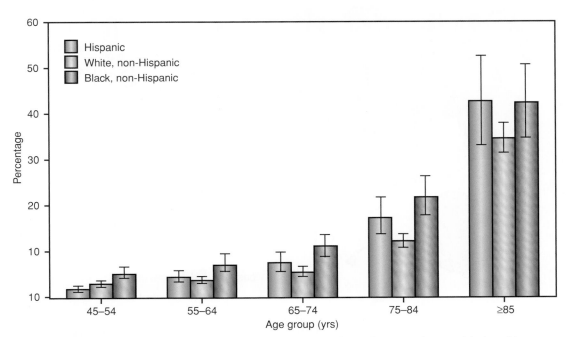

FIGURE 7.4 Percentage of adults aged greater than or equal to 45 years who need help with routine activities by age group and selected race/ethnicity—National Health Interview Survey, United States, 2011. (Available from https://www.cdc.gov/nchs/data/series/sr_10/sr10_255.pdf.)

need help with routine activities. However, the pattern changes among adults aged 75 years and over. Hispanics and non-Hispanic blacks were both more likely to need help with routine activities than non-Hispanic whites. Studying figures such as this one can give public health practitioners data that is needed to institute primary, secondary, and tertiary interventions to enhance the health of these groups (CDC, 2013).

Facts are stubborn, but statistics are more pliable. **Mark Twain**

Place: Where

Examining the differences in the rates of illness or disability and determining where they are highest or lowest assists in determining health needs, planning prevention and control measures, and allocating resources. Natural boundaries, political boundaries, and environmental characteristics are taken into consideration in this process.

Variations in incidence and prevalence rates can be examined by continent, nation, states, city, census tract, city block, or other geographic area. Differences between urban and rural areas or among smaller localities may be helpful in investigating specific health needs for communities. Place of occurrence is almost always examined when investigating outbreaks, both in the community and within institutions. Rates can be compared among institutions, among units in a single institution, or among different groups within any healthcare facility. This

information indicates where prevention and control measures and health resources should be concentrated to decrease incidence and prevalence of a particular problem.

Evidence for Practice

The CDC monitored the 2015–2017 outbreak of salmonella related to exposure to pet guinea pigs, the fourth such outbreak since 2006 (CDC, 2018). A total of nine cases have occurred in eight states and the District of Columbia, but many more unreported illnesses likely occurred. This is similar to the 2008 outbreak, demonstrated in Figure 7.5, which caused a multistate outbreak of salmonella related to exposure to pet turtles (CDC, 2010c). In this third outbreak in 2015–2017, a total of 135 cases occurred in 25 states and the District of Columbia. Figure 7.5 shows the distribution of the confirmed cases by state. The first known (index) case was a 2-year-old girl who was brought to a physician's office in Philadelphia after 3 days of diarrhea and fever. *Salmonella typhimurium* was isolated from her stool specimen. Three weeks earlier, the family had purchased two pet turtles with shell lengths less than 4 in from a street vendor. Within weeks, more clients in Pennsylvania were diagnosed with the same strain of the organism, and matching isolates had been found in cases from 10 states. Most ill people reported

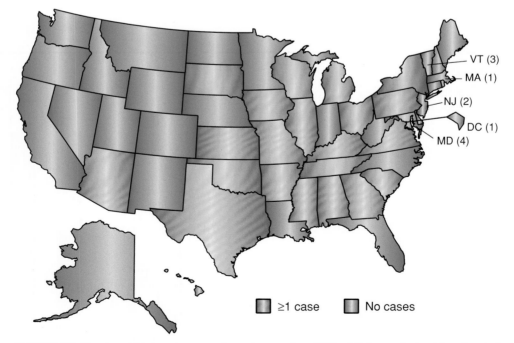

FIGURE 7.5 Number of laboratory-confirmed cases (*n* = 135) of *Salmonella typhimurium* infection with the outbreak strain, involving pet turtles in the United States, March 13 through November 17, 2008. (Data from Centers for Disease Control and Prevention. [2010]. Multistate outbreak of human *Salmonella typhimurium* infections associated with pet turtle exposure—United States, 2008. *Morbidity and Mortality Weekly Report*, 59[07], 191–196. Retrieved from http://www.cdc.gov/mmwr/preview/mmwrhtml/mm5907a2.htm.)

exposure to turtles with shell lengths less than 4 in that had been acquired from flea markets, street vendors, and souvenir shops. It is important to note that small turtles pose a greater risk to young children because they are perceived as safe pets, but are small enough to be placed in the mouth or handled inappropriately.

Investigation of the salmonella outbreak documented that young children without direct turtle exposure are at risk for turtle-associated salmonellosis through person-to-person transmission in child care settings. This investigation reinforced the need for continuing the existing prevention and control measures. Increasing enforcement of the existing local, state, and federal regulations against the sale of small turtles, increasing penalties for illegal sales, and enacting more state and local laws regulating the sale of small turtles could enhance federal prevention efforts and facilitate a more rapid public health response (CDC, 2010d).

Time: When

Variations in time can be short-term, periodic, or long-term. **Short-term changes** are measured in hours, days, weeks, or months. They are commonly found in outbreaks of infectious disease. Figure 7.6 illustrates an **epidemic curve** created from study of an outbreak of mumps that occurred from June 2009 to January 2010 in New York and New Jersey. Cases of reported confirmed or probably mumps ($n = 1,494$) are shown by week of illness onset and age group during the outbreak. At the time of the report, local transmission continued to occur (CDC, 2010e).

More recently, reports on an increase in newborn microcephaly in northeast Brazil demonstrated an emerging epidemic of the Zika virus. Infants born with a small head, measured by circumference, and those whose head circumference fails to increase in infancy have a condition called microcephaly (WHO, 2016). This is a rarity and usually

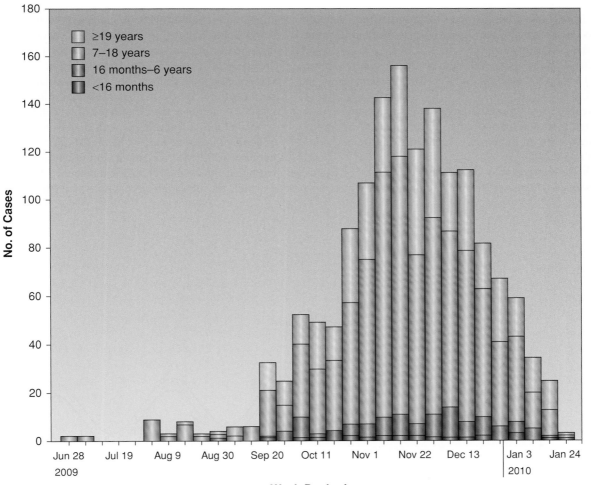

FIGURE 7.6 Number ($n = 1,494$) of reported confirmed or probable mumps cases, by week of illness onset and age group in New York and New Jersey, June 2009 through January 2010. (Data from Centers for Disease Control and Prevention. [2010]. Update: Mumps outbreak—New York and New Jersey, June 2009–January 2010. *Morbidity and Mortality Weekly Report*, 59[05], 125–129. Retrieved from http://www.cdc.gov/mmwr/preview/mmwrhtml/mm5905a1.htm.)

TABLE 7.3 Zika Information From Brazil: Date, Total Cases, Locations, and Deaths

Date	Total # Cases	Locations	Reported Deaths
As of October 2015	Increase # cases	Northeastern Brazil	0
As of 17 November 2015	399	Northeastern Brazil Seven states	0
As of 21 November 2015	739	Northeastern Brazil Nine states	1
As of 05 December 2015	1761	Nationally across 42 municipalities across 14 federal units The Northeastern region continued to report the highest number	19
As of 02 January 2016	3,174	Nationally across 684 municipalities of 21 federal units. The Northeastern region continued to report the highest number of suspected cases	38

Source: World Health Organization. (2017). Microcephaly Brazil. Retrieved from http://www.who.int/csr/don/8-january-2016-brazil-microcephaly/en.

occurs in one case among several thousand births. The outcome of microcephaly is severe, with physical and learning disabilities occurring.

In 2016, the Ministry of Health of Brazil reported to the World Health Organization (WHO, 2017) the data shown in Table 7.3.

In response to this emerging data, the World Health Organization and Brazilian public health agencies responded with an increase in vector prevention and control (WHO, 2017).

Periodic changes may be seasonal or cyclic. For example, respiratory diseases are more common in winter and spring, and infectious hepatitis increases in incidence every 7 to 9 years. Figure 7.7 shows the percentage of all deaths attributed to pneumonia and influenza for 122 cities in the United States between 2009 and 2013. The seasonal variation in death rates reflects the seasonal variation in respiratory infections. When studying these mortality statistics, it is possible to compare the percentage of all deaths attributable to pneumonia and influenza with a seasonal baseline and epidemic threshold value calculated for each week. An increase of 1.645 standard deviations above the seasonal baseline deaths is the "epidemic threshold." This is the point at which the observed proportion of deaths attributed to

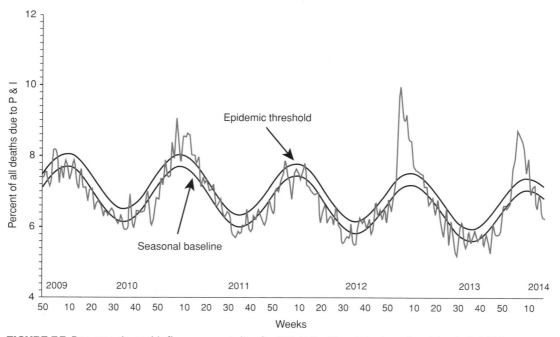

FIGURE 7.7 Pneumonia and influenza mortality for 122 U.S. cities: Week ending March 8, 2014. (Available at http://www.cdc.gov/flu/weekly.)

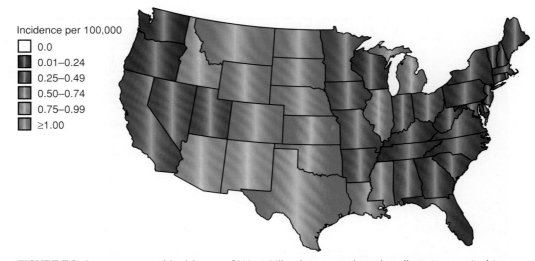

FIGURE 7.8 Average annual incidence of West Nile virus neuroinvasive disease reported to CDC by state, 1999 to 2012. (*Source:* ArboNET, Arboviral Diseases Branch, Centers for Disease Control and Prevention. Retrieved from http://www.cdc.gov/westnile/statsMaps/cumMapsData.html.)

Incidence per 100,000
- 0.0
- 0.01–0.24
- 0.25–0.49
- 0.50–0.74
- 0.75–0.99
- ≥1.00

pneumonia or influenza is significantly higher than would be expected at that time of the year. **Long-term changes** extend over decades and reflect gradual changes. An interesting example follows the tracking of West Nile virus infection, a disease that is transmitted by a mosquito vector. Figure 7.8 follows the progression of the illness from one state to another after it was first reported in New York in 1999. This figure combines variation in both place and time over a period of 15 years (CDC, 2014b).

Figure 7.9 shows that variations in trends of the mortality of various cancers can be seen when examined over many years. Overall, the age-adjusted cancer rates between 1930 and 2010 have fluctuated but are decreasing slowly. Cancer of the lung and bronchus leads all cancers as the cause of mortality in both men and women. It is interesting to note that the mortality rate for cancer of the stomach has decreased steadily since 1930, that cancer of the lung rose steadily until the 1990s, and that cancer of the colon and rectum continues to decrease (American Cancer Society, 2018). This is likely a result of primary prevention measures such as education and increased awareness as well as secondary prevention measures such as colonoscopy screening.

TYPES OF INCIDENCE RATES

Mortality Rates

Mortality rates or death rates are common incidence rates that are calculated for public health purposes. Crude mortality rates indicate the probability of death from any cause among the entire population in a designated geographic area. **Cause-specific** (disease-specific) **mortality rates** indicate the probability of death from a specific cause; the number of deaths from a specific disease is divided by the number of people in the population at midyear and multiplied by 100,000. In calculating the **case fatality rate**, the number of people with a specific disease such as lung cancer becomes the subgroup being studied out of the entire population in a designated geographic area. For example, the case fatality rate is calculated by dividing the number of deaths from lung cancer by the number of people living with lung cancer during the year, and multiplying by 100. Further breakdown into specific subgroups might involve age, sex, occupation, tobacco use, or other characteristics for calculation of mortality rates.

It is possible to confuse the **proportional mortality ratio (PMR)** with the cause-specific mortality rate. The PMR compares deaths from a specific illness to deaths from all other causes; it reflects the proportion of deaths due to a specific cause. The PMR is not a rate. The denominator includes all deaths within a given time period rather than the entire population under study. In contrast, the cause-specific mortality rates indicate the risk of death from a specific disease for a given living population. Both the PMR and cause-specific mortality rates should be calculated when death statistics are being examined for public health purposes.

Incidence Density

When there are unequal periods of observation for study subjects, it may be necessary to use a person-time denominator in the calculation of incidence rates. This technique provides a measure of **incidence density**. In healthcare, people often enter a study period at different times and therefore contribute unequal periods of time to the study. To identify the precise period of observation for each person and weigh that period of observation properly in calculating rates, a person-time unit, such as person-day or person-year, can be constructed. A person-day represents one person at

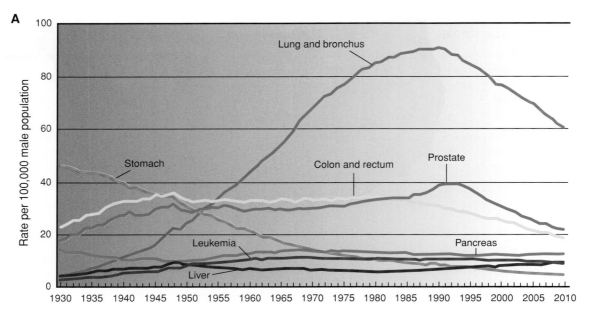

Per 100,000, age adjusted to the 2000 U.S. standard population

Note: Due to changes in ICD coding, numerator information has changed over time. Rates for cancer of the liver, lung and bronchus, and colon and rectum are affected by these coding changes.

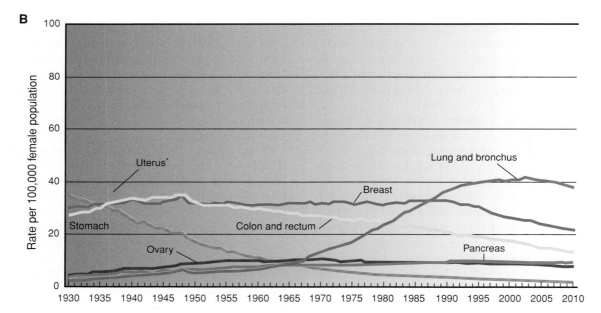

Per 100,000, age adjusted to the 2000 U.S. standard population
*Uterus refers to uterine cervix and uterine corpus combined.

Note: Due to changes in ICD coding, numerator information has changed over time. Rates for cancer of the liver, lung and bronchus, and colon and rectum are affected by these coding changes.

FIGURE 7.9 **A:** Age-adjusted cancer death rates, males by site, United States, 1930 to 2010. **B:** Age-adjusted cancer death rates, females by site, United States, 1930 to 2010. Rates are per 100,000 age-adjusted to the 2000 U.S. standard population. (Data from American Cancer Society. [2018]. *Cancer Facts & Figures 2018*. Atlanta: American Cancer Society. Retrieved from https://www.cancer.org/content/dam/cancer-org/research/cancer-facts-and-statistics/annual-cancer-facts-and-figures/2018/incidence-and-mortality-rates-for-selected-cancers-by-race-and-ethnicity-us-2010-2015.pdf.)

TABLE 7.4 Incidence Rates of Institution-Associated Pneumonia in an Acute and Long-Term Care Setting

Setting	No. of Cases	No. at Risk	Client or Patient Days	Crude Incidence (%)	Incidence (Density/ 100 Patient Days)
Acute care	33	2,249	19,102	1.5	1.75
Long-term care	27	366	37,064	7.4	0.73

Source: Data from Harkness, G. A., Bentley, D. W., & Roghmann, K. (1990). Nosocomial pneumonia in the elderly. *American Journal of Medicine, 89,* 459.

risk for 1 day, and a person-year represents one person at risk for 1 year. Incidence density can be calculated as:

$$\text{Incidence Density} = \frac{\begin{array}{c}\text{New cases}\\\text{occuring during}\\\text{the study period}\end{array}}{\begin{array}{c}\text{Person-time units}\\\text{accumulated by subjects}\\\text{during the study period}\end{array}} \times \text{Base multiple of 10}$$

Table 7.4 demonstrates the difference between the calculation of crude incidence rates and incidence density in a study that examined the development of hospital- and institution-associated pneumonia in both an acute care facility and a long-term care facility. These incidence data illustrate the need to calculate and compare both crude incidence and incidence density rates when comparing different settings with varying lengths of stay. In this example, the incidence rate in long-term care was almost five times that of the acute care setting. However, when the researchers included client days in the denominator, the acute care setting reflected twice the incidence density of the long-term care setting. More clients contributed shorter periods of time in the acute care setting, whereas there was relatively little turnover in residents in the long-term care setting.

Measures of incidence density can account for those persons who die, those who are lost to follow-up, or those who have acquired the illness and are therefore not at risk for the entire study period. Normally, it is assumed that the risk of acquiring the illness is constant throughout the entire period of the study.

Attributable Risk

Attributable risk is the difference between the incidence rates in an exposed group of people and an unexposed group of people. It measures the risk of a condition occurring in an exposed group that is attributable to a specific exposure but not to other factors. In almost any health-related event, some risk occurs normally in a population without a specific exposure. In calculating attributable risk, the risk of the event that would have occurred under normal circumstances is subtracted from the risk of the event in the exposed group:

Attributable Risk = Incidence rate in the exposed − The incidence rate in the nonexposed

Relative Risk Ratio

Incidence rates indicate the occurrence of a health-related event in a population in a given period of time. It is an indicator of the probability that people without a specific condition will develop the condition within a designated period of time. Therefore, it is a measure of the risk of developing the condition. Often, incidence rates for groups exposed to a certain risk factor are compared with the incidence rates for people who are not exposed. This procedure results in a **relative risk ratio**. It is a ratio of the incidence rate in the exposed group and the incidence rate in the nonexposed group.

$$\text{Relative Risk} = \frac{\text{Incidence rate in the exposed group}}{\text{Incidence rate in the nonexposed group}}$$

A relative risk of 1.0 indicates that the risk is equal for both groups, and conversely, a relative risk greater than 1.0 indicates that the risk is greater in the exposed group. For example, a relative risk of 6.0 can be interpreted to mean that people who are exposed to a disease are six times more likely to develop it. The CDC used this technique to develop an educational chart for use in HIV prevention programs (Fig. 7.10). This chart shows how the relative risk for transmission from a person living with HIV to a person without the infection varies according to sexual activity and condom use. For example, it is possible to contrast insertive oral sex while using a condom, which has a low risk for HIV transmission, with receptive anal sex without a condom, which is 2,000 times more risky. This kind of information regarding HIV transmission can influence decisions about sexual activity and condom use (CDC, 2007).

A relative risk less than 1.0 indicates that the risk is less in the exposed group; the factor in question may possibly protect against the condition under study. Although this finding is not very common, it may signify that further study is warranted. Statistical tests, such as the calculation of the chi-square statistic, are used to determine whether the relative risk ratios are different from those that would be expected by chance. In this way, the statistical significance of the findings can be established.

SENSITIVITY AND SPECIFICITY

Sensitivity and specificity are statistical measures that evaluate the validity and reliability of a test. **Sensitivity** is the ability of the test to identify correctly people who have the

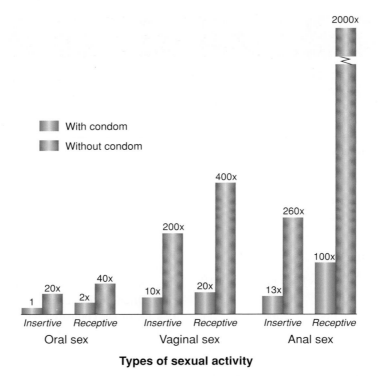

FIGURE 7.10 Relative risk for transmission from a person living with HIV. (Data from CDC. *Relative risk for transmission from a person living with HIV.* Retrieved from http://www.cdc.gov/hiv/topics/treatment/PIC/pdf/chart.pdf.)

health problem under study. It is the probability of testing positive if the health problem is truly present. **Specificity** is the ability of the test to correctly identify people who do not have the health problem. It is the probability of testing negative if the health problem is truly absent. Increasing the sensitivity of a test causes a decrease in specificity, and conversely, increasing the specificity of a test decreases sensitivity. The formulas for calculation of sensitivity and specificity are found in Box 7.2. To obtain sensitivity and specificity values, it is necessary to perform research studies that obtain the values of screening tests and then determine whether the health problem truly exists in each subject.

In an ideal situation, a screening test is able to identify the presence or absence of a health problem correctly in every person screened with a sensitivity and specificity of 100%. However, this is almost impossible to achieve in actual practice. One way to address this problem is to use several screening tests to make health decisions.

Before screening projects are undertaken, it is important to determine carefully the screening levels or test values. Much depends on the consequences of leaving some cases undetected (false negatives) or classifying healthy people as having a health problem (false positives). When the disease being studied is rare, the specificity of a test is rarely high enough to give an adequate positive predictive value. Only the sensitivity of a test is useful in the case of a rare disease. The choice of screening levels is subjective and based on the severity of the disease, cost, time factors, advantages of early treatment, and other screening criteria.

7.2 How to Calculate Sensitivity and Specificity

$$\text{Sensitivity} = \frac{\text{(true positive results)}}{\text{(true positive results + false negatives)}}$$

$$\text{Specificity} = \frac{\text{(true negative results)}}{\text{(true negative results + false positives)}}$$

The outreach program promotes HIV testing in the African American population. Lindsay examines the types of tests available and finds that rapid, same-day testing has a high sensitivity and specificity. She reviews the below example to understand what this means.

This is perhaps best illustrated by example. Imagine a population of 100,000 people, of whom 10,000 are actually HIV-infected and 90,000 HIV-uninfected. The goal of a screening procedure would be to correctly identify all 10,000—and only those 10,000—HIV-positive individuals. A test with 99% sensitivity would correctly identify 9,900 of the 10,000 infected individuals (99%). One hundred infected people would test falsely negative (a false-negative rate of 1%).

If the same test procedure had a specificity of 90% (an unrealistically low value used to simplify this example), it would correctly identify 90% (81,000) of the HIV-uninfected individuals as HIV-negative. However, 9,000 HIV-uninfected persons would test falsely positive (a false-positive, http://www.aidsmap.com/Sensitivity-and-specificity/page/1322984/ rate of 9,000/90,000=10%). Box 7.2 for the equations used to calculate sensitivity and specificity.

essential in determining the rationale for an experimental or intervention study.

Researchers design descriptive studies to acquire more information about the occurrence of health problems or, alternatively, the factors that keep people well. The specific rates calculated in these studies describe people who have or do not have the health problem in terms of person, place, and time. These studies provide a picture of the events as they naturally occur. Therefore, this type of data is very helpful for nurses involved in health planning or administration in both community and institutional settings. Knowledge of people who are the most or least susceptible to a health problem can help when deciding to implement programs for prevention or control of health problems and to allocate resources.

USE OF RATES IN DESCRIPTIVE RESEARCH STUDIES

Epidemiologic descriptive studies include the descriptions of health conditions, case reports, and correlational studies. Descriptive studies are very useful in describing the characteristics of disease occurrence and in generating hypotheses for further study. They are the first studies to be performed in investigating the determinants of a health problem and are

Lindsay develops a plan to evaluate the effectiveness of the outreach program. Using the HIV/AIDS Outreach Survey, decide what statistics should be calculated for each of the 10 questions. Include the calculation of both general (crude) rates and specific rates where appropriate.

KEY CONCEPTS

- Measuring the magnitude or frequency of a state of health determines the characteristics of those who are at high risk.
- Epidemiologic descriptive studies have determined measurable risk factors for major illnesses.
- Calculation of rates provides the best indicators of the probability that a specific state of health will occur.
- Indexes of the health of a community, region, or country include comparisons of general mortality rates and maternal infant rates.
- A variety of rates can be calculated according to need, including incidence, prevalence, adjusted, and specific rates.

- Specific rates calculated by person, place, and time provide the best description of a health condition.
- Prevalence is influenced by the number of people who have developed the condition in the past and the duration of their illness. Prevalence rates provide essential data for implementing prevention measures.
- Before screening projects are undertaken, the sensitivity and specificity of screening levels or test values should be carefully reviewed.

CRITICAL THINKING QUESTIONS

1. Between January 1 and December 31, 35 new cases of tuberculosis were diagnosed in a city. There were a total of 300 active cases among the population of 400,000 on December 31 of that year. Twenty deaths from tuberculosis were recorded during the 1-year period.
   a. What was the incidence rate per 100,000 people for tuberculosis during the year?
   b. What was the prevalence rate of tuberculosis per 100,000 on December 31?

   c. What is the cause-specific death rate per 100,000 for tuberculosis during the year?

2. A recent report from a state health department included a map indicating the distribution and number of rabid animals for each of the 167 towns in the state between January 1 and October 31. What type of information about the occurrence of rabies does this report include? Why were rates not calculated? How might this information be used to control rabies?

CRITICAL THINKING QUESTIONS *(Continued)*

3. A community nurse uncovers the following statistics regarding HIV infection in African Americans in two rural counties in the United States:

  a. What is the incidence rate in black males and black females per 10,000 people in the 1-year period?

  b. What is the prevalence rate in black males and black females per 10,000 people in the 1-year period?

  c. Interpret the incidence and prevalence rates. Which statistics provide the best information to use for program planning?

d. What population group should be targeted for the HIV/AIDS outreach program? Why?

	New HIV Infection	Living With HIV	Population Total
Males	150	838	29,560
Females	234	1,312	28,315
African American population	384	2,150	57,875

REFERENCES

American Cancer Society. (2018). *Cancer facts & figures 2018.* Atlanta: American Cancer Society. Retrieved from https://www.cancer.org/content/dam/cancer-org/research/cancer-facts-and-statistics/annual-cancer-facts-and-figures/2018/incidence-and-mortality-rates-for-selected-cancers-by-race-and-ethnicity-us-2010-2015.pdf.

Bernacki, J. M., & Davies, W. H. (2012). Prevention of the Choking Game: parent perspectives. *Journal of Injury and Violence Research, 4*(2), 73.

Brown, E. J., & Brown, J. S. (2003). HIV prevention outreach in black communities of three rural North Florida counties. *Public Health Nursing, 20*(3), 204–210.

Brown, K., Williams, D. B., Kinchen, S., Saito, S., Radin, E. Patel, H., … Voetsch, A. C. (2018). Status of HIV epidemic control among adolescent girls and young women aged 15–24 years—Seven African countries (2015-2017). *Morbidity and Mortality Weekly, 67*(1), 29–32.

Centers for Disease Control and Prevention. (2007). Relative risk for transmission from a person living with HIV. Retrieved from http://www.cdc.gov/hiv/topics/treatment/PIC/pdf/chart.pdf.

Centers for Disease Control and Prevention. (2010a). Healthy People 2020. Retrieved from https://www.healthypeople.gov/.

Centers for Disease Control and Prevention. (2010b). "Choking game" awareness and participation among 8th graders—Oregon, 2008. *Morbidity and Mortality Weekly Report, 59*(1), 1–5.

Centers for Disease Control and Prevention. (2010c). Multistate outbreak of human Salmonella typhimurium infections associated with pet turtle exposure—United States, 2008. *Morbidity and Mortality Weekly Report, 59*(7), 191–196.

Centers for Disease Control and Prevention. (2010d). Multistate outbreak of human Salmonella typhimurium infections associated with pet turtle exposure—United States, 2008. *Morbidity and Mortality Weekly Report, MMWR News Synopsis.* Retrieved from https://www.cdc.gov/media/mmwrnews/2010/n100225.htm.

Centers for Disease Control and Prevention. (2010e). Update: Mumps outbreak—New York and New Jersey, June 2009–January 2010.

Morbidity and Mortality Weekly Report, 59(5), 125–129. Retrieved from http://www.cdc.gov/mmwr/preview/mmwrhtml/mm5905a1.htm.

Centers for Disease Control and Prevention. (2012) NCHS fact sheet: NCHS data on injuries. Retrieved from http://www.cdc.gov/nchs/data/factsheets/factsheet_injury.htm.

Centers for Disease Control and Prevention. (2013). QuickStats: Percentage of adults aged ≥45 years who need help with routine activities by age group and selected race/ethnicity—National Health Interview Survey, United States, 2011. *Morbidity and Mortality Weekly Report, 62*(33), 683. Retrieved from http://www.cdc.gov/mmwr/preview/mmwrhtml/mm6233a7.htm?s.

Centers for Disease Control and Prevention. (2014a). NCHS data on injuries: NCHS fact sheet. Retrieved from http://www.cdc.gov/nchs/data/factsheets/factsheet_injury.htm.

Centers for Disease Control and Prevention. (2014b). West Nile virus disease cases and deaths reported to CDC by year and clinical presentation, 1999–2012. Final cumulative maps & data for 1999–2012. Retrieved from http://www.cdc.gov/westnile/statsMaps/cumMapsData.html.

Centers for Disease Control and Prevention (CDC). (2016). Age-adjusted death rates, by race, Hispanic origin, state, and territory. Retrieved from https://www.cdc.gov/nchs/data/hus/2016/016.pdf.

Centers for Disease Control and Prevention. (2018). Multistate outbreak of salmonella enteritidis infections linked to pet guinea pigs. Retrieved from https://www.cdc.gov/salmonella/guinea-pigs-03-18/index.html.

World Health Organization. (2015). The top 10 causes of death. Retrieved from http://www.who.int/mediacentre/factsheets/fs310/en/.

World Health Organization. (2016). Microcephaly. Retrieved from http://www.who.int/mediacentre/factsheets/microcephaly/en/.

World Health Organization. (2017). Microcephaly Brazil. Retrieved from http://www.who.int/csr/don/8-january-2016-brazil-microcephaly/en/.

WEB RESOURCES

Please visit thePoint® for up-to-date web resources on this topic.

Gathering Evidence for Public Health Practice

Barbara A. Goldrick

Of course we don't know what we're doing, that's why it's called research.
Albert Einstein

1. Statistical significance is not the same thing as practical importance.
2. The more complex the test required to show statistical significance, the less important to an individual the association is likely to be.
3. The word "significant" without the prefix "statistical" is usually a coward's way of implying "important" without mathematical evidence.

Cowden's Three Rules of Statistics; John M. Cowden, English epidemiologist

People commonly use statistics like a drunk uses a lamppost: for support rather than for illumination.
Mark Twain

CHAPTER HIGHLIGHTS

- Epidemiologic/public health research defined
- Observational studies: Descriptive versus analytical research

- Strengths and limitations of epidemiologic research methodology
- Applying epidemiologic research to public health nursing practice

OBJECTIVES

- Describe the difference between descriptive and analytical research.
- Discuss the strengths and weaknesses of retrospective, prospective, case–control, and experimental designs.

- Generate research questions related to problems identified in community and public health nursing practice.

KEY TERMS

Analytical study: Investigation that uses comparisons between groups to determine the role of various risk factors in causing the problem.

Association: Statistical relationship between two or more events, characteristics, or other variables.

Case–control study: Observational analytic study that enrolls one group of persons with a certain health problem (case patients) and a group of persons without the health problem (control subjects). It compares differences in exposures,

behaviors, and other characteristics to identify and quantify associations, test hypotheses, and identify causes.

Case study: Research method that involves an in-depth analysis of an individual, group, or institution.

KEY TERMS (continued)

Causality: Relationship between two variables in which the presence or absence of one variable (the "cause") determines the presence or absence of the other (the "effect").

Clinical trial: Experimental study in which the investigator specifies the type of exposure for each study participant and then follows each person's health status to determine the effects of the exposure.

Cohort study: Observational analytic study in which enrollment is based on status of exposure to a certain factor or membership in a certain group.

Controls: Subjects in an experiment who do not receive the "treatment" and provide baseline data against which the effects of the treatment can be measured.

Cross-sectional study: Study in which a sample of persons from a population is enrolled and their exposures and health outcomes are measured simultaneously.

Demographic variables: Characteristics or attributes that are collected to describe the sample.

Dependent variable: The response, behavior, or outcome presumed to be affected by the independent variable(s).

Descriptive study: Study in which information is collected to characterize and summarize a health event or problem.

Epidemiologic research: The study of the distribution and determinants of health conditions or events among populations. The studies may be descriptive or analytic.

Extraneous variables: Variables outside of the study that can affect (confound) the measurement and relationship among study variables. These can be intrinsic to the subjects (e.g., stress) and/or external factors (e.g., environment). Randomization is the most

effective method to control for extraneous variables in study subjects. Control over variables external to the study generally take place in an artificial environment such as a laboratory setting.

Hypothesis: Statement of the expected outcome between two or more variables in a specific population.

Independent variable: The treatment or experimental activity that is manipulated by the researcher to test its effect on the dependent variable.

Intervention study: Investigation designed to test a hypothesized relationship by modifying an identified factor in a population. Studies may be therapeutic (clinical) or preventive.

Null hypothesis: Statement that there is no difference between/ among the variables under study.

Observational study: Study in which the investigator observes rather than influences exposure and disease among participants.

Odds ratio (OR): Measure of association used in comparative studies, particularly case–control studies, which quantifies the association between an exposure and a health outcome.

p value: In statistical testing, the probability that the obtained results are not due to chance alone. Generally, the significance level set by the researcher is less than or equal to 0.05.

Preventive trial: Study in which the investigator provides a specific preventive measure to the group under study and follows the group to determine the effects of the intervention.

Prospective study: Analytic study in which participants are enrolled before the health outcome of interest has occurred.

Quasi-experimental study: Study with limited control where the subjects cannot be randomly assigned to an intervention. However, the researcher can still manipulate the dependent variable.

Relationship: See association; the two terms are often used interchangeably.

Relative risk (RR): Ratio of the risk of disease or death among those exposed to the risk among the unexposed; synonymous with risk ratio.

Retrospective study: Analytic study in which participants are enrolled after the health outcome of interest has occurred.

Sample: Selected subset of a population; a sample can be random or nonrandom and representative or nonrepresentative.

Survey research: Systematic canvassing of persons to collect information, often from a representative sample of the population. Studies may use questionnaires and/or interviews to collect data.

Therapeutic trial: Clinical trial in which the investigator provides a specific intervention/ treatment (therapy) to the group under study and follows the group to determine the effects of the treatment.

Type I error: An error created by rejecting the null hypothesis when it is true; that is, a difference is seen to exist when in fact it does not.

Type II error: An error created by accepting the null hypothesis when it is false; that is, it is concluded that no difference exists when in fact it does.

Variables: Qualities or characteristics of persons, things, or situations that change and can be manipulated or measured in research. Extraneous variables can affect the measurement and relationship among study variables.

CASE STUDIES

References to the case studies are found throughout this chapter (look for the case study icon). Readers should keep the case studies in mind as they read the chapter.

CASE 1

A *Healthy People 2020* goal is to increase the proportion of adults aged 65 years and older who are vaccinated against pneumococcal disease, which is caused by *Streptococcus pneumoniae*, to at least 90% (USDHHS, 2010). However, data from the Centers for Disease Control and Prevention (CDC)/National Center for Health Statistics (NCHS) found that only 61% of persons 65 years of age or older had ever received pneumococcal polysaccharide vaccine in 2014 (CDC, NCHS, 2014b).

A group of community health nurses learn that their state is not on target to meet the *Healthy People 2020* objective to increase the proportion of persons aged 65 years or older vaccinated against pneumococcal disease to 90% (USDHHS, 2010). In addition, the state health department has reported the occurrence of four cases of multidrug-resistant *S. pneumoniae* in the state within the past several months.

CASE 2

In 2014 the World Health Organization (WHO) updated its 2011 report and confirmed that noncommunicable diseases (NCDs) are still the leading cause of mortality worldwide. Cardiovascular diseases account for most NCD deaths, at 17.7 million people annually, followed by cancers (8.8 million), respiratory diseases (3.9 million), and diabetes (1.6 million). These four groups of diseases account for 81% of all NCD deaths and share four common risk factors:
- Physical inactivity
- Tobacco use
- Poor diets
- Harmful use of alcohol

Seventeen million people die from a NCD before the age of 70, with 87% of these "premature" deaths occurring in low- and middle-income countries (WHO, 2014).

In Chapter 6, epidemiology was defined as the study of the distribution and determinants of states of health and illness in human populations. This information provides the data necessary to justify the establishment of health services designed to maintain and improve health. Epidemiologic surveillance is then conducted to monitor and evaluate these health services. The purposes of **epidemiologic research**, on the other hand, are to: (1) identify community/public health problems; and (2) describe natural history and etiology of diseases. Community/public health nurses use a variety of epidemiologic research methods to generate new knowledge and provide evidence for best practice. As can be seen in Figure 8.1, the epidemiologic research cycle includes both experimental or intervention studies and observational studies.

OBSERVATIONAL STUDIES

Observational studies may be either descriptive or analytical. In **descriptive studies**, the researcher collects information to characterize and summarize the health event or problem when little is known about the phenomenon. Descriptive studies provide the foundation for the development and testing of **hypotheses**.

As can be seen in see Figure 8.1, observational studies can be hypothesis-generating and hypothesis-testing studies.

1. Descriptive studies

2. Model-building/hypotheses formulation

3. Analytic/hypotheses-testing studies

4. Analysis of results, further descriptive studies/new hypotheses

FIGURE 8.1 Epidemiologic study cycle.

Hypothesis-generating research includes case studies and cross-sectional studies. Hypothesis-testing studies, on the other hand, include analytical studies that test the relationship between two or more **variables** in a specified population (see further discussion below).

In **analytical studies**, the researcher relies on comparisons between groups to determine the role of various risk factors in causing the problem.

Descriptive Studies

Descriptive studies are fundamental to public health research and practice (CDC, 2012a). Descriptive research identifies the characteristics of individuals, situations, or groups and the frequency with which certain phenomena (risks) occur (Gray, Grove, & Sutherland, 2017). The concept of risk was defined in Chapter 6 as it relates to person, place, and time. Therefore, descriptive studies, which are frequently used in public health, are designed to acquire more information about characteristics of health (or disease) as they pertain to person, place, and time. People in the study population will all have some characteristic in common; therefore, some restrictions to this broad definition must be made. For example, research is limited to considering people of the same age range, sex, or geographic location.

Many descriptive studies are observational; that is, no intervention or treatment is included. However, descriptive studies provide the foundation for the development and testing of hypotheses.

> If it looks like a duck, and quacks like a duck, we have at least to consider the possibility that we have a small aquatic bird of the family Anatidae on our hands. **Douglas Adams, science fiction writer**

Case Studies

Case studies involve an in-depth analysis of an individual, group, or social institution (Gray, Grove, & Sutherland, 2017). In epidemiologic and public health research, the case study often is the first clue that a problem may exist. A case series is a group of people with the same, or similar, illness or injury and with the same, or similar, factors that may be importantly related to the disease or injury. A historic example of a case series was the first cases of young men who presented with Kaposi sarcoma and *Pneumocystis carinii* pneumonia in California and New York in the early 1980s. What these young men had in common was having sex with other men. In June 1981, the CDC published the first report about AIDS in the United States, which alerted the medical and public health communities 4 months before the first peer-reviewed article on the subject of AIDS was published. For more information on the history of HIV/AIDS, see the CDC website at http://www.cdc.gov/hiv/topics/basic/#origin and AVERT website at http://www.avert.org/history-aids-1986.htm.

Survey Research

Another method used in public health to collect data is **survey research**. Survey research focuses on the collection of information regarding the status quo of some situations by questionnaire or by interviews with a sample of respondents (Gray, Grove, & Sutherland, 2017). The main principle of survey research is that the **sample** of respondents must represent the population from which it was drawn.

An example of survey research was conducted by nurse researchers using existing data from a larger study. The purpose of the study was to determine the predictors of smokers' participation in a smoking cessation program among patients with head and neck cancer from three Veterans Affairs medical centers. All participants who agreed to participate ($N = 136$) had smoked within the past 6 months and were classified as currently smoking, having quit in the past month, or having quit in the past 6 months. The **dependent variable** for the analysis was the smoker's participation (yes/no) in the smoking cessation program (intervention). The major **independent variables** of interest included perceived difficulty in quitting, health behaviors (smoking and problem drinking), clinical characteristics (depression and cancer site and stage), and **demographic variables**.

More than half of the participants believed it would be very to extremely difficult to quit smoking. More than 60% were currently smoking and were smoking a pack a day or less. The remaining 40% of participants had quit smoking within the past 1 to 6 months. Significant associations were found between participation in the smoking-cessation program and high perception that it would be difficult to quit, miles traveled to the clinic, and hospital site ($p < 0.05$). No significant associations were found between participation status and alcohol use problems, greater symptoms of depression, time since diagnosis, age, or educational level.

The authors cited several limitations to the study. Although depressive symptoms and alcohol use were measured by a validated screener, they were not confirmed by a medical evaluation, which may have resulted in an overestimation of drinking problems and depressive symptoms. Despite the researchers' efforts to recruit from three Veterans Affairs medical centers with a large number of minorities, the sample was predominantly white. The original sample included 286 patients with approximately equal numbers of participants and nonparticipants; however, only 136 (48%) agreed to participate. Therefore, some of the studied variables may have reached significance had the sample size been larger (Duffy et al., 2010).

Another example of survey research is the National High Blood Pressure Education Program, coordinated by the National Heart, Lung and Blood Institute (NHLBI) of the National Institutes of Health. Established in 1972, the program has succeeded in increasing awareness, prevention, treatment, and control of hypertension. Considerable success has been achieved in the National High Blood Pressure Education Program. The last hypertension

TABLE 8.1 2017 Guideline for the Prevention, Detection, Evaluation, and Management of High Blood Pressure in Adults[a]

BP Category	SBP		DBP
Normal	<120 mm Hg	and	<80 mm Hg
Elevated	120–129 mm Hg	and	<80 mm Hg
Hypertension			
Stage 1	130–139 mm Hg	or	80–89 mm Hg
Stage 2	≥140 mm Hg	or	≥90 mm Hg

[a]Individuals with SBP and DBP in 2 categories should be designated to the higher BP category.
BP indicates blood pressure (based on an average of ≥2 careful readings obtained on ≥2 occasions); DBP, diastolic blood pressure; SBP, systolic blood pressure; mm Hg, millimeters of mercury.
Source: Whelton, P. K., et al. (2017). ACC/AHA/AAPA/ABC/ACPM/AGS/APhA/ASH/ASPC/NMA/PCNA Guideline for the Prevention, Detection, Evaluation, and Management of High Blood Pressure in Adults. *Hypertension, 70*(5), 1–283. Retrieved November 30, 2017 from http://hyper.ahajournals.org/content/guidelines2017.

guidelines published by NHLBI Joint National Committee (JNC) on Blood Pressure in Adults was in 2014 (James et al., 2014). However, in 2017, the American College of Cardiology/American Heart Association Task Force on Clinical Practice Guidelines developed new high blood pressure clinical practice guidelines, which update prior JNC reports (Whelton, P. K., et al., 2017). The 2017 hypertension guidelines, presented in Table 8.1, used an evidence-based approach to the management of hypertension in adults. Table 8.2 outlines the 2013 American Heart Association/American College of Cardiologists recommendations for lifestyle management to lower blood pressure and cardiovascular risk (Eckel et al., 2014).

Evidence for Practice

Hepatitis C virus (HCV) infection is the most common bloodborne infection in the United States. According to a 2015 study, it is estimated that 3 to 4 million people are currently infected with hepatitis C in the United States. Based on the CDC data, an additional 800,000 individuals are estimated to be infected each year (CDC, 2018).

More than 75% of adults infected with HCV are baby boomers (those born from 1945 to 1965). It is believed that most boomers became infected in the 1970s and 1980s when rates of hepatitis C were the highest. People with hepatitis C can live for decades without symptoms, and approximately half are unaware that they were infected with HCV many years ago (CDC, 2018).

The following persons are known to be at increased risk for HCV infection and should be tested:

- Current or former injection drug users, including those who injected only once many years ago
- Recipients of clotting factor concentrates made before 1987, when more advanced methods for manufacturing those products were developed
- Recipients of blood transfusions or solid organ transplants before July 1992, when better testing of blood donors became available
- Chronic hemodialysis patients
- Persons with known exposures to HCV, such as healthcare workers after needlesticks involving HCV-positive blood, recipients of blood or organs from a donor who tested HCV-positive
- Persons with HIV infection
- Have persistently abnormal alanine aminotransferase levels (ALT)
- Children born to HCV-positive mothers (CDC, 2018)

TABLE 8.2 Recommendations for Lifestyle Management to Lower Blood Pressure

	Recommendations	NHLB Strength of Evidence
Diet	1. Consume a dietary pattern that emphasizes intake of vegetables, fruits, and whole grains	Strong
	2. Include low-fat dairy products, poultry, fish, legumes, nontropical vegetable oils and nuts	Strong
	3. Limit intake of sweets, sugar-sweetened beverages and red meats	Strong
	4. Achieve this by following the USDA food pattern, or the ADA diet	Strong
	5. Lower sodium intake to 1,500 mg/day	Moderate
	6. Combine the DASH dietary pattern with lower sodium intake	Strong
Physical Activity	Engage in aerobic physical activity three to four times a week, lasting on average 40 minutes, and involves moderate-to-vigorous physical activity	Moderate

Adapted from Eckel, R. H., Jakicic, J. M., Ard, J. D., de Jesus, J. M., Houston Miller, N., Hubbard, V. S., … Tomaselli, G. F. (2014). 2013 AHA/ACC guideline on lifestyle management to reduce cardiovascular risk: A report of the American College of Cardiology/American Heart Association task force on practice guidelines. *Circulation, 129*(25 suppl 2), S76–S99. Retrieved July 10, 2017, from http://circ.ahajournals.org/content/129/25_suppl_2/S76.

Who should be tested for HCV?

One-time HCV testing is recommended for adults born from 1945 through 1965 (without prior ascertainment of HCV risk factors and regardless of country of birth).

There is no vaccine against HCV infection, but research into the development of a vaccine is under way.

The Food and Drug Administration (FDA) has approved several antiviral drugs to treat chronic HCV infection. These medications have proven efficacy when used as a component of a combination antiviral regimen to treat HCV-infected adults with compensated liver disease, cirrhosis, HIV co-infection, and hepatocellular carcinoma awaiting liver transplant (CDC, 2018).

Guidance for hepatitis C treatment in adults is changing constantly with the advent of new therapies and other developments. The Infectious Diseases Society of America (IDSA) and American Association for the Study of Liver Diseases (AASLD), in collaboration with the International Antiviral Society–USA (IAS–USA), developed a web-based process for the rapid formulation and dissemination of evidence-based, expert-developed recommendations (CDC, 2018). For the latest published recommendations for testing, managing, and treating hepatitis C, see their website at http://www.hcvguidelines.org.

Cross-Sectional Studies

Cross-sectional studies (prevalence studies) are another example of public health survey research. In this type of study, the population to be studied is defined, and data are collected from members of the group about their disease and exposure status. The data represent a point in time; therefore, they provide a "snapshot" of the population. Cross-sectional studies are good for examining the **relationship** between a variable and a disease/condition but not for determining cause and effect, which requires the collection of data over time. Cross-sectional studies may be designed to gather data from two or more groups with different characteristics or with different exposure risk.

An example of cross-sectional studies is the Behavioral Risk Factor Surveillance System (BRFSS) established by the CDC in the early 1980s when scientific research clearly indicated that personal health behaviors played a major role in premature morbidity and mortality. The BRFSS is an efficient method that takes a cross-section of the population at a single point in time and monitors the prevalence of the major behavioral risks in adults associated with premature morbidity and mortality at the state level. These data are useful for planning, initiating, supporting, and evaluating health promotion and disease prevention programs. Several states use these data to determine progress toward achievement of *Healthy People 2020* objectives (USDHHS, 2010). For more information on the BRFSS, see the CDC's BRFSS website at http://www.cdc.gov/brfss/.

TABLE 8.3 Assessment of Selected *Healthy People 2020* Objectives, 2014		
Objective	**Year 2014 (%)**	**Target 2020 (%)**
Reduce the proportion of adults (aged ≥18 years) who are obese	28.9	30
Increase the proportion of adults (aged ≥18 years) who engage in leisure-time physical activity	47.5	47.9
Reduce cigarette smoking by adults (aged ≥18 years)	17.0	12
Increase the proportion of adults (aged ≥65 years) who are vaccinated annually against influenza	70.1	90
Increase the proportion of adults (aged ≥65 years) who are vaccinated against pneumococcal disease	61.3	90

Sources: Centers for Disease Control and Prevention, National Center for Health Statistics. (2014). *Health, United States, 2014.* Retrieved July 14, 2017, from https://www.cdc.gov/nchs/data/hus/hus14_inbrief.pdf.; U.S. Department of Health and Human Services. *Healthy People 2020.* Retrieved July 14, 2014, from http://www.healthypeople.gov/2020/topicsobjectives2020/default.aspx.

Table 8.3 outlines an assessment of how progress was being made on selective objectives of *Healthy People 2020* in 2014. These data are based on the CDC National Center for Health Statistics (NCHS) 2014 (CDC, NCHS, 2014b). As can be seen in see Table 8.3, the prevalence of obesity among U.S. adults aged 18 and over was lower than the 2020 objective for obesity in this age group. Also, the percentage of adults (18 years and older) who had participated in federal guidelines for physical activity in 2014 was closer to the 2020 target of 47.9%. However, the percentage of adults who were current smokers in 2014 was more than the targeted 12% by 2020 (USDHHS, 2010).

Healthy People 2020 targets to increase influenza and pneumococcal vaccination in adults, which had been retained from *Healthy People 2010*, still had not been met as of 2014 (CDC, NCHS, 2014b). The percentage of adults aged 65 and older who had received influenza and pneumococcal vaccinations in 2014 remained well below the targets of 90%, respectively. It will be interesting to see how many of the objectives proposed for *Healthy People 2020* are met by the target date (USDHHS, 2010).

Case 1: In an attempt to increase the number of people aged 65 years or older who are vaccinated against pneumococcal disease, the community health

nurses in Case 1 decide to conduct the following:

- An assessment of baseline knowledge, attitudes, and practices among healthcare providers in the community regarding pneumococcal vaccination to identify barriers to providing pneumococcal vaccination
- An assessment of baseline knowledge, attitudes, and beliefs among community residents aged 65 years or older to determine barriers to receiving pneumococcal vaccination
  1. What research method could the nurses use to perform these assessments?
  2. How would you go about gathering the data for these assessments?

Analytical Studies

As can be seen in Figure 8.2, research study designs are on a continuum, ranging from strongest to weakest designs.

There are two general types of nonexperimental designs used in epidemiologic studies: cohort (prospective) studies and case–control (retrospective) studies. These nonexperimental studies may be "weaker" on the continuum; however, they can lead to hypothesis testing based on established associations (correlations).

The research design continuum in Figure 8.2 is designed to be used as a tool to help researchers, practitioners, and policymakers better understand best available research evidence. On a practical level, the continuum can be used to help practitioners and policymakers make decisions about which prevention strategies to adopt in their communities. It also can be used by researchers and practitioners to identify which aspects of a prevention program, practice, or policy can be improved to better demonstrate the evidence of its effectiveness.

Cohort Studies

Cohort studies, sometimes referred to as longitudinal studies, are **prospective studies** that monitor subjects over time to find associations between risk factors and health outcomes (Porta, 2014). Although they are stronger in design methodology than are case–control studies when well executed (see later discussion), cohort studies also are more

expensive. In their simplest form, a sample (cohort) of subjects who are exposed to the risk factor(s) is matched with a sample of subjects not exposed to the risk factor(s). Some prospective studies, such as the Framingham Heart Study, which were designed to estimate the lifetime risk of coronary heart disease, lasted for decades. Many recommended public health guidelines for BP, total cholesterol, and low-density lipoprotein cholesterol resulted from the Framingham Heart Study (Shortreed, Peeters, & Forbes, 2013).

Practice Point

A biased sample will result in a biased study with biased results. Randomization is crucial to obtaining a representative sample. The larger the sample, the greater the chances of a true representation of the population.

The advantages of cohort studies are that they minimize selection bias, a threat to internal validity, and provide preliminary evidence of the incidence of a risk factor with which the **relative risk (RR)** can be established. Internal validity is the degree to which the effects detected in a study are real rather than from confounding or **extraneous variables** (Gray, Grove, & Sutherland, 2017). See Box 8.1 for threats to internal validity.

Relative risk is defined as the ratio of disease incidence (or death) in an exposed population to that in an unexposed population. The assumption is that the underlying risk without the exposure is the same in both groups:

$$RR = \frac{\text{Incidence rate in people exposed}}{\text{Incidence rate in people not exposed}}$$

Relative risk is a ratio ranging from zero to infinity that indicates the strength of the **association** between the risk factor and the outcome. It is calculated by dividing the risk in the group exposed to a risk factor by the risk in the unexposed group.

An RR significantly greater than 1 (statistically) indicates that the exposure is associated with increased risk of disease. An RR significantly less than 1 (statistically) indicates that the exposure is associated with decreased risk of disease;

True experimental	Quasi-experimental	Nonexperimental Descriptive	Exploratory
Pre-/posttest control group Posttest-only control group	One group pre-/posttest Two group pre-/posttest	Survey Observation	Prospective Retrospective
(Strongest, most control)	**(Less control)**	**(Weakest, less control)**	

FIGURE 8.2 Research design continuum.

8.1 Threats to Internal Validity

History: Refers to events that are occurring during the study, which could influence participants' responses to the intervention.

Maturation: Refers to unplanned and unrecognized changes in the participants that could affect the findings of the study, such as fatigue, hunger, or increased knowledge.

Testing: Refers to the effect of multiple measurements of participants' responses that could influence the participants' responses thereby altering the outcome of the study.

Selection: Refers to the process by which participants are selected and grouped for a study. This threat is more likely to occur when randomization is not possible.

Instrumentation: Refers to changes in the measurement instrument used in the study, which result in inconsistent data collection.

Mortality: Refers to loss of subjects from the study. When those who drop out of the study differ significantly from those who remain in the study, and if there is a difference in those who remain in experimental and control groups, the outcome of the study would be affected.

Source: Gray, J. R., Grove, S. K., & Sutherland, S. (2017). *Burns and Grove's the practice of nursing research: Appraisal, synthesis, and generation of evidence* (8th ed.). St. Louis, MO: Elsevier.

8.2 Criteria for Causality

The relationship must be clear (strength of association).
Observation of the association must be repeatable in different populations at different times (consistency).
The cause must precede the effect (temporality).
The explanation must make sense biologically (plausibility).
There must be a dose–response relationship (biological gradient).

Source: Adapted from Hill, A. B. (1965). The environment and disease: Association or causation. *Proceedings of the Royal Society of Medicine*, 58(5), 295–300.

that is, the exposure is protective. An RR not significantly different from 1 (statistically) indicates that there is no association between the exposure and the risk of disease (Washington State University, n.d.).

Epidemiologic cohort studies are developed to examine **causality** among variables in illnesses. Causal associations found in this manner are known as inferred causality. Repeated, multiple studies strengthen the causal link. This strategy may not be as powerful as experimental designs; however, in many epidemiologic studies, a true experimental study would not be ethical. For example, a researcher would not deliberately expose one group to an infectious microorganism to study its effect. An important finding of inferred causality came from the well-known cohort study, the Harvard Nurses' Health Study, which has followed female registered nurses from 14 states since 1976. A 1994 landmark study established an association between breast cancer and long-time use of hormone replacement therapy (Colditz et al., 1995). The Nurses' Health Study, considered the "grandmother" of women's health studies, is the world's largest, longest-running study of women's health. The study, which is now in its third phase (Nurses' Health Study 3, n.d.), has also provided other valuable information on women's health (e.g., increased dietary calcium intake does not protect against fractures of the hip and wrist among postmenopausal women; birth control pills do not increase the risk of heart disease among nonsmoking women). More information on the Harvard Nurses' Health Study can be found at http://www.channing.harvard.edu/nhs/.

Cohort studies attempt to find cause-and-effect **relationships**; however, to find statistically meaningful data

(i.e., causality), a large number of cases are needed. There may also be threats to internal validity due to loss of subjects from the study (mortality). Nonetheless, data from cohort studies may be used as the basis for hypotheses generation for stronger experimental studies, such as randomized controlled trials (CDC, 2012a). The five criteria listed in Box 8.2, which are based on the historical Bradford Hill criteria (1965) have been used in assessing the quality of research evidence and include considerations arising to establish a cause-and-effect relationship.

To every complex question there is a simple answer … and it is wrong. **H. L. Mencken, writer and wit**

Case-Control Studies

Case–control studies, also known as **retrospective studies**, work backward from the effect to the suspected cause (Porta, 2014). Subjects are selected on the basis of the presence or absence of the disease or outcome in question: one group of people (case subjects) with the health problem and another group without the health problem (**controls**). The two groups are then compared to determine the presence of specific exposures or risk factors.

For example, diethylstilbestrol (DES) was thought to be a safe and effective way to prevent miscarriages or premature deliveries. It has been estimated that between 5 and 10 million people were exposed to DES in the United States between 1938 and 1971. However, landmark case-controlled epidemiologic studies have found health risks associated with DES in women for whom it was prescribed during pregnancy and the offspring born of those pregnancies (DES sons and daughters). DES daughters and sons are defined as women or men who were exposed to DES in utero. Research has confirmed that daughters of mothers who took DES are at risk for clear cell adenocarcinoma, a rare kind of vaginal and cervical cancer that may affect females from their early teens to their 40s. Studies have also demonstrated that sons of mothers who took DES are at risk for epididymal cysts and other genital abnormalities, including testicular hypoplasia, cryptorchidism, and microphallus (CDC, 2012b).

In addition, research is underway to determine whether the offspring of sons and daughters of mothers who took DES might have health effects related to DES exposure. These grandchildren of women prescribed DES during pregnancy are sometimes called the "third generation" (CDC, 2012b). More detailed information about DES can be found at the CDC website DES Update Home at http://www.cdc.gov/des/hcp/nurses/index.html.

The relationship between exposure and outcome in a case–control study is quantified by calculating the **odds ratio (OR)**. The OR is an estimate of RR that is interpreted in the same manner as RR. When a disease is relatively rare (e.g., a cumulative annual incidence of less than 5% in the unexposed population), the OR is similar to the RR. Otherwise, the OR overestimates RR. An OR significantly greater than 1 (statistically) indicates that the exposure is associated with increased risk of disease, and an OR not significantly different from 1 statistically indicates there is no association between the exposure and the risk of disease (CDC, 2012a).

Case–control studies have several advantages: they (1) allow for the examination of multiple exposures for a single outcome; (2) are suitable for studying rare diseases and those with long latency periods; (3) require fewer case subjects; and (4) generally are quicker and less expensive to conduct than cohort studies, making them well suited for an outbreak investigation (see Chapter 14). They have several disadvantages: (1) they are not appropriate for studying rare exposures, (2) they are subject to bias because of the method used to select controls, and (3) they do not allow the direct measure of the incidence of disease. Also, because they look backward, case–control studies may create uncertainty about the temporal relationship between exposure and disease (CDC, 2012a).

INTERVENTION (EXPERIMENTAL) STUDIES

True experiments that control all factors other than the one under investigation are rare when studying human populations. Many studies, although experimental in design, are not able to either randomize selection of subjects or exert the same degree of control of the study variables that would be found in true experimental studies. Manipulation of the independent variable occurs, but it may not be possible to control influencing or confounding factors.

Case 2: Data from the 2016 National Health and Nutrition Examination Survey indicate that adults aged 20 years and older in the United States had at least one of the following preventable cardiovascular disease risk factors: obesity, diabetes, or smoking. For 2016,

30.6% of U.S. adults aged 20 and over were obese. Also, in 2016, 9.4% of adults aged 18 and over have been diagnosed with diabetes. The prevalence of current cigarette smoking among U.S. adults declined from 24.7% in 1997 to 15.8% in 2016. However, the percentage of adults aged 18 and over who were current cigarette smokers was still higher than the 12% target for 2020 (CDC, 2016). The incidence of heart disease is increased in persons who are overweight or obese (BMI >25), while high blood pressure is twice as common in adults who are obese than in those who are a healthy weight. And obesity is associated with elevated triglycerides, diabetes, and decreased HDL cholesterol (USDHHS, 2013).

The Framingham Heart Study estimated the lifetime risks for cardiovascular disease, which account for most noncommunicable diseases worldwide, at 17.7 million (WHO, 2014).

1. What type of epidemiologic study was conducted in the Framingham Heart Study?
2. What does a "more-than-twofold increase in RR for cardiovascular disease" mean?

Student Reflection

Public health practitioners strive for comprehensiveness in characterizing an epidemiologic event, whether it be a pandemic of influenza or mammograms to detect early breast cancer. Descriptive epidemiology covers time, place, and person.

The 5Ws in descriptive epidemiologic research include:

What: health issue of concern
Who: person
Where: place
When: time
Why/how: causes, risk factors, modes of transmission

In epidemiologic research public health professionals tend to use synonyms for the 5Ws: diagnosis or health event (what); person (who); place (where); time (when); and causes, risk factors, and modes of transmission (why/how). Community and public health nurses reviewing and/or conducting research should keep these five essential components of a study in mind.

Adapted from CDC. (2012a). *Principles of epidemiology in public health practice.* 3rd ed. Retrieved July 6, 2017 from, https://www.cdc.gov/ophss/csels/dsepd/ss1978/index.html.

Practice Point

When gathering evidence for practice, nurses should consider the *strength* of the evidence as follows:

High: There are consistent results from good-quality studies. Further research is very unlikely to change the conclusions.

Moderate: Findings supported, but further research could change the conclusions.

Low: There are very few studies, or the existing studies are flawed.

Insufficient: Research is either unavailable or does not permit estimation of a treatment effect.

Source: Agency for Healthcare Research and Quality. (2012). *Treatment to prevent osteoporotic fractures: An update.* Retrieved July 14, 2017, from http://www.effectivehealthcare.ahrq.gov/ehc/products/160/1048/lbd_clin_fin_to_post.pdf.

Intervention studies in public health are categorized as preventive trials and therapeutic trials, and both can be either quasi-experimental studies or true experimental studies. **Quasi-experimental** study designs are weaker because assignment of subjects into groups is not randomized, the researcher is unable to manipulate the variable under study (see Fig. 8.2), or because of situations where it may be unethical or impractical to randomize subjects. The quasi-experimental design is used in preventive trials that focus on primary prevention (i.e., during the prepathogenesis stage to reduce the incidence of disease).

Preventive Trials

An example of a **preventive trial** using a quasi-experimental design is a study of a school district participating in a smoking prevention program. The sample is divided into two groups: some schools receive a health education program on smoking ("treatment"), and the others receive nothing ("control"). The two groups are then assessed for the incidence of smoking at 3 months, 6 months, and 1 year following the program. In this case, assignment to the treatment and comparison groups was not randomized; therefore, it is considered a quasi-experimental study. The greatest strengths of quasi-experimental studies are their practicality, feasibility, and, to some extent, their generalizability (external validity) to similar groups. External validity is the degree to which the results of a study can be generalized to other settings or samples other than the ones studied (Gray, Grove, & Sutherland, 2017). Box 8.3 for threats to external validity.

When a quasi-experimental design is used, control over other factors (confounding variables) may result in statistical differences due to competing hypotheses (**type I error**) or result in no statistical difference when it does exist (**type II error**). Also, if a quasi-experimental design is used, it cannot be assumed that the treatment and control groups were equal. However, the design can be made stronger by

8.3 Common Threats to External Validity

Reactivity: Also known as the "Hawthorne effect;" this threat occurs when participants behave in a certain way because they know they are being studied, affecting the generalizability of the findings.

Novelty: Occurs when a new intervention affects the outcome of the study because of either enthusiasm or skepticism by the researchers or the participants.

Experimenter/participant effect: Occurs when the researcher or subject has preconceived expectations of the intervention, resulting in bias and affecting generalizability of the findings.

Interaction of selection and intervention: Occurs when subjects willing to participate in the study are not representative of the target population, thus limiting the generalizability of the results.

Interaction of setting and intervention: Occurs when the characteristics of the study setting influence the outcome of the study, limiting the generalizability of the findings to other settings.

Interaction of history and intervention: Occurs when the circumstances (history) of the study influence the results of the study, and decrease the generalizability of the findings.

Source: Gray J. R., Grove, S. K., & Sutherland, S. (2017). *Burns and Grove's the practice of nursing research: Appraisal, synthesis, and generation of evidence* (8th ed.). St. Louis, MO: Elsevier.

pretesting both groups before the intervention. If both groups respond similarly on the pretest, then information obtained after the intervention can be assumed to be the result of the intervention (Gray, Grove, & Sutherland, 2017).

Practice Point

Although statistical analysis is beyond the scope of this text, it is important to know that the sample size in intervention trials should be large enough for adequate statistical power to prevent a type II error. In addition, the researcher should set the expected statistical *p* value, generally at 0.05, to ensure that the study results are not due to chance alone and to avoid committing a type I error.

A type I error occurs when the null hypothesis (Ho, a theory that has been put forward, either because it is believed to be true or because it is to be used as a basis for argument) is rejected when it is true. A type II error occurs when one accepts the **null hypothesis** when it is false (i.e., the alternative hypothesis [Ha] is true). For example, in a clinical trial of a new drug, the null hypothesis might be that the new drug is no better than the current drug. The null hypothesis and alternative hypothesis, respectively, would be:

Ho: there is no difference between the two drugs.
Ha: there is a difference between the two drugs.

From error to error, one discovers the entire truth.
Sigmund Freud

Evidence for Practice

Falling is a significant problem among community-living older adults in the United States. Liu and Frank (2010) examined 19 published longitudinal studies that studied the effects of the Chinese art of Tai Chi on reducing the risk of falling among the elderly through regular exercise. They found that Tai Chi exercise duration of 12 weeks or longer, with frequencies of twice a week or more, and session lengths of at least 45 minutes had the following outcomes: reduced fear of falling, increased single-leg stance, decreased rate of falling, increased flexibility, and improved walking. The authors concluded that Tai Chi could be an economic and effective exercise program for improving balance and balance confidence in older adults.

Properly executed experimental studies provide the strongest empirical evidence. The hallmark of the experimental study is random assignment of subjects to treatment (intervention) and control groups, which controls for potential unknown **extraneous** (confounding) variables. Randomization also provides a better foundation for statistical procedures to prevent type I and type II errors than do observational and quasi-experimental studies. The research continuum in Figure 8.2 indicates that experimental study designs are the strongest because they control for all factors except that which is under investigation. The "gold standard" for experimental studies is the prospective, double-blind, placebo control group design, also referred to as **clinical trials** or therapeutic trials. In double-blind experimental studies, neither the researchers nor the subjects are aware to which group they are randomly assigned.

Therapeutic Trials

Therapeutic trials are based on secondary prevention, which focuses on limiting the spread of disease (see Chapter 14), and where the treatment (independent variable) is manipulated by the researcher. For example, the 1994 landmark study conducted between 1991 and 1993 enrolled 477 HIV-infected pregnant women between 14 and 34 weeks of gestation. In this double-blind, placebo-controlled, randomized therapeutic trial, the women were stratified according to gestational age (14 to 26 weeks or greater than 26 weeks) and were randomly assigned to receive either zidovudine (AZT) or placebo. There were no significant differences between the characteristics of the AZT group and the placebo (control) group (Connor et al., 1994).

The AZT regimen consisted of antepartum AZT (100 mg orally five times daily) plus intrapartum AZT (administered intravenously every hour until delivery), as well as AZT for the newborn beginning 8 to 12 hours after birth (2 mg/kg orally every 6 hours for 6 weeks). During the study period, 409 women gave birth to a total of 415 live infants. The infants were evaluated by cultures and HIV serologic tests both at birth and at several weekly intervals until 78 weeks of age. At the 18-month analysis for AZT efficacy, there was a two-thirds reduction (67%) in the risk of HIV transmission from mother to infant in the AZT group. Because of these rather dramatic findings, the study was halted, and all mothers were given AZT (Connor et al., 1994). Recent studies of antiretroviral prophylaxis in the prevention of mother-to-child HIV transmission have found similar results (Sturt, Dokubo, & Sint, 2010; Tudor-Car et al., 2013).

The U.S. Public Health Service Task Force recommends the use of antiretroviral therapy to reduce perinatal HIV transmission, universal prenatal HIV counseling, and HIV testing with consent for all pregnant women in the United States. As a result, the number of HIV-infected infants born each year in the United States has decreased from approximately 1,750 (in the mid-1990s) to approximately 143 in 2010 (CDC, 2013). For more information regarding the prevention of maternal–child transmission of HIV, see CDC, Eliminating Perinatal HIV Transmission at http://www.cdc.gov/primarycare/materials/hivtransmission/.

In both preventive trials and therapeutic trials, planning includes sample selection, protocol methodology, data collection, and data analysis. Sample selection is taken from the target population, the population to which the results of the intervention are applicable. In the Connor and colleagues (1994) AZT trial described above, the target population was HIV-infected pregnant women. The sample consisted of HIV-infected pregnant women who were randomly assigned to the treatment (AZT) group or the placebo (control) group. The study was a double-blind study, in which neither the researchers nor the participants knew who was receiving AZT treatment until the study was ended. A double-blind study is one method to prevent observation bias. In a single-blind study, only the investigator knows which participants are receiving the treatment and which are not. In unblinded studies, both the investigator and the participants know who is in the treatment group and the control group. Nonetheless, measures should be taken to prevent observation bias in both single-blind and unblinded studies.

Chance favors the prepared mind. **Harlan Ellison, American author**

Practice Point

Do not evaluate all research studies at the *p* value of 0.05. No researcher has a fixed level of significance that accepts or rejects hypotheses from year to year, and in all circumstances. Rather, consider each finding according to its usefulness in clinical situations. Studies may have clinical significance and not be statistically significant.

KEY CONCEPTS

- Epidemiologic research identifies community/ public health problems and describes the natural history and etiology of diseases.
- Epidemiologic/public health research can be descriptive or analytical. Study designs are based on the problem under study and range in strength on a continuum, with the weakest design being the retrospective design and the strongest being the experimental design.
- Descriptive studies are most frequently used in public health research. They may be observational or analytical.
- Findings from descriptive epidemiologic studies lead to hypotheses for future research.
- The case study provides an in-depth examination of a single unit, such as a person, family, community, or institution.
- Case–control studies retrospectively compare subjects (cases) with a condition (disease) and matched subjects/control without the condition/disease (e.g., those with a foodborne infection compared with those without an infection).
- Cohort studies, also called longitudinal studies, examine phenomena prospectively to observe presumed effects over time (e.g., effects of diet and exercise on heart disease).
- Cross-sectional studies examine the relationship of health-related characteristics and other variables of interest (e.g., age, gender) in a defined population at a particular point in time.
- Quasi-experimental and experimental designs are used to examine causality.
- The "gold standard" for research design is the randomized, control group design.
- Preventive trials focus on primary prevention to reduce the incidence of disease.
- Therapeutic trials are based on secondary prevention, which focuses on limiting the spread of disease.
- Community health nurses are the consumers of health-related research, which is the foundation of **evidence-based nursing practice** and also is used to inform and educate the public.
- *Healthy People 2020* has identified several objectives that have not met their targets. These provide opportunities for community health programs to meet these objectives.

CRITICAL THINKING QUESTIONS

1. Read the following report: Qaseem, A., Forciea, M. A., McLean, R. M., Denberg, T. D. Treatment of low bone density or osteoporosis to prevent fractures in men and women: A clinical practice guideline update from the American College of Physicians. *Annals of Internal Medicine*, 2017, *166*(11), 818-839. Retrieved July 14, 2017 from http://annals.org/aim/article/2625385/treatment-low-bone-density-osteoporosis-prevent-fractures-men-women-clinical.
   a. Is the report evidence-based?
   b. Identify the strengths and weaknesses of evidence in the report.
   c. What prevention strategies would you recommend for patients at risk for osteoporotic fractures?

2. There is a high increase in teenage smoking in your community, and community leaders are developing a plan to decrease the incidence of smoking to reach the *Healthy People 2020* target of 12%.
   a. Develop a research question to address the problem.
   b. Design a study to decrease the incidence of smoking in teenagers.

   c. Would the study be descriptive or analytical?
   d. Where on the research design continuum (see Fig. 8.2) would the study fall?

3. In 2014, the CDC found that the percentage of adults (18 years and older) who had participated in federal guidelines for physical activity was closer to the *Healthy People 2020* target of 47.9%. However, the percentage of obesity among adults in your community has not reached more than 40%. A cross-sectional study of this population would include:
   a. A representative sample
   b. A survey questionnaire
   c. Demographics
   d. All of the above

4. Read three studies of your interest using the following link: http://journals.lww.com/nursingresearchonline/Pages/issuelist.aspx.
   a. What type of studies were conducted? Descriptive? Analytical?
   b. What additional research questions would you develop based on the studies?
   c. Did they provide evidence for best practice?
   d. Were nurse researchers identified in the studies?

REFERENCES

Agency for Healthcare Research and Quality. (2012). Treatment to prevent osteoporotic fractures: An update. Retrieved July 14, 2017, from http://www.effectivehealthcare.ahrq.gov/ehc/products/160/1048/lbd_clin_fin_to_post.pdf.

American Association for the Study of Liver Diseases and the Infectious Diseases Society of America. (2017). HCV guidance: Recommendations for testing, managing, and treating hepatitis C. Retrieved July 14, 2017 from http://hcvguidelines.org/sites/default/files/full-guidance-pdf/HCVGuidance_April_12_2017_b.pdf.

Centers for Disease Control and Prevention. (2012a). *Principles of epidemiology in public health practice*. 3rd ed. Retrieved July 6, 2017 from, https://www.cdc.gov/ophss/csels/dsepd/ss1978/index.html.

Centers for Disease Control and Prevention. (2012b). DES, updated bibliographies. Retrieved July 5, 2017, from https://www.cdc.gov/des/bibliographies/index.html.

Centers for Disease Control and Prevention. (2013). Hepatitis C: Testing baby boomers saves lives. Retrieved July 6, 2017, from https://www.cdc.gov/features/vitalsigns/hepatitisc/.

Centers for Disease Control and Prevention. (2014a). CDC's behavioral risk factor surveillance system (BRFSS). Retrieved July 6, 2017, from https://www.cdc.gov/brfss/index.html.

Centers for Disease Control and Prevention. (2014b). National Center for Health Statistics. Health, United States, 2014. Retrieved July 10, 2017, from https://www.cdc.gov/nchs/hus/index.htm.

Centers for Disease Control and Prevention. (2015). Testing recommendations for hepatitis C virus infection. Retrieved July 6, 2017, from http://www.cdc.gov/hepatitis/HCV/GuidelinesC.htm.

Centers for Disease Control and Prevention. (2016). National Center for Health Statistics. Health, United States, 2016. Retrieved July 29, 2017, from https://www.cdc.gov/nchs/data/hus/hus16.pdf

Centers for Disease Control and Prevention. (2017a). Hepatitis C FAQs for health professionals. Retrieved July 29, 2017, from https://www.cdc.gov/hepatitis/hcv/hcvfaq.htm.

Centers for Disease Control and Prevention. (2017b). HIV among pregnant women, infants, and children. Retrieved July 10, 2017, from https://www.cdc.gov/hiv/group/gender/pregnantwomen/index.html.

Centers for Disease Control and Prevention (2018). Hepatitis C FAQs for Health Professionals. Retrieved June 23, 2018, from http://www.cdc.gov/hepatitis/hcv/hcvfaq.htm#a5

Colditz, G. A., Hankinson, S. E., Hunter, D. J., Willett, W. C., Manson, J. E., Stampfer, M. J.,... Speizer, F. E. (1995). The use of estrogens and progestins and the risk of breast cancer in postmenopausal women. *New England Journal of Medicine, 332*(24), 1589–1593.

Connor, E. M., Sperling, R. S., Gelber, R., Kiselev, P., Scott, G., O'Sullivan, M.,...Jacobson, R. L. (1994). Reduction of maternal-infant transmission of human immunodeficiency virus type 1 with zidovudine treatment. Pediatric AIDS Clinical Trials Group Protocol 076 Study Group. *New England Journal of Medicine, 331*(18), 1173–1180.

Duffy, S. A., Scheumann, A. L., Fowler, K. E., Darling-Fisher, C., & Terrell, J. E. (2010). Patients with head and neck cancer. *Oncology Nursing Forum, 37*(3), 349–356.

Eckel, R. H. Jakicic, J. M., Ard, J. D., de Jesus, J. M., Houston Miller, N., Hubbard, V. S.,...Tomaselli, G. F. (2014). 2013 AHA/ACC guideline on lifestyle management to reduce cardiovascular risk: A report of the American College of Cardiology/American Heart Association task force on practice guidelines. *Circulation, 129*(25 Suppl 2), S76–S99. Retrieved July 10, 2017, from http://circ.ahajournals.org/content/129/25_suppl_2/S76.

Gray, J. R., Grove, S.K., & Sutherland, S. (2017). *Burns and Grove's The Practice of Nursing Research* (8th ed.). Philadelphia, PA: Saunders.

Hill, A. B. (1965). The environment and disease: Association or causation. *Proceedings of the Royal Society of Medicine, 58*(5), 295–300 [PMC free article] [PubMed]

Infectious Disease Society of America/American Association for the Study of Liver Disease. HCV guidelines. Retrieved July 29, 2017, from http://www.hcvguidelines.org

James, P. A., Oparil, S., Carter, B. L., Cushman, W. C., Dennison-Himmelfarb, C., Handler, J.,...Ortiz, E. (2014). 2014 Evidence-based guideline for the management of high blood pressure in adults. Report from the panel members appointed to the eighth joint national committee (JNC 8). *JAMA, 311*(5), 507–520. Retrieved July 14, 2017, from http://jamanetwork.com/journals/jama/fullarticle/1791497.

Liu, H., & Frank, A. (2010). Tai chi as a balance improvement exercise for older adults: A systematic review. *Journal of Geriatric Physical Therapy, 33*(3), 103–109.

Nurses' Health Study 3. (n.d.). Retrieved from http://www.nhs3.org/

Porta, M. (Ed.). (2014). *A dictionary of epidemiology* (6th ed.). New York: Oxford University Press.

Qaseem, A., Forciea, M. A., McLean, R. M., Denberg, T. D.; Clinical Guidelines Committee of the American College of Physicians. (2017). Treatment of low bone density or osteoporosis to prevent fractures in men and women: A clinical practice guideline update from the American College of Physicians. *Annals of Internal Medicine, 166*(11), 818–839.

Shortreed, S. M., Peeters, A., & Forbes. (2013). Estimating the effect of long-term physical activity on cardiovascular disease and mortality: Evidence from the Framingham Heart Study. *Heart, 99*(9), 649–654. doi: 10.1136/heartjnl-2012-303461.

Sturt, A. S., Dokubo, E. K., & Sint, T. T. (2010). Antiretroviral therapy (ART) for treating HIV infection in ART-eligible pregnant women. *The Cochrane Database of Systemic Reviews, 17*(3), CD008440.

Tudor-Car, L., Brusamento, S., Elmoniry, H., van Velthoven, M. H., Pape U. J, Welch, V., ... Atun, R. (2013). The uptake of integrated perinatal prevention of mother-to-child HIV transmission programs in low- and middle-income countries: a systematic review. *Public Library of Science, 8*(3), e56550. Retrieved July 6, 2017, from http://www.plosone.org/article/info%3Adoi%2F10.1371%2Fjournal.pone.0056550.

U.S. Department of Health and Human Services. (2010). *Healthy People 2020*. Retrieved July 10, 2017, from http://www.healthypeople.gov/2020/topicsobjectives2020/default.aspx.

U.S. Department of Health and Human Services. (2013). *Overweight and obesity: Health consequences*. Retrieved July 29, 2017, from http://www.surgeongeneral.gov/library/calls/obesity/fact_consequences.html.

Washington State University (n.d.). Clinical epidemiology & evidence-based medicine glossary: Terminology specific to epidemiology. Retrieved July 29, 2017, from http://www.vetmed.wsu.edu/cources-jimgay/Glossary.htm.

Whelton, P. K., Carey, R. M., Aronow, W. S., Casey, D. E., Collins, K. J., Dennison Himmelfarb, C., ... Wright JT. (2017). ACC/AHA/AAPA/ABC/ACPM/AGS/APhA/ASH/ASPC/NMA/PCNA Guideline for the Prevention, Detection, Evaluation, and Management of High Blood Pressure in Adults. *Hypertension, 70*(5), 1–283. Retrieved on November 30, 2017 from http://hyper.ahajournals.org/content/guidelines2017.

World Health Organization. (2014). Global status report on noncommunicable diseases, 2014. Retrieved July 29, 2017, from http://www.who.int/nmh/publications/ncd-status-report-2014/en/.

Part | 3

Implementing Nursing Practice in Community Settings

Planning for Community Change

Stephanie M. Chalupka and Cheryl L. Hersperger

> Change will not come if we wait for some other person or some other time. We are the ones we've been waiting for. We are the change that we seek.
> **Barack Obama**
>
> Never believe that a few caring people can't change the world. For indeed, that's all who ever have.
> **Margaret Mead**
>
> For time and the world do not stand still. Change is the law of life. For those who only look to the past or the present are certain to miss the future.
> **John Fitzgerald Kennedy**

CHAPTER HIGHLIGHTS

- Health planning at the state, national, and global level
- Social and environmental determinants of health
- Social ecologic model and multilevel interventions
- Community coalitions
- Community empowerment
- Health impact pyramid
- Health equity and social justice
- Lewin's change theory, force field analysis, and levers of change
- Logic models
- Role of the community health worker
- Funding community health interventions
- Evaluating community health interventions
- Nurse-managed health centers

OBJECTIVES

- Explain social determinants of health and how they contribute to the health status of a community.
- Describe social justice and health equity.
- Apply force field analysis as a technique for managing change at the community level.
- Explain the importance of changing the social and environmental context to improve health promotion and interventions through community empowerment.
- Use a logic model as a planning and communication tool for community programs.
- Develop community program objectives that are specific, measurable, achievable, relevant, and time-bound (SMART).
- Describe the role of the community health worker in providing services for poor, underserved, and diverse populations.
- Explain why multilevel interventions are needed to achieve change in complex community health conditions that have multiple determinants.
- Identify sources of funding for community health intervention programs.
- Describe the contributions made by nurse-managed health centers.

KEY TERMS

Coalition: Group of consumers, health professionals, policy-makers, and others working together to improve community health status or to solve a specific community health problem.

Community empowerment: Community ownership and action for social and political change. A process of gaining more community control to address social, cultural, political and social determinants of health.

Key informant: Person knowledgeable about specific aspects of a problem and the community's current and past attempts to address it.

Logic model: Visual representation of how a program is organized, including activities, resources, short-term and intermediate outcomes, and program goals.

Population aggregate: A defined subset of the population such as people with or at risk for a specific health problem or having specific social or demographic characteristics.

Stakeholder: An individual, organization, or group that has an interest (stake) in a specific community health issue or the outcome of a community-level intervention.

Sustainability: Establishing the conditions for the health improvements achieved by an intervention to continue beyond the period of a formal community health program or for a program to continue after grant funding ends.

CASE STUDIES

References to case studies are found throughout this chapter (look for the case study icon). Readers should keep the case studies in mind as they read the chapter.

Helen, a public health nurse, is the coordinator of Health Promotion for Children for the prevention of asthma in the city of Rockville. A federally funded health study of the school-aged children in Rockville revealed a very high rate of childhood asthma. The rate was especially high in the more economically challenged neighborhoods in the city. A program for assessment and interventions for the prevention and the reduction of morbidity and mortality in childhood asthma was established between the department of public health and the local children's hospital. Helen's role is to supervise her lay workers who assist with the home exposure risk evaluations and coordinate prevention education throughout the school district. The goal of the program is to reduce hospitalizations for severe asthma in children by 10% in 3 years through a grant from the U.S. Department of Housing and Urban Development.

HEALTH PLANNING

Health planning is an organized and systematic process in which problems are identified, priorities selected, and objectives set for the development of community health programs on the basis of the findings of community health assessments (CHAs) and health surveillance data. Health planning occurs at the global, national, regional, state, county, and local levels. Ideally, health planning is coordinated and consistent among each of these levels.

Health Planning at the Global Level

WHO Description of Community Empowerment

The World Health Organization (WHO) defines **community empowerment** as "the process of enabling communities to increase control over their lives" (1998a). The model identifies forces from the individual and the community as influencing the options available to them when planning a program of intervention for a community. The goal in using the model is to develop plans of care interventions for communities with lay workers toward more effective health for the individuals and the community (WHO, 1998).

OTTAWA CHARTER

In 1986, the Ottawa Charter was developed during the first international conference on health promotion held in Canada (WHO, 1986). The strategies to promote action for better health in communities include the following: building healthy public policy, strengthening community action, developing personal skills, and reorienting health services (WHO, 1986). The model directs communities to increase awareness and ownership for their health decisions and consequences by increasing responsibility in which a community is more empowered to effect change. The charter assumes that people and the community are willing to learn and develop strategies for the betterment of their health. Another assumption of the charter is the existence of a collaborative approach within and throughout health promotion systems and the healthcare system toward similar goals. An effective approach for the application of health promotion is demonstrated with the ecologic approach to health promotion assessment, planning, and interventions (see Chapter 5). The charter speaks to community empowerment through skill development, enabling community change, mediating for solutions, and advocating for vulnerable populations.

SUSTAINABILITY DEVELOPMENT GOALS

The Sustainability Development Goals (SDGs) are an evolution of the original Millennium Developmental Goals (MDGs) ratified by the United Nations in 2000. The MDGs sought to reduce morbidity and mortality while promoting health in areas including child and maternal mortality; to halt the epidemics of HIV, malaria, and tuberculosis; to increase sustainable access to safe drinking water and sanitation; to reduce violence and injuries; and to decrease tobacco use and chronic disease, including cardiovascular disease (UN, 2012). Data from the participating countries for the SDGs demonstrated much progress but many areas lacking. For instance, target goals were met by many countries in the areas of poverty, gender parity, and improvement in water sources. However, several target goals were seriously unmet for many countries in the areas of maternal morbidity and mortality, sanitation, and infant mortality and malnourishment (UN, 2015a).

To address the ongoing health and well-being goals the MDGs are transitioning to the SDGs. The SDGs include 193 countries working with the United Nations toward sustainable actions for health and well-being by the year 2030.

Principles underlying the SDGs include investing in universal health and health coverage, sustainability, participation by all to recognize determinants of health, and increase the equality of health and well-being throughout the world (UN, 2015).

SHANGHAI DECLARATION

In 2016, the ninth global conference on health promotion was held in Shanghai China. A declaration was promulgated in support of the SDGs of the United Nations SDGs. The declaration committed to support cities to promote policies for health using the most up to date innovations and technologies. The declaration includes a focus on fairness in access and inclusion in the healthcare system and community services through vigorous community engagement with key **stakeholders**. The declaration recognizes that health literacy is a key component in the determination of health investments and program development. Community empowerment through local control and citizen involvement in their own health in an environment that provides and promotes healthy choices is a key to **sustainability** (Shanghai Declaration, 2016).

In 2008, the WHO Commission on Social Determinants of Health (CSDH) issued their report *Closing the Gap in a Generation*, calling on all nations to address such social issues as poverty, lack of access to education and job opportunities, poor infrastructure, and environmental pollution, which all have a significant impact on health. The three

overall recommendations of the CSDH are to (1) improve the conditions under which all people are born, grow, live, work, and age to minimum standards; (2) ensure more equitable distribution of power, money, and resources; and (3) expand knowledge of the social determinants of health and establish a system to measure and monitor health inequity. These national and international health planning documents recognize the need to promote health and prevent disease by addressing their underlying political, economic, and social causes and to ensure health equity.

Health Planning at the National and State Levels

Ongoing health planning occurs within state health departments, the Centers for Disease Control and Prevention (CDC), and the U.S. Department of Health and Human Services (HHS) through initiatives such as *Healthy People 2020* and the National Prevention Strategy (NPS). This ongoing planning is driven by trends in health outcomes and health behavior identified from disease surveillance by the states and the CDC; data produced by the National Center on Health Statistics (NCHS) from the Behavioral Risk Factor Surveillance System (BRFSS), National Health Interview Survey (NHIS), and other sources; claims data from the Centers for Medicare and Medicaid Services (CMS); and data from the U.S. Census Bureau from the ongoing American Community Survey. Such data are used for the periodic evaluation of progress toward meeting the objectives of *Healthy People 2020* and for identifying trends in the incidence or prevalence of health problems such as diabetes, asthma, or Alzheimer disease; of health behaviors such as binge drinking or smoking; or of communicable diseases such as influenza or chlamydia. Trends identified in these data may lead the CDC, HHS, and other federal agencies or state health departments to develop new initiatives or to change health polices or programs.

Healthy People 2020

Healthy People 2020 are national objectives for improved health outcomes that guide the health promotion and disease prevention efforts in the United States. *Healthy People 2020* objectives are 10-year targets for health improvement that build on four decades of health improvement efforts that began with the publication of *Healthy People: The Surgeon General's Report on Health Promotion and Disease Prevention* in 1979. The overall goals of *Healthy People 2020* are to:

- Attain high-quality, longer lives free of preventable disease, disability, injury, and premature death
- Achieve health equity, eliminate health disparities, and improve health of all groups
- Create social and physical environments that promote good health for all
- Promote quality of life, healthy development, and healthy behaviors across all life stages (HHS, 2012, para. 5)

There are 26 leading health indicators (LHIs) that represent strategic opportunities to address high-priority health issues that contribute to preventable death and health disparities across the lifespan (HHS, 2010). The *Healthy People 2020* objectives are organized into 42 topic areas, including many new topics such as genomics, LGBT health, and healthcare-associated infections. *Healthy People 2020* objectives and resources are available on an interactive website that includes links to data sources, evidence-based practice guidelines, and state-level plans. The *Healthy People 2020* website also includes historical data on progress toward meeting prior *Healthy People* objectives. *Healthy People 2020* objectives provide a framework for assessing the health status of a community and can serve as the benchmark against which to compare the health status of a population aggregate when conducting a CHA. The *Healthy People 2020* objectives can also serve as the long-term goals of a community health intervention.

The goals for *Healthy People 2030* are under evaluation and public feedback at the time of the writing of this chapter.

Practice Point

When conducting a CHA, think of the target level within the *Healthy People 2020* objective as the ideal goal for health improvement. For example, the *Healthy People* target for the reduction of adult obesity is 10% by 2020. Using state or local data for the total population of adults aged 18 to 79 in your community or population aggregate, compare the percentage with type 2 diabetes in the city and to the *Healthy People* target goal in the reduction of type 2 diabetes to set your goal. The aggregate data total provides a context for interpreting the percentage rate reduction in obesity for your population and for setting health improvement goals.

National Prevention Strategy

The Patient Protection and Affordable Care Act (ACA) of 2010 (see Chapter 4) created the National Prevention Council which was charged with developing the NPS, published by the Office of the Surgeon General in 2011. The goal of the NPS and several other initiatives embedded in the ACA is to focus the nation's healthcare system on population health through initiatives and funding to prevent disease and to support health promotion and wellness across the lifespan (HHS, 2016a; Koh & Sebelius, 2010).

The overall goal of the NPS is to increase the number of Americans who are healthy at every stage of life. The NPS has four strategic directions for national prevention efforts that form the foundation for the plan and its recommendations. These are (1) creating healthy and safe community environments, (2) integrating clinical and community preventive services, (3) empowering people in making healthy choices, and (4) eliminating health disparities. The NPS also makes evidence-based recommendations for actions in seven priorities which have the greatest potential to improve the health of the U.S. population and to reduce the burden of preventable chronic disease, disability, and death. The seven original priorities are as follows:

- Tobacco-free living
- Preventing drug abuse and excessive alcohol use
- Healthy eating
- Active living
- Injury- and violence-free living
- Reproductive and sexual health
- Mental and emotional well-being

Detailed recommendations for policies, programs, and system changes at the local, state, and national levels are included for each of the priorities (National Prevention Council, 2011).

Recently, the advisory board for the National Prevention and Health Promotion Council has issued an overview of the strategies of the council and recommendations moving forward. The council identified the need to add a focus to health equity throughout the NPS. They also note that not all populations are insured with health coverage despite the intention of the ACA. They have noted the value of other healthcare workforces that should be included to create a more holistic approach to care recognizing traditional, and nontraditional healthcare providers who are licensed or nationally recognized through certification. They reiterate that the lead-tainted water in Flint, MI, was a herald call to investigate and mitigate health disparities.

Through community engagement, the advisory board is focused on the following strategies: (1) the opioid crisis; (2) core surveillance and response for older long-standing issues like tuberculosis and emerging infectious diseases like Ebola and Zika; (3) climate change and its effect on health through water, agriculture, food production, and air quality; (4) and bridging the political and social divisions regarding violence in the use of guns (HHS, 2016a). An example provided by the advisory board is the city of Minneapolis's "Blueprint for Action to Prevent Youth Violence" (HHS, 2016a, p. 8).

State Departments of Public Health

In the United States, state departments of public health have a central role in health planning. These departments coordinate planning at many levels—with federal agencies, including the CDC, with other agencies of state government, with local or county health departments, and with health providers. Most states have adopted state health plans that build on the national objectives in *Healthy People 2020*. HHS and state departments of public health use state-level data from the BRFSS, Youth Risk Behavior Survey (YRBS), NHIS, and the National Health and Nutrition Examination Survey (NHANES), as well as vital statistics and disease surveillance information, to monitor progress toward meeting the

Healthy People 2020 objectives and other health improvement goals.

Practice Point

Each state and territory has a *Healthy People* coordinator who is responsible for coordinating with the HHS Office of Disease Prevention and Health Promotion to ensure that the state's health plan is in line with *Healthy People 2020*. To find the *Healthy People* coordinator for your state, go to www.healthypeople.gov and search for state-specific plans.

Community Health Improvement Planning Process

Community health improvement planning is a systematic process that involves all sectors of a community to conduct a comprehensive CHA, identify priorities for action, develop and implement a CHIP, and guide future community decisions and resource allocations. Although similar to several other public health and community organizing models (Box 9.1), the CHIP emphasizes accountability and includes specific performance measures for improvement. Hospitals, community health centers, schools, employers, public officials, housing authorities, faith communities, and many other sectors of a community are included in the planning and implementation process. Nurses working in the community in public health, community health centers, clinics, home care, schools, and occupational settings are often actively involved.

Planning health promotion or prevention interventions at the community level can be a complex process. Several models and frameworks help organize some or all of the steps in the planning process (see Box 9.1). One model developed specifically for public health nursing is the intervention wheel that describes 17 public health nursing interventions at the individual, community, and systems levels (see Chapter 1).

COMMUNITY ASSESSMENT

Community health assessment is a systematic process that may use several approaches, including **key informant** interviews, analysis of data on health status and health behavior indicators, observation, and community surveys. The goal of a CHA is to identify the community health problems that are the priorities for intervention, as well as community resources available to address each health problem or need. Assessment of a community includes identification of community assets and strengths, as well as specific health problems or health needs. Assessment of community readiness and community capacity to address the identified health problems is also an important part of the process. The process of community assessment is discussed in Chapter 11.

9.1 Models and Tools for Community Health Planning

MAP-IT is a framework developed by HHS to help communities to implement *Healthy People 2020*. http://www.healthypeople.gov/2020/implement/MapIt.aspx

Mobilizing for Action through Planning and Partnerships (MAPP) is a framework for community health assessment and strategic planning developed by the National Association of County and City Health Officials (NACCHO). MAPP focuses on community engagement to help communities identify and address public health priorities (Lenihan, 2005). http://www.naccho.org/topics/infrastructure/MAPP/index.cfm

Community Toolbox is an online set of tools and practical suggestions for community health assessment, coalition-building, logic models, and the community health improvement process (CHIP) from the University of Kansas. http://ctb.ku.edu/en/default.aspx

Guideline and Template for Community Health Improvement Planning was developed by the Connecticut Department of Public Health to develop comprehensive prevention and control plans for specific diseases or conditions such as HIV, smoking, or lead poisoning. http://www.naccho.org/topics/infrastructure/accreditation/upload/CHIP-Guide.pdf

Lifestyle Medicine Institute explains, reviews, and educates on the history of the CHIP model for health improvement. https://www.chiphealth.com/About-CHIP/ProgramOutline/

Precede–Proceed Model was developed for planning health promotion programs to address health behaviors. A toolkit to help use this model in practice is included in the community toolkit. http://ctb.ku.edu/en/tablecontents/sub_section_main_1008.aspx

Community Health Assessment and Group Evaluation (CHANGE) is a tool developed by the CDC to help communities focus on changes in policies, systems, and environments to improve population health. Includes a CHANGE tool to track progress. http://www.cdc.gov/healthycommunitiesprogram/tools/change.htm

Data from the Rockville City Department of Public Health indicate that the schools reported a total of 18.4% of absences of 1 to 5 days for asthma attacks. The reported prevalence rate for Hispanic children is 14.9%, black non-Hispanics 24.1%, and white non-Hispanics lower at 7.6%. What social determinants of health may contribute to the significant variation in the prevalence of childhood asthma? How can the community engage and empower the population toward health promotion and prevention strategies?

Helen has used health status data to identify higher asthma rates among school-aged Hispanics and blacks as the community health problem her program will address. What community assets and strengths might be available to address this priority health problem and how might Helen identify them? How can she apply the framework of Persily and Hildebrand to address the CHA needs of the children of Rockville?

SYSTEMS THEORY

A community is a complex system of human activity conducted within the context of the social and ecologic environment. Every family, neighborhood, workplace, school, and recreational facility is itself a system with its own boundaries, rules, and purpose. These systems overlap to the extent that individual people in each family system participate in the activities or are affected by the decisions made within other systems. Social systems engage in reciprocal exchange or flows of information, energy, resources, and goods or services. Systems within the community are interdependent and interconnected. Change in one system leads to reciprocal changes in interconnected systems (McLeroy, Norton, Kegler, Burdine, & Sumaya, 2003). This interconnectedness means that bringing about change in the community often requires influencing systems at multiple levels because the conditions within one system, such as the family or workplace, are influenced by and reflect the broader social, economic, environmental, or political systems. It also means that changes made within one system, such as the school or workplace, may have an impact on other areas with reciprocal exchange of information or resources such as the family or the broader community.

WORKING WITH THE COMMUNITY

Just as the nurse would engage an individual patient or family in their plan of care, the community health nurse seeks the participation of community members and institutions as partners in planning and implementing programs, or changing policies, to achieve desired health outcomes at the community level. One strategy to enlist the community as a partner in the change process is the formation of a **coalition**, task force, committee, consortium, or community advisory board. (Although each has a distinct meaning, the term coalition is used in this chapter to mean any of these types of community partnership.)

Coalitions bring together consumers, health professionals, policymakers, and other constituencies to work together to improve community health status. The strategy of using coalitions to bring about change recognizes that (1) population health results from the interaction of social, cultural, economic, and political determinants in the overall community and (2) both the problems and the solutions are embedded in the community system. Systems change and an

increase in community capacity are often necessary to improve the health status of the community (Emshoff et al., 2007; McLeroy et al., 2003).

Research to increase the social accountability in engaging and empowering communities through coalitions and partnerships recommend that the information shared in the community is actionable, that there is a concerted effort to identify the community partners, an assessment is conducted that specifically indicates how the environment can be improved, and how accountability and sustainability goals will be met (Fox, 2015).

Great things are done by a series of small things brought together. **Vincent Van Gogh**

Evidence for Practice

The Allies Against Asthma initiative used community coalitions to improve the quality of care and health outcomes of low-income children in seven communities with high prevalences of asthma. These coalitions included diverse groups of stakeholders and focused on systems-level changes in homes and schools to help families manage asthma better and to improve the indoor and outdoor air quality. The odds of hospitalizations and emergent treatment for asthma among children under age 18 on Medicaid for the seven communities where these coalitions intervened, was significantly lower than in a matched group of control communities. The evaluation of this program indicated that "...ongoing consumer voices in coalition processes and decisions likely increased the quality of policy and systems changes ...[because] they reflected the actual needs of families attempting to manage asthma" (Clark et al., 2013, p. e4).

Defining the Population of Interest

To develop a plan for a community program or initiative, first identify the population of interest that will be affected by, benefit from, or participate in the planned change. The population of interest may be an entire nation, state, county, or city on the basis of geographical or political boundaries. This may be the case, for example, when planning responses to pandemic influenza or programs to reduce carbon emissions at all levels, even global, where the objective is to protect the health of all people. The population of interest may also be a **population aggregate** such as adults aged 50 and older for an initiative to increase the rate of screening for colon cancer. It is important for the community health nurse who is planning a program to know, for example, whether the population of interest is the population of adults aged 55 to 74 living in Wisconsin; the panel of patients served by a large group medical practice; families of migrant farm workers in Broward County, FL; or the students in kindergarten through sixth grade in the Chicago public schools.

Coalitions

When forming a coalition, it is important to be clear about the nature and scope of responsibility of the group. A common mistake is to ask people to serve on a coalition to satisfy the requirements of a grant or government agency without providing the coalition with a "real job" (Box 9.2). The reasons for a coalition's failure may include lack of a clear mission, goals, objectives, and expectations; lack of leadership; and lack of accountability for meeting expectations. Poor management of meetings and lack of consideration for the time and expertise of members can also lead to the failure of a coalition (Zakocs & Edwards, 2006). Organizers should do the following (see Box 9.2):

- Make use of the expertise of individual members by asking for their help and input on matters directly related to their field.
- Seek out people with a range of opinions and roles in the community. Find out who has been a valuable member of previous community coalitions or teams.
- Consider how each member of a coalition and the organization or group they represent will benefit from the work of the coalition.
- Understand group dynamics and remember that people agree to serve on coalitions in exchange for more than feeling good about helping address a community issue.
- Try to have a heterogeneous group but one in which members are able to show mutual respect and listen to each other's ideas without criticism of the person.

> When we turn to one another for counsel we reduce the number of our enemies. **Khalil Gibran**

9.2 How to Be a Valuable Member of a Coalition or Program Team

Only say "yes" to invitations to serve when you are really interested and have time to do the work. Do not agree and fail to participate.

Come to meetings on time, and stay for the entire meeting.

If you are leading a meeting, start and end on time.

Come to meetings prepared. Read any material sent to you in advance.

Come to meetings undistracted—no texting or multitasking.

Practice active listening and ask questions.

Show respect for differing opinions and suggestions—listen without interrupting, and look for ways to build on the strengths of all ideas.

Observe group dynamics to learn how group leaders achieve consensus, maintain momentum, and make progress toward goal achievement.

Keep your commitments. Complete your assignments.

Exchange business cards and network with colleagues.

Practice Point

To run meetings efficiently, it helps to:

- Know the purpose of the meeting (to make a decision, generate ideas, communicate something, or to plan).
- Show respect for the time and expertise of coalition members.
- Begin and end on time.
- Send an agenda and background materials in advance.
- Get the right people to attend. Know who your resources are and the role that they play.
- Invite only key stakeholders.
- Stay on topic.
- Communicate results.
- Learn how to resolve conflicts and reach consensus.

Stakeholders and Opinion Leaders

The people and organizations that are stakeholders (Box 9.3) are commonly included in coalitions. Factors to consider in forming a coalition include the history of the stakeholders working together (successfully or unsuccessfully); success or failure of prior attempts to resolve the community health problem being addressed, including the reasons for these results; and the degree to which prior improvements were sustained. As part of the community assessment, it is helpful to discuss factors that contribute to the problem, and other issues that may need to be addressed, with community leaders. These community leaders may include formal and informal leaders from faith organizations, schools, and employers. It is important to consider whose opinion counts most with the population group(s) expected to participate in the program. Such "opinion leaders" often make good members of coalitions or may recommend others to participate.

9.3 Questions to Help Identify Community Stakeholders

Who is most affected by this community health problem or issue? Who is most concerned?

Who are the "opinion leaders" in the community who would be interested in this health issue? Who may have different views?

Who stands to "gain" or "lose" if this community health problem is addressed? How can they be engaged in finding solutions?

Whose help will be needed to address this community health problem?

Who needs to be "on board" or "invested" for this intervention to be successful and for the changes to be sustained after the intervention?

Who are the stakeholders in the Rockville City initiative? Who would you suggest Helen ask to serve on a community coalition to achieve the goals of this program? Why?

SOCIAL ECOLOGIC MODEL

The social ecologic model is based on general systems theory and health promotion theory. Multiple determinants of health interact at different levels to affect the health status of individual people, population aggregates, or communities (Bopp, Kaczynski, & Campbell, 2013; McLeroy et al., 2003; Smedley & Syme, 2002). Planning for change at the community level is often based on a social ecologic approach with interventions at multiple levels. The social ecologic model includes consideration for how social, cultural, economic, political, environmental, organizational, and neighborhood factors influence health behaviors and health status within a community (refer to the discussion of the ecologic model in Chapter 5). Although people may change their health behavior or receive services as part of a community-level program, the concern of public health professionals is primarily the health status of the community as a whole or of a population aggregate. "[T]he goal of community-based interventions is not only to change individual perceptions and behavior but also to embed public health values in our social ecology..." (McLeroy et al., 2003, p. 532).

Even small changes in health behavior at the community or population level have the potential to significantly affect health status. The overall impact of interventions implemented at the community level is greater than the sum of the changes made by individuals or families as a result of community-level programs (Smedley & Syme, 2002). Change in health behavior or health status at one level produces changes at other levels of the community system (McLeroy et al., 2003). For example, a community-level intervention that results in 200 people quitting smoking may also lead to changes in community or family norms that affect future levels of smoking initiation or reduce the number of cigarettes smoked each day because of new restrictions at work and public places. A person or family who brings unwanted pharmaceuticals to a community take-back program instead of flushing them down the toilet contributes to environmental health by preventing contamination of drinking water supplies. A city or town that contracts for curbside pickup of recycled materials and charges residents a fee for each bag of trash collected may achieve a greater impact.

Interventions at institutional or societal levels may achieve significant changes in public health without the need for behavior change on the part of individual people. Examples abound. Fluoridation of water and advances in preventive dentistry improved dental health and dramatically reduced the incidence of dental caries in children. Laws banning trans fats in foods served to the public in New York City led to reformulation of foods throughout the fast food and snack food industry. Folic acid supplementation of cereals reduced the incidence of neural tube birth defects.

Practice Point

Sometimes, the most important action that the community health nurse may take is to advocate for a change in public policy or to collaborate with officials with responsibility for environmental health or elder services. It is important to consider the range of social, cultural, economic, or policy forces that influence the health behavior or health condition of concern and then to work at multiple levels to bring about change.

HEALTH IMPACT PYRAMID

Figure 9.1 presents the health impact pyramid. Developed by Frieden (2010), this is a framework that describes the public health impact of interventions at different levels in the social ecologic model.

At the base of the pyramid are interventions to address socioeconomic conditions such as poverty, lack of education, and lack of access to clean water or sanitation. At the next level are interventions that change the environment or options available so that making the choice for a healthy behavior is the "default" or easy choice while choosing a less healthy option would require a person to spend more time, effort, or money. Examples include food and drug safety, iodization of salt, elimination of trans fats in food, and restrictions on smoking in public places and work sites. Changing food manufacturing to eliminate trans fats, for example, will have a positive impact on the health of the entire population without people having to change their buying or eating habits and would be sustained over time. "Changing the environmental context so that individuals can easily take heart-healthy actions in the normal course of their lives can have a greater population impact than clinical interventions that treat individuals" (Frieden, 2010, p. 592). Interventions to improve socioeconomic conditions and to make the healthy choice the default choice may yield large returns in population health without requiring individuals to change health behaviors, but some may be politically difficult to achieve or require significant investment of time, money, or political capital.

At the middle of the pyramid are community health interventions such as immunizations that have a long-term protective effect as well as periodic screenings such as colonoscopy. At the next highest level are clinical interventions such as treatment of hypertension, hyperlipidemia, and diabetes. While clinical interventions can have an important impact on the prevention or control of disease at the individual level,

Population Impact
Increases

Individual Effort
Increases

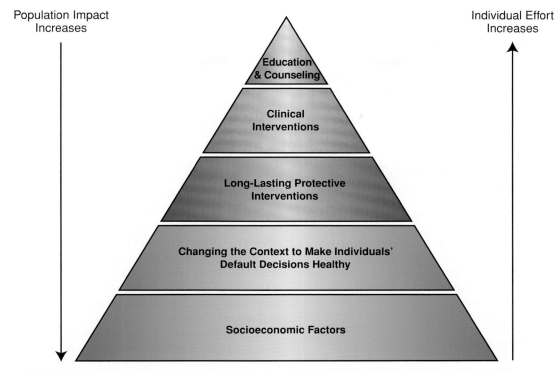

FIGURE 9.1 Health impact pyramid. (From Frieden, T. R. [2010]. A framework for public health action: The health impact pyramid. *American Journal of Public Health*, *100*[4], 590–595. Used with permission.)

the benefits may be limited because not everyone has access to primary care, people often do not adhere to treatment regimens over the long term, and treatments are not always effective. At the top of the pyramid are counseling and health education. These interventions require the largest effort by individuals, and achieving sustained health behavior change is the exception rather than the rule. In addition, counseling and health education reaches a limited number of people and may have little effect if used as the sole intervention. Health counseling may be helpful in individual and family interventions, but must be repeated with each new client and may have little effect at the population level. "Nevertheless, educational interventions are often the only ones available, and when applied consistently and repeatedly may have considerable impact" (Frieden, 2010, p. 592).

The health impact pyramid is a useful framework for community health nurses when planning health promotion interventions at multiple levels. While we often think about health education and screening interventions, these require the greatest effort on the part of individuals and have the least population impact. In addition to these interventions, we should think about what changes could be made in the environment, in policy, and in programs to make it easier for people to make healthy choices.

MULTILEVEL INTERVENTIONS

Because of the complexity of the problems that most community-level interventions are designed to address and the

multiple determinants or causes of such problems, the most successful interventions are those that combine interventions at more than one system level. Even when changes in individual health behaviors such as smoking, exercise, or healthful eating are the desired outcomes of an intervention, it is important to focus efforts on higher levels to change the social and cultural norms or context within which the behavior occurs (Frieden, 2010; McLeroy et al., 2003; Smedley & Syme, 2002). Interventions directed at different system levels can be described as follows:

- Upstream: at the societal, environmental, or policy level
- Mainstream: at the population or community level
- Downstream: at the individual level

Downstream one-on-one interventions do little to address the social or environmental determinants of population health and require continued and repeated efforts as new people continue to experience the relevant health problem. Prevention of disease by intervening upstream at the social or environmental levels or mainstream at the community level amplifies the impact of such interventions on population health (Bekemeier, 2008; Eisen, 2012). "The ways that behavior is institutionalized (organizational-level change), normalized (community-level change), and legally bound (policy-level change) are essential "social facts," without which individual behavioral change is not easily sustained" (McLeroy Norton, Kegler, Burdine & Sumaya, 2003, p. 533).

Bekemeier (2008) points out that practitioners of public health nursing in the early 20th century, including Lillian

Wald and visiting nurses, recognized that their most important work was to reform "...the conditions that create and exacerbate disease" (p. 50) and call on nurses to focus their practice and research on primary prevention and the root causes of ill health. "Focusing...on the underlying causes of poor health and health disparities requires an upstream perspective that brings nursing (back) into the realm of policy analysis, social reform, environmental health, sociology, and international health" (p. 50).

Practice Point

Remember to always "look upstream" when thinking about where to target interventions. Dr. Richard Jackson at the UCLA School of Public Health explains that "public health needs to look at the cause of the cause." He gives the example of a person struck by a car and killed. That death is recorded as the result of an accident. Dr. Jackson suggests looking upstream: Why was the person hit by the car? Was there a way to walk along the road safely? Was there a sidewalk? Dr. Jackson asks if the cause of death was actually the poor design of the community or the lack of a place to walk in an area without the risk of being hit by a car (Brown, 2012).

How can we apply this same thinking of upstream causes to the primary prevention of chronic disease? What are the "causes of the cause" of diabetes, cancer, or heart disease? How can we better address these upstream determinants of health?

SOCIAL DETERMINANTS OF HEALTH

The circumstances in which people are born, grow up, live, work, and age, and the systems put in place to deal with illness are termed the *social determinants of health*. These circumstances are in turn shaped by the wider context, including economics, social policies, and politics (WHO, 2017).

The social ecologic model recognizes that the determinants of health are complex and multidimensional. The health status of a community, a population aggregate, a group, or an individual person results from a complex interaction of social, economic, environmental, and behavioral factors. Chronic diseases, including cardiovascular disease, diabetes, cancer, and chronic respiratory disease, are among the leading causes of morbidity and mortality in developed nations. These diseases have multiple interactive causes that accrue over the course of the lifespan, including diet, physical activity levels, smoking, alcohol intake, exposure to toxic environments, genetic and familial factors, socioeconomic status, and demographics (Gostin & Powers, 2006; Smedley & Syme, 2002; Stokols, 1992). Community health nurses may construct a web of causation (see Chapter 5) to help identify the multiple factors that contribute to the chronic disease or community problem of interest as part of the planning process.

Obesogenic and Salutogenic Environments

Understanding the impact of the social, economic, and political systems on the factors that contribute to childhood obesity, for example, reframes the problem. Obesity is not just an issue of personal or family responsibility but one created by an *obesogenic* environment—defined as an environment promoting or contributing to obesity (Schwartz & Brownell, 2007; Smedley & Syme, 2002). Rather than directing interventions toward individual behavior change by families whose children are overweight or obese, the goal of community-level interventions is to change the environment to one that creates the conditions where healthy choices are the default or norm. Making school a *salutogenic* environment, where only healthy food choices are available and physical activity is incorporated into school curricula, benefits all children (Schwartz & Brownell, 2007). Salutogenic environments are ones "...that reduce vulnerability to illness and promote enhanced levels of well-being" (Stokols, 1992, p. 12).

Healthy people require healthy environments to live in, work, and play. The *built environment* is broadly defined as human-made surroundings that include buildings, public resources, land use patterns, the transportation system, and design features. Research is increasingly demonstrating links between the built environment and eating and physical activity behaviors, which in turn affect health outcomes (Prevention Institute, 2008). Environments should be designed in ways that help people access healthy foods and easily incorporate physical activity into their daily routines. The creation of healthy environments is not accomplished by any single group or entity. It requires coordinated and comprehensive efforts by stakeholders, community leaders, multiple sectors, professional organizations, and leaders. Healthy community design integrates evidence-based health strategies into community planning, transportation, and land-use decisions. Toolkits for healthy community design can guide the planning for improving people's health by increasing physical activity, reducing injury; increasing access to healthy food; improving air and water quality; minimizing the effects of climate change; decreasing mental health stresses; strengthening the social fabric of a community; and providing fair access to livelihood, education, and resources (CDC, 2013).

Student Reflection

We attended one of the public hearings for the city's community health improvement plan. One of the people that provided testimony was Gina, a public health nurse for the city. She was advocating for the adoption of a "complete streets" policy. She explained that complete streets are focused on safe access without exceptions across population groups and their needs (Smart Growth America, 2018). Pedestrians, bicyclists, motorists, and public transportation users of all ages and abilities are able to safely move along and across a complete street. Complete streets make it easy to cross the street, walk to shops, and bicycle to work. It was interesting to see evidence-based practice in action because Gina provided data from research that demonstrated that residents who live in communities with pedestrian- and bicycle-friendly infrastructure are more physically active. She also provided evidence that residents in a highly walkable neighborhood have been shown to engage in about 70 more minutes per week of moderate and vigorous physical activity than residents in a low-walkability neighborhood.

Health Impact Assessment

A health impact assessment (HIA) helps communities make informed choices about improving public health through community design. HIA is a process that helps evaluate the potential health effects of a plan, project, or policy before it is built or implemented. A HIA can provide recommendations to increase positive health outcomes and minimize adverse health outcomes. HIA brings potential public health impacts and considerations to the decision-making process for plans, projects, and policies that fall outside the traditional public health arenas, such as transportation and land use (CDC, 2012).

HIA is usually voluntary, although several local and state laws support the examination of health impacts in decision-making and a few explicitly require the use of the HIA. Outside the United States, HIA is more widely used. Some countries have mandated HIA as part of a regulatory process. In the United States, HIA is a rapidly emerging practice among local, state, and federal jurisdictions, mostly on a voluntary basis.

HIA holds promise for incorporating aspects of health into decision-making because of its applicability to a broad array of policies, programs, plans, and projects; consideration of adverse and beneficial health effects; ability to consider and incorporate various types of evidence; and engagement of communities and stakeholders in a deliberative process (CDC, 2012).

Health Disparities, Health Equity, and Social Justice

The WHO CSDH wrote that the "unequal distribution of health-damaging experiences is not in any sense a "natural" phenomenon but is the result of a toxic combination of poor social policies and programs, unfair economic arrangements, and bad politics" (WHO, 2008, p. 1). Differences in health status exist at the population level between nations or within nations; the basis of these differences is age, race or ethnicity, gender, socioeconomic status, or other characteristics. "Health disparities become health inequities when they are unnecessary, unfair, and preventable resulting from social injustices that become engrained in the fabric of society through its social, economic, and political structures, laws, policies, and culture so as to become largely invisible" (Falk-Rafael & Betker, 2012, p. 98).

Achieving health equity is the overarching goal established in *Healthy People 2020*, WHO *Millennium Declaration and the WHO* 2030 Agenda for Sustainable Development. The Sustainable Development Goals (SDGs) build on the Millennium Development Goals (MDGs) universally apply to all; countries will mobilize efforts to end all forms of poverty, fight inequalities, and tackle climate change to ensure that no one is left behind. The SDGs are unique in that they call for action by all countries, poor, rich, and middle-income to promote prosperity while protecting the planet. They recognize that ending poverty must go hand-in-hand with strategies that build economic growth and address a range of social determinants of health including education, health, social protection, and employment opportunities while tackling climate change and environmental protection (United Nations, 2015).

Health inequities are *avoidable* inequalities in health between groups of people within countries and between countries. These inequities arise from inequalities within and between societies. Social and economic conditions and their effects on people's lives determine people's risk of illness and the actions taken to prevent them becoming ill or to treat illness when it occurs (WHO, 2013). There are numerous examples of health inequality within the United States. The United States has the world's highest per capita spending on healthcare, but it ranks 50th in global life expectancy with a very significant gap in life expectancy between the rich and poor. The gap is as large as 20 years between rich whites living in Maryland and poor African Americans living only 20 miles away in Washington, D.C. (Eisen, 2012). Health equity requires the elimination not only of health disparities, but also of health inequalities resulting from disparities in the living and working conditions that are the social determinants of health. Health equity is based on the principles of fairness and social justice, as well as the belief that all people have an equal value.

Villeneuve (2008) of the Canadian Nurses Association issued a call to action to the world's nurses to rally around a vision of eliminating health disparities and to understand the importance of population health. Nurses need to be informed about the dynamics of economics, global demographics, and access to healthcare and begin to learn to frame health status indicators and health disparities "as examples of *system-level vital signs*" (italics in the original; p. 335). Villeneuve suggests that nurses need to "find policy levers with which to weave these dynamics into their work in order to influence the development of healthy public policy based on broad determinants of health" (2008, p. 339).

Social justice is a value central to the practice of nursing and public health. Social justice refers to an equitable sharing of both the common burdens and the common benefits or advantages in society. The basis of social justice is a value system in which healthcare is a right and achieving health equity and population health are goals. Social justice holds that all individuals are entitled to equal protection from health hazards in the environment produced by the powerful (Beauchamp, 1976). In contrast, in the value system of "market justice," which characterizes modern American society, health is one of personal individual responsibility, and healthcare and other social goods are treated as commodities or economic goods (Beauchamp, 1976; Budetti, 2008; Gostin & Powers, 2006). Achieving social justice requires addressing the root causes of ill health, including "poverty, substandard housing, poor education, unhygienic and polluted environments, and social disintegration…[that] lead to systemic disadvantage not only in health, but also in nearly every aspect of social, economic, and political life" (Gostin & Powers, 2006, p. 1054).

The gross inequalities in health that we see within and between countries present a challenge to the world. That there should be a spread of life expectancy of 48 years among countries and 20 years or more within countries is not inevitable. A burgeoning volume of research identifies social factors at the root of much of these inequalities in health…[The Millennium Declaration] goals challenge the world community to tackle poverty in the world's poorest countries. Included in these goals is reduction of child mortality, the health outcome most sensitive to the effects of absolute material deprivation. **Marmot, 2005, p. 1099**

Practice Point

Nurses are in a unique position in society to act as role models, advocates, and champions of community health change. They should identify an issue about which they are passionate and let others know of their interest. They should seek out a mentor and look for opportunities to help bring about changes they want to see in the community. Read the inspirational stories of nurses working in their communities to improve human health and make a difference at the Luminary Project at http://www.theluminaryproject.org.

Philosophical, Theoretical, and Ethical Basis for Practice for Nurses in Public Health

Cynthia Persily and Eugenie Hildebrandt developed a middle range theory to describe community empowerment in 2003. The purpose of the theory was to answer questions in research and clinical practice for ways to offer effective interventions to communities (Persily & Hildebrandt, 2008). Early in her career, Persily conducted research using other disciplines to help provide needed services for high-risk pregnant woman living with diabetes (Persily, 1995). She noticed in her study that inventions of care could be provided by not only the nurse but effectively by others as well.

This conclusion led to a study providing services to pregnant women in a rural setting with lay persons. The conclusion of a need for community involvement became evident with the research of the pregnant women in a rural community. She began a literature search to see if a model of community involvement existed. In her search she came across the work of Hildebrandt who worked with a cohort of 100,000 people in a South Africa city to test her model of community-based participatory research (CBPR) (Hildebrandt, 1996). The two then worked on the original model developing the middle range theory of community empowerment (Persily & Hildebrandt, 2008).

The theoretical model includes three critical concepts: (1) lay workers, (2) involvement, and (3) reciprocal health. By definition, community empowerment is defined as "the involvement or participation of community-based lay workers in the promotion of reciprocal health" (Persily & Hildebrandt, 2008, p. 132). The lay worker is viewed in relationship between the community, the involvement, and actions within the community while focusing on their role and the relationship of health in the community which is termed "reciprocal health" (Persily & Hildebrandt, 2008).

Community Empowerment Model: Empowering Neighborhoods and Communities

A neighborhood engagement study in Philadelphia by Alicea-Alvarez and colleagues (2016) utilized the local medical community in an intervention to engage low-income, minority neighborhoods with local healthcare education within their own neighborhoods. The study indicated improving education to the population with a focus on health literacy has the potential to impact the health of urban community dwellers. The study notes a lack of a framework for eliminating health disparities exists. Future plans to provide specific local financial resources in realignment of how resources are currently allocated for community education for health promotion and preventions are in step with the goals of the ACA (Alicea-Alvarez et al., 2016).

In 2015, a qualitative study in Africa of the children of Uganda regarding childhood mortality before the age of 5 was conducted using the concept of community empowerment. Deaths are due primarily related to infectious diseases, pneumonia, diarrhea, and malaria. A project with UNICEF called the Community and District Empowerment for Scale-Up (CODES) project assessed the priorities and barriers or bottlenecks to bringing services together and engaging the community to discuss and find solutions for their local health challenges. The CODES project used a combination of a four-tool analysis approach to identify needed interventions. Prioritizing interventions is a determined key component to engage and empower the community. With the primary intention to improve childhood mortality, the health team (1) identified bottlenecks, (2) analyzed root causes, (3) identified solutions and strategies, and (4) consulted stakeholders (Katahoire et al., 2015). Continuing community communication with the local population, stakeholders, and government proved critical. A focus on health literacy using images and peer-to-peer learning helped to create a dialogue to identify the barriers, challenges, and successes within the communities in the study. Prioritizing interventions within each community rather than a blanket approach improves the use of resources and creates an environment for better outcome measures (Katahoire et al., 2015).

CHANGE THEORY

Bringing about change in the health status of a community and its members may come through change in health behaviors, as well as through change in the environment, public policy, social or cultural norms, or healthcare delivery. Theories of health behavior change at the individual, family, and community levels have been discussed in Chapter 5. Such theories of health behavior change are embedded in many interventions to bring about change at the community level. In addition to changing health behavior, interventions at the community level use theories and techniques designed to bring about change in complex systems, including theories of organizational change.

Lewin's Model of Change

The field theory developed by Karl Lewin, an organizational and social psychologist in the 1950s, is one useful change theory. In recent years, the discussion of change has been largely dominated by the issue of power and politics. This has resulted in diminished interest in Lewin's planned approach to change, with its ethical basis and stress on democratic participation. The emergent approach, which is consistent with the free market approach and focuses on use of power and politics to bring about change, has been in ascendency. However, we are in an era where ethical and socially responsible behavior is becoming more important than profit maximization and self-interest; therefore, Lewin's work is even more relevant (Burnes, 2009).

Lewin envisioned planned organizational change as a three-step process of unfreezing, changing, and refreezing (Shirey, 2013). Understanding the three steps of Lewin's theory, the technique of force field analysis, and the levers of change are useful in visualizing and creating change at the community level.

Unfreezing

Unfreezing the status quo is a necessary precursor to change. This may occur either gradually, through generational changes in beliefs, language, and group norms, or rapidly through a paradigm shift (e.g., the terrorist attacks of September 11, 2001). Gradual, incremental change in attitudes and behaviors related to drinking and driving have led to new community norms such as "designated drivers" and the hiring of limousines for prom nights. Rapid unfreezing of a community's indifference about bicycle helmets may occur when a local child riding without a helmet dies or is seriously injured in an accident when a helmet could have prevented injury.

Unfreezing moves a community from the stage of denial or lack of awareness of the need to change a condition or to address an issue, to a stage of preplanning or preparation for change. Education about the extent of the problem or condition and its consequences may begin the process of unfreezing a community's state of denial of a health problem or acceptance of current unhealthy behaviors or norms. Nurses can play a role as change agents during this stage to help mobilize the community by helping to highlight discrepancies between current and desired community health status, or creating a sense of urgency about a health issue (Shirey, 2013). Public policies requiring restaurants and fast food outlets to display the calories and fat grams of menu items or requiring public schools to send parents a periodic "health report card," including a body mass index (BMI) calculation, are examples of interventions intended to begin the process of unfreezing the status quo. Creating dissatisfaction with the current state and raising awareness of a need for change are catalysts for unfreezing (Shirey, 2013).

> A round man cannot be expected to fit in a square hole right away. He must have time to modify his shape. **Mark Twain**

Changing

Once a community has become sufficiently aware of the need for change, or sufficiently dissatisfied with the current conditions through increasing awareness of an issue or as the result of a crisis, the process of changing or transition may begin. Change is a dynamic process that may be more successful when it is actively managed rather than allowed to happen haphazardly. It is seldom a neat, linear process. Change is more often achieved incrementally through repeated cycles or steps than it is by large paradigm shifts. Changing requires an understanding of what needs to be changed, how the change will take place, and an idea of what the change will "look like" when the desired state has been achieved (Shirey, 2013).

Refreezing

Refreezing is the process of stabilizing once a change has occurred with the goal of sustaining the change in the community's systems, policies, and customs. Making the new behaviors the community norms helps ensure that the change toward more positive health status will remain in place once the intervention or program is completed. Refreezing establishes a new status quo from which further change may be possible in the future (Shirey, 2013).

Sustainability must always be a concern when planning changes in health beliefs, knowledge, behavior, or social conditions. New behaviors are difficult to maintain until they become habitual. Part of the process of planning community health change is to anticipate the support system that must be in place when a program ends so that the positive changes in health are maintained. Involvement of the community as a partner in the change process is a key to such sustainability. Community members and stakeholders must be involved in all stages of the planning process so that they have "ownership" of the process or program and feel engaged and empowered by the changes that are accomplished (Cyril, Smith, Possamai-Inesedy, & Renzaho, 2015; MacDuffie & DePoy, 2004). If change is imposed from outside the community or embraced only by the health professional, lasting change is unlikely.

Force Field Analysis

Force field analysis is a change management technique developed by Lewin. Force field analysis involves identifying factors within a community or organization that are driving or reinforcing change in the desired direction, as well as those that are restraining or resisting change. When the driving forces and restraining forces are relatively equal, a state of equilibrium exists. Knowing the direction and strength of each force helps identify which can be increased or decreased to allow the process of unfreezing to occur. It is also important to identify which forces are not possible to change due to political, structural, cultural, organizational, financial, or other constraints so that the plan for change is realistic and achievable. It is not necessary or possible to change every force that is driving or restraining change. Ideally, force field analysis is a participatory process involving the major stakeholders in the community (MacDuffie & DePoy, 2004).

The key is to identify those forces that will require the investment of a reasonable amount of time or resources yet yield the greatest opportunity to effect change in the situation. The primary value of a force field analysis is to help one select the most appropriate targets for intervention(s). Reducing restraining forces and/or strengthening driving forces may create the unfreezing, disequilibrium, and dissatisfaction with the status quo necessary to bring about change in community beliefs, behaviors, social and environmental conditions, and health status.

An example of a force field analysis applied to the case study is shown in Figure 9.2. If you were Helen, which of the restraining forces would you try to decrease and which of the driving forces would you try to increase? Why? What strategies might Helen use to unfreeze the status quo to create an environment conducive to change?

Levers of Change

The purpose of using levers of change is to increase driving forces and/or to decrease restraining forces—leverage points

identified in the force field analysis. Just as physical levers amplify the force applied to move a physical object and allow a person to move a larger object with a smaller expenditure of energy or effort, levers of change are tools or techniques that achieve the largest changes with the least investment of resources. Policymakers can strategically use these levers in public policy or social marketing to bring about desired change in the health status of the community (Berenson, Li, Lynch, & Pagán, 2017).

Examples of public policy levers used to reduce the rates of smoking were laws requiring workplaces, restaurants, and other public places to be smoke-free; ordinances against the sale of cigarettes to minors; and significant taxes on tobacco products. Levers to change social norms about smoking have included social marketing concerning the detrimental effect of secondhand smoke on children and the value of smoke-free homes. These "levers" have helped amplify the impact of health education and smoking cessation programs designed to change individual health behaviors on smoking rates in the United States (Smedley & Syme, 2002).

Community Readiness for Change

Planning programs or interventions to change community health status includes an assessment of the community's readiness to undertake the change process related to a specific health issue. Communities may be at different states of readiness, ranging from not being aware of a problem or denying that a problem exists to having already initiated or undergone changes (Åhström, Larsson, & Lindberg, 2016).

A community's readiness for change is issue-specific (Åhström, Larsson, & Lindberg, 2016). The community readiness model (CRM) is a tool used to measure a community's readiness to change in six dimensions through key informant interviews. Developed by the Tri-Ethnic Center for Prevention Research at Colorado State University for drug and alcohol use prevention programs, researchers have shown that the CRM is a useful framework in planning prevention programs addressing such issues as intimate partner violence, HIV/AIDS, breast cancer education, needle exchange programs (York & Hahn, 2007), and childhood obesity (Findholt, 2007). York and Hahn extended the evaluation of the CRM beyond community-based prevention programs to study its usefulness in developing and implementing public policies to limit exposure to smoking (York, Hahn, Rayens, & Talbert, 2008). A handbook for using the CRM, including a set of questions for key informant interviews, is available at the CRM website and is included in the Community Toolbox at the University of Kansas (see Box 9.1).

Evidence for Practice

Findholt (2007) evaluated the readiness of a county in Oregon to address the problem of childhood obesity and found the community had no awareness of the

Forces Driving Change   Status
                              Quo   Forces Restraining Change

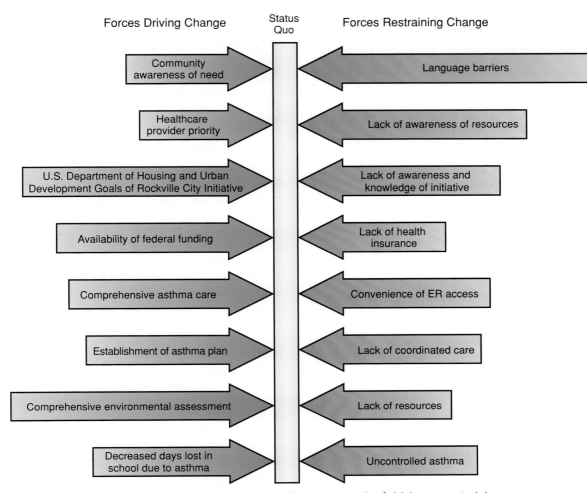

FIGURE 9.2 Force field analysis: Length of arrow indicates strength of driving or restraining force.

problem. Rather than implementing a program, Findholt worked with community leaders to establish a childhood obesity prevention coalition and to implement activities to increase community awareness and level of readiness to address the problem. The process of conducting key informant interviews as part of applying the CRM "...stimulated community interest in the problem of childhood obesity and generated support for a community-wide prevention effort, even before strategies were implemented to increase readiness" (p. 570). Findholt's evaluation of community readiness resulted in "unfreezing" and the first steps toward change in this community health problem.

PLANNING COMMUNITY-LEVEL INTERVENTIONS

The success of community health programs depends on well-conceived interventions and implementation plans. Selecting the most appropriate intervention(s) requires consideration of the resources available, including people,

money, facilities, and time. The types of interventions available to address childhood obesity will be different for the staff of an individual school working within their current budget for one school year than for a community-wide coalition with a large foundation grant for a 3-year demonstration project. Trying to do too much with limited resources may result in failure to achieve stated objectives when a more realistic plan with achievable objectives and the same results would be judged a success.

Guide to Community Preventive Services

The Task Force on Community Preventive Services (TFCPS) conducts systematic reviews of research for evidence of the effectiveness of community-based prevention and health promotion programs and practices. The goal of the TFCPS is to make recommendations for translation of research into practice. The work of this task force parallels that of the U.S. Preventive Services Task Force, which conducts similar work related to clinical prevention services in primary care.

9.4 Sources of Evidence for Community Health Interventions

Healthy People 2020—Each section of the *Healthy People 2020* Topics & Objectives has a tab for "interventions and resources" with links to the major evidence that supports the objectives. www.healthypeople.gov

National Prevention Council with information on the evidence supporting the recommendations in the National Prevention Strategy. https://www.surgeongeneral.gov/priorities/prevention/strategy/index.html

National Council on Aging Center for Healthy Aging—evidence-based health promotion programs for chronic disease management, fall prevention, and other programs for older adults. http://www.ncoa.org/improve-health/center-for-healthy-aging/

The Guide to Community Preventive Services, known as the "Community Guide." http://www.thecommunityguide.org/index.html

U.S. Preventive Services Task Force (USPSTF) recommendations. https://www.uspreventiveservicestaskforce.org/Page/Name/recommendations

AHRQ Guide to Clinical Preventive Services. http://www.ahrq.gov/professionals/clinicians-providers/guidelines-recommendations/guide/index.html

National Guideline Clearinghouse. http://www.guideline.gov/

The Cochrane Library of systematic reviews. http://www.cochrane.org/

Research and systematic reviews published in *Public Health Nursing, American Journal of Public Health, Preventing Chronic Disease*, and other nursing, public health, and health promotion journals.

The work of the TFCPS is published online as the Guide to Community Preventive Services, also known simply as the Community Guide. New systematic reviews are published periodically in the *American Journal of Preventive Medicine* and *Morbidity and Mortality Weekly Report (MMWR)* and summarized on the task force website.

The Community Guide is organized by topics such as injury prevention, obesity, and diabetes. Interventions within each topic are listed either as recommended or as not yet having sufficient evidence from research to support a recommendation. Other sources of evidence for community-based interventions are identified in Box 9.4.

Helen consults the local CHIP and the state data on asthma in school-aged children for recommendations on asthma prevention and respiratory health promotion. She finds that multiple interventions implemented in combination with community healthcare workers and engaging a wide variety of organizations that touch the school-aged child such as school, the health clinic, the emergency room, and local social areas where community leaders may be identified. Interventions conducted in a silo without community engagement had limited impact for outcome changes and sustainability. What does this tell Helen about how she should plan her intervention?

Logic Model

A **logic model**—also known as a program model, theory of change, or theory of action—is a graphic illustration of how a program or intervention is expected to produce desired outcomes. It shows the relationships among the inputs and resources available to create and deliver an intervention, the activities the intervention offers, and the expected results (Petersen, Taylor, & Peikes, 2013). A logic model for a community health program illustrates *who* will receive services (target population), *what* will be done (activities), *when* it will happen (timeline), *where*, and *why* (program theory) (Taylor-Powell & Henert, 2008).

The model is usually a formal process map or flow diagram (Fig. 9.3) but can be more informal using graphics or pictures. The logic model is a tool for both planning and communication. It helps the community health nurse identify available and needed resources, plan the sequence and timeframe for program implementation, develop a budget, and identify how results will be measured. The logic model also informs community leaders, program staff, stakeholders, and decision-makers on the operation of the program and how it will achieve the desired results (Petersen, Taylor, & Peikes, 2013).

Logic will get you from A to B. Imagination will take you everywhere. **Albert Einstein**

A program's theory or logic is evidence-based and derived from epidemiologic and program research using sources of evidence such as those listed in Box 9.5 and a critical review of relevant literature. The program theory may also be one of those described in Chapter 5, such as the health belief model or the ecologic model. It may be important to adapt or modify the program theory or assumptions to the specific community by using information from the community assessment, such as a community's capacity, resources, results of previous efforts to address the problem, and community readiness to change. Step-by-step guides to developing and using logic models are provided in the community toolkit (see Box 9.1) and the resources for program evaluation listed in Box 9.6.

Practice Point

Logic models are great tools for communicating with decision-makers and grant sources. Proposals that include a well-constructed logic model are more likely to be approved and funded.

Mission: The mission of the Welford City Access to healthy foods is to ensure that healthy fresh produce is available conveniently. The project is consistent with the CDC guidelines and *Healthy People 2030*.

INPUTS/RESOURCES	ACTIVITIES	OUTPUTS/MEASURES	INTERMEDIATE OUTCOMES
Coalition members	Conduct interview with key informants in the community	Number of families accessing markets	Program becomes self-sustaining
Social marketing plan	Meet with opinion leaders and potential spokespersons	Number of meals per week that include fresh produce	Maximize opportunities to purchase fresh produce
Public health nurses			
Students nurses and faculty	Identify barriers to and facilitators healthy eating	Number of locations available where fresh foods are available over 12 months	GOALS
Translators			Reduce the number of cases of new onset type 2 diabetes to meet objective in Healthy People 2030.
Volunteers	Establish Welford City coalition	Accessible transportation to markets	
Healthy food			
Farmers and other markets	Recruit locations for markets and eliminate food deserts	Number of translators	Eliminate barriers to healthy eating in the city of Welford.
Expand market access	Coordinate with nursing faculty at university	Number of volunteers	
Funding to increase local produce availability	Contract for translators	Number of participating local farms (within 100-mile radius)	Eliminate food deserts in the city of Welford.
Food stamps value expansion for healthy choices	Schedule staff volunteers, translators, and students		
CONSTRAINTS	Schedule and publicize markets		
Food deserts			
Food habits			
Fast food access and cost			
Transportation			

CONTEXT or CONDITIONS: The services are targeted to families in the city of Welford who need access to healthy food. Adapted from Taylor-Powell, E., and Henert, E. (2008). Developing a logic model: teaching and training guide.

FIGURE 9.3 Logic model for healthy food program. (Adapted from Taylor-Powell, E., & Henert, E. [2008]. *Developing a logic model: Teaching and training guide*. Retrieved from http://www. uwex.edu/ces/pdande/evaluation/pdf/lmguidecomplete.pdf. Used with permission.)

9.5 Writing SMART Program Objectives

Specific: What behaviors, knowledge, skill, change in health status indicators or outcome will result from the program?

Measurable: How will the outcome be measured and how will one know if the objective is achieved? Are the data available?

Achievable: Is it realistic to reach the desired outcome with the resources and time available to the program?

Relevant: Is the objective related to the program's goals and activities?

Time-bound: When will the objective be achieved?

Not SMART: The program will reduce teen pregnancy.

SMART: The number of births to girls aged 19 and younger in Springfield will be reduced by 20% from 40 births in 2010 to 32 or fewer in 2015.

Not SMART: Fewer teens will start smoking.

SMART: The proportion of high school sophomores in the state of Georgia who report having ever smoked a cigarette on the Youth Behavioral Risk Factor Survey in 2020 will be no more than 7%.

Not SMART: The number of older minority residents of River City receiving a flu shot will double.

SMART: The number of people aged 50 and older who receive a flu shot at a clinic sponsored by RC3-I and who identify themselves as Hispanic or Latino will increase 50% in the fiscal year (FY) 2015 over the baseline number in FY 2012.

9.6 Resources for Program Evaluation

CDC Framework for Program Evaluation including steps and standards. http://www.cdc.gov/eval/framework/index.htm

CDC Introduction to Program Evaluation for Public Health Programs: A Self-Study Guide. http://www.cdc.gov/eval/guide/index.htm

CDC Division for Heart Disease and Stroke Prevention Evaluation Guides include step-by-step instructions and examples for writing SMART objectives, developing and using a logic model, writing an evaluation plan, and other skills. https://www.cdc.gov/dhdsp/evaluation_resources/index.htm

University of Wisconsin Extension. Program development and evaluation website including tools and resources for developing program evaluations and logic models. http://www.uwex.edu/ces/pdande/evaluation/index.html

Helen reviews the theory and assumptions underpinning the statewide asthma initiative based on the goals of *Healthy People 2020*. She learns that the goals for decreasing emergency room visits for acute asthma exacerbations and more effective asthma management in school-aged children are based on the research data found in the state data registry for hospital data and collected state data for attendance and absences from school.

The reported prevalence rate of asthma for the city of Rockville's Hispanic children is (14.9%), black non-Hispanics (24.1%), and white non-Hispanics lower at (7.6%). The identified need for asthma attack management and prevention dovetails with top indicator goals for promoting respiratory health in the *Healthy People 2020* data (HealthyPeople.gov). Community empowerment theory informs Helen that she will need community leaders, community health workers who are bilingual, the support of nurses in other disciplines, and the healthcare providers in local clinics and the hospital. Reciprocal health potential for the community involves actualizing accountability and action to increase health. Indeed, it is a delicate balance to build an environment that supports coalitions, promotes trust, and maximizes rapport to increase and improve communication for better outcomes.

Using the logic model in Figure 9.3 and information provided in the case, write three objectives for the asthma program in the SMART format.

Smart Objectives

SMART is an acronym for program objectives that are *sp*ecific, *m*easurable, *a*chievable, *r*elevant, and *t*ime-bound. Program objectives written in the SMART format help in planning interventions and establishing measurement systems to evaluate programs and outcomes (see Box 9.5).

COLLABORATION AND TEAMWORK

Rarely does the community health nurse work alone. The practice of public health and community health nursing requires a willingness and readiness to work on a collegial basis with community members from all walks of life and with other professionals from a wide range of fields. Other members of a team may include social workers, policymakers, elected officials, public health professionals, school officials, senior center directors, educators, community health workers (CHWs), and researchers.

Respect for the abilities and appreciation for the contributions of community members and other health and social service professionals are essential to the success of team building and collaboration. Depending on the specific needs and composition of the group, the community health nurse may play many different roles—team leader, team member, consultant, educator, or facilitator. Active listening is just as important a nursing skill when working with community members as it is when caring for an individual person. CHWs and community members have much to teach health professionals about how to provide services that are concordant with the unique social, cultural, and linguistic needs of the community.

One of the tests of leadership is the ability to recognize a problem before it becomes an emergency. **Arnold Glasgow**

Practice Point

Nurses should seek input and feedback from community members using focus groups and key informant interviews to tailor an intervention to the unique needs, culture, and priorities of the community of interest.

Community Health Workers

Community health workers (CHWs), also called lay health advisors, outreach workers, promotores(as) de salud (promoters of health), peer educators, patient navigators, and community health advocates, are essential to effective and comprehensive health systems globally (Fig. 9.4). Over the past five decades, CHWs have been a growing force for extending healthcare and improving the health of populations. CHWs frequently work in communities outside of health facilities and have some type of formal, but limited, training for the tasks they are expected to perform (Perry, Zulliger, & Rogers, 2014). CHWs are recognized in the

FIGURE 9.4 Promotora de salud providing diabetic instruction. (Photo courtesy of the Migrant Clinician's Network.)

Patient Protection and ACA as important members of the healthcare workforce. CHWs have unique access and local knowledge. They are therefore able to provide a cultural and language bridge to the members of the target population (Islam, Nadkarni, Zahn, Skillman, Kwon, & Trinh-Shevrin, 2015; Pérez & Martinez, 2008). CHWs work with community health nurses and other members of the program team in both urban and rural areas to provide health education, outreach and assistance in accessing services, translation, and specific interventions. Generally recruited from the community of interest and trained by program staff, CHWs make an important contribution to providing patient-centered care and decreasing health inequalities. The evidence shows that they can help improve healthcare access and outcomes; strengthen healthcare teams; and enhance quality of life for people in poor, underserved, and diverse populations and communities (Rosenthal et al., 2010). In addition to connecting patients to existing services and improving outreach, communications, and adherence, CHWs can also have an important impact on healthcare costs and on the prevention and control of both chronic and infectious disease. The successes of the CHW model have resulted in broader use of CHWs into the health delivery system (Sabo et al., 2013).

Evidence for Practice

In October 2010, New York-Presbyterian Hospital in association with the Columbia University Medical Center launched an integrated network of patient-centered medical homes that were linked to other providers and community-based resources and formed a "medical village" to address the health needs of the Washington Heights-Inwood section of Manhattan. Washington Heights-Inwood is a Hispanic and low-income community with disproportionately high rates of chronic disease, including diabetes, asthma, and congestive heart failure.

Three years later, among 5,852 patients some combination of diabetes, asthma, and congestive heart failure, researchers found a 29.7% reduction in that emergency department visits and a 28.5% reduction in hospitalizations, compared to the year before implementation of the network. In addition, researchers noted a 36.7% decrease in 30-day readmissions and a 4.9% decrease average length-of-stay. Patient satisfaction scores improved across all measures.

New York-Presbyterian also had fiscal gains through a short-term return on investment of 11%. A portion of this gain was the result of increased reimbursements from New York State. However, these findings demonstrate that academic medical centers can improve outcomes for low-income communities by building regional care models centering on medical homes that incorporate patient-centered processes and are linked through information systems and service collaborations to hospitals, specialty practices, and community-based providers and organizations (Carillo, Carillo, Guimento, Mucaria, & Leiman, 2014).

Although CHWs have much to teach healthcare professionals about their communities, the CHWs need a structure within which to work and training to develop skills and to understand the activities and strategies of the specific community health program. Building relationships, mutual respect, and trust between the CHWs, community or public health nurses, and other members of the program team is critical to success. Written job descriptions, step-by-step intervention guidelines, scripts for health education, and ongoing training and supervision for CHWs are required to ensure the fidelity and consistency of interventions as well as to support CHW job satisfaction and job performance (HRSA, 2007; Pérez & Martinez, 2008).

What skills and knowledge might CHWs recruited to work on the Rockville asthma prevention program bring to the program that Helen may not have? How can Helen work with the CHWs to make the best use of their talents?

EVALUATING COMMUNITY-LEVEL INTERVENTIONS

Evaluation begins as a program is being planned. The activities and intermediate outcomes identified in the logic model and the SMART program objectives are the start of an evaluation plan. It is critical to make plans for evaluating a program at the time of initial program planning to ensure the development of the necessary tools and methods for collection of data to measure the impact of the program in advance of the intervention. Planning for the evaluation of a program also includes, when possible, measuring preintervention levels of health status or behavior using the same evaluation criteria to establish a baseline for comparison with program results.

The evaluation plan often includes both process and outcome evaluations. Process evaluations focus on how well the program was implemented and looks at processes, activities, and capacity building. Outcome evaluation focuses on the extent to which the intervention achieved its objectives for changes in knowledge, skills, or health behavior and for improvement in community health status. Measures used for evaluation include both quantitative and qualitative data (CDC, n.d.).

Steps in developing the evaluation plan include the following:

1. Develop evaluation questions "focused on what happened, how well it happened, why it happened the way it did, and what the results were" (CDC, n.d., p. 5).
2. Determine indicators or measures you will use to answer your evaluation questions.
3. Identify where you will find the data you need to measure your indicators and answer your questions.
4. Decide what method you will use to collect data.
5. Specify the time frame for when you will collect data.
6. Plan how you will analyze your data based on the type of data you are using.
7. Decide how you will communicate your results (CDC, n.d.).

In addition to evaluation done by the program staff or consultants, foundations or government agencies funding the program may hire outside evaluators to conduct process and outcome evaluations. This often happens with large multisite demonstration projects in which the results of evaluation research are important outcomes used to determine the efficacy and impact of new intervention strategies.

The RE-AIM framework was developed to evaluate health behavior research and has helped to establish the evidence base of many health promotion programs. The RE-AIM framework includes five dimensions that together represent the elements that a health promotion program needs to have an overall impact on population health. The dimensions are *r*each, *e*ffectiveness, *a*doption, *i*mplementation, and *m*aintenance and are measured at both the participant and organizational levels.

- *Reach* is based on how well the intervention reaches its target audience. This includes the number and percent of people in the target population who are served.
- *Effectiveness* is the impact of the intervention on health behaviors, health status, quality of life, and other outcome measures. This includes a consideration of any negative effects or consequences of the intervention.
- *Adoption* looks at the extent to which the community-based organizations or providers who were expected to participate actually implemented the program.

- *Implementation* evaluates intervention fidelity or the extent to which the program was carried out as it was intended and how consistently service delivery was given between providers.
- *Maintenance* evaluates how well the behavior change or health improvements are maintained by the participants as well as the extent to which the program is continued by the participating providers (Belza, Toobert, & Glasgow, n.d.; Gaglio, Shroup, & Glasgow, 2013).

"The overall goal of the RE-AIM framework is to encourage program planners, evaluators, readers of journal articles, funders, and policy-makers to pay more attention to essential program elements that can improve the sustainable adoption and implementation of effective evidence-based health promotion programs" (Belza et al., n.d., p. 2). More information and resources on using the RE-AIM framework are available at www.re-aim.org.

Practice Point

It is important to include short-term and intermediate objectives and evaluation measures in the logic model and evaluation plan. Most community-level interventions require many years before there are measurable changes in community health status or health outcomes.

The public health nurse has a directive to provide specific measures for part of the outcome analysis according to the federal grant. An evaluation subcommittee has developed process and outcome measures that each entity within the community coalition of school, hospital and community health clinics has agreed to use to facilitate cross-city comparative analysis. In addition, each person attending an education session for asthma prevention and respiratory health promotion will be asked to complete a card that asks their reason for attending the program if they ever had education about asthma before, how they heard about the public health clinic, and if they required language assistance. Why did the evaluation committee include these questions?

FUNDING COMMUNITY-LEVEL INTERVENTION PROGRAMS

Planning and implementing community health programs includes finding and securing funding. Funding for a new program may come from the internal budgets of the sponsoring organization and its collaborative partners or may require outside funding from a foundation or government grant. To address a community health problem, some initiatives may not need additional funds but simply the reconfiguration of current programs or creation of a coalition to use existing resources. Additional funding may come from other sources such as community benefit programs of local health providers or insurance companies, in-kind contributions from business enterprises, and sponsorship of specific aspects of a program by a local bank or business.

Accountability

Whether a program is funded by one's own agency or an outside grant, the community health nurse will have to be accountable for how the program was implemented. Accountability includes regular communication about how funds were used, details of program activities, and progress toward achieving program goals. Large foundations and government agencies often expect logic models and formal evaluation plans as part of grant proposals. Performance in meeting the expectations for regular and meaningful progress, outcome, and financial reports is an important factor in decisions about renewal of grant funding.

Sustainability

Sustainability is an important consideration in program planning and a key factor in grant making. Most funding agencies expect programs to give a clear and convincing plan outlining how efforts started with grant funding will be continued after the grant ends. For example, is there a written commitment from the participating agencies that they will maintain changes in the delivery of services brought about by the program if those changes prove effective and produce the desired results? Developing a strategy for how a program will continue after initial funding ends should begin early in the planning process.

Helen is planning to decrease the number of emergency room visits for acute asthma attacks, and increase prevention strategies in the homes of the vulnerable populations targeted by the program through community engagement. The sustainability of the program relies on effective education measures that become part of common knowledge among the populations of the neighborhoods most at risk. How does Helen engage the leaders of the communities to promote health and prevention strategies in order that emergency room acute attack care measures are not the treatment plan of choice for the parents who have children with asthma? How does the socioeconomic status effect the outcome of sustainability?

Program Replication

What may have succeeded in one location may reflect how ready the community was to change, not how well a program was designed and/or how well it was implemented. The ability to replicate or reproduce a successful program within a different community or with a new population aggregate is a test of the strength of the design of an intervention. When an intervention has yielded positive results in one community, the next step in establishing evidence for practice is to test the intervention by replication.

Student Reflection

The elementary school where I am doing my community health nursing practicum has just begun an "Andrews Elementary Walking School Bus" program. The program began in the fall, during International Walk to School Month. There is a structured walking route with meeting points, a timetable, and a schedule of trained volunteers. It sounds simple, and it is. It can be as informal as two families taking turns walking their children to school or something larger and more structured such as a route with meeting points, a timetable, and a regularly rotated schedule of trained volunteers. Many other communities have used the "walking school bus" program, and the school was able to take advantage of information available from the CDC and other schools to help the program get off to a good start.

Project Funding

Government Agencies

Funding of community health programs by state or federal government agencies usually involves a formal competitive request for proposal (RFP) process. Most often grants from the NIH, CDC, or HRSA are categorical (e.g., targeted to a specific disease or health behavior such as childhood obesity or smoking initiation by teens), with a limited set of target populations and program models. Grants from federal agencies are usually made to a state's department of health or human services, universities, or large regional service providers with an established track record. Grants from state and local government agencies are often made using a combination of federal funds granted to the state and funds allocated from the state or local government budget.

The ACA has created new opportunities for federal and state funding of health promotion and prevention programs. These opportunities include community transformation grants that will fund programs to improve nutrition, physical activity, and wellness with priority given to strategies to reduce healthcare disparities. Grants will be available to small business to provide comprehensive workplace wellness programs. New funding will be available to expand the services of community health centers and to expand Medicaid. The ACA established the Prevention and Public Health Fund with the purpose of targeting health outcomes and quality of care values by the public. This particular fund targets the use of evidence in public health practice and includes programs, research, data analyses, and tracking as well as sustainability through capacity building in the workforce. Some states have also established similar prevention funds. The planned use of Prevention and Public Health Fund resources, including funding to be targeted at $931,000,000 in fiscal year 2017 and beyond to invest in new prevention and wellness initiatives, brings many new opportunities for funding community health nursing programs and interventions (U.S. DHHS, 2016b).

Private Foundations

Private foundations of all sizes provide grants for community health services. Most foundations publish guidelines that identify their program interests, proposal guidelines, range of grant amounts, and eligible grantees. It is important to learn as much as possible about a foundation before submitting a proposal, to select a foundation or foundations whose interests align closely with the proposed program, and to follow guidelines carefully. If an applicant is submitting proposals to more than one foundation for the same program, it is important to indicate this fact in the cover letter and proposal budget.

Local Resources

Local banks and other businesses, faith communities, civic groups such as Rotary International or the Junior League, and other local resources may provide seed money, matching funds, or in-kind support for community health programs. In-kind support such as donating items for a silent auction, volunteering hours at a food bank, or printing program materials are valuable contributions that local businesses can make in addition to, or instead of, cash. Even if the amount of funds from local groups is not large, it is important to seek local support. Not only does the support of the program by local groups demonstrate community engagement to larger funding sources, the interest and involvement of local leaders helps ensure program success and increases the likelihood of sustainability.

Community Benefit Programs

Community benefit programs of local or regional hospitals and health maintenance organizations (HMOs) may be valuable partners to the public health department or community health nurse in planning, implementing, and funding programs to improve population health. Each nonprofit hospital is required to provide and document community benefits as the basis for their tax exemption. Community benefits are programs and services designed to improve health in communities and increase access to healthcare (Barnett, 2009). Hospital community benefit programs can provide both leverage and resources to increase the effect of regional health initiatives. While community benefit programs are most commonly focused on services related to direct patient care (e.g., free care or unreimbursed services), redirecting only a portion of the community benefit contributions

toward high-leverage community health improvement initiatives could have a significant impact on the health of vulnerable populations and build community capacity to access other potential funding sources (Corrigan, Fisher, & Helser, 2015). More information and tools for community benefit programs are available on the website of the Association for Community Health Improvement (ACHI).

> ### Practice Point
>
> Develop long-term relationships with funders by thanking them, providing regular progress reports on the program they have funded, and acknowledging their support in each press release about the program. Foundations and businesses are more likely to fund proposals from organizations that have communicated well and have been accountable for funds previously provided than from organizations that only contact them when funding is needed (Box 9.7).

9.7 Community Benefit Programs in Action

The Care-A-Van

The Bon Secours Care-A-Van is a free medical service that provides primary care to uninsured adults and children of the Greater Richmond community. Often, an uninsured individual may wait to access care until their health gets to an emergency level. Care-A-Van services are designed to provide medical care in a timely manner to those who need it. Bon Secours Care-A-Van has been operating in Richmond since 1994. The program currently serves 21 different locations.

The Care-A-Van team is bilingual (Spanish/English) and composed of physicians, nurse practitioners, registered nurses, patient care technicians, licensed practical nurses, drivers, registrars, trained medical interpreters, registered dieticians, licensed clinical social workers, and outreach workers.

Healthy Dollar

St. John Providence Health System/Ascension Health Alliance, Detroit, MI, Enterprising Health Ascension Health Holdings, a subsidiary of Ascension Health Alliance, is a sponsor of Enterprising Health (EH), a program to help new or potential entrepreneurs build the skills necessary to develop and operate sustainable businesses, which must be focused on improving the health of Detroit and the surrounding communities. One of the selected projects is a project called "Healthy Dollar," a strategically located storefront and meeting space that creates a hub for health in the city of Flint by providing access to low-cost fresh fruits and vegetables, and a setting for health education and community health events. Other supported projects include a web-based grocery store that makes home deliveries of fresh food to make healthy eating more convenient for families, professionals, students. It is an innovative approach to improving the health literacy of Detroit-area mothers with the goal of reducing infant mortality.

Helen planned a launch event for the asthma initiative with the nurse program coordinators from the hospital, the schools, and the community health workers along with two identified community leaders in the targeted neighborhoods. A local news crew and local community papers in both English and Spanish were invited to attend. After the start of the program Helen recorded outcomes data and reported this to the Chief of the Public Health department, the medical director of the hospital, the chief of the emergency room, the Superintendent of the targeted school, the selected community leaders, the health clinic director, and the manager of the community health workers. Why is outcomes data collection important? What is the value of communicating the success and challenges of a program?

SOCIAL MARKETING

Social marketing (Box 9.8) is the use of marketing principles and practices to change health behaviors or beliefs, social or cultural norms, or community standards to improve health or benefit society (CDC, 2011b). Social marketing is used primarily to design, develop, use, and evaluate initiatives specifically in the area of communicable diseases such as sexually transmitted infections (CDC, 2011). It has also been effective in meeting noncommunicable disease challenges such as smoking and other social challenges such as safety and environmental issues. Social marketing approaches add value to public health programs by providing systematic ways of active engagement with individuals and communities end-users (European Centre for Disease Prevention and Control, 2014). Examples include the use of social marketing to promote health behavior change related to eating fruits and vegetables (five a day), breast-feeding, active play by children, and following guidelines for cancer screenings. It has also been used to change social and cultural norms related to smoking, texting while driving, condom use, and consumption of transfats. Social marketing is an increasingly important tool in bringing about change in individual and population health (Crawshaw, 2013; Hoek, 2011). Several resources are available to help the community health nurse learn to use social marketing through the CDCynergy Lite: Social Marketing Made Simple website (https://www.cdc.gov/health-communication/pdf/CDCynergyLite.pdf).

Social marketing is more than just media communication or health education. The goal is to change behavior. All people are exposed to commercial and social marketing each day. Marketing may look easy and seem intuitive but it is really very challenging to do well. Most public health programs lack the resources to develop social marketing campaigns; fortunately, it is not necessary to "recreate the wheel." Many social marketing programs and materials that can be adapted for local use are available through the CDC, HHS, and national associations such as the American Heart Association and the National Dairy Council. These programs are available free or for a nominal fee (CDC, 2011).

9.8 Social Marketing

Take a look at these sentences. What do the **bold** words have in common?

- **Fasten** your seat belt.
- **Eat** more fruit.
- **Pull over** to use your cell phone.
- **Don't** litter.
- **Get** a mammogram.
- **Talk** to your doctor

These words describe problems to be addressed by changing behavior. Research may help to describe what your audience is currently doing or thinking, which can help shape realistic goals for behavior change. Social marketing is about identifying the specific target audience segment(s), describing the benefits you will offer, and the creating interventions that will influence or support the desired behavior change.

Social marketing planning requires us to understand and incorporate the "The Four Ps of Marketing," into our program planning. Social marketing is critical because it looks at the "Four Ps" and the provision of health services from the viewpoint of the consumer. The "Four Ps of Marketing" are:

1. PRODUCT represents the desired behavior you are asking your audience to do, and the associated benefits, tangible objects, and/or services that support behavior change.
2. PRICE is the cost (financial, emotional, psychological, or time-related) of overcoming the barriers the audience faces in making the desired behavior change.
3. PLACE is where the audience will perform the desired behavior, where they will access the program products and services, or where they are thinking about your issue.
4. PROMOTION stands for communication messages, materials, channels, and activities that will effectively reach your audience.

Sometimes there is a fifth P — policy. POLICIES are the laws and regulations that influence the desired behavior, such as requiring sidewalks to make communities more walkable or prohibiting smoking in shared public spaces.

Adapted from Gateway to Health Communication and Social Marketing Practice (2011).

Student Reflection

When I was in high school, the school nurse showed us an empty soft drink bottle half filled with sugar. She said there are 10 tsp of sugar in a 12-oz (350-mL) bottle. Can you imagine eating that much sugar with a spoon? The nurse said that diet drinks are no better because they change your metabolism and make you crave sweets. I stopped drinking soft drinks that day and started drinking water and diluted fruit juice and lost 10 lb in 6 months without trying. The visual aid that nurse used did more to convince me than anything I had read.

NURSE-MANAGED HEALTH CENTERS

Nurse-managed health centers (NMHCs) are a unique model of community health services led by advanced-practice nurses and providing a wide range of services and programs to vulnerable and underserved populations. The communities served by NMHCs are usually geographically defined and are most often vulnerable and underserved population aggregates such as the rural poor, migrant farm workers, low-income mothers and children, inner-city neighborhoods, and immigrant communities. The NMHC may offer services in subsidized housing projects, homeless shelters, correctional institutions, schools, faith communities, storefronts, and other locations easily accessible to the population aggregate being served. The NMHCs emphasize health promotion, disease prevention, and health education. Many provide specialized programs to meet the needs of specific population aggregates such as pregnant and parenting women, teens, or homeless people. Primary prevention is a core component of the care provided, and the range of services varies from health promotion programs to a full range of primary care and chronic disease management programs (Esperat, Hanson-Turton, Richardson, Debisette, & Rupinta, 2012).

Many NMHCs are academic nursing centers established by colleges of nursing to provide service to the community as well as clinical practice and research opportunities for students and faculty, and to prepare students with skills to

9.9 *Healthy People 2020*—Indicator Nutrition, Physical Activity, and Obesity

Nutrition, physical activity, and obesity are a top goal for *Healthy People 2020*. The obesity rate of adults remains high at 36.2% and 16.1% in children and youths aged 2 to 19 years. Physical activity guidelines recommend aerobic and muscle-strengthening exercises totaling 150 minutes for a lighter work out or 75 minutes for very intense activity per week. Targets for increased physical activity are met with a 10% improvement over the baseline. Several determinants of health may influence the outcome of success in this indicator based on an assessment of environmental, social, and nutritional barriers to healthy weight and activity.

1. How would you calculate the percentage of improvement expected in the adult group? In the children and youth group?
2. Go to the website below and click the top tab named "Life Stages and Determinants." How does the built environment inform the populations ability for increasing health for this *Healthy People*, indicator?

https://www.healthypeople.gov/2020/leading-health-indicators/2020-lhi-topics/Nutrition-Physical-Activity-and-Obesity/data.

work in medically underserved areas. Other NMHCs are federally qualified health centers of federally qualified look-alikes or are clinics within the structure of a hospital or health system. HRSA has funded some NMHCs, particularly those at schools of nursing, and NMHCs are included in provisions for expanded funding of safety-net providers and community health centers under the ACA. NMHCs belong to the National Nursing Centers Consortium, where you can find more information about these community health nursing programs that build on the legacy of Lillian Wald in meeting the needs of vulnerable and underserved communities (Esperat et al., 2012).

KEY CONCEPTS

- Common themes of current national and international health plans include providing health promotion and disease prevention at the population level, addressing social determinants of health, and achieving health equity.
- Social justice and health equity are key values in community health and public health nursing.
- Changing the social and environmental context to make healthy choices the default is an effective strategy for improving the health of a community.
- Even small changes at the community or population level have the potential to create significant change in the health status of a community.
- Logic models provide a visual representation of how a program is organized: what it will do (activities), what resources are needed (inputs),

how short-term and intermediate outcomes will be measured, and how the program goals will be achieved.
- The change process can be visualized as three steps of unfreezing the status quo, changing or moving to a new state, and refreezing to sustain the change or changes made.
- Force field analysis is a tool used to identify the forces driving or restraining change.
- The health status of a community and its members is the result of a complex interplay of social, economic, environmental, behavioral, political, and cultural forces.
- Health behavior change, whether at the individual or community level, requires sustained effort, and results may not be evident in the short term.

- Community participation through engagement and empowerment in all steps of the change process helps to increase the potential for program success and sustained change in community health status.
- Community readiness to change needs to be considered in selecting the most appropriate types and levels of interventions.
- Multilevel interventions are needed to achieve change in complex community health conditions that have multiple determinants.
- Public policies such as tax increases on tobacco, alcohol, or soft drinks can serve as policy levers to bring about change in community health status.

- Nurses can play an important role in their professional and personal lives as advocates and champions for health improvement, social justice, and health equity at the local, regional, national, and global levels.
- Community health workers can help bridge the gap between the community health nurse and the community, especially when there are cultural and language differences.
- Nurse-managed health centers provide health promotion and primary care services to vulnerable and underserved population aggregates.

CRITICAL THINKING QUESTIONS

1. Think about the factors (social, developmental, environmental, and policy) that contribute to the problem of binge drinking on college campuses. Use a force field analysis to think about how the change process could be applied to reduce binge drinking on your campus.
   a. Which driving force(s) would you want to strengthen? What approach would you use to accomplish this? Why?
   b. Which restraining force(s) would you want to decrease? What approach would you use to accomplish this? Why?
2. Can you think of recent changes in public policy, the environment or social context that have made it easier to make healthy choices in your own health behaviors? How might you apply the concept of making healthy choices the default choice to your nursing practice to support healthier behaviors among your clients?

3. How can community empowerment and engagement effect health behavior changes?
4. Based on community-level data, you have identified the need to increase immunization rates in the refugee and immigrant population in your community. Who might you enlist as partners in planning and implementing programs to achieve desired health outcomes at the community level? Why did you select these partners?
5. Bekemeier, Villeneuve, and Falk-Rafael all suggest that nurses need to actively work to bring about change upstream in the social and environmental determinants of health. How might this vision for the role of nurses in population health manifest itself in your practice?
6. How does the Persily and Hildebrand model offer a framework for community engagement in the following case?

REFERENCES

Åhström, M., Larsson, N., & Lindberg, L. (2016). Change of community readiness over time: Measurements of reduction of parental support and availability of alcohol in seven communities. *Health Promotion Practice, 17*(4), 586–595.

Alicea-Alvarez, N., Reeves, K., Lucas, MS., Huang, D., Ortiz, M., Burroughs, T., & Jones, N. (2016). Impacting health disparities in urban communities: Preparing future healthcare providers for "Neigborhood-Engaged Care" through a community engagement course intervention. *Journal of Urban Health, 93*(4), 732–743. doi: 10.1007/s11524-016-0057-6.

Barnett, K. (2009). Beyond the numerical tally: Quality and stewardship in community benefit. Retrieved from http://www.phi.org/uploads/application/files/yddicgszozcnwkoo2fdzqr9a5r61ixcdcky-wu9d8cqxgutptoi.pdf

Beauchamp, D. E. (1976). Public health as social justice. *Inquiry, 13*, 3–14.

Bekemeier, B. (2008). "Upstream" nursing practice and research. *Applied Nursing Research, 21*, 50–52.

Belza, B., Toobert, D. J., & Glasgow, R. E. (n.d.). *RE-AIM for program planning: Overview and applications.* Washington, DC: National Council on Aging. Retrieved from https://www.ncoa.org/wp-content/uploads/IssueBrief_ReAim_Final-2.pdf

Berenson, J., Li, Y., Lynch, J., & Pagán, J. A. (2017). Identifying policy levers and opportunities for action across states to achieve health equity. *Health Affairs, 36*(6), 1048.

Bopp, M., Kaczynski, A. T., & Campbell, M. E. (2013). Social ecological influences on work-related active commuting among adults. *American Journal of Health Behavior, 37*(4), 543–554.

Brown, J. (2012). Wellness and sustainability. *Greenhealth Magazine.* Retrieved from http://greenhealthmagazine.org/wellness-and-sustainability/

REFERENCES *(Continued)*

Budetti, P. P. (2008). Market justice and US health care. *JAMA, 299*(1), 92–94.

Burnes, B. (2009). Reflections: Ethics and organizational change—time for a return to Lewinian values. *Journal of Change Management, 9*(4), 359–381.

Carrillo, J. E., Carrillo, V. A., Guimento, R., Mucaria, J., & Leiman, J. (2014). The New York-presbyterian regional health collaborative: A three-year progress report. *Health Affairs, 33*(11), 1985–1992.

Centers for Disease Control and Prevention. (2011a). CDCynergy: Gateway to health communications and social marketing practice. Retrieved from http://www.cdc.gov/healthcommunication/CDCynergy/

Centers for Disease Control and Prevention. (2011b). Gateway to Health Communication and Social Marketing Practice (2011). Retrieved from https://www.cdc.gov/healthcommunication/healthbasics/whatishc.html

Centers for Disease Control and Prevention. (2012). Designing and building health places. Retrieved from http://www.cdc.gov/healthyplaces/default.htm.

Centers for Disease Control and Prevention. (2013). Health community design checklist toolkit. Retrieved from https://www.cdc.gov/healthyplaces/toolkit/

Centers for Disease Control and Prevention. (2016). CDC Evaluation Documents, Workbooks and Tools. Retrieved from https://www.cdc.gov/eval/tools/index.htm

Children's Hospital of Philadelphia. (n.d.). Community asthma prevention program (CAPP). Retrieved from http://www.chop.edu/centers-programs/community-asthma-prevention-program-capp

Clark, N. M., Lachance, L. L., Benedict, M. B., Doctor, L. J., Gilmore, L., Kelly, C. S.,...Wilkin, M. (2013). Improvements in health care use associated with community coalitions: Long-term results of the allies against asthma initiative. *American Journal of Public Health, 103*(6), 1124–1127.

Corrigan, J., Fisher, E., & Heiser, S. (2015). Hospital community benefit programs: Increasing benefits to communities. *JAMA, 313*(12), 1211–1212.

Crawshaw, P. (2013). Public health policy and the behavioural turn: The case of social marketing. *Critical Social Policy, 33*(4), 616–637.

Cyril, S., Smith, B. J., Possamai-Inesedy, A., & Renzaho, A. M. N. (2015). Exploring the role of community engagement in improving the health of disadvantaged populations: A systematic review. *Global Health Action, 8*(1), 29842.

Eisen, J. (2012). Sick people or sick societies? *Canadian Dimension, 46*(4), 40–44.

Emshoff, J. G., Darnell, A. J., Darnell, D. D., Erickson, S. W, Schneider, S., & Hudgins, R. (2007). Systems change as an outcome and a process in the work of community collaborative for health. *American Journal of Community Psychology, 39*, 255–267.

Esperat, M. C., Hanson-Turton, T., Richardson, M., Debisette, A. T., & Rupinta, C. (2012). Nurse-managed health centers: Safety-net care through advanced nursing practice. *Journal of the American Academy of Nurse Practitioners, 24*, 24–31.

European Centre for Disease Prevention and Control. (2014). Social marketing guide for public health managers and practitioners. Retrieved from https://ecdc.europa.eu/sites/portal/files/media/en/publications/Publications/social-marketing-guide-public-health.pdf

Falk-Rafael, A., & Betker, C. (2012). Witnessing social injustice downstream and advocating for health equity upstream: "The trombone slide" of nursing. *Advances in Nursing Science, 35*(2), 98–112.

Findholt, N. (2007). Application of the community readiness model for childhood obesity prevention. *Public Health Nursing, 24*(6), 565–570.

Fox, J. (2015). Social accountability: What does the evidence really say? *World Development, 72*, 346–361. Retrieved from http://dx.doi.org/10.1016/j.worlddev.2015.03.011

Frieden, T. R. (2010). A framework for public health action: The health impact pyramid. *American Journal of Public Health, 100*(4), 590–595.

Gaglio, B., Shoup, J. A., & Glasgow, R. E. (2013). The RE-AIM framework: A systematic review of use over time. *American Journal of Public Health, 103*(6), e38–e46.

Gostin, L. O., & Powers, M. (2006). What does social justice require for the public's health? Public health ethics and policy imperatives. *Health Affairs, 25*(4), 1053–1060.

Haviland, A. M., Elliott, M. N., Hambersoomian, K., & Lurie, N. (2011). Immunization disparities by Hispanic ethnicity and language preference. *Archives of Internal Medicine, 171*(2), 158–165.

Health Resources and Services Administration. (2007). Community health worker national workforce study. Retrieved from https://bhw.hrsa.gov/sites/default/files/bhw/nchwa/projections/communityhealthworkforce.pdf

Healthy People 2020. (2017). Diabetes Prevention. Interventions involving community healthcare workers. Retrieved from https://www.healthypeople.gov/2020/tools-resources/evidence-based-resource/diabetes-prevention-interventions-engaging-community

Hildebrandt, E. (1996), Building Community Participation in Health Care: A Model and Example from South Africa. *Image: The Journal of Nursing Scholarship, 28*, 155–159.

Hoek, J., & Jones, S. C. (2011). Regulation, public health and social marketing: A behaviour change trinity. *Journal of Social Marketing, 1*(1), 32–44.

Hope Street Group. (n.d.) Grow your family strong. Retrieved from http://hopestreetgroup.org/wp-content/uploads/2015/01/HSG-GYFS-Pilot_5.pdf

Islam, N., Nadkarni, S. K., Zahn, D., Skillman, M., Kwon, S. C., & Trinh-Shevrin, C. (2015). Integrating Community Health Workers Within Patient Protection and Affordable Care Act Implementation. *Journal of Public Health Management and Practice: JPHMP, 21*(1), 42–50.

Katahoire, A. R., Henriksson, D. K., Ssegujja, E., Waiswa, P., Ayebare, F., Bagenda, D.,...Peterson, S. S. (2015). Improving child survival through a district management strengthening and community empowerment intervention: Early implementation experiences from Uganda. *BMC Public Health, 15*, 797.

Koh, H. W., & Sebelius, K. G. (2010). Promoting prevention through the Affordable Care Act. *New England Journal of Medicine, 363*(14), 1296–1299.

Lenihan, P. (2005). MAPP and the evolution of planning in public health practice. *Journal of Public Health Management Practice, 11*(5), 381–386.

Lochner, K. A., & Wynne, M. (2011). Flu shots and the characteristics of unvaccinated elderly Medicare beneficiaries. *Medicare & Medicaid Research Review, 1*(4). http://doi.org/10.5600/mmrr.001.04.b01

MacDuffie, H., & DePoy, E. (2004). Force field analysis: A model for promoting adolescents' involvement in their own health care. *Health Promotion Practice, 5*, 306–313.

Marmot, M. (2005). Social determinants of health inequalities. *Lancet, 365*, 1099–1104.

McElroy, J. A., Haynes, S. G., Eliason, M. J., Wood, S. F., Gilbert, T., Barker, L. T., & Minnis, A. M. (2016). Health weight in lesbian and bisexual women aged 40 and older: an effective intervention in 10 cities using tailored approaches. *Women's Health Issues, 26* Suppl 1, S18–S35. Retrieved from http://www.whijournal.com/article/S1049-3867(16)30037-8/pdf

McLeroy, K. R., Norton, B. L., Kegler, M. C., Burdine, J. N., & Sumaya, C. V. (2003). Community-based interventions. *American Journal of Public Health*, 93(4), 529–533.

National Prevention Council. (2011). *National Prevention Strategy*. Washington, DC: U.S. Department of Health and Human Services, Office of the Surgeon General. Retrieved from https://www.surgeongeneral.gov/priorities/prevention/strategy/report.pdf

Nichol, K. L., Nordin, J. D., Nelson, D. B., Mullooly, J. P., & Hak, E. (2007). Effectiveness of influenza vaccine in the community-dwelling elderly. *New England Journal of Medicine*, 357(14), 1373–1381.

O'Malley, A. S., & Forrest, C. B. (2006). Immunization disparities in older Americans. *American Journal of Preventive Medicine*, 31(2), 150–158.

Ottawa Charter. (1986). Image. Retrieved from https://www.med.uottawa.ca/sim/data/Models/Ottawa_Charter.htm

Ottawa Charter for Health Promotion. (1986). https://www.med.uottawa.ca/sim/data/Health_Promotion_e.htm#Ottawa_Charter

Persily, C. (1995). Help seeking in high risk pregnancy. The role of the CNS. *CNS: The Journal of Advanced Practice*, 9, 207–220.

Persily, C. A., & Hildebrandt, E. (2008). *Theory of community empowerment* (2nd. ed.). New York: Springer Publishing Company. Retrieved from https://gold.worcester.edu/login?url=https://search.proquest.com/docview/189456204?accountid=29121

Perry, H. B., Zulliger, R. & Rogers, M. (2014). Community health workers in low-, middle-, and high-income countries: An overview of their history, recent evolution, and current effectiveness. *Annual Review Public Health*, 35:399–421.

Pérez, L., & Martinez, J. (2008). Community health workers: Social justice and policy advocates for community health and well-being. *American Journal of Public Health*, 98(1), 11–14.

Prevention Institute. (2008). Strategies for enhancing the built environment to support healthy eating and active living. Retrieved from https://2f9312f7-a-a7546207-s-sites.googlegroups.com/a/calendow.org/resource-library/home/philanthropy-reports/TCE%20Strategies%20Enhancing%20BE.pdf?attachauth=ANoY7cqsg18Fy1Q2r6xbBWjLezB6mfmKGjlH_Ia2QDGl_Jxd2HJWvPAsVqDSZ-V4l0EwB9EJSS3w0p_K4VcFNX6mV-Sa5R0Nr4RqHH-vOk5qP04ujOvTkNuYDmDYz-BZpI5QNTLlTCXZWb-p346vYL8P2uOhPHbJUOrYBVhXapGD3nnAK6vi8XM0xRULb-huw2mUWvcaUlL_WKPR3wGdR7d4FxNOIarUXpNru45G2Ory-nPBkpjburmFOPMIbyqcHmEMeaHJFp-0lcJ1HJiOVAoskJFchGpRNzS6Q%3D%3D&attredirects=0

Petersen, D., Taylor, E. F., Peikes, D. (2013). The logic model: The foundation to implement, study, and refine patient-centered medical home models (AHRQ). Retrieved from https://pcmh.ahrq.gov/sites/default/files/attachments/logic-model-brief.pdf.

Robert Wood Johnson Foundation. (n.d.). How do we empower communities to get healthy? Retrieved from http://www.rwjf.org/en/culture-of-health/2014/07/how_do_we_empowerco.htmlhttp://www.rwjf.org/en/culture-of-health/2014/07/how_do_we_empowerco.html

Rosenthal, E. L., Brownstein, J. N., Rush, C. H., Hirsch, G. R., Willaert, A. M., Scott, J. R., Fox, D. J. (2010). Community health workers: Part of the solution. *Health Affairs*, 29(7), 1338–1342.

Sabo, S., Ingram, M., Reinschmidt, K. M., Schachter, K., Jacobs, L., Guernsey de Zapien, J., … Carvajal, S. (2013). Predictors and a framework for fostering community advocacy as a community health worker core function to eliminate health disparities. *American Journal of Public Health*, 103(7), e67–e73.

Schmid, P., Rauber, D., Betsch, C., Lidolt, G., & Denker, M. L. (2017). Barriers of Influenza Vaccination Intention and Behavior— A Systematic Review of Influenza Vaccine Hesitancy, 2005–2016. *PLoS ONE*, 12(1), e0170550. http://doi.org/10.1371/journal.pone.0170550

Schwartz, M. B., & Brownell, K. D. (2007). Actions necessary to prevent childhood obesity: Creating the climate for change. *Journal of Law, Medicine & Ethics*, 35, 78–89.

Shaw, J. E., Sicree, R. A., & Zimmet, P. Z. (2010). Global estimates of the prevalence of diabetes for 2010 and 2030. *Diabetes Research and Clinical Practice*. Retrieved from http://www.diabetesresearchclinicalpractice.com/article/S0168-8227(09)00432-X/fulltext. http://dx.doi.org/10.1016/j.diabres.2009.10.007

Shirey, M. R. (2013). Lewin's theory of planned change as a strategic resource. *The Journal of Nursing Administration*, 43(2), 69–72.

Smart Growth American (2018). National complete streets coalition. Retrieved on June 7, 2018, from https://smartgrowthamerica.org/program/national-complete-streets-coalition/

Smedley, B. D., & Syme, S. L. (2002). *Promoting health: Intervention strategies from social and behavioral research. Institutes of Medicine*, Washington, DC: National Academies Press.

Stokols, D. (1992). Establishing and maintaining healthy environments. *Toward a social ecology of health promotion American Psychologist*, 47(1), 6–20.

The Community Guide. (2016). Diabetes Prevention: Interventions engaging community health workers. Retrieved from https://www.thecommunityguide.org/findings/diabetes-prevention-interventions-engaging-community-health-workers

Taylor-Powell, E., & Henert, E. (2008). Developing a logic model: Teaching and training guide. Retrieved from https://fyi.uwex.edu/programdevelopment/files/2016/03/lmguidecomplete.pdf

United Nations. (2012). *Millennium Development Goals Report, 2012*. New York, NY: Author. Retrieved from http://www.un.org/millenniumgoals/pdf/MDG%20Report%202012.pdf

United Nations. (2015a). Transitioning from the MDGs to the SDGs. Retrieved from http://www.undp.org/content/undp/en/home/librarypage/sustainable-development-goals/transitioning-from-the-mdgs-to-the-sdgs.html

United Nations. (2015b). Transforming our world: the 2030 Agenda for Sustainable Development Retrieved from http://www.un.org/ga/search/view_doc.asp?symbol=A/RES/70/1&Lang=E

U.S. Department of Health and Human Services. (2010). *Healthy People 2020*. Retrieved from https://www.healthypeople.gov/2020/topics-objectives

U.S. Department of Health and Human Services. (2012). About Healthy People. Retrieved from http://www.healthypeople.gov/2020/about/default.aspx

U.S. Department of Health and Human Services. (2016a). Advisory Group on Prevention, Health Promotion, and Integrative and Public Health, Fulfilling the Legacy Report. Retrieved from https://www.surgeongeneral.gov/priorities/prevention/advisorygrp/2016-12-20-fulfilling-the-legacy-report.pdf

U.S. Department of Health and Human Services. (2016b). Prevention and Public Health Fund. Retrieved from https://www.hhs.gov/open/prevention/index.html

Villeneuve, M. J. (2008). Yes we can! Eliminating health disparities as part of the core business of nursing on a global level. *Policy, Politics, & Nursing Practice*, 9(4), 334–341.

World Health Organization. (1998a). Health promotion. Track 1: Community empowerment. Retrieved from http://www.who.int/healthpromotion/conferences/7gchp/track1/en/

World Health Organization. (1998b). Health promotion glossary. Retrieved from http://www.who.int/healthpromotion/about/HPR%20Glossary%201998.pdf

World Health Organization. (2008). *Closing the gap in a generation: Health equity through action on the social determinants of health*. Geneva, Switzerland: Author. Retrieved from http://whqlibdoc.who.int/hq/2008/WHO_IER_CSDH_08.1_eng.pdf

World Health Organization. (2013). Social determinants of health: Key concepts. Retrieved from http://www.who.int/social_determinants/thecommission/finalreport/key_concepts/en/index.html

REFERENCES *(Continued)*

World Health organization. (2015). The global action plan for influenza vaccines: Report of the tenth meeting of the Advisory Group of the WHO Global Action Plan for Influenza Vaccines. 2015. Retrieved from http://www.who.int/influenza_vaccines_plan/advisory_group/members/Report_GAPAG_10th_SaoPaulo_FINAL.pdf

WHO, Health Promotion (The Ottawa Charter for Health Promotion). (2017). Retrieved from https://www.who.int/healthpromotion/conferences/previous/ottawa/en/.

WHO, Shanghai Declaration (2016). Shanghai Declaration on promoting health in the 2030 Agenda for Sustainable Development. Retrieved on December from https://www.who.int/healthpromotion/conferences/9gchp/shanghai-declaration/en/.

Xakellis, G. C. (2005). Predictors of influenza immunization in persons over age 65. *Journal of the American Board of Family Practice*, *18*(5), 426–433.

York, N. L., & Hahn, E. J. (2007). The community readiness model: Evaluating local smoke-free policy development. *Policy, Politics & Nursing Practice*, *S*(3), 184–200.

York, N. L., Hahn, E. J., Rayens, M. K., & Talbert, J. (2008). Community readiness for local smoke-free policy change. *American Journal of Health Promotion*, *23*(2), 112–120.

Zakocs, R. C., & Edwards, E. M. (2006). What explains community coalition effectiveness? A review of the literature. *American Journal of Preventive Medicine*, *30*(4), 351–361.

WEB RESOURCES

Please visit thePoint® for up-to-date web resources on this topic.

Chapter 10

Cultural Competence: Awareness, Sensitivity, and Respect

Teresa Eliot Roberts

I don't think things are moving toward an omega point; I think they're moving toward more diversity.

Clifford Geertz

Preservation of one's own culture does not require contempt or disrespect for other cultures.

Cesar Chavez

I do not want my house to be walled in on all sides and my windows to be stuffed. I want the cultures of all the lands to be blown about my house as freely as possible. But I refuse to be blown off my feet by any.

Mohandas Gandhi

CHAPTER HIGHLIGHTS

- Culture in community settings
- Cross-cultural nursing
- Cultural competence and related concepts
- How culture affects health
- Cultural health assessment

OBJECTIVES

- Define culture and describe ways in which it is propagated.
- Define cross-cultural nursing practice.
- Explain how culture can affect health.
- Explain ways in which a nurse can be culturally competent.
- Define subculture and explain how it may come into play in a clinical encounter.
- Describe the limitations and possible pitfalls of cultural competence.

KEY TERMS

Culture: Knowledge, values, practices, customs, and beliefs of a group.

Cross-cultural or transcultural nursing: Any nursing encounter in which the client and nurse are from different cultures.

Cultural competence: Openness to and respect for others' ideas and ways of life; curiosity, patience, and self-awareness of one's own culture and culturally mediated ideas.

Cultural safety: Culturally appropriate health services to disadvantaged groups while stressing dignity

and avoiding institutional racism, assimilation (forcing people to adopt a dominant culture), and repressive practices.

Ethnocentrism: The assumption that others believe and behave as one's own culture does, or the belief that one's own culture is superior to others.

Subculture: A group sharing some practices, language, or other characteristics in common, within a larger society that does not share those characteristics.

CASE STUDY

References to the case study are found throughout this chapter (look for the case study icon). Readers should keep the case study in mind as they read the chapter.

Susan, who works in a community health clinic, is explaining to her client, Nilda, why she needs a colposcopy. She tells her that her Papanicolaou (Pap) smear shows cell changes that could, if left untreated, develop into cervical cancer. A colposcopy and biopsies are necessary to determine a more exact diagnosis and guide treatment. To Susan's surprise, Nilda looks stricken and begins to cry quietly.

After further conversation, Susan realizes that Nilda, who is from Brazil, believes that she has cancer. Nilda understands English very well; therefore, Susan has not used an interpreter. However, even if she had, her remarks may still have been confusing, because language is not the only difference between people from different countries. Their cultural assumptions may not be the same.

What Susan does not know is that in Brazil serious diagnoses such as cancer are generally not given directly and bluntly; the clinician brings the conversation slowly around to the illness and hints at the serious diagnosis (Graça & Barry, 2016). In Anglo-American culture, clinicians tend to be both direct and blunt. Values such as time efficiency during an appointment and the patient's right to know all the possible differential diagnoses make Anglo-American culture feel impersonal and confusing to many people from other cultures. When Susan explains that cancer is a *possibility*, Nilda assumes that this is a gentle way of saying she probably *has* cancer. So, it is a cultural misunderstanding that makes Susan's first nursing intervention fail.

This chapter introduces the reader to culture as a health mediator, especially as it relates to community health. Aspects of culture that directly affect health and health decision-making are discussed, as well as specific challenges that face nurses and patients when they come from different cultures. Nurses and nursing students face challenges when they consider their cultural origins and assumptions; they need to remain respectful, open, and curious when interacting with patients from cultures different from their own. First, though, an analysis of what culture is will help focus the discussion.

CULTURE AND NURSING

What Is Culture?

Culture has been defined in many different ways, yet it remains hard to describe. A basic definition of culture could be the music, language, economy, fashion, religion, and art of a community. A more thorough analysis reveals, however, that although culture encompasses those phenomena, it also includes intangibles that are even more subtle and sometimes abstract. Culture is "a set of practices and behaviours defined by customs, habits, language, and geography that groups of individuals share" (Napier et al., 2014, p. 1609). Culture has been described as that which occupies the space between people in the world. Anthropologist Renato Rosaldo explains that *"[c]ulture lends significance to human experience by selecting from and organizing it. It refers broadly to the forms through which people make sense of their lives, rather than more narrowly to the opera or art museums.... All human conduct is culturally mediated. Culture encompasses the every*

day and the esoteric, the mundane and the elevated, the ridiculous and the sublime. Neither high nor low, culture is all-pervasive" (1993, p. 26).

Culture includes language, religion, occupation, economics, art, politics, and philosophy. It affects practices of individuals, families, and institutions. Culture is how people approach the world. One difficulty in discussing culture, though, is that because of its nature, people often fail to recognize its influence on themselves. Generally, only when we are outside our own culture do we even recognize that it exists, when "the fish becomes aware of the water in which it swims" (Rahmawati & Taylor, 2017).

Nurses and other human service professionals have come to realize what anthropologists have long known, that culture affects how people view health, illness, treatment, regaining and maintaining health, as well as death and dying. For these reasons, culture has become a major nursing concern. It is a fundamental and important issue in evidenced-based practice in community settings.

Properties of Culture

Dynamic, Not Static

Culture is an ever-changing phenomenon. Culture changes over time. For example, the culture of 19th-century Egypt is related to that of present-day Egypt, but it is not the same. The language has lost a few words and gained new ones. Social media, climate change, and other 21st-century concerns have affected Egyptian work, communication, agriculture, and education. Egyptian religion, language, values, and family dynamics are closely linked to what they used to be but have evolved over time.

Culture also adapts to new circumstances. For example, in and around Houston, the culture changed dramatically after Hurricane Harvey in 2017. Evacuations, damage to infrastructure, housing, and flooding radically changed how residents lived and thought about their communities. The cultures of individual people and families also evolve with changes in home life, illness, or migration to a new country, although these changes are usually less dramatic.

Shared, Not Private

The definition of culture can vary among anthropologists, but all agree that one characteristic of culture is that it is something that is shared among people. Families and peers are the source of the first cultural sharing for most children. When a parent explicitly explains a value system to his or her children or cooks food for them or even teaches them their primary language, that parent is sharing cultural knowledge. A similar process happens in schools and neighborhoods, through online social media, or in any place where people interact. Individual people may have cultural values, beliefs, and practices, but the sharing of these among people is the process of culture.

I have always felt that the action most worth watching is not at the center of things but where edges meet. **Anne Fadiman**

Learned, Not Inherited

A person is not born *with culture* the way he or she is born *with genes*. Thus, if a Honduran newborn is adopted by an English couple and raised in London, that child will be culturally British. Usually, culture is first "learned" from parents and siblings and then from peers, teachers, neighbors, books, television, and other media. A Hungarian parent may teach a child that rich food is fundamental to a healthy diet and that Christianity is the best religion, for example, whereas a Japanese parent may teach that fish and rice are a healthy diet and that studiousness and selflessness are virtues. These lessons may be explicit, as in when a parent explains his or her own values, or parents or peers may teach cultural norms implicitly, as when they model or reward certain behaviors.

Cross-Cultural Nursing

Cross-cultural nursing is any nursing work in which the nurse and patient have different cultures. **Transcultural nursing** is sometimes used as a synonym but can also refer specifically to the work and model of Leininger (2002), a nurse-anthropologist who sought to focus nursing attention on culture.

 In the case of Nilda and Susan, their different cultural assumptions contributed to a misunderstanding. However, the experiences of cross-cultural clinical encounters are also potentially enriching, showing each participant new ways of looking at the world and providing opportunities for introspection.

How can nurses working in communities develop a non–self-blaming and nondefensive posture when they make mistakes based on cultural assumptions and misunderstandings? How can mistakes like this be used and turned into learning experiences?

It is critical that nurses understand that culture is neither static nor deterministic (Usher, Mills, West, & Power, 2017). For example, just because a client is Indonesian, Mayan, Angolan, or French, that person does not necessarily act or believe like most people from the same culture. Moreover, an individual's culture does not necessarily have the same importance to that person at all times or in every situation. Rather than assuming anything, "communicate a recognition that people live their ethnicity differently, that the experience of ethnicity is complicated but important, and that it bears significance in the healthcare setting" (Kleinman & Benson, 2006).

 Student Reflection

During my first clinical rotation in home care, I was visiting a 50-year-old Vietnamese lady recovering from pneumonia. While I was assessing her respiratory status, I noticed several round brown bruises down her back, bilaterally. I was a little shocked, not knowing what it was. I could not think of anything about her infection that would cause that. But she told me that when she came from the hospital, her sister-in-law had given her a "fire cupping" treatment. I went home and did some research. It turns out that people in many countries treat some respiratory conditions by trapping hot air in little cups on the skin of the back, which can cause bruising. I wrote a paper about it and did a presentation to my community health class. My instructor said that even she had not really known much about cupping until she read my paper!

Cultural Competence

Nurses in an ethnically diverse society, then, should strive to serve their clients in a culturally sensitive, respectful, and effective manner. In other words, they should demonstrate cultural competence. In nursing, **cultural competence** means considering cultural aspects of health, illness, and treatment for each client or community, as well as doing so at each stage of the nursing process. Giger describes cultural competence as "A dynamic, fluid, continuous process whereby an individual, system, or healthcare agency finds meaningful and useful care delivery strategies based on knowledge of the cultural heritage, beliefs, attitudes and behaviors of those to whom they render care" (2017, p. 7).

Institutional Cultural Competence

Nurses and other health professionals should take culture into account in providing client-centered care, but to promote community health and well-being, healthcare organizations must also strive for cultural competence and be aware of and seek to minimize *structural* hindrances to cultural openness and respect. For community and public health agencies to be culturally competent, they must "provide effective, equitable, understandable and respectful quality care and services that are responsive to diverse cultural health beliefs and practices, preferred languages, health literacy and other communication needs," through governance, leadership, workforce, communication, engagement, continuous improvement, and accountability (Office of Minority Health, 2016).

Proponents of cultural competence also conceptualize it as a process, which is to say that as people, groups, and cultures change, nurses will never arrive at one point of mastery but should continue striving for culturally sensitive care (Jeffreys, 2015; Smith, 2017).

In Susan's case, especially if she has many Brazilians in her community service area, it would be good nursing practice to find out more about Brazilian culture. The facility in which Susan works should consider hiring Brazilian staff and/or consultants, find out whether there are health concerns specific to this population (a form of community health assessment; see Chapter 11), have a strong and professional interpretation department, and continuously ask in what ways the facility can improve services to this population, including ongoing self-assessment to consider how the nurses' cultures affect care.

How could nurses organize a descriptive research study that could answer some of these questions? How could Susan investigate how nurses feel about hiring practices? How could she design a study to answer if interpreter services are adequate?

It is crucial that nurses expand their views beyond the individual practitioner and client. Nurses must be culturally knowledgeable and sensitive, but they should also be critical of the systems and policies in society that perpetuate health disparities among groups. Healthcare professionals who have tolerant nondiscriminatory attitudes will not necessarily be culturally competent if they are not also trained to recognize when behavior unintentionally supports the status quo or a business-as-usual mentality and favors some over others (Rajaram & Bockrath, 2014). Indeed nurses must be actively critical to best promote the wellness of their clients.

Evidence for Practice

Silvestri-Elmore and colleagues (2017) surveyed new nurses across the United States and several factors to see which, if any, perceived level of cultural competence. Among this group of 126, being at least 10 months postgraduation statistically predicted increased cultural competence, as did Hispanic ethnicity and participation in a cultural immersion experience.

Practice Point

Memorizing a list of cultural traits of clients is simplistic; it may facilitate stereotyping and obscure the fact that each client is a multifaceted human for whom culture can play unique roles. It is incumbent that nurses approach their clients as individuals who may be more or less acculturated and should not be prejudged.

Some cross-cultural nursing texts list traits of various cultures, implying that memorizing these will make a person sensitive cross-culturally. However, human beings are complex, and culture is just one of the many factors that influences how they view health and illness. Indeed, using lists of common cultural themes can be seen as reductionist, demeaning, and too simplistic, given that all cultures are ever-changing, and that every individual has his or her own life experiences, feelings, and viewpoints.

Principles of Cultural Competence

There are thousands of cultures in the world, countless because they are always changing. A nurse cannot have encyclopedic knowledge about every culture a client might come from. But as a nurse is focusing on a certain community, it is advisable to learn what major cultural groups comprise that community and what facets of the community give it its own unique subculture as well. Indeed, nurses should do this while they are doing the general community health assessment (see Chapters 9 and 11). Although the nurses will not be fluent in all cultures at all times, certain principles will make nurses more culturally competent: openness to others' ideas and ways of life; respect, curiosity, patience, and self-awareness of one's own culture and culturally mediated ideas; and the humility to know that one can always learn more about a certain client's culture and that person as an individual. Individual nurses must work toward cultural awareness and competence to help erase health disparities and power imbalances among groups.

In such diffused changes of culture two factors are necessary: contact and understanding. **Hu Shih, Chinese philosopher**

Cultural Safety

Historically, many practices of healthcare institutions and clinicians have been discriminatory and hurtful to minority groups. **Cultural safety** refers to providing culturally appropriate health services to disadvantaged groups while stressing dignity and avoiding institutional racism, assimilation, and repressive practices. "Fundamental to cultural safety theory are issues of social justice and the significance of nurses' power, prejudice and attitudes. This requires the recognition of power disparities within the nurse/patient relationship as well as at the level of social structures, policies and processes" (Richardson, Yardwood, & Richardson, 2017).

For the community health nurse, this means ongoing learning about the health beliefs and practices of their clients and never dismissing or disrespecting folk traditions. For instance, communities in the United States that use healing practices of Vodou (or Voodoo), a Haitian religion, often feel that they have to hide their practices because the dominant society considers the religion unacceptable or even evil. A nurse who is not familiar with these practices might at first be shocked or scared by Vodou, but providing culturally safe care means that he or she would need to analyze those feelings and instead approach Vodou with respect and openness, encouraging clients to use Vodou if they see it as beneficial.

Evidence for Practice

A survey of 358 Ethiopian immigrants in the United States showed that more than 57% had recently used herbs and supplements, mostly for respiratory illnesses. They also used acupuncture, chiropractic, holy water, incense, prayer, and *wegesha* (traditional physiotherapy and bone-setting). Though the majority of this group did have health insurance, most did not discuss their alternative therapies with their primary care practitioners (Hailemeskel, Habte, Fullas, & Al-Matari, 2017).

Cultural Humility

Because "competency" implies mastering a finite task, "cultural humility" has been proposed as another, perhaps more appropriate, goal (Fisher-Borne, Cain, & Martin, 2015). If nurses treat patients' cultures as atypical behavior that needs to be learned and mastered, "this approach can further reinforce existing stereotypes and cultural essentialism" (Rajaram & Bosckrath, 2014). Cultural humility requires nurses to continually self-evaluate and critique their own cultural

assumptions and to advocate for their clients in a nonpaternalistic way. To do the latter, they should:

- Ask open-ended questions about beliefs and practices of the client and family and
- Ask about traditions. What does the client think may have caused an illness, and how has the client already tried to address it?

Rather than trying only to learn tricks or nuggets of cultural knowledge, it is better to have an ongoing, humble attitude and commitment to self-awareness and client-centered care.

For example, a school nurse interacting with students from many cultural groups finds it impossible to be an expert on the health beliefs and practices of all the cultures. However, he or she understands the common health practices of some of the cultures. A teacher complains that a boy is wearing small magnets on his ears, which is against the dress code. After interviewing the child, the school nurse learns that he has been experiencing headaches in class. It turns out that the magnets have been placed on his ears by a traditional Chinese medicine practitioner as treatment for his headaches. The school nurse should explain to the teacher that this is a valid therapeutic technique and that Chinese medicine is a legitimate healthcare system 10 times older than Western allopathic medicine. Also, the therapy is likely to make the child more comfortable in class and better able to learn.

Ethnocentrism

Ethnocentrism refers to two related phenomena. First, ethnocentrism means the tendency of people to assume that everyone else thinks the same way they do, and has the same worldview, logic, and culture. For instance:

- A family that eats a big Christmas dinner of ham and sweet potatoes in the afternoon of Christmas day might assume that everyone celebrates the Christmas holiday that way—even that everyone celebrates the holiday. Christmas as a holiday at all, as well as specific Christmas rituals, differ significantly across cultural groups, even for those living near each other.
- Nurses often assume that they can reach clients by phone or e-mail, but if their clients are indigent, they may have neither phones nor internet access.
- A woman drives to work and has an office job, and she forgets that many other people commute on foot, or have an occupation that requires them to be physically active.
- A student nurse asks a client, "What do you usually eat for dinner?" The client answers, "Oh, regular food." The client is assuming that most people eat the same things he or she does and does not even know how to describe it, perceiving his or her own diet as the norm.

Ethnocentrism can also refer to the tendency of people to view their way of doing things and their culture as superior to the cultures and ways of others. For instance, someone may feel that a "real" marriage requires a wedding in a certain religious denomination. This may reflect ignorance about or even disdain for hundreds of other ways of creating marriages that occur across the world. If people think that their own regions' fashions or medicines or languages are *better* than those of another region (as opposed to just personally preferring them), they are thinking ethnocentrically.

> Perhaps Nilda would like to consult an herbalist about ways to treat her cervical cellular changes. Susan can ethnocentrically reject the idea, telling Nilda that herbalism is primitive and dangerous, or she can find out more about it, offering to work together with Nilda's chosen herbalist to develop a complementary treatment plan.
>
> What would be some concrete first steps in finding an herbalist? How could a nurse build community-collaborative relationships from small-scale relationships with patients in communities?

Subculture

Just as any group of people from a certain place may share a culture, any group of people who share a certain characteristic can share a smaller culture, or **subculture**. For instance, within the United States, Methodists share a subculture of their religion and religious practices. Just as with larger cultures, there is plenty of heterogeneity within Methodism, and not all Methodists are the same or have exactly the same religious beliefs. We can say, however, that it is likely that they share certain beliefs, practices, experiences, and/or religious discourse.

Subcultures might be groups of an occupation, age cohort, sexual orientation, avocation, socioeconomic status, region, or some other characteristic that the individuals share. It is reasonable to assume that construction workers from Tampa to Seattle share some experiences, language, and practices. Similarly, motorcycle enthusiasts have interests and knowledge in common that make them a subcultural group, as are nurses, skiers, lesbians, cancer survivors, and café owners. A subculture may be large or small, clustered together or scattered, but its members share some cultural facets such as experience, belief, language (or "lingo"), practices, and values.

> It is time for parents to teach young people early on that in diversity there is beauty and there is strength. **Maya Angelou**

> Nilda's original culture was Brazilian, but the fact that she has had a new experience of migrating to the United States means that she also belongs to a smaller

subculture of Brazilians living in the United States. These people have shared certain experiences. She also probably belongs to other subcultures, such as her church, neighborhood, and occupational group. Nilda and Susan also share subcultures; for example, they are both women, they live in the same city, and may be of the same age or love the same television program.

Race

Race can also be thought of as a subculture because people of the same race often share experiences, such as how they are treated by and reflected in a larger society. What is important to understand is that race is a social construct, not a biologic entity. Because there is more genetic variation within a "race" (e.g., black, white, Hispanic) than there is *between* races and because its use can actually contribute to discrimination, some scientists have decried using the concept of race in biologic sciences at all (Perez-Rodriguez & de la Fuente, 2017; Yudell, Roberts, DeSalle, & Tishkoff, 2016). Racism is certainly a reality and can have devastating effects on health (Brondolo, Libretti, Rivera, & Walsemann, 2012), but race itself is based on social ideas and not on biologic determinants. Indeed, there are significant health disparities among races in the United States (United States Department of Health and Human Services, 2016). It is important to know that although a nurse may use a client's appearance to consider what diseases he or she may be susceptible to, appearance may not be a good indicator of genetic propensity, and there are many more factors that are probably more predictive of risk than what apparent race a client might belong to. Similarly, a person's eye shape, skin tone, or hair texture does not tell very much about that person's cultural practices or lifestyle, and not even a great deal about his or her genes.

WESTERN BIOMEDICINE AS "CULTURED"

For many years, anthropologists (scientists who study culture) approached culture in a one-sided way. That is, they studied their subjects, the Maori in New Zealand or the Maasai in Kenya, and did not realize that they themselves were viewing the world from a certain cultural lens. The truth is that no one is "normal" or views the world from a blank slate of neutrality. Every person comes from a certain cultural background. However, people from some cultures, having enjoyed more dominance in the world, may feel more "normal" because their culture is well reflected in world and local media.

Similarly, and importantly, nurses also belong to a cultural subset. The common educational experience, working conditions, such as shift work, and views of health and illness, based on a belief in microbial theory, all contribute to a shared cultural perspective among nurses. In addition, nurses who are from or were educated in the United States share much in common with American national culture and are infused with "Western" values in addition to the values and outlooks shared with medicine and allied health professions. All nurses should recognize and acknowledge this special cultural perspective and the ways in which it influences nursing care of clients.

The first imperative of cultural competence is to be competent in one's own cultural heritage. The nurse should ask himself or herself, "Where are my ancestors and current family from? What traditions and health beliefs did I explicitly inherit and what subtler assumptions were implicitly handed down to me? With what major cultural groups do I identify and which other ones have also affected my worldview?" Answering these questions can be extremely difficult because the nature of culture is that we grow up with it without identifying it. It is, by its nature, assumed. "Indeed, the hardest thing to know in a relative and comparative sense might be one's own culture: what anthropologists call the anthropological paradox … to critique objectively the subjective nature of our own practices" (Napier et al., 2014, p. 1610).

After personal understanding come respect and appreciation for the values and behaviors of others. Knowledge of cultural differences is essential if sensitivity and competence are to occur. Only when self-awareness combines with insight about others can nurses and other healthcare professionals demonstrate true sensitivity (Napier et al., 2014). This concept is important to keep in mind as nurses approach their clients, especially those who come from cultures different from their own. Culture is not a curiosity or a phenomenon that "exotic" clients have, unrelated to the nurses themselves. Indeed, clients from different cultures can just as easily view their clinicians as exotic. In reality, every clinical encounter is a cultural exchange.

ASPECTS OF CULTURE DIRECTLY AFFECTING HEALTH AND HEALTHCARE

Attribution of Illness

Different cultural world views tend to reflect different ideas about what causes disease. Anglo-American culture, for instance, emphasizes infection, genetics, and personal responsibility as factors in disease and health. Illness is seen as something inside or inherent to an individual (Brown & Closser, 2016). Other cultures may be "macroreligious," meaning there is more emphasis on divine influence on health and illness. Likewise, luck, fatalism, curses or piety may be seen as mediating disease.

Evidence for Practice

A multinational group of scientists conducted an ethnography about birthing practices and beliefs in Akwa Ibom, Nigeria (Mboho, Furber, & Waterman, 2013). They found that traditional birth attendants were considered to have supernatural powers. Women often preferred to labor in the homes of traditional birth attendants or even churches, rather than in hospitals, because they felt that there they would be protected from malevolent witchcraft. Additionally, if labor was particularly difficult, it was believed to be an indication of past sin, and a confession of infidelity would be required before traditional birth attendants would intervene.

Diet

What and how people eat vary tremendously among cultures, the understanding of which is crucial to good nursing care. Perhaps a nurse needs to teach a client who is newly diagnosed with diabetes or hyperlipidemia about dietary restrictions. The nurse will be much more effective if he or she chooses examples that resonate with that particular client. For instance, a new immigrant from India is more likely to eat rice and legumes than is a fourth-generation Midwesterner whose staples are red meat and bread. A nurse teaching an anemic client about iron-rich foods would want to use food examples that might appear in the client's own diet. Buddhism, Judaism, Hinduism, Islam, and other religions have dietary restrictions about various meats, for instance, and nursing interventions are more successful if the nurse is sensitive to a client's predilections. Often, various cultures and religions incorporate certain herbs, teas, and honeys into their diets, and the potential medicinal effects should be noted (Fig. 10.1).

Evidence for Practice

Researchers were interested in finding out more about how Korean immigrants to the United States viewed diabetes, in order to formulate effective strategies to prevent and treat the disease in this group. They held focus groups in a Korean community center, asking adult Korean Americans with type 2 diabetes about the disease. They found that diabetes held a significant social stigma and that, before their own diagnoses, many participants had believed that diabetes happened to "lazy" people and those who "cannot control" themselves (Nam, Song, Park, & Song, 2013).

Communication

Verbal Communication

Culture also has a significant impact on communication, in terms of verbal as well as nonverbal language, and style of

FIGURE 10.1 A: Examples of herbs used for medicinal purposes, from Dominican botánica. *Clockwise, from bottom left*: mastuerzo (vining nasturtium, spitfire, *Tropaeolum majus*)—used as an antimicrobial, source of vitamin C, and to fight coughs and colds; ajenjo (wormwood)—used against intestinal worms and for gallbladder maladies; tilo (linden)—used for anxiety, colds, hypertension, and fevers; guatapanal (divi-divi)—used against infections, especially of the tonsils, for hemorrhoids, and to dress sores. **B:** Medicinal teas for sale in a Brazilian store (Somerville, MA). Boldo (*Peumus boldus*)—for stomach and digestive ailments; Laxante— laxative; Hepatico—liver maladies. **C:** Honeys with medicinal supplements, Brazilian store (Somerville, MA).

communication. "Health communication has to be sensitive to the cultural background of the message receiver to maximize its effectiveness… a 'one-size-fits-all' approach will not be sufficient" (Betsch & Böhm, 2016, p. 795). Clinical encounters should always be held in a language in which the client is fluent, and if interpretation is necessary, a professional interpreter should be used. Interpretation should never be conducted by family or friends of a client, except in emergencies. Use of family or friends as interpreters subverts privacy and confidentiality. Further, professional interpreters are not only fluent in both languages and technical healthcare terms, they are also trained in issues of ethics and cultural brokerage. "Cultural brokerage" means mediating an interaction between people of different cultures. A broker may point out and/or explain cultural differences to the participants, in order for the parties to understand each other better. A professional interpreter knows how and when to carefully add context, as opposed to invisibly translating word for word.

Practice Point

Lack of fluency in English implies nothing about a client's level of education. Bilingual nurses or those with professional interpreters can aim their teaching at the appropriate educational level for each client, regardless of the client's English language skills.

Nonverbal Communication

Nonverbal language also varies significantly with culture, and misinterpretation of body language can lead to clinical misunderstandings. Some examples are as follows:

- Eye contact: In many cultures (e.g., Native American, Chinese, Haitian), a younger client meeting the gaze of a clinician is a sign of disrespect. However, in other cultures (e.g., white American or German), eye contact is a

necessary sign of respect. A clinician from those cultures might misinterpret lack of eye contact as signifying inattention, depression, or noncompliance.

- Personal space: Clients from cultures in which people normally stand close together (e.g., Italian, many Latin American cultures) may feel that a nurse who sits or stands further away is cold and unfriendly. However, people from a Nordic-influenced culture may be more comfortable with larger spaces between people.

For clinical encounters with refugees and survivors of war or torture, the nurse should conduct interviews gently and pleasantly so that it does not seem like an interrogation. The client should feel in control, and the nurse should explain all procedures. Sometimes, medical devices or procedures reminiscent of healthcare practices are used in torture (shock, acid, excisions, sharps). Gynecologic procedures may invoke memories of rape or sexual assault, especially if the refugee has not had similar gynecologic care in the past. Also, it may be necessary to have interpretation needs more closely regulated by the client if he or she is a refugee of violence or war. The Yugoslav and the Rwandan conflicts of the 1990s, for instance, pitted people who spoke the same languages against each other, and a client may not feel safe with certain groups of people who speak their own language.

Style of Communication

Cultures are often described as communicating either linearly or nonlinearly. People from Western European and U.S. cultures generally favor direct narrations with a beginning, middle, and end (in that order). American medical and nursing cultures may be among the most linear and direct of all, with our emphasis on time efficiency and concise documentation. Many other cultures use nonlinear narratives, communicating ideas in more subtle and, arguably, more sophisticated ways. Interactions between clients from those cultures and U.S. acculturated care providers can sometimes be jarring for the client and frustrating for the clinician.

Nilda might start explaining her symptoms with a story about her job back in Brazil, only coming slowly around to how this relates to her current condition. Although this could feel frustrating and ambiguous to Susan, Nilda is contextualizing her symptoms, albeit slowly, while also providing quite a bit more detailed information about herself and her illness. If Susan realizes that this style of communication is culturally valid and listens attentively, she may get much more helpful information about her client.

If time constraints on the part of the nurse interfere with giving individuals the culturally relevant time they need to explain their symptoms, what may be some creative options to support this style and use the time of the nurse wisely?

Time Orientation

Cross-cultural studies refer to "past-," "present-," and "future-oriented" cultures. Although this may be somewhat simplistic, it is true that different cultures do view time differently. For instance, people from highly industrialized and western cultures tend to plan ahead, be stricter in their concept of time, plan, and behave in the present with an eye toward the future (Fulmer, Crosby, & Gelfand, 2014). Some cultures, for instance some East Asian ones, focus more on the past, consulting history to help make decisions now (Gao, 2016). Other cultures, such as agricultural-based or less industrialized ones, focus more on the present, meaning that people focus on the activity more than the clock (Fulmer et al., 2014).

Differences in how people view time can create a clash of expectations in clinical encounters. For Anglo-American culture, for instance, time is thought of as linear and perishable. This is especially true in the healthcare world, in which time is considered a scarce commodity. In contrast, a Hispanic immigrant may view 10:00 AM as a suggested time for a clinic appointment and will arrive when other responsibilities are accomplished. If this patient reports to the appointment at 11:00 AM, an Anglo-American provider is likely to view this negatively. It is also necessary to consider a client's orientation to time when teaching about medication dosing.

When Susan tells Nilda to "take your medication at the same time every day" she may mean to take it when the clock says 8:00 AM every day, whereas Nilda may infer that anytime between 5:00 and 11:00 AM is OK, because *morning* is the "same time every day."

Can you think of some creative ways to make Susan's message clear to Nilda?

Evidence for Practice

Researchers in the Midwest United States examined homelessness using transcultural nursing theory and found several ideas and strategies for nurses caring for homeless patients (Woith, Kerber, Astroth, & Jenkins, 2017). They found strong themes of wanting to be "listened to," "taken seriously," and treated with compassion, empathy, respect, and fairness. Participants very often felt judged by care providers, and, interestingly, felt strongly that they wanted nurses to show that they enjoyed their work.

Roles

Cultures around the world have different expectations of the roles of children, young adults, and elderly adults; of men versus women; and of the role of a sick person. For instance, some children speak for themselves; others are taught to remain silent. In some cultures, such as American and British ones, a sick person makes decisions for him or herself; in others, such as many Asian and Latin American ones, the family makes treatment decisions as a group. Some cultures expect difficult prognoses and test results to be discussed with the family first and the patient later, if at all, which explicitly conflicts with the U.S. values of confidentiality and autonomy.

Practice Point

No matter what culture your clients are from, you want to know what roles they fulfill at home or in their families, because that will affect the significance of their illness and treatment in their lives. For instance, many clients are the primary caregivers in their families, and an illness may have ramifications in their families or communities, or in the patient's own sense of self, that might not be immediately apparent to you as the nurse or nursing student.

Religion

One central facet of culture is religion, and this also directly affects health, illness, and treatment (Fig. 10.2). Some religions attribute disease to divine forces, for instance. Some cultures are relatively fatalistic, affecting health behaviors (Brittain, Christy, & Rawl, 2016; Hayward, Krause, Ironson, & Pargament, 2016). *Insha'Allah* ("if God wills") is a common refrain for many Muslims, although they may mean it more or less literally. Some congregations practice faith healing and may reject secular treatment plans. Prayer and other religious practices can also amicably complement nursing interventions. Prayers, especially for a client who believes in a supportive god, may be advantageous to health (Simão, Caldeira, & de Carvalho, 2016). Indian yoga and

FIGURE 10.2 Religion and spirituality bear directly on health, illness, and treatment. **A:** Buddha statuette, from Puerto Rican botánica (Boston, MA). **B:** Saints, Italian storefront (Somerville, MA). **C:** Candelas from a Boston supermarket. *Left to right:* Siete Potencias Africanas—seven African powers; black candle—against negative spirits; Yamaya Olocun—the ocean goddess Yamaya. **D:** Spiritual remedial oils from a Caribbean botánica (Boston, MA). *Left to right:* Healing Curativo—healing curative; La Milagrosa—the miracle; Oil San Lazaro—Saint Lazarus oil; Jinx Killer Contra El Mal—jinx killer against evil.

Chinese Tai Chi are popular health promotion practices that grew out of ancient religious traditions.

All religions have traditions and rituals around death and dying, and although an individual client and family may or may not desire traditional practices, culture has a tremendous impact on end-of-life issues (Irish, Lundquist, & Nelsen,

2014). The nursing process has a history of acknowledging and incorporating some spiritual interventions, although most nurses could learn more about specific religious beliefs. In a nursing home that serves mostly Jewish clients, for instance, the nurses learn the Jewish death ritual of washing the body after death so that they are ready to do so if the family requests it. Buddhist monks, who come to chant for dying people, may join hospice nurses who serve Burmese clients, or a Hindu family may request that a deceased patient be constantly attended until and after the body leaves the hospital.

 If Nilda belongs to a Christian denomination that believes that God regulates health and illness, she may be less likely to make changes in her own health behaviors, such as getting a colposcopy and subsequent Pap smears.

Evidence for Practice

To investigate the beliefs about and uses of salt of Mexican and Central American farm workers in California, researchers conducted individual interviews as well as focus groups. They found that salt was ingested not only for gustatory purposes, but also because it is believed to restore balance, prevent disequilibrium, and reduce vulnerability to disease. Participants described beliefs illustrating hot/cold humoral balance dichotomy, a worldview long identified in Latin America. Though the farm workers did view excess salt as dangerous for the cardiovascular system, it was also thought to be beneficial for certain symptoms, like dizziness, stomach ache, fever blisters, and insect bites (Barker, Guerra, Gonzalez-Vargas, & Hoeft, 2017).

Folk Medicine

Herbs and other home remedies are used in every culture around the world (Fig. 10.3). However, some folk healing traditions are currently more robust, whereas others were marginalized in the 20th century with the dominance of professional biomedicine. Clients may be self-prescribing or going to folk practitioners such as Curandero(as), Santero(as), Shamans, or Ayurvedic practitioners. There are myriads of folk remedies a client might be using, some of which can have very powerful effects (Box 10.1). Just as nurses ask about over-the-counter medication use, they should also inquire, respectfully, about what other preparations or nonpharmacologic strategies their clients may be using to maintain or regain health.

FIGURE 10.3 A: Supplements for sale in a Brazilian store (Somerville, MA). Óleo de Copa'ba—antiinflammatory and antimicrobial; Castanha da India—astringent, analgesic, vasoconstrictor, and antiinflammatory; Alcachofra com Beringela—for problems of the liver and gallbladder as well as diabetes and high cholesterol; Cáscara Sagrada—laxative; Ginkgo Ginseng—(thought to have) numerous beneficial effects; Ginkgo biloba—circulation and memory aid. **B:** Tiger balm from Vietnamese store (Boston, MA). Tiger balm, applied topically, is used for muscle strains and soreness as well as for respiratory congestion.

10.1	**Examples of Folk Remedies and Healing Practices**	
Foods	**Herbs**	**Methods**
Chicken soup	Comfrey	Coining
Garlic	Ginger	Cupping
Ginger tea	Ginseng	Exorcism
Honey	Lavender	Holy candle burning
Lemon	Rosemary	Massage
Pepper	St. John's wort	Protective jewelry

Evidence for Practice

Health researchers conducted a systematic review of the literature to investigate the prevalence of medicinal herbs (or "botanicals") by racial and/or ethnic minorities in the United States (Gardiner et al., 2013). They reviewed 108 studies and found that African Americans used herbs for health reasons at a rate of 17%, 30% of Hispanics and 30% of Asians used botanicals, although regional and smaller studies tended to find higher rates of use than did national or larger studies. Patients were using herbs for cancer, menopause, diabetes, arthritis, and HIV-related diseases, and many groups rarely disclosed their herb use to their healthcare providers.

CULTURAL HEALTH ASSESSMENT

Individual Clinicians

There are several ways to approach cultural health assessment. Kleinman and Benson (2006) recommend using Kleinman's explanatory models. These researchers prefer using this individualist method (a "mini ethnography"), tailored to each client, as opposed to the concept of generalized cultural competence. Kleinman's explanatory models are a set of questions that explore the clients' view of illness and treatment, including what they think caused it, how serious they think it is, and what they fear about it. These questions can often uncover cultural ideas that the provider would not otherwise have known. They may also show, of course, that the client views his or her illness and treatment much the same way as the provider does. Others suggest using a cultural genogram to explore and illustrate how a client's heritage affects his or her health perspectives. Whatever method is chosen, it is important to create an atmosphere that encourages the client to tell his or her own story, with all its cultural nuances.

Healthcare Organizations

As mentioned above, it is also imperative that healthcare organizations such as hospitals and visiting nurses agencies conduct ongoing cultural assessments of their service areas. Douglas and team (2014, p. 113) contend that "healthcare organizations should provide the structure and resources necessary to evaluate and meet the cultural and language needs of their diverse clients." The Office of Minority Health (2016) recommends that healthcare organizations "[c]onduct regular assessments of community health assets and needs and use the results to plan and implement services that respond to the cultural and linguistic diversity of populations in the service area."

Cultural competence requires ongoing self-assessment by both individual nurses and by healthcare organizations (Jeffreys, 2015). "Understanding one's own cultural values and beliefs as well as the culture of others is essential if nursing care is to be not only appropriate but deemed effective by the patient, family, and community. Self-awareness, as the initial step, is the...process of identifying one's own values and beliefs" (Douglas et al., 2014, p. 112).

KEY CONCEPTS

- Culture is dynamic, shared, and learned.
- "Cultural competence" is an attitude of openness to, respect for, and curiosity about different cultural values and traditions, and ideally includes a broader critical analysis of power relations affecting health disparities. For community health nurses, it necessitates familiarizing oneself with (and continuing to learn about in an ongoing way) cultures that are represented in the communities they serve. In this way, "culture" could mean a national culture (e.g., Vietnamese or Honduran culture), a religious culture (e.g., Jewish culture), the culture of homelessness, a school's culture, or that of any other subculture. Further, "inherent in culturally competent nursing is the moral obligation to advocate for and protect the rights of the most vulnerable through social justice" (Douglas et al., 2014).
- Advocates for groups that have been sociopolitically marginalized promote "cultural safety," the ideal of considering cultural aspects of groups while working against assimilation and repression.
- "Cultural humility" is an acknowledgment that *everyone's* views are culturally influenced, that our own are not inherently better than those of our clients, and that our clients can teach us.
- Ethnocentrism can be defined as an assumption that everyone shares your cultural values, or an opinion that your culture is superior to others.
- Subcultures, or smaller subgroups of a larger society, have characteristics in common that may impact health beliefs or practices.

CRITICAL THINKING QUESTIONS

1. Do you think that the notion of cultural competence risks stereotyping? If so, how, and if not, why not?
2. How can nurses strive for cultural competence without pigeonholing or prejudging clients?
3. What are some of the main cultural groups in the region or city in which you live? What are some of the smaller cultural groups in your city or region?
4. Think for a while about cultural practices and how they affect health or illness in your own family. They may be difficult to identify as such at first, but they do exist. What ideas about illness prevention does your family adhere to? What do you do when someone gets sick? What rituals does your family practice when someone dies?

REFERENCES

Barker, J. C., Guerra, C., Gonzalez-Vargas, M. J., & Hoeft, K. S. (2017). An ethnographic study of salt use and humoral concepts in a Latino farm worker community in California's Central Valley. *Journal of Ethnobiology and Ethnomedicine*, *13*(1), 11.

Betsch, C. & Böhm, R. (2016). Cultural diversity calls for culture-sensitive health communication. *Medical Decision Making*, *36*(7), 795–797.

Brittain, K., Christy, S. M., & Rawl, S. M. (2016). African American patients' intent to screen for colorectal cancer: Do cultural factors, health literacy, knowledge, age and gender matter? *Journal of Health Care for the Poor and Underserved*, *27*(1), 51–67.

Brondolo, E., Libretti, M., Rivera, L., & Walsemann, K. M. (2012). Racism and social capital: The implications for social and physical well-being. *Journal of Social Issues*, *68*(2), 358–384.

Brown, P. J., & Closser, S. (Eds.). (2016). *Understanding and applying medical anthropology*. New York: Routledge.

Douglas, M. K., Rosenkoetter, M., Pacquiao, D. F., Callister, L. C., Hattar-Pollara, M., Lauderdale, J., … Purnell, L. (2014). Guidelines for implementing culturally competent nursing care. *Journal of Transcultural Nursing*, *25*, 109–121.

Fisher-Borne, M., Cain, J. M., & Martin, S. L. (2015). From mastery to accountability: Cultural humility as an alternative to cultural competence. *Social Work Education*, *34*, 165–181.

Fulmer, C. A., Crosby, B., & Gelfand, M. J. (2014). Cross-cultural perspectives on time. *Time and Work*, *2*, 53–75.

Gao, X. (2016). Cultural differences between East Asian and North American in temporal orientation. *Review of General Psychology*, *20*, 118.

Gardiner, P., Whelan, J., White, L. F., Filippelli, A. C., Bharmal, N., & Kaptchuk, T. J. (2013). A systematic review of the prevalence of herb usage among racial/ethnic minorities in the United States. *Journal of Immigrant and Minority Health*, *15*(4), 817–828.

Giger, J. N., (2017). *Transcultural nursing: Assessment and intervention*. (7th ed.). St. Louis, MO: Elsevier.

Graça, S. S., & Barry, J. M. (2016). Culture impact on perceptions of communication effectiveness. *International Business Research*, *10*, 116.

Hailemeskel, B., Habte, A., Fullas, F. & Al-Matari, R. A. (2017). A survey on the use of complementary and alternative medicine among Ethiopian immigrants in the USA. *Journal of Complementary Medicine and Alternative Healthcare*, *1*(4), 555–568.

Hayward, R. D., Krause, N., Ironson, G., & Pargament, K. I. (2016). Externalizing religious health beliefs and health and well-being outcomes. *Journal of behavioral medicine*, *39*(5), 887–895.

Irish, D., Lundquist, K., & Nelsen, V., eds. (2014). *Ethnic variations in dying, death and grief: Diversity in universality*. Washington, DC: Taylor & Francis.

Jeffreys, M. R. (2015). *Teaching cultural competence in nursing and health care: Inquiry, action, and innovation*. New York: Springer Publishing Company.

Kleinman, A., & Benson, P. (2006). Anthropology in the clinic: The problem of cultural competency and how to fix it. *Public Library of Science Medicine*, *3*(10), e294.

Leininger, M. (2002). Culture care theory: A major contribution to advance transcultural nursing knowledge and practices. *Journal of Transcultural Nursing*, *13*(3), 189–192; discussion 200–201.

Mboho, M., Furber, C. & Waterman, H. (2013). Social-cultural practices and beliefs influencing maternal mortality. *African Journal of Midwifery and Women's Health*, *7*(1). doi: http://dx.doi.org/10.12968/ajmw.2013.7.1.26

Nam, S., Song, H. J., Park, S. Y., & Song, Y. (2013). Challenges of diabetes management in immigrant Korean Americans. *The Diabetes Educator*, *39*(2), 213–221.

Napier, A. D., Ancarno, C., Butler, B., Calabrese, J., Chater, A., Chatterjee, H., … Macdonald, A. (2014). Culture and health. *The Lancet*, *384*(9954), 1607–1639.

Perez-Rodriguez, J., & de la Fuente, A. (2017). Now is the time for a postracial medicine: Biomedical research, the National Institutes of Health, and the perpetuation of scientific racism. *The American Journal of Bioethics*, *17*(9), 36–47.

Rahmawati, Y., & Taylor, P. C. (2017). "The fish becomes aware of the water in which it swims": revealing the power of culture in shaping teaching identity. *Cultural Studies of Science Education*, *13*(2), 1–13.

Rajaram, S. S., & Bockrath, S. (2014). Cultural competence: New conceptual insights into its limits and potential for addressing health disparities. *Journal of Health Disparities Research and Practice*, *7*(5), 6.

Richardson, A., Yarwood, J., & Richardson, S. (2017). Expressions of cultural safety in public health nursing practice. *Nursing inquiry*, *24*, e12171.

Rosaldo, R. (1993). *Culture & truth: The remaking of social analysis*. Boston, MA: Beacon Press.

Silvestri-Elmore, A. E., Alpert, P. T., Kawi, J., & Feng, D. (2017). The predictors of cultural competence among new baccalaureate degree nursing graduates: Implications for nursing education. *Journal of Nursing Education and Practice*, *7*, 33–44.

Simão, T. P., Caldeira, S., & de Carvalho, E. C. (2016). The effect of prayer on patients' health: systematic literature review. *Religions*, *7*(1), 11.

Smith, L. S. (2017). Cultural competence: A guide for nursing students. *Nursing 2017*, *47*(10), 18–20.

United States Department of Health and Human Services. (2016). *National Healthcare Disparities Report, 2016 (AHRQ Publication No. 17-0001)*. Rockville, MD: Agency for Healthcare Research and Quality. Retrieved from https://minorityhealth.hhs.gov/omh/browse.aspx?lvl=2&lvlid=53

United State Department of Health and Human Services, Office of Minority Health, (2016). National CLAS Standards. Retrieved

REFERENCES *(Continued)*

from https://minorityhealth.hhs.gov/omh/browse.aspx?lvl=
2&lvlid=53

Usher, K., Mills, J., West, R., & Power, T. (2017). Cultural safety in
nursing and midwifery. In Daly, J., Speedy, S. & Jackson, D.,
(Eds.) *Contexts of Nursing*. (5th ed). New South Wales: Elsevier;
337–350.

Woith, W. M., Kerber, C., Astroth, K. S., & Jenkins, S. H. (2017).
Lessons from the homeless: Civil and uncivil interactions with
nurses, self-care behaviors, and barriers to care. *Nursing Forum*,
52(3), 211–220.

Yudell, M., Roberts, D., DeSalle, R., & Tishkoff, S. (2016). Taking
race out of human genetics. *Science*, *351*(6273), 564–565.

WEB RESOURCES

Please visit thePoint® for up-to-date web resources on this topic.

Chapter 11

Community Assessment

Rosanna F. DeMarco

> Never doubt that a small group of thoughtful, committed citizens can change the world. Indeed, it is the only thing that ever has.
> **Margaret Mead**
>
> One of the signs of passing youth is the birth of a sense of fellowship with other human beings as we take our place among them.
> **Virginia Woolf**
>
> I don't even know what street Canada is on.
> **Al Capone**

CHAPTER HIGHLIGHTS

- Components of a community assessment
- Defining a community
- Frameworks of community assessment
- Different approaches to community assessment

OBJECTIVES

- Define and describe types of communities.
- Describe the process of a community assessment.
- Identify biologic, psychological, and sociocultural indicators of community health.
- Conduct a systematic community assessment using a specific framework or a combination of frameworks.
- Explain how community health nurses can affect change within a community based on conclusions drawn from assessment.

KEY TERMS

Asset-based assessment: Attention is directed to community strengths and resources as a primary approach to community assessment.

Collaborative models: An approach to assessment that begins with planning that includes representative parties of a population, including service organizations, corporations, and government officials.

Community: A group of people sharing common interests, needs, resources, and environment; an interrelating and interacting group of people with shared needs and interests.

Community as partner: Within the process of community assessment, considering the expertise of community dwellers as central to the task of understanding the health and well-being of the community.

Developmental model: A retrospective, historical analysis of system parameters such as the physical environment, education, safety and transportation, politics and government, health and social services, communication, economics, and recreation in a community.

Epidemiologic model: A process used to assess a community using data collected from descriptions and statistical relationships to evaluate the level of health and well-being within a community to address identified healthcare needs.

KEY TERMS *(continued)*

Framework: A model or a road map that assists the direction toward a goal.

Functional health pattern: A systematic and deliberate approach to community assessment, evaluating patterns of behaviors of community dwellers that occur sequentially across time.

Geopolitical community: Group of people who live within identified boundaries and governing systems.

Phenomenologic community: Group of people who have interpersonal and intrapersonal connections.

Windshield survey: Observation of a community while driving a car or riding public transportation to collect data for a community assessment.

CASE STUDY

References to the case study are found throughout this chapter (look for the case study icon). Readers should keep the case study in mind as they read the chapter.

In many circumstances, communities undertake in-depth assessments to understand what the needs of the community may be and how members of the community who have ways of assisting (health, business, religious, mental health, policing agencies, for example) can be part of a solution for the needs that are uncovered. Some recent examples of this approach include (1) using a participation of community dwellers to understand the health needs of the community (DeMarco & Lanier, 2014); (2) healthcare providers evaluating barriers to colorectal cancer screening in high-risk populations (Patel et al., 2012); and (3) community leaders against violence evaluating threat assessment related to mental health indicators of potential violence in communities (Interdisciplinary Group on Preventing School and Community Violence, 2013).

Similarly, a classic and seminal example of a detailed, step-by-step assessment undertaken more than 10 years ago used a report card approach to assessment. The population of San Diego County is the second largest in California and the fourth largest in the United States. The 2.7 million residents represent diverse racial and ethnic backgrounds, and present many challenges to those providing public health and social services. Many recent social changes, such as welfare reform, managed care, and restructuring of healthcare services, have affected healthcare delivery in the region. The San Diego County Board of Supervisors, along with members of the community, wanted to know what impact these changes might have on the health and well-being of children and families. To address this issue, the board ordered that a monitoring system be developed, and the San Diego County Child

and Family Health and Well-Being Report Card was created to monitor community-level outcomes.

The San Diego Health and Human Services Agency (HHSA), which was in the process of creating performance measures for its operations, partnered with Children's Hospital and Health Center in San Diego to develop the components of the community "report card." There were five key stages of development:

- An evaluation of other community report cards
- A literature review
- An extensive community information–gathering process
- Reviews by technical and community advisory groups and a national consultant
- Final approval from the board

The resulting report card reflected a broad definition of health and well-being. Data sources ranged from local health, education, and law enforcement entities to state and federal agencies. Included were 3 to 5 years of historical data, state and national comparative data, and, where available, race/ethnicity data. Compilation of these comprehensive statistics created a population-based, data-driven monitoring system (Simmes, Blaszcak, Kurtin, Bowen, & Ross, 2000).

In examining the San Diego case study, we can see that many people representing many groups needed to be identified, be organized with a particular mission, and then be encouraged to work together to establish key indicators that eventually became a report card for health in their community. The information obtained can then be used to design health programs to address the needs that were identified from the assessment data. Thus, the effort has a very practical and important end.

INTRODUCTION

Understanding the interactions between people, health, and environment is a primary concern of nursing practice. Community assessment has been called a critical process for the future which can be used as a means for understanding these interactions, as well as for finding a way to improve both the health status of at-risk populations, and outreach activities.

Most recently, we have seen the value of community assessment as a key contributor to advancing humanitarian aid to communities in times of emergency need (Kirsch et al., 2012). In addition to providing information that is essential to understanding the community, community assessment allows for critical thinking about its strengths, weaknesses, assets, and deficits. Whenever nurses conduct an assessment of a community, they examine biologic, psychological, and sociocultural influences of the environment of a group of people who share specific characteristics. Initially, the idea of conducting a community assessment might seem overwhelming. However, knowledge gained from this endeavor provides valuable insight into the ways that people's health behaviors directly and indirectly influence the overall health and well-being in their community.

> A man of a right spirit is not a man of narrow and private views, but is greatly interested and concerned for the good of the community to which he belongs, and particularly of the city or village in which he resides, and for the true welfare of the society of which he is a member. **Edgar Allan Poe**

The principles of epidemiology that are described in Chapter 6 provide a valuable framework to begin community assessment. In addition, information about communities can be expanded beyond the context of community health nursing and applied to other areas of nursing practice. This chapter defines communities and identifies a variety of methods and tools that can be used to assess communities. Community assessment is a comprehensive evaluation of the status of a community. It identifies vulnerable populations, determines unmet needs, and documents community resources. The information is then used to set goals, plan programs for intervention, and evaluate outcomes. The approach that is used for community assessment depends on the type and characteristics of community. Most frameworks described will be feasible for the assessment of geopolitical communities, yet using some frameworks with phenomenologic communities or specific aggregates can present challenges. When data are collected, combinations of frameworks can be integrated if it makes sense. The methods of community assessment that will be described are all useful but are not equally appropriate in all settings.

Community assessment is an integral function that supports all aspects of nursing practice. The approaches to assessment that will be described provide a foundation to develop and implement interventions that build and maintain healthy communities. Although community assessment presents some challenges, the information yielded from the assessment is invaluable in accomplishing health-related goals. Within the context of a greater healthcare team, and with the community members as partners, a community assessment assists community health nurses to maintain wellness and prevent illness in a population. An overview of the community assessment process is found in Box 11.1.

DEFINING THE COMMUNITY AND ITS BOUNDARIES

Geopolitical Communities

The word **community** has several meanings that are relevant to the process of assessment. Community can be a group of people who live in the same area, or can be the area in which

---

11.1 | How to Complete a Community Assessment

1. Establish a working group, including community members.
2. Define the composition of the community.
3. Identify the information that needs to be collected.
4. Identify an organizing framework for collecting data.
5. Use existing data to describe the community's strengths and weakness, assets, and liabilities.
   - Collect demographic data from national, state, county, and city or town from the internet.
   - Collect local data from libraries, service organizations, municipal records, newspapers, phonebooks, and other local sources.
6. Gather new data as necessary.
   - Community forums
   - Focus groups
   - Key informants
   - Participant observation
   - Surveys
7. Analyze the data, looking for similarities, differences, and inconsistencies.
8. Develop a profile of the community.
9. Identify vulnerable populations, unmet needs, resources, and unique characteristics.
10. Outline a plan for intervention based on findings.
11. Prepare a report and disseminate it to others.
12. Design, implement, and evaluate a project based on findings.

---

they live. Types of communities that commonly come to mind are municipalities or townships with identifiable geographic or other designated boundaries. These communities may be cities, towns, neighborhoods, or locales. A community that is described as a specific area, possessing geographic boundaries and sharing the same governing structure, is often called a **geopolitical community**.

The group of people, or an *aggregate* as it is often called in the literature, consists of those who live within the boundary of the geopolitical community. However, these borders are really ambiguous. The aggregate could also include people who work within the community but who do not necessarily live there and could include those living close to community boundaries who visit the communities to purchase goods or use facilities for nonwork activities.

Practice Point

Seek data about people who funnel in and out of the community. These are often overlooked by students who are trying to understand who constitutes the community. Local town or city employment data may direct you to companies that employ large numbers of people. For example, most of the population from a metropolitan area may work for three or four large corporations. By approaching these corporations, you can find data about employee residence. Interviewing some employees may tell you where they are receiving healthcare. In addition, you may identify these peoples' concerns related to their health and well-being while working for this particular corporation.

Evidence for Practice

A community health education center, which was affiliated with an academic institution, recognized that a way to invest in the professional development of students was to develop a project called "Creating Community Connections." This project was designed to characterize the evolving community landscape following Hurricane Katrina while providing opportunities for students to engage in experiential learning. Students in the project gained skills in program planning and community assessment, as well as in leadership and communications. Twenty-three students worked on the project during its 2 years, developing data collection tools, organizing and conducting key informant interviews, facilitating focus groups and community forums, managing data, and summarizing project findings for community presentations. Participation in this project allowed the students to grow as public health leaders and researchers while gaining a greater appreciation for community collaboration (Martin, Cunningham, & Magnus 2011).

Phenomenologic Communities

Another way to understand or describe a community is to think of it as a group of persons who share common interests or beliefs. For example, neighbors interested in enhancing their property to maintain the unique qualities of a neighborhood have a common interest but not necessarily a formal organizational structure, whereas members of a church congregation do have a formal structure and interests that bind them together. The term **phenomenologic community** (Maurer & Smith, 2013) refers to members of a community with common interests who have interpersonal and intrapersonal connections. Community members share common interests, beliefs, or goals, and together they identify what activities, structures, and outcomes are meaningful specifically to them. Phenomenologic communities frequently exist within a geopolitical community, although their borders are often less well defined. Examples of phenomenologic communities include groups such as the homeless or persons with disabilities.

Phenomenologic communities also include groups that are referred to as "communities of solution" (Maurer & Smith, 2013). A community of solution is formed by an aggregate specifically to address health concerns within a particular area. Communities of solution are not only composed of persons from the area of need, but also include members of neighboring communities who have a vested interest in a challenge the community faces. These communities can form in response to a health threat, such as contaminated water or industrial air pollution. Other examples include certain political action groups or the formation of ad hoc task force groups.

Underserved populations can also be regarded as a phenomenologic community. Social connections between members are likely to be loose and not integrated, and without an organized structure. Often, members of these aggregates are disenfranchised in many ways. Also, members of these communities might be included within other larger groups. Examples are undocumented immigrants, women living with HIV/AIDS, or teens at risk for being involved in violent crimes.

I would never belong to a group that would accept someone like me as a member. **Groucho Marx**

Student Reflection

One of the most rewarding things I have realized is that my dormitory floor could be a community of solution. I was very concerned for a long time about the drinking behavior of some of the students who lived around me. Three students got drunk beyond belief after a hockey game one week and pulled a fire alarm in the dorms to be funny. All of them were suspended. I talked with some of the students on the floor about this, and we began to plan how we could try to address this situation. The first step involved obtaining accurate information about the rate and severity of the drinking behavior on the floor, what was causing the behavior, and how the behavior compared to that on other floors and to the campus as a whole. It was really interesting to see how many of us banded together out of concern and shared the same valued concerns about the well-being of our colleagues and ourselves while attending school.

Evidence for Practice

The topic of this research report was the role of promotoras (health promoters in Spanish language) briefly trained in depression care at community health centers. Community assessment revealed the need to understand and develop interventions within the world of those living in the community. The intervention focused on four contextual sources of depression in underserved, low-income communities: underemployment, inadequate housing, food insecurity, and violence. A multimethod design included quantitative and ethnographic techniques to study predictors of depression. A community assessment was completed to evaluate the intervention's impact. On the basis of an intake interview, 120 patients with depression were randomly assigned to enhanced care plus the promotora contextual intervention, or to enhanced care alone. All four contextual problems emerged as strong predictors of depression (χ^2, $p < 0.05$). Logistic regression revealed housing and food insecurity as the most important predictors (odds ratios [ORs] both 2.40, $p < 0.05$). Research that assessed both ethnic and geographic factors demonstrated a predominantly positive response to the intervention among stakeholders, which included patients, promotoras, primary care practitioners (PCPs), nonprofessional staff workers, administrators, and community advisory board members (Waitzkin et al., 2011).

Evidence for Practice

To understand differences and similarities in demographics, health, and healthcare access in Chinese and Vietnamese adults, this study used a cross-sectional participatory community health assessment in an urban city in Massachusetts. The researchers collected qualitative data from community stakeholders to create a community health assessment tool that addressed information on healthcare access, health status, behavioral health, and chronic disease history and treatment. Areas of concern were issues of healthcare access and poor health status, particularly among Chinese participants, and mental health symptomology in both groups. These findings revealed important health concerns in two Asian ethnic groups. Studies like this one are needed to better understand these concerns and inform programs and policies to improve health outcomes in these Asian ethnic groups and other groups (Tendulkar et al., 2012).

Societal, National, or International Communities

In its broadest context, community is used to describe society in general, or a nation. For example, U.S. citizens have a common federal government and share ideals, whereas individual communities within the country have different state and local governments and priorities in relation to individual needs and interests. Recently, however, references have been made to the international community or global community, which encompasses nations outside the United States. Although the overall composition of these communities may differ, some have strikingly similar characteristics, with shared interests and goals, including members' health and safety. To continue to advance the goals of health and safety, there must be a thorough way of understanding each of the communities described, especially if nurses are to accurately target ways to address goals for change. The first step in any plan to help a community is to assess the community's needs. These needs should be assessed in multiple ways.

Practice Point

Different navigational techniques have evolved over the ages in different cultures, but all involve locating one's position compared to known locations. Patterns are derived from multiple perspectives. Triangulation, which comes from navigation methodology, is defined as the process of planning, recording, and controlling the movement of a craft or vehicle from one place to another. Specifically, triangulation involves finding coordinates and distance to a point by calculating the length of one side of a triangle, using measurements of angles and sides of the triangle formed by that point, and two other known reference points. In summary, triangulation is the use of multiple methods or perspectives to collect and interpret data about some phenomenon, and is used to come together for an accurate representation of reality (Grove, Burns, & Gray, 2013). In other words, whenever you are trying to find an accurate answer to a question you may have about a community, consider looking at the question in different ways or finding more than one way to address it.

The amorphous nature of the community can create some challenges to the identification of its members and to the assessment of their immediate needs. In thinking about the nursing process, the initial phase of gathering data to develop a diagnosis, problem statement, or challenge needs to be addressed. Establishing goals, objectives, and key interventions seems formidable if nurses do not consider how they are defining the community that is to be assessed.

What type of community was described in the case study about San Diego? Was more than one type of community represented? If so, what kinds?

How did the working group define who was and who was not a member of the community?

Student Reflection

I was scared to death when trying to figure out how to complete my community assessment assignment. However, after a while I realized how exciting it was to feel like a private investigator on a quest of trying to solve a problem (i.e., figuring out the truth about the health of the community in which I was serving: elders in their homes). After I was able to understand where to look for health information data on the internet and in city records, what I really liked was interviewing members of the community about what they thought about living in this city, what was good about it, and what was not so good. After a while, I was able to take all sorts of information I had found and merge it together—like finding hidden pieces of a jigsaw puzzle. What really helped me was organizing a plan of how to do this, and what areas I wanted to investigate, into a priority list. It was a really cool assignment.

How community health nurses conduct a community assessment varies depending on the overall purpose of the assessment. Each setting, and those who are part of the setting, defines the context within which a plan can be developed. The plan should include appropriate ways to access and assess data, validate the findings develop a plan to address challenges, and include a plan to evaluate interventions that are instituted.

Often, community assessments are related to a specific practice setting. Some examples of an assessment in a school setting might include the following:

- Learning about the outbreak of a specific communicable infectious disease (lice)
- Learning about healthcare practices associated with a specific chronic disease (asthma)
- Learning how best to protect children and adolescents, as well as their families, from the spread of infectious disease in a school setting

Therefore, school health nurses must be familiar with information about the disease, such as the organism that causes it, incubation periods, mode of transmission, symptoms, protective measures, and necessary treatment.

Knowing these parameters helps these nurses devise a plan to assess the numbers of students and family members who may have symptoms of a disease, and to identify those who are at risk for acquiring the infection. The school nurse can then assist them in understanding how they can care for themselves or access resources. The evidence that follows is an example of the principles and processes of gathering health-related information related to obesity, and an intervention to address this issue in children.

Evidence for Practice

This study evaluated a school nurse–delivered intervention in improving diet and activity, and in reducing body mass index (BMI) among overweight and obese adolescents. Six high schools were randomly assigned to either a six-session, school nurse–delivered counseling intervention that utilized cognitive–behavioral techniques or contact with a nurse who provided information. Eighty-four overweight or obese adolescents in grades 9 through 11 completed behavioral and physiologic assessments at baseline and at 2- and 6-month follow-ups. At 2 months, participants who received the counseling intervention ate breakfast on more days per week (difference = 1.01 days; 95%

CI: 0.11, 1.92) and had a lower intake of total sugar (difference = −45.79 g; 95% CI: −88.34, −3.24) and added sugar (difference = −51.35 g; 95% CI: −92.45, −10.26), compared to control participants. At 6 months, they were more likely to drink soda once a day or less frequently (OR: 4.10; 95% CI: 1.19, 16.93) and eat at fast food restaurants once a week or less frequently (OR: 4.62; 95% CI: 1.10, 23.76) compared to control participants. There were no significant differences in BMI, activity, or caloric intake (Pbert et al., 2013).

Evidence for Practice

One program (Allegheny County Immunization Coalition, 2017) is a great example of school nurses developing a coalition between clinician pharmacists, physicians, and students to design a true collaborative solution to increasing uptake of immunizations in school-aged children. School nurses caring for children learned five key lessons that are examples of what these nurses need to assess when considering how to plan for the needs of these children in their school community:

- Establish strong links with clinicians. Immunization as primary prevention helps decrease morbidity, but without ongoing follow-up and communication and coordination with clinicians in the community, primary care becomes inconsistent.
- Target students and parents who are most affected by decreased access to prevention care. School nurses should assess their school community for those children who may be at risk for not having immunizations addressed in a timely manner or who may have parents who are unable or unwilling to address immunization needs.
- Identify an appropriate mix of resources (videos, immunization schedules, web links, and vaccine manufacturers' information) which should include an immunization champion at the school, appropriate school nurse staffing, and the involvement of parents.
- Use a collaborative approach, which is critical. Collaboration in this sense means identifying at risk children.
- Support evaluating this combination of efforts by measuring outcomes.

This approach allows for adjustment and readjustment of interventions to make the outcomes more successful over time.

Assessments made by community health nurses are often informal. They use the **windshield survey** to learn about the neighborhoods in which their clients live. Many community health providers use this method, but it has its limitations. It is a subjective process which nurses may use to understand the community by viewing surroundings. It is a descriptive way of understanding what appears to be the physical expression of the community as it is viewed on foot or through the windshield of a car. Anderson and McFarlane (2015) suggest that a community assessment can be accomplished this way by observing the level of economic development through physical environment, educational systems, safety and transportation, health and social services, communication, and recreation. Anderson and McFarlane refer to this approach as "learning about the community on foot."

Practice Point

A windshield survey is a great way to get a subjective idea of what a community is like. When you decide to either walk or ride through a community (keeping safety precautions in mind at all times and being alert to the level of crime or danger), try to plan the experience by first consulting a map. Get a sense of the physical boundaries that define the community, and explore not only residential spaces, but also recreational open space and businesses. Look at all the details and observe closely. Look at the quality of streets, bridges, types of house materials (e.g., wood, brick), people, light, air quality, and stores, especially grocery stores. Make the survey an adventure.

FRAMEWORKS FOR COMMUNITY ASSESSMENT

Community assessment is not unique to community or public health nursing practice. Epidemiologists, genetic counselors, and social workers also conduct assessments to understand which people are at risk of acquiring a specific illness, or to identify those who may need social support as they experience a traumatic event. Understanding and appreciation for community strengths, deficits, resources, and needs through community assessment is the objective that community health nursing shares with other disciplines (Jackson et al., 2014; Piper, 2011; Wessells, 2016).

There is recent criticism that community assessments have often emphasized what was missing in communities to address health and safety, rather than looking at the strengths and resources the community may have to address these issues (Piper, 2011).

In the examples presented, nurses followed identical underlying principles and processes to gather health-related data about communities. The nurses developed a planned community assessment to determine how people who share social or spatial relationships respond to internal and/or external influences on health. Identifying patterns of response to these influences can help planning interventions to preserve or improve the health of the community. However, it is always difficult to know how to start and the best way to approach this process. Previously defined **frameworks** are examples of successful ways to assess communities. They provide direction for the assessment. The following

frameworks serve as methods that can be used to develop assessments. The approach to the assessment will require considerable organization and a sequential plan.

Most nursing perspectives on community assessment incorporate concepts used in **epidemiologic models** to identify areas that affect the health of communities. The scope of nursing assessment also includes identification of communities' assets and capacity to create and implement changes from within the aggregate. There are two main reasons to conduct a community assessment: (1) to gain information and clarify the need for change and (2) to empower those responsible for implementing that change (Piper, 2011). The following section includes several frameworks for community assessment that can be used individually or in combination to identify key strengths and weakness in a community's health and well-being.

Epidemiologic Approach to Community Assessment

Healthy People 2020, the broad-based collaborative effort among federal, state, territorial, and private and nonprofit organizations, has established the leading health indicators and priorities for action in the United States (Box 11.2). These 10 public health indicators are tracked, measured, and reported regularly using epidemiologic methods and a wide variety of data-collection techniques. Although these objectives can be applied to the nation as a whole, or to populations of a state, county, region, city, or town, it is the practical impact at the individual and family level that is most important. For many reasons, communities vary in their ability to reach targeted objectives. Therefore, investigating the community's status in reaching these objectives is a part of any community assessment.

Community report cards provide a snapshot of the overall health and well-being of a community through the use of indicators or measurements of local social and health trends. Such reports are used increasingly across the United States to communicate critical information concerning local issues

11.2 Leading Health Indicators: 10 High-Priority Public Health Issues in the United States

Physical activity
Overweight and obesity
Tobacco use
Substance abuse
Responsible sexual behavior
Mental health
Injury and violence
Environmental quality
Immunization
Access to healthcare

Source: Healthy People 2020. From https://www.healthypeople.gov/2020/leading-health-indicators.

to community members, service groups, and policymakers. Developing a community report card helps articulate the community's desired goals—to establish means of measuring the condition of the community in relation to what is desired, and to collect data to measure progress toward goals. Members of the community and professional groups then decide how to create programs to address needs, change the circumstances that exist, or maintain those activities that have created a healthy community.

In developing the San Diego County community report card, indicators were developed to assess the community. Technical, community, and scientific advisory groups were established to firmly ground the development process in local technical and political realities. More than 20 local data experts reviewed and helped refine a list of indicators from secondary sources that would require no primary data collection. In addition, a scientific advisory committee of eight local leaders from the fields of public health, social work, pediatrics, and medicine provided scientific oversight throughout the development process. These two committees reviewed the preliminary list of indicators and made recommendations for refinement of five domains: economics, health, safety, education, and access to services. Twenty-nine scientifically based or consensus-driven indicators are listed according to their domain (Table 11.1).

TABLE 11.1 Community Report Card Indicators: San Diego County, California

Economics

Average percentage unemployed

Percentage of children living in poverty

Rate of public assistance to children

Percentage of parents receiving public assistance who are working or involved in work-related activities

Rate at which children receive food stamps

Rate at which children are identified as homeless

Health

Infant mortality rate

Percentage of infants born with low birth weight

Rate of births to teenagers

Rate of youth suicides

Rate of hospitalization of children and youth for mental illness

Percentages of adolescent health risk behaviors: cigarette use, binge drinking, marijuana use

Access to Services

Number of subsidized child care spaces

Average wait time for publicly funded outpatient alcohol and drug treatment services for adolescents

Average wait time for publicly funded nonemergency outpatient mental health services for children and youth

Percentage of children who are adequately immunized

Percentage of children with health insurance

Safety

Rate of delinquency petitions filed in juvenile court

Rate of child and youth homicides

Rate of children living in out-of-home placement owing to abuse/neglect

Number of domestic violence reports

Rate of unintentional injuries and unintentional injury–related deaths

Rate at which children and youths are killed or injured in alcohol/drug-related motor vehicle crashes

Education

Annual percentage of students who drop out of high school

Percentage of students who attend school daily

School suspension rate

School expulsion rate

> What are the epidemiologic methods that have been used to develop the community report card? Explain how these indicators relate to (1) describing the *who*, *what*, *where*, and *when* and (2) the descriptions of person, place, and time that are necessary components of a community report card (see Chapter 6).

Principles of epidemiology are used throughout the development, planning, implementation, and evaluation phases of the community assessment process. Epidemiologic methods can help identify patterns of health and social inequity and can be used to determine trends in three ways: (1) by describing the disease or disability, (2) by determining relationships that can predict health or health disparities, and (3) by developing and testing interventions.

Describing the Disease or Disability

Before engaging in any data collection, the members of the community must be defined. It should be very clear who is a member of the community and who is not. The organizing framework and resulting plan of action should articulate what information needs to be collected and how it will be obtained. Then, the working group can begin the assessment (see Box 11.1).

Existing (secondary) data can often be used to identify the community's strengths and weakness, to determine assets and liabilities, and to describe, along with available community resources, the amount of disease/disability or health in a population. (Box 11.3 provides resources for this data.) Finding data that identify the "who, what, where, and when" related to disease, disability, and exemplars of health must then be systematically organized and analyzed. Plans for collecting new (primary) data may include community forums, focus groups, key informants, participant observation, and surveys. (For more information on developing and using these methods, please refer to a nursing research textbook.)

By exploring data available on the internet, community health nurses can not only describe trends but can also identify resources that address the trends and determine where gaps may exist. The aggregate data from these resources include local demographics, such as death rates, causes of death, marital status, gender, age, ethnicity, and density of the population. Depending on the purpose of the community assessment, records in health facilities may be examined. This information can provide a sense of what the people living or working in the community face in terms of health problems, and can assess what happens to them over time in terms of follow-up and wellness. The local chamber of commerce can help identify and describe the physical environment, health and social services, economy, transportation/safety, politics and government, communication, education, and recreation facilities available to the population. In addition, census tract data and the perceptions of informants

11.3 Resources for Community Assessment

Administration for Children and Families
Agency for Healthcare Research and Quality
Alcoholics Anonymous
Alzheimer's Association
American Association of Retired Persons
American Cancer Society
American Dental Association
American Diabetes Association
American Heart Association
American Public Health Association
American Red Cross
American School Health Association
Association for Children and Adults with Learning Disabilities
Asthma and Allergy Foundation
Centers for Disease Control and Prevention
Healthy People 2010
Indian Health Services
March of Dimes
National Alliance for the Mentally Ill
National Association for HealthCare
National Association of Rural Health Clinics
National Center for Farmworker Health
National Council of the Aging
National Hospice and Palliative Care Organization
National Kidney Foundation
National Wellness Institute
Occupational Safety and Health Administration
Planned Parenthood
Real Solutions to Gun Violence
Substance Abuse and Mental Health Administration
World Health Organization
Women's Health (Health and Human Services)
Youth Risk Survey

(people who live in the community) about how they experience the physical environment, health and social services, economy transportation/safety, politics and government, communication, education, and recreation can all be considered descriptive data relative to the community and the way it is experienced by those who live in it. Census tract maps are often electronically produced and accessible by state, city, county, and town. These maps include an option to click and zoom in on a specific area of interest. Embedded in the maps is the capacity to access specific data related to the earlier mentioned areas of interest.

For example, a Massachusetts census tract and statistical site (Massachusetts Public Health Statistics, 2017) provides the opportunity to access specific city data, including health data: birth rate, birth weight rate, teen birth rate, birth rate changes by year, lead poisoning rate, cancer incidence, and presence of hospitals. As shown in Figure 11.1, the city of Brockton, Massachusetts, a suburb of the major metropolitan city of Boston, demonstrates higher-than-normal premature mortality. The color legend for Brockton indicates a

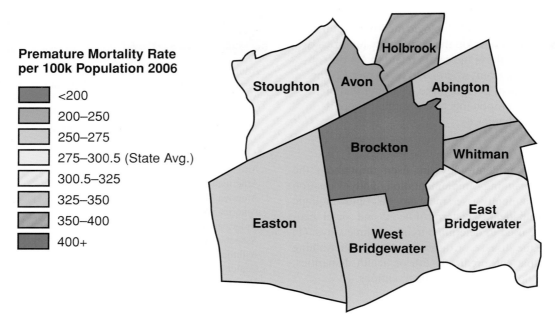

FIGURE 11.1 Premature mortality rate in Brockton, Massachusetts, and surrounding communities. (Data from MassStats, 2013. *Premature mortality rate: Brockton, Massachusetts.* Retrieved from http://www.caliper.com/Maptitude/MassStats/Map.aspx.)

higher-than-normal premature mortality rate (>400 per 100,000 people), whereas the town of Avon, which borders Brockton, has a less-than-normal rate (<200 per 100,000 people). Similarly, in a more rural setting in the United States, epidemiologic data may reveal high levels of farm machine fatalities, but may also reveal equally high levels of family instability related to intrafamilial conflict and mental health.

Determining Relationships That Can Predict Health Status

Data can be analyzed in such a way that relationships that predict health status (i.e., illness) can be defined. This information can be very helpful to community health nurses in planning programs and/or interventions. In Chapter 7, measures of association are described as statistical measures which are used to investigate the degree of relationship between events and/or circumstance of illness/disability in cases and cohorts of the population. The idea of association means that events or illness/disability may have a strong tendency to occur together rather than just by chance. In more recent years, statistical information has been transferred graphically so that assessment can be seen as concentrations on maps of cities, towns, counties, and states. The relationships that occur can be vividly portrayed as an association.

CHOLESTEROL AND CARDIOVASCULAR DISEASE

It is known that there is a strong relationship between high levels of cholesterol and cardiovascular disease. The Centers for Disease Control and Prevention (CDC) provide state-by-state information about the rate of screening for cholesterol by providing the percentage of individual responses (Table 11.2). These data, which can be gathered at the state, county, or city level, help to assess the use of prevention in health behaviors of citizens. This helps target education and support programs that can help members of populations obtain the information they need to make decisions that promote health. In addition, it assists healthcare providers in making sure that citizens have access to resources where reasonably inexpensive screening and follow-up are available.

Practice Point

Scrutinize your data carefully for similarities and differences. For example, using see Table 11.2, determine which state has the lowest percentage of cholesterol screening within the past 5 years. If you were going to target an age group for a screening program in this state, what age group would you choose? If you had to choose a state that did the best job of cholesterol screening of its residents within the past 5 years, which state would you choose?

Using the list of San Diego community health indicators, suggest some relationships that could be examined to develop further information about the population.

TABLE 11.2 Cholesterol Screening Among Adults by Selected State, 1997–2005											
	≤5 yr				>5 yr				Never			
Location	18+, Age-adjusted	18–44	45–64	65+	18+, Age-adjusted	18–44	45–64	65+	18+, Age-adjusted	18–44	45–64	65+
Alabama	72.0	58.7	85.4	90.2	3.1	3.6	3.2	1.6	24.6	37.3	11.3	8.1
Arkansas	67.7	51.2	83.5	91.5	4.4	4.8	4.8	2.5	27.7	43.8	11.6	5.8
California	71.8	57.5	84.6	94.0	3.6	3.9	4.0	1.9	24.6	38.6	11.4	4.0
Colorado	71.5	56.2	86.5	92.7	4.7	4.8	5.2	3.2	23.6	38.6	8.2	4.0
Washington, D.C.	80.7	71.7	89.2	94.0	3.0	3.6	2.7	a	16.1	24.4	8.1	4.5
Florida	76.2	64.5	88.0	92.1	2.2	2.4	2.4	1.4	21.4	33.0	9.5	6.3
Georgia	75.6	62.7	88.2	93.4	3.5	4.1	3.5	1.9	20.7	32.9	8.2	4.6
Hawaii	71.4	57.4	85.1	90.9	3.2	3.4	3.7	1.7	25.1	38.8	11.1	7.3
Idaho	66.5	50.4	81.4	90.7	5.9	5.9	7.0	3.6	27.5	43.5	11.6	5.7
Illinois	70.6	56.3	84.5	91.0	3.7	4.0	4.2	1.7	25.4	39.3	11.2	7.2
Iowa	69.9	54.8	84.0	92.2	4.7	4.5	6.0	2.9	25.0	40.1	9.9	4.8
Kansas	69.0	53.4	83.8	91.4	3.9	4.2	4.5	2.1	26.9	42.1	11.7	6.4

Geographic Information Systems

Geographic information systems (GISs) are another example of drawing relationships and associations that are important in community assessments. An example of a United States Geological Survey (USGS, 2017) GIS map outlining water deficiencies (hydrologic drought) in the United States is found in Figure 11.2, with noted visual comparisons of drought in Tucson, Arizona, from 1942 to 1989. The GIS system takes the physical knowledge of drought change to another level of comparison in a map system. GIS is a system of hardware and software used for storage, retrieval, mapping, and analysis of geographic data. Spatial features are stored in a coordinate system that refers to a particular place on the earth. Spatial data and associated attributes can be layered together for mapping and analysis. GIS can be used for scientific investigations, resource management, and development planning.

The use of GIS in health sciences is relatively new, but it appears to be expanding faster than any other area of GIS application. Health scientists have long used geographic information conceptually, but the availability of user-friendly GIS tools for community health research is recent. The GIS tools assist in determining locations of disease incidence, characteristics of surrounding environments, location of healthcare facilities, identification of the geographic boundaries of the communities, and other essential community infrastructures (CDC, 2017)

Developing and Testing Interventions

Using both descriptive data and relational data, nurses can develop interventions that can empower communities and effect change. These are then evaluated according to the results or outcomes of the interventions. As in the case study, the report card's indicators are now being used as outcome measures for county health and human services programs.

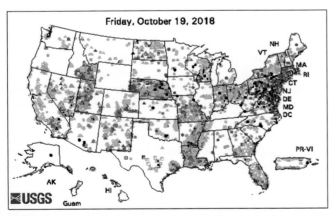

FIGURE 11.2 United States Geological Survey (USGS, 2017) GIS map outlining water deficiencies (hydrologic drought), with noted visual comparisons of drought in Tucson, Arizona, from 1942 to 1989.

Evidence for Practice

Children with attention-deficit/hyperactivity disorder (ADHD) often exhibit psychiatric comorbidities, which may impact interventions because of how psychiatric comorbidities can affect illness presentation, diagnosis, and treatment outcomes. Guidelines exist for dealing with these complex cases but little is known about how comorbidities are being handled in community pediatric settings. This study explored 319 medical charts of children presenting at primary care community clinics for ADHD-related issues. Assessment and treatment behaviors were identified and parents rated ADHD symptoms at the time of diagnosis and at 3, 6, and 12 months. Fifty percent of the sample met screening criteria for a comorbid mental health condition. It was concluded that children with ADHD and mental health comorbidities, particularly internalizing disorders, exhibit less robust response to ADHD medication and may require additional testing before starting medication and/or alternative treatment approaches in community primary care (Al Ghriwati et al., 2017).

Community as Partner Framework

Anderson and McFarlane (2015) use a wheel to represent a core surrounded by eight subsystems (Fig. 11.3). The core represents people as central members of the community. The eight parts of the community that interact with the various members of the community are physical environment, health and social service, economy, transportation and safety, politics and government, communication, education, and recreation. Anderson and McFarlane (2015) have proposed that it is necessary to consider the history, demographics, ethnicity, and values and beliefs of the entire community. "Flexible lines of defense" (buffer zones), "normal lines of defense" (health), and "lines of resistance" (strengths) are identified and surround the wheel, as well as separate each subsystem. These lines of defense represent a dynamic level of health after stressors have impinged on the system and can be used as a systems approach by teams to effectively assess a community. The word "partner" and particularly "**community as partner**" is key, because it demonstrates the equity of the nurse's relationship with the community.

The development of the San Diego Community Report Card used a partnership approach. Members of the Child Well-Being Subcommittee, composed of 13 people from diverse professional backgrounds, served as community ambassadors and provided broad policy guidance. To gain the trust and support of the large, diverse San Diego community, the project team solicited extensive feedback from more than 40 community groups. They distributed an information packet and survey in Spanish, English, and Vietnamese. After evaluating the input from the community, the list of indicators was modified to reflect comments made during this process.

Functional Health Status Approach

Functional health patterns (FHPs) assessment (Gordon, 1994) is designed to be used for individual, family, or community assessment. FHP assessment involves a systematic and deliberate format. Gordon defines assessment as a form of evaluation. Pattern, according to Gordon, represents "a configuration of behaviors that occur sequentially across time" (p. 70). Understanding community patterns provides insight into how groups respond to problems and take action.

Gordon includes questions that are applicable to community assessment for 11 FHPs (Box 11.4). Because the FHPs were designed for use with nursing diagnoses, clinicians are expected to identify defining characteristics from each pattern and assign relevant diagnoses. Although the FHPs are arranged in numerical order, the assessment format is intended to be used as a guide. Questions for community assessment are open-ended, specifically to elicit responses that provide depth and breadth to inquiries. Gordon acknowledged that because the community encompasses a number of systems, completion of the assessment requires time.

Community and public health nurses will appreciate the format, which is adaptable for use in most communities (Gordon, 1994). Assessment questions are not limited to informants' responses but also include clinicians' descriptions of the community. Novice nurses, especially if they have some familiarity with FHP, might find the model easy to follow as they learn about community assessment. The questions are clear and direct. The FHP community assessment also calls on students to use a variety of means to collect data.

Using Box 11.4, identify five FHP assessments that would be helpful in developing the San Diego Community Report Card.

Developmental Models and Approaches

An effective way to assess a community can be a retrospective, historical approach; this is a **developmental model**. Using system parameters, a community health nurse could travel back in history through historical documents, data, figures, and images, and piece together the stages a population or community has experienced. These system parameters can include the physical environment, education, safety and transportation, politics and government, health and social services, communication, economics, and recreation as segments of community life that are shared between those that live and work in a community (see Fig. 11.3). This approach could include gathering historical reports from interviews with community members who could describe their experiences in their own words. Both historical informants and mined data (i.e., data that are examined through extensive and rigorous searches) can help

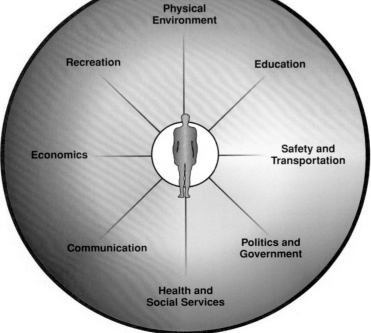

FIGURE 11.3 Communities as interdependent systems.

11.4 Functional Health Patterns

I. Health Perception/Health Management Pattern:
1. History (community representatives)
   a. In general, what is the health/wellness level of the population on a scale of 1 to 5, with 5 being the highest level of health/wellness? Any major health problems?
   b. Any strong cultural patterns influencing health practices?
   c. People feel that they have access to health services?
   d. Demand for any particular health services or prevention programs?
   e. People feel that fire, police, safety programs are sufficient?
2. Examination (community records)
   a. Morbidity, mortality, disability rates (by age group, if appropriate)
   b. Accident rates (by district, if appropriate)
   c. Current operating health facilities (types)
   d. Ongoing health promotion/prevention programs; utilization rates
   e. Ratio of health professionals to population
   f. Laws regarding drinking age
   g. Arrest statistics for drugs, drunk driving by age groups

II. Nutritional/Metabolic Pattern:
1. History (community representatives)
   a. In general, do most people seem well nourished? Children? Elderly?
   b. Food supplement programs? Food stamps: rate of use?
   c. Foods at a reasonable cost in this area relative to income?
   d. Stores accessible for most? "Meals on Wheels" available?
2. Examination
   a. General appearance (nutritional appearance; teeth; clothing appropriate to climate)? Children? Adults? Elderly?
   b. Food purchases (observations of food store checkout counters)
   c. "Junk" food machines in schools?
   d. Specific nutritional risk factors: socioeconomic status (SES), culture, gender, and age

III. Elimination Pattern:
1. History (community representatives)
   a. Major kinds of wastes (industrial, sewage, etc.)? Disposal systems? Recycling programs? Any problems perceived by community?
   b. Pest control (type, method, frequency)? Food service inspection (restaurants, street vendors)?
   c. Water supply source and quality; testing services; water usage costs; drought restrictions?
   d. Concern that community growth will exceed good water supply?
   e. Heating/cooling costs manageable for most? Help programs?
   f. Air pollution sources and control?
2. Examination
   a. Communicable disease statistics
   b. Air pollution statistics

IV. Activity—Exercise Pattern:
1. History (community representatives)
   a. How do people find the transportation here? To work? To recreation? To healthcare?
   b. People have/use community centers (seniors, others)? Recreation facilities for children? Adults? Seniors?
   c. Is housing adequate (availability, cost)? Public housing?
2. Examination
   a. Recreation/cultural programs
   b. Aids for the disabled
   c. Residential centers, nursing homes, and rehabilitation facilities relative to population needs
   d. External maintenance of homes, yards, and apartment houses
   e. General activity level

V. Sleep—Rest Pattern:
1. History (community representatives)
   a. Generally quiet at night in most neighborhoods?
   b. Usual business hours? Industries round the clock?
2. Examination
   a. Activity-noise levels in business district? In residential districts?

VI. Cognitive—Perceptual Pattern:
1. History (community representatives)
   a. Most groups speak English? Bilingual?
   b. Educational level of population?
   c. Schools seen as good/need improving? Adult education desired/available?
   d. Types of problems that require community decisions? Decision-making process? What is the best way to get things done/changed here?
2. Examination
   a. School facilities (type and condition); dropout rate

VII. Self-Perception/Self-Concept Pattern:
1. History (community representatives)
   a. Good community to live in? Going up in status, down, about the same?
   b. Old community? Fairly new?
   c. Any age group predominates?
   d. Peoples' moods in general: enjoying life, stressed, feeling "down?"
   e. People generally have the kind of abilities needed in this community?
   f. Community/neighborhood functions?
2. Examination
   a. Racial, ethnic mix (if appropriate)
   b. Socioeconomic level
   c. General observations of mood

VIII. Role—Relationship Pattern:
1. History (community representatives)
   a. People seem to get along well together here? Places where people tend to go to socialize?
   b. Type of government? Do people feel they are heard by government? High/low participation in meetings?
   c. Enough work/jobs for everyone? Wages good/fair? Do people seem to like the kind of work available (happy in their jobs/job stress)?

d. Any problems with riots, violence in the neighborhoods? Family violence? Problems with child/spouse/elder abuse?

e. Get along with adjacent communities? Collaborate on any community projects?

f. Do neighbors seem to support each other?

2. Examination

a. Observation of interactions (generally or at specific meetings)

b. Statistics on employment, income/poverty

c. Divorce rate

IX. Sexuality—Reproductive Pattern:

1. History (community representatives)

a. Average family size?

b. Do people feel there are any problems with pornography, prostitution? Other?

c. Do people want/support sex education in schools/community?

2. Examination

a. Family size and types of households

b. Male-to-female ratio

c. Average maternal age, maternal mortality rate, infant mortality rate

d. Teen pregnancy rate

e. Abortion rate

f. Sexual violence statistics

g. Laws/regulations regarding information on birth control

X. Coping—Stress Pattern:

1. History (community representative)

a. Any groups that seem to be under stress?

b. Need/availability of phone helplines? Support groups (health related, other)?

2. Examination

a. Delinquency, drug abuse, interpersonal violence, alcoholism, suicide, psychiatric illness statistics

b. Unemployment rate by race/ethnicity/sex

XI. Value—Belief Pattern:

1. History (community representative)

a. Community values: What seem to be the top four things that people living here see as important in their lives (note health-related values, priorities)?

b. Do people tend to get involved in causes/local fund-raising campaigns?

c. Religious groups in community? Churches available?

d. Do people tend to tolerate/not tolerate differences/socially deviant behavior?

2. Examination

a. Zoning laws

b. Scan of community health department reports (goals, priorities)

c. Health budget relative to total budget

Source: Used with permission from Gordon, M. (1994). *Nursing diagnosis: Process and application* (3rd ed.). St. Louis, MO: Mosby.

describe the cultural changes within a community or aggregate over time, and help to plan for the future. In this way, developmental data are obtained, and then compared, to determine what variables may have enhanced or detracted from development, and what resources were available at the time.

One generation plants the trees; another gets the shade. **Chinese proverb**

In the San Diego County case, 3 to 5 years' worth of historical data, as well as comparisons with other areas that were geographically comparable, were used in the development of the report card.

What data do you think would be particularly helpful in understanding the historical movement of a community in this particular case, and what do you think would be the strategies to obtain this information?

COMMUNITY ASSESSMENT ASSETS-BASED APPROACH

More than a decade ago, Ammerman and Parks (1998) observed that those who assess communities often approach community assessment with a distinct bias toward traditional deficit-based models. Despite good intentions, the focus of assessment even today is often on numerous problems, grim health statistics, and widening gaps in services. In an effort to build collaboration between a particular university and community, although it could be another institution in another area, an assets model can change the perspective on how one conducts an assessment within a community. When attention is directed to community strengths and resources, better relationships can be developed between all those working on the assessment, especially when the community is part of the process. Working relationships are enhanced when community members realize that the assessment process has the potential to be an empowering experience; the strengths and positive aspects of the community are measured in conjunction with what is needed or not actualized.

Use of the **asset-based assessment** model led to development of the community-based public health initiative (CBPHI) for research, practice, and teaching (Ammerman & Parks, 1998). A key factor of the CBPHI is building coalitions and active partnerships with the community during the assessment phase. Collaboration with community members shifts the focus from dependency on experts to empowerment of all, working together toward a goal. Using an assets model requires taking a different philosophic approach to the assessment process. Interaction with the community is the primary approach.

 Using the San Diego Community Report Card indicators as a guideline, create a list of indicators for assessing the strengths and resources of the community.

Evidence for Practice

Historically, Gerberich, Stearns, and Dowd (1995) supported the idea that overemphasis on statistics and other data resources could divert assessment attention away from opportunities to know a community's "personality." To support a level of understanding, the Community Assessment Instrument for Baccalaureate Learners (CAIBL) was developed, which continues to be used today. Based on Benner's model of skill acquisition, the CAIBL was designed for the novice nurse. The overall purpose of the CAIBL is to allow students to develop observation skills and learn to apply abstract concepts and principles of community health nursing practice. The authors outlined the four-part instrument in detail. Part I of the tool was used to identify and describe the community for assessment. Part II consisted of a windshield assessment. Here, 14 categories for data collection were detailed: housing; zoning; space use; boundaries; common areas; transportation; service centers; stores; street scene; community growth; race, ethnicity and religion; politics; media; and "community personality." The students' task in part III was to review documents and begin to summarize data. Students gathered data by visiting agencies and interviewing key informants. Students were encouraged to share data with other students during postconference. Part IV is divided into three phases. First, students reviewed the 14 systems to decide whether each was an "important asset," "problem or deficit," or "no effect" in relation to the community (p. 242). Next, to improve community health, students identified goals at a health status, health structure and function, or process level. The final step in this phase included students recommending nursing interventions for each goal on the basis of community assets and resources.

Collaborative Model

A **collaborative model** of assessment is an integral function of community health nursing practice. To develop the skill of collaboration, public health experts can work in partnership in a community assessment model that emphasizes the interdisciplinary nature of the task (Campbell, Whitcomb, Culver, & McClanahan, 2015). Assessment includes nurses as well as social workers in collaboration with community residents. Beyond interdisciplinary expert collaboration, another approach used in community assessment is collaboration between experts and those with health concerns. It is important to ensure that members of a population have an active voice in identifying issues and in making decisions about what is needed. Engaging participants with a "we can do it together" approach is more effective than using a "we/they" approach.

This process, however, has distinct drawbacks. This form of assessment is time-consuming, and logistical, systematic approaches must be pre-established to maintain clarity in the process for all those involved.

Evidence for Practice

Focus groups provide an effective means of incorporating the perspectives of "hidden" populations in assessments of community health needs and assets. In the study reported by Yoshida, Craypo, and Samuels (2011), researchers conducted a series of focus groups with youth in specifically targeted segments of a community to develop a comprehensive picture of community health. Despite differences in age, length of residence, and ethnicity, the focus groups were remarkably similar regarding the issues raised. Leadership capacity was facilitated through teamwork, community assessments, and policy work. Conclusions included that youth gained leadership confidence while successfully advocating for community-level change. Focus group findings have been used to initiate activities which address identified community problems. Focus group participation has the added benefit of increasing community members' participation in other community endeavors.

KEY CONCEPTS

- Community assessment includes examination of biologic, psychological, and sociocultural influences of the environment that surrounds a specific group of people.
- Community can be defined as follows:
  - Geopolitical, sharing geographic boundaries and governing structures
- Phenomenologic, sharing common interests or beliefs
- Communities of solution, formed by a group of people to address common interests, beliefs, or needs
- A society, nation, or international or global communities

- The epidemiologic approach to community assessment includes the following:
  - Describing the health of a population
  - Determining relationships that can predict health and illness
  - Developing and testing interventions to empower communities and affect change
- The community as partner framework uses a systems approach with a focus on partnerships to affect change.
- The functional health status approach evaluates health patterns in the community.

- The developmental approaches use a retrospective historical approach to understand cultural changes over time to provide information for future initiatives.
- The assets-based approach identifies community resources and strengths along with community needs.
- The collaborative model involves assessment by an interdisciplinary term and members of the community.
- The approach used depends on the type of community that is to be assessed. Combinations of frameworks can often be used.

CRITICAL THINKING QUESTIONS

Use the following scenario when answering the six questions given below. Use a group format so that sharing can occur across and between students and faculty.

In conducting a community assessment targeting information about women of color at risk for or living with HIV/AIDS, you gather key collaborative stakeholders together. You want to begin the process by engaging everybody's goodwill for the project. You start the process by having a 2-day retreat where you discuss and educate everybody as to the parameters of this process. You need to consider many things before the retreat. Please answer them as a way of preparing for the retreat by using a critical thinking approach that raises vital questions, offers relevant information, develops well-reasoned conclusions, and fosters open-minded communication by recognizing assumptions. Feel free to use information from websites, such as the Centers of Disease

Control and Prevention, which discusses GIS and mapping; the United States Census, which includes expansive census tract data; and local city halls or areas where data are collected statewide describing the community activities and statistics, as resources for answering these questions.

1. What does this assessment involve?
2. How do those in a partnership conduct a community assessment?
3. How can a community assessment engage families and community members?
4. What factors are involved in understanding community assets?
5. How should assessment information be used and by whom?
6. How can a partnership use assessment results to move from planning to action?

REFERENCES

Al Ghriwati, N., Langberg, J. M., Gardner, W., Peugh, J., Kelleher, K. J., Baum, R.,…Epstein, J. N. (2017). Impact of mental health comorbidities on the community-based pediatric treatment and outcomes of children with attention deficit hyperactivity disorder. *Journal of Developmental and Behavioral Pediatrics*, 38(1), 20–28.

Allegheny County Immunization Coalition. (2017). Retrieved June 26, 2017, from http://www.immunizeallegheny.org/for-health-pros/for-school-nurses/

Ammerman, A., & Parks, C. (1998). Preparing students for more effective community intervention: Assets assessment. *Family and Community Health*, 21(1), 32–45.

Anderson, E. T., & McFarlane, J. (2015). *Community a partner: Theory and practice in nursing* (7th ed.). Philadelphia, PA: Lippincott, Williams, & Wilkins.

Campbell, L. A. Whitcomb, K., Culver, C. M., & McClanahan, C. (2015). Community engagement: Leveraging resources to improve health outcomes. *Nursing Administration*, 39(3), E26–E30.

Centers for Disease Control and Prevention (CDC). (2017). GIS and public health at the CDC. Retrieved June 27, 2017, from https://www.cdc.gov/gis/index.htm

DeMarco, R. F. & Lanier, L. R. (2014). The Concept of "Silencing the Self" in low income, aging, HIV-infected Black women: A

ten-year community-based participatory program of research with results. *Journal of the Association of Nurses in AIDS Care*, 25(2), 112–122.

Gerberich, S. S., Stearns, S. J., & Dowd, T. (1995). A critical skill for the future: Community assessment. *Journal of Community Health Nursing*, 12, 239–250.

Gordon, M. (1994). *Nursing diagnosis: Process and application* (3rd ed.). St. Louis, MO: Mosby.

Grove, S. K., Burns, N., & Gray, J. R. (2013). *The practice of nursing research: Appraisal, synthesis, and generation of evidence* (7th ed.). St. Louis, MO: Elsevier Saunders.

Interdisciplinary Group on Preventing School and Community Violence. (2013). December 2012 Connecticut school shooting position statement. *Journal of School Violence*, 12(2), 119–133.

Jackson, F. M., Saran, A. R., Ricks, S., Essien, J., Klein, K., Roberts, D., & Worthy, N. (2014). Save 100 Babies©: engaging communities for just and equitable birth outcomes through photovoice and appreciative inquiry. *Maternal Child Health*, 18(8), 1786–1794.

Kirsch, T. D., Perrin, P., Burkle, F. M., Canny, W., Purdin, S., Lin, W., & Sauer, L. (2012). Requirements for independent community-based quality assessment and accountability practices in humanitarian assistance and disaster relief activities. *Prehospital & Disaster Medicine*, 27(3), 280–285.

REFERENCES *(Continued)*

Martin, A. E., Cunningham, S. C., & Magnus, J. H. (2011). Professional development using student-led, community-based activities. *Journal of Public Health Management & Practice*, *17*(4), 354–357.

Massachusetts Public Health Statistics. (2017). Retrieved June 26, 2017, from http://www.mass.gov/eohhs/docs/dph/commissioner/health-mass.pdf

Maurer, F. A. & Smith, C. S., & (2013). *Community/public health nursing practice: Health for families and populations* (5th ed.). St. Louis, MO: Saunders Elsevier.

Patel, K., Hargreaves, M., Liu, J., Kenerson, D., Neal, R., Takizala, Z.,...Blot, B. (2012). Factors influencing colorectal cancer screening in low-income African Americans in Tennessee. *Journal of Community Health*, *37*(3), 673–679.

Pbert, L., Druker, S., Gapinski, M. A., Gellar, L., Magner, R., Reed, G.,...Osganian, S. (2013). A school nurse-delivered intervention for overweight and obese adolescents. *Journal of School Health*, *83*(3), 182–193.

Piper, S. M. (2011). Community empowerment for health visiting and other public health nursing. *Community Practitioner*, *84*(8), 28–31.

Simmes, D. R., Blaszcak, M. R., Kurtin, P. S., Bowen, N. L., & Ross, R. K. (2000). Creating a community report card: The San Diego experience. *American Journal of Public Health*, *90*(6), 880–882.

Tendulkar, S. A., Hamilton, R. C., Chu, C., Arsenault, L., Duffy, K., Huynh, V.,...Friedman, E. (2012). Investigating the myth of the "Model Minority": A participatory community health assessment of Chinese and Vietnamese adults (includes abstract). *Journal of Immigrant & Minority Health*, *14*(5), 850–857.

United States Geological Survey. (2017). Hydrologic unit runoff graphs and maps in the United States. Retrieved from https://water.usgs.gov/ogw/drought/

Waitzkin, H., Getrich, C., Heying, S., Rodríguez, L., Parmar, A., Willging, C.,...Santos, R. (2011). Promotoras as mental health practitioners in primary care: A multi-method study of an intervention to address contextual sources of depression. *Journal of Community Health*, *36*(2), 316–331.

Wessells, M. G. (2016). Strength's-based community action as a source of resilience for children affected by armed conflict. *Global Mental Health*, *21*(3):e1.

Yoshida, S. C., Craypo, L., & Samuels, S. E. (2011). Engaging youth in improving their food and physical activity environments. *Journal of Adolescent Health*, *48*(6), 641–643.

Chapter 12

Care Management, Case Management, and Home Healthcare

Rosanna F. DeMarco

> Without a sense of caring, there can be no sense of community.
> **Anthony J. D'Angelo**
>
> Care is the state in which something does matter; it is the source of human tenderness.
> **Rollo May**
>
> We can all make a difference in the lives of others in need, because it is the most simple of gestures that make the most significant of differences.
> **Miya Yamanouchi**

CHAPTER HIGHLIGHTS

- Defining care management and case management
- Situating case management as a key component to home visiting
- Historical overview and definition of home care practice
- Description of the home care provision of services
- Examining types of home care agencies, services, and reimbursement
- Exploring role and scope of home care nursing practice during a home visit
- Identifying interprofessional roles in models of care delivery and use of telehealth
- Describing types of chronic care conditions found in home care patients
- Review of current healthcare reform and home healthcare delivery

OBJECTIVES

- Identify the relationship between care and case management as a philosophical underpinning to the care given by community health nurses in the home.
- Define home care nursing practice.
- Identify the role of the home care nurse as part of an interdisciplinary team.
- Describe the key components of a home visit.
- Identify common care situations and interventions in home care.

KEY TERMS

Assisted living: A model of care for the elderly or disabled that includes services such as home care to maintain the independence of patients.

Balanced Budget Act: The historical federal act of 1997 that made significant cuts in home care budgets on the basis of the enactment of prospective reimbursement.

Care management: Coordination of a plan or process to bring health services together as a common whole in a cost-effective way.

Case management: Development and coordination of care for a selected patient and family.

Family caregiver: A member of the patient's family, as defined by the patient, who has voluntary

KEY TERMS *(continued)*

responsibility to assist with the care of a patient.

Homebound: A condition in whicha patient cannot leave his or her home without significant effort.

Home healthcare: A provision of healthcare that occurs in the setting patients consider their home.

Hospital-based agency: A home health agency that is not freestanding in the community, one of many specialty services offered at a hospital setting.

Interprofessional collaboration: Sharing of evidence-based practice and skills by several disciplines as an integration strategy with patients and families in homes and other healthcare settings.

Intermittent care: Care that is not required continuously.

Managed care: A framework of fiscal management that emphasizes cost containment.

Medical home: A model of organization of primary care that includes care and case management and home care.

Medical necessity: Home care service given by a home care agency is reasonable on the basis of the status of the patient.

Official agency: A home health agency that exists at the bequest of local, state, or federal legislation.

Parish nursing: A model of care for members of a faith community that can include wellness care through home visiting.

Patient outcomes: Measurable objectives related to specific patient care interventions.

Plan of care: An agency-generated written document that is guided by a lengthy assessment of patient and family needs.

Population health management: The aggregation of patient data across multiple health

information technology resources.

Proprietary agency: A home health agency that is motivated by a for-profit philosophy.

Reimbursement: The form of financial payment offered to home health agencies, among others, for services rendered to patients and families.

Skilled care: The requirement for reimbursement of services in home care (specifically, Medicare, but also Medicaid).

Skilled needs: Refer to the needs of the patient that are accomplished through the professional abilities of a registered nurse or his or her supervised designee (e.g., a home health aide).

Telehealth: A form of electronic communication used to deliver healthcare information.

Voluntary agency: A home health agency that is motivated by a not-for-profit philosophy.

CASE STUDY   *References to the case study are found throughout this chapter (look for the case study icon). Readers should keep the case study in mind as they read the chapter.*

Eleanor is an 85-year-old woman who lost her husband a year ago. She never learned to drive, and she was dependent on her husband. Now she must rely on her family, both functionally and financially. Eleanor owns a single-family home, and with the support of local family members, she has chosen to live alone there. She has savings of $20,000.

Eleanor is receiving Medicare benefits, including Medicare supplements for prescription drugs at extra cost. On the advice of an internal medicine physician whom she trusts, she takes several prescription drugs and sees a podiatrist. Her blood glucose level has been so high that she requires insulin therapy. She has been unable to leave her home without much effort. A home

care nurse who came for two months helped find a homemaker and home health aide to provide assistance with bathing, meals, and light housekeeping. (This is a state-funded project for the elderly.)

Even with the help of her family and services, it is becoming less and less safe for Eleanor to live at home alone, and she needs to have more home health aide care for her safety. She has been told that to qualify for more services she would need to become eligible for Medicaid by "spending down" the $20,000 to $2,000. However, before Eleanor could become eligible for Medicaid services, she falls and is admitted to the local hospital with a hairline fracture in her upper humerus.

Increased longevity and improvements in the ability to care for people with chronic illness have led to an enormous increase in healthcare needs for people older than 65 years, as well as for younger people with chronic or life-threatening conditions. Even though 47 million Americans have no health insurance, the United States spends more on

healthcare than other industrialized nations where all citizens are insured (California Health Care Foundation, 2018). Despite the increasing quality of life seen in older people and others who are disabled in some way, experts agree that excessive administrative costs, inflated prices, and inappropriate care are some of the many complicated reasons healthcare costs so much in the United States (Elder Care in the United States, 2014). These are the key demographic factors behind the need to address a multigenerational complex of healthcare management, both globally and locally. Preventing illness and promoting health has often been given a lower priority financially in the United States, as described in Chapter 2. However, on an optimistic note, recent data do suggest that there is (1) a decrease in the prevalence of chronic disability, (2) an earlier diagnosis and treatment of disease, and (3) improved treatment of health problems (National Coalition on Health Care [NCHC], 2013).

Health-related quality of life and well-being is a key objective of *Healthy People 2020* (HP 2020, 2018). As such, this chapter emphasizes the need to create, develop, and continue to invest in the evolution of an infrastructure that allows diverse populations to create the best place and circumstances for them to stay well in terms of how they define relevant and sensitive "quality." The following unravels key components of the efforts being made across all three levels of prevention to allow quality of life and well-being to be defined and addressed.

CARE MANAGEMENT

Care management is a term coined to define the evaluation of healthcare interventions, including need and appropriateness of care, and the actions taken to attain effective and efficient outcomes. The Utilization Review Accreditation Commission (URAC, 2018), an independent, not-for-profit organization committed to promoting healthcare quality, identifies health utilization management as a key component in the care of patients because of continued rising medical costs. Care management and utilization management are often used as synonyms. In many cases, advances in technology, including the use of predictive modeling and other methods of data analysis, are creating opportunities for utilization management to be targeted to specific disease management areas more precisely.

 In the case of Eleanor, care management or utilization management is the process by which her physician's office designates a nurse utilization manager to review patient records along with her physician. Eleanor has Medicare coverage and has chosen to be part of a health provider system that offers inpatient and outpatient care directly or by referral. Her care is centralized by electronic record, so the utilization manager or care manager can easily track use of services within the approved system. The tracking is completed not just to keep statistical trends, but to understand the trends and costs associated with them. Once the trends and costs are understood, ways to give quality care at the best cost are offered to Eleanor. Care management and utilization management will inevitably benefit her by helping caregivers anticipate her needs, like home care, as more disability evolves from her advancing chronic comorbid conditions.

CASE MANAGEMENT

The Case Management Society of America (2018) defines **case management** as "an integrated collaborative process of assessment, planning, facilitation and *advocacy* for options and services to meet an individual's health needs through communication and available resources to promote quality cost-effective outcomes." Advocacy in case management is significant, as is the case with all levels of patient care across the lifespan, because it requires health professionals and others to bring private needs to the level of public awareness. Advocacy is always moving the needs of patients, families, and communities to a point of awareness that will advance change and increase quality of a life and experience.

According to the URAC (2018), case management was first practiced by public health service providers early in the last century. The concept has been integrated into other systems over time and has become associated with the care of low-income patients and families who are considered at risk. The chief motivation in this integration is the need for a healthcare professional who advocates for the resources needed by patients. Care management is related to case management; without case management, care management could not be successful. Thus, case management can be considered a building block of care management.

Case management involves an intensive process called disease management. Disease management is a system of coordinated healthcare interventions and communications for groups of people with conditions in which patient self-care efforts are significant. Disease management emphasizes prevention at the secondary and tertiary level using evidence-based practice guidelines. Collaborative practice models are a key to the success of disease management programs. These programs include physicians, nurses, and support-service providers, patient and family, self-management education, process, and outcomes measurement, evaluation, and management; there is a routine reporting/feedback loop (Disease Management Association of America-The Care Continuum Alliance, 2018). Disease management often focuses on the care of populations in the context of a continuum of care such as chronic illnesses like heart disease, heart failure, diabetes, pulmonary disease, urinary incontinence, and asthma.

In disease or care continuum management programs, in addition to medications, there is strong emphasis on the use of telephone coaching, internet resources, and intensive patient and family teaching to advance self-care and adherence to wellness care. Recently, to help patients and families manage their health problems in an effective and efficient manner, there has been an effort to bundle disease states together in light of many comorbidity patterns.

Eleanor's care and case management takes the form of a home care nurse, who uses a disease management approach to Eleanor's diabetes, congestive heart failure (CHF), and hypertension. This disease management approach involves these three conditions because they are all interrelated.

Other examples of management approaches may not be disease oriented at all. For example, case management programs may evolve uniquely for pregnancy or postpartum care (County Health Rankings and Roadmaps, 2018).

Evidence for Practice

According to the County Health Rankings and Roadmaps (2018), case management for pregnant or parenting teens provides a range of services that is "needs"-based. Caseworkers provide support and counseling, assist in creating plans with specific goals such as finishing high school, work to create support networks among a teen's family, friends, and partner, or connect teen parents to healthcare or social services. Case management typically takes place in schools or other community locations, and may be utilized into dropout prevention programs for teen mothers. Expected outcomes that have been evaluated based on this type of intervention management include (1) reduced teen pregnancy, (2) reduced rapid repeat pregnancies, (3) increased use of contraception, (4) improved social networks, (5) increased academic achievement, and (6) increased graduation rates. In particular, there is some evidence that intensive case management (increased frequency of interventions over a shorter period of time) reduces repeat pregnancies among black and Hispanic adolescent mothers while they participate in the intervention (Tolma, 2014). A South Carolina-based study indicated that case management programs may also strengthen support networks, improve academic outcomes, and increase graduation rates among black teen mothers in rural areas. Research suggests that programs to reduce repeat pregnancy among pregnant and parenting teens are more likely to be effective when easy access to services, contraceptive education, home visiting, and tailored messages are included and when programs are presented in individual rather than group formats (Kan et al., 2012). For case management programs that include home visits, more frequent visits appear to reduce repeat pregnancy more effectively than usual care (Kan et al., 2012); frequent visits can also increase use of long-acting reversible contraception (LARCs) (Kan et al., 2012).

To be a case or disease manager, one need not be a nurse. Although the American Nurses Credentialing Center (2018)

12.1 Case Managers' Role

A case manager's responsibilities include the following functions:
- Advocacy and education—ensuring that the client has a representative who can speak up and represent their needs for needed services and education
- Clinical care coordination/facilitation—coordinating multiple aspects of care to ensure that the client progresses
- Continuity/transition management—transitioning of the client to the appropriate level of care needed
- Utilization/financial management—managing resource utilization and reimbursement for services
- Performance and outcomes management—monitoring and, if needed, intervening to achieve desired goals and outcomes for both the client and the hospital
- Psychosocial management—assessing and addressing psychosocial needs, including individual, familial, and environmental
- Research and practice development—identifying practice improvements and using evidence-based data to influence needed practice changes

Source: Data from Kongstvedt, P. R. (2001). *The managed healthcare handbook* (4th ed.). New York: Aspen.

does certify nurses in this specialty, social workers and public health experts may also serve in this role. The role is complex, and the many responsibilities include addressing the direct and immediate needs of patients and families and achieving quality improvement in the future (Box 12.1).

Care management and case management can be used across the continuum of health from acute care to care within communities. One important area where practices of care management and case management occur is in the home. The rest of this chapter is devoted to discussing home healthcare.

HOME HEALTHCARE

People spend most of their time in their neighborhoods and communities to which they belong. When they are ill and need care, they continue to spend most of their time in those same neighborhoods and communities. Home care nurses are challenged in many ways in caring for patients in their own homes. Home care nurses continue a historical legacy of autonomy, creativity, connection, and talent in advancing nursing practice using research and professional experience as their guides. If there is one thought that comes to mind when one says, "home care," it is the place where the fainthearted need not apply. Home care is a place where nurses practice in the extremes of complexity. It takes a competent and knowledgeable professional to make home care their professional "home."

People facing an acute or chronic illness or a new health-related situation may be candidates for **home healthcare**. This service involves caring for patients and their families wherever they may call "home," regardless of economic and class divisions. Home healthcare is part of a continuum of care to which nurses contribute. It has evolved over time on the basis of three distinct needs: (1) quality healthcare in places and spaces where people live most of their lives (homes and communities), (2) continued development of ways to inform healthcare providers what realities affect health promotion and prevention in the diverse, complex lives of people and families, and (3) cost containment in the healthcare industry. The development of health insurance, rising costs in healthcare in general, and medical and nursing specialization all have played a part in the development of home healthcare as it is today.

History of Home Healthcare

In the United States, home healthcare began in the early 1800s. Key historical points are listed in Box 12.2. The last historical event in this list, the establishment of Medicare, has set a pattern for payment for home services for the next 40 years. The federal government and its fiscal intermediaries at the state level established Medicare's initial payment protocol. This protocol involved fee-for-service (i.e., a set fee for a particular service) charges. Home health agencies such as visiting nurse associations (VNAs) and other agencies established the cost for a particular service and then billed Medicare for that service. Unfortunately, this payment approach left Medicare and patients vulnerable to a blossoming industry where some home care services fraudulently inflated costs and service billing frequency to increase profit margins (National Center for Policy Analysis, 2013).

In the past 20 years, Medicare regulations have served as the basis for Medicaid programs, as well as for other health insurance protocols for payment or **reimbursement**. In this

context, payment for healthcare costs was scrutinized because of its inflationary nature. As patients aged and became more seriously ill with chronic illnesses, the system of **managed care** was introduced to encourage healthcare providers to hold costs down through the streamlining of services (Kongstvedt, 2001). Managed care efforts included the idea of prospective reimbursement. Prospective reimbursement is a system in which reimbursement rates are set for a given period of time prior to the circumstances giving rise to actual reimbursement claims (Prospective Reimbursement, 2008). In response to this payment approach, hospitals began to reduce the stays of patients and more patients went home earlier and sicker than before. In a continued effort to decrease costs in home health industry, in 1997, Congress passed the **Balanced Budget Act** (DeMarco & O'Brien, 1999). Congress cut $16 billion in payments to the home health industry over five years; that is, it slashed reimbursement rates. As a result, home health agencies closed or began to merge because they could not keep up with the costs. In 1997, there were 10,000 home care agencies. After the Balanced Budget Act of 1997, there were 7,000 such agencies (Magee, 2007). Agencies were forced to develop so-called care mixes, where the incentive based on reimbursement encouraged them not to take care of the sickest or the most costly "cases"—patients.

As the previous discussion indicates, many home care agencies depend on reimbursement trends, and trends in payment for home care are beginning to change again. In 2003, the Medicare Modernization and Improvement Act included a provision to eliminate what would have been an inflation increase in home health rates (Centers for Medicare & Medicaid Services [CMS], 2018). Medicare is exploring reimbursement based on performance (i.e., successful outcomes) (Rosenthal & Frank, 2006). However, home care agencies continue to be needed for the aging population of the United States because most people continue to want to be cared for in their own homes, whether they are facing acute or chronic illness or death. The saying "there is no place like home" is truly a reality.

Types of Agencies

Because of the variety of reimbursement mechanisms that have evolved over time in home healthcare, many different forms of services have evolved based on levels of philanthropy; profit-making needs; and federal, state, and city funding. There are four distinct types of home healthcare agencies: private/voluntary (not-for-profit), hospital-based, proprietary (for-profit), and public (Medline Plus, 2013).

Private/Voluntary Agencies

Voluntary agencies are generally established as not-for-profit entities, although they operate with the same fiscal objectives as "for-profit agencies." The difference is that they are often governed by a voluntary board of directors and community-based advisory boards that are interested in fiscally sound, high-quality care for patients they decide will

---

12.2	**History of Home Healthcare**

- 1800s—Large wave of immigration to the United States with poverty and poor health facing families and professional caregivers
- 1859—William Rathbone, a wealthy Quaker philanthropist business man, with the help of Florence Nightingale, sent trained nurses into the homes of the sick poor in Liverpool, England
- 1885—First Visiting Nurse Associations established in Buffalo (NY), Boston (MA), and Philadelphia (PA)
- 1893—Henry Street Settlement established by nurse Lillian Wald in New York City
- 1894—VNAs are established and grow rapidly
- 1909—Metropolitan Life Insurance Company offers homecare services as a benefit
- 1910—Columbia University offers the first university course in public health nursing
- 1929—Crash of the stock market occurs, and federal government allocates funds to help those in need of home care
- 1940s—Hospitals interested in home care because of chronic illness rates
- 1966—Medicare established

Source: Data from Buler-Wilkerson, K. (2001). *No place like home.* Baltimore, MD: The Johns Hopkins University Press.

be their service population. Any profit margin that is acquired is reinvested in the operations of the home health-care service. The advisory and legislative members of the boards direct the chief executive and fiscal officers in how home healthcare should be offered to the service population. A good example is a VNA.

Hospital-Based Agencies

Hospital-based agencies have developed within the past 25 years to save money and maintain control of patient care costs. In addition, a key objective is to maintain levels of quality and increase collaboration by establishing home healthcare services as part of a continuum of care offered by the hospital. As a healthcare system, hospitals embraced an approach to care that included prevention and health promotion through divisions that offer primary care, emergency care, acute care, and chronic care in various onsite or offsite facilities. The home is one such site. The principal idea was to establish plans of care that were congruent with a hospital system philosophy. Hospital-based home healthcare agencies are governed by not only the same board that governs the hospital but also an advisory board similar to that of a VNA; this helps match their care initiatives to the realities of the population they serve. Depending on the hospital, hospital-based agencies can be "for-profit" or "not-for-profit."

An example of a home healthcare agency associated with a hospital is the Home Health Care Department of Boston General Hospital. All Boston General Hospital patients who need skilled nursing care at home are referred to the home healthcare department of the hospital and followed over time. People that have been readmitted and others may also be referred to this group.

> Eleanor receives all of her home care services, including skilled nursing, physical therapy, and occupational therapy, through a hospital-based hospice program that is part of a hospital system made up of five hospitals. The hospitals are owned by the Catholic diocese of the city in which Eleanor lives.

Proprietary Agencies

Proprietary agencies are private agencies that plan to and want to make a profit. They can be part of a local, national, or international chain of home healthcare agencies directed toward any group of patients with particular healthcare problems or challenges. For example, an agency that has as its goal the provision of home health aides and homemaking services to people in need of personal care and housekeeping services will provide for profit trained home health aides and homemakers to assist people and families with these needs. Their services are often paid for privately by families, and any profit margin is used to benefit the owner of the agency or chain of agencies.

Official Agencies

Official agencies are supported by public monies that often come from taxes. The public monies can come from local, state, or federal governments. Essentially, citizens and legislators identify a need for home health services that are often part of a larger public health approach to certain populations. For example, a county health department may be established with several goals and objectives to promote the health of people in the area for which they are responsible. This may include lead paint screening for children, tuberculosis treatment and follow-up, well-child clinics, water-testing facilities, and a public home care agency. Generally, there is a mandate to serve all people without exception. Thus, public home health programs often care for many patients that may not be admitted to private, voluntary, or proprietary home health programs. However, with the constant rise in public health problems such as obesity, diabetes, human immunodeficiency virus/acquired immunodeficiency syndrome (HIV/AIDS), low–birth-weight births, and infant mortality, many public home health agencies are supported financially for the care they give to citizens who may have little access to any other care.

Financing and Regulation of Home Care

Home healthcare services are reimbursed by local, state, and federal funds; private insurance; and private individuals. Government funding for home healthcare includes Medicare (federal) and Medicaid (state) (CMS, 2018) as well as monies from TRICARE (federal funds for military personnel and their dependents) and the Veterans Administration (federal funds for those who are currently serving or have served in the armed services of the United States [TRICARE, 2014]). Insurance companies that pay for home healthcare can be independent (e.g., State Farm Insurance) or can be part of a health maintenance organization (HMO) or a case management organization. Medicare, Medicaid, TRICARE, and Veterans Administration coverage is generated from monies that citizens contribute to the state or federal government through taxes. Insurance companies, HMOs, and case management organizations give coverage based on monies that are paid directly to them in monthly or annual increments for the purpose of giving home healthcare when and if they are needed. What is common in the latter type of insurance is these organizations coordinate with home healthcare agencies from which the patients are able to obtain care.

Home healthcare is regulated by the state and federal government. Insurance companies generally align themselves with the regulations stipulated by these governments but may have their own rules and regulations. Home health agencies are certified through a process in which stipulated conditions must be present for the agency to give services to the public and receive payment for those services. For example, Medicare has the following criteria for eligibility: homebound, a plan of care, skilled needs, intermittent care needs, and necessity.

Homebound refers to a condition based upon how difficult it is for a patient to leave the home. To leave home must require a taxing effort and must be related to maintaining health and personal care. This may include attending a medical day care program where the patient would receive medications and therapy while family members may be at work. It may also include only leaving home when going to an appointment with a healthcare provider. There may be variations in why a patient must leave home (church, a family birthday event, to buy a pair of shoes), but the key stipulation is the taxing effort required to do this and the infrequency of the event. Determining a patient's homebound status is primarily a way reimbursement systems qualify the severity level of an illness for which they will pay for services.

Eleanor manages to move from a chair in the kitchen to a chair in the living room and to the bathroom with a walker. She requires great effort in ambulating with a walker. In the past, if she had to leave the house, she used to need two people to descend eight steps. Eventually, her family installed an exterior elevator lift to help her access a car to go to physician appointments or family gatherings. By definition, she is homebound because of the taxing effort required to leave her home.

A **plan of care** is an agency-generated written document that is guided by a lengthy assessment. The assessment that is currently used across the United States is called the Outcome and Assessment Information Set (OASIS, 2018). This assessment tool represents items that help home care professionals assess adult home care patients. The items in OASIS assessment include sociodemographic, environmental, health, functional health, personal support data, and the status of adult patients who are in a pre- or postnatal state. The OASIS data are reported to the state where the home health agency exists to create a larger database that can be used for state comparisons across the United States. The accuracy needed to complete this assessment is critical because each assessment item becomes the standard from which **patient outcomes** are measured. In addition, the OASIS data are used by Medicare to help determine how home healthcare agencies are paid for their services (CMS, 2014).

Evidence for Practice

O'Connor and Davitt (2012) recognized that the OASIS is the patient-specific, standardized assessment used in Medicare home healthcare to plan care, determine reimbursement, and measure quality in home care settings. The authors studied the debate over the reliability and validity of the OASIS as a research tool and outcome measure. They undertook a systematic literature review of English-language articles and identified 12 studies published in the last 10 years examining the validity and reliability of the OASIS. Empirical findings indicated the validity and reliability of the OASIS range from low to moderate but vary depending on the item studied. Limitations in the existing research include nonrepresentative samples; inconsistencies in methods used, items tested, measurement, and statistical procedures; and the changes to the OASIS itself over time. The inconsistencies suggest that additional research is needed to confirm the value of the OASIS for measuring patient outcomes, research, and quality improvement.

The home health nurse completes the assessment and establishes the functional needs of the patient and the services required. What is important to understand is that, like many areas of healthcare, home healthcare is progressing toward a system of reimbursement that will be based not just on prospective reimbursement (diagnosis and presumed trajectory of care) but on outcomes of care. Therefore, a plan of care based on an accurate assessment with identified activities leading to outcomes will be critical to sustaining all types of home healthcare agencies in the future.

Another very well-known system that assists healthcare providers in organizing clinical data in the context of assessment is called the Omaha System (Omaha System, 2013). This model of organizing data includes three relational components: a problem classification scheme (patient assessment), an intervention scheme (care plans and services), and a problem rating scale of outcomes (patient change/evaluation). The work on creating this model began in the 1970s by the Visiting Nurse Association of Omaha, Nebraska, while adopting a problem-oriented approach as a guide to practice and documentation and management (Omaha System, 2013). The idea was conceived and developed so that an information system could be used that was standardized (written or now computerized) based on an integrated, valid, reliable clinical approach which was organized for patients who received services, and their specific needs. Over 10 years of nationally funded research yielded consensus on standardized language used in patient assessment, care plans, and outcomes. This system currently meets Medicare/Medicaid, Joint Commission, and Children's Health Care Assistance Plan (CHAP) guidelines and regulations. It has been recognized by the American Nurses Association (ANA) since 1992 and passed the Healthcare Information Technology Standards Panel (HITSP) Tier 2 selection criteria for Use Cases in 2007. It is integrated into the National Library of Medicine's Metathesaurus; CINAHL; ABC Codes; NIDSEC; Logical Observation Identifiers, Names, and Codes (LOINC); and SNOMED CT. It is registered (recognized) by Health Level Seven (HL7), and is congruent with the reference terminology model for the International Organization for Standardization (ISO). It is being mapped to the International Classification of Nursing

Practice (ICNP) (Omaha System, 2013). Current users are mostly in the United States and include home care, public health, and school health practice settings, nurse-managed center staff, hospital-based and managed care case managers, educators and students, occupational health nurses, faith community staff, acute care and rehabilitation hospital/ long-term care staff, researchers, members of various disciplines, and computer software vendors (Omaha System, 2013). In each instance, the focus of care is **skilled needs** provided by these professionals and directed to patients, families, and communities. See Box 12.3 for domains, intervention schemes, and outcome rating scales of the Omaha System.

12.3 | Omaha System (Domains, Intervention Schemes, and Outcome Rating Scale) (Omaha System, 2013)

Domains and Problems of the Problem Classification Scheme

Environmental domain: Material resources and physical surroundings both inside and outside the living area, neighborhood, and broader community
Income
Sanitation
Residence
Neighborhood/workplace safety

Psychosocial domain: Patterns of behavior, emotion, communication, relationships, and development
Communication with community resources
Social contact
Role change
Interpersonal relationship
Spirituality
Grief
Mental health
Sexuality
Caretaking/parenting
Neglect
Abuse
Growth and development

Physiological domain: Functions and processes that maintain life
Hearing
Vision
Speech and language
Oral health
Cognition
Pain
Consciousness
Skin
Neuromusculoskeletal function
Respiration
Circulation
Digestion–hydration
Bowel function
Urinary function
Reproductive function
Pregnancy
Postpartum
Communicable/infectious condition

Health-related behaviors domain: Patterns of activity that maintain or promote wellness, promote recovery, and decrease the risk of disease
Nutrition
Sleep and rest patterns

Physical activity
Personal care
Substance use
Family planning
Healthcare supervision
Medication regimen

Intervention Categories

Teaching, guidance, and counseling: Activities designed to provide information and materials, encourage action and responsibility for self-care and coping, and assist the individual/family/ community to make decisions and solve problems

Treatments and procedures: Technical activities such as wound care, specimen collection, resistive exercises, and medication prescriptions that are designed to prevent, decrease, or alleviate signs and symptoms of the individual/family/community

Case management: Activities such as coordination, advocacy, and referral that facilitate service delivery, improve communication among health and human service providers, promote assertiveness, and guide the individual/family/community toward use of appropriate resources

Surveillance: Activities such as detection, measurement, critical analysis, and monitoring intended to identify the individual/ family/community's status in relation to a given condition or phenomenon

Targets

Anatomy/physiology
Anger management
Behavior modification
Bladder care
Bonding/attachment
Bowel care
Cardiac care
Caretaking/parenting skills
Cast care
Communication
Community outreach worker services
Continuity of care
Coping skills
Day care/respite
Dietary management
Discipline
Dressing change/wound care
Durable medical equipment use
Education
Employment
End-of-life care
Environment

Exercises
Family planning care
Feeding procedures
Finances
Gait training
Genetics
Growth/development care
Home
Homemaking/housekeeping
Infection precautions
Interaction
Interpreter/translator services
Laboratory findings
Legal system
Medical/dental care
Medication action/side effects
Medication administration
Medication coordination/ordering
Medication prescription
Medication setup
Mobility/transfers
Nursing care
Nutritionist care
Occupational therapy care
Ostomy care
Other community resources
Paraprofessional/aide care

Personal hygiene
Physical therapy care
Positioning
Recreational therapy care
Relaxation/breathing techniques
Respiratory care
Respiratory therapy care
Rest/sleep
Safety
Screening procedures
Sickness/injury care
Signs/symptoms—mental/emotional
Signs/symptoms—physical
Skin care
Social work/counseling care
Specimen collection
Speech and language pathology care
Spiritual care
Stimulation/nurturance
Stress management
Substance use cessation
Supplies
Support group
Support system
Transportation
Wellness
Other

Concepts and Ratings of the Problem Rating Scale for Outcomes

Concept	1	2	3	4	5
Knowledge: Ability of the client to remember and interpret information	No knowledge	Minimal knowledge	Basic knowledge	Adequate knowledge	Superior knowledge
Behavior: Observable responses, actions, or activities of the client fitting the occasion or purpose	Not appropriate behavior	Rarely appropriate behavior	Inconsistently appropriate behavior	Usually appropriate behavior	Consistently appropriate behavior
Status: Condition of the client in relation to objective and subjective defining characteristics	Extreme signs/ symptoms	Severe signs/ symptoms	Moderate signs/ symptoms	Minimal signs/ symptoms	No signs/ symptoms

Skilled needs refer to the needs of the patient that are accomplished through the professional abilities of registered nurses or their supervised designees (e.g., home health aides). This includes skilled observation, assessment, teaching, management, and evaluation of a variety of conditions and situations. Examples of skilled nursing needs versus nonskilled nursing needs are presented in Table 12.1.

stabilized. For example, one admission occurred after a hospitalization for CHF. When her weight, breathing patterns, medication adherence, and blood pressure stabilized, she was discharged to the care of her daughters, and the local elder services provided her with home health aides to help with meals, bathing, and housekeeping needs.

Intermittent care refers to a situation in which skilled care is usually provided over several hours during the day several days during the week for a specified time period. Medicare requires the specified time period to be 60 days with appropriate renewals if skilled needs continue to exist.

 Eleanor has had several admissions for home care. Each admission stopped after a 60-day period (required by Medicare guidelines), when her **skilled care** condition

TABLE 12.1 Comparison of Skilled and Nonskilled Nursing Care

Skilled	Nonskilled
Assessment of lungs and weight of a client diagnosed with congestive heart failure	Changing a dry dressing
Teaching a newly diagnosed diabetic client how to fill insulin syringes or use an insulin pen	Teaching the client's significant other/spouse how to pay healthcare bills
Management of care given to a client postcerebrovascular accident by speech therapy, physical therapy, and home health aide services	Managing care of a home health aide after all healthcare skilled needs have been stabilized
Changing a complicated wet-to-dry dressing on a client's abdomen	Pouring medications in plastic labeled container
Monitoring the fluctuating blood pressure of an elderly man who has just started taking antihypertensive medication	Visiting the client to decrease loneliness

Medical necessity means that the service given by a home care agency is reasonable based on the status of the patient. For example, it would be unreasonable to schedule daily visits to the home of patients who have learned to use a glucometer to test their blood glucose levels effectively. It would be reasonable to visit twice a week for two weeks to see if the patient is conducting the blood glucose test correctly and accurately.

Role and Scope of Home Health Practice

The ANA has provided nurses in home health practice with an official document called the *Scope and Standards of Home Health Nursing Practice* (American Nurses Association, 2014). It provides guidelines for nurses involved in home healthcare practice, including standards of care and standards of professional practice. The standards of care include the key elements of the nursing process:

1. Assessment by collecting data about home care patients
2. Diagnosis through the analysis of data
3. Outcome identification that helps home care nurses identify nurse-sensitive measures
4. Planning in the form of nurse-sensitive interventions directed to the identified outcomes
5. Implementation-identified, nurse-centered actions in collaboration with patients and families
6. Evaluation outcome accomplishment through nurse-sensitive interventions

Although this may sound familiar in view of the standards of care in many areas of the continuum of nursing practice, Medicare, Medicaid, and private insurance agencies are moving in the direction of using these standards of practice as reimbursement strategies for agencies based on successful outcome management. Thus, fiscal rewards in the future may be related to identifying nurse-sensitive outcomes as described in this process.

Standards of professional performance described in the ANA document are areas that home care nurses must address in the context of their practice. They include the following:

- Evaluating quality of care
- Evaluating their performance in the agency or home care work in which they are involved, maintaining current competency
- Helping develop nursing students and other colleagues who aspire to become home care nurses, as well as collaborating with others in the care of home care patients
- Being ethical in their practice, as well as using evidence-based practice in their encounters with patients and families

One of the most powerful professional performance standards, unique to home care because of patient and family engagement in patients' own world (their home), is the emphasis on helping patients and families be consumers of healthcare. This may take the form of helping patients and families receive information about their health conditions, health promotion, and disease prevention, as well as the risks and benefits of receiving healthcare in the home.

Student Reflection

I absolutely loved my clinical rotation in home care. One of my patients was an older man. I really liked traveling to his home and meeting him in his own living space. I could really teach and apply principles of medical-surgical care by adapting them to his world. For example, I needed to figure out where the cleanest and most optimal place for him to sit and bend over to change a small dressing on his leg would be, and I managed to do this successfully by observing the cleanest and safest place during the home visit. We together decided that the first floor bathroom would work because he could sit on the elevated toilet, reach the sink to wash his hands, and bend effectively without becoming hypotensive.

I have to admit that despite having a cell phone and easy access for help and advice, when I was allowed to visit my patient without my instructor for the first time, I was nervous. There is a lot of autonomy in this role, and many people say that before you take a job in home care, you should have two years of hospital experience. If I really wanted to concentrate in home care, I would need to figure out how to be mentored as a new graduate so my confidence would be supported by a system that would help me learn to think critically while being a solitary practitioner of nursing care in the community.

Interprofessional Care

Home care, like many areas of healthcare, is made up of workgroups where **interprofessional collaboration** occurs. Various members of the healthcare team, not just nurses, contribute their expertise to patient management in the home. Generally, the following groups receive care from home health agencies: adults with acute or chronic illnesses, older adults, mothers and newborns, and children and their parents. Nurses are often the clinical leaders who manage the necessary care. Often, this care is highly specialized and requires the expertise of other members of the healthcare team. Often, physical therapists, occupational therapists, speech therapists, recreational therapists, social workers, nutritionists, and home health aides assist the nurse in meeting patient-centered outcomes. Home health aide assistants and home care nurses follow through with delegated tasks that are legally appropriate in terms of the standards of practice designated by the ANA and the local board of registration of nursing. Other members of the home health team are members of different disciplines—professionals who have a special and unique knowledge about an area of clinical science, such as physicians or nurse practitioners in specific fields. It is not uncommon for clinicians on these teams to work together on particular outcomes that benefit the patient and family as a whole (Lehning & Austin, 2011).

The challenge of interprofessional work and teams is to be able to work together in a complementary way to help patients and families on the basis of their assessed needs. This is not always easy because many members of various healthcare disciplines see only the unique contribution they make as an isolated involvement with patients and families (Chatfield, Christos, & McGregor, 2012). In reality, all healthcare professionals, regardless of discipline, must work together and find common outcomes so that patients and families can achieve wellness. For example, a woman diagnosed with a cerebrovascular accident may be a patient of a home health agency. In this case, she may have speech difficulties and restricted use of her upper and lower extremities. Together with coping with the loss of control, she also needs to make healthier food choices directly related to the pre-existing condition that is thought to have caused the "stroke" (hypertension). The nurse who makes the home visit would immediately consult with a speech and language expert, physical therapist, occupational therapist, and a nutritionist in conjunction with a physician as a team. The home care nurse, acting as a clinical leader, would talk together formally at case conferences, or informally with a group of experts, about the need to change or to maintain the plan of care to meet identified outcomes.

An example and extension of interprofessional collaboration with shared outcomes that includes the use of home care services is the "**medical home**" model. This model of care delivery has five components: (1) comprehensive care, (2) patient-centered care, (3) coordination of care, (4) accessible services, and (5) quality and safety. According to Agency for Healthcare Research and Quality (AHRQ) of the U.S. Department of Health and Human Services (AHRQ, 2018 https://pcmh.ahrq.gov/page/defining-pcmh), comprehensive care refers to the accountability of meeting each patient's physical and mental health needs including prevention and wellness, acute care, and chronic care. An interprofessional team of providers that includes physicians, advanced practice nurses, physician assistants, home care nurses, pharmacists, nutritionists, social workers, educators, and care coordinators work together to build teams to link themselves and patients to providers and services in communities. Patient-centered care means that the care is relationship-based. Partnership with patients and families to learn to manage their care with consideration of their values and culture is central to the care given. Coordinated care is an effort to organize care across services that can include home care, hospitals, and other community services. The key skill for successful coordination is clear and open communication. Accessible services refers to every effort to be responsive in terms of timing (shorter waiting periods to see a care provider on the team), availability (24/7), and responsive to the particular preference patients and families request. Quality and safety is a comprehensive commitment to the use of evidence-based clinical care and decision-making with attention to outcomes and the practice of population health management.

Population health management as defined as a component of a medical home is a system within any model of delivery of care that creates a way to manage care comprehensively. Population health management is focused on the analysis of data from patients that are organized in a record where providers and researchers can make efforts to understand and improve health and financial outcomes. Telehealth is an operational component of a population health management approach that gathers data to contribute to the larger system or aggregate of data to help nurses and other health professionals understand effectiveness and efficiencies of care for the better. The following discusses at length telehealth and how it is used to advance quality and safety.

Telehealth

Telehealth is a form of electronic communication used to deliver (1) acute care and specialty consultations, (2) home telenursing, and (3) electronic referrals to specialists in expert health facilities. According to Sewell (2016), telehealth as a form of informatics involves the use of electronic or digital communications for transmitting healthcare information such as health promotion, disease prevention, professional or lay education, diagnosis, or actual treatment to people located at a different geographical areas. Telehealth relates to two kinds of approaches that are applicable in home care. The first involves electronically stored information that can be shared with others using technology, and the second involves a real interaction between a patient and a healthcare provider. The latter telehealth approach is called real-time technology (Sewell, 2016), which can include the use of diagnostic instruments that can transmit images or sounds to professionals in other areas. For example, an otoscope can be used in a patient's home to send images electronically to an otolaryngology expert for evaluation. In another instance, monitoring devices can be installed in homes to record the blood pressure, pulse, and weight of a patient who has been diagnosed with CHF. Telecommunication and informatics sent to home health agencies allows interprofessional teams to enhance their responsiveness related to subtle changes in patient's conditions (Omboni, Gazzola, Carabelli, & Parati, 2013). The goal is for the patients to be stable and well at home and for the home health system to have electronically stored and shared information that be useful to others in the larger scope of healthcare practice have information at their fingertips to help individuals, families, and communities.

Evidence for Practice

Antonicelli, Mazzanti, Abbatecola, and Parati (2010) undertook a research study addressing the needs of the elderly diagnosed with CHF. Despite evidence showing that administration of β-blockers (β-adrenoceptor antagonists) can improve the clinical status of CHF patients, use of these agents in adequate dosages is not routine at home because of the possible risk of bradyarrhythmia. Telecardiology has recently been investigated as a means of constantly monitoring the heart rate of CHF patients in their homes, and may be a solution to increase use of β-blockers (β-adrenoceptor antagonists) while decreasing the risk of bradyarrhythmia. Antonicelli and colleagues assessed the impact of telemonitoring on patients' adherence to prescribed therapeutic regimens, particularly β-blockers, and whether use of home telemonitoring reduced mortality and rate of readmission to hospital in elderly CHF patients compared with normal specialized CHF team care. A total of 57 patients with CHF (31 New York Heart Association [NYHA] class II, 23 NYHA class III, and 3 NYHA class IV), with a mean ± SD age of 78.2 ± 7.3 years, were randomized to a control group who received standard care, or to a home telemonitoring

(TM) group. Patients were followed up over 12 months. Compared with the control group, the TM group had a significant increase in the use of β-blockers, HMG-CoA reductase inhibitors (statins) and aldosterone-receptor antagonists. A reduction in nitrate administration compared with baseline was also seen in the TM group. The 12-month occurrence of the primary combined endpoint of mortality and hospital readmission for CHF was significantly lower in the TM group than in the control group ($p < 0.01$). This study showed that a home care model, including telemonitoring of relevant clinical parameters, may provide useful support in the management of patients with CHF.

Telehealth can also be used in other ways. Information that is stored electronically and shared with others using electronic devices is another way home care providers can keep records of patient and family progress, but it can also be a way to share patient education information (Sewell, 2016). For example, slide presentations can be transferred to help patients and families learn about an intervention that may help with their care or help them learn more about a chronic illness and the usual care practices offered to help their situation. Other examples are programs that allow downloadable information with dynamic pictures and multimedia effects to help patients understand their illness, or transition to a new role (new mothers), or adjust to changes in mobility (Sewell, 2016).

Home Care Models
Assisted Living

Long-term supportive services have evolved and currently include assisted living and continuing care communities, as well as nursing homes.

Assisted living is a type of community-based long-term care that combines quasi-independent living with the availability of nursing care onsite and through home care visits (CDC Long Term Care Services, 2018). It generally is a level of care for people who cannot live on their own, but are not yet ready for a nursing home. This type of living arrangement is different from living independently in one's own apartment, such as living in a senior living facility, in that many activities are provided communally (e.g., eating, recreation). There is an organized effort to create a "caring community" where residents are supervised and help is available for day-to-day living tasks. Many older community dwellers find assisted living or continuing care communities to be places where gradual changes in physical, cognitive, and emotional abilities can be addressed with centralized services. In many cases, this choice is made on the basis of financial ability to support such an option. Many people may want to stay in their own homes as a way to protect long-term investments financially and emotionally.

Eleanor does not want to leave her home. She is willing to "spend down" her $20,000 in the bank to become eligible for Medicaid so that she can receive more services in her home and not have to move to an assisted living or retirement community. But this decision to live alone, despite having family nearby, puts her in jeopardy for falls and other possible emergencies. The decision is an autonomous one because she has no cognitive deficits. Once she was "admitted" to home care for a skilled need, a social worker came to visit her and tried to convince her to think about a safer way to live, but she adamantly refused.

in conjunction with environmental determinants have a different impact on people at different ages. These researchers refer to retirement or assisted living communities as naturally occurring retirement communities (NORCs). Health benefits to living within NORCs have been observed and likely vary depending on where the specific NORC exists on the healthy NORC spectrum. Some NORC environments are healthier than others for seniors. Health benefits within healthy NORCs are higher where physical and social environments facilitate greater activity and promote feelings of well-being. Compared with the provision of additional medical or social services, healthy NORCs are a low-cost, community-level approach to facilitating healthy aging. Municipal governments should pursue policies that stimulate and support the development of healthy NORCs.

Home health nurses see many patients in assisted living communities. The care they give is congruent with the standards of care described previously, but often the other members of the assisted living community become the patient's "family"—and rightfully so. Retirement community dwellers consistently live an ethic of caring for each other and are involved with each other's care. Interdisciplinary teams from home care agencies have developed, with great success, extensive resources to support community elders in assisted living units (Flatt, Agimi, & Albert, 2012). There is a growing belief that not only do patients (particularly elders experience chronic care issues), families, and communities benefit from the contributions of the many healthcare professionals (physicians, nurses, midwives, dietitians, pharmacists, podiatrists, mental health and addiction professionals, physiotherapists occupational therapists, and chiropractors among others), but these professions themselves benefit in the context of case and care management. Interdisciplinary collaboration improves patient care and outcomes, access to care, recruitment and retention of health providers, and improved satisfaction among patients and health providers. Family health teams are evolving in effectively providing comprehensive primary healthcare as well as long-term care for elders for improved health-related quality of life (Zubritsky et al., 2012). The opportunity to be part of an interdisciplinary team can expand the scope of services by allowing teams to evolve with unique cultures and skill sets.

The patient-centered medical home (PCMH) is an evolving model that improves access to care by increasing coordination between patients, families, and their interdisciplinary team. Emerging data show that an integrated approach from a professional team to care of the whole person improves management of chronic illnesses wherever the patient lives (National Committee for Quality Assurance, 2018).

Home Visits to the Homeless

The thought of making a home visit to a person who may not have a home seems counterintuitive, but home care nurses do visit many homeless people (Pijl-Zieber & Kalischuk, 2011). There are unique challenges related to timing, location, and clean conditions in making a visit and providing care to someone who is homeless, but it is possible and quite rewarding. Many facilities provide shelter to homeless patients, including shelters devoted to post-hospitalization care, until the patients are strong enough to return to their usual way of surviving in the community. These shelters may be where the home visit occurs. "Home" care for stasis ulcer care or follow-up related to tuberculosis or HIV is not unusual. There are also groups of interprofessional caregivers who make visits to patients throughout the streets of the community, especially at times when many homeless people are at great risk for injury and may need care. This includes during very cold or hot weather, natural disasters, and during unstable conditions related to violence in communities. The comorbidities that are often present pose challenges (National Health Care for the Homeless Council, 2012). Many homeless people have two or more medical and/or surgical conditions, along with mental health problems or addiction histories, including smoking (Okuyemi et al., 2013). For example, people may have mental health problems as well as alcoholism and other addictions. Special skills are required to understand how to assist these people while trying to obtain affordable and safe housing for them.

Other underserved adults and older adults, including uninsured, underinsured, and racially and ethnically diverse populations, are being treated in hospitals, or are receiving extended care in long-term care facilities because they face serious, chronic illness that require palliative care. Many clinical management issues are pertinent to caring for seriously ill patients and their families, including the need to integrate *Healthy People 2020* objectives, such as those that specifically address the epidemic of HIV, cancer, kidney disease, diabetes, chronic and disabling health conditions, respiratory illness, heart disease and stroke, dementia, drug safety,

Evidence for Practice

Ivery and Akstein-Kahan (2010) used a collaborative health model to hypothesize that health management mental health, nutrition, and preventive services. Home care nurses who specialize in the area of palliative care may visit these areas specifically because they offer the patient and staff expertise in comfort care as a patient's condition deteriorates. Hospice home care is one example of a "home visit" made to facilities that care for the serious and chronically ill who are choosing to stop all curative interventions. Hospice home care is discussed in more detail in Chapter 23.

Parish/Faith Community Nursing

According to Carson and Koenig (2011), **parish nursing** is an approach to holistic care for patients and families in the community. The seminal work of Westberg (1999) identified seven key roles of the parish or faith community nurse: (1) health educator, (2) personal health counselor, (3) referral agent, (4) coordinator of volunteers, (5) developer of supportive groups, (6) integrator of faith and health, and (7) health advocate. Faith community nursing can be delivered in several ways in communities. One aspect of faith community nursing is that of home visiting. The home visits are focused on care given in the context of the seven roles identified by Westberg (1999) and are often negotiated with a faith leader in a community parish, congregation, or synagogue. In many cases, these roles are not reimbursed by insurance, but serve as ways to coordinate care to families as needed.

> Tis not enough to help the feeble up, but to support them after. **William Shakespeare**

The Home Visit

There are five phases to a home visit: (1) initiating the visit, (2) preparation, (3) the actual visit, (4) termination of the visit, and (5) post-visit planning. In the context of each of these phases, attention must be paid to safety for the nurse as well as for the patient.

Initiating the Visit

Community health nurses initiate home visits for a variety of reasons. Many home care agencies receive referrals from physicians or their designees (discharge planners from other healthcare institutions). Referrals can be sent to home health agencies at any time (24/7). Generally, home care agencies make sure that an initial visit is made within 24 hours after receiving a referral. The patient's situation must satisfy the reimbursement criteria mentioned earlier if Medicare funding is to be used. Often, these conditions are validated during the first home visit, and plans or alternatives are discussed if these are not met. When receiving a referral, it is particularly important to make sure that the orders and directions for care are clear and accurate. If necessary, a clarifying phone call should be made prior to the visit to the person who has referred the patient to the agency.

Preparation

Documentation is critical. All appropriate paperwork required for the assessment of the patient and family must

be available in electronic format if the nurse plans to use a laptop computer for charting, or as hard copy.

EQUIPMENT

The home care nurse must bring supplies and equipment that may be needed for the visit, depending on the patient's diagnosis and specific skilled need. Examples include sterile or clean dressings, urinary catheters, a walker, sterile saline solution, and distilled water, as well as antimicrobial agents and paper towels that can be used for handwashing. A home care nurse does not use patient sink areas to wash his or her hands in order to decrease the chance of cross-contamination. Many nurses use alcohol-based cleansers as a reasonable and aseptic way to cleanse their hands in home situations. In addition, the nurse must keep equipment that is often used and may be needed unexpectedly (e.g., dressings, sterile solutions if weather permitting, catheters) in his or her vehicle. These articles should be secured in the trunk or hatch of the car so that they are not visible; this decreases the potential for theft and damage to the vehicle used for the home visit.

DIRECTIONS AND VISIT VERIFICATION SYSTEMS

Getting directions for the home visit is very important. Portable or vehicle-installed global positioning systems (GPSs) are available, which work via a satellite, or generic maps or hard copy maps in areas where there is little or poor connectivity can help home care nurses locate patients. However, becoming familiar with the directions of routes (north, south, east, west), using landmarks, and making sure that unusual locations are explained before one leaves for a visit are important. More sophisticated systems are evolving currently in the form of apps. These include electronic visit verification tracking the type of service once it occurs. The term "Electronic Visit Verification" with respect to personal care services or home healthcare services is a system under which visits conducted as part of such services are electronically verified with respect to type of service, patient receiving the service, as well as date, time, delivery and provider giving the service (my Geo Tracking, 2018). Geofences also known as geozones can predefine areas on a map and assist with finding patients' homes in communities and verifying a visit that has been made to decrease fraudulence (my Geo Tracking, 2018).

PERSONAL SAFETY

Safety prevention for home care nurses is part of preparing for a home visit. Many issues need to be considered. Some key advice is given in Box 12.4. Home care nurses must think about questions such as, "When and where will I go to the bathroom? When and where will I eat? What will I do if I get lost? What will I do if I am involved in an automobile accident?" Generally, home care nurses locate public restrooms in the community where they can stop for a bathroom break safely. Stopping in the community for eating breaks is also a decision that requires familiarity and safety as part of a process during the average work day, although many nurses bring their own break food from home. In both cases, this not only allows the nurse privacy but also does not expose them to conditions where they could contaminate patients and their families and vice versa. Carrying a functioning cell phone and having a list of emergency numbers to call is critical. A cell phone can also help if directions are lost or if an accident occurs.

The In-Home Visit

The actual home visit includes introducing home care services to the patient and family, as well as the process of obtaining help from the home care agency when a planned home visit is not occurring. Details are given orally and in writing about when, whom, and how to call in an emergency or nonemergency. It also includes the application of the standards of care for home care practice, which includes the use of the nursing process with defined initial outcomes. The key component of the first in-home visit is assessment. The home care nurse is a guest in the patient's home, and must obtain the patient's permission and ask for the patient's guidance about how to carry out the initial assessment in the context of the home. It is necessary to carry out an overall assessment of the patient's and family's strengths, weaknesses, and challenges. In addition, it is also essential to assess home safety risks—medication errors, falls, and abuse and neglect.

ASSESSING FOR RISK OF MEDICATION ERRORS

The risk of errors associated with medications is inherently high. Medications may be taken incorrectly (wrong medication, wrong route, wrong dose) and may have adverse effects or interactions. These negative side effects include hypotension/bradycardia/syncope, dizziness, ataxia, adverse bleeding, confusion/sedation, and urinary urgency (Romagnoli, Handler, Ligons, & Hochheiser, 2013). Taking the wrong medication/wrong dose/wrong route can occur because of errors in prescribing, errors in transcribing during the referral phase of the home care visit process, and

errors in hearing the medication order; patient and family confusion; pharmacy errors; and cultural beliefs. Although all of the various kinds of medication errors can occur in hospitals as well as homes, there are some unique circumstances that make home care medication safety particularly challenging. Sometimes, in the freedom of their own home, patients refuse to take medications, forget to take medications, do not fill prescriptions because of cost, lack of knowledge about how to renew a prescription, or lack of access to a pharmacy. Sometimes, medication errors occur because of multiple physician involvement in care, transitions from hospital to home, patient or family error, or the use of over-the-counter (OTC) drugs in addition to prescribed medication that may cause adverse reactions.

On average, community-dwelling elders use 4.5 prescription medications at any giving time in addition to OTC drugs. Corbett, Setter, Daratha, Neumiller, and Wood (2010) found a mean of 10.4 medications prescribed to patients at time of hospital discharge, supporting the frequency with which polypharmacy is occurring at time of hospital discharge (Box 12.5). Adverse reactions included death, falls/confusion/sedation, adverse bleeding, inappropriate/ineffective treatment, disease exacerbation, emergency department visits and/or rehospitalizations, and ineffective pain control (Romagnoli et al., 2013). At the initial home visit, it is important for the home care nurse to develop a medication profile that is accurate and will be reviewed at each visit. It is critical to talk about the use of prescribed medications with OTCs and herbal supplements, and develop a plan that includes the patient and family being vigilant about medication safety (Box 12.6).

ASSESSING FOR RISK OF FALLS

Falls are a major health problem in home care. One-third of older adults fall every year with serious consequences that include death, fractures, and head injuries. For the elderly, there are even more consequences when a fall is sustained. These include an ongoing fear of falling, loss of function and mobility, disability, restriction of activity, decreased independence, increased social isolation, depression, and nursing home placement (Leveille et al., 2009)).

Fifty-five percent of fall-related injuries occur inside the home (Greene, Sample, & Fruhauf, 2009). The most

12.6 Herbal Medications and Adverse Interactions

Ginkgo biloba
Used as an antioxidant and natural blood thinner
Adverse interactions with anticoagulants, OTC pain relievers (causes adverse bleeding), anticonvulsants, and antidepressants

Ginseng
Decreases stress and effects of aging
Adverse interactions with digoxin, anticoagulants, antidepressants, and analgesics

St. John's Wort
Used as antidepressant
Adverse interactions with chemotherapy, indinavir, cyclosporine, digoxin, and theophylline

Source: Data from Salmond, S. (2002). Polypharmacy and phytotherapy: Issues of herb/drug interactions in the elderly. *Australian Journal of Medical Herbalism*, *14*(1), 12–14.

Eleanor and her family obtain a "fall alert" bracelet from their local hospital. This encourages them. The technology works very much like other wireless systems, alerting emergency services and the police if needed. This alert system is connected electronically to Eleanor's home phone with a special piece of equipment that always allows a person to converse with her if she pushes the alert bracelet and needs help. During two occasions in the early evening, Eleanor uses the alert bracelet when she slips off the side of her bed and cannot get up. This effectively allows her to stay at home and have the psychological feeling of being connected to someone who could help her in an emergency when her children are not available.

common rooms where people fall include the living room (31%), bedroom (30%), kitchen (19%), bathroom (13%), and hallway (10%). Fall rates for the elderly are related to intrinsic and extrinsic factors (Table 12.2). In the context of the first home visit, many of these factors are modifiable. For example, the home care nurse can make plans with the family or home care agency to make environmental modifications that can decrease the chance of a fall. For example, this may involve having handrails installed in the bathroom and removing scatter rugs or putting nonskid pads under them. The initiation of an exercise program, medication adjustments, and the management of pain, orthostatic hypotension, and corrected vision all can begin at this first visit (multimodal exercise programs for older adults [Baker, Atlantis, & Fiatarone-Singh, 2007]).

ASSESSING FOR RISK OF ABUSE AND NEGLECT

Unfortunately, in community settings, there can be instances when patients and family members can be victims of abuse and neglect. This is often hidden until home care nurses or other home care personnel enter the home and observe the potential, or actual, abuse, or neglect. In thinking about the difference between abuse and neglect, there are not only subtle differences between the two conditions but also differences in motivating factors behind the situations. Some authors define *abuse* as blatant disregard for the safety and welfare of a patient versus neglect as a chronic, eroding lack of physical, psychosocial, and spiritual support of another (Stark, 2011). Abuse can be physical, emotional (often in the form of verbal abuse), and, especially with the elderly, financial. This is often true when caregivers are responsible for the financial management of the household. Neglect is not always the responsibility of others. Some patients, for a variety of reasons that

TABLE 12.2 Intrinsic and Extrinsic Factors Related to Falls in the Home	
Intrinsic	**Extrinsic**
Age	Poor or inadequate lighting
Previous history of falls	Changes in floor surface or slippery surface
Cognitive impairment	High-gloss floors
Muscle weakness, decreased lower extremity strength	Lack of handrails on stairs
Female	Inappropriate chair height
Taking four or more medications a day	Clutter, throw rugs, electrical cords, loose carpeting
Taking psychotropic medications	Poor sidewalk and pavement conditions, snow and ice
Vision impairment	Pets
Peripheral neuropathy	
Parkinson disease	
History of a stroke (cerebrovascular accident)	
Arthritis	

include diagnosed and undiagnosed depression, can be victims of self-neglect (Underwood et al., 2013). Self-neglect can take the form of not taking care of personal hygiene, refusing to take medications that may improve their physical or mental condition(s), and refusing to eat.

Abuse and neglect are sometimes motivated intentionally, but more often they can be unintentionally present as issues for patients. This is the case particularly with neglect and self-neglect. Extenuating circumstances may involve a lack of knowledge (not being aware of the resources in the community that are available to help with a situation) (Johannesen & LoGiudice, 2013).

One important cautionary note is that home care nurses need to be careful about making judgments related to identifying abuse and neglect involving patients and families. Consideration must be given to cultural beliefs, lack of caregiver knowledge and/or skill, caregiver burden or lack of support, well-intended but misguided care, and patient autonomy and the right to self-determination (Johannesen & LoGiudice, 2013).

Termination

In terminating the initial visit, it is critical to make sure that patients and families know how to reach the home care nurse at any time of the day, and that an emergency plan is understood by the patient and the family. This understanding may involve the neighbors. It is equally important to establish an initial plan of care, and to make a plan for the next scheduled visit. If there are any circumstances that would impede future visits, it is important to address these at this time. For example, if the patient or family members smoke, and the home care nurse is allergic to smoke or cannot tolerate smoking, the home care nurse should make a contract related to a "no smoking" visit policy. If there are pets that disrupt the visit, the home care nurse needs to make a contract that the pet will be put in another area during future home visits.

 Student Reflection

I have to admit, with the short length of stay in hospital settings, caring for patients in the community over many months, depending on their skilled needs, and recertification of care by members of a physician team, makes it difficult to discharge the patient. It is not just the patient but the family that is missed because they are often caregivers that make the care a possibility. So the goodbye is doubly hard sometimes. As a student, I became much more aware of the realities facing patients when they left the hospital and now often wonder why there is such a separation in practice from the hospital to the home. Wouldn't it be great if nurses in the hospital could visit or check in on patients at home after they left?

Post-Visit Planning

After the initial visit, the home care nurse establishes, through the nursing process and the use of the initial assessment protocol, a specific plan of care that may include other healthcare disciplines and home health aide services. Outcome goals are established, and a schedule of planned visits is organized. The most crucial post-visit activity is the establishment of outcome measures, so that the home health team can plan an intervention approach that allows reasonable time and effort for healthcare providers and the patient and family to achieve these measures. This is accomplished through the expert judgment of the home care nurse, who manages the home care effort, and consideration of the constraints of Medicare, Medicaid, and other health insurance policies.

Nurse–Family Interactions in Home Care

Professional boundaries in the home care setting are an important consideration because home care nurses are guests in a patient's home (Rowem & Kellam, 2011). Home care nurses are very aware that dealing with the three Cs— culture, contracts, and confidentiality—is important and that they have unique applications in nonhospital settings.

Culture

In Chapter 10, culture and cultural competency are addressed extensively. However, it is important to reiterate that in home visiting, it is important to converse with patients and families about cultural patterns with which the home care nurse may not be familiar. This includes assessing the degree of acculturation, religious or spiritual needs, the patient and family understanding of the health problem that brought the home care nurse to the home, etiquette, and social customs and rituals and practices.

Contracting

In many home care patient and family situations, one of the roles of the home care nurse is to develop a plan of care that is mutually accepted so that health outcomes can be met, and at a variety of levels of prevention (primary, secondary, and tertiary; see Chapter 5). In many instances, a patient- or family-centered approach leads to differences in levels of motivation to meet outcomes. For example, the home care nurse established positive glycemic control as an outcome for a patient who is living with type 2 diabetes at the age of 85. There are instances when the patient and family find it difficult to accomplish this mutually agreed-upon activity, related to exercise, food portion control, types of food selections, and medication scheduling. On the surface, it may seem as though a patient or family is "fighting against" needed lifestyle changes that are highly connected with health outcomes. On the other hand, a patient may say that he wants to get well and be healthy, which results in two conflicting and ambivalent positions. Thus, finding a way to make a contract that is mutually binding between the patient, family, and nurse is crucial.

Motivation to change behaviors may be related to ambivalence. Motivational interviewing is a patient-centered, directive method for enhancing intrinsic motivation to change by exploring and resolving ambivalence (Wilcox, Kersh, & Jenkins 2017). There are four principal approaches used in motivational interviewing: express empathy, support self-efficacy, roll with resistance, and find a discrepancy (Motivational Interviewing, 2013).

An empathetic approach involves identifying with the emotional aspects of the patient's experiences, attempting to understand those experiences from the patient's perspective. When patients perceive empathy on a counselor's part, they become more open to gentle challenges about lifestyle issues and beliefs about substance use. Patients become more comfortable fully examining their ambivalence about change and less likely to defend unhelpful attitudes, such as the denial of problems (Wilcox, Kersh, & Jenkins 2017).

Self-efficacy is the belief on the part of the patient that change is possible. Self-efficacy by definition is a critical motivator to operational change in health behaviors. A person who has a high sense of self-efficacy regarding a particular behavior is more likely to engage in that behavior. For example, people with stronger perceived self-efficacy for carrying out safer healthcare behaviors will be more likely to persist with these behaviors in the face of interpersonal pressure to behave otherwise (Bandura, 1997). Home care nurses can help patients believe that they can make a change by asking about other changes they have made in their lives in the past and how they were particularly successful. This approach emphasizes the ability of the patient to accomplish a goal successfully.

In motivational interviewing, the home care nurse does not fight patient resistance but "rolls with it." Statements demonstrating resistance are not challenged. Instead the home care nurse lets the patient take the lead. Using this approach, resistance tends to be decreased rather than increased. Patient's argumentative resistance to suggestions is not reinforced and the "devil's advocate" role is minimized.

Home care nurses also work to develop opportunities for patients to discover discrepancies between their current behavior and what they want to accomplish through changed behaviors. When patients perceive that their current behaviors are not leading toward some important future goal, they become more motivated to make important life changes. This approach is accomplished gently and gradually to help patients see that the way they approach health issues may be leading them away from accomplishing their stated goals.

Privacy, Confidentiality, and Security

In 1997, the Health Insurance Portability and Accountability Act (HIPAA) was passed in the United States (United States Department of Labor, 2018). The law assures that personal healthcare information will be kept private and secure. Home care as an industry has strived to maintain privacy of patients and families since its inception. However, new challenges arise related to longitudinal medical records and the numerous healthcare professionals who will have access to healthcare information over a continuum of care. In recent years, the increased use of portable internet systems to document patient and family information brings new challenges to the rights of patients and confidentiality (Sewell, 2016). Protecting patient and family privacy is a nursing responsibility. Home care nurses must be careful to do the following:

1. Conduct assessment interviews in environments that protect privacy (i.e., a place where conversation may not be overheard, if applicable).
2. When using a computer to access or document data, be mindful that no one else can view the screen.

In addition, home care computerized records must be maintained with an organizational commitment to allow only those with an appropriate identification and password to "log in." This approach is associated with ethical responsibility. Confidentiality also is an issue when healthcare data are transmitted. Much data is transferred electronically through facsimiles (faxes) or computer transfers. Encryption is often used as a way of protecting information so that only persons with special "keys" can decrypt messages that are sent (Sewell, 2016). The best way to enhance a commitment to confidentiality in a home care agency is to maintain written policies about the use of patient and family data. This includes an orientation and annual updates with staff to ensure that the policies are understood.

Finally, it is the responsibility of all home health agencies to keep all the data they collect secure. Data must be checked for accuracy. Decisions must be made at the organizational level as to (1) who are the personnel that absolutely need access to the information, (2) what type of firewalls will be established on computerized documents to protect patient data from outside intruders, and (3) when and how data will be backed up to prevent loss of information.

Key Chronic Conditions and Quality Improvement in Home Care

In many healthcare situations, there are several chronic diseases and conditions that are often managed in the home by nurses in collaboration with other healthcare providers. Because of the management of this care by nurses, they often are involved with quality improvement related to these key conditions. Quality improvement simply means that nurses are interested in developing and managing healthcare interventions of a home health team that can improve or stabilize chronic conditions in the home. Common diseases and conditions include diabetes (Hartman, Litchman, Reed, & Burr, 2009), incontinence (Flanagan et al., 2012), pain (Duke, Botti, & Hunter, 2012), hypertension, and CHF (Taylor & Campbell, 2007). It is important to understand that, although these conditions are studied by nursing students in adult healthcare or medical–surgical nursing class and clinical settings, they take on a new complexity when patients leave a controlled environment such as an acute care hospital or rehabilitation facility.

During in-home care, complexity of care may include such issues as (1) family, (2) environment, and (3) even the home care nurse's capacity to attend consistently to assessment and intervention criteria. Complexity of care also arises from the fact that many patients cared for in homes live with multiple healthcare problems and conditions (comorbidities). For example, a patient living with diabetes at home who has a problem with chronic incontinence needs a **family caregiver** to be informed of nutritional needs. If a family caregiver does not collaborate or participate, the interactive effects of glycemic and incontinence control through diet will be defeated. Although incontinence may have many complex etiologies in and of itself, often the bundling of interventions can help patients have positive outcomes in several areas of concern as long as a principal caregiver participates in the plan of care.

In the same way, if the household environment is not safe, the patient with diabetes or dyspnea from CHF may suffer falls and unexpected injuries that could lead to nonhealing wounds, further dyspnea, and unnecessary pain. Careful analysis of safety within the home, and interventions directed toward making the home environment safer through physical adjustments or through the assistance of ambulation strengthening, are key in keeping patients healthy at home.

Finally, home care nurses must be exacting and consistent in their assessment and follow-up with patients and their family caregivers. Because patients are in their own homes, many times home care nurses are faced with trying to balance the need to expeditiously care for patients when they are often fully dressed. This is different than in the hospital setting where patients are often in hospital gowns. In caring for patients living with diabetes, it is critical for home care nurses to ask patients to take off their socks and shoes so that full neurovascular assessments can be completed consistently over time. Symptoms such as subtle changes in sensation may be ignored or overlooked in the context of a chronic health condition, although these same symptoms would warrant immediate care in a more acute illness (Centers for Disease Control and Prevention [CDC], 2012; Hartman et al., 2009).

CASE MANAGEMENT, HOME HEALTHCARE, AND CURRENT HEALTHCARE REFORM

According to the Medicare Payment Advisory Committee (MedPAC, Home Health Care Services, 2016), in 2014 about 3.4 million Medicare beneficiaries received home care, and the Medicare program spent about $18.4 billion on home health services (MedPAC, Home Health Care Services, 2016). The number of agencies participating in Medicare reached 12,199 in 2011 where indicators of payment adequacy for home healthcare were seen as generally positive (MedPAC, Home Health Care Services 2016). However,

almost one in five Medicare patients will be readmitted to the hospital within 30 days of discharge, at a cost of $15 billion and which does not include the heavy emotional and health toll on the patients and their families (MedPAC, Home Health Care Services, 2016). Avoidable hospital readmissions are typically caused by insufficient posthospitalization care, failure to adhere to recommended medication or therapy regimens, and lack of physical support for the discharged patient.

The federal government's Medicare program has created initiatives and incentive programs in a broad effort to lower the costs of avoidable utilization and to improve the quality of care that is delivered and received at healthcare institutions nationwide (MedPAC, Home Health Care Services, 2016). The healthcare home model is an evolving, comprehensive, and cost-saving model that includes home care and case management. This model was introduced originally in the late 1960s as a model of healthcare delivery for children with special needs and was a way to coordinate multiple services to children with complex developmental and physical challenges. Outcomes of the model, beyond family-centered comprehensive care, included a way to coordinate care effectively while being culturally relevant and sensitive. This model is currently referred to as the PCMH and includes a chronic care model congruent with home care services described in this chapter. The distribution of services was originally introduced as a way to address those populations who were underserved and at high risk who needed coordinated care when they could not access primary care easily. The current terminology referring to this model is "healthcare home" versus "medical home" so that the true nature of the coordination is interprofessional with nursing as a central role (American Nursing Association, 2014). The healthcare home model intends to reduce barriers to access by providing services such as enrollment into healthcare services, transportation, and coordination with service providers that include home care services.

Currently pilot projects and efficacy and efficiency studies are underway that use this approach to develop a reimbursement structure. Projects are particularly looking at care coordination for patients with chronic conditions where decreased emergency room and hospital use, in terms of rehospitalization, brought notable savings per year (National Partnership for Women and Families, Side-by-Side Summary of State Medical Home Programs, 2013).

Challenges related to adopting and implementing healthcare home approaches continue to be formidable because current reimbursement rates do not cover the larger scope of services that are meant to be provided. The accountable care organization (ACO) model now utilized by hospital systems was created to coordinate care with an emphasis on prevention, and provide incentive structures in the context of the provisions of the Affordable Care Act (ACA) in which the healthcare home model would be seen as a key component in partnership with those hospital systems utilizing the ACO approaches (McClellan, McKethan, Lewis, Roski, & Fisher,

2010). For many, the need to reform the current primary care model in partnership with case management and home care is critical so that collaborations between ACOs and healthcare home models can truly coordinate care for individuals, families, and communities (Child and Adolescent Health Initiative, 2013).

Evidence for Practice

The National Partnership for Women and Families (2013) last updated a list of all those states that have used medical home programs. Factors include organizational leadership, populations served, provider requirements, payment policies, and outcome measures of success. Please refer to http://www.nationalpartnership.org/research-library/general/standing-up-for-women-families-in-2013.pdf

Look up your state or regional location for ongoing information/evidence of success.

In the final analysis, it is the home care nurse who has a significant role in reducing acute care emergency department and hospital use. As healthcare reform continues, the home care nurse will play a significant role in reducing emergency department and hospital use by improving outcomes in chronic care. In a recent study of all home healthcare agencies, Medicare-certified agencies offered training in outcome-based quality improvement to their professional staff, particularly nursing, as a way to ensure outcomes that did not involve expensive and unnecessary interventions (Pace & Johnson, 2006). Those that addressed (1) pain interfering with activity, (2) improvement in transferring, (3) improvement in managing oral medications, and (4) improvement in ambulation and locomotion demonstrated improved outcomes in comparison with national rates. Improvement continues to be needed in (1) emergent care needs, (2) dyspnea, (3) acute care hospitalization, (4) care of surgical wounds, (5) bathing, and (6) incontinence as home care progresses in its scope and standards of care to the public.

Healing is a matter of time, but it is sometimes also a matter of opportunity. **Hippocrates**

KEY CONCEPTS

- Home care is part of a continuum of care on which patients have the opportunity to live and move through the experiences of subacute, chronic, and end-of-life care.
- The care given in home care settings is often managed and directed by a registered nurse.
- Many aspects of the care in both generic and hospice home care are part of a larger care management plan that is individualized using a case management approach.
- The care given in home care settings is interdisciplinary in nature.
- Caregivers are often family members and friends. They must be considered members of the home care team and offered appropriate support if their commitment to care for a loved one at home is to be successful.

CRITICAL THINKING QUESTIONS

1. You are caring for a home care patient with a large venous stasis wound on her left calf. She is obese and also suffers from CHF and osteoarthritis. She has trouble transferring out of her recliner chair due to pain and shortness of breath. Her physician has recommended daily cleansing of her venous ulcer in the shower. Her bathroom is fully handicapped-accessible with grab bars, a handheld shower head, and a transfer bench, but her pain and shortness of breath prevent her from using the shower. What would you do first?

   a. Explain to the physician that given the patient's limitations, showering is not a possibility.

   b. Order a Hoyer lift for the patient to assist with transfers.

   c. Consult with a physical therapist about getting the patient an electric scooter to facilitate transfers.

   d. Consult with the physician about a better regimen to manage the patient's arthritis pain and add a home health aide to her home care services.

2. Look through several major newspapers for articles that discuss care of the elderly in the community or care of those at the end stage of a life-threatening illness.

   a. What is the role of a community health nurse in assisting families in the care of these citizens in their homes?

   b. What are some of the barriers related to the initiation of home care services in communities?

   c. How does living in an urban area versus a rural area affect home care services?

3. There is an increased use of drugs with elderly populations raising concerns related to adverse outcomes, falls, and hospitalizations. The following list of references represent published manuscripts

that may be of interest to nurses interested in addressing this serious and complex situation facing healthcare practice in the home and other locations of care. Choose three articles of interest from the list, and share your insights with your class.

4. Go to the National Association for Home Care and Hospice website (http://www.nahc.org/) and choose a legislative issue that affects home care.

What are the key issues related to the political efforts made by promoters of home care? What are the political barriers that affect home care?

5. In thinking of five social determinants of health as identified in *Healthy People 2020*, identify the social determinants specifically that may be barriers to home care and case or care management services, and explain why.

COMMUNITY RESOURCES

- Local hospitals that have hospital-based generic or hospice home care programs
- Visiting nurse associations

- Elder affairs organizations
- Local and state health departments
- State offices of Medicare and Medicaid

REFERENCES

Agency for Healthcare Research and Quality (AHRQ). (2018) Retrieved from https://pcmh.ahrq.gov/page/defining-pcmh

American Nurses Association. (2014). *Home health nursing: Scope and standards of practice*. Washington, DC: American Nurses Publishing.

American Nurses Credentialing Center. (2018). Retrieved from http://nursecredentialing.org/NursingCaseManagement

Antonicelli, R., Mazzanti, I., Abbatecola, A. M., & Parati, G. (2010). Impact of home patient telemonitoring on use of β-blockers in congestive heart failure. *Drugs Aging*, 27(10), 801–805.

Baker, M. K., Atlantis, E., & Fiatarone-Singh, M. A. (2007). Multimodal exercise programs for older adults. *Age Ageing*, 36(4), 375–381.

Bandura, A. (1997). *Self-efficacy: The exercise of control*. New York: W. H. Freeman.

California Health Care Foundation. (2013). Retrieved from http://www.chcf.org

California Health Care Foundation. (2018). *US Health Care Spending*. Retrieved November 9, 2018 from https://www.chcf.org/wp-content/uploads/2018/01/HealthCareCostsQRG201801.pdf

Carson, V. B., & Koenig, H. G. (2011). *Parish nursing: Stories of service and care*. West Conshohocken, PA: Templeton Press.

Case Management Society of America. (2018). Retrieved on January 13, 2018, from http://www.cmsa.org/education/icm/

Centers for Disease Control and Prevention (CDC). (2012). Diabetes complications. Retrieved from http://www.cdc.gov/diabetes/statistics/complications_national.htm

Centers for Disease Control and Prevention CDC. (2018). Long term care providers and users services in the United States. Retrieved from https://www.cdc.gov/nchs/data/series/sr_03/sr03_038.pdf

Centers for Medicare & Medicaid Services (CMS). (2018). Retrieved from http://www.cms.gov/Medicare/Quality-Initiatives-Patient-Assessment-Instruments/HomeHealthQualityInits/index.html?redirect=/homehealthqualityinits/

Centers for Medicare and Medicaid Services (CMS). (2014). OASIS data set. Retrieved from http://www.cms.gov/Medicare/Quality-Initiatives-Patient-Assessment-Instruments/HomeHealthQuality-Inits/HHQIOASISDataSet.html

Chari, A. V., Engberg, J., Ray, K. N., & Mehrotra, A.(2014). The Opportunity Costs of Informal Elder-Care in the United States: New Estimates from the American Time Use Survey. *Health Services Research*. doi: 10.1111/1475-6773.12238. Available at http://www.rand.org/pubs/external_publications/EP66196.html

Chatfield, L., Christos, S., & McGregor, M. (2012). Interdisciplinary therapy assessments for the older adult. *Perspectives on Gerontology*, 17(1), 11–16.

Child and Adolescent Health Measurement Initiative. (2013). 2005–2006 National survey of children with special health care needs.

Data Resource Center for Child and Adolescent Health. Retrieved from http://www.cshcndata.org/DataQuery/DataQueryResults.aspx

Cooney, D., & Pascuzzi K. Polypharmacy in the elderly: focus on drug interactions and adherence in hypertension. *Clin Geriatr Med*, 2009; 25(2):221–233.

Corbett, C., Setter, S., Daratha, K., Neumiller, J., & Wood, L. (2010). Nurse identified hospital to home medication discrepancies implications for improving transitional care. *Geriatric Nursing*, 31(3), 188–196.

County Health Rankingss and Roadmaps. (2018). Intensive case management for pregnant and parenting teens. Retrieved on January 13, 2018 from http://www.countyhealthrankings.org/take-action-to-improve-health/what-works-for-health/intensive-case-management-for-pregnant-parenting-teens

DeMarco, R., & O'Brien, L. (1999). Home health care in Massachusetts: The impact of reductions in medicare spending on lay caregivers. *Massachusetts Nurse*, 69(6), 12.

Disease Management Association of America-Care Continuum Alliance. (2013). Retrieved from http://www.carecontinuum.org/about_us.asp

Disease Management Association of America-The Care Continuum Alliance. (2018). Retrieved November 9, 2018 from http://www.carecontinuum.org/about_our_mission.asp

Duke, M., Botti, M., & Hunter, S. (2012). Effectiveness of pain management in hospital in the home programs. *Clinical Journal of Pain*, 28(3), 187–194.

Flanagan, L., Roe, B., Jack, B., Barrett, J., Chung, A., Shaw, C., & Williams, K. S. (2012). Systematic review of care intervention studies for the management of incontinence and promotion of continence in older people in care homes with urinary incontinence as the primary focus (1966–2010). *Geriatrics & Gerontology International*, 12(4), 600–611.

Flatt, J. D., Agimi, Y., & Albert, S. M. (2012). Homophily and health behavior in social networks of older adults. *Family & Community Health*, 35(4), 312–321.

Greene, D., Sample, P., & Fruhauf, C. (2009). Fall-prevention pilot: Hazard survey and responses to recommendations. *Occupational Therapy in Health Care*, 23(1), 24–39.

Hartman, A., Litchman, M. L., Reed, P., & Burr, R. E. (2009). In-home chronic disease management in diabetes: A collaborative practice model for home health care and endocrinology providers. *Home Health Care Management & Practice*, 21(4), 246–254.

Healthy People 2020. (2018). 2020 Topics and objectives. Retrieved from http://www.healthypeople.gov/2020/topicsobjectives2020/default.aspx

REFERENCES *(Continued)*

Ivery, J. M., & Akstein-Kahan, D. (2010). The Naturally Occurring Retirement Community (NORC) Initiative in Georgia: Developing and Managing Collaborative Partnerships to Support Older Adults. *Administration in Social Work, 34*(4), 329–343.

Johannesen, M., & LoGiudice, D. (2013). Elder abuse: A systematic review of risk factors in community-dwelling elders. *Age and Aging, 42*(3), 292–298.

Kan, M. L., Ashley, O. S., LeTourneau, K. L., Williams, J. C., Jones, S. B., Hampton, J., Scott, A. R. (2012). The adolescent family life program: A multisite evaluation of federally funded projects serving pregnant and parenting adolescents. *American Journal of Public Health, 102*(10):1872–1878.

Killick, C., & Taylor, B. J. (2009). Professional decision making on elder abuse: Systematic narrative review. *Journal of Elder Abuse & Neglect, 21*(3), 211–238.

Kongstvedt, P. R. (2001). *The managed health care handbook* (4th ed.). New York: Aspen.

Lehning, A. J., & Austin, M. J. (2011). On Lok: A pioneering long-term care organization for the elderly (1971–2008). *Journal of Evidence-Based Social Work, 8*(1/2), 218–234.

Leveille S. G., Jones R. N., Kiely, D. K., Hausdorff, J. M., Shmerlin, R. H., Guralnik, J. M., … Bean, J. F. (2009). Chronic musculoskeletal pain and the occurrence of falls in an older population. *JAMA,302*, 2214–2221.

Magee, M. (2007). *Home-centered health care*. New York: Spencer.

McClellan, M., McKethan, A. N., Lewis, J. L., Roski, J., & Fisher, E. S. (2010). A national strategy to put accountable care into practice. *Health Affairs, 29*(5), 982–990. doi:10.1377/hlthaff.2010.0194

MedPAC. (2016). Home Health Services Report (Chapter 8). Retrieved from http://www.medpac.gov/docs/default-source/reports/chapter-8-home-health-care-services-march-2016-report-.pdf?sfvrsn=0

Medicare Payment Advisory Committee. (2013). Retrieved from http://www.medpac.gov/documents/Mar13_EntireReport.pdf

Medline Plus. (2013). *Home Care Services*. Retrieved on November 9, 2018 from https://medlineplus.gov/homecareservices.html

Medline Plus. (2018). Retrieved from https://medlineplus.gov/homecareservices.html

Motivational Interviewing. (2013). Retrieved from http://www.motivationalinterview.org

My Geo Tracking. (2018) Electronic verification app for home care business-What to look for. Retrieved from https://www.mygeo-tracking.com/blog/electronic-visit-verification-app-for-home-care/

National Center for Policy Analysis. (2013). Retrieved from http://www.ncpa.org/sub/dpd/index.php?Article_ID=18680

National Coalition on Health Care. (2013). Retrieved from http://nchc.org/blog/nchc-white-paper

National Committee for Quality Assurance. (2018). Patient-centered medical homes. Retrieved from http://www.ncqa.org/Programs/Recognition/PatientCenteredMedicalHomePCMH.aspx

National Health Care for the Homeless Council. (2012). Managing complex co-morbidities in individuals experiencing homelessness. Retrieved from http://www.nhchc.org/wp-content/uploads/2011/10/Managing-Complex-Comorbidities-in-Individuals-Experiencing-Homelessness.pdf

National Partnership for Women and Families. (2013). Side by side summary of state medical home programs. Retrieved from http://www.nationalpartnership.org/site/DocServer/HC_Summary_State-MedicalHomePrograms_081028.pdf?docD=4262

OASIS. (2018). Outcome and Assessment Information Set. Retrieved November 9, 2018 from https://www.cms.gov/Medicare/Quality-Initiatives-Patient-Assessment-Instruments/OASIS/index.html

O'Connor, M., & Davitt, J. K. (2012). The Outcome and Assessment Information Set (OASIS): A review of validity and reliability. *Home Health Care Services Quarterly, 31*(4), 267–301.

Okuyemi, K. S., Goldade, K., Whembolua, G. L., Thomas J. L., Eischen, S., Guo, H., … Jarlais, D. D. (2013). Smoking characteristics and comorbidities in the power to quit randomized clinical trial for homeless smokers. *Nicotine & Tobacco Research, 15*(1), 22–28.

Omaha System. (2013). Retrieved from http://www.omahasystem.org/overview.html

Omboni, S., Gazzola, T., Carabelli, G., & Parati, G. (2013). Clinical usefulness and cost effectiveness of home blood pressure telemonitoring: Meta-analysis of randomized controlled studies. *Journal of Hypertension, 31*(3), 455–468.

Pace, K. B., & Johnson, K. E. (2006). Nursing counts. *American Journal of Nursing, 106*(1), 38.

Pijl-Zieber, E. M., & Kalischuk, R. G. (2011). Community health nursing practice education: Preparing the next generation. *International Journal of Nursing Education Scholarship, 8*(1), 1–13.

Prospective Reimbursement. (2008). Retrieved from http://www.online-medicaldictionary.org/Prospective+Reimbursement.asp?q=Prospective+Reimbursement

Romagnoli, K. M., Handler, S. M., Ligons, F. M., & Hochheiser, H. (2013). Home-care nurses' perceptions of unmet information needs and communication difficulties of older patients in the immediate post-hospital discharge period. *BMJ Quality & Safety, 22*(4), 324–332.

Rosenthal, M. B., & Frank, R. G. (2006). What is the empirical basis for paying for quality in health care? *Medical Care Research and Review, 63*(2), 135–157.

Rowem, J., & Kellam, C. (2011). Ethics and moral development: Core ingredients of a compliance culture. *Home Health Care Management & Practice, 23*(1), 55–59.

Sewell, J. (2016) *Informatics and nursing: Opportunities and challenges* (5th ed.). Philadelphia, PA: Lippincott, Wolters Kluwer.

Stark, S. W. (2011). Blind, deaf, and dumb: Why elder abuse goes unidentified. *Nursing Clinics of North American, 46*(4), 431–436.

Taylor, J. R., & Campbell, K. M. (2007). Home monitoring of glucose and blood pressure. *American Family Physician, 76*(2), 255–260.

Tolma, E. L., Stoner, J. A., McCumber, M., Montella, K., Douglas, T., & Digney, S. A. (2014). Longitudinal evaluation of a teenage pregnancy case management program in Oklahoma. *Journal of Family Social Work, 17*(5):457–479.

TRICARE. (2014). *Military Health System Review-Final Report*. Retrieved November 9, 2018 from file:///C:/Users/rosanna.demarco/Downloads/File%202%20MHS%20Review%20%20Section%201%20Introduction%20and%20Section%202%20Overview%20of%20the%20MHS.pdf

Underwood, M., Lamb, S., Eldridge, S., Sheehan, B., Slowther, A., Spencer, A., … Taylor, S. J. (2013). Exercise for depression in care home residents: A randomized control trial with cost-effectiveness analysis (OPERA). *Health Technology Assessment, 17*(18), 1–281.

United States Department of Labor. (2018). HIPAA. Retrieved from https://www.dol.gov/agencies/ebsa/laws-and-regulations/laws/hipaa

URAC. (2018) Health utilization management. Retrieved January 13, 2018 from https://www.urac.org/accreditation-and-measurement/accreditation-programs/case-management-programs/health-utilization-management/

Westberg, G. (1999). A personal historical perspective of whole person health and the congregation. In P. A. Solari-Twadell, & M.A. McDermott (Eds.). *Parish nursing: Promoting whole person health within faith communities*. Thousand Oaks, CA: Sage.

Wilcox, J., Kersh, B. C., & Jenkins, E. A. (2017). *Motivational Interviewing for Leadership: MI-LEAD*. Gray Beach Publishing.

Zubritsky, C., Abbott, K. M., Hirschman, K. B., Bowles, K. H., Foust, J., & Naylor, M. D. (2012). Health-related quality of life: Expanding a conceptual framework to include older adults who receive long-term services and support. *Gerontologist, 53*(2):205–210.

Chapter 13

Family Assessment

Judith Healey-Walsh

> The family is one of nature's masterpieces.
>
> **George Santayana**

> Feelings of worth can flourish only in an atmosphere where individual differences are appreciated, mistakes are tolerated, communication is open, and rules are flexible—the kind of atmosphere that is found in a nurturing family.
>
> **Virginia Satir**

> If we are peaceful, if we are happy, we can smile, and everyone in our family, our entire society, will benefit from our peace.
>
> **Thich Nhat Hanh**

CHAPTER HIGHLIGHTS

- Family nursing practice
- Definitions of family
- Theoretical perspectives of family
- Descriptions of current family configurations
- Family Systems Nursing: Calgary Family Assessment and Intervention Models
- Family-focused home visiting
- Family caregivers

OBJECTIVES

- Define family nursing practice competencies.
- Compare three theoretical perspectives of family nursing.
- Analyze contemporary family issues
- Apply the Calgary Family Assessment and Calgary Intervention Clinical Practice Models
- Examine evidence-based maternal-child health home visiting programs
- Analyze components of family caregiving.

KEY TERMS

Calgary Family Assessment Model (CFAM): A clinical practice model linked to Family Systems Nursing developed to assist nurses in performing a family assessment in an organized, systematic manner. The CFAM is a multidimensional model comprised of three basic assessment categories: *structural, functional, and developmental.*

Calgary Family Intervention Model (CFIM): A clinical practice model linked to Family Systems Nursing developed to assist nurses in family-focused interventions. The model address three domains: cognitive, affective, and behavioral and focuses on enhancing, improving, and sustaining family functioning through the establishment of

KEY TERMS *(continued)*

a collaborative partnership between the nurse and the family, the use of therapeutic conversations, and a focus on family strengths and resiliency.

Caregiver burden: Fatigue or frustration expressed by persons who care for convalescing or chronically ill persons on a daily basis.

Ecomap: A diagram used to identify the direction and intensity of family relationships between members and/or community institutions of importance to the family (e.g., schools, workplaces, places of worship).

Family: Two or more persons who share emotional closeness and identify themselves as members of a family.

Family Systems Nursing: A conceptual framework developed to promote family nursing practice. It emphasizes the reciprocal relationship between individual members and the family as a whole. Nurses provide care for the family as a unit.

Genogram: A diagram of family relationships between blood relatives that can span two or more generations. Life events such as marriages, divorces, births, and deaths are included

in the diagram. The genogram is used to identify relationships as well as possible patterns of disease.

Intrafamily strain: The effect of stressors on families that can interfere with effective family communication, interaction, and functioning, and negatively impact family well-being.

System: A group that works on the principle that each part contributes to the way the whole functions.

Theory: A system of interrelated statements that is used to explain, predict, control, or understand a phenomenon.

CASE STUDIES

References to case studies are found throughout this chapter (look for the case study icon). Readers should keep the case studies in mind as they read the chapter.

CASE 1

Lucy, a public health nurse in a mid-sized city, has been following the Barnes family for two years. Eight-year-old Tanya and her 6-year-old brother Luke have asthma, and Lucy has been helping the family control asthma triggers at home. Tanya and Luke's 51-year-old grandmother, Elsa Morris, is their guardian. The children's mother is in the military and is now overseas. She sends e-mails with photos to the children almost daily. The children's father, who never married their mother, has had no contact with the children for more than four years.

At Lucy's most recent home visit, Elsa tells Lucy that Tanya has been unable to sleep through the night. Lucy also learns that the children have "too many treats" between meals and after dinner. Mrs. Morris tries to get the children to go to bed around 8 p.m., but they like to watch television. Elsa says that she knows she needs to be stricter, but the children miss their mother and she wants to avoid upsetting them.

Elsa's husband has been unemployed for several months. Although he received a generous severance payment from his company, he has had to apply for unemployment. He is generous and caring to the children and to their mother. Elsa works part-time and only makes enough money to cover expenses. She tells Lucy that the cost of the children's medications

is "adding up." She also wants to enroll the children in extracurricular activities, but they are "too expensive."

- What three priorities for this family can you identify?
- What additional information would you want from Mrs. Morris?
- What types of community resources to support this family would you recommend?

CASE 2

Agnes and Mark Thomas are 83 and 84 years of age, respectively. They have four adult children and eight grandchildren; all live within 25 miles of the couple. Mrs. Thomas likes the family to have dinner together at least twice a month at her home. Over the past six months, her children have noticed that their mother often forgets her grandchildren's names. Mr. Thomas, a retired firefighter and once avid swimmer, has arthritis in his spine, which has decreased his mobility.

The Thomases' elder daughter, 58-year-old Arlene, is developmentally delayed and has lived in various state-run residential facilities since she was 5 years old. Arlene's siblings had little contact with her when she was growing up except on birthdays and holidays. Recently, the director of the facility sent the Thomases a letter to inform them that the state is closing the facility and that they need to find housing for Arlene.

Laura, a nurse from the residential facility where Arlene lives, phones Agnes to arrange a home visit. Agnes tells Laura that Arlene cannot live with her and Mark, and she asks Laura to talk to her youngest son Jim, 47 years old. Although Jim has had minimal contact with his sister, he agrees to meet with Laura. He tells her that his parents' health is declining, especially his mother's, and proposes that Arlene might be able to move into the in-law apartment in his home. Jim and Laura arrange another meeting that includes Arlene, as well as Jim's wife and their adolescent twin daughters.

- What potential conflicts can arise in this family?
- What information about the family's resources could help to offset their anxiety about Arlene's change in housing?
- Who else should be included in any plans?

INTRODUCTION

Nursing is defined as the "protection, promotion, and optimization of health and abilities, prevention of illness and injury, alleviation of suffering through the diagnosis and treatment of human response, and advocacy in the care of individuals, families, communities, and populations" (ANA, 2010, p. 10). Therefore, working with families is an inevitable and integral aspect of nursing practice. However, much emphasis in clinical practice is on individual problems and needs. Family care is frequently the focus of concern in particular clinical situations, such as nursing sick children, family-centered maternity care, and home health and hospice nursing care. Learning about the complex nature of family can provide insight into the ways that family life, interactions, and practices influence individual health, and how individual health and illness impact the family. In many cases, family connections play a vital role in providing support to members. Yet, at other times, family influences can be perceived less positively, and can cause challenges to both family members and the healthcare providers who care for them. This chapter explores family-focused care and family nursing practice. It includes a discussion of the expanded definition of family, and the comparison of three theoretical perspectives of family nursing. The current diversity of family forms is explored. The Calgary Family Assessment Model (CFAM) and Calgary Family Intervention Model (CFIM) are described as evidence-based clinical practice models that guide family nursing practice. Maternal-child health home visiting programs and the role of family caregivers are presented to exemplify how community health nurses apply family-focused nursing practice. The case studies at the beginning of the chapter illustrate how complex issues can affect families and their health management, and how a family-focused approach is necessary for both assessment and intervention.

FAMILY NURSING PRACTICE

Family nursing practice asserts that there is a reciprocal relationship between a family and its individual members, and between the family and illness. The health and illness of individual members impacts the family, and the family affects the health and illness of individual members (Bell & Wright, 2015; IFNA, 2013; Kaakinen, Hanson, & Denham, 2010). Wright and Leahey (2013) explain that health and "illness are a family affair" (p. ix). The International Family Nursing Association's position statement (2013) explains that "A family's life world is therefore an integrative experience of individual and collective health and illness. In response nurses must accommodate both an individual and collective focus to meet health and illness needs" (p. 2). The holistic nature of nursing supports the inclusion of the family when providing nursing care to individuals of all ages and in varied settings (Abraham & Moretz, 2012). Although family nursing is frequently associated with maternity and pediatric practice, IFNA emphasizes that family nursing is appropriate and effective within many nursing specialties including home health and palliative care (Ferrell & Whittenberg, 2017; Harding, 2014; Imanigoghary, Peyrovi, Nouhi, & Kazemi, 2017; Norinder, Goliath, & Alvariza, 2017). IFNA proposes that family-focused nursing care should be the standard of practice across the lifespan. In 2015, to support this goal, the IFNA published a Position Statement on Generalist Competencies for Family Nursing Practice. The identified competencies are listed in Box 13.1. To be competent in the provision of quality family nursing, community health nurses need to have a theoretical understanding of family.

13.1 Family Nursing Competencies: Generalist

1. Enhance and promote family health.
2. Focus nursing practice on families' strengths; the support of family and individual growth; the improvement of family self-management abilities; the facilitation of successful life transitions; the improvement and management of health; and the mobilization of family resources.
3. Demonstrate leadership and systems thinking skills to ensure the quality of nursing care with families in everyday practice and across every context.
4. Commit to self-reflective practice based on examination of nurse actions with families and family responses.
5. Practice using an evidence-based approach.

Source: IFNA. (2015). Position statement on generalist competencies for family nursing practice. Retrieved from https://internationalfamilynursing.org/wordpress/wp-content/uploads/2015/07/GC-Print-friendly-PDF-document-in-black-white-no-photos-English-language1.pdf.

UNDERSTANDING FAMILY

Family is a complex phenomenon. The concept of family is
dynamic, as it is impacted by sociocultural and economic
factors. Therefore, varied definitions and theoretical perspectives exist, which can assist the community health nurse
in acquiring a broad and deep understanding of the universal
characteristics and changing nature of family. Looking at
different definitions of and theories relevant to family is a
good place to begin exploring this concept.

Definitions of Family

For demographic use and purposes, the U.S. Census Bureau
narrowly defines family as "people living together and are
related by birth, adoption, or marriage" (Vespa, Lewis, &
Keide, 2013). The concept of family is not static and evolves
over time influenced by cultural and societal changes. Historically, the nuclear family was defined as comprised of a
mother, father, and children. Families today assume a variety of forms. Factors such as delayed marriage and childbearing, increased divorce rates, remarriage rates, increased
co-habitation, smaller family size, grandparenting, and the
same-sex marriage ruling have all influenced family structures, A nurse's own family of origin is usually a frame of
reference for what comprises family and how its members
relate to one another.

One broad definition of family is "two or more persons
who are joined together by bonds of sharing and emotional
closeness . . . who identify themselves as being part of the
family" (Friedman, Bowden, & Jones, 2003, p. 10). This
definition characterizes the range of families in 21st-century
America and covers a wide range of relationships, including
those outside the genetic and legal definitions of family.
Another definition is that families decide who they are, and
family boundaries are not limited to traditional definitions
(Wright & Leahey, 1999, 2009). Although this definition
might seem simplistic, it draws attention to individual group
needs to affirm identity as family and establish connection
to others within that group.

Overall, both definitions of family have characteristics of
living in a diverse society that includes groups of different
ethnic, religious, or political backgrounds. Both definitions
clearly indicate that individual people determine their status
as family. An advantage to these definitions is that the ideal
of what constitutes family includes groups that 50 years ago
would not be recognized as such (e.g., gay and lesbian families, cohabiting partners, and single-parent families).
However, sociologic trends make describing families based
solely on their attributes difficult (Wright & Leahey, 1999,
2009).

Theoretical Perspective of Family

Generally speaking, a **theory** presents a systematic view of
related statements to describe, explain, predict, or prescribe
a phenomenon of interest (Walker & Avant, 2010). A range
of theoretical frameworks has been used to analyze and
describe family composition, roles, interactions, and behaviors. Given the complexity of the concept of family, no one
theory is broad enough to explain all the aspects of family.
Therefore, several theoretical perspectives must be considered. Family theories use a specific perspective to provide a
guide to analyze and understand the concept of family. Family systems theory, family structural-functional theory, and
family developmental theory are frequently used to provide
an understanding of typical characteristics of family.

Family Systems Theory

Family theorists have applied general systems theory principles to explain how families interact with their members
and with society. From a systems perspective, the family
social system is comprised of interacting subsystems (individual members) and is also a part of and in constant interaction with suprasystems in the external environment
(neighborhood, community, and societal institutions). The
family is defined as a system characterized by continual
interaction between its members and with the environment.
A central tenet of systems theory is that the system, as a
whole, is greater than its parts. The interrelationships and
interactions in the family system, are such that a change in
one member affects a change in all other members. In nursing practice, the word *system* is often used to describe families. A **system** works on the principle that each part
contributes to the functioning of the whole. Its structure,
personal history, and patterns of communication affect how
well the system operates. Family systems are groups of individual people whose functioning depends on one another
(Wright & Leahey, 1999, 2009, 2013). Therefore, to understand the family, interrelationships of the members with
each other and with the larger society must be analyzed.

Family Structural-Functional Theory

Structural-functional theory views the family as a social system, but emphasizes the organization or structure of the family and how this structure facilitates its functioning. Family
structure refers to the ordered set of relationships among the
parts and between the family and other social systems. The
structure serves to facilitate the achievement of the functions. The functions serve both the individual family members, the community, and society. Societal and cultural
norms also affect changes in family structure.

Traditionally, family structure was distinguished between what constituted the nuclear family and the extended family. Nuclear families consist of first-degree relatives—that is, two generations who live together. Commonly, the two generations include parents and children. Extended families include both first- and second-degree relatives and can include grandparents, aunts, uncles, and cousins. Traditional definitions of extended family indicate that the family shares a dwelling, but members can live in the same neighborhood or in relatively close proximity to one another. The time that an extended family spends together depends not only on geographic closeness to one another but also on family customs. Extended family can also include persons who are not blood relatives, but who share a common locale of origin or culture. This situation is common in immigrants or in persons whose own families live elsewhere. To determine family structure, the community health nurse must identify the individuals that make up the family, their relationships to each other, and the relationships between the family and other social systems. Family structure is evaluated based on how effectively it accomplishes the functions that are essential to its members and society.

From a sociological perspective the family serves as the basic sociocultural and economic unit in society. The family provides the initial context in which children learn, grow, and develop. Therefore, families provide essential functions including all basic needs such as food, shelter, and clothing. In addition, five critical functions of the family have been identified that are important for community health nurses to understand (Friedman, 1998):

- Reproductive: addition of new members through procreation or adoption
- Affective: provision of nurturance, love, and sense of belonging
- Socialization and social placement: transmission of culture, values, rules, social norms, and social identity
- Economic: production, consumption, and distribution of goods and services
- Healthcare: promotion and protection of health and well-being, coordination of care and health services

Family Developmental Theory

The developmental or life-cycle theory proposes that families progress through typical stages. Stages begin with marriage followed by childbirth and child-rearing. Duvall (1977) and Duvall and Miller (1985) were major contributors toward the advancement of family developmental theory. The stages from their work are based on the traditional, nuclear, heterosexual middle class family experience, which was the predominant and widely accepted family structure at the time. The theorists identified eight stages within the family life cycle. The first stage viewed the young adult, typically in their early 20s leaving their family of origin to get married and start a career (primarily to support their family). The following four stages focused on childbearing and child-rearing in a heterosexual two-parent family. The sixth stage involved the parents launching their adult children to begin their married life and career. And the final two stages involved middle-aged and aging families with a focus on the empty nest, establishing new intergenerational relationships, retirement, coping with the loss of a spouse and living alone. The stages assume homogeneity (two parents, husband and wife), presenting a middle class bias. Given the sociocultural and economic factors, which have prompted variations in family structure and the timing of family developmental tasks over the past 30 years, these life-cycle stages have limitations. The timing of leaving home, getting married, and having children has changed. The stages are not as predictable and do not fit as well with the changing structure of contemporary families. A familiarity with family theories provides nurses with a foundational understanding of the concept of family. However, community health nurses must be attentive to the changing definition, structure, and life cycle of families, so that the diversity of family forms is respected and that family health and well-being is promoted for all families (McGoldrick, Garcia-Preto, & Carter, 2016). To accomplish this, community health nurses need to understand the contemporary family configurations and the sociocultural and economic factors that have shaped these changes.

> ### ✎ Practice Point
>
> An understanding of theoretical perspectives of the concept of family can guide community health nurses in promoting family nursing practice and addressing family health and well-being.

Family isn't something that's supposed to be static, or set. People marry in, divorce out. They're born, they die. It's always evolving, turning into something else. **Sarah Dessen**

Contemporary Family Issues

A range of sociocultural and economic factors has prompted family configurations that vary from the traditional family and historically were not accepted by major social institutions. Community health nurses are in a position in which they can advocate for wider acceptance of and policies that support diversity of family forms.

Changes in Family Life Cycle

Timing of developmental tasks in the traditional family life cycle has changed significantly, impacting contemporary families. In the past, young adults were expected to have completed school, started a career, and moved out usually with a spouse, in their 20s, with the arrival of their first child to soon follow. Unlike their parents, young adults are leaving home at an older age, and many return home after living independently. In addition, young adults are delaying marriage and childbearing, or having children outside of marriage (Vespa, 2017). Schondelmyer (2017) reported that that there were fewer married households (down to 44%) and more individuals living alone (20%), or with a partner (8%), which represents the biggest change in households in the last five decades. The United States has seen a rise in both males and females delaying marriage. Since 1967, the median age for first marriage for women has increased from 20.6 to 27.4 years of age and from 23.1 to 29.6 years of age for men (Schondelmyer, 2017). Delaying marriage can delay childbirth. In 1967, 53.3% of 18- to 24-year-olds had children living with them, and by 2016, only 31.2% of the same age group had children living with them. An even greater change was reported among 25- to 34-year-olds. In 1967, only 23.9% in that age group did not have their own children living with them, whereas by 2016, the number more than doubled with 61.5% not having their own children living with them.

In 1960, 88% of children were living in two-parent families (America Counts, 2017). By 2016, this percentage had dropped to 69%, with 65% of children living with two married parents and 4% with two unmarried, cohabitating parents (America's Children, 2017). The birth rate among unmarried women ages 15 to 44 peaked at 52 births per 1,000 in 2007 and decreased to 43 births per 1,000 in 2015. The largest decline occurred to adolescents aged 15 to 17, with the birth rate for this age group declining from 33 live births per 1,000 females in 1980 to a record low of 10 per 1,000 in 2015.

Divorce, which has increased in prevalence, is a major variation in the family life cycle that can compound the complexity of developmental tasks (Friedman et al., 2003). It affects families at every stage of development (U.S. Census Bureau, 2005). Most importantly, divorce has far-reaching effects for family members at every generational level in both the nuclear and extended families. The sequelae of divorce depend on the family. For example, divorce in a family without children is substantially different from one with children. A child's age and stage of development determines his or her perception of the change in marital relationship, and the resolution of any conflicts. For the married couple, the stage of their relationships helps determine the level of loss and bereavement. For example, divorce that occurs after 25 years of marriage can be devastating and cause "couple identity" crisis as shared financial investments and possessions are dissolved (Friedman et al., 2003). In the same way, divorce that occurs in marriages of shorter duration can be equally upsetting; marital identity is in process and may leave members of the family unit with a sense of unfinished process or a sense of abject failure that may impact other relationships in the future.

McGoldrick and colleagues (2016), have identified specific family life-cycle phases for divorcing and remarrying families, which include the divorce, the post-divorce family, and the remarriage. During the divorce phase, families are working through the actual decision, planning for the separation and changes in the family system. During this time, family members, both nuclear and extended, are dealing with many emotions including anger, sadness, guilt, and fear, along with practical issues such as living arrangements, finances, custody issues, and restructuring relationships. All of these stressors impact family health and well-being. In the post-divorce family with children, adjusting to a single-parent structure and some form of shared custody or visitation schedule are focal issues. Developing respectful co-parenting relationships and processes is important in assisting children's adjustment to new living arrangements and family dynamics. Remarriage leads to complexity and the formation of multiple new relationships and structural changes within the family system. Adjustment to these changes requires time and patience, as family membership, roles, functions, and boundaries evolve.

> The bond that links your true family is not one of blood, but of respect and joy in each other's life. **Richard Bach**

Changes in Family Structure

In 2016, the majority (69%) of American children under the age of 18 still lived in two-parent families, yet this reflected a significant decrease from 88% in 1960 (America Counts, 2017). The concept of family has broadened and become more inclusive, and extends beyond the two-parent traditional nuclear family. Families share some common traits, but structural configurations have become more varied. Single-parent, blended, cohabitating, gay and lesbian, and homeless families are all more prevalent contemporary family configurations. The assessment and clinical approach to families and family health, now and in the future, require expanding the traditional notions of family.

SINGLE-PARENT FAMILIES

Single-parent families can form due to divorce or widowhood (death of a spouse). However, as more women have become pregnant outside of a marital relationship, this family form has become more prevalent and accepted. Between 1980 and 2015, the percentage of all births to unmarried women increased by 22% points, from 18% to 40%. In 2015, the birth rate among unmarried women ages 15 to 44 was 43 births for every 1,000 women, down from 52 per 1,000 in 2007, when rates had reached their peak. In 2017, 27% of children under the age of 18 lived with one parent, 23% with their mothers, and 4% with their fathers. Of the almost 20 million children under 18 who lived with one parent in 2017, 83.9% lived with their mothers (down from 87.5% in 2007) and 16.1% lived with their fathers (up from 12.5% in 2007) (U.S. Census, 2017). Forty-nine percent of single mothers have never been married, whereas the most common marital status of single-parent fathers is divorced. Between 1960 and 2015, the birth rate among adolescents aged 15 to 17 declined from 33 live births per 1,000 females to 10 live births per 1,000, a record low for the United States (Forum on Child and Family Statistics, 2017).

BLENDED FAMILIES

Blended families form when two single-parents either marry or cohabitate and raise their children from previous relationships together. This type of family has become widespread as more divorced or widowed people remarry. The Pew Research Center (2011) found that four in 10 Americans currently have at least one step-relative, and three in 10 have a step or half sibling. Thirteen percent of adults have at least one stepchild. Survey respondents showed higher levels of commitment and obligation to biological parents, grown children, and siblings over those with stepparents, stepchildren, or step/half siblings (85% vs. 56%; 78% vs. 62%; and 64% vs. 42%, respectively).

COHABITING COUPLES AND FAMILIES

Marriage is a valued institution in most cultures. In American culture, the decision to marry or not is regarded as individual and personal. Couples might choose to cohabit either before they marry, or instead of marrying. According to U.S. Census Bureau (2017) figures, 7.8 million unmarried opposite-sex couples comprise households. Of the unmarried opposite-sex couples living together, 37% live with children under the age of 18. Families often form when couples in a group of people cohabit. They consider themselves to be a family, as they have formed committed emotional bonds and share possessions and possibly home ownership.

GAY AND LESBIAN FAMILIES

As the prevalence of marriage in the general population continues to decline, marriage between same-sex couples has substantially increased in the past decade as same-sex marriage was initially recognized in some states and then established in all 50 states (June, 2015) as a result of the Supreme Court ruling. There are now more than 547,000 married same-sex couples in the United States (Romero, 2017). In addition, there are about 400,000 unmarried same-sex partners living together. Approximately 220,000 children in the United States are being raised by same-sex couples. While same-sex couples have the right to marry in all states, anti-LGBTQ discrimination and social stigma remains. Despite substantial evidence of successful parenting by same-sex couples and increasing societal acceptance of sexual minorities (Gates, 2013; Miller, 2017; Richards, Rothblum, Beauchaine, & Balsam, 2017), some negative attitudes toward same-sex parenting continue to exist with opponents contending that the parents' sexual orientation is detrimental to their children. Same-sex couples may be raising their families in a heteronormative community where their family status is devalued and possibly discriminated against (Ollen & Goldberg, 2016).

HOMELESS FAMILIES

Family homelessness has become a major national problem. Families with children comprise 35% of the homeless population in the United States. The 2017 federal point-in-time-count reported that on any given night, almost 60,000 families with children are homeless. Almost 16,000 people in families were living on the streets or in a car. During 2016, about half a million people in families stayed at a homeless shelter or in a transitional housing program, including 292,166 children, of whom about 145,000 were younger than 6 years of age (National Alliance to End Homelessness, 2017). Poverty contributes to homelessness as families struggle with incomes that are too low to pay for housing and other basic financial needs. Precipitating factors to homelessness can include lost jobs or work hours, eviction, overcrowding, a catastrophic illness, unanticipated major bills, interpersonal violence or natural disaster (Brush, Gultekin, Dowdel, Saint Arnault, & Satterfield, 2017; Grant, Gracy, Goldsmith, Shapiro, & Redlener, 2013; Sandel, Sheward, & Sturtevant, 2015).

Young single mothers (with young children) with limited education head a majority of homeless families (Bassuk & Beardslee, 2014). Homeless families are at greater risk for illness and disability, substance use disorder, violence-related injuries, and mental health problems. Living in shelters or temporary facilities is associated with depression, anxiety, and sadness (Gultekin, Brush, Bairidi, Kirk, & VanMaldehem, 2014). Homelessness impacts children's physical and mental health, education, sense of safety, and overall development (Bassuk & Beardslee, 2014).

Evidence for Practice

As the majority of homeless families with young children are headed by single mothers, it is important for community health nurses to understand what the experience of homelessness is like, how it impacts family health, and what services are needed to support these families.

Gultekin, Brush, Baiardi, Kirk, and VanMaldenhem (2014) conducted a qualitative descriptive study using focus groups at a Michigan service agency, which provided case management services to homeless families. The study aims were to (a) explore individual pathways into homelessness, (b) understand the day-to-day experience of living in an emergency shelter and the process of re-housing, (c) identify real and perceived barriers for families attempting to reestablish stable housing, and (d) understand the impact of homelessness on families' overall health and well-being. The researchers' intent was to use the focus groups "to capture the *how* and *why* of individuals' lives as either homeless mothers or caseworkers" (Gultenkin et al., 2014, p. 394). The sample included five caseworkers and 13 homeless mothers (who met the inclusion criteria of female, 18 or over, caring for at least one dependent child). Semi-structured interview questions guided the four focus groups (one with caseworkers and three with homeless mothers). The questions for the mothers centered on (a) causes for homelessness, (b) experiences in the shelter and with re-housing, (c) health impacts on the family's health, and (d) hopes for the future. Whereas, questions for the caseworkers concentrated on (a) their roles in case management, (b) their perceptions of barriers to assisting families, and (b) their impressions of the health risks for the homeless families. The mothers were single, separated, or divorced with children ranging in age from 4 months to 16 years; two were pregnant.

Transcribed digital recordings and field notes of nonverbal communication and interactions were analyzed for themes. Four main themes, each with subthemes were identified. Perceptions of the mothers and caseworkers included both similarities and differences. Under the theme of "pathways to and meaning of homelessness," mothers expressed pride in their roles as mothers but also identified pride as blocking them for reaching out when they needed help. They acknowledged that they were on their own, lacking a safety net as family relationships were broken, and they expressed family legacies of poverty, violence, and substance use disorders. In the second them, "daily shelter life and the rehousing process," participants expressed that they felt labeled and misunderstood about the complicated choices that they faced. They wanted to be viewed as more than homeless and acknowledged for their commitment to their children and the value they put on education and job training. They expressed frustration with many rules of the shelter that did not account for individual needs or circumstances and frequently felt disrespected. "What women need and want" formed the third theme, and the women reported that being homeless made them think about the future, and begin to focus on goals that would support their education, employment, and healthier lives for themselves and their children. The final theme addressed "impact on health and well-being," with the women admitting to physical and emotional exhaustion from dealing with their difficult circumstances. They described their struggles dealing with stress, anxiety, and depression, and frustration with the lack of accessible mental health services. Despite the difficulties that they faced, they expressed a sense of hope and optimism in trying to plan for a better future for their family. Their spirituality was identified as a strength that helped them with their daily struggles.

The caseworkers' responses mirrored the mothers' in many areas but diverted around the mothers' motivation and actions toward change. They did not view the mothers as making reasonable plans for education or job training. They worried that their interventions did not push the mothers to achieve independence and may have been disempowering, rendering the mothers unable to self-identify actions that could improve their lives and those of their children. The caseworkers realized that all shelter workers need to be trained in acknowledging the trauma these families experienced and that trauma-sensitive care needed to be integrated into the program.

Practice Point

Families form when a group of persons has strong emotional bonds, and they may simply proclaim themselves to be families. Sociocultural and economic factors have influenced changes in family structure and life cycle.

Happiness is having a large, loving, caring, close-knit family in another city. **George Burns**

FAMILY NURSING THEORY

Family Systems Nursing (FSN) is a conceptual framework developed by Wright and Leahey (1990) to promote family nursing practice. At its core, FSN emphasizes "a focus on the interaction, reciprocity, and relationships among several systems levels, that is, individual, family, and larger systems" (Bell & Wright, 2015, p. 180). The intent of FSN is to focus on the family as the unit of care. Wright and Leahey (2009, 2013) emphasize the importance of concentrating on both the individual and the whole family simultaneously. FSN is theoretically rooted in systems theory, communication theory, and change theory (Bell & Wright, 2015). In FSN practice, the nurse must assess the interaction between and impact of health, illness suffering, and family functioning. A central belief in the FSN framework is that there are relationships and an interconnectedness among systems and subsystems (individual, family, and community), which have a strong reciprocal effect on health and illness. Community health nurses provide care to individuals, families, and the community, and therefore need to employ a conceptual framework, such as FSN, to understand the relationships, interactions, and reciprocity at multiple systems levels. A central tenet of the framework is the primacy of the relationship between the individual/family and a nonjudgmental nurse. The relationship between the nurse and the family must be nonhierarchical, meaning that the nurse does not approach the family as the expert, but forms an authentic, respectful collaborative partnership with the family. FSN accepts that family members can have multiple perspectives of the family's health and illness, which needs to be explored through a nurse-guided therapeutic conversation with the family. Although problems, needs, and concerns are addressed, family strengths are openly acknowledged and resiliency is emphasized. FSN recognizes that the family "suffers" when they are dealing with an illness, injury, or disability of a family member and the suffering needs to be examined, and forms of relief, such as maximizing family strengths and connecting with needed resources, can be identified (Ostlund and Persson, 2014). The overall goal is to restore, enhance, and sustain family health and well-being (Bell, 2009).

To operationalize this broad conceptual framework in nursing practice, Wright and Leahey (2009, 2013) developed two clinical practice models: the Calgary Family Assessment Model (CFAM) and the Calgary Family Intervention Model (CFIM) to link FSN to nursing practice, in a practical and understandable manner. The models were initially conceptualized from their extensive experience in family nursing practice, and have continued to evolve, reflective of changes in family structure, functioning, and development, and in response to widespread use, evaluation, and research findings. Having a clinical practice model to guide family assessment is essential for the community health nurse to provide high quality, individualized care to families who vary in structure, function, and developmental stage, access to resources, and health and illness experiences. For example, the community health nurse may be providing care to a family whose teenage daughter is pregnant, or a young family that is adjusting to the realities of the father's (primary breadwinner) slow recovery from a major stroke, or an extended family trying to arrange care of an older adult declining quickly from Alzheimer disease. Using the CFAM, which is described in detail in the next section, can help the nurse obtain a thorough and focused assessment of both individuals, the family as a whole, and the family's relationship with community-based resources. The assessment findings will then provide insight to and guidance in the selection of the necessary, individualized family interventions.

Family Assessment: Calgary Family Assessment Model

Families are complex social systems and there are multiple factors that influence their health and illness experiences. To understand and intervene with families to promote their health and soften their illness experiences, a detailed assessment needs to be completed. The **CFAM** was developed to assist nurses in performing a family assessment in an organized, systematic manner. The CFAM is a multidimensional model comprised of three basic assessment categories: *structural, functional, and developmental*, and the multiple subcategories of each that combine the elements needed to gain a multilayered understanding of family components. The model is comprehensive and can initially seem impractical and somewhat overwhelming given time constraints, however the nurse is responsible for selecting and prioritizing which subcategories are most relevant to the family. Not all subcategories will need to be addressed with every family; it is up to the nurse's clinical judgment. For example, a community nurse whose practice involves home visits and an ongoing relationship may complete a comprehensive assessment, while a community nurse working in a clinic setting and seeing the family in a more episodic manner may have to prioritize and focus the assessment more specifically.

Structural Assessment

Three aspects of family structure can be assessed using identified subcategories: (a) internal structure (family composition, gender and sexual orientation of the members, birth order of children, subsystems including couple, parent–child, and sibling, and boundaries; (b) external structure (extended family, larger systems which include social and community connections such as schools, work, religious and healthcare organizations) and (c) context (culture, race, social class, spirituality and/or religion, environment) (Wright & Leahey, 2013). Identifying family relationships can be complicated. Diagrams are a useful visual aid to identify these relationships. Community health nurses encounter family health concerns in a wide range of circumstances. Attention to the dimensions and influence of family helps identify ways to support everyone involved. Identifying key relationships, both within and outside the family, is a good starting point. Two structural assessment tools, the genogram and the ecomap, are frequently used to provide a graphic portrayal of the internal and external structure of a family. Although they are similar, each highlights different aspects of family connections and relationships.

The **genogram** provides a diagram of the family constellation, and can provide substantial information about family structure in a clear and simple format. It should include the information that is most important in assessing the particular family unit. Typically it will include at least two generations, highlighting family members' age, gender, relationship, birth order, marital status, and mortality (Tavernier, 2009) (Fig. 13.1). However, it can be expanded to include other areas, such as health status, education, and occupation. Genograms show how interdependent family members are related to each other. Nurses can use genograms to help families identify common traits as well as unique attributes of various members. **Ecomaps** outline the influence that other systems or groups have on families (Fig. 13.2). They illustrate family relationships and show vital connections, which can include religious, work, educational, cultural, healthcare and social organizations and groups. Solid or hatched lines plot the strength of connections. Community health nurses often find that ecomaps are especially helpful to identify social supports and to show families whether resources are available to assist them (Rempel, Neufeld, & Kushner, 2007).

> Sister is probably the most competitive relationship within the family, but once the sisters are grown, it becomes the strongest relationship. **Margaret Mead**

Practice Point

Genograms and ecomaps are graphic representations of family relationships. Nurses can use genograms to identify key events and relationships within families, and ecomaps can be used to identify interactions between families and the communities in which they live.

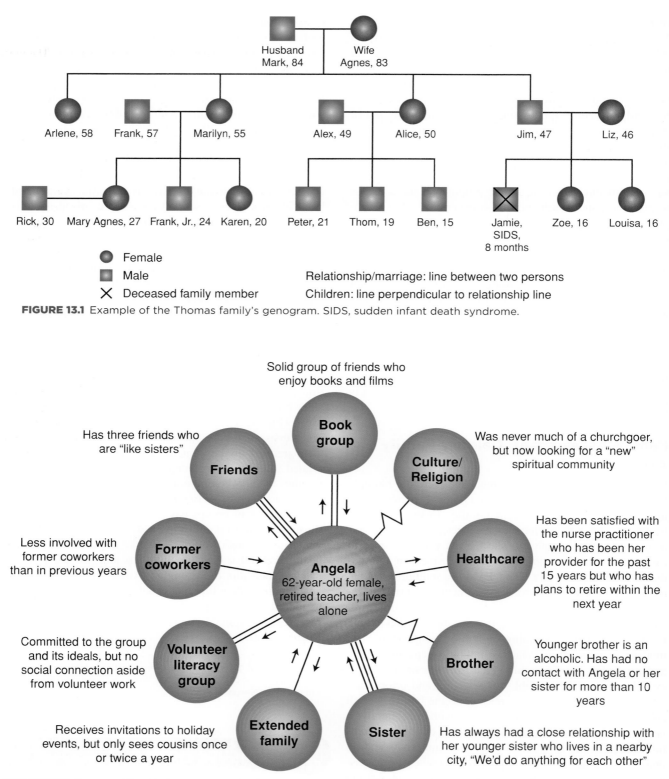

FIGURE 13.1 Example of the Thomas family's genogram. SIDS, sudden infant death syndrome.

FIGURE 13.2 Ecomap. The circles represent both persons and institutions or organizations to which a person or family is connected. The number of lines indicates the strength of the relationship, the *jagged line* indicates a negative relationship, and *arrows* indicate the direction or reciprocity of the relationship.

Functional Assessment

The functional assessment emphasizes the interaction among family members, assessing how members actually behave with each other. It focuses on the present, how the family is functioning now, although past history can be considered. The model includes two basic aspects of family functioning: instrumental and expressive. The instrumental aspect includes both activities of daily living (ADLs) and instrumental activities of daily living (IADLs). The nurse assesses the routines, patterns, behaviors, and interactions related to typical daily activities, such as hygiene, grooming, meal prep, laundry, sleeping, shopping, housework, medication administration, and how the family's current state of health and illness(es) are impacting instrumental family functioning. During the assessment, the nurse is identifying who is responsible for certain tasks, how well the tasks are being performed, if all family members ADLs and IADLs are being met, and if the division of labor is fair and reasonable.

The CFAM identifies several key subcategories of expressive function. A focal area is on family communication, which is influenced by culture, socioeconomic status, and family history. The community health nurse should use observations and effective questioning to assess the communication patterns of the family, including verbal and nonverbal behaviors. The nurse should be sensitive to how emotions are expressed among the family members, observing during interactions if a healthy range of emotions are accepted and supported or if emotional expression limited and suppressed. Additionally, the nurse should assess the meanings and messages in verbal communication: are they clear and direct, or are there concealed meanings, vague responses, and frequent misunderstandings? Nonverbal communication, such as facial expressions, body posture, and gestures can be detrimental to or supportive of family interactions and functioning. Table 13.1 describes each of the subcategories of expressive function and includes sample questions that could be used during the family assessment.

Developmental Assessment

The developmental assessment explores the evolving path the family goes through and the tasks that need to be addressed at key periods. Wright and Leahey (2013) distinguish between family development which "emphasizes the *unique* path constructed by a family" and "is shaped by predictable and unpredictable events" (p. 91) and family life cycle, which "refers to the *typical* path most families go through" (p. 91). Typical life-cycle events include birth, child-rearing, departure of children, retirement, and death. Historically, the sequence of stages had been fairly predictable, even with individual, cultural, and ethnic variations. However, more recently, sociocultural, economic, and other societal factors have increased the variety of family constellations and influenced family development and life cycle. Given that families present in various forms, community nurses should avoid a focus on universality and an expectation of smooth progression through stages. Family life is dynamic, filled with expansion and contraction (as members join or leave), joys and satisfactions, as well as stresses and conflicts. During these critical transitions, roles change resulting in a distinct change in the family life patterns. The nurse should individualize the assessment of the family's current stage and its ability to accomplish the tasks that will allow the family to continue on its unique developmental path.

Family Interventions: Calgary Family Intervention Model

The CFAM and the CFIM are closely integrated with areas of assessment and intervention overlapping. The therapeutic relationship established between the nurse and the family is central to both models. The **CFIM** focuses on enhancing, improving, and sustaining family functioning through the establishment of a collaborative partnership between the nurse and the family, the use of therapeutic conversations, and the focus on family strengths and resiliency (Bell, 2013, 2016; Ostlund & Persson, 2014; Persson & Benzein, 2014; Wright, 2015; Wright & Leahey, 2013). Interventions are not standardized or pre-planned; they are specific to each family context and are directed by the family's beliefs, preferences, behaviors, and experiences, as shared during nurse–family interactions and conversations. The nurse–family relationship, which is based on respect and trust, is integral to the interventions. The focus of interventions is on needed changes within three domains of family functioning, which would support the lessening of family suffering (difficulty) and the promotion of family healing and well-being related to the family experience of illness, injury, or disability. The three domains include cognitive, affective, and behavioral.

Cognitive domain is related to thinking and the need to gain new information and knowledge about a health problem affecting the family. The desired outcome of the cognitive domain is to change the way a family perceives its health problem so that members can discover new solutions. Studies found that family nursing interventions improved family members' understanding and increased their confidence and capability to live with illness. Families gained new and multiple perspectives and an enhanced adjustment (Bell, 2013, 2016; Ostlund & Persson, 2014; Persson & Benzein, 2014)

Affective domain is related to feelings and the need to reduce emotions that may be interfering with a family's ability to problem solve, cope, and heal, or the need to increase emotions that support family functioning within the illness experience. Studies found that family systems interventions softened suffering and increased a sense of individual and family well-being. The therapeutic conversation enhanced families' emotional engagement in problem solving as well as feelings of closeness and affirmation within family relationships (Bell, 2016; Bell & Wright, 2015; Ostlund, Backstrom, Lindh, Sundin, & Saveman, 2014; Perrson & Benzein, 2014).

Behavioral domain is related to action and doing and involves helping families change behaviors that may be detrimental to family functioning and promote behaviors that support healthy coping, adjustment, and family functioning.

TABLE 13.1 Calgary Family Assessment Model: Assessing Key Areas of Expressive Functions

Expressive Functions	Explanation	Questions to Ask
Emotional Communication	Range of emotions that family expresses, wide or narrow	How does your mother react when your father is angry? How do you know when your brother who has diabetes is happy? How is your family coping with the loss of your grandmother? Are you and your family members comfortable crying when you are sad?
Verbal Communication	The clarity and directness or masked meaning in a verbal interaction	When discussing family rules, who is the clearest and most direct? How do you respond when your father accuses you of being late?
Nonverbal Communication	Influenced by culture: eye contact, body posture, personal space, gestures, facial expressions, linked to emotional communication	How do you feel when your stepsister rolls her eyes when you are telling your mom that your migraine headaches have gotten worse?
Problem Solving	Involves behaviors, patterns, and resources the family uses to respond to and solve its own problems	What do you do when your baby won't fall asleep each night? How are you dealing with your mother's safety as her Alzheimer disease progresses? How did you respond when your brother told you he was being bullied at school?
Roles	Behaviors and responsibilities that serve to fulfill family functions	Who is most responsible for managing the house (shopping, cooking, cleaning)? When things go wrong, who usually gets blamed? You described your foster daughter as a perfect child; can you tell me what you mean? Who takes care of you when you are sick?
Influence and Power	Refers to the ability of one family member to persuade, pressure, negotiate, or control responses and behaviors of another member; relationship can be hierarchical or collaborative	Who is responsible for financial decisions? Who makes the decisions about mealtime, bedtime, use of electronic devices? Who decides on discipline for any family infractions? How are decisions made on things that affect most family members?
Beliefs	Refers to the values, attitudes, assumptions, and premises that guide individuals' and family's thoughts and behaviors; culture, socioeconomic status, and life experience influence beliefs	What is important to do to maintain your health? What do you think is the cause of your son's illness? How does your chronic pain affect the family? What do you think will improve your partner's asthma control?

Source: Wright, L. M., & Leahey, M. (2013). *Nurses and families: A guide to family assessment and intervention* (6th ed.). Philadelphia, PA: F.A. Davis.

Interventions are directed to help family members interact with and behave differently when relating to each other. Studies have found outcomes of family members acting in a more caring manner and being more supportive of each other, improving family communication, and identifying improved methods in coordinating care and completing family activities (Bell, 2016; Bell & Wright, 2015; Ostlund et al., 2014).

The therapeutic conversation provides family members the opportunity to hear each other's concerns, challenges, and strengths. The purpose of the conversation is to "create a context for change and to support the creation of new beliefs, new meanings, and opportunities in relation to problems described by the family, that is things hampering the family's health" (Ostlund et al., 2014, p. 582). The nurse's openness and interest encourages family members to ask questions and to share their experience. Each family member present is given time to describe his or her experience and perspective of the illness experience within the family context. The nurse's role is to listen and observe to gain a broad and deep understanding of the concerns, questions, emotions, behaviors, and interactions among family members. The family members and the nurse work collaboratively, identifying family strengths, resiliency, and resources. The nurse provides information, education, training and referral to community resources as indicated and found acceptable by the family.

Table 13.2 provides examples of interventions for each of the three domains of family functioning: cognitive, affective, and behavioral.

TABLE 13.2 Calgary Family Intervention Model

Domain of Family Functioning	Interventions	Advice for Interventions	Outcomes
Cognitive Domain	(a) Commend family and individual strengths by observing positive patterns of behavior (b) Offer information and opinions, including new ideas, and education on a specific health problem or risk	(a) Observe family for strengths in coping with health problems Communicate sincerity Begin and end family conversation with commendations (b) Use clear, relevant, understandable language Provide easily readable, written information Provide information on community services and resources Encourage family to respond to the information and opinions shared	(a) Focus on strengths and resiliency to promote families' positive self-view and self-efficacy Foster nurse–family relationship (b) Provide new ideas, information, and education to change the way the family thinks about the health problem and finds new and effective solutions
Affective Domain	(a) Acknowledge, validate, and normalize emotional (b) Encourage family members to share their unique experience with the illness or health condition (c) Establish emotional support to respond to family members' concerns and feelings	(a & b) Establish a safe environment and facilitate a family conversation in which all members can express their feelings, find support, and understand any negative impact (b) During the family conversation, ask each member to tell their specific experience in dealing with an illness in the family (c) Listen intently to family members' feelings and concerns, and observe for emotional support that family members are able to offer each other	(a) Reduce intense emotions that may be interfering with the family's ability to communicate and problem-solve (b) Gain a broad understanding of the illness experience for the family beyond the specific diagnosis and treatment (c) Identify emotional strengths that can support healthy coping and adjustment
Behavioral Domain	(a) Identify family caregivers and provide caregiver education and support (b) Encourage self-care and respite for the family caregiver (c) Assist the family in developing helpful daily rituals and routines	(a) Provide education on the illness Provide training on all caregiving tasks Observe the interactions between the care recipient and caregivers (b) Inform family of available community services (support groups, home health aids, daycare, respite facilities) Teach components of self-care (c) Assess typical pre-illness routines and rituals Work with family members to identify adjustments and new routines needed to deal with the illness or problem	(a) Improve understanding of the caregiver role, performance of caregiver tasks, and care for the recipient (b) Decrease caregiver burden and support caregiver health and well-being (c) Routines and rituals provide structure and organization and decrease stress

Source: Wright, L. M. & Leahey, M. (2013). *Nurses and families: A guide to family assessment and intervention* (6th ed.). Philadelphia, PA: F.A. Davis.

Practice Point

Establishing a nonhierarchical, nonjudgmental nurse–family relationship is foundational to the Calgary Family Assessment and Intervention Models and essential to family nursing practice.

Family Interview

As in other areas of clinical practice, community health nurses frequently have limited time for family assessments because of demanding caseloads or staffing shortages. It may not be reasonable or necessary to complete a comprehensive assessment following the CFAM. Additionally, focused family interviews of 15 minutes or less can yield a wealth of information (Box 13.2). The 15-Minute Family Interview, which is based on the CFAM and CFIM, offers a pragmatic framework for nurses to engage families in a purposeful, therapeutic interaction. Wright and Leahey (1999, 2005, 2009, 2013); (Duhamel, Dupuis, & Wright, 2009) suggest the following five leading principles, which maximize information gleaned in a 15-minute family interview:

- *Manners*: Common courtesies, such as the nurse introducing himself or herself to the family, indicate a desire to connect with the family and to instill trust in family members.
- *Use of therapeutic conversation*: When time is limited, purposeful and focused conversation helps build a relationship. Nurses validate family concerns with their active listening.
- *Ecomaps and genograms*: These tools are invaluable, especially when family members are likely to be involved with the care of another member.
- *Use of therapeutic questions*: Asking family members therapeutic questions helps them not only identify their expectations about nursing care but also assign priorities to their most urgent needs.
- *Commendations acknowledging family strengths*: Informing families about the assets and resources they already possess leads them to view their situation differently and makes them more likely to move toward more effective problem-solving.

Studies have supported the components of the 15-Minute Family Interview as a purposeful, effective, and efficient means of providing support to families (Bell, 2016; Holtslander, 2005; Holtslander, Solar, & Smith, 2013; Moules, & Johnstone, 2010; Ostlund et al., 2014; Ostlund, Backstrom, Saveman, Lindh, & Sundin, 2016; Persson & Benzein, 2014; Sveinbjarnardottir, Svaavarsdottir, & Wright, 2013; Yarwood, Richardson, & Watson, 2016). The guidelines for the 15-minute assessment (Wright & Leahey, 2005, 2009) are useful to help keep the interview focused and family-centered.

13.2 Key Points for a 15-Minute Family Assessment

- Show interest throughout.
- Keep body language relaxed.
- Face the family member when asking a question.
- Try to minimize writing while listening.
- Acknowledge the family's strengths.
- Share any genograms and ecomaps that illustrate relationships with family members.
- Ask family members for their interpretations/impressions (shared between the family and clinician).
- Avoid offering advice prematurely.
- Allow everyone present to voice observations, insights, or concerns before offering how they could change the situation.
- Ask the family if they see an area that could be changed.
- Plan goals and outcomes with the family.
- Forge a partnership with the family's full participation.
- Collaborate with the family to set priorities, plan care, and evaluate goals.

Source: Adapted from Wright, L., & Leahey, M. (2005). The three most common errors in family nursing: How to avoid or sidestep. *Journal of Family Nursing, 11*(2), 90–101.

Evidence for Practice

Holtslander and team (2013) wanted to find an effective educational strategy to integrate classroom learning in a family nursing course to a clinical practicum and to provide an authentic opportunity for student nurses to engage with families. To promote students' ability to develop interpersonal relationships and therapeutic communication, they implemented the use of the 15-Minute Family Interview in a clinical practicum. Students used all five components of the interview, and were surprised that families were willing and enthusiastic about participating in the interview. Students evaluated the use of this educational strategy through reflective papers and a course survey. By intentionally focusing on using manners, students realized that their respectful, thoughtful, and courteous approach developed a trusting relationship with the family that remained throughout the day. Students reported being more conscientious about not interrupting the family members as they spoke and interacted. They were surprised that simple gestures, such as calling each member by name, were so appreciated. While establishing a brief therapeutic conversation, students realized the value of listening actively, giving undivided attention, showing genuine concern, and making an effort to connect with the family and understand the suffering that the illness has caused throughout the family. Completing the genogram and ecomap at the beginning of the interview engaged all members of the family and provided foundational information that guided the remainder of the interview.

One family was hesitant to complete the tools, and the student learned that they were afraid as they felt that their family structure varied from the norm and that they might be judged harshly. One mother who was quite fearful and stressed about her daughter's illness felt reassured after completing the genogram and ecomap that she had many family and community supports that could assist her with her daughter's care. Students are frequently concerned about asking the right questions, and faculty reminded them that a primary goal of the therapeutic questions were to "meet the family's needs for information, referrals, acknowledgement, and involvement as caregivers" (Holtslander et al., 2013, p. 240). Using a variety of questions (direct, open-ended and circular), students gained confidence in facilitating the interview, making it individualized to the family's context and needs.

Students also realized that the interview provided a valuable opportunity to observe family communication and differences in their personality and perspectives. Family members can be quite fatigued, distressed, and demoralized as they struggle to deal with the multiple stressors that accompany a family member's illness or injury. Acknowledging the challenges the family faces while also recognizing the strengths and resources that the family possesses provided family members with a sense that they had the ability to cope, change, and find solutions to the current problems they were facing. In their reflection papers, students reported that following the interview components provided a deeper understanding of the family's needs and priorities, which then guided their ability to provide therapeutic family-focused intervention and care. Clinical faculty found that use of the interview helped move students from only focusing on and providing care to the individual patient to addressing the needs and concerns of the whole family.

Review the components of the 15-Minute Family Interview, is this something that you could use in your community health clinical setting to provide more family-focused care?

FSN and the CFAM and CFIM emphasize the centrality of the nurse–family relationship and how the relationship can be used therapeutically to improve and sustain family development and functioning, and ultimately family health and well-being. The typical settings in which community health nurses practice (home, schools, public health departments, and community-based clinics and organizations), support a family focus and allow more continuing care and the structure to establish a committed and longer-term relationship.

HOW COMMUNITY HEALTH NURSES SUPPORT FAMILIES

Focusing on individual illness or health needs often obscures or omits the influence of the family. Community health nurses encounter family health concerns in a wide range of circumstances. Therefore, community health nurses provide family-focused care to family units, for example, who are dealing with pregnancy and childrearing, an acute illness or injury of a family member, a chronic illness of a family member, or end-of-life care to a family member. Community health nurses have an advantage in providing family-focused care as many community health nurses make home visits. Home visiting allows the nurse to observe and assess the family in their natural setting. Several generations may live in a single household. For example, a teen mom might share a home with her parent(s), or a grandparent with early signs of dementia might live with his or her children and their families. Observation of interpersonal dynamics in these intergenerational households during family assessment can provide much insight into patterns of coping and communication within the family.

Diversity embraces every aspect of family life and finds expression in family history, heritage, and language, as well as in the ways that families manifest and maintain health. Understanding diversity in individual families emphasizes the need for community health nurses to pay close attention to various dimensions of family life. Patterns of everyday family life are likely to change if a family member has to assume full-time or part-time responsibility for the care of another family member. Cultural considerations related to ethnicity, religion, and language figure prominently; however, generational difference and lifestyle choices also contribute significantly to diversity among and within families.

Home visiting programs by community and public health nurses have proven beneficial for family nursing provided to vulnerable populations, such as pregnant women and their young children (Davis, & Gufstafson, 2014; Dmytryshyn et al., 2015; Garcia, McNaughton, Radosevich, Brandt, Monsen, 2013; Jack et al., 2015; Jean-Baptiste et al., 2017; Olds, 2006, 2012). Community and public health nurses are strong advocates for maternal-child and family health.

Your children are not your children. They are the sons and daughters of Life's longing for itself. They came through you but not from you and though they are with you yet they belong not to you. **Khalil Gibran**

Family-Focused Home Visiting in Community-Based Maternal-Child Health

Pregnancy is a developmental event in families. Whether a pregnant woman is an adolescent or an adult, accessible high-quality prenatal and postpartum care is essential to prevent a host of negative short- and long-term outcomes. Infant mortality rates in the United States are considered high for an industrialized country, and low birth weight continues to be directly related to poverty more than any other variable (Meade & Ickovics, 2005). Prevention initiatives are essential to respond to situations that are threatening to the mother, child, father, and extended family engaged in the prospective birth and in learning nurturing parenting skills. Efforts to prevent substance use, including alcohol, during pregnancy are vitally important (Koniak-Griffin, Anderson, Verzemnieks, & Brecht, 2000). Finally, pregnant adolescents need support from their families and schools because teen pregnancy is a distinct predictor of poverty, intrafamily conflict, substance use disorder, and violence (Pickett, Mookherjee, & Wilkinson, 2005). Early intervention programs in which nurses establish a trusting relationship and provide prenatal care, emotional support and counseling, and parenting skill education have promoted individual and family health and positive development.

Nurse–Family Partnership is an evidence-based, community health program focused on promoting maternal and child health for vulnerable low-income expectant first-time mothers (including adolescent mothers) and their newborns. Each expectant mother is paired early in her pregnancy with a community health nurse, who provides ongoing home visits until the child's second birthday. The program design and implementation is based on over 30 years of research, including several randomized controlled trials, which have examined both short- and long-term outcomes in mother, child, and family health and well-being. Based on the evidence of success, the program has been replicated throughout the United States (Olds, 2006, 2012; Olds et al., 2013) and also internationally in Canada (Dmytryshyn et al., 2015; Jack et al., 2015), the United Kingdom (Rowe, 2013; Smyth & Anderson, 2014), Australia, and New Zealand (Fowler et al., 2012).

The following are the three major goals for the Nurse–Family Partnership Program:

- To improve pregnancy outcomes by helping women engage in good preventive health practices
- To improve child health and development by helping parents provide responsible and competent care
- To improve the economic self-sufficiency of families by helping parents develop a vision for their own future, plan future pregnancies, continue their education, and find work

The program is funded by a range of private and public sources (services are free), and it is offered in 42 states in the United States. It has served 280,487 families since its inception in 1996 and currently has 33,804 families enrolled with 1,888 nurses providing the home visits (Nurse-Family Partnership [NFP], 2018). Throughout the home visits, the nurses focus on three major interventions: (a) promoting behaviors (new mother and other family members) which positively affect pregnancy outcomes, the child's health and development, and the parents' life course (future pregnancy decisions, education, and work); (b) guiding the women in establishing supportive relationships with family members and friends; and (c) connecting the women and their family members with needed health, educational, work-related, and social services. The program is family-centered and strength-based such that the nurses approach the interventions in ways that are consistent with the parents' values, beliefs, and aspirations and build on the parents' and family's assets. The nurse facilitates the parents' belief in their ability to change while focusing on understanding the family circumstances and views.

Multiple studies have revealed positive multigenerational outcomes that benefit individuals, families, and communities, and reduce the costs of long-term social service programs. Positive outcomes reported when compared to a control group include decreased pre-term and low-weight births, increased breastfeeding, improvements in up-to-date immunizations by 6 months of age (NFP, 2018); improved prenatal nutrition and decrease in smoking, increased informal support and improved use of formal community services (Olds, 2006); sensitive, competent care of the child with a decrease in injuries, emergency room visits, and child maltreatment (Olds, 2006), and regarding the parental life course, fewer subsequent pregnancies with longer intervals between the first and second children, greater participation in the workforce, and less dependence on entitlement programs (welfare, food stamps).

> What is home? My favorite definition is "a safe place," a place where one is free from attack, a place where one experiences secure relationships and affirmation. It's a place where people share and understand each other. Its relationships are nurturing. The people in it do not need to be perfect; instead, they need to be honest, loving, supportive, recognizing a common humanity that makes all of us vulnerable. **Gladys M. Hunt**

 ## Evidence for Practice

The family–nurse relationship, which is developed through respect and trust and focused on strengths and collaboration, is foundational to family nursing practice. The relationship is critical to guiding the family through the necessary changes to promote positive family functioning and health. Aston and colleagues (2015) explored how public health nurses (PHNs) supported mothers and families during postpartum home visits. The researchers recruited 16 nurses who worked in the postpartum home visiting program (range 2.5 to 12 years working in the program) and 16 mothers who received the home visits. The mothers ranged in age from 18 to 38 years of age, were first-time mothers, and most lived in urban areas. Individual semi-structured interviews were conducted in a private office at work for the PHNs and in their home for the mothers. Open-ended questions were used to encourage participants to share their perspective on the home visiting experience. A core finding was the importance of establishing a positive relationship beginning with the initial phone call and continuing throughout all the home visits. The nonhierarchical, therapeutic relationship fostered the formation of trust and allowed significant learning, acquisition of parenting skills, and necessary changes to occur within a supportive environment. The mothers admitted that they were initially fearful of being judged by an authority figure as inadequate as a new mother.

The findings provided insight into the "how to" of relationship development. It was important that the PHNs present as friendly and approachable, not as distant and controlling. Being aware of the power dynamic was critical so that the PHNs did not use a directive, invasive approach as the expert but genuinely were open to and fostered an authentic, collaborative relationship. The nurses encouraged the mother to lead the visits so that the focus was on her needs at the time, and that she was viewed as the expert of her baby. Although the program had specific topics that had to be addressed during the visits, the nurses did not present them in a prescriptive manner but remained flexible and let the mothers' and the families' needs dictate what was addressed at each visit. The PHNs reported using a strength-based interactional process, as opposed to a deficit model, and the mothers verified the significance of this. They never felt criticized or demeaned. The PHNs intentionally chose the words they used, the timing of interventions, and teaching strategies employed so that they built confidence, competence, and self-esteem and promoted positive family functioning and development. The study's findings supported the major premises of family systems nursing practice and the Calgary Family Models.

I sustain myself with the love of family. **Maya Angelou**

Family Caregivers: In Need of Education and Support

When illness or disability becomes part of a family experience, community health nurses distinguish themselves as facilitators by helping both the family unit and individual family members to find balance. Whether caring for an older adult who has functionally declined due to chronic comorbidities such as diabetes and heart failure or a neurodegenerative condition, such as Alzheimer's disease, **caregiver burden** has been well documented in the literature as a significant stressor on the family member who assumes primary responsibility for care (Easom, Cotter, & Ramos, 2018; Spurlock, 2005). In most cultures, women (mothers, wives, sisters, daughters, or female in-laws) have assumed this role, usually by default. Caregiver burden is a significant issue for families because it can cause the development of physical or emotional illness in the caregiver over time (Blair & Perry, 2017; Caceres & Perez, 2018; Friedemann, & Buckwalter, 2014). Caregivers might express feeling trapped, isolated, and overwhelmed with no possible help with care. In addition, caring for a family member can lead to financial and work strain in some circumstances. An important consideration is that, although caregiver burden

does exist, caregivers articulate their desire to provide caregiving in grateful appreciation for what the recipient has done for them in the past. Expression of positive feelings and the privilege connected with caring for another is plentiful in the literature (Baker, 2018; Lund, 2005). Yet, caregiver burden inevitably affects the dynamic of the entire family unit and is considered **intrafamily strain** (Baker, 2018; Friedemann, & Buckwalter, 2014).

Family Caregiver Characteristics and Needs

More attention is being directed at the role and challenges related to informal family caregiving, as the older adult population, many of whom suffer from debilitating chronic conditions, continues to increase. Family members are expected to assume more responsibility in their care. To help understand the complexity of caregiving in the U.S. population, the American Association of Retired Persons completed an extensive study, which provided valuable findings for healthcare providers and public policy makers (AARP, 2015). An estimated 43.5 million adults in the United States provide unpaid care to an adult or a child. The estimated prevalence of caring for an adult is 16.6%, or 39.8 million Americans, of whom approximately 34.2 million provide unpaid care to an adult aged 50 or older. The majority of caregivers are female (60%), but male family caregivers are increasing and now account for 40%. Almost half (48%) of family caregivers are providing care to a parent or parent-in-law. On average, caregivers spend 24 hours a week providing care to the family member, however, spouse/partner caregivers, considered higher-hour caregivers, typically provide 45 hours a week (AARP, 2015). Higher-hour caregivers are a vulnerable population as they characteristically experience higher levels of emotional stress, physical impact, and financial strain, which collectively affect their health and well-being (Cohen, Cook, Sando, Brown, & Longo, 2017). Family caregivers perform a wide range of care tasks, including personal hygiene and grooming, meal preparation, housework, errands, transportation, coordination of healthcare, and complex nursing tasks. Many care providers are also trying to balance other aspects of their life, such as work, child care, and their own home maintenance. In addition, care providers report feeling ill-prepared to assume all the responsibilities, particularly coordinating healthcare and assuming responsibility to perform nursing tasks. They report that information and teaching from healthcare providers were lacking or inadequate.

Reinhard, Levine, and Samis (2012) published results from their survey of 1,677 family caregivers that exposed the challenges they faced in providing more complex care to family members suffering from serious chronic conditions. The findings of this report prompted public policy and legislative action in the form of the Caregiver Advise, Record, and Enable (CARE) Act. Within three years of the publication of this report, 39 states had enacted this legislation that involves the family caregiver from the point of hospital admission, through adequate notice of and preparation for discharge home (Gould, 2018). This act stipulates that hospitals participate in very specific exchanges with family caregivers on the patient's behalf in order to collect information and provide education. Under this law, hospitals must do the following:

1. Record the name of the family caregivers in the patient's medical record at the point of admission.
2. Inform the identified family caregivers when the patient is to be discharged, providing adequate notice.
3. Provide the family caregivers with education and live instruction to prepare them for undertaking medical/ nursing tasks on behalf of the discharged patient. (Gould, 2018)

This may seem like a simple or even obvious addition to standard healthcare practices, but it represents an acknowledgement that caregivers are significant and relevant to a person's transition home and overall health management. Family caregivers need detailed discharge teaching related to coordination of care and the specific tasks that they will be providing.

Home Health Nurses and Family Caregivers

The *American Journal of Nursing* has assumed a leadership role in efforts toward educating nurses to provide improved support to family caregivers through the development and dissemination of *Supporting Family Caregivers: No Longer Home Alone*, a series of articles with the purpose of helping nurses provide caregivers with the tools they need to manage their family member's healthcare at home. The series includes topics such as discharge planning and teaching, medication administration and management, home safety and fall prevention, ostomy, skin, and wound care, and was produced in cooperation with the AARP Public Policy Institute. Each article includes an informational handout and links to instructional videos. The series was published between 2017 and 2018, and is available at https://journals.lww.com/ajnonline/pages/collectiondetails.aspx?TopicalCollectionId=38.

Family caregivers are critical to the ability of family members to remain at home and to have their ADLs and specific healthcare needs met. However, assuming this role can put a strain on individual family members and overall family communication and functioning. Home health nurses can serve an essential role in providing education, training, and support to family caregivers. In addition to teaching family members how to provide the needed care, home health nurses can assist families dealing with challenging caregiving issues to avoid or resolve family conflict, stress, burden, and burnout. Caregivers are diverse, varying in age, gender, race, ethnicity, and socioeconomic status (Cohen et al., 2017). Although they may share some commonalities in the challenges they face and the positive aspects they experience, caregivers may encounter different burdens based on their circumstances. Based on the care recipient's condition and needs and the caregiver's own problems and resources, different education, services, and support may be required. A recent study demonstrated that family caregivers beyond expending substantial time and effort in providing care, also spend significant amount of their own money, adding financial stress (Rainville, Skufca, & Mehegan, 2016). The authors found that in 2016, family caregivers spent approximately $7,000 on caregiving expenses, accounting on average to 20% of their total income. In addition, caregivers experience work strain and personal strain related to their finances. More than half of the caregivers in the study reported at least one work-related strain, such as reducing or changing their hours and taking paid or unpaid time off. To meet these additional financial obligations, caregivers were decreasing their own personal spending, using savings, and reducing retirement contributions (Rainville et al., 2016).

Certain groups of caregivers face a disproportionate burden in caregiving. Community health nurses need to be aware of these higher-risk caregivers. For example, there has been increased interest in and concern for Latino family caregivers. Latino older adults experience health disparities, suffering from a disproportionate burden of chronic illnesses, such as diabetes, cardiovascular diseases, and an increasing prevalence of Alzheimer disease and other dementias. Latino older adults are also economically disadvantaged; 70% of Latino adults who are 65 and older have incomes less than two times the supplemental poverty threshold (Gould & Cooper, 2013). Many Latino older adults live with their children or extended family. Twenty-one percent of the estimated 40 million family caregivers are Latino (AARP, 2017). Given cultural values and expectations, Latino older adults are typically cared for by Latina female family members and are much less apt to be aware of or to seek assistance outside of the family (Caceres & Perez, 2018; Cruz-Oliver, Parikh, Wallace, Malmstrom, Sanchez-Reilly, 2018). These family caregivers spend 44% of their annual income on caregiving related expenses (more than double the average) and provide 52% more time on weekly caregiving when compared to the caregiver population (Rainville et al., 2016). The National Hispanic Council on Aging (2017) completed a survey on caregiving in the Latino population and asked about the challenges the caregivers face. The top three challenges included (a) balancing family caregiving and personal responsibilities (64%), (b) problems understanding governmental insurance and assistance programs (56%), and (c) locating information and resources that would assist with their caregiving (47%). Half of the respondents reported that they lacked training and would benefit from formal information and training on caregiving, and stress management. The nurse needs to be aware that the needs of family caregivers can vary based on race, ethnicity, gender, and socioeconomic status, with some groups at risk for higher burden and burnout.

Through family assessment, home health nurses can identify areas of teaching, training and referral, which will benefit both the care recipient and the caregiver and overall family functioning. Using the 15-Minute Family Interview could help the nurse establish trust and rapport; encourage

13.3 Resources for Family Caregivers and Care Recipients

Caregiver support groups
Stress management programs
Individual and family counseling
Home delivered meals
Adult daycare programs
Homemakers
Home health aides
Companions
Assisted living
Nursing homes
Transportation services
Information on Medicare and Medicaid
Information on fuel assistance and SNAP benefits
   (food stamps)
Grocery delivery services
Mail order pharmacy services

family members (care recipient and care provider) to openly share their needs, concerns, and frustrations; prioritize needs (information and training); and acknowledge their strengths and efforts. Using the genogram, the nurse and family could recognize other family members who may be able to assist and how roles and responsibilities could be better distributed. Using the ecomap would reveal any external resource connections that the family may have and then assist the nurse in making recommendations and referrals for other services that could assist the family. Improving a family's understanding of available services and community resources and how to apply for them is an important aspect of the home health nurse's role. Box 13.3 lists several of the important services and resources of which the home health nurse should be knowledgeable and able to discuss with family members.

The nurse could facilitate periodic family meetings and conversations that allow family members to express their feelings about the caregiving, assess the effectiveness of their communication related to caregiving needs, prioritize the multiple demands, organize the required tasks, develop a caregiving schedule (that avoids duplication and gaps), and identify helpful community resources.

During home visits, the nurse could provide teaching on the family member's condition so that the caregiver is aware of signs and symptoms of decline, how to follow the plan of care, and who to contact when a symptom occurs. In addition, the nurse is able to provide training on home safety, medication administration, personal care, specialized feedings, wound and ostomy care, and any other typical nursing tasks that the caregiver is now providing. Providing feedback on the caregiver's performance of the skills and expressing confidence in his or her ability to learn and safely perform the needed nursing tasks will promote the caregiver's sense of self-efficacy.

Helping family caregivers understand that self-care is essential for them to maintain their physical and emotional well-being, to balance all of their responsibilities, and to sustain their role and functioning as a care provider. The family caregiver needs to understand the importance of period of respite, when he or she can have a break from responsibilities, either through in-home services (homemaker, home health aid) or out-of-home services (adult daycare, overnight residential facilities). The home health nurse can encourage both the caregiver and the care recipient of the need for respite services, and facilitate the referral for the appropriate ones.

The home health nurse is well positioned to address the needs of family caregivers through the provision of emotional support, care coordination, didactic teaching, task training, and resource referral.

Evidence for Practice

All caregivers, and in particular caregivers for family members who have dementia, need respite from their caregiving functions. Caregiving for a family member with dementia has a lengthy trajectory (five years or more) and involves continual functional decline, with increasing occurrence of difficult behaviors. Understanding the need for and seeking respite is essential for continued caregiving survival.

Easom and team (2018) studied self-efficacy, defined as "the degree to which one is motivated to take action" (p. 16) in relation to seeking respite care among a sample of family caregivers of family members with Alzheimer's disease. The researchers wanted to examine if an intervention led to any differences in self-efficacy between African American and Caucasian caregivers. The study was based on the Resources for Enhancing Alzheimer Caregiver Health (REACH II), a randomized controlled trial that evaluated a multicomponent, evidence-based intervention for caregivers of individuals with dementia. The intervention involved individualized education, support and stress management skills through home visits, and telephone contact over a six-month period.

The current study is a translation of the clinical trial in a community setting, which followed all the previous study's protocols and measurements but did not include a control group. The researchers used a pre- and post-test design with self-efficacy measured using the Revised Scale for Caregiving Self-Efficacy, at the first home visit (baseline) and at the last home visit (program's end). The scale has a 15-item checklist used to measure caregiver confidence in caregiving skills. The higher the score, the higher self-efficacy. The subscale for self-efficacy included obtaining respite. The intervention was completed by 123 caregivers, including 66 African American and 49 Caucasian participants. Both groups showed significant improvements in self-efficacy related to obtaining respite. Of note, although the percentage of change in self-efficacy score was the same in both groups, the African American caregivers both began the study and ended it with higher levels of self-efficacy. The study demonstrates that self-efficacy in obtaining respite, an important skill relative to maintaining the caregiver's well-being and ability to sustain caregiving can be enhanced for different racial groups through a tailored intervention. The authors recommend further research to study individual components of the intervention to determine if improvement is related to specific components.

CASE STUDY 1

Both Tanya and Luke Barnes have been sleeping poorly at night. They have not received any e-mails or phone calls from their mother for 10 days. Lately, they show little interest in school or other activities they usually enjoy. They constantly ask Elsa and her husband when they will hear from their mother. One afternoon before the children returned from school, an army chaplain visits the home to inform the family that Elaine has been severely wounded in a mortar attack. Elsa phones Lucy immediately and asks, "What do I do now?"

- Thinking about the Calgary Family Assessment Model, which areas would be most important for the nurse to assess?
- Using the Calgary Family Intervention Model" Affective Domain, what therapeutic questions and interventions could the nurse use to help Tanya and Luke express and cope with their emotions, after hearing about their mother's injury?
- Use an ecomap to identify the family's probable connections with the community (school, medical care, church, etc.). Which connections should be aware of the children's situation? What community resources could the nurse identify to assist the family?

CASE STUDY 2

Laura arranged a meeting at Jim's home with his family, Arlene, and Nancy, the social worker assigned to the case. Jim took everyone to see the new facility. Arlene would eat breakfast and lunch at a day program from 7:30 to 4:00 on weekdays and have dinner with the family. Arlene was unhappy with the plan because she does not want to leave her "home." Jim's daughters were also upset about their aunt moving into their home and said their life will not be "normal" anymore.

Later that week, Laura phoned Jim and Liz to tell them that several vacancies have opened in a residential community. Several of Arlene's friends are moving there. Although Arlene would receive a small subsidy to move into the facility, the family would have to pay approximately $2,000 a month for expenses.

Jim wants to talk to his sisters, especially because their parents' health is declining. The elder Thomases receive homemaker services through their town's council on aging. Mrs. Thomas's dementia is advancing, and she might need placement in an Alzheimer care facility. Mr. Thomas receives a monthly pension, and his savings are limited.

The three Thomas siblings have had difficulty trying to agree on care arrangements for both their parents and older sister. The elder of the two, Marilyn, 55 years old, strongly opposes placement. Their sister Alice, 50 years old, is relatively indifferent. Use the Calgary Family Assessment and Intervention Models and 15-Minute Family Interview as guides when thinking about your responses to the following questions:

- Describe strategies for an open conversation at a family meeting. How would the nurse intervene in the cognitive, affective, and behavioral domains (to provide information, address feelings and emotions, and identify needed actions).
- What are the family caregiver issues related to Arlene and Mrs. Thomas? How can the nurse assist the family with distributing the tasks, and assuring quality care?
- Identify the factors that will affect the Thomas siblings' decisions about placement for their mother and sister.
- What approaches could help the Thomas family learn about possible placement options?
- Identify social factors that might influence the Thomas family's decision-making.
- What type of community resources could help the Thomas family cope with care and financial issues?
- How would you support Arlene during the decision-making process?

As illustrated in the two case studies, illness, disability, and death can affect family structure (the head of the household), function (decision-making), and outcomes (economic stability) both positively and negatively, in a variety of ways, (Mactavish & Schleien, 2004; Maes, Broekman, Dosen, & Nauts, 2003; McIntyre, Blacher, & Baker, 2002; Williams et al., 2002).

Happy families are all alike; every unhappy family is unhappy in its own way. **Leo Tolstoy**

Practice Point

Education, training, and support by nurses are essential to effective family caregiving. Family caregivers need encouragement to use community and respite services to reduce their burden and allow for self-care so that they can continue their caregiving responsibilities.

 Student Reflection

Throughout my nursing program, I have struggled to find a balance between being a student and a nurse. After my community health clinical practice, I am struck by the difficulty families have in making decisions for one another, even if it's in their best interest. Today, I worked with an 84-year-old woman who was discharged from the hospital after treatment for a fall at home. She cannot remember what happened right before she fell, but her doctors suspected that she had a mild seizure or stroke. The nurse at the center let me come along on a visit to the woman's home last week to assess home safety. The woman's children are concerned about her living alone, and until now, they have been reluctant to talk about alternative living arrangements.

At the family meeting, the woman's doctor said that it was in the family's best interest to consider assisted living arrangements because of Mrs. J.'s impaired mobility and decreased cognitive status. Both her social worker and community health nurse expressed that the family needed more time to make a decision. Her adult children said that they could see the advantages of assisted living. They worry about their mother's safety living alone and want to make sure that she is safe and has some independence, and they would like to visit a local facility. As a student nurse, I thought this situation was difficult. Clearly, the decision to move a parent into an assisted living facility is complicated, but I observed that the goal of the meeting was to help them make an informed decision and support them through the process. I realized how difficult it was for adult children to make decisions on their parents' behalf. I can't imagine having to do that for my mom or dad. Every family has a different way of dealing with difficult situations. As I develop as a nurse, I have to remember that everyone I care for has someone to call family, and learn how to meet individual and family needs. Experience will help me master this skill.

COMMUNITY HEALTH NURSES' RESPONSIBILITY TO FAMILIES

Family configurations and life cycles have changed due to the influence of sociocultural and economic factors. Community health nurses need to gain a theoretical understanding of family and of the contemporary changes in family structure, function, and development. In fulfilling their responsibility to provide family-focused care, community health nurses must develop family nursing competencies, provide care to the family as a unit, and understand the critical importance of the nurse–family relationship in family nursing practice.

Working with families frequently requires community health nurses to be creative when planning interventions. Family assessment, using a structured guide, such as the 15-Minute Family Interview, provides a good starting point, which enables nurses to explore a family's practices and priorities related to health and wellness. The ultimate goal should be to enable the family to identify its health needs and to help them choose the best way they can meet the needs and any required change. In this instance, a community health nurse's responsibility is to listen and facilitate building consensus within the family. The Calgary Family Assessment and Intervention Models provide evidence-based guidance on completing a family assessment and offering family interventions.

Community health nurses are known for being resourceful. Sharing information about available agencies and relevant resources will help families meet their health goals. Actions could be as simple as providing internet websites or as complex as finding all the resources needed by family caregivers.

Most importantly, community health nurses have a responsibility to advocate for families. A primary challenge is to promote health and wellness within the family. The two overarching goals of *Healthy People 2020* (CDC, 2011) are to improve the quality and years of healthy life and to eliminate health disparities. Community health nurses often intervene on a family's behalf to make sure that families receive access to optimal healthcare. Families often need assistance to navigate the healthcare system, especially when the family is unfamiliar with the setting or trying to cope with illness or crisis that disrupts everyday life.

 Practice Point

The responsibilities of community health nurses to families are to provide theory-guided and evidence-based family assessment and intervention to promote family health and well-being.

KEY CONCEPTS

- Family nursing practice acknowledges the interrelatedness of the health of the family and its individual members. In providing care for both the family and its individual members, a therapeutic nurse–family relationship is essential.
- Community health nurses need to be knowledgeable about changes in family structure and lifestyle based on sociocultural and economic factors.
- The Calgary Family Assessment and Intervention Clinical Models and 15-Minute Family Interview provide theoretical and practical guidance for providing family nursing care.

- Home visiting programs by nurses support nurse–family relationships, and promote maternal-child family health.
- Family caregiver burden and stress is a major problem for families. Home health nurses can provide the education, training, referral and support necessary to improve care for the recipient, sustain family caregiving, and promote self-care for the caregiver.

CRITICAL THINKING QUESTIONS

1. Consider a family from your clinical practice that is different in some way from your own. Discuss the challenges of working with the family and describe how you were able to support them. Write a short paragraph about something you learned from that experience. Include an action that you might approach differently if you were in a similar situation again.

2. Draw an ecomap for a family that you recently encountered. Identify what could be an obstacle to that family's health. Discuss how limitations in a family could be made more positive, and how using the ecomap would be helpful.

3. Family assessment can be challenging, often because of time constraints. Describe how you could gather valuable information about a family in the following situations, use the 15-Minute Family Interview to guide you:

   a. A student's aunt who comes to the school health office to take her nephew home because of head lice

   b. A single father who brings his toddler to the clinic because of an earache

   c. Two married adult daughters of an elderly woman with dementia during a home visit

   d. An elderly man who never married visits the local senior center for a blood pressure check

4. Describe a situation from clinical experience in which a family's culture influenced how they approached healthcare. Include factors that affected interaction, for example, language barriers.

5. Discuss how unexpected life crises, catastrophic illness, and chronic illness affect families. Use examples from your clinical experience to illustrate the ways that the nurse–family relationship can support family coping and functioning with these events.

6. Use pertinent components of the Calgary Family Assessment and Intervention Models to assess and intervene with a family from your clinical practice.

REFERENCES

American Association of Retired Persons (AARP). (2015). *Caregiving in the U.S.* Retrieved from https://www.aarp.org/content/dam/aarp/ppi/2015/caregiving-in-the-united-states-2015-report-revised.pdf

American Association of Retired Persons (AARP). (2017). AARP launches major effort to raise awareness on the impact of family caregiving on U.S. Latinos. Retrieved from https://states.aarp.org/aarp-to-raise-awareness-about-latino-family-caregiving/

Abraham, M., & Moretz, J. G. (2012). Implementing patient-and family-centered care: Part I-understanding the challenges. *Pediatric Nursing, 38*(1), 44.

America's Children. (2017). Key national indicators of well-being. *Federal Interagency Forum on Child and Family Statistics.* Retrieved from https://www.childstats.gov/pdf/ac2017/ac_17.pdf

America Counts Staff. (2017). Living with mothers only is second-most common. US Census. Retrieved from https://www.census.gov/library/stories/2017/08/majority-of-children-live-with-two-parents.html

American Nurses Association (ANA). (2010). Nursing's social policy statement: The essence of the profession. Silver Spring, MD: ANA Publishing.

Aston, M., Price, S., Etowa, J., Vukic, A., Young, L., Hart, C., … Randel, P. (2015). The power of relationships: Exploring how public health nurses support mothers and families during postpartum home visits. *Journal of Family Nursing, 21*(1), 11–34.

Baker, K. A. (2018). Focus on family caregivers [Editorial]. *Society of Gastroenterology Nurses, 41*(1), 10–12.

Bassuk, E. L., & Beardslee, W. R. (2014). Depression in homeless mothers: Addressing and unrecognized public health issue. *American Journal of Orthopsychiatry, 84*(10), 73–81.

Bell, J. M. (2009). Family systems nursing: Reexamined [Editorial]. *Journal of Family Nursing, 15*(2), 123–129.

Bell, J. M. (2013). Family nursing is more than family centered care. *Journal of Family Nursing, 19*(4), 411–417.

Bell, J. M. (2016). The central importance of therapeutic conversations in family nursing: Can talk be healing? *Journal of Family Nursing, 22*(4), 439–449.

Bell, J. M., Wright, L. M. (2015). The illness beliefs model: Advancing practice knowledge about illness beliefs, family healing, and family interventions [Editorial]. *Journal of Family Nursing, 21*(2), 179–185.

Blair, M., & Perry, B. (2017). Family caregiving and compassion fatigue: A literature review. *The Journal of Gerontological Nursing Association, 39*(2), 14–19.

Brush, B. L., Gultekin, L. E., & Grim, E. C. (2016). The data dilemma in family homelessness. *Journal of Health Care for the Poor and Underserved, 27*(3), 1046–1052.

Brush, B. L., Gultekin, L. E., Dowdell, E. B., Saint Arnault, D. M., & Satterfield, K. (2017). Understanding trauma normativeness, normalization, and help seeking in homeless mothers. violence against women. *Violence Against Women, 24*(13):1523–1539.

Caceres, B. A., & Perez, A. (2018). Implications of the CARE act for Latino caregivers. *Journal of Gerontological Nursing, 44*(3), 9–14.

Centers for Disease Control and Prevention (CDC). (2011). Healthy People 2020. Retrieved from http://www.cdc.gov/nchs/healthy_people/hp2020.htm

Cohen, S. A., Cook, S. K., Sando, T. A., Brown, M. J., Longo, D. R. (2017). Socioeconomic and demographic disparities in caregiving intensity and quality of life in informal caregivers. *Journal of Gerontological Nursing, 43*(6), 17–24.

Cruz-Oliver, D. M., Parikh, M., Wallace, C. L., Malmstrom, T. K., Sanchez-Reilly, S. (2018). What did Latino family caregivers expect and learn from education intervention: "Caregivers like me"? *American Journal of Hospice and Palliative Care Medicine, 35*(3), 404–410.

Davis, R. A., & Gustafson, D. T. (2014). Academic-practice partnerships in public health nursing: Working with families in a village-based collaboration. *Public Health Nursing, 32*(4), 327–338.

Dmytryshyn, A. L., Jack, S. M., Ballantyne, M., Wahoush, O, MacMillan, H. L. (2015). Long-term home visiting with vulnerable young mothers: Am interpretive description of the impact on public health nurses. *BMC Nursing, 14*(12), 1–14.

Duhamel, F., Dupuis, F., & Wright, L. (2009). Families' and nurses' responses to the "One question": Reflections for clinical practice, education and research in family nursing. *Journal of Family Nursing, 15*(4), 461–485.

Duvall, E. M. (1977). *Marriage and family development*. Philadelphia, PA: J.B. Lippincott.

Duvall, E. M., & Miller, B. (1985). *Marriage and family development* (6th ed.). New York: Harper & Row.

Easom, L., Cotter, E., & Ramos, A. (2018). Comparison of African American and Caucasian caregiver self-efficacy. *Journal of Gerontological Nursing, 44*(3), 16–21.

Ferrell, B., & Wittenberg, E. (2017). A review of family caregiving intervention trials in oncology. *CA: Cancer Journal for Clinicians, 67*(4), 318–325.

Forum on Child and Family Statistics. (2017). America's Children. Retrieved from https://www.childstats.gov/americaschildren/index.asp

Fowler, C., Rossiter, C., Bigsby, M., Hopwood, N., Lee, A., & Dunston, R. (2012). Working in partnership with parents: The experience and challenge of practice innovation in child and family health nursing. *Journal of Clinical Nursing, 21*(21–22), 3306–3314.

Friedemann, M. L., & Buckwalter, K. C. (2014). Family caregiver role and burden related to gender and family relationships. *Journal of Family Nursing, 20*(3), 313–336.

Friedman, M. M. (1998). *Family nursing practice*. Stamford, CT: Appleton & Lange.

Friedman, M. M., Bowden, V. R., & Jones, E. G. (2003). *Family nursing: Research, theory and practice* (5th ed.). Upper Saddle River, NJ: Prentice Hall.

Garcia, C., McNaughton, D., Radosevich, D. M., Brandt, J, Monsen, K. (2013). Family home visiting outcomes for Latina mothers with and without mental health problems. *Public Health Nursing, 30*(5), 427–438.

Gates, G. J. (2013). *LGBT parenting in the United States*. Retrieved from http://williaminstitute.law.ucla.edu/wp-comtent/uploads/LGBT-Parenting.pdf

Gould, E., & Cooper, D. (2013). Financial security of elderly Americans at risk: Proposed changes to social security and Medicare could make a majority of seniors "economically vulnerable." Retrieved from https://www.epi.org/publication/economic-security-elderly-americans-risk/

Gould, J. A. (2018). The CARE act: Identifying and supporting family caregivers from hospitals to home [Editorial]. *Dimensions of Critical care Nursing, 37*(2), 59–61.

Grant, R., Gracy, D., Goldsmith, G., Shapiro, A., & Redlener, I. E. (2013). Twenty-five years of child and family homelessness: Where are we now? *American Journal of Public Health, 103*(Suppl. 2), e1–e10.

Gultekin, L, Brush, B. L., Baiardi, J., Kirk, K., & VanMaldehem, K. (2014). Voices from the street: Exploring the realities of family homelessness. *Journal of Family Nursing, 20*(4), 390–414.

Harding, R. (2014). Caregivers of people at the end of life: emerging evidence. *Current Opinion in Supportive and Palliative care, 8*(4), 391–393.

Holtslander, L. (2005). Clinical application of the 15-minute family interview: Addressing the needs of postpartum families. *Journal of Family Nursing, 11*(1), 5–18.

Holtslander, L., Solar, J., & Smith, N. R. (2013). The 15-Minute Family Interview as a learning strategy for senior undergraduate nursing students. *Journal of Family Nursing, 19*(2), 230–248.

Imanigoghary, Z., Peyrovi, H., Nouhi, E., & Kazemi, M. (2017). The role of nurses in coping process of family caregivers of vegetative patients: A qualitative study. *International Journal of Community Based Nursing and Midwifery, 5*(1), 70–81.

International Family Nursing Association (IFNA). (2013). Position statement on pre-licensure family nursing education. Retrieved from https://internationalfamilynursing.org/wordpress/wp-content/uploads/2015/07/FNE-Complete-PDF-document-in-colour-with-photos-English-language1.pdf

International Family Nursing Association (IFNA). (2015). Position statement on generalist competencies for family nursing practice. Retrieved from https://internationalfamilynursing.org/wordpress/wp-content/uploads/2015/07/GC-Print-friendly-PDF-document-in-black-white-no-photos-English-language1.pdf

Jack, S. M., Catherine, N, Gonzalez, A, MacMillan, H. L, Sheehan, D, Waddell, D. (2015). Adapting, piloting, and evaluating complex public health interventions: lessons learned from the nurse-family partnership in Canadian public health settings. *Health Promotion and Chronic Disease Prevention in Canada, 35*(8–9), 151–158.

Jean-Baptiste, E., Alitz, P, Birriel, P. C, Davis, S, Ramakrishnan, R, Olson, L, Marshall, J. (2017). Immigrant health through the lens of home visitors, supervisors, and administrators: The Florida maternal, infant, and early childhood home visiting program. *Public Health Nursing, 34*(6):531–540.

Kaakinen, J. R., Hanson, S. M. H., & Denham, S. A. (2010). Family health care nursing: An introduction. *In Family Health Care Nursing: Theory, Practice and Research*. (4th ed.). Philadelphia, PA: F. A. Davis Company, 3–33.

Koniak-Griffin, D., Anderson, N. L., Verzemnieks, I., & Brecht, M. L. (2000). A public health nursing early intervention program for adolescent mothers: Outcomes from pregnancy through 6 weeks postpartum. *Nursing Research, 49*(3), 130–138.

Lund, M. (2005). Caregiver, take care. *Geriatric Nursing, 26*(3), 152–153.

Mactavish, J. B., & Schleien, S. J. (2004). Re-injecting spontaneity and balance in family life: Parents' perspectives on recreation in families that include children with developmental disability. *Journal of Intellectual Disabilities Research, 48*(Pt 2), 123–141.

REFERENCES *(Continued)*

Maes, B., Broekman, T. G., Dosen, A., & Nauts, J. (2003). Caregiving burden of families looking after persons with intellectual disability and behavioral or psychiatric problems. *Journal of Intellectual Disabilities Research, 47*(Pt 6), 447–455.

McGoldrick, M., Garcia-Preto, N., & Carter, B. (2016). *The expanded family life cycle: Individuals, family and social perspectives* (5th ed.). Upper Saddle River, NJ: Prentice Hall.

McIntyre, L. L., Blacher, J., & Baker, B. L. (2002). Behavior/mental health problems in young adults with intellectual disability: The impact on families. *Journal of Intellectual Disabilities Research, 46*(Pt 3), 239–249.

Meade, C. S., & Ickovics, J. R. (2005). Systemic review of sexual risk among pregnant and mothering teens in the USA: Pregnancy as an opportunity for integrated prevention of STD and repeat pregnancy. *Social Sciences & Medicine, 60*(4), 661–678.

Miller, B. G. (2017). No differences? Meta-analytical comparisons of psychological adjustment of children of gay fathers and heterosexual parents. *Psychology of Sexual Orientation and Gender Diversity, 4*(71), 14–22.

Moules, N. J., & Johnstone, H. (2010). Commendations, conversations, and life-changing realizations: Teaching and practicing family nursing. *Journal of Family Nursing, 16*(2), 146–160.

National Alliance to End Homelessness. (2017). Children and families. Retrieved from https://endhomelessness.org/homelessness-in-america/who-experiences-homelessness/children-and-families/

National Hispanic Council on Aging. (2017). Results of the national Hispanic council on aging's 2017 national caregiving survey. Retrieved from http://www.nhcoa.org/results-of-the-national-hispanic-council-on-agings-2017-national-caregiving-survey/

Norinder, M., Goliath, I., & Alvariza, A. (2017). Patients' experiences of care and support at home after a family member's participation in an intervention during palliative care. *Palliative and Supportive Care, 15*(3), 305–312.

Nurse-Family Partnership (NFP). (2018). Nurse-family partnership. Retrieved from https://www.nursefamilypartnership.org/about/

Olds, D. L. (2006). The nurse-family partnership: An evidence-based preventive intervention. *Infant Mental Health Journal, 27*(1), 5–25.

Olds, D. L. (2012). Improving the life chances of vulnerable children and families with prenatal and infancy support of parents: The nurse-family partnership. *Psychosocial Intervention, 21*(2), 129–143.

Olds. D. L., Donelan-McCall, N., O'Brien, R., MacMillan, H., Jack, S., Jenkins, T. (2013). Improving the nurse-family partnership in community practice. *Pediatrics, 132*(2), S110–S117.

Ollen, E. W., & Goldberg, A. E. (2016) Parent-child conversations about legal inequalities in gay-and lesbian families in Florida. *Journal of GLBT Family Studies, 12*(4), 365–385.

Ostlund, U., & Persson, C. (2014). Examining responses to family systems nursing interventions: An integrated review. *Journal of Family Nursing, 20*(3), 259–286.

Ostlund, U., Backstrom, B., Lindh, V., Sundin, K., & Saveman, B. I. (2014). Nurses' fidelity to theory-based components when implementing family health conversations: A qualitative inquiry. *Scandinavian Journal of Caring Sciences, 29*(3), 582–590.

Östlund, U., Bäckström, B., Saveman, B. I., Lindh, V., & Sundin, K. (2016). A family systems nursing approach for families following a stroke: Family health conversations. *Journal of Family Nursing, 22*(2), 148–171.

Persson, C., & Benzein, E. (2014). Family health conversations: How do they support health. *Nursing Research and Practice*, 1–11.

Pew Research Center. (2011). A portrait of stepfamilies. Retrieved from http://www.pewsocialtrends.org/subjects/stepfamilies/

Pickett, K. E., Mookherjee, J., & Wilkinson, R. G. (2005). Adolescent birth rates, total homicides, and income inequality in rich countries. *American Journal of Public Health, 95*(7), 1181–1183.

Rainvill, C., Skufca, L., & Mehegan, L. (2016). Family caregiving and out-of-pocket costs: 2016 report. Retrieved from https://www.aarp.org/content/dam/aarp/research/surveys_statistics/ltc/2016/family-caregiving-costs.doi.10.26419%252Fres.00138.001.pdf

Reinhard, S. C., Levine, C., & Samis, S. (2012). *Home alone: Family caregivers providing complex chronic care*. Washington, DC: AARP Public Policy Institute & United Hospital.

Rempel, G. R., Neufeld, A., & Kushner, K. E. (2007). Interactive use of genograms and ecomaps in family caregiving research. *Journal of Family Nursing, 13*(4), 403–419.

Richards, M. A., Rothblum, E. D., Beauchaine, T. P., Balsam, K. (2017). Adult children of same-sex and heterosexual couples: Demographic "thriving." *Journal of GLBT Family Studies, 13*(1), 1–15.

Romero, A. P. (2017). 1.1 million LGBT adults are married to someone of the same sex. Retrieved from https://williamsinstitute.law.ucla.edu/wp-content/uploads/Obergefell-2-Year-Marriages.pdf

Rowe, A. (2013). Family Nurse Partnership: Theories, principles and practice methods. *Journal of Health Visiting, 1*(2), 117–121.

Sandel, M., Sheward, R., & Sturtevant, L. (2015). Compounding stress: The timing and duration effects of homelessness on children's health. *Insights from Housing Policy Research*. Retrieved from https://www.issuelab.org/resources/21731/21731.pdf

Schondelmyer, E. (2017). Fewer married household and more living alone. Retrieved from https://www.census.gov/library/stories/2017/08/more-adults-living-without-children.html

Smyth, S., & Anderson, G. (2014). Family nurse partnership: Meeting the needs of teenage mothers. *British Journal of Midwifery, 22*(12), 870–875.

Spurlock, W. R. (2005). Spiritual well-being and caregiver burden in Alzheimer's caregivers. *Geriatric Nursing, 26*(3), 154–161.

Sveinbjarnardottir, E. K., Svavarsdottir, E. K., & Wright, L. M. (2013). What are the benefits of a short therapeutic conversation intervention with acute psychiatric patients and their families? A controlled before and after study. *International Journal of Nursing Studies, 50*(5), 593–602.

Tavernier, D. L. (2009). The genogram: Enhancing student appreciation of family genetics. *Journal of Nursing Education, 48*(4), 222–225.

U.S. Census. (2017). America's families and living arrangements. Retrieved from https://www.census.gov/data/tables/2017/demo/families/cps-2017.html

U.S. Census Bureau. (2005). *Health Insurance Data*. Retrieved from http://www.census.gov/hhes/www/hlthins.html

Vespa, J., Lewis, J. M., Krider, R. M. (2013). America's families and living arrangements: 2012 population characteristics. Retrieved from https://www.census.gov/prod/2013pubs/p20-570.pdf

Vespa, J. (2017). The changing economics and demographics of young adulthood: 1975–2016. Retrieved from https://www.census.gov/library/stories/2017/08/young-adults.html

Walker, L. O., & Avant, K. C. (2010). *Strategies for Theory Construction in Nursing* (5th ed) Upper Saddle River, NJ: Pearson.

Williams, P. D., Williams, A. R., Graff, J. C., Hanson, S., Stanton, A., Hafeman, C., … Sanders, S. (2002). Interrelationships among variables affecting well siblings and mothers in families of children with a chronic illness or disability. *Journal of Behavioral Medicine, 25*(5), 411–424.

Wright, L. M. (2015). Brain science and illness beliefs: An unexpected explanation of the healing power of therapeutic conversations and the family interventions that matter. *Journal of Family Nursing, 21*(2), 186–205.

Wright, L. M., & Leahey, M. (1990). Trends in nursing of families. *Journal of Advanced Nursing, 15*(2), 148–154.

Wright, L., & Leahey, M. (1999). Maximizing time, minimizing suffering: The 15-minute (or less) family interview. *Journal of Family Nursing, 5*, 259–274.

Wright, L., & Leahey, M. (2005). The three most common errors in family nursing: How to avoid or sidestep. *Journal of Family Nursing, 11*(2), 90–101.

Wright, L., & Leahey, M. (2009). *Nurses and families: A guide to family assessment and intervention* (5th ed.). Philadelphia, PA: F. A. Davis Co.

Wright, L., & Leahey, M. (2013). *Nurses and families: A guide to family assessment and intervention* (6th ed.). Philadelphia, PA: F. A. Davis Co.

Yarwood, J., Richardson, A., & Watson, P. (2016). Public health nurses endeavors with families using the 15 minute interview. *Nursing Praxis in New Zealand, 32*(3), 20–30.

WEB RESOURCES

Please visit thePoint® for up-to-date web resources on this topic.

Part 4

Challenges in Community and Public Health Nursing

Chapter 14

Risk of Infectious and Communicable Diseases

Barbara A. Goldrick

WE ARE LEGEND

We are HIV. Our family is ancient.
Out of Africa,
Monkey to man,
From the trees and forests,
To the towns and cities.
We are here.
For we are HIV, we are legion.
Our children are billions,
Our home, in your defenses,
In your blood, your brain,
Your saliva, your semen.
We are everywhere.
For we are HIV, we are immortal.
We are part of you,
And you of us,
We live with you, but
May not die with you.
We go on.

For we are HIV, we are travelers.
From lover to lover,
Mother to baby,
Donor to blood bank,
Blood bank to patient,
We follow you.
For we are HIV, we evolve.
NRTIs, NNRTIs, PIs, INIs,
New designs, new drugs,
Bring it on, bring it on,
Q151M, K103 N, L90M.
We adapt, we survive.
We are HIV. We consume.
Your resources, your time,
Your hope, your lives,
Your new drugs are easy.
Where are your vaccines?
Can you stop us? We will see.

—Julian W. Tang

CHAPTER HIGHLIGHTS

- Infectious versus communicable disease
- Outbreak investigation: person, place, time
- Healthcare-associated infections
- Public health surveillance
- Foodborne and waterborne illnesses
- Sexually transmitted diseases

OBJECTIVES

- Explain the difference between infectious and communicable diseases.
- Examine the agent, host, and environmental characteristics of healthcare-associated infections and common community-acquired infections.
- Describe the major means of transmission of communicable diseases.
- Define an outbreak investigation by person, place, and time.
- Describe public health surveillance.
- Differentiate between foodborne and waterborne illnesses.
- Outline prevention and control measures for sexually transmitted diseases.

KEY TERMS

Agent: Infectious agents are biological in nature and are capable of producing an infection or infectious disease and include bacteria, viruses, rickettsiae, fungi, protozoa, and helminths.

Carrier: A person or animal that harbors an infectious organism and transmits the organism to others, although having no symptoms of the disease.

Colonization: The presence and multiplication of infectious organisms without invading or causing damage to tissue.

Common source outbreak: An outbreak characterized by exposure to a common, harmful substance.

Contagious: Communicable by direct or indirect contact.

Endemic: The constant or usual prevalence of a specific disease or infectious agent within a population or geographic area.

Epidemic: Significant increase in the number of new cases of a disease than past experience would have predicted for that place, time, or population; an increase in incidence beyond that which is expected.

Healthcare-associated infection: Originating in a healthcare facility; formerly called nosocomial infection.

Incubation period: Time period between initial contact with the infectious agent and the appearance of the first signs or symptoms of the disease.

Infectious disease: Presence and replication of an infectious agent in the tissues of a host, with manifestation of signs and symptoms. An infectious disease need not be contagious or communicable.

Pathogenicity: Ability of the agent to produce an infectious disease in a susceptible host.

Propagated outbreak: Outbreak resulting from direct or indirect transmission of an infectious agent from an infected person to a susceptible host; secondary infections can occur.

Reservoir: Location where an infectious agent is normally found, where it lives and reproduces under normal circumstances.

Secondary infection: Infections that occur within the accepted incubation period following exposure to a primary case.

Surveillance: A continual dynamic method for gathering data about the health of the general public for the purpose of primary prevention of illness.

Transmission: The transfer of an infectious agent from one person or place to another.

CASE STUDIES

References to case studies are found throughout this chapter (look for the case study icon). Readers should keep the case studies in mind as they read the chapter.

CASE 1

In 2008–2009, contamination of the municipal drinking water supply occurred in Alamosa, CO. At that time, the city's drinking water was not chlorinated for disinfection due to a waiver from the statewide requirement for disinfection granted to the city in 1974. In 2007, the city was in compliance with all health-based drinking water standards, with the exception of the arsenic standard (Adapted from Falco & Williams, 2009).

CASE 2

Megan is a high school senior who moved into the community several months ago with her parents and younger brother. She has been sexually active for 2 years. She has had unprotected intercourse with three classmates since her arrival in town. For the past 2 weeks, she has had an urge to urinate frequently. Her vaginal secretions have increased, and the mucus has an unusual odor. She has made an appointment with the school nurse to discuss her symptoms.

INTRODUCTION

Infectious disease is universal, and any attempt to imagine how it arose…will inevitably take us back to the very earliest phases of life. **Frank MacFarlane Burnet and D. O. White**

According to the World Health Organization (WHO), more than half (54%) of the 56.4 million deaths worldwide in 2015 were due to the following top 10 causes: ischemic heart disease, stroke, lower respiratory infections, chronic obstructive pulmonary disease, lung cancer (along with trachea and bronchus cancers), diabetes, dementias/ Alzheimer disease, diarrheal diseases, tuberculosis (TB), and road injuries. Lower respiratory infections remained the most deadly communicable disease, causing 3.2 million deaths worldwide in 2015. The death rate from diarrheal diseases almost halved between 2000 and 2015, but still caused 1.4 million deaths in 2015. Similarly, TB killed fewer people during the same period, but was still among the top 10 causes of disease, with a death toll of 1.4 million (WHO, 2015). As populations age in middle- and low-income countries over the next 20 years, the proportion of deaths due to noncommunicable diseases will rise significantly. Globally, noncommunicable disease deaths from cancer will increase to 12.6 million by 2030, and deaths from cardiovascular diseases will rise to 22.2 million during the same period (WHO, 2013).

Although HIV/AIDS is no longer among the world's top 10 causes of death, it killed 1.1 million people in 2015 (compared with 1.5 million in 2000), but it is projected to fall to less than 400,000 by 2030 (WHO, 2013).

Almost half of the world population was still at risk for malaria in 2015, with 214 million cases and 438,000 deaths; two-thirds of these deaths occurred in children under 5 years of age. The global target is to reduce this number by 90% by 2030 (WHO, 2013). In addition, new pathogenic microorganisms have emerged, new strains of known organisms have developed that are more virulent, microorganisms have become resistant to many antibiotics, and infectious diseases have now become a means of terrorism. The characteristics of infectious diseases have changed, but they still are a significant health burden in most of the world.

This is true despite the great advances during the 20th century in the prevention and control of infectious diseases. These advances primarily occurred in developed countries and included purified drinking water, waste control, plentiful foods, immunizations, and drug therapy. This was preceded, however, by the need to prevent and control epidemics of infectious diseases, such as cholera, typhus, and influenza, which killed many people in Europe, America, and much of the rest of the world in the later part of the 19th century. By 1900, infectious diseases were the leading cause of death in the United States. Today, changes in health patterns in the world's more developed countries reflect an increased lifespan, with associated chronic diseases such as heart disease, cancer, and cardiovascular accidents.

Nonetheless, influenza and pneumonia remained in the top 10 causes of death in the United States in 2015 (National Center for Health Statistics, 2016). The *Healthy People 2020* (U.S. Department of Health and Human Services [USDHHS], 2010) initiative in the United States provides science-based, 10-year national objectives for improving the health of all Americans. For three decades, *Healthy People* has established benchmarks and monitored progress over time regarding established goals and objectives. Specific goals and objectives for prevention and control of infectious diseases are designed to reduce morbidity, mortality, and costs associated with infectious diseases. Selected objectives from *Healthy People 2020* for immunization and infectious diseases are found in Box 14.1.

Several new and reemerging infectious diseases have been identified in the past 40 years. Some examples are briefly described below.

1. In the 1970s, toxic shock syndrome (TSS) killed several women before it was linked to the use of high-absorbency tampons that provided a moist, warm home where the bacteria could thrive. It was also found to be associated with the contraceptive sponge and diaphragm birth control methods. TSS is caused by a well-known organism, *Staphylococcus aureus*. Streptococcal TSS, a related infection, is caused by *Streptococcus* bacteria.

2. Legionnaires disease, which is caused by the Legionella pneumophila bacterium, was first recognized among hotel guests during an outbreak in Philadelphia, PA in 1976. Between 8,000 and 18,000 people are hospitalized with Legionnaires disease in the United States each year.

3. Another infectious disease that occurred in the last century is acquired immunodeficiency syndrome (AIDS), which was first observed in a few young men in 1981. Infection with HIV, largely transmitted through sexual contact, is now a major cause of morbidity and mortality throughout the world. Today, 35 years after the first cases were reported, HIV is still a leading cause of death and a health threat to millions worldwide. Each year, HIV claims more than a million lives, and about 2 million people become newly infected with the disease. The U.S. Centers for Disease Control and Prevention (CDC) provides support to over 75 countries to strengthen their national HIV/AIDS programs and build sustainable public health systems through the U.S. President's Emergency Plan for AIDS Relief (PEPFAR). PEPFAR is supporting life-saving antiretroviral treatment (ART) for nearly 11.5 million people, exceeding its 2016 target of 11.4 million, and up from the 50,000 individuals who were receiving ART in sub-Saharan Africa prior to when PEPFAR began.

4. Lyme disease began in 1975 when a cluster of children and adults residing in the Lyme, CT area experienced uncommon arthritic symptoms. By 1977, the first 51 cases of Lyme arthritis were described, and the Ixodes scapularis (black-legged) tick was linked to the transmission of the disease. In 1982, *Borrelia burgdorferi*, the tick-borne spirochete that causes Lyme disease, was discovered. Lyme disease is focally endemic in North America, Europe, and Asia and is probably the most common tick-borne bacterial disease in the world. Lyme disease is the most commonly reported vector-borne illness in the United States; in 2015, it was the sixth most common nationally notifiable disease. However, this disease is concentrated heavily in the northeast and upper Midwest, and so far, it has not occurred nationwide (CDC, *Lyme disease*). See Chapter 15, Emerging Infections, for more on Lyme disease.

5. A new respiratory disease appeared in May 1993, when several healthy young members of the Navajo Nation in New Mexico died within a short period of time from an unexplained respiratory condition. This cluster of strange, unexplained deaths caught the attention of the world, resulting in rapid diagnosis of what was later called hantavirus pulmonary syndrome (HPS). As of November 1, 2012, the National Park Service had announced a total of 10 confirmed cases of hantavirus infection in people who recently visited

14.1 *Healthy People 2020* Objectives for Immunization and Infectious Diseases

Reduce, eliminate, or maintain elimination of cases of vaccine-preventable diseases.

Reduce early-onset group B streptococcal disease.

Reduce meningococcal disease.

Reduce invasive pneumococcal infections.

Achieve and maintain effective vaccination coverage levels for universally recommended vaccines among young children.

Increase the percentage of children aged 19 to 35 months who receive the recommended doses of DTaP, polio, MMR, Hib, hepatitis B, varicella and pneumococcal conjugate vaccine (PCV).

Decrease the percentage of children in the United States who receive 0 doses of recommended vaccines by age 19 to 35 months.

Maintain vaccination coverage levels for children in kindergarten.

Increase routine vaccination coverage levels for adolescents.

Increase the percentage of children and adults who are vaccinated annually against seasonal influenza.

Increase the percentage of adults who are vaccinated against pneumococcal disease.

Increase the percentage of adults who are vaccinated against zoster (shingles).

(Developmental) Increase hepatitis B vaccine coverage among high-risk populations.

(Developmental) Increase the scientific knowledge on vaccine safety and adverse events.

Increase the percentage of providers who have had vaccination coverage levels among children in their practice population measured within the past year.

Increase the percentage of children under 6 years of age whose immunization records are in a fully operational, population-based immunization information system (IIS).

Increase the number of states collecting kindergarten vaccination coverage data according to CDC minimum standards.

Increase the number of states that have 80% of adolescents with two or more age-appropriate immunizations recorded in an IIS among adolescents aged 11 to 18 years.

Increase the number of states that use electronic data from rabies animal surveillance to inform public health prevention programs.

Increase the number of public health laboratories monitoring influenza virus resistance to antiviral agents.

Reduce hepatitis A.

Reduce chronic hepatitis B virus infections in infants and young children (perinatal infections).

Reduce hepatitis B.

Reduce new hepatitis C infections.

Increase the proportion of persons aware they have a hepatitis C infection.

(Developmental) Increase the proportion of persons who have been tested for hepatitis B virus within minority communities experiencing health disparities.

Reduce tuberculosis (TB).

Increase treatment completion rate of all tuberculosis patients who are eligible to complete therapy.

Increase the percentage of contact to sputum smear–positive cases who complete treatment after being diagnosed with latent tuberculosis infection.

Reduce the average time for laboratories to confirm and report tuberculosis cases.

Source: U.S. Department of Health and Human Services. *Healthy People 2020: Immunization and infectious diseases objectives.* Retrieved April 29, 2013, from http://healthypeople.gov/2020/topicsobjectives2020/objectiveslist.aspx?topicId=23.

Yosemite National Park (CDC, *Outbreak of hantavirus infection in Yosemite National Park*).

6. About this same time, a toxic strain of *Escherichia coli* (O157:H7), an organism that normally inhabits the intestines of animals, caused illness and death in children in many parts of the United States. When there are news reports about foodborne outbreaks of "*E. coli*" infections, they are usually talking about *E. coli* O157.

7. Also, a virulent strain of *Streptococcus pyogenes* (Group A strep), known for its ability to evade the normal walling-off process by human immune systems, was named a "flesh-eating bacteria" (necrotizing fasciitis) because of the serious consequences of the infection.

8. In 1996, the possible transmission of mad cow disease (bovine spongiform encephalopathy, or BSE) to humans resulted in the slaughter of thousands of cattle in England. This is a particularly interesting disease, because the infectious agent is a protein (prion) rather than a microorganism.

9. Ebola hemorrhagic fever was initially recognized in 1976, with two simultaneous outbreaks in Nzara, Sudan,

and in the Democratic Republic of Congo in Africa. The latter outbreak occurred in a village near the Ebola River, from which the disease takes its name. Ebola hemorrhagic fever outbreaks, with a case-fatality rate of 50% or more, have appeared sporadically since its initial recognition. The most recent Ebola outbreaks occurred in 2018, where by mid-December 2108, 529 cases of Ebola virus disease (EVD) were reported to the WHO. In total, at that time, there were 311 reported deaths due to EVD, for a case-fatality rate of 58.8% (ISID, 2018).

Researchers believe that the virus is zoonotic (animalborne) and is normally maintained in an animal host that is native to the African continent. The Ebola virus is transmitted through close contact with the blood, other body fluids, or organs of infected animals. It also is transmitted by contact with blood or other body fluids (including semen) from persons infected with EVD. See Chapter 15, Emerging Infections, for more on Ebola.

10. In 2003, newspapers, television, and the internet were full of frightening articles and images about an outbreak of severe acute respiratory syndrome (SARS), a

viral illness, in Asia. At that time, the possibility of a SARS pandemic was worldwide news.

11. Shortly thereafter, also in 2003, fear of a bird flu (avian influenza virus H5N1) outbreak captured the attention of the world. Avian viruses do not usually infect humans, which means that the risk for avian influenza is generally low for most people. However, since 2003, the WHO has reported a total of 859 laboratory-confirmed cases of human infection with avian influenza A(H5N1) virus, including 453 deaths, from 16 countries (WHO, 2017). Most cases of H5N1 avian influenza infection in humans have resulted from contact with infected poultry. See Chapter 15, Emerging Infections, for more on H5N1 avian influenza.

12. In 2009, H1N1, a new influenza virus, was identified that caused illness in people. This new virus, which was first detected in Mexico and the United States in April 2009, caused the first flu pandemic in more than 40 years. The virus spread from person to person worldwide, in much the same way that regular seasonal influenza viruses spread. In mid-2009, the WHO had declared a pandemic of 2009 H1N1 influenza. By August 2010, worldwide more than 214 countries and territories had reported laboratory-confirmed cases of pandemic influenza H1N1 2009, including over 18,449 deaths. The CDC estimated that the total number of 2009 H1N1 cases in the United States between April 2009 and April 2010 ranged between 43 and 89 million, with an estimated 12,469 related deaths (Shrestha et al., 2011; WHO, *Pandemic (H1N1) 2009*). For more information on the 2009 H1N1 virus, see Chapter 15, Emerging Infections, for more on H1N1.

13. Avian influenza A(H7N9) had not previously been seen in either animals or people until it was found in March 2013 in China. As of September 2018, a total of 1,567 laboratory-confirmed human cases, including at least 615 deaths, had been reported to the WHO. The 2018 wave of A(H7N9) was the sixth wave of the outbreak. However, only three new human cases had been detected as of September 2018. Also, there had been fewer A(H7N9) virus detections in poultry and environmental samples. See Chapter 15 for more on Avian influenza A(H7N9).

14. In late 2012, the WHO received reports of two clusters of human infection with a novel coronavirus (CoV) in the Middle East. Although this new coronavirus is distantly related to SARS-CoV, it is different, and this particular strain of CoV had not been previously identified in humans. However, the WHO and the CDC recognized that the emergence of a new coronavirus was capable of causing severe disease and raised concerns due to the recent experience with SARS. Because of the location of the discovery of the new coronavirus, it was named Middle East respiratory syndrome coronavirus (MERS-CoV). As of September 2018, 27 countries had reported a total of 2,229 laboratory-confirmed cases of MERS-CoV to WHO, including at least 798 deaths (case-fatality rate, 35.8%). The majority of cases had occurred in Saudi Arabia, as well as in multiple other countries of the Arabian Peninsula. See Chapter 15 for more on Middle East respiratory syndrome coronavirus.

15. The Zika virus, a mosquito-borne virus, was first discovered in 1947 in the Zika Forest in Uganda. The first human cases of Zika virus infection were detected in 1952. Since 2015, outbreaks of Zika virus infection have reported evidence of mosquito-borne Zika virus transmission to the WHO from 73 countries and territories, including the United States. Twelve countries, including the United States also have reported evidence of person-to-person transmission of the Zika virus. Pregnant women are at increased risk for congenital infection, and 23 countries and territories reported microcephaly, or suggestive congenital infection, and other CNS malformations potentially associated with Zika virus infection. See Chapter 15 for more on Zika virus.

With the global mobility of humans, animals, food, and feed products greater than ever before, the spread of dangerous pathogens has and will continue to increase. Infectious diseases are a growing threat to all nations, although the burden is greatest in the developing world. To address these issues, the CDC and a network of international public health partnerships have been formed. These partnerships, which include WHO, the United Nations, the World Bank, and the Bill & Melinda Gates Foundation, are contributing to the increased availability of drugs and vaccines, and providing better public health education programs worldwide (CDC, *CDC's Global health partnerships*).

 Student Reflection

When I was a teenager, I went to summer camp for 2 weeks. We cooked our own meals over a campfire. It was great. However, by the second week, several of us went to the camp nurse for help with diarrhea and/or vomiting. After several days, 23 of us were ill with these symptoms. As a result, the local health department was notified, the camp was closed, and environmental disinfection was undertaken. Hand hygiene was emphasized. Stool samples were obtained from symptomatic campers and tested for bacterial and viral pathogens. Fifteen out of the 23 (65%) stool samples were positive for norovirus. All the campers recovered from their gastroenteritis. Although the cause of this outbreak was never identified, the encounter stayed with me and made me aware of how important sanitation and hand hygiene is to public health.

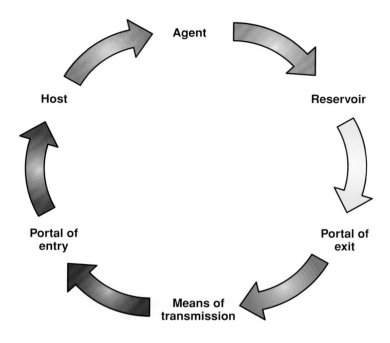

FIGURE 14.1 Chain of infection.

EPIDEMIOLOGY OF THE INFECTIOUS PROCESS: THE CHAIN OF INFECTION

According to the germ theory of disease, specific microorganisms cause specific diseases. As described in Chapter 6, the epidemiologic triangle is a model that scientists have developed for studying health problems. It helps us understand infectious diseases and how they spread. The **agent**, or the microbe that causes the disease, is the "what" of the triangle. The *host*, or the human, animal, or insect that is harboring the infectious agent, is the "who" of the triangle. The *environment*, which includes those external factors that cause or allow disease transmission, is the "where" of the triangle.

An **infectious disease** in a human (or animal) host is one caused by the growth of pathogenic microorganisms in the body. Other necessary elements that add to the epidemiologic triangle are in the so-called chain of infection, which include a portal of exit from the host, environmental reservoirs, transmission, and a portal of entry to a new host (McKenzie, Pringer, & Kotecki, 2014) (Fig. 14.1). For a disease to be communicable, or **contagious**, there must be a portal of exit from the infected person (or animal), a means of transmission, and a portal of entry to a susceptible host.

Agent

Infectious agents are biologic agents capable of producing an infection or infectious disease and include bacteria, viruses, rickettsiae, fungi, protozoa, and helminths (Heymann, 2014). An infectious disease need not be contagious or communicable.

Case 1: A month-long investigation found that there were 442 reported cases of *Salmonella typhimurium*, including 122 laboratory-confirmed cases, 20 hospitalizations, and one death. An epidemiological investigation estimated that up to 1,300 people may have become ill from the city's water supply. Residents were advised to drink bottled water while the entire water system was flushed and hyperchlorinated. A boil water order followed the bottled water order, and it remained in place until tests confirmed that the city's water was safe to drink again (Adapted from Falco & Williams, 2009).

In this case, what was the "where" of the epidemiologic triangle?

In addition to the interaction between the infectious agent, the host, and the environment, the progression of an infectious agent depends on its pathogenicity. **Pathogenicity** is the ability of an infectious agent to cause disease in a susceptible host (Heymann, 2014). It depends on the infectivity of the infectious agent, its ability to invade and destroy body cells (invasiveness), produce toxins (toxicity), and its virulence.

Infectivity varies depending on the route of entry of the infectious agent and the susceptibility of the host. For example, if *Clostridium tetani* (tetanus bacilli) gains entry into the body through a puncture wound, and the person has current tetanus immunization, the person (host) is not susceptible to infectivity by *C. tetani*. Various characteristics of an infectious agent are found in Box 14.2.

14.2 Properties of Infectious Agents Influenced by the Host and the Environment

Pathogenicity: Ability of the agent to produce an infectious disease in a susceptible host

Infectivity: Ability of the agent to invade the host and replicate

Virulence: Severity of the infectious disease that results from exposure to the agent

Toxicity: Ability of the agent to produce toxins

Immunogenicity: Ability of the agent to produce specific immunity within the host

Invasiveness: Ability of the agent to destroy body cells

Practice Point

An understanding of the pathogenicity of an infectious agent is important in a decision to initiate prevention and control measures. It is necessary to break the chain of infection. For example, good hand hygiene breaks this chain by preventing the transmission of infectious agent from one person to another.

But however secure and well-regulated civilized life may become, bacteria, Protozoa, viruses, infected fleas, lice, ticks, mosquitoes, and bedbugs will always lurk in the shadows ready to pounce when neglect, poverty, famine, or war lets down the defenses.
Hans Zinsser

Host

The second component of the epidemiologic triad is the susceptible host. In infectious disease epidemiology, just the presence of an infectious agent is not sufficient to produce an infectious disease. The process requires a susceptible host. There are several host factors that determine whether a person is at risk for an infection or an infectious disease. These include age, sex, race, physical and emotional health, and immune status.

Portals of Entry and Exit

Infectious agents both enter and leave the body in multiple ways. Portals include the skin, respiratory tract, alimentary tract, genital tract, conjunctiva, and vertical transmission from parent to offspring. An example is the fecal–oral transmission of hepatitis A through indirect contact with infected fecal material.

Incubation Period

If an infectious agent enters the host and begins to multiply, an infection occurs. The time between exposure to an infectious agent and the manifestation of symptoms in the host is called the **incubation period**. Each infectious disease has its own incubation period, but it can also vary in different hosts. For example, the incubation period for influenza is 24 to 72 hours after the virus enters the body, when symptoms start. However, some people can be infected with the influenza virus but have no symptoms. The period of communicability varies. Adults can begin spreading the influenza virus one day before they have any symptoms and for 3 to 7 days after symptoms start. Children can transmit the virus after more than 7 days (Heymann, 2014).

Case 1: *Salmonella typhimurium* is transmitted via the fecal–oral route and the time when the strength of the transmission increases is 12 to 72 hours after infection. Over a period of 4 to 7 days, the majority of people infected feel better even if not treatment but one of the severe effects of the infection is losing electrolytes through fluid loss in diarrhea and this symptom and losses can require hospitalization. It typically takes 2 to 4 weeks from the start of a person's illness to confirming that they are part of an outbreak.

1. Is *Salmonella typhimurium* a communicable (contagious) disease?
2. Who were the susceptible hosts?

Some diseases have longer incubation periods. For example, hepatitis B has an average incubation period of 60 to 90 days, but it can be as short as 2 weeks and as long as 6 to 9 months. A person infected with hepatitis B virus (HBV) may be asymptomatic but still can transmit the virus to others. Asymptomatic people with chronic hepatitis antigenemia (the presence of HBV antigen in the blood) are **carriers** of the HBV and can transmit the virus to others through percutaneous inoculation, exposure to mucous membranes, and sexual contact (Heymann, 2014). More information about hepatitis can be found in medical–surgical textbooks.

When an infectious agent is present and there are no clinical signs of disease, **colonization** with the infectious agent is said to have occurred, and the infected person is capable of transmitting the agent. An example is methicillin-resistant *S. aureus* (MRSA), which has become increasingly common in many healthcare facilities over the past decade. A person can carry MRSA in his or her nose and throat and can then shed the bacteria. For example, a healthcare worker colonized with MRSA can transmit the organism to neonates or to postoperative patients (surgical wounds), causing severe morbidity and mortality. In recent years, MRSA has become a community-acquired infection (CA-MRSA), with outbreaks in athletes, schoolchildren, military recruits, and prison inmates. Factors that have been associated with the spread of CA-MRSA skin infections include close skin-to-skin contact, openings in the skin such as cuts or abrasions, contaminated items and surfaces, crowded living conditions, and poor hygiene. CA-MRSA most often presents as skin or soft tissue infection such as a boil or abscess (CDC, *MRSA*). Asymptomatic, subclinical, or occult infections are identifiable only by certain laboratory tests, such as serology or skin tests. An example of a skin test to identify infection is the purified protein derivative (PPD) skin test used to identify TB infection. Screening for specific conditions such as TB is also a form of secondary prevention.

Infection with HIV is unapparent in its early stages and may be transmitted from one person to another when infected blood, semen, or vaginal secretions come in contact with an uninfected person's broken skin or mucous membranes. In addition, an infected pregnant woman can transmit HIV to her infant during pregnancy or delivery, as well as through breastfeeding. At the end of 2014, the most recent year for which data are available, an estimated 1,107,700 adults and adolescents were living with HIV. An estimated 166,000 (15%) had not been diagnosed, and young people were the most likely to be unaware of their infection. Among people aged 13 to 24, an estimated 51% (31,300) of those living with HIV at the end of 2013 didn't know they were infected (CDC, 2017).

Environment: Reservoir

The third component in the epidemiologic triad, the environment, provides reservoirs of infectious agents (microbes); these **reservoirs** can be humans, animals, plants, insects, water, and soil. Microbes live everywhere and their habitats expand as humans alter the environment and extend contact with them. Microbes are adept at adaptation and change under selective pressures for survival and replication. For example, influenza viruses continually evolve, resulting in annual epidemics and an ongoing need to develop new influenza vaccines each year. Another example is antibiotic-resistant strains of microorganisms, such as MRSA.

> Infectious disease, then, is not nature's tantrum against humanity. Often it is an argument in what becomes a long marriage.
> **Arno Karlen**

Infections transmitted from animal reservoirs to humans are known as *zoonoses*. Examples of zoonoses are rodent-transmitted plague, hantavirus, and monkeypox. Although rare, zoonotic infections occur in the United States. Hantavirus pulmonary syndrome (HPS), a severe, sometimes fatal, respiratory disease in humans, is caused by an infection with a hantavirus. Anyone who comes into contact with rodents or their droppings that carry hantavirus is at risk for HPS (CDC, *Hantavirus pulmonary syndrome*). In November 2012, the National Park Service announced a total of 10 confirmed cases of hantavirus infection in people who recently visited Yosemite National Park. Three of the confirmed cases were fatal (CDC, 2012a).

Changes in the environment tend to have the greatest influence on the transmission of microbial agents that are waterborne, airborne, foodborne, or vector-borne, or those that have an animal reservoir. Transformation of forest to agricultural land in Venezuela led to emergence of a new disease in 1989: Venezuelan hemorrhagic fever. Reforestation of abandoned farmlands in the northeast was a factor in the emergence of Lyme disease in the United States.

> In **Case 1**, at the time of the outbreak, the Alamosa's community public water system infrastructure consisted of seven deep artesian wells, from an aquifer considered to be a protected groundwater source, two elevated storage tanks, and one ground-level storage reservoir. Over 75% of the water pumped to the city's water system was from the Weber well through the Weber reservoir at the time of the outbreak.
>
> Although the Safe Drinking Water Program had increased in recent years, the city of Alamosa had not addressed integrity issues at the Weber Reservoir, and were not detected during previous inspections of the water system (Adapted from Falco & Williams, 2009).
>
> What environmental factors contributed to this outbreak?

Transmission

Mechanisms of **transmission** of an infectious agent from a reservoir to another host include airborne transmission, direct contact, indirect contact, and droplet transmission.

Airborne Transmission

Airborne transmission occurs when microorganisms are carried in the air in small particles, called droplet nuclei, at distances that exceed a few feet. TB is an example of an airborne infection transmitted by droplet nuclei. A person with active TB disease of the lungs or throat releases TB bacteria into the air when he or she coughs, sneezes, speaks, or sings. People nearby may breathe in these bacteria and become infected. TB bacteria also may spread by droplet nuclei to persons who are not nearby (e.g., through air-conditioning units).

Bacterial spores (e.g., *Aspergillus* spores) can spread by airborne transmission through dust when they are mixed in with dry soil (Heymann, 2014).

Direct Contact

Direct contact occurs through direct body surface-to-body surface contact and physical transfer of microorganisms between a susceptible host and an infected or colonized person (or animal). For example, sexually transmitted diseases (STDs) are transmitted by direct contact with an infected person.

An example of direct contact with an animal reservoir is the transmission of the H5N1 avian influenza virus, which was transmitted from poultry to humans in the "bird flu" epidemic that occurred between 2004 and 2008. Recently published papers indicate that we are only three genetic changes away from a pandemic of H5N1 influenza (Enserink, 2012). See Chapter 15 for more information on avian influenza viruses.

Indirect Contact

Indirect contact involves contact of a susceptible host with a contaminated intermediate inanimate object, called a vehicle, such as a contaminated surgical instrument, needle, toy, soiled clothing, or bed linen. Vehicles also include food, water, and contaminated hands that are not washed (Heymann, 2014). Indirect contact also includes vector transmission. Vectors are animal or insect carriers of infectious agents. Mechanical vector-borne transmission occurs when an insect carries the microorganisms on its feet or proboscis, or through its gastrointestinal tract. Biologic vector-borne transmission occurs when propagation of the microorganism is required within the insect before it can be transmitted to another host. Malaria is an example of biologic vector-borne infectious disease, which is transmitted by mosquitoes (Heymann, 2014).

Evidence for Practice

The CDC has reported an increasing number of outbreaks of enteric disease associated with animals at fairs and petting zoos. Investigators found the route of transmission was usually from direct hand-to-mouth contact with animal feces. Guidelines to reduce the risk of disease are designed to interrupt this route. They include recommendations to wash hands after touching animals, to keep food and drinks outside of animal areas, and to prevent children from putting their hands or objects (such as pacifiers or sippy cups) in their mouths while interacting with animals. Most petting zoos provide hand hygiene facilities, but handwashing compliance varies. The CDC has published measures to prevent infection associated with animals at fairs and petting zoos. See CDC (2011a)—Compendium of measures to prevent disease associated with animals in public settings, 2011 at http://www.cdc.gov/mmwr/pdf/rr/rr6004.pdf

Droplet Transmission

Although droplet transmission theoretically is a form of contact transmission, the mechanism of transfer of the pathogen to the host is quite distinct from either direct or indirect transmission. Therefore, droplet transmission is considered a separate route of transmission. Droplets are generated from the source person primarily during coughing, sneezing, and talking, and are propelled a short distance (less than 3 ft) through the air and deposited on the conjunctivae, nasal mucosa, or mouth of another person. Measles and influenza are examples of communicable diseases transmitted by droplet spread (Heymann, 2014).

In **Case 1**, Salmonella survival studies indicate that a low infective dose of 10 to 100 organisms in drinking water may be sufficient to cause illness. Also, the bacteria can survive in drinking water or biofilms for at least a week, depending on the level of contamination. Based on all the information gained during the investigation, the likelihood that fecal matter from an animal source (e.g., avian source) of Salmonella bacteria entered the Weber reservoir and then contaminated the remainder of the Alamosa drinking water system was supported (Adapted from Falco & Williams, 2009).

1. How is *Salmonella typhimurium* transmitted?
2. What was the portal of entry to the new host(s)?

OUTBREAK INVESTIGATION

An **endemic** disease, infection, or infectious agent occurs when it becomes prevalent within a population or geographic area. For example, chloroquine-resistant malaria is endemic in most of Africa, the Middle East, Asia, and all of the South Pacific islands (CDC, *The yellow book 2017*). An **epidemic** refers to a significant increase in an infection or infectious disease beyond the expected (endemic) level in a certain population and/or geographic area. Epidemics also occur when a new infectious agent emerges or reemerges. A pandemic is an epidemic that generally spreads worldwide. An example of a pandemic is the H1N1 influenza outbreak that occurred in 2009 to 2010. Outbreak carries the same definition of epidemic, but is often used for a more limited geographic area (Porta, 2014). The steps of an outbreak investigation are outlined in Box 14.3.

14.3 | Steps in an Outbreak Investigation

- Establish and verify diagnosis of reported cases; identify agent.
- Search for additional cases; collect critical data and specimens.
- Characterize cases by person, place, and time.
- Formulate and test tentative hypotheses regarding possible causative factors.
- Implement control measures to control the outbreak.
- Evaluate efficacy of control measures.
- Communicate findings; prepare written report.

Source: Association for Professionals in Infection Control and Epidemiology. (2009). *APIC text of infection control and epidemiology* (3rd ed.). Washington, DC: Author.

Establishing the Existence of an Outbreak

To establish that an outbreak exists, a comparison of the current incidence of cases with baseline or endemic status is essential. If local data are not available, the incidence (described in Chapter 7) of cases should be compared with that in the literature. Observed rates should be greater than the expected level. In some situations, a single case of a communicable disease long absent from the population, or the first occurrence of an infection not previously recognized in that geographic area, requires immediate reporting and epidemiologic investigation; two such cases associated in time and place may indicate the start of an epidemic (Heymann, 2014). For example, two cases of smallpox in the United States are above the expected level, because smallpox was eradicated worldwide in 1977.

The criteria used for defining a case are important aspects of an outbreak investigation; however, the case definition may change as more data are collected. Once the criteria have been established, the suspected cases are grouped into definite cases, probable cases, and possible cases categories.

Describing Cases by Person, Place, and Time

As was discussed in Chapter 6, person, place, and time characterize the description of an epidemiologic problem. As data are collected on individual cases in an outbreak investigation, attack rates can be calculated according to demographic variables such as age, sex, and other factors or attributes like occupation or exposure to the suspected agent. These data are helpful in comparing the characteristics of those who develop the infection with the characteristics of those who do not when conducting case-control studies (Chapter 8). This occurs when epidemiologists test tentative hypotheses to explain the outbreak and identify the population at risk (CDC, 2012b).

When describing an outbreak by place, it may be necessary to use spot maps to identify concentrations of cases within certain areas, and this may show clustering of cases. The use of maps also further defines the population at risk. The use of time in describing an outbreak requires that investigators go back to the first case or indication of outbreak activity. These data graphically provide a histogram of the epidemic curve, which helps determine whether the outbreak is from a common source or from a propagated (continuous) source. The epidemic curve also helps determine the incubation period of the infection and if the problem is ongoing. As a general rule, a unit of time used in an outbreak investigation is one-fourth (0.25) of the average incubation period for the illness under investigation (CDC, 2012b).

The data in Figure 14.2 illustrate an epidemic curve from the well-known common source outbreak of cholera in London in 1854, which was investigated by John Snow, the "father of epidemiology." Dr. Snow established that cholera was spread by water from the contaminated Broad Street well. When the pump handle was removed and people could no longer obtain water from the well, the epidemic subsided. Note that although the typical incubation period for cholera is 1 to 3 days, the outbreak lasted more than one month, because of the contaminated water supply, before the Broad Street pump handle was removed. Figure 14.3 is an example of a propagated epidemic curve of a measles outbreak. The incubation period for measles is typically 10 days, but may be as short as 7 days and as long as 18 days (CDC, 2012b). The secondary infections, which are spread from person to person, show intervals in the

FIGURE 14.2 Common source epidemic curve: Broad Street pump cholera outbreak, London, 1854. (*Source:* Centers for Disease Control and Prevention.)

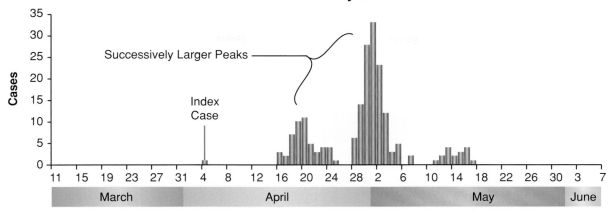

FIGURE 14.3 Propagated epidemic curve: Measles outbreak. (*Source:* Centers for Disease Control and Prevention. Retrieved from http://www.cdc.gov/epo/dih/Epidemic_Curve/page06.htm.)

epidemic curve, indicating that the outbreak is not from a common source.

A **common source outbreak** is one that has the same origin (i.e., same person or vehicle as the reservoir or means of transmission). A **propagated (continuous) outbreak** is one in which the infection is transmitted from person to person over a longer period of time than with a common source outbreak, and it can generate secondary infections with intervals between peaks that approximate the usual incubation period for the infection. An example of measles cases is outlined in see Figure 14.3. **Secondary infections** are those that occur within the accepted incubation period following exposure to a primary case (Porta, 2014). Characterizing an outbreak by person, place, and time is called descriptive epidemiology (see Chapter 8), because it describes the population under study. This step is critical for several reasons. First, by becoming familiar with the data, it is possible to learn what information is reliable and informative (e.g., the same unusual exposure reported by many of the people affected) and what may not be as reliable (e.g., many missing or "don't know" responses to a particular question). Second, a comprehensive description of an outbreak is provided by showing its trend over time, its geographic extent (place), and the populations (people) affected by the disease and the time period in which it occurs. This description lets an epidemiologist begin to assess the outbreak in light of what is known about the disease (e.g., the usual source, mode of transmission, risk factors, and populations affected) and to develop causal hypotheses (CDC, *Principles of Epidemiology*, 2012). In turn, these hypotheses can be tested using the techniques of analytic epidemiology (see Chapter 8).

HEALTHCARE-ASSOCIATED INFECTIONS

Healthcare-associated infections (HAIs) (previously called nosocomial infections) are a significant cause of morbidity and mortality in the United States. It is estimated that about one in every 20 inpatients has an infection related to healthcare. These infections cost the U.S. healthcare system billions of dollars each year and lead to the loss of tens of thousands of lives. In addition, HAIs can have devastating emotional, financial, and medical consequences. The majority of HAIs are urinary tract infections (UTIs), surgical-site infections (SSIs), bloodstream infections, and pneumonia (CDC, *Estimates of Healthcare-Associated Infections*). The U.S. Department of Health and Human Services' (USDHHS) ultimate goal of eliminating all HAIs has identified the reduction of central line-associated bloodstream infections (CLABSIs), SSIs, and catheter-associated urinary tract infections (CAUTIs) as a primary goal in 2013 (USDHHS, 2013).

The CDC's National Healthcare Safety Network (NHSN) is a public health surveillance system that maintains and supports the USDHHS national HAI prevention priorities. Since its inception in 2005, NHSN has collected HAI data from nearly all U.S. hospitals. NHSN data are reported annually to measure progress toward the HHS goal of HAI prevention. As of 2014, a 50% reduction occurred in CLABSIs, up from the 32% reduction reported in 2010; a 17% reduction in SSIs since 2008, up from the 7% reduction reported in 2010; and a 5% reduction in CAUTIs since 2009 (CDC, 2016c).

An estimated 1 to 3 million HAIs occur among residents in long-term care settings each year. In addition to infections that are largely endemic, such as UTIs and lower respiratory tract infections, outbreaks of respiratory and gastrointestinal infections are also common. Pneumonia and other lower respiratory tract infections are the most frequent reasons for transferring residents of long-term care facilities to the hospital (CDC, *Tracking infections in long-term care facilities*). When an outbreak occurs in a healthcare setting, an epidemiologic investigation is conducted, using the same criteria outlined above. Applying the basic principles of infection control, which include hand hygiene, aseptic technique, and isolation precautions, can prevent HAIs. Community/public health nurses also can prevent and control infections in the home by using appropriate aseptic techniques, attention to good hand hygiene, and educating family members in the principles of infection control.

Evidence for Practice

In September 2012, an alert clinician notified the Tennessee Department of Health of a patient who had developed culture-confirmed *Aspergillus fumigatus* meningitis after he had received an epidural steroid injection in July at an ambulatory surgical center. The patient was admitted to the hospital in late August. The Tennessee Department of Health notified the CDC, and within days, the CDC had identified the source of the largest multistate healthcare-associated outbreak to be an injectable steroid medication prepared by a New England Compounding Center (NECC). At that time, the CDC and the Food and Drug Administration (FDA) recommended that all healthcare professionals discontinue use and remove from their pharmaceutical inventory any product produced by that compounding center. A massive effort to contact nearly 19,000 potentially exposed patients and their physicians was undertaken by the CDC.

By May 2013, there were 753 cases and 64 deaths reported among patients in 20 states who received injections of the contaminated steroid medication associated with the outbreak. A probable case was defined as a person who received a methylprednisolone acetate (MPA) injection, linked to injectable steroids from three recalled lots of preservative-free MPA distributed by NECC after May 21, 2012, and subsequently developed any of the following: meningitis of unknown etiology; posterior circulation stroke without a cardioembolic source; osteomyelitis, abscess, or other infection of unknown cause at or near the site of injection; osteomyelitis or worsening inflammatory arthritis of a peripheral joint (e.g., knee, shoulder, or ankle) of unknown cause. A confirmed case included identification of a fungal pathogen (by culture, histopathology, or molecular assay) associated with a clinical syndrome listed above.

In the early stages of the outbreak, the majority of patients were diagnosed with meningitis. However, the majority of patients developed a localized infection following exposure to contaminated injections, including epidural abscess, arachnoiditis (a disorder caused by the inflammation of the arachnoid membrane that surrounds and protects the nerves of the spinal cord), discitis (an infection in the intervertebral disc space), or vertebral osteomyelitis.

Most of the cases occurred in Michigan (*n* = 264), followed by Tennessee (*n* = 153). The predominant fungus identified in the outbreak was *Exserohilum*

rostratum. One patient, the index case from Tennessee, had a laboratory-confirmed *A. fumigatus* infection. These fungi are common in the environment, and fungal infections are not transmitted from person to person. In October 2015, CDC updated its web resources for patients and clinicians. Patients affected by tainted steroid injections from NECC continue to receive treatment for their infections and clinicians continue to monitor patient recovery (CDC, *Multistate outbreak of fungal meningitis and other infections*).

This is an example of the importance of public health preparedness to identify rare pathogens and implement measures to control them.

PUBLIC HEALTH SURVEILLANCE

At the federal level, the USDHHS is the U.S. public health infrastructure that develops policies to protect the nation's health. The CDC is a major USDHHS agency that protects the nation's health by developing guidelines that promote health and quality of life by preventing and controlling disease, injury, and disability (CDC, *About CDC*).

Surveillance for infectious and/or communicable diseases in the United States consists of a variety of efforts at both the state and federal levels. At the state level, healthcare providers and healthcare facilities are required to report certain infectious diseases to state health departments. State public health departments that monitor disease incidence and identify possible outbreaks within their states report these data to the CDC. Certain infectious and/or communicable diseases must be reported to the CDC. For the current list of notifiable diseases, see the CDC's Nationally Notifiable Diseases website at http://wwwn.cdc.gov/nndss/default.aspx

The CDC is also a partner with the WHO through the Global Outbreak Alert and Response Network and the WHO Surveillance and Response System, which provide international epidemic alerts and responses (WHO, *CSR and global team*).

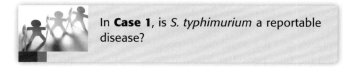

In **Case 1**, is *S. typhimurium* a reportable disease?

At the U.S. federal level, the CDC maintains surveillance systems to analyze data for disease trends and outbreaks. For example, one such surveillance system is FoodNet (Foodborne Disease Active Surveillance Network), which is a collaborative effort among the FDA, the U.S. Department of Agriculture, and the CDC. Specific states, which report cases and outbreaks of foodborne illnesses, are selected to participate in the CDC Emerging Infections Program (CDC, *FoodNet*). The Department of Defense (DoD) also has an electronic surveillance system for the early notification of community-based epidemics

(ESSENCE), which has been in operation since 2001 to detect infectious disease outbreaks (DoD, *Global emerging infections system*).

SPECIFIC COMMUNICABLE DISEASES

Foodborne Diseases

Foodborne diseases involve biologic and nonbiologic agents and can be caused by microorganisms and their toxins, marine organisms and their toxins, fungi and their related toxins, and chemical contaminants. Raw and undercooked foods of animal origin are the most likely to be contaminated. The CDC estimates that each year roughly one in six people in the United States (or 48 million people) get sick, 128,000 are hospitalized, and 3,000 die of foodborne diseases. The top five pathogens contributing to domestically acquired foodborne illnesses in 2016 were noroviruses, *Salmonella*, *Clostridium perfringens*, *Campylobacter*, and *Staphylococcus aureus* (CDC, *Estimates of foodborne illness in the United States*).

Recent changes in human demographics and food preferences, changes in food production and distribution systems, microbial adaptation, and lack of support for public health resources and infrastructure have led to the emergence of novel as well as traditional foodborne diseases. With increasing travel and trade opportunities, it is not surprising that the risk of contracting and spreading a foodborne disease now exists locally, regionally, and even globally.

Foodborne diseases monitored through the CDC FoodNet include infections caused by bacteria: *Campylobacter, Listeria, Salmonella*, Shiga toxin–producing *Escherichia coli* (STEC) O157 and non-O157, *Shigella, Vibrio, Yersinia*; and parasites: *Cryptosporidium* and *Cyclospora*. According to the most recent FoodNet surveillance data for 2016, compared to 2013–2015, the average annual incidence of confirmed *Campylobacter* infections was lower, incidences of confirmed STEC, *Yersinia*, and *Cryptosporidium* infections were higher, and for incidences of confirmed or culture-independent diagnostic tests positive, only STEC and *Yersinia* infections were higher (Marder et al., 2017). *Salmonella* infections have not declined for nearly two decades, and the incidence of 15.40 per 100,000 population in 2016 was nearly higher than the *Healthy People 2020* target of 11.4 cases per 100,000 population (Box 14.4 for *Healthy People 2020* objectives for food safety). These findings highlight the need to continue to identify and address food safety gaps that can be targeted for action by the food industry and regulatory authorities. Effective measures include preventing contamination of meat during slaughter and of all foods, including produce, during processing and preparation; cooking meat thoroughly; vigorously detecting and investigating outbreaks; and recalling contaminated food (CDC, *CDC and food safety*). Nurses and other healthcare providers should educate their patients about the

14.4	*Healthy People 2020 Objectives for Food Safety*

Reduce infections caused by key pathogens commonly transmitted through food.

Reduce the number of outbreak-associated infections due to Shiga toxin–producing *E. coli* O157, or *Campylobacter, Listeria,* or *Salmonella* species associated with food commodity groups.

Prevent an increase in the proportion of nontyphoidal *Salmonella* and *Campylobacter jejuni* isolates from humans that are resistant to antimicrobial drugs.

Reduce severe allergic reactions to food among adults with a food allergy diagnosis.

Increase the proportion of consumers who follow key food safety practices.

(Developmental) Improve food safety practices associated with foodborne illness in food-service and retail establishments.

Source: U.S. Department of Health and Human Services. *Healthy People 2020 food safety objectives.* Retrieved July 11, 2013, from http://healthypeople.gov/2020/topicsobjectives2020/objectiveslist.aspx?topicId=14.

hazards of potentially life-threatening foodborne diseases and the preventive measures to reduce them.

Noroviruses

Noroviruses are common foodborne pathogens. Norovirus infections are often called "stomach flu"; however, this is a misnomer, because the norovirus is not an influenza virus. Noroviruses are recognized as the most common cause of acute infectious gastroenteritis in people of all ages, and are the leading cause of disease outbreaks from contaminated food in the United States (CDC, *Vital signs: Preventing norovirus outbreaks*). Each year on average in the United States, norovirus causes 19 to 21 million cases of acute gastroenteritis (inflammation of the stomach or intestines or both); leads to 1.7 to 1.9 million outpatient visits and 400,000 emergency department visits, primarily in young children; and contributes to about 56,000 to 71,000 hospitalizations and 570 to 800 deaths, mostly among young children and the elderly (CDC, *Norovirus*).

Noroviruses are spread primarily from one infected person to another by the fecal–oral route through contaminated hands, contaminated food or water, or by contact with contaminated objects in the environment. In some cases, aerosolized vomitus has been implicated in transmission of noroviruses. The incubation period for norovirus gastroenteritis is 12 to 48 hours; it causes more vomiting than diarrhea, is self-limited, and usually resolves within 48 hours. However, the elderly, children, and those with severe underlying medical conditions are at increased risk due to fluid volume depletion and electrolyte imbalance (CDC, *Norovirus*).

Nearly two-thirds of all norovirus outbreaks reported in the United States occurred in long-term care facilities.

Outbreaks of norovirus illness also have occurred in restaurants, cruise ships, schools, banquet halls, summer camps, and even at family dinners. These are all places where people often eat food handled or prepared by others. Outbreaks of noroviruses on cruise ships and continuation of the outbreaks with the same strains on consecutive cruises in new passengers suggest that noroviruses have high infectivity (CDC, *Norovirus*).

Oral hydrating solutions should be given for attacks of norovirus, and in severe cases, intravenous fluid and electrolyte replacement may be necessary. At the first signs of this acute gastroenteritis outbreak, good handwashing, thorough and immediate disinfection with appropriate solutions, and isolation of sick people until 72 hours after they are symptom-free are critical (CDC, *Norovirus*).

Campylobacter

Campylobacteriosis is a leading cause of foodborne illness in the United States, and was not nationally notifiable until 2015. It also is an important cause of diarrheal illness throughout the world regardless of people's age. It is often implicated in traveler's diarrhea. The annual median number of *Campylobacter* outbreaks had increased in the United States from 28 in 2004–2006 to 56 in 2010–2012. Antimicrobial susceptibility testing of isolates from 4,793 domestic and 1,070 travel-associated infections revealed that, comparing 2004–2009 to 2010–2012, ciprofloxacin resistance increased among domestic infections (12.8% vs. 16.1%) (Geissler et al., 2017).

Consumption of contaminated poultry is the most common source of *Campylobacter* infection, although undercooked meats, ground beef, pork, cheese, eggs, shellfish, unpasteurized milk, and direct exposure to pets and farm animals have been implicated. Generally, the incubation period ranges from 2 to 5 days. The resulting diarrheal illness usually lasts no more than a week. Typical symptoms include nausea, vomiting, abdominal pain, fever, headache, and muscle pain. Occasionally, a severe case may last longer, and about 25% of the people affected may experience a relapse.

Campylobacter infection is usually a self-limited illness, diagnosed by stool culture, and treated by antidiarrheal medications such as loperamide. In more severe cases, antibiotics are prescribed. It is essential that affected people drink plenty of fluids, such as oral rehydration solutions, and wash hands carefully to prevent transmission to others (CDC, *Campylobacter*).

Listeria Monocytogenes

Listeria monocytogenes can cause listeriosis, an uncommon but potentially fatal foodborne bacterial disease. The disease primarily affects older adults, pregnant women, newborns, and adults with weakened immune systems, and can result in miscarriage, stillbirth, or severe illness and death in newborn infants. However, rarely, persons without these risk factors can also be affected. The risk may be reduced by recommendations for safe food preparation, consumption, and storage (CDC, *Listeria*).

Practice Point

Nurses and other healthcare providers should suspect listeriosis in high-risk patients (e.g., pregnant women) who become ill with diarrhea and/or flu-like symptoms, and have a recent history of eating delicatessen food, soft cheeses, or smoked seafood.

Nontyphoid Salmonella

Nontyphoid *Salmonella* is a bacterial disease transmitted by contaminated food and water, or contact with infected animals and reptiles. Because many milder cases are not diagnosed or reported, the actual number of infections may be 30 times greater. There are many kinds of *Salmonella* bacteria. *Salmonella* serotypes *Typhimurium* and *Enteritidis* are the most common in the United States. People at risk for severe or complicated illness include infants, the elderly, people with compromised immune systems, and organ transplant recipients. Salmonellosis is characterized by diarrhea, fever, and abdominal cramps 12 to 72 hours following exposure, and generally lasts 4 to 7 days. The majority of those infected recover without treatment.

However, in some cases, the diarrhea may be so severe that the patient needs to be hospitalized. Each year, 19,000 hospitalizations and 380 deaths from salmonellosis occur in the United States. A small number of persons with *Salmonella* develop pain in their joints. This is called reactive arthritis, and it can last for months or years. It also can lead to chronic arthritis which is difficult to treat. Treatment of dehydration and electrolyte imbalance is essential. Antibiotics are not usually necessary unless the infection spreads from the intestines. The CDC has identified *Salmonella* bacteria that have become resistant to antibiotics, largely as a result of the use of antibiotics to promote the growth of food animals (CDC, *Salmonella*).

Practice Point

An efficient and effective homemade oral rehydration solution is to stir one level teaspoon of salt and eight level teaspoons of sugar into one quart or liter of clean drinking water or water that has been boiled and cooled.

Salmonella enteritidis, generally found in shell eggs, has been decreasing as a source of foodborne illness during the past decade, attributed in part to farm-based egg control programs, as well as education of farm worker and consumers. Nonetheless, outbreaks continue to occur. For example, the CDC recently reported a multistate outbreak caused by *Salmonella oranienburg* infections linked to an egg company (CDC, *Salmonella oranienburg* infections linked to Good Earth Egg Company Shell Eggs: Final update, 2016). Outbreaks of *Salmonella* also have been associated with direct or indirect contact with live poultry, frogs, and turtles (CDC, *Salmonella*). In 2017, the CDC was conducting an on-going investigation of a multistate outbreak of human *Salmonella* infections linked to live poultry in backyard flocks. There were 790 cases reported in 48 states and the District of Columbia. Illnesses started on dates ranging from January 4, 2017 to June 20, 2017. Of 580 people with available information, 174 ill people had been hospitalized. However, no deaths had been reported. Figure 14.4 for map of the outbreak (CDC, 2017b).

Escherichia Coli O157:H7

Shiga toxin–producing *Escherichia coli* O157 is a deadly form of *E. coli*, which produces symptoms of severe abdominal cramps, bloody and nonbloody diarrhea, and vomiting that generally resolve within 7 to 10 days. In the very young and the elderly, infection with STEC O157:H7 can cause fatal hemolytic–uremic syndrome and renal failure (CDC, *E. coli*). This severe complication includes temporary anemia, profuse bleeding, and kidney failure.

Several outbreaks of *E. coli* O157:H7 have been associated with commercially packaged *foods* and fresh produce (CDC, *Multistate Foodborne Outbreak Investigations*). A recent multistate outbreak of *E. coli* O157:H7 involved I. M. Healthy Brand Soy Nut Butter products (CDC, 2017c). See Chapter 15 for a further discussion of *E. coli* O157:H7. Foodborne infections should be considered in people with diarrheal illness who are residents of, or travelers to an area where foodborne outbreaks have been reported. A careful history also should consist of contact with animals and reptiles as a source of infection.

Waterborne Diseases

In the United States, Canada, United Kingdom, and much of Europe, the drinking water supply is normally safe. The United States has one of the safest public water supplies in the world. The year 2008 marked the 100th anniversary of one of the most significant public health advances in U.S. history, the disinfection of drinking water. However, millions of people worldwide do not have access to safe water. In 2015, 71% of the global population (5.2 billion people) used a safely managed drinking-water service—that is, one located on premises, available when needed, and free from contamination. However, 884 million people lack even a basic drinking-water service, including 159 million people who are dependent on surface water. Globally, at least 2 billion people lack access to adequate sanitation and use a drinking water source contaminated with feces. Diarrheal diseases such as cholera kill more children than AIDS, malaria, and measles

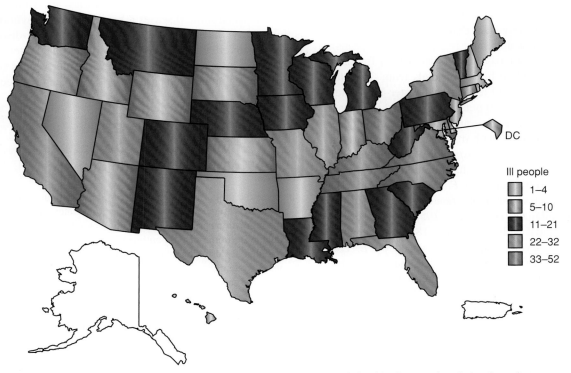

FIGURE 14.4 Multiple outbreaks of human salmonella infections linked to live poultry in backyard flocks, 2017. (*Source:* CDC. Retrieved August 2, 2017, from https://www.cdc.gov/salmonella/live-poultry-06-17/index.html.)

combined, making it the second leading cause of death among children less than 5 years of age. The majority of these deaths are attributable to unsafe water, poor sanitation, and inadequate hygiene (WHO, *Drinking-water fact sheet*).

In the United States, state and local governments establish and enforce regulations for protecting recreational water from naturally occurring and human-made contaminants. No federal regulatory agency has authority over treated recreational water (e.g., pools and interactive fountains), and no minimum federal design, construction, operation, disinfection, or filtration standards exist. The Environmental Protection Agency (EPA) sets water quality guidelines for natural, untreated recreational water (e.g., lakes, rivers, and oceans). Despite drinking water treatment advances, it is estimated that millions of annual diarrheal illness episodes still occur in the United States from exposure to contaminated municipal drinking water. In addition, we face emerging public health concerns such as chlorine-tolerant pathogens and the increasing complexity of waterborne diseases.

In surveillance data for 2011–2012, 32 drinking water–associated outbreaks were reported, accounting for at least 431 cases of illness, 102 hospitalizations, and 14 deaths. *Legionella* was responsible for 66% of outbreaks and 26% of illnesses, and viruses and non-Legionella bacteria together accounted for 16% of outbreaks and 53% of illnesses. The two most commonly identified deficiencies leading to drinking water–associated outbreaks were *Legionella* in building plumbing systems (66%) and untreated groundwater (13%) (CDC, 2015a).

Outbreaks of illness associated with recreational water use result from exposure to chemicals or infectious pathogens in recreational water venues that are treated (e.g., pools and hot tubs or spas) or untreated (e.g., lakes and oceans). For 2011–2012, the most recent years for which finalized data were available, public health officials from 32 states and Puerto Rico reported 90 recreational water–associated outbreaks to the CDC. The 90 outbreaks resulted in at least 1,788 cases, 95 hospitalizations, and one death. Among 69 (77%) outbreaks associated with treated recreational water, 36 (52%) were caused by *Cryptosporidium*. Among the 21 (23%) outbreaks associated with untreated recreational water, seven (33%) were caused by *E. coli* (*E. coli* O157:H7 or *E. coli* O111). These outbreaks resulted in at least 479 cases and 22 hospitalizations. Twenty (95%) of these outbreaks were associated with fresh water; 18 (86%) began in June–August; and seven (33%) were caused by *E. coli* O157:H7 or O11 (CDC, 2015b). The CDC has deficiency classifications for drinking water, and water not intended for drinking used during waterborne outbreak investigations (CDC, 2011b). These are outlined in Table 14.1.

The U.S. EPA and the CDC set national standards to protect drinking water and its sources against naturally occurring or human-made contaminants. In the United States, all public water systems must be monitored for total coliform bacteria (fecal contamination), which is 0 (or no) total coliform per 100 mL of water at a prescribed frequency.

TABLE 14.1 Estimates of People Affected by Global HIV/AIDS Epidemic, End of 2010	
HIV/AIDS Epidemic 2010	**Estimate**
People living with HIV/AIDS	34 million
Adults living with HIV/AIDS	30.6 million
Women living with HIV/AIDS	15.3 million
Children living with HIV/AIDS	3.4 million
People newly infected with HIV	2.7 million
Children newly infected with HIV	369,000
AIDS-related deaths in adults and children	1.8 million

More than 30 million people have died of AIDS since 1981.
Africa has more than 15 million AIDS orphans.
At the end of 2010, women accounted for 50% of all adults living with HIV worldwide.
Most countries aspire to expand antiretroviral treatment access to around 80% of those in need. However, this target has not been met, with current global treatment coverage at 54%.
Source: UNAIDS/WHO. *AIDS epidemic statistics 2010.* Retrieved April 30, 2013, from http://www.avert.org/worldstats.htm#.http://www.avert.org/ worldstats.htm.

State and local governments establish and enforce regulations to protect recreational water against naturally occurring or human contaminants. Standards for operating, disinfecting, and filtering public swimming and wading pools are regulated by state and local health departments and, as a result, vary throughout the United States. Reports of outbreaks in the states and territories are voluntary. However, waterborne diseases associated with recreational activities have been added to the CDC waterborne-disease outbreak surveillance system. Most recreational water outbreaks have been associated with treated water venues such as swimming pools or spas. Box 14.5 presents selected

---

14.5 *Healthy People 2020* Environmental Objectives Related to Water Quality

Increase the proportion of persons served by community water systems who receive a supply of drinking water that meets the regulations of the Safe Drinking Water Act.

Reduce waterborne-disease outbreaks arising from water intended for drinking among persons served by community water systems.

Reduce per capita domestic water use.

Maintain the percentage of days that beaches are open and safe for swimming.

Reduce the global burden of disease due to poor water quality, sanitation, and insufficient hygiene.

U.S. Department of Health and Human Services. *Healthy People 2020 environmental objectives: Water quality.* Retrieved April 29, 2013, from http://healthypeople.gov/2020/topicsobjectives2020/objectiveslist. aspx?topicId=12#364.

Healthy People 2020 objectives for environmental health and water quality.

Two criteria must be met for an event to be defined as a water-associated disease outbreak. First, two or more people must be linked epidemiologically by time, location of exposure to water, and illness characteristics. Second, the epidemiologic evidence must implicate recreational water or volatilization of water-associated compounds into the air surrounding the water as the probable source of illness. Multiple etiologic agents should be considered when waterborne disease is suspected and might be related to sewage or septic contamination (CDC, 2015a). The CDC has distributed guidance for assisting state and local health departments, aquatic facility inspection programs, building officials, the aquatics industry, and other interested parties in improving the health and safety at public aquatic facilities (CDC, 2016a).

As noted above, Legionnaires' disease was first recognized among hotel guests during an outbreak in Philadelphia, PA, in 1976. Between 8,000 and 18,000 people are hospitalized with Legionnaires disease in the United States each year. However, many infections are not diagnosed or reported, so this number may be higher. More illness is usually found in the summer and early fall, but it can happen any time of year. Outbreaks of this disease have been associated with potable water sources, air-conditioning cooling towers, and cruise ships. *Legionella* bacteria are not transmitted from person to person (CDC, *Legionella*).

Case 1: Examine Figure 14.5
1. Did the Alamosa, CO, contaminated water supply meet the definition of an outbreak?
2. If so, what type of outbreak was it?
3. Following the CDC Deficiency Classification for Drinking Water outlined in see Table 14.1, how many deficiencies did the Alamosa water supply have?

Evidence for Practice

The Shelby County Health Department in Tennessee received laboratory confirmation of nine cases of Legionnaires' disease among guests at the aquatics facilities and Guest House at the Graceland Hotel in Memphis, TN. It was estimated that the *Legionella* exposure extended from May 15 through June 27, 2017, with the first cases becoming symptomatic between July 1 and July 6, 2017. The last four cases were reported on July 14, 2017. The aquatic facilities were closed on June 27, 2017. Legionnaires' disease has an incubation period of 2 to 10 days, but can extend for about 2 weeks after exposure. Therefore, those

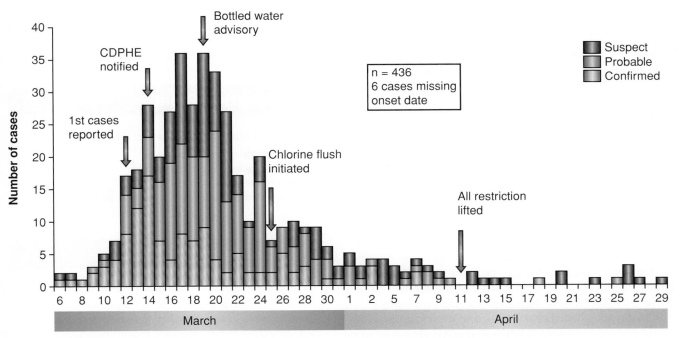

FIGURE 14.5 Epidemic curve for the waterborne outbreak in Alamosa, CO, 2008. (Falco, R. & Williams, S. I. [2009]. *Waterborne salmonella outbreak in Alamosa, Colorado, March and April 2008*. Retrieved August 5, 2017, from https://colorado.gov/pacific/sites/default/files/WQ-DW-Publications-Alamosa-Outbreak-Investigation-Report.pdf.)

exposed to the source could become symptomatic up to 2 weeks after remediation at the aquatic facilities took place. The Guest House at Graceland opened in October 2016, with 450 rooms and an aquatic area consisting of a hot tub and an outdoor pool. Unfortunately, no information was provided if the species and genotypes of *Legionella* that were isolated from the nine patients matched isolates from environmental sources.

Source: International Society for Infectious Diseases, July 20, 2017. *Legionellosis—USA (Tennessee) hotel, hot tub/pool.*

Sexually Transmitted Diseases (Sexually Transmitted Infections)

Sexually transmitted diseases (STDs) or sexually transmitted infections (STIs) affect men and women of all backgrounds and economic levels. Despite the fact that a great deal of progress has been made in STD prevention over the past four decades, the CDC estimates that there are about 20 million new STDs in the United States each year, with a cost of nearly $16 billion in direct medical costs alone. Almost half of the new cases occur in young people aged 15 to 24 years. It has been estimated that the actual rate of infection may be twice that of the reported rate, because many cases are undiagnosed and untreated. In addition, the CDC data suggest that there are more than 110 million total STDs among men and women across the nation. Its analyses included eight common STDs: chlamydia, gonorrhea, hepatitis B, herpes simplex (caused by herpes simplex virus type 2 [HSV-2]), HIV infection, human papillomavirus (HPV) infection, syphilis, and trichomoniasis (CDC, *STD fact sheet*).

Each of these infections is a potential threat to an individual's immediate and long-term health and well-being. In addition to increasing a person's risk for acquiring and transmitting HIV infection, STDs can lead to chronic pain and severe reproductive health complications, such as infertility and ectopic pregnancy. Many cases of chlamydia, gonorrhea, and syphilis continue to go undiagnosed and unreported, and data on several additional STDs, such as HPV, herpes simplex virus, and trichomoniasis, are not routinely reported to CDC. As a result, the annual surveillance reports capture only a fraction of the true burden of STDs in America (CDC, *STD fact sheet*).

Although the consequences of untreated STDs often are worse among young women, new data reveal that the annual number of new infections to be roughly equal among young women and young men, but young women are heavily affected by STDs since they face the most serious long-term health consequences. It is estimated that undiagnosed STDs cause infertility in more than 20,000 women each year.

Chlamydia, gonorrhea, syphilis, and trichomoniasis are easily treated and cured if diagnosed early. However, too many of these infections go undetected because they often have no symptoms. But even STDs without symptoms can have serious health consequences. Undiagnosed and untreated chlamydia or gonorrhea, for example, can put a woman at increased risk of chronic pelvic pain, life-threatening ectopic pregnancy, and an increase in infertility (CDC, *STD fact sheet*).

Any genital symptoms such as discharge or burning during urination or unusual sore or rash should be a signal for a person to stop having sex and to see a healthcare provider immediately. Infections caused by bacteria can be treated and usually cured with antibiotics, but those caused by viruses cannot be cured this way. All partners must be notified so that they can be examined and treated, if necessary. Other than abstinence, a long-term mutually monogamous relationship with a partner who has been tested and is known to be uninfected is the best way to avoid STDs. Sexual partners should talk to each other about their STDs so that preventive action can be taken. Prevention of STD transmission does not include washing the genitals, urinating, and/or douching after sex. Latex condoms can reduce the risk of transmission but only when used consistently (every time) and correctly. However, genital ulcer diseases, such as syphilis, can occur anywhere within the male and female genital areas, whether or not they are covered by a latex condom. Correct and consistent use of latex condoms can reduce the risk of STDS *only* when the infected area or site of potential exposure is protected. Condoms lubricated with spermicides (especially nonoxynol-9 or N-9) are no more effective than other lubricated condoms in protecting against the transmission of STDs. Based on the findings from several research studies, N-9 may itself cause genital lesions, providing a point of entry for HIV and other STDs. Therefore, since 2010, the CDC has recommended that N-9 not be used as a microbicide or lubricant during vaginal or anal intercourse since 2010), and remains in its updated 2015 guidelines (CDC, 2015c). The *Healthy People 2020* objectives for STDs are presented in Box 14.6.

Practice Point

Any person is in a high-risk group for STDs if they

- Have multiple sexual partners.
- Do not use a condom during sex.
- Have other STDs.
- Have a sexual partner who has had an STD.

Evidence for Practice

The clinical treatment guidelines for STDs typically recommend antibiotic therapy to cover common infections. However, overtreatment and under treatment of STDs are common during emergency department (ED) visits. Huppert and colleagues (2013) examined a quality improvement (QI) project that aimed to improve follow-up care for STDs in the ED. They compared the

14.6 *Healthy People 2020 Objectives for Sexually Transmitted Diseases*

Reduce the proportion of females aged 15 to 44 years who have ever required treatment of pelvic inflammatory disease (PID).

Reduce congenital syphilis.

Reduce the proportion of adolescents and young adults with *Chlamydia trachomatis* infections.

Reduce gonorrhea rates.

Reduce sustained domestic transmission of primary and secondary syphilis.

Reduce the proportion of adults with genital herpes infection due to herpes simplex type 2.

Reduce the proportion of females with human papillomavirus (HPV) infection.

Increase the proportion of sexually active females aged 24 years and younger enrolled in commercial health insurance plans who are screened annually for genital *Chlamydia* infections.

Increase the proportion of sexually active females aged 24 years and younger enrolled in Medicaid who are screened annually for genital *Chlamydia* infections.

Increase the proportion of HIV-infected persons who know they are infected.

Source: U.S. Department of Health and Human Services. *Healthy People 2020 sexually transmitted diseases objectives.* Retrieved April 29, 2013, from http://healthypeople.gov/2020/topicsobjectives2020/objectiveslist. aspx?topicId=37.

point-of-care (POC) treatment patterns for gonorrhea and trichomoniasis among young women seen in an ED over an 18-month period. Of the 1,877 visits, 8.8% of women had gonorrhea and 16.5% had trichomoniasis. Overtreatment was higher for women with gonorrhea than with trichomoniasis (54% vs. 23%, $p < 0.001$). However, overtreatment for gonorrhea decreased from 58% to 47% ($p < 0.01$) and overtreatment for trichomoniasis decreased from 24% to 18% ($p < 0.01$), which corresponded to improvements in patient follow-up for the QI project. Undertreatment was higher for women with gonorrhea than with trichomoniasis (29% vs. 21%, $p = 0.03$), and did not change over time. An unanticipated benefit of the QI project to improve patient follow-up was the decrease in antibiotic usage in the ED. Given the ability of gonorrhea to develop antibiotic resistance, Hubbert and colleagues recommended that future studies focus on the development of an accurate POC test for gonorrhea.

In **Case 2**, Megan discussed her urinary frequency and abnormal vaginal discharge with the school nurse. What advice might the school nurse have given her?

Chlamydia

Chlamydia, caused by infection with *Chlamydia trachomatis*, is the most common notifiable disease in the United States. It is among the most prevalent of all STDs, and since 1994, has comprised the largest proportion of all STDs reported to the CDC, with 1,526,658 cases reported in 2015 at a rate of 478.8 per 100,000 population. Studies also demonstrate the high prevalence of chlamydial infections in the general U.S. population, particularly among young women. The rate of reported cases of chlamydia is highest among adolescents and young adults aged 15 to 24 years. In 2015, the rate of reported cases of chlamydia among 15- to 19-year-olds was 1,857.8 cases per 100,000 population and the rate among 20- to 24-year-olds was 2,574.9 cases per 100,000 population. From 2011 to 2013, the rate of reported cases decreased to 443.5 cases per 100,000 population. The rate of reported cases then increased in 2014 at 452.2 and up 5.9% again in 2015 at 478.8 (CDC, *Chlamydia*).

Substantial racial/ethnic disparities in chlamydial infection exist, with prevalence among non-Hispanic blacks approximately 5.9 times the prevalence among non-Hispanic whites. Chlamydia is also common among men who have sex with men (MSM) (CDC, *Chlamydia fact sheet*). Chlamydia is a nationally notifiable disease, and CDC 2016 data indicated that the *Healthy People 2020* objective to reduce *C. trachomatis* infections among females 15 to 24 years of age attending family planning clinics to 6.7% had been met (CDC, 2017). Chlamydial infection is caused by a bacterium, *C. trachomatis*, which is transmitted during vaginal, oral, or anal sexual contact with an infected partner.

Chlamydia is known as a "silent" infection because most infected people are asymptomatic and lack abnormal physical examination findings. In women, the bacteria initially infect the cervix, where the infection may cause signs and symptoms of cervicitis (e.g., mucopurulent endocervical discharge, easily induced endocervical bleeding), and sometimes the urethra, which may result in signs and symptoms of urethritis (e.g., pyuria, dysuria, urinary frequency). Infection can spread from the cervix to the upper reproductive tract (i.e., uterus, fallopian tubes), causing pelvic inflammatory disease (PID), which may be asymptomatic and is a major cause of infertility among women of childbearing age. A pregnant woman may pass chlamydial infection to her newborn during delivery, resulting in subsequent neonatal eye infection or pneumonia. Men who are symptomatic typically have urethritis, with a mucoid or watery urethral discharge and dysuria. A minority of infected men develop epididymitis (with or without symptomatic urethritis), presenting with unilateral testicular pain, tenderness, and swelling (CDC, *Chlamydia fact sheet*, 2018).

Screening programs have been demonstrated to reduce rates of adverse sequelae in women. There are a number of diagnostic tests for chlamydia, including cell culture (the criterion standard) and nucleic acid amplification tests (NAATs), and others. NAATs are the most sensitive tests and can be performed on easily obtainable specimens such as vaginal swabs (either clinician- or patient-collected) or urine (CDC, *Chlamydia fact sheet*, 2018). Urine is the specimen of choice for males. Self-collected vaginal swab specimens perform at least as well as other approved specimens using NAATs. Generally, girls in adolescent phase of development may collect their own urine or swab their own vagina to screen for Chlamydia especially if they are not having symptoms. Persons with chlamydia should abstain from sexual activity for 7 days after single-dose antibiotics or until completion of a 7-day course of antibiotics, to prevent spreading the infection to partners. Chlamydia can be easily cured with antibiotics. HIV-positive persons with chlamydia should receive the same treatment as those who are HIV-negative (CDC, *Chlamydia fact sheet*). A number of antibiotics such as azithromycin (Zithromax), doxycycline, or erythromycin may be prescribed for treatment (CDC, *Chlamydia curriculum*).

Evidence for Practice

The CDC and the U.S. Preventive Services Task Force (USPSTF) recommends yearly chlamydia screening of all sexually active women aged 25 or younger and older women with risk factors for chlamydial infections (e.g., women who have a new or more than one sex partner). Pregnant women should be screened during their first prenatal care visit. Pregnant women under 25 or at increased risk for chlamydia (e.g., women who have a new or more than one sex partner) should be screened again in their third trimester. Any woman who is sexually active should discuss her risk factors with a healthcare provider who can then determine if more frequent screening is necessary. Routine screening is not recommended for men. However, the screening of sexually active young men should be considered in clinical settings with a high prevalence of chlamydia (e.g., adolescent clinics, correctional facilities, and STD clinics) when resources permit and will decrease screening programs for women (CDC, *Chlamydia fact sheet*; Agency for Health Research and Quality [AHRQ], 2014).

Gonorrhea

Gonorrhea is second only to chlamydia in number of cases reported to the CDC. In 2015, persons aged 15 to 44 years accounted for 92.7% of reported gonorrhea cases with known age (CDC, *Gonorrhea*). Infections with *Neisseria gonorrhoeae*, like those resulting from *C. trachomatis*, cause several clinical syndromes, including urogenital, pharyngeal, and rectal infections in males and females, and conjunctivitis in adults and neonates. If untreated, gonorrhea can cause PID, tubal infertility, ectopic pregnancy, and chronic pelvic pain (CDC, *Gonorrhea fact sheet*).

Like chlamydia, gonorrhea is substantially underdiagnosed and underreported; the number of reported cases is suspected to underestimate incidence by approximately 50%. In 2009, the gonorrhea rate decreased to 98.1 cases per 100,000 population. This was the lowest rate since recording of gonorrhea rates began in the 1970s. Between 2009 and 2012, the rate increased slightly each year to 106.7 cases per 100,000 population in 2012. In 2013, the rate decreased slightly to 105.3 cases per 100,000 population and then during 2013–2015, the rate increased each year. By 2015, a total of 395,216 cases were reported for a rate of 123.9 cases per 100,000 population. The rate of reported gonorrhea cases among males was higher than the rate among females. Reported gonorrhea cases continued to be highest among adolescents and young adults, with persons aged 15 to 44 years accounting for 92.7% of reported gonorrhea cases in 2015 (CDC, *Gonorrhea*). These data indicate that the rate of gonorrhea still remained higher in 2015 than the *Healthy People 2020* target of 251.9 new cases of gonorrhea among females aged 15 to 44 years per 100,000 population, and 194.8 new cases of gonorrhea among males aged 15 to 44 years per 100,000 population (CDC, 2017a) (see Box 14.6 for *Healthy People 2020* STD objectives).

Patients infected with *N. gonorrhoeae* frequently are coinfected with *C. trachomatis*. Therefore, patients with gonorrhea should be tested for other STDs. Because of findings that chlamydial and gonorrheal infections often coexist led to the recommendation that patients treated for gonococcal infection also be treated routinely with a regimen that is effective against uncomplicated genital *C. trachomatis* infection. In addition, because most gonococci in the United States are susceptible to doxycycline and azithromycin, routine co-treatment hinder the development of antimicrobial-resistant *N. gonorrhoeae* (CDC, 2015c).

Drug-resistant strains of gonorrhea are increasing in many areas of the world, including the United States, making successful treatment of gonorrhea more difficult. Antimicrobial susceptibility patterns of *N. gonorrhoeae* have been closely monitored since 1986 through the Gonococcal Isolate Surveillance Project (GISP), and the information has been used to update treatment recommendations. The increased prevalence of fluoroquinolone resistance in *N. gonorrhoeae* became widespread in the United States in the 1990s and 2000s, when the proportion of *N. gonorrhoeae* isolates in MSM that were resistant to ciprofloxacin (a fluoroquinolone antimicrobial) increased significantly. While the first fluoroquinolone-resistant *N. gonorrhoeae* cases were detected among heterosexuals, fluoroquinolone resistance became widespread in the continental United States among MSM with gonorrhea before becoming widespread among heterosexuals. By 2011, the CDC no longer recommended the use of fluoroquinolones for the treatment of gonococcal infections and associated conditions such as PID. Therefore, currently, the CDC recommends dual therapy with ceftriaxone (an injectable cephalosporin) 250 mg intramuscularly as a single dose plus azithromycin 1 g orally as a single dose given together for 7 days as the most effective treatment for uncomplicated gonorrhea. However, in the case of azithromycin allergy, doxycycline (100 mg orally twice a day for 7 days) can be used in place of azithromycin as an alternative second antimicrobial when used in combination with ceftriaxone (or cefixime) (CDC, 2015c).

People who have had gonorrhea and have been treated can get the disease again if they have sexual contact with people infected with gonorrhea. Every person who has been diagnosed and treated for gonorrhea should notify all recent sex partners so that they can see a healthcare provider and be treated. This will reduce the development of serious complications from gonorrhea and also reduce the possibility of reinfection. All people involved must avoid sex until they have completed their treatment of gonorrhea.

In **Case 2**, following the suggestion of the school nurse, Megan saw a nurse practitioner at a local women's health clinic. After taking a history, the nurse suspected an STD. A pelvic examination revealed mucopurulent cervicitis, and a tissue culture was taken. A dipstick urine analysis of a urine sample was positive for bacteria. A chlamydial infection was suspected, and a UTI was diagnosed.

1. What other information should the nurse practitioner consider in this case?
2. What treatment is indicated in this case?
3. What additional recommendations would you make?

Evidence for Practice

The United States Preventive Services Task Force (USPSTF), an independent panel of experts supported by the Agency for Healthcare Research and Quality (AHRQ), recommends that clinicians routinely screen all sexually active women, including pregnant women, for gonorrhea and chlamydia infections if they have a history of previous STDs, new or multiple sexual partners, inconsistent condom use, sex work, and drug use. Currently, the USPSTF concludes that the current evidence is insufficient to assess the balance of benefits and harms of screening for chlamydia and gonorrhea in men (USPSTF, 2014). Also, the USPSTF recommends prophylactic ocular topical medication for all newborns for the prevention of gonococcal ophthalmia neonatorum (USPSTF, 2014).

In **Case 2**, within a few days, Megan's tissue culture that was collected before treatment came back positive for *N. gonorrhoeae* in addition to *C. trachomatis*.
Does the nurse practitioner need to report these infections to the local health authorities?

Syphilis

Syphilis has often been called "the great imitator," because many of the signs and symptoms are indistinguishable from those of other diseases. This genital ulcerative disease is caused by the bacterium *Treponema pallidum*. It is transmitted from person to person through direct contact with a syphilitic sore. These sores occur mainly on the external genitals, vagina, anus, or in the rectum, although they can occur on the lips or in the mouth. Transmission occurs during vaginal, anal, or oral sex, and the organism can pass the placental barrier and infect the fetus.

Syphilis causes significant complications if untreated and facilitates the transmission of HIV infection. Primary and secondary syphilis rate has increased almost every year since 2000–2001. In 2015, a total of 23,872 primary and secondary syphilis cases were reported. During 2014–2015, the national primary and secondary syphilis rate increased 19.0% to 7.5 cases per 100,000 population, the highest rate reported since 1994 (CDC, *Syphilis*). Primary and secondary syphilis are the most infectious stages of the disease, and if not adequately treated, can lead to visual impairment, stroke, and in rare cases, even death. The primary stage of syphilis consists of a single sore or multiple sores. The sore(s) appears at the location where syphilis entered the body.

The sore is usually firm, round, and painless. Because the sore is painless, it can easily go unnoticed. The sore lasts 3 to 6 weeks and heals regardless of whether the person is treated. However, if the infected person does not receive adequate treatment, the infection progresses to the secondary stage. Skin rashes and/or sores in the mouth, vagina, or anus (also called mucous membrane lesions) mark the secondary stage of symptoms. This stage usually starts with a rash on one or more areas of the body. Rashes associated with secondary syphilis can appear from the time when the primary sore is healing to several weeks after the sore has healed. The rash usually does not cause itching. This rash may appear as rough, red, or reddish brown spots both on the palms of the hands and/or the bottoms of the feet. However, this rash may look different on other parts of the body and can look like rashes caused by other diseases. The latent (hidden) stage of syphilis begins when primary and secondary symptoms disappear. Without treatment, the infected person can continue to have syphilis in their body, even though there are no signs or symptoms. This latent stage can last for years (CDC, *Syphilis, Fact sheet*). Untreated early syphilis in pregnant women results in perinatal death in up to 40% of cases and, if acquired during the 4 years before pregnancy, can lead to infection of the fetus in 80% of cases (CDC, *Syphilis, Fact sheet*).

Syphilis cases had been declining significantly in the United States since reporting began in 1941. For example, the overall rate of primary and secondary syphilis in the United States had declined 90% between 1990 and 2000. However, the syphilis rate in the United States had increased each year from 2001 to 2008. But, the overall rate of syphilis infection had been falling since 2008. In 2010, the overall rate decreased for the first time in 10 years, and the rate of primary and secondary syphilis in 2011 remained unchanged. Nonetheless, by 2015, there were 74,702 reported new diagnoses of syphilis (all stages), with 23,872 of the cases being primary and secondary syphilis. The majority of these cases occurred among gay, bisexual, and other men who have sex with men (MSM). In 2015, MSM accounted for 81.7% of all primary and secondary syphilis cases among males in which sex of sex partner was known and 60% of all primary and secondary syphilis cases overall. However, in recent years, the rate of primary and secondary syphilis has been increasing among heterosexual men and women as well as among MSM (CDC, *Fact sheet*).

Congenital syphilis (syphilis passed from pregnant women to their babies) continues to be a concern in the United States. After a steady decline from 2008 to 2012, data show a sharp increase in congenital syphilis rates. In 2015, the number of cases was the highest it's been since 2001. In 2015, 487 cases of congenital syphilis were reported, with rates 8.0 times and 3.5 times higher among infants born to black and Hispanic mothers (35.2 and 15.5 cases per 100,000 live births, respectively) compared to white mothers (4.4 cases per 100,000 live births). The rates of congenital syphilis remained higher than the *Healthy People 2020* objective of 9.6 new cases of congenital syphilis per 100,000 live births) (CDC, 2017a).

Penicillin G, administered parenterally, is the preferred drug for treatment of all stages of syphilis. The preparation or preparations used (i.e., benzathine, aqueous procaine, or aqueous crystalline), the dosage, and the length of treatment depend on the stage and clinical manifestations of the disease. Treatment for late latent syphilis and tertiary syphilis requires a longer duration of therapy, because organisms theoretically might be dividing more slowly although the scientific community has not been able to prove systematically if this is really true. Treating people diagnosed with latent syphilis for a more extensive time is indicated for adequate treatment if they were exposed in the previous year. Selection of the appropriate penicillin preparation is important, because *T. pallidum* can reside in sequestered sites (e.g., the CNS and aqueous humor) that are poorly accessed by some forms of penicillin. The recommended regimen for early latent Syphilis is benzathine penicillin G, 2.4 million units IM in a single dose. For late latent syphilis, the recommended regimen is benzathine penicillin G, at weekly doses of 2.4 million units for 3 weeks. The recommended regimen for tertiary syphilis

with a normal CSF examination is benzathine penicillin G 7.2 million units, total, administered as three doses of 2.4 million units IM each at 1-week intervals. Persons with HIV infection, who have primary or secondary syphilis should be treated as those without HIV infection. Parenteral penicillin G is the only therapy with documented efficacy for syphilis during pregnancy. Pregnant women with syphilis in any stage who report penicillin allergy should be desensitized and treated with penicillin. As of 2017, Pfizer, the sole manufacturer of penicillin G benzathine (Bicillin L-A) in the United States, continued to experience a manufacturing delay of this product. Penicillin G procaine also was unavailable. CDC is working with FDA's Drug Shortage Staff and Pfizer to address this situation (CDC, *Syphilis*).

Because effective treatment is available, it is important that people be screened for syphilis on an ongoing basis if their sexual behaviors put them at risk for STDs. People who are diagnosed and treated for syphilis must abstain from sexual contact until the syphilitic sores are completely healed. All persons who have syphilis should be tested for HIV infection. The USPSTF recommendations screening of all pregnant women at the first prenatal visit, retest early in the third trimester and at delivery, if at high risk. In geographic areas in which the prevalence of HIV is high, sexually active individuals should be screened at first HIV evaluation, and at least annually thereafter. More frequent screening might be appropriate depending on individual risk behaviors and the local epidemiology (USPSTF, 2015).

> ### ◎ Evidence for Practice
>
> In addition to all pregnant women, the USPSTF strongly recommends that clinicians screen people at increased risk for syphilis infection; this includes MSM, commercial sex workers, people who exchange sex for drugs, and people in correctional facilities (USPSTF, 2015).

Human Papillomavirus

Genital HPV infection is one of the most common causes of STDs in the world. It is estimated that 100% of sexually active men and women acquire genital HPV infection at some point in their lives. With an estimated annual incidence of 14.1 million cases, the CDC estimates that HPV accounts for the majority of newly acquired STDs in the United States. There is an estimated $1.7 billion annual cost in direct medical costs to treat conditions associated with genital HPV infection (e.g., warts, cervical dysplasia, cancer). An estimated 79 million women aged 14 to 59 years are infected with HPV, with the highest prevalence in those between the ages of 20 and 24 years. While the vast majority (90%) of HPV infections will go away on their own within 2 years and cause no harm, some of these infections will take hold and potentially lead to serious disease, including cervical cancer. Although rare, genital HPV infection with low-risk types can be transmitted from mother to newborn during delivery and can cause respiratory tract warts in the child, known as juvenile-onset recurrent respiratory papillomatosis (CDC, *CDC curriculum HPV*).

More than 100 types of HPV exist, more than 40 of which can infect the genital area. Genital HPV types are divided into two groups: low-risk types and high-risk types. Low-risk (nononcogenic) types can cause genital warts and benign or low-grade cellular changes (e.g., mild Pap test abnormalities), but are not associated with increased risk of cancer. High-risk (oncogenic) types can cause cervical dysplasia (both low-grade and high-grade cervical cellular changes), moderate to severe Pap test abnormalities, and in rare cases, cancers of the cervix. In addition, these types of HPV infection have been associated with cancers of the vulva, vagina, anus, penis, and oropharynx. Infection is predominantly associated with sexual activity, including vaginal and anal intercourse, oral sex, and nonpenetrative sexual activity (genital–genital contact); therefore, it requires contact with viable HPV and microtrauma to skin or mucous membranes to establish infection, but transmission can occur from asymptomatic and subclinically infected persons. The natural history of HPV infection is usually benign. Low-risk genital HPV types are associated with mild Pap test abnormalities and genital warts. High-risk types are associated with mild to severe Pap test abnormalities, and rarely, cancers of the cervix, vulva, vagina, anus, penis, and oropharynx. Most women infected with HPV infection do not develop cervical cancer. Recurrence of genital warts within the first several months after treatment is common (CDC, *curriculum HPV*).

Three HPV vaccines are licensed for use in the United States. Quadrivalent and 9-valent HPV vaccines (4vHPV and 9vHPV, Gardasil and Gardasil 9, Merck and Co, Inc., Whitehouse Station, NJ) are licensed for use in females and males aged 9 through 26 years. Bivalent HPV vaccine (2vHPV, Cervarix, GlaxoSmithKline, Rixensart, Belgium) is licensed for use in females aged 9 through 25 years. However, as of late 2016, only 9vHPV is being distributed in the United States. The majority of all HPV-associated cancers are caused by HPV 16 or 18, types targeted by all three vaccines. In addition, the 4vHPV vaccine targets HPV 6 and 11, types that cause genital warts. The 9vHPV vaccine protects against these and five additional types: HPV 31, 33, 45, 52, and 58. All three vaccines have been approved for administration in a three-dose series at intervals of 0, 1, or 2, and 6 months. In October 2016, after considering new clinical trial results, the Food and Drug Administration (FDA) also approved 9vHPV for use in a two-dose series for girls and boys aged 9 through 14 years. In October 2016, the Advisory Committee on Immunization Practices (ACIP) recommended a two-dose schedule for adolescents initiating

HPV vaccination in this age range (Meites, Kempe, & Markowitz, 2016) The CDC recommends that all teenage girls and women through age 26 receive HPV vaccines, as well as all teenage boys and men through age 21 (and through age 26 for gay, bisexual, and MSM). Also, immunocompromised persons (including those with HIV infection) should be vaccinated through age 26 years. Neither vaccine is recommended for persons over age 26. Ideally, the vaccines should be administered before onset of sexual activity (CDC, *curriculum HPV*; *STD fact sheet*). The American Academy of Pediatrics (AAP) has developed a "HPV Champion Toolkit" to help educate healthcare professionals discuss HPV vaccination with parents and make changes in practice to improve HPV vaccination rates (AAP, *HPV champion toolkit*).

Treatment of warts or cervical cellular abnormalities may reduce, but likely does not eliminate infectiousness of HPV. Most genital HPV infections, whether caused by low-risk or high-risk types, are transient, asymptomatic, and have no clinical consequences. CDC-recommended patient-applied and provider-administered treatment regimens are available. Choice of treatment should be guided by location of the lesion(s), patient preference, experience of the healthcare provider, available resources, and pregnancy status. Healthcare providers should identify warts for patient-applied treatment and teach patients how to apply substances. Patient-applied treatments consist of podofilox 0.5% solution or gel, imiquimod 5% cream, or sinecatechins 15% ointment. Podofilox, an antimitotic drug that destroys warts, is relatively inexpensive, easy to use, and safe. Imiquimod 5% cream is a topically active immune enhancer that stimulates production of interferon and other cytokines. The safety of podofilox, imiquimod, and sinecatechins during pregnancy has not been established. Also, the safety of sinecatechins has not been established in HIV- or HSV-coinfected individuals. CDC-recommended provider-administered regimens for external genital warts include cryotherapy with liquid nitrogen or cryoprobe, podophyllin resin 10% to 25% in compound tincture of benzoin, trichloroacetic acid (TCA) or bichloroacetic acid (BCA) 80% to 90%, or surgical removal (CDC, *curriculum HPV*).

Practice Point

It is important to incorporate issues of HPV management into well visits for young men and women of all ages. All boys and girls ages 11 or 12 years should get vaccinated, and they need to know that the current HPV vaccine can reduce their risk of being infected by four types of HPV. They also need to know that although condom use does not completely prevent the transmission of HPV, it can significantly decrease it.

Most HPV infections usually go away by themselves, but having an HPV infection can cause certain kinds of cancer to develop. These include cervical cancer in women, penile cancer in men, and anal cancer in both women and men. The virus also can cause cancer in the back of the throat, including the base of the tongue and tonsils (called oropharyngeal cancer). All of these cancers are caused by HPV infections that did not go away. Cancer develops very slowly and may not be diagnosed until years, or even decades, after a person initially gets infected with HPV. Currently, there is no way to know who will have only a temporary HPV infection, and who will develop cancer after getting HPV. Screening should continue, even in vaccinated women, to look for abnormal changes in cells. The vaccine is a series of injections of a noninfectious virus-like particle. Young men and women need to know that they cannot develop an HPV infection from the vaccine.

Source: CDC. *Human Papillomavirus (HPV).* Retrieved August 9, 2017, from https://www.cdc.gov/std/hpv/default.htm.

Human Immunodeficiency Virus

HIV is a retrovirus that infects cells of the human immune system, impairing and destroying their function. Symptoms may be absent in the early stages of infection. However, as the infection progresses, the immune system becomes more compromised, and the person becomes more susceptible to opportunistic infections. In addition, HIV infection increases the risk of reactivation of latent TB (CDC, *HIV and tuberculosis*). The most advanced stage of HIV infection is AIDS (stage 3). It can take 10 to 15 years for an HIV-infected person to develop AIDS, but antiretroviral therapy (ART) can slow down the process even further. Before the highly active ART (HAART) era, the median time from HIV seroconversion to the development of AIDS was 7.7 to 11.0 years, with a median survival rate from 7.5 to 12 years. These effective drug therapies keep HIV-infected persons healthy longer and significantly reduced the death rate in 20 years by 50%. AIDS is now considered a chronic and controlled disease. According to the United Nations Program on HIV/AIDS (UNAIDS), 19.5 million people globally are now on life-saving treatment, with AIDS-related deaths halved since 2005. Therefore, the number of people living with HIV is increasing in countries where HAART treatment is available (AVERT, 2017).

Still, according to the most recent CDC data, 39,513 HIV infections were diagnosed in the United States in 2015. Gay, bisexual, and other men who have sex with men bear the greatest burden by risk group, representing an estimated 26,200 of these new HIV infections (*CDC, HIV/AIDS*) (Table 14.2).

HIV continues to be a major global public health issue. In 2015, an estimated 36.7 million people were living with HIV (including 1.8 million children), with a global HIV prevalence of 0.8%. The vast majority of this number live in low- and middle-income countries. An estimated 40% don't know their infection status. In the same year, 1.1 million people died of AIDS-related illnesses (AVERT, 2017).

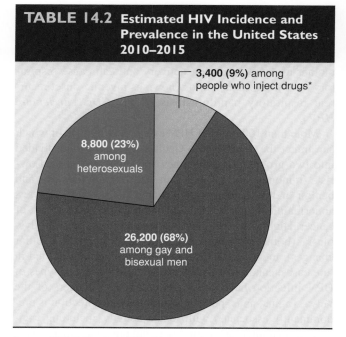

TABLE 14.2 Estimated HIV Incidence and Prevalence in the United States 2010–2015

3,400 (9%) among people who inject drugs*

8,800 (23%) among heterosexuals

26,200 (68%) among gay and bisexual men

Source: CDC. Estimated HIV incidence and prevalence in the United States, 2010–2015. *HIV Surveillance Supplemental Report* 2018;23(1).

Since the start of the epidemic, an estimated 78 million people have become infected with HIV and 35 million people have died of AIDS-related illnesses. In 2015, there were roughly 2.1 million new HIV infections, 150,000 of which were among children. Most of these children live in sub-Saharan Africa and were infected via their HIV-positive mothers during pregnancy, childbirth, or breastfeeding. Progress in decreasing new HIV infections among adults has slowed in recent years. Since 2010, the annual number of new infections among adults (age 15 years and over) has remained static at 1.9 million. However, significant progress has been made in the prevention of mother-to-child transmission of HIV. In 2015, 77% of all pregnant women living with HIV accessed treatment to prevent HIV transmission to their babies. By the end of 2015, 46% of all adults and 49% of all children living with HIV were accessing ART (AVERT, 2017).

A comparison of country data shows huge discrepancies in efforts to slow the spread of new HIV infections. Some countries have achieved a decline of 50% or more in new HIV infections among adults over the last 10 years, while many have made no measurable progress. Yet others are experiencing worrying increases in new HIV infections (AVERT, 2017). According to UNAIDS (2016), the number of new HIV infections in 2015 are down an overall 6% from 2010. The WHO reports that as of 2015, the global number of people living with HIV was 36.7 million (range: 34.0 to 39.8 million), compared to 31.8 million (range: 29.4 million to 34.5 million) in 2005. This reflects continued transmission of HIV despite reductions in incidence, and the benefits of significantly expanded access to antiretroviral, which have helped to reduce the number of people dying from

Number of people, by WHO region

- Eastern Mediterranean: 330 000 [240 00–490 000]
- Western Pacific: 1 400 000 [1 100 000–2 000 000]
- Europe: 2 500 000 [2 300 000–2 700 000]
- Americas: 3 400 000 [3 000 000–3 900 000]
- South-East Asia: 3 500 000 [3 000 000–4 100 000]
- Africa: 25 500 000 [23 00 000–28 400 000]

Total: 36 700 000 [31.40–35.90]

FIGURE 14.6 Adults and children estimated to be living with HIV by WHO region, 2015. (Data from WHO. [2016]. *Global summary of the HIV epidemic, 2015*. Retrieved August 2, 2017 from http://gamapserver.who.int/mapLibrary/Files/Maps/HIV_all_2015.png.)

AIDS-related causes, especially since 2004–2005. These data reflect not only the number of people newly infected (incidence) with HIV, but the prevalence (total number of infections, as defined in Chapter 7) of all cases of HIV due in part to the expanded access to ART, which has helped to reduce the number of people dying from AIDS-related causes. Sub-Saharan Africa still bears an inordinate share of the global HIV burden. Although the rate of new HIV infections has decreased, the total number of people living with HIV continues to rise. In 2015, that number reached 25.5 million, about 70% of the global total (Fig. 14.6) (WHO, *Number of people living with HIV*).

HIV targets predominantly young- and middle-aged adults who are the mainstay of the economy and the principal support of their families. As the loss of productive people in a society gradually increases, poverty also increases; there are fewer resources to cope with the situation, and fewer options for change whether at family, community, or national level. Economic growth is compromised, and the very fabric of society can be destroyed (CDC, *Global HIV/AIDS*).

The CDC estimates an estimated 1.1 million people in the United States were living with HIV at the end of 2014, the most recent year for which this information is available. Of those people, about 15%, or 1 in 7, did not know they were infected. Gay, bisexual, and other MSM are most seriously affected by HIV. In 2014, gay and bisexual men accounted for 70% of all new HIV infections. In the same year, individuals infected through heterosexual sex made up 23% of all new HIV infections. Within the overall estimates, however, some groups are affected more than others. If we look at HIV diagnoses by race and ethnicity, African Americans are most affected by HIV. In 2015, African Americans made up only 12% of the U.S. population but had 45% of all new HIV diagnoses. Additionally, Hispanic/Latinos are also strongly affected. They made up 18% of the U.S. population but had 24% of all new HIV diagnoses in 2015. Young people aged 13 to 24 are especially affected by HIV. In 2015, they comprised 16% of the U.S. population but accounted for 22% of all new HIV diagnoses. All young people are not equally at risk, however. Young gay and bisexual men accounted for 84% of all new HIV diagnoses in people aged 13 to 24 in 2015, and young African American gay and bisexual men are even more severely affected (CDC, *HIV Basic Statistics*).

> As for AIDS, it's a plague. We are human, we get plagues. They come along every so often, kill off two-thirds of the population; in the next generation it's a quarter; after that it's a childhood disease. **Larry Niven**

From 2010 to 2014, the annual number and rate of diagnoses of HIV infection in the United States decreased to 39,513 and 12.3, respectively. However, numbers and rates of diagnoses of HIV infection increased in some subgroups and decreased in others. From 2010 to 2014, the rate for persons aged 25 to 29 years increased, with the highest rate among persons aged 25 to 29 years (33.4), followed by persons aged 20 to 24 years (31.2). Nonetheless, the rates for persons aged 20 to 24 years remained stable. The rates for children (aged less than 13 years) and persons aged 13 to 19, 30 to 64 years, and 65 years and older decreased. The rates for male and female adults and adolescents decreased, with males accounting for 81% of all diagnoses of HIV infection among adults and adolescents. The highest rate was for blacks/African Americans at 44.3, followed by 16.4 for Hispanics/Latinos. Transmission from 2010 through 2014, among male adults and adolescents, the annual number of diagnosed HIV infections attributed to injection drug use, to male-to-male sexual contact and injection drug use, or to heterosexual contact decreased. The number of infections attributed to male-to-male sexual contact remained stable. Among female adults and adolescents, the number of infections attributed to injection drug use or to heterosexual contact decreased.

The 2014 revised surveillance case definition for HIV was used to classify cases diagnosed in 2014 and later. The term *diagnosis of HIV infection* is defined as a diagnosis of HIV infection regardless of the stage of disease (stage 0, 1, 2, 3 or unknown) and refers to all persons with a diagnosis of HIV infection. The term HIV infection, stage 3 (AIDS) and its condensed version, stage 3 (AIDS), refer specifically to persons with diagnosed HIV whose infection was classified as stage 3 (AIDS) during a given year (for diagnoses) or whose infection has ever been classified as stage 3 (AIDS) (for prevalence and deaths). By 2015, the rate of infections classified as stage 3 (AIDS) was 5.7 (CDC, 2015b).

Healthy People 2020 objectives focused on HIV are outlined in see Box 14.8. A major objective in this category is to *increase the proportion of persons living with HIV who know their serostatus* (*Healthy People 2020 HIV objectives*). HIV is spread by unprotected sexual contact with an infected person, by sharing needles and/or syringes with someone who is infected, or, very rarely in countries where blood is not screened for HIV antibodies, through transfusions of infected blood or blood clotting factors. Also, infants born to HIV-infected women may become infected before or during birth or through breastfeeding after birth (CDC, *HIV/AIDS fact sheets*). There are many misconceptions about HIV transmission. Scientists and medical authorities agree that HIV does not survive well in the environment, making the possibility of environmental transmission remote. HIV is not transmitted through insects or insect bites. There is no known risk of HIV transmission to coworkers, clients, or consumers from incidental contact in industries such as food-service establishments. Although HBV has been transmitted through tattooing or body piercing, HIV has not been transmitted in this manner. Casual contact through closed-mouth or "social" kissing is not a risk factor for transmission of HIV. The CDC recommends against engaging in "French" or open-mouth kissing with a person known to be infected, although the risk of acquiring HIV in this manner is believed to be very low. Contact with saliva, tears, or sweat has never been shown to result in transmission of HIV. Biting is a risk factor only when there is severe trauma with

14.7 Measures for Preventing HIV Exposure and Transmission When Caring for an Infected Person

Wear gloves during contact with blood or other body fluids such as urine, feces, or vomit.

Cover cuts, sores, or breaks on both the caregiver's and the patient's exposed skin with a bandage.

Wash hands and other parts of the body immediately after contact with blood or other body fluids.

Disinfect surfaces soiled with blood with a bleach solution.

Avoid practices that increase the likelihood of blood contact, such as sharing of razors and toothbrushes.

Use and dispose of needles and other sharp instruments appropriately.

extensive tissue tearing and damage and presence of blood (CDC, *HIV transmission*). Box 14.7 presents guidelines for prevention of exposure to the blood of persons who are HIV infected, at risk for HIV infection, or whose infection and risk status are unknown.

Strategies for preventing infection with HIV emphasize testing to identify infected people and ensuring access to appropriate medical care, treatment, and prevention services. The only way to know whether someone has HIV infection is to be tested for HIV. More than 1.1 million people in the United States are living with HIV today, and one in seven of them don't know it. To increase awareness of HIV status, the CDC established its Expanded Testing Initiative, which is aimed at (1) significantly increasing the number of persons tested in jurisdictions with a high rate of HIV among disproportionately affected populations, and (2) supporting implementation of the *revised recommendations for HIV testing of adults, adolescents, and pregnant women in healthcare settings* (CDC, *Expanded Testing Program*). The 2006 CDC *Revised Recommendations for HIV Testing* advocates routine HIV screening as a normal part of clinical practice *and are targeted to* subpopulations of persons at higher risk for HIV, typically defined on the basis of behavior, clinical, or demographic characteristics. The revised recommendations *include* HIV screening for persons aged 13 to 65 years in all healthcare settings (e.g., hospitals, acute-care clinics, and STD clinics) after the patient is notified that testing will be performed, unless he/she declines (opt-out screening). In 2013, the USPTF also recommended HIV screening for persons aged 15 to 65, as well as pregnant women. Younger and older who are at increased risk should also be screened (USPTF, 2013). HIV screening in the routine panel of prenatal screening for all pregnant women after the patient is notified that testing will be performed, unless she declines (opt-out screening) (CDC, *HIV among pregnant women, infants, and children*).

HIV infection can be diagnosed by serologic tests that detect antibodies against HIV-1 and HIV-2 and by virologic tests that can detect HIV antigens. Antibody testing begins with a sensitive screening test (e.g., the conventional or rapid enzyme immunoassay [EIA]). Currently available serologic tests are both highly sensitive and specific and can detect all known subtypes of HIV-1. Most also can detect HIV-2 and uncommon variants of HIV-1. The advent of HIV rapid serologic testing has enabled clinicians to make an accurate presumptive diagnosis of HIV infection within half an hour, which could potentially facilitate the identification of those who are living with HIV and are unaware of their serostatus. In addition to screening, prevention counseling should be offered and encouraged in all healthcare facilities that serve patients at high risk (e.g., STD clinics), because these facilities routinely gather information that places persons at high risk for HIV. Prevention counseling need not be explicitly linked to HIV testing. However, some patients might be more likely to think about HIV and consider their risk-related behavior when undergoing an HIV test. HIV testing presents an excellent opportunity to provide prevention counseling to assist with behavior changes to reduce the risk for acquiring HIV infection (CDC, *HIV infection: Detection, counseling, and referral*). In addition to the strategies outlined above, barriers to HIV prevention and screening programs can be eliminated by making these programs culturally sensitive. Box 14.8 presents *Healthy People 2020* objectives for HIV infection.

> HIV does not make people dangerous to know, so you can shake their hands and give them a hug: Heaven knows they need it.
> **Larry Niven**

 In **Case 2**, when Megan was seen by the nurse practitioner, a rapid HIV test was performed. The results were negative. What primary prevention measures would you recommend?

Caring for the HIV/AIDS patient in the community is a challenge. Because the disease is chronic and there is no cure, infected people continue to live, work, and socialize as they normally have in the past. However, appropriately timed interventions in HIV-positive persons can reduce risks for clinical progression, complications or death from the disease, and HIV transmission.

Evidence for Practice

The USPSTF 2013 guidelines recommended that clinicians screen for HIV infection in adolescents and adults aged 15 to 65 years. Younger adolescents and older adults who are at increased risk should also be screened This includes MSM; men and women having unprotected sex with multiple partners; past or present injection drug users; men and women who exchange sex for money or drugs; individuals whose

14.8 *Healthy People 2020 Objectives for HIV*

Diagnosis of HIV Infection and AIDS

(Developmental) Reduce new HIV diagnoses among adolescents and adults.

(Developmental) Reduce new (incident) HIV infections among adolescents and adults.

Reduce the rate of HIV transmission among adolescents and adults.

Reduce new AIDS cases among adolescents and adults.

Reduce new AIDS cases among adolescent and adult heterosexuals.

Reduce new AIDS cases among adolescent and adult men who have sex with men.

Reduce new AIDS cases among adolescents and adults who inject drugs.

Reduce perinatally acquired HIV and AIDS cases.

Death, Survival, and Medical Healthcare after Diagnosis

(Developmental) Increase the proportion of new HIV infections diagnosed before progression to AIDS.

(Developmental) Increase the proportion of HIV-infected adolescents and adults who receive HIV care and treatment consistent with current standards.

Increase the proportion of persons surviving more than 3 years after a diagnosis with AIDS.

Reduce deaths from HIV infection.

HIV Testing

Increase the proportion of persons living with HIV who know their serostatus.

Increase the proportion of adolescents and adults who have been tested for HIV in the past 12 months.

Increase the proportion of adults with tuberculosis (TB) who have been tested for HIV.

HIV Prevention

Increase the proportion of substance abuse treatment facilities that offer HIV/AIDS education, counseling, and support.

Increase the proportion of sexually active persons who use condoms.

(Developmental) Reduce the proportion of men who have sex with men (MSM) who reported unprotected anal sex in the past 12 months.

Source: U.S. Department of Health and Human Services. *Healthy People 2020 HIV objectives.* Retrieved 29, 2013, from http://healthypeople.gov/2020/topicsobjectives2020/objectiveslist.aspx?topicId=22.

sex partners were HIV infected, bisexual, or injection drug users; people being treated for STDs; people who have had a blood transfusion between 1978 and 1985. In addition, the USPSTF recommended that clinicians screen all pregnant women for HIV.

Source: USPSTF. (2013). *Immunodeficiency Virus (HIV) Infection: Screening.* Retrieved July 31, 2017, from https://www.uspreventiveservicestaskforce.org/Page/Document/UpdateSummaryFinal/human-immunodeficiency-virus-hiv-infection-screening.

OTHER SEXUALLY TRANSMITTED DISEASES

Herpes Simplex Virus

There are two types of herpes simplex virus (HSV), both of which can cause genital herpes. HSV type 1 (HSV-1) most commonly causes sores on the lips (known as fever blisters or cold sores), but it also can cause genital infections. HSV-2 most often causes genital sores, but it also can infect the mouth. The CDC estimates that 15.7% of persons aged 14 to 49 years in the United States have HSV infection, but the overall prevalence is likely higher because an increasing number of genital herpes infections are caused by HSV-1. HSV-2 infection is more common among women than men (20.3% vs. 10.6% in 14- to 49-year-olds), and is more common among non-Hispanic blacks (39.2%) than non-Hispanic whites (12.3%). This disparity remains even among persons with similar numbers of lifetime sexual partners (e.g., two to four partners). Annually, 776,000 people in the United States acquire new herpes infections. HSV-2 prevalence has changed very little since 2004, and increases in genital HSV-1 infections have been found in patient populations worldwide (CDC, *Fact sheet: genital herpes*).

Most individuals infected with HSV-1 or HSV-2 are asymptomatic, or have very mild symptoms that are mistaken for another skin condition. As a result, most persons infected with HSV-2 may be unaware of their infection; in the United States, an estimated 87.4% of 14- to 49-year-olds infected have never received a clinical diagnosis. Generally, HSV-2 infection is transmitted during sexual contact with someone who has a genital HSV-2 infection, and most commonly occurs from an infected partner who does not have a visible sore and may not know that he or she is infected. The average incubation period after exposure is 4 days (range, 2 to 12). The vesicles break and leave painful ulcers that may take 2 to 4 weeks to heal. Experiencing these symptoms is referred to as having an "outbreak," or episode. Although the infection can stay in the body indefinitely, the number of outbreaks tends to decrease over time. Recurrences are much less frequent for genital HSV-1 infection than for genital HSV-2 infection. Genital ulcerative disease caused by herpes makes it easier to transmit and acquire HIV infection sexually. There is an estimated two- to fourfold increased risk of acquiring HIV, if exposed to virus when genital herpes is present. Type-specific HSV tests may be useful among persons with HIV infection and MSM at increased risk for HIV acquisition. Healthcare providers should also screen pregnant women if they have a history of genital herpes, as the virus can be passed from mother to child, resulting in a potentially fatal infection (neonatal herpes), one of the most serious complications of genital herpes. However, the CDC does not recommend screening for HSV-1 or HSV-2 in the general population (CDC, *Fact sheet: Genital herpes*).

Hepatitis Viruses

The rate of new HBV infections in the United States has declined by approximately 82% since 1991, when a national strategy to eliminate HBV infection was implemented in the United States. The decline has been greatest among children born since 1991, when routine vaccination of children was first recommended. In 2014, a total of 2,953 cases of acute hepatitis B were reported from 48 states to the CDC. The overall incidence rate for 2014 was 0.9 cases per 100,000 population. After adjusting for under-ascertainment and under-reporting, an estimated 19,200 acute hepatitis B cases occurred in 2014. However, because many HBV infections are either asymptomatic or never reported, the actual number of new infections was estimated to be approximately 10-fold higher. Rates were highest among adults, particularly males aged 25 to 44 years. An estimated 850,000 to 2.2 million persons in the United States have chronic HBV infection. Chronic infection is an even greater problem globally, affecting approximately 240 million persons. It also is estimated that 786,000 persons worldwide die from HBV-related liver disease each year (CDC, *Hepatitis B FAQs for health professionals*).

Hepatitis B viral infection becomes an STD when it is transmitted through mucosal contact with infectious blood or body fluids (e.g., semen, saliva) during sex with an infected partner. Those at increased risk of becoming infected with HBV include sexually active persons who are not in a long-term, mutually monogamous relationship (e.g., more than one sex partner during the previous 6 months) and MSM. Although 95% of adults recover completely from HBV infection and do not become chronically infected, 15% become chronically infected and die prematurely from cirrhosis or liver cancer; the majority remain asymptomatic until onset of cirrhosis or end-stage liver disease. In the United States, chronic HBV infection results in an estimated 1,800 deaths per year. Therefore, the ACIP recommends that hepatitis B vaccination also include the following:

- Susceptible sex partners of hepatitis B surface antigen (HBsAg)–positive persons
- Sexually active persons who are not in a long-term, mutually monogamous relationship
- Persons seeking evaluation or treatment for an STD
- Men who have sex with men (CDC, *Hepatitis B FAQs for health professionals*).

In addition to hepatitis B, other types of hepatitis viruses, such as hepatitis C and D, can be transmitted sexually; however, sexual transmission is not the primary means of spread as with HBV.

PREVENTION AND CONTROL OF SPECIFIC INFECTIOUS DISEASES

Nurses can intervene in the infectious process through primary, secondary, and tertiary prevention strategies that address the specific characteristics and transmission patterns of the infectious agents. Methods of prevention make it possible to reduce the risk of exposure. The use of vaccines can reduce the risk of infection before exposure to an infectious agent; this is termed primary prevention. The CDC recommends vaccinations for children, adolescents, and adults. The latest recommendations for vaccination can be found at the CDC website: https://www.cdc.gov/vaccines/index. html. Postexposure prophylaxis can reduce the risk of an infectious disease after exposure, if the prophylactic treatment is provided shortly after the exposure; this is called secondary prevention. An example of tertiary prevention is treating opportunistic infections among HIV-infected adults and adolescents. The CDC periodically updates its guidelines for treating opportunistic infections. The latest guidelines can be found at the CDC website. Chapters 5 and 6 discuss the natural history of disease and the levels of prevention (primary, secondary, and tertiary) that are appropriate to each stage of the illness.

Practice Point

Nurses can reduce the risk of infection through primary and secondary prevention measures that are specific to the characteristics of the infectious disease. For example, use of insect repellants and wearing light-colored long pants tucked inside socks is a primary prevention measure for tick-borne Lyme disease. Examining a "bull's eye" lesion, prescribing antibiotics, and performing ELISA testing of serum at a later date are secondary prevention measures.

 Case 1. What measures should be taken to protect the citizens of Alamosa, CO, following the report of fecal contamination of a well that supplied water to the community public water system infrastructure?

Prevention of Foodborne Diseases

Making food safe is a major undertaking, involving all steps in moving from the farm or fishery to the table. Many different organizations and regulatory agencies are involved in preventing or limiting food contamination. Consumers can do their part by purchasing foods that have been processed for safety, such as juices and ciders that have been pasteurized. *Basics for Handling Food Safely*, guidelines for shopping, storage, preparation, thawing, cooking, serving, handling leftovers, and refreezing food safely can be found at the United States Department of Agriculture, Food Safety and Inspection Service website. Other precautions include good handwashing after handling raw eggs, meat and poultry, pets, and farm animals. Also, use soap and hot water to wash utensils and other surfaces that might have come in contact with raw or undercooked meat, poultry, or eggs (CDC, *CDC and Food safety*). Consumers should be advised to avoid eating fresh produce irrigated with water of unknown quality (CDC, *Hepatitis B FAQs for health professionals*). Illnesses that primarily cause diarrhea or vomiting can lead to dehydration if the person loses more electrolytes than he or she takes in. Replacing lost fluids and electrolytes and keeping up with fluid intake are important. Medical treatment is necessary for a diarrheal illness that is accompanied by fever (temperature of more than 101.5°F), prolonged vomiting, bloody stools, or dehydration.

Prevention of Waterborne Diseases

It is important to know where drinking water comes from, how it has been treated, and if it is safe to drink (e.g., a septic tank should not be too close to a private well). Although most community water systems use groundwater for their water supply, more people actually depend on community water systems that use surface water. Community water systems supply water to the same population year-round and are regulated by the EPA. The Safe Drinking Water Act (SDWA) requires EPA to establish and enforce standards that public drinking water systems must follow (EPA, *Water topics*). Transient noncommunity water systems provide water to 25 or more people for at least 60 days/year, but not to the same people and not on a regular basis (e.g., campgrounds).

The EPA has published guidelines for microbiologic water quality for recreational freshwater (e.g., lakes and rivers) and marine water (EPA, *Water topics*). States have latitude regarding their guidelines or regulations and can post warning signs to alert potential bathers until recreational water quality improves. Unlike treated areas, where disinfection can be used to address most problems with the microbiologic quality of water, contaminated freshwater can require weeks or months to improve or return to normal. However, swimming pools might need to be closed until the water has been adequately treated and filtered or the swimming pool drained and refilled to remove contamination. Prompt identification of potential sources of contamination and remedial action are necessary to return bathing water to an appropriate quality for recreational use.

Swallowing, breathing, or having contact with contaminated water from swimming pools, spas, lakes, rivers, or oceans spreads recreational water illnesses. Contamination of recreational water can be avoided when nurses educate the public to remember the following:

- Do not swim if you have diarrhea.
- Do not swallow the pool water.
- Wash hands with soap and water after using the restroom or changing diapers.
- Take children to the bathroom often. Change diapers in the bathroom and not at poolside.
- Wash children thoroughly with soap and water before swimming (CDC, *12 Steps for prevention of recreational water illnesses*).

Prevention of Sexually Transmitted Infections

At the time of the 1997, Institute of Medicine (IOM) report, *The hidden epidemic: Confronting sexually transmitted diseases* (Eng & Butler, 1997), an effective national system for STD prevention did not exist in the United States. However, the CDC's efforts to implement the recommendations of the IOM 1997 report resulted in the development of Comprehensive STD Prevention Systems and publication of the STD Program Operation Guidelines. The purpose of the guidelines is to further STD prevention by providing a resource to assist in the design, implementation, and evaluation of STD prevention and control programs. The target audience for the guidelines is public health personnel and other persons involved in managing STD prevention programs (CDC, *Program operations guidelines for STD prevention*).

STDs are among the leading causes of morbidity and mortality in the United States. They affect men and women of all backgrounds and economic levels, and account for substantial healthcare spending. Data suggest the direct cost of treating STDs in the United States is nearly $16 billion annually (Owusu-Edusei et al., 2013). Nearly 20 million new STDs occur each year in the United States, with half of them among young people aged 15 to 24. With more than 110 million total (new and existing) infections occurring across the nation, at any given time, there are opportunities to focus on prevention and wellness and support the development of national strategies to improve the nation's health through evidence-based clinical and community prevention and wellness activities. The updated CDC *Guidelines for the Treatment of Sexually Transmitted Diseases* integrates recommendations on the most effective treatment regimens, screening procedures, and prevention strategies for STDs. The CDC revised these guidelines in 2015, based on scientific evidence-based review (CDC, 2015c).

KEY CONCEPTS

- The epidemiology of the infectious disease process adds other elements to the epidemiologic triad (agent, host, and environment): a portal of exit for the infectious agent, a means of transmission, and a portal of entry to a new host.
- The environment/reservoirs of infectious agents can be humans, animals (zoonotic), plants, insects, water, and soil.
- Mechanisms of transmission of an infectious agent from one host to another include direct contact, indirect contact, droplets, and airborne transmission.
- An infectious disease may or may not be contagious or communicable.
- An epidemic refers to a significant increase in an infection or infectious disease beyond the expected (endemic) level in a certain population and/or geographic area.
- Nurses play an important role in the prevention of healthcare-associated infections and represent the first line of defense for such adverse outcomes.
- The CDC is a major agency that protects the nation's health by developing guidelines that promote health and quality of life by preventing and controlling disease, injury, and disability. It also maintains surveillance systems to analyze data for infectious disease trends and outbreaks.
- *Healthy People 2020* has outlined objectives for immunizations and infectious diseases.
- Foodborne illnesses include biologic and nonbiologic agents and can be caused by microorganisms and their toxins.
- Waterborne illnesses are associated with drinking water and recreational water.
- *Healthy People 2020* has outlined objectives for food and water safety.
- The EPA sets standards for drinking water.
- The CDC has deficiency classifications for drinking water, and water not intended for drinking used during waterborne outbreak investigations.
- STDs are among the leading causes of morbidity and mortality in the United States. The CDC reports that an estimated 1.1 million people in the United States were living with HIV at the end of 2014, the most recent year for which this information is available. Of those people, about 15%, or 1 in 7, did not know they were infected. HPV is one of the most common causes of STD in the world. It is estimated that 100% of sexually active men and women acquire genital HPV infection at some point in their lives, and can lead to cancer of the cervix in women.
- The CDC provides an effective system for STD prevention to assist community/public health professionals in the design, implementation, and evaluation of STD prevention and control programs.
- *Healthy People 2020* has outlined objectives for the prevention and control of STDs and HIV/AIDS.

CRITICAL THINKING QUESTIONS

1. In the outbreak outlined earlier, 23 campers became ill with gastroenteritis over a period of 7 days. An outbreak of norovirus is defined by the CDC as an occurrence of two or more similar illnesses resulting from an exposure that is either suspected or laboratory-confirmed to be caused by norovirus.

   a. Given that the incubation period for norovirus gastroenteritis is 12 to 48 hours, was this a common source or a propagated outbreak?

   b. What is a major means to prevent the transmission of a communicable disease like norovirus?

2. There is a planned community health project to decrease the incidence of HPV.

   a. Who is/are the target population? Why?

   b. What are some key factors to consider when planning an HPV prevention program?

3. Check the *Healthy People 2020* objectives for HIV website at https://www.healthypeople.gov/2020/topics-objectives/topic/hiv/objectives

   a. How close to the 2020 target is the objective to increase the proportion of persons living with HIV who know their serostatus?

   b. How close to the 2020 target is the objective to reduce newly diagnosed perinatal-acquired HIV cases?

REFERENCES

Agency for Health Research and Quality (AHRQ). (2014). *Guide to Clinical Preventive Services, 2014*. Retrieved August 8, 2017, from https://www.ahrq.gov/sites/default/files/wysiwyg/professionals/clinicians-providers/guidelines-recommendations/guide/cps-guide.pdf

American Academy of Pediatrics (AAP). *HPV champion toolkit*. Retrieved from https://www.aap.org/en-us/advocacy-and-policy/aap-health-initiatives/immunizations/HPV-Champion-Toolkit/Pages/HPV-Champion-Toolkit.aspx

AVERT. *Global HIV and AIDS statistics*. Retrieved August 5, 2017, from https://www.avert.org/global-hiv-and-aids-statistics

Centers for Disease Control and Prevention (CDC). (2006). Revised recommendations for HIV testing of adults, adolescents, and pregnant women in health-care settings. *Morbidity & Mortality Weekly Report Recommendations and Reports*, 55(RR-14), 1–17.

Centers for Disease Control and Prevention (CDC). (2011a). Compendium of measures to prevent disease associated with animals in public settings, 2011. *Morbidity & Mortality Weekly Report*. Retrieved August 10, 2017, from http://www.cdc.gov/mmwr/pdf/rr/rr6004.pdf

Centers for Disease Control and Prevention (CDC). (2011b). Surveillance for waterborne disease outbreaks associated with drinking water—United States, 2007–2008. Surveillance Summaries. *Morbidity & Mortality Weekly Report*, 60(SS12), 38–68. Retrieved August 17, 2017, from https://www.cdc.gov/mmwr/preview/mmwrhtml/ss6012a4.htm

Centers for Disease Control and Prevention (CDC). (2012a). *Principles of epidemiology* (3rd ed.). Retrieved August 11, 2017, from https://www.cdc.gov/ophss/csels/dsepd/ss1978/ss1978.pdf

Centers for Disease Control and Prevention (CDC). (2014). Vital Signs: Foodborne Norovirus Outbreaks—United States, 2009–2012. *Morbidity & Mortality Weekly Report*, 63(22), 491–495. Retrieved August 7, 2017, from https://www.cdc.gov/mmwr/preview/mmwrhtml/mm6322a3.htm

Centers for Disease Control and Prevention (CDC). (2015a). Surveillance for waterborne disease outbreaks associated with drinking water—United States, 2011–2012. *Morbidity & Mortality Weekly Report*, 64(31), 842–848. Retrieved August 7, 2017, from https://www.cdc.gov/mmwr/preview/mmwrhtml/mm6431a2.htm

Centers for Disease Control and Prevention (CDC). (2015b). Outbreaks of illness associated with recreational water—United States, 2011–2012. *Morbidity & Mortality Weekly Report*, 64(24), 668–672. Retrieved August 11, 2017, from https://www.cdc.gov/mmwr/preview/mmwrhtml/mm6424a4.htm

Centers for Disease Control and Prevention (CDC). (2015c). Sexually Transmitted Diseases Treatment Guidelines, 2015. *Morbidity & Mortality Weekly Report, Recommendations and Reports*, 64(3), 1–40. Retrieved August 5, 2017, from https://www.cdc.gov/std/tg2015/tg-2015-print.pdf

Centers for Disease Control and Prevention (CDC). (2016a). Model aquatic health code. Retrieved August 11, 2017, from https://www.cdc.gov/mahc/pdf/2016-mahc-annex-final.pdf

Centers for Disease Control and Prevention (CDC). (2016b). HIV surveillance report, 2015; vol. 27. Retrieved August 12, 2017, from https://www.cdc.gov/hiv/pdf/library/reports/surveillance/cdc-hiv-surveillance-report-2015-vol-27.pdf

Centers for Disease Control and Prevention (CDC). (2017a). Chapter 37: Sexually Transmitted Diseases. *Healthy People 2020 Midcourse Review*. Hyattsville, MD: National Center for Health Statistics. Retrieved August 10, 2017, from https://www.cdc.gov/nchs/data/hpdata2020/HP2020MCR-C37-STD.pdf

Centers for Disease Control and Prevention (CDC). (2018). Estimated HIV incidence and prevalence in the United States, 2010–2015. *HIV Surveillance Supplemental Report, 23*(No. 1). Retrieved April 4, 2018 from http://www.cdc.gov/hiv/library/reports/hiv-surveillance.html

Centers for Disease Control and Prevention (CDC). *12 Steps for prevention of recreational water illnesses*. Retrieved August 11, 2017, from https://www.cdc.gov/healthywater/swimming/aquatics-professionals/twelve-steps-for-prevention-rwi.html

Centers for Disease Control and Prevention (CDC). *About CDC*. Retrieved August 8, 2017, from https://www.cdc.gov/about/default.htm

Centers for Disease Control and Prevention (CDC). *Campylobacter*. Retrieved August 7, 2017, from https://www.cdc.gov/foodsafety/diseases/campylobacter/index.html

Centers for Disease Control and Prevention (CDC). *Chlamydia*. Retrieved August 10, 2017, from https://www.cdc.gov/std/stats15/chlamydia.htm

Centers for Disease Control and Prevention (CDC). *Chlamydia curriculum*. Retrieved August 10, 2017, from https://www2a.cdc.gov/stdtraining/ready-to-use/chlamydia.htm

REFERENCES *(Continued)*

Centers for Disease Control and Prevention (CDC). Chlamydia fact sheet. Retrieved August 10, 2017, from https://www.cdc.gov/std/Chlamydia/STDFact-Chlamydia.htm

Centers for Disease Control and Prevention (CDC). *CDC curriculum: HPV.* Retrieved August 12, 2017, from https://www2a.cdc.gov/stdtraining/ready-to-use/hpv.htm

Centers for Disease Control and Prevention (CDC). *CDC and food safety.* Retrieved August 7, 2017, from https://www.cdc.gov/foodsafety/cdc-and-food-safety.html

Centers for Disease Control and Prevention (CDC). *CDC's global health partnerships.* Retrieved August 5, 2017, from https://www.cdc.gov/globalhealth/partnerships.htm

Centers for Disease Control and Prevention (CDC). *CDC's role in global HIV control.* Retrieved August 5, 2017, from https://www.cdc.gov/globalhivtb/who-we-are/about-us/globalhiv/globalhiv.html

Centers for Disease Control and Prevention (CDC). *E. coli.* Retrieved August 8, 2017, from https://www.cdc.gov/ecoli/index.html

Centers for Disease Control and Prevention (CDC). *Estimates of foodborne illness in the United States.* Retrieved August 8, 2017, from https://www.cdc.gov/foodborneburden/index.html

Centers for Disease Control and Prevention (CDC). *Estimates of healthcare-associated infections.* Retrieved August 12, 2017, from https://www.cdc.gov/hai/surveillance/index.html

Centers for Disease Control and Prevention (CDC). *Fact sheet: Genital herpes.* Retrieved August 12, 2017, from https://www.cdc.gov/std/herpes/stdfact-herpes-detailed.htm

Centers for Disease Control and Prevention (CDC). *Gonorrhea.* Retrieved August 10, 2017, from https://www.cdc.gov/std/Gonorrhea/

Centers for Disease Control and Prevention (CDC). *Gonorrhea fact sheet.* Retrieved August 10, 2017, from https://www.cdc.gov/std/gonorrhea/stdfact-gonorrhea.htm

Centers for Disease Control and Prevention (CDC). *Global HIV/AIDS.* Retrieved August 11, 2017, from https://www.cdc.gov/globalaids/global-hiv-aids-at-cdc/default.html

Centers for Disease Control and Prevention (CDC). *Hantavirus pulmonary syndrome.* Retrieved August 10, 2017, from https://www.cdc.gov/hantavirus/hps/index.html

Centers for Disease Control and Prevention (CDC). *Hepatitis B FAQs. Information for health professionals.* Retrieved August 10, 2017, from https://www.cdc.gov/hepatitis/hbv/hbvfaq.htm#overview

Centers for Disease Control and Prevention (CDC). *HIV/AIDS.* Retrieved August 6, 2017, from https://www.cdc.gov/hiv/basics/index.html

Centers for Disease Control and Prevention (CDC). *HIV basic statistics.* Retrieved August 11, 2017, from https://www.cdc.gov/hiv/basics/statistics.html

Centers for Disease Control and Prevention (CDC). *HIV and tuberculosis.* Retrieved August 11, 2017, from https://www.cdc.gov/hiv/pdf/library/factsheets/hiv-tb.pdf

Centers for Disease Control and Prevention (CDC). *HIV expanded testing program.* Retrieved August 10, 2017, from https://www.cdc.gov/hiv/pdf/library/factsheets/hiv-expanded-testing-program.pdf

Centers for Disease Control and Prevention (CDC). *HIV infection: Detection, counseling, and referral.* Retrieved July 31, 2017, from https://www.cdc.gov/std/tg2015/hiv.htm

Centers for Disease Control and Prevention (CDC). *HIV transmission.* Retrieved August 12, 2017, from https://www.cdc.gov/hiv/basics/transmission.html

Centers for Disease Control and Prevention (CDC). *Legionella.* Retrieved August 8, 2017, from https://www.cdc.gov/legionella/index.html

Centers for Disease Control and Prevention (CDC). *Listeria.* Retrieved August 7, 2017, from https://www.cdc.gov/listeria/index.html

Centers for Disease Control and Prevention (CDC). Lyme disease. Retrieved August 10, 2017, from https://www.cdc.gov/lyme/index.html

Centers for Disease Control and Prevention (CDC). *MRSA.* Retrieved August 10, 2017, from https://www.cdc.gov/mrsa/community/index.html

Centers for Disease Control and Prevention (CDC). *Multistate foodborne outbreak investigations.* Retrieved August 9, 2017, from https://www.cdc.gov/foodsafety/outbreaks/multistate-outbreaks/outbreaks-list.html

Centers for Disease Control and Prevention (CDC). *Multistate outbreak of fungal meningitis and other infections.* Retrieved August 12, 2017, from https://www.cdc.gov/hai/outbreaks/meningitis.html

Centers for Disease Control and Prevention (CDC). (2017b). *Multistate outbreaks of human salmonella infections linked to live poultry in backyard flocks, 2017.* Retrieved August 8, 2017, from https://www.cdc.gov/salmonella/live-poultry-06-17/index.html

Centers for Disease Control and Prevention (CDC). (2017c). *Multistate outbreak of shiga toxin-producing Escherichia coli O157:H7 infections linked to I. M. Healthy Brand Soy Nut Butter: Final update.* Retrieved August 9, 2017, from https://www.cdc.gov/ecoli/2017/o157h7-03-17/index.html

Centers for Disease Control and Prevention (CDC). (2016c). *National and state healthcare associated infections progress report, 2016.* Retrieved August 12, 2017, from https://www.cdc.gov/HAI/pdfs/progress-report/hai-progress-report.pdf

Centers for Disease Control and Prevention (CDC). *Norovirus.* Retrieved August 10, 2017, from https://www.cdc.gov/norovirus/index.html

Centers for Disease Control and Prevention (CDC). (2012b). *Outbreak of hantavirus infection in Yosemite National Park.* Retrieved August 10, 2017, from https://www.cdc.gov/hantavirus/outbreaks/yosemite/index.html

Centers for Disease Control and Prevention (CDC). *Primary and secondary syphilis.* Retrieved from https://www.cdc.gov/std/stats15/syphilis.htm

Centers for Disease Control and Prevention (CDC). *Program operations guidelines for STD prevention.* Retrieved August 11, 2017, from https://www.cdc.gov/std/program/overview.pdf

Centers for Disease Control and Prevention (CDC). *Salmonella.* Retrieved August 7, 2017, from https://www.cdc.gov/salmonella/index.html

Centers for Disease Control and Prevention (CDC). *Salmonella oranienburg infections linked to Good Earth Egg Company Shell Eggs: Final update, 2016.* Retrieved August 8, 2017, from https://www.cdc.gov/salmonella/oranienburg-10-16/map.html

Centers for Disease Control and Prevention (CDC). *STD fact sheet.* Retrieved August 7, 2017, from https://www.cdc.gov/nchhstp/newsroom/docs/factsheets/std-trends-508.pdf

Centers for Disease Control and Prevention (CDC). *Syphilis.* Retrieved August 12, 2017, from https://www.cdc.gov/std/tg2015/syphilis.htm

Centers for Disease Control and Prevention (CDC). *Syphilis fact sheet.* Retrieved August 12, 2017, from https://www.cdc.gov/std/syphilis/stdfact-syphilis-detailed.htm

Centers for Disease Control and Prevention (CDC). *The yellow book, 2017.* Retrieved August 11, 2017, from https://wwwnc.cdc.gov/travel/page/yellowbook-home

Centers for Disease Control and Prevention (CDC). *Tracking infections in long-term care facilities.* Retrieved August 12, 2017, from https://www.cdc.gov/nhsn/ltc/index.html

Centers for Disease Control and Prevention (CDC). *Vital signs: Preventing norovirus outbreaks.* Retrieved August 7, 2017, from https://www.cdc.gov/vitalsigns/norovirus/index.html

Centers for Disease Control and Prevention (CDC). *Chlamydia-CDC Fact Sheet.* Retrieved June 7, 2018, from https://www.cdc.gov/std/chlamydia/stdfact-chlamydia-detailed.htm

Department of Defense (DoD). *Global emerging infections system.* Retrieved August 5, 2017, from https://www.health.mil/Military-Health-Topics/Health-Readiness/Armed-Forces-Health-Surveillance-Branch/Global-Emerging-Infections-Surveillance-and-Response

Eng, T. R., & Butler, W. T. (Ed.). Institute of Medicine (1997). *The hidden epidemic: confronting sexually transmitted diseases.* Washington, DC: National Academy Press. Retrieved August 4, 2017, from http://www.nap.edu/catalog/5284.html

Enserink, M. (2012). Public at last, H5N1 study offers insight into virus's possible path to pandemic. *Science, 336,* 1494–1497.

Environmental Protection Agency. *Water topics.* Retrieved August 1, 2017, from https://www.epa.gov/environmental-topics/water-topics

Falco, R., & Williams, S. I. (2009). *Waterborne salmonella outbreak in Alamosa, Colorado, March and April 2008.* Retrieved August 5, 2017, from https://colorado.gov/pacific/sites/default/files/WQ-DW-Publications-Alamosa-Outbreak-Investigation-Report.pdf

Geissler, A. L., Bustos, F., Swanson, K., Patrick, M. E., Fullerton, K. E., Bennett, C.,...Mahon, B. E. (2017). Increasing campylobacter infections, outbreaks, and antimicrobial resistance in the United States, 2004–2012, *Clinical Infectious Diseases,* 65(10):1624–1631. published July 20, 2017. Retrieved August 7, 2017, from https://doi.org/10.1093/cid/cix624

Heymann, D. L. (2014). *Control of communicable diseases manual* (20th ed.). Washington, DC: American Public Health Association.

Huppert, J. S., Taylor, R. G., St. Cyr, S., Hesse, E. A., & Reed, J. L. (2013). Point-of-care testing improves accuracy of STI care in an emergency department -of care. *Sexually Transmitted Infections,* 89(6), 489–494.

International Society for Infectious Diseases (ISID). (2017). *Legionellosis—USA (12): (TN) hotel, hot tub/pool susp. ProMed Mail,* July 20, 2017. Retrieved on August 10, 2017 from http://www.promedmail.org

International Society for Infectious Diseases (ISID). (2018). Ebola update (150): Democratic republic of Congo. *ProMed Mail,* December 15, 2015. Retrieved on December 15, 2018 from http://www.promedmail.org

Marder, E. P., Cieslak, P. R., Cronquist, A. B., Dunn, J., Lathrop, S., Rabatsky-Ehr, T.,...Geissler, A. L. (2017). Incidence and trends of infections with pathogens transmitted commonly through food and the effect of increasing use of culture-independent diagnostic tests on surveillance—Foodborne diseases active surveillance network, 10 U.S. sites, 2013–2016. *Morbidity & Mortality Weekly Report,* 66(15), 397–403. Retrieved August 9, 2017, from https://www.cdc.gov/mmwr/volumes/66/wr/mm6615a1.htm

McKenzie, J. F., Pringer, R. R., & Kotecki, J. E. (2014). *An introduction to community health* (8th ed.). Boston, MA: Jones & Bartlett.

Meites, E., Kempe, A., & Markowitz, L. E. (2016). Use of a 2-dose schedule for human papillomavirus vaccination—Updated recommendations of the Advisory Committee on Immunization Practices. *Morbidity & Mortality Weekly Report,* 65(49), 1405–1408. Retrieved August 9, 2017, from https://www.cdc.gov/mmwr/volumes/65/wr/mm6549a5.htm

National Center for Health Statistics. (2016). *Health United States, 2016.* Retrieved August 6, 2017, from https://www.cdc.gov/nchs/data/hus/hus16.pdf

Owusu-Edusei, K., Chesson, H. W., Gift, T. L., Tao, G., Mahajan, R., Ocfemia, M. C. B., & Kent, C. K. (2013). The estimated direct medical cost of selected sexually transmitted infections in the United States, 2008. *Sexually Transmitted Diseases,* 40(3), 197–201. Retrieved August 15, 2017, from http://journals.lww.com/std-journal/Fulltext/2013/03000/The_Estimated_Direct_Medical_Cost_of_Selected.3.aspx

Porta, M. (Ed.) (2014). *A dictionary of epidemiology* (6th ed.). New York: Oxford University Press.

President's Emergency Plan for AIDS Relief (PEPFAR). *Fact Sheet,* 2016. Retrieved August 5, 2017, from https://www.pepfar.gov/documents/organization/264882.pdf

Shrestha, S. S., Swerdlow, D. L., Borse, R. H., Prabhu, V. S., Finelli, L., Atkins, C. Y., ... Meltzer MI. (2011). Estimating the burden of 2009 pandemic influenza A (H1N1) in the United States (April 2009-April 2010). *Clin Infect Dis, 52*(Suppl 1):S75–S82.

United Nations AIDS Program (UNAIDS). (2016). *Global AIDS update.* Retrieved August 8, 2017, from http://www.who.int/hiv/pub/arv/global-AIDS-update-2016_en.pdf?ua=1

U.S. Department of Health and Human Services. (2010). *Healthy People 2020. Topics and objectives.* Retrieved August 5, 2017, from https://www.healthypeople.gov/2020/topics-objectives

U.S. Department of Health and Human Services (USDHHS). (2013). *National Action Plan to Prevent Health Care-Associated Infections: Road Map to Elimination.* Retrieved on August 11, 2017 from: http://www.health.gov/hai/prevent_hai.asp#hai_plan

U.S. Department of Health and Human Services. *Healthy People 2020 environmental objectives related to water quality.* Retrieved August 11, 2017, from https://www.healthypeople.gov/2020/topics-objectives/topic/environmental-health

U.S. Department of Health and Human Services. *Healthy People 2020 objectives for food safety.* Retrieved August 8, 2017, from https://www.healthypeople.gov/2020/topics-objectives/topic/food-safety

U.S. Department of Health and Human Services. *Healthy People 2020 objectives for HIV.* Retrieved August 8, 2017, from https://www.healthypeople.gov/2020/topics-objectives/topic/hiv/objectives

U.S. Department of Health and Human Services. *Healthy People 2020 objectives for immunization and infectious diseases.* Retrieved August 6, 2017, from https://www.healthypeople.gov/2020/topics-objectives/topic/immunization-and-infectious-diseases

U.S. Department of Health and Human Services. *Healthy People 2020 objectives for STDs.* Retrieved August 14, 2017, from https://www.healthypeople.gov/2020/topics-objectives/topic/sexually-transmitted-diseases

United Nations AIDS Program (UNAIDS). (2016). *Global AIDS update.* Retrieved August 8, 2017, from http://www.who.int/hiv/pub/arv/global-AIDS-update-2016_en.pdf?ua=1

U.S. Preventive Services Task Force. (2013). *Immunodeficiency virus (HIV) infection: Screening.* Retrieved July 31, 2017, from https://www.uspreventiveservicestaskforce.org/Page/Document/UpdateSummaryFinal/human-immunodeficiency-virus-hiv-infection-screening

U.S. Preventive Services Task Force. (2014). *Chlamydia and Gonorrhea: Screening.* Retrieved August 12, 2017, from https://www.uspreventiveservicestaskforce.org/Page/Document/UpdateSummaryFinal/chlamydia-and-gonorrhea-screening

U.S. Preventive Services Task Force. (2015). *Recommendations for screening in adults and adolescents ages 15 to 65.* Retrieved August 12, 2017, from https://www.cdc.gov/std/tg2015/screening-recommendations.htm

World Health Organization (WHO). *Adults and children living with HIV by region, 2015.* Retrieved August 14, 2017, from http://www.who.int/gho/hiv/epidemic_status/cases_all/en

World Health Organization (WHO). *Drinking-water fact sheet.* Retrieved August 14, 2017, from http://www.who.int/mediacentre/factsheets/fs391/en/

REFERENCES *(Continued)*

World Health Organization (WHO). *Global outbreak alert and response*. Retrieved August 9, 2017, from http://www.who.int/csr/alertresponse/en/

World Health Organization (WHO). *HIV/AIDS fact sheet*. Retrieved August 11, 2017, from http://www.who.int/mediacentre/factsheets/fs360/en

World Health Organization (WHO). (2017). *HIV data*. Retrieved August 11, 2017, from http://www.who.int/hiv/data/en/

World Health Organization (WHO). *Influenza at the human-animal interface. Summary and assessment, 17 May 2017 to 15 June 2017*. Retrieved August 3, 2017, from http://www.who.int/influenza/human_animal_interface/Influenza_Summary_IRA_HA_interface_06_15_2017.pdf?ua=1

World Health Organization (WHO). *Number of people living with HIV, 2015*. Retrieved August 14, 2017, from http://www.who.int/hiv/en/

World Health Organization (WHO). *Pandemic (H1N1) 2009, Update 112*. Retrieved August 6, 2017, from http://www.who.int/csr/don/2010_08_06/en/

World Health Organization (WHO). (2013). *Projections of mortality and causes of death, 2015 and 2030*. Retrieved August 10, 2017, from http://www.who.int/healthinfo/global_burden_disease/projections/en/

World Health Organization (WHO). (2015). *The top 10 causes of death: Fact sheet*. Retrieved August 2, 2017, from http://www.who.int/mediacentre/factsheets/fs310/en/index2.html

WEB RESOURCES

Please visit thePoint® for up-to-date web resources on this topic.

(PEPFAR. *Fact Sheet, 2016* https://www.pepfar.gov/documents/organization/264882.pdf.)

Chapter 15

Emerging Infectious Diseases

Barbara A. Goldrick

FANTASTIC VOYAGE: INFLUENZA

Time to go! Time to go!
An influenza virus,
Hiding in saliva, buried in a cell,
Antibodies and T cells are coming.
Get out! But how?
Induce a sneeze? Kickstart a cough?
Ah yes, here we go…
Aahhh-choo! Freedom at last!
Where are we?
A quick look around
A hospital? I see children,
Very thin, sick children,
Must be the cancer ward.
No B cells or T cells—a virus paradise!
Let's travel, find a breeze and float.
Where's my next victim?
My previous young doctor host
Walking quickly away
Head down, embarrassed
Scolded by a nurse—where was his mask?

Too busy and careless, poor fool
He still serves me well, dragging me into his wake.
Here I go, following and floating
A door nearby opens—negative pressure!
In I go, but on a cancer ward,
This should be positive pressure!
To keep bugs out, not draw them in.
I cannot complain
All good for me, for now I can see
A young girl with leukemia
Sitting in bed, watching TV
Laughing, inhaling, bringing me close.
But wait, what's this? Her mother!
Opening the toilet door,
Even greater negative pressure in there.
And worse, wet surfaces glistening inside,
Cleaned by her mother with chlorhexidine.
No! Not yet! Not now! I'm so close!
Being pulled in. No escape. Falling, falling…
The young girl is laughing. Now her mother is too.

—JT Tang, National University Hospital, Singapore

CHAPTER HIGHLIGHTS

- Emerging versus reemerging infectious diseases
- Factors that influence the emergence/reemergence of infectious diseases
- Recent emerging/reemerging infectious diseases
- Prevention and control of emerging and reemerging infectious diseases
- Reemergence of vaccine-preventable diseases

OBJECTIVES

- Identify factors that influence emerging and reemerging infectious diseases.
- Describe recent emerging and reemerging infectious diseases from a global perspective.
- Relate the methods of transmission of emerging and reemerging infectious diseases to methods of control and prevention.
- Explain prevention and control of reemergence of vaccine-preventable diseases.
- Identify antimicrobial-resistant threats in the United States.

KEY TERMS

Antigenic drift: Slow and progressive genetic changes that take place in DNA and RNA as organisms replicate in multiple hosts.

Antigenic shift: Sudden change in the molecular structure of DNA and RNA in microorganisms, resulting in a new strain of the microorganism.

Antibiotic stewardship: Refers to a set of coordinated strategies to improve the use of antimicrobial medications with the goal of enhancing patient health outcomes, reducing resistance to antibiotics, and decreasing unnecessary costs.

Convergence model: Model illustrating the interaction of 13 factors that contribute to the emergence and reemergence of infectious diseases.

Directly observed therapy (DOT): Observation of clients to ensure that they ingest each dose of anti-TB medication to maximize the likelihood of completion of therapy.

Ecosystem: Natural unit consisting of all living things (plants, animals, bacteria, viruses) interacting with, and dependent on, one another for survival within their nonliving environment.

Emerging infectious disease: Newly identified, clinically distinct (novel) infectious disease.

Herd immunity: Type of immunity in which a large proportion of people in a population are not susceptible to a communicable disease and the few people who are susceptible will not likely be exposed and contract the illness.

Microbial adaptation: Process by which organisms adjust and change to their environment.

Pandemic: Epidemic occurring worldwide.

Reemerging infectious disease: The reappearance (reemergence) of a known infectious disease after its decline, with an incidence that is increasing in a certain geographic area or among a specific population.

Vaccine-preventable diseases: Dangerous or deadly diseases that are preventable by vaccination.

CASE STUDIES

References to case studies are found throughout this chapter (look for the case study icon). Readers should keep the case studies in mind as they read the chapter.

CASE 1

Pandemic influenza is different from other infectious diseases, due to the ability of influenza viruses to change and spread easily from person to person. Influenza pandemics have led to widespread morbidity and mortality over the past 100 years. As a result, past pandemic influenza plans have focused on severe pandemics, like the first pandemic of A (H1N1), known as the "Spanish flu," which occurred between 1918 and 1919. It was very deadly, spread across the globe within 6 months, affected young healthy adults, and resulted in 1,400,000 deaths worldwide; 99% of deaths occurred in persons aged ≤65 years.

In June 2009, the World Health Organization (WHO) declared an A (H1N1) influenza pandemic, the first global pandemic in 40 years as well as the first in the 21st century. At that point, the pandemic was in phase 6, the highest WHO alert level, which meant that a global epidemic was underway. By August 2010, more than 214 countries and overseas territories or communities had reported laboratory-confirmed cases of pandemic influenza H1N1 2009, including at least 18,449 deaths. However, the A (H1N1) influenza pandemic experienced in 2009 was less severe than originally thought. Nonetheless, by preparing only for severe pandemics, the former plans did not include specific guidance for H1N1 2009 pandemic (CDC [2010a]. *2009 H1N1: Overview of a pandemic*).

CASE 2

Despite the overall decline in tuberculosis (TB) incidence in the United States, outbreaks of TB among homeless persons continue to challenge TB control efforts. In January 2010, public health officials recognized an outbreak of TB after three overnight guests at a homeless shelter in Illinois received diagnoses of TB disease caused by *Mycobacterium tuberculosis* isolates with matching genotype patterns. In April 2007, a 55-year-old man received a diagnosis of sputum smear–positive TB disease caused by an *M. tuberculosis* isolate with a particular genotype pattern not documented previously in that County. The man had been a frequent overnight guest at a particular county facility that provided short-term shelter each night for approximately 180 persons whose housing situation was unstable. Subsequent case finding among other guests and staff members at the shelter identified no additional cases.

However, in October 2009 and January 2010, two additional cases with the index patient's TB genotype pattern were identified among overnight shelter guests, alerting public health officials to a potential outbreak.

By March 2010, three additional cases with the outbreak genotype pattern had been identified among shelter guests, leading county and state officials to request on-site epidemiologic assistance from the Centers for Disease Control and Prevention (CDC). Because all patients had been guests at the shelter, the CDC recommended on-site case finding among guests and staff members at the shelter.

Source: Adapted from Centers for Disease Control and Prevention (CDC). (2012). Tuberculosis outbreak associated with a homeless shelter—Kane County, Illinois, 2007–2011. *Morbidity and Mortality Weekly Report, 61*(11), 186–189.

Infants, children, adolescents, teens, and adults need different vaccinations, depending on their age, location, job, lifestyle, travel schedule, health conditions, or previous vaccinations.

INTRODUCTION

Infectious organisms have been with humanity since the dawn of civilization; a basic part of life, they are universal. Diseases will continue to emerge and reemerge. **Emerging infectious diseases** and their basic causes are a global threat that affects the stability of nations and the entire planet. Developing nations, which have the fewest resources to respond to this emergence and reemergence, bear the greatest burden of this threat. However, infectious diseases, which may spread rapidly and indiscriminately, present a significant risk to the health and development of all nations. No country or population is immune. In its 1992 report, the Institute of Medicine (IOM, 1992) defined an emerging infectious disease as either (1) a newly identified clinically distinct infectious disease or (2) the reappearance (or reemergence) of a known infectious disease after its decline with an incidence that is increasing in a certain geographic area or in a specific population. An example of a new infectious disease, first recognized by a World Health Organization (WHO) physician in Hanoi, Vietnam, in 2003, was made very clear when severe acute respiratory syndrome (SARS) appeared worldwide in 2003.

Practice Point

Astute clinicians can detect a possible emerging infectious disease by taking a careful history that includes travel history, which may reveal travel to an area where an emerging infection has been reported.

FACTORS THAT INFLUENCE EMERGING INFECTIOUS DISEASES

Factors that influence the emergence/reemergence of infectious diseases are complex and interrelated. In *The Coming Plague* (1995), Pulitzer Prize–winning author Laurie Gar-

rett pointed out that by the end of the 20th century, microbes were no longer confined to remote ecosystems but had transformed the planet into a global village. Although a global village provides social and economic opportunities, it also gives emerging infectious diseases a chance to spread.

More than 36 new emerging infectious diseases have been identified worldwide in the past 40 years. Figure 15.1 illustrates recent infectious diseases identified by the WHO and the Centers for Disease Control and Prevention (CDC) (Morens, Folkers, & Fauci, 2008). A 2003 IOM report illustrated that "health protection and disease prevention among the U.S. population requires global awareness and collaboration with domestic and international partners to prevent the spread of infectious diseases" (Smolinski, Hamburg, & Lederberg, 2003). In *Microbial Threats to Health: Emergence, Detection, and Response*, the IOM identified 13 factors that affect emerging and reemerging infections. These are listed in Box 15.1. The IOM **convergence model** (Fig. 15.2) demonstrates how these 13 factors are grouped and overlap. There are four types of interrelated and overlapping microbe–human interactions, which can lead to **emerging/reemerging infectious diseases:** (1) genetic and biologic; (2) physical/environmental; (3) ecologic; and (4) social, political, and economic. The ability of microbes to adapt and the dynamic interaction between microbes and humans are central to the IOM convergence model. Several of these interactions are discussed below.

Microbial Adaptation and Change

Microbes live everywhere and are very adept at adaptation. They are constantly interacting with other living organisms and changing in response to their environment. Their habitats expand as humans alter the environment, extending their contact with a wider variety of microbes. As microbes reproduce, genetic changes may result in pathogens that are immunologically distinct from their parental strains. For example, **antigenic drift**, the slow and progressive genetic changes that take place in DNA and RNA as organisms replicate in multiple hosts, causes changes in influenza viruses each year. **Antigenic shift** occurs when there is a sudden change in the DNA and RNA, resulting in a new strain of the microorganism, and people have little or no acquired immunity.

FIGURE 15.1 Examples of recent emerging and reemerging infectious diseases.

Three stages of **microbial adaptation** and change occur over varying periods of time. During stage I, an epidemic occurs. The microbes enter a "virgin" population where hosts have no prior exposure to the organism and have few defenses. This leads to further spread in the population. Ultimately, survivors are usually left with improved defenses against reinfection. During stage II, the infection becomes endemic or continuously present in a geographic area or population of people. Routine childhood diseases are an example of such infections. During stage III, symbiosis is possible. Further adaptation occurs, resulting in mutual tolerance and sometimes mutual benefit for both the microorganism and the host. This is the preferred outcome.

> Our relationship to infectious pathogens is part of an evolutionary drama. Here we are. Here are the bugs.
> **Joshua Lederberg, molecular biologist**

As microbes adapt over the centuries, the illnesses they produce become less acute. Symptoms become milder, and fewer organs are involved as immunity develops. Syphilis first appeared in the late 15th century in Europe, causing repulsive pustules over the entire body. Many internal organs were involved, and death occurred within a few years. Just 50 years later, symptoms were limited to the genitals, face, and nervous system, and people could live with the disease for decades, thus having an opportunity to transmit it. Even the mode of transmission can change over time. For example, the "black plague," or bubonic plague, that devastated the European population in the 12th and 13th centuries was transmitted through the bites of fleas that lived on rats. Centuries later, a new form of the disease emerged. The organism, normally trapped in the lymph nodes, was released and the lungs became infected. As a result, an even more deadly form of the disease, the pneumonic plague, emerged. Transmission was now airborne, and the disease was transmitted from person to person. Pneumonic plague was fatal in 95% of its victims and remains resistant to antibiotic treatment today.

15.1   Factors That Contribute to the Emergence and Reemergence of Infectious Diseases

- Microbial adaptation and change
- Human susceptibility to infection
- Climate and weather
- Changing ecosystems
- Human demographics and behavior
- Economic development and land use
- International travel and commerce
- Technology and industry
- Breakdown of public health measures
- Poverty and social inequality
- War and famine
- Lack of political will
- Intent to harm (bioterrorism)

Source: Smolinski, M. S., Hamburg, M. A., & Lederberg, J. (2003). *Microbial threats to health: Emergence, detection, and response.* Washington, DC: Institute of Medicine, The National Academies Press.

> ...a flea has smaller fleas that on him prey; And these have smaller still to bite 'em, And so proceed ad infinitum. **Jonathan Swift, On Poetry: A Rhapsody (1733)**

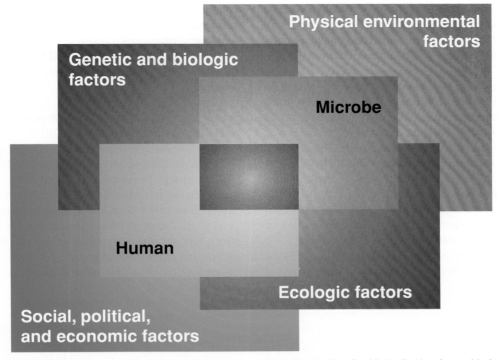

Physical environmental factors

Genetic and biologic factors

Microbe

Human

Ecologic factors

Social, political, and economic factors

FIGURE 15.2 Institute of Medicine convergence model. (From Smolinski, M. S., Hamburg, M. A., & Lederberg, J. [2003]. *Microbial threats to health: Emergence, detection, and response.* Washington, DC: Institute of Medicine, The National Academies Press.)

Fortunately, a new acute illness is usually the exception rather than the rule. Relatively few potentially pathologic microbes enter humans, and few survive. Actually, to cause disease, microbes must beat enormous odds. There is a "parasite's dilemma." If the microbe proliferates rapidly, it may kill the host. If it cannot be transmitted quickly to a new host, the microbe dies. However, if the microbe proliferates slowly, within a week the host's immune system will recognize the microbe as foreign, form antibodies, and destroy the microbe. If microbes survive and cause disease, the reason is usually due to changes illustrated by the epidemiologic triad: (1) a change in the behavior of humans—the host, (2) a change in the behavior of the microbes—the agent, or (3) a change in the environment.

Human Susceptibility to Infection

Many characteristics of the human body and the physical environment determine whether a microbe will cause a disease. For infections to occur, people must be susceptible to infection. If the host has not been exposed to the microbe in the past, there is no acquired immunity to the organism. Immunity can be impaired because of environmental stresses, poor nutrition, medication, or the presence of other illnesses. Normal defense mechanisms can be bypassed through injury or deliberate medical or surgical procedures. Diseases persist only if the population is dense enough to allow continued transmission of germs and large enough to produce a continual supply of susceptible hosts. If a

substantial proportion of people in a population are not susceptible to a communicable disease, the few people who are susceptible are not likely to be exposed and contract the illness. This is a process called **herd immunity**.

Infectious diseases introduced with Europeans, like smallpox and measles, spread from one Indian tribe to another, far in advance of Europeans themselves, and killed an estimated 95% of the New World's Indian population. **Jared Diamond, scientist and author**

Climate, Changing Ecosystems, and Human Behavior

Many infectious diseases have characteristic geographic distributions and seasonal variations. Probably the most common is the influenza virus that peaks each fall and winter. Factors such as temperature, precipitation, and humidity affect the life cycle of many disease pathogens and their vectors, and consequently they can affect disease outbreaks. Natural changes in climate, such as the effects of El Niño ocean current, global warming, and natural disasters, result in a change in environmental conditions. These changes are not always beneficial to infectious organisms. However, the relationships between climate and infectious disease are a complicated web of causation that includes almost all of the factors that underlie the emergence of these diseases. Dr. Claire Heffernan, a trained veterinarian and a specialist in global health and disease interaction between animals and humans, is concerned that as the climate warms in Arctic regions, more and more diseases from around the world are spreading there, threatening both animal and human populations (International Society for Infectious Diseases [ISID], 2013).

Ecologic changes are one of the most frequently identified factors in the emergence of infectious diseases. **Ecosystems** are groups of interacting living things (e.g., plants, animals, bacteria, and viruses) that depend on each other for survival. Ecosystems become unstable with climate change, and throughout history, humans have contributed to ecologic flux. Humans are responsible for land use changes, which are often associated with economic development, with the accompanying dislocation of indigenous animals, plants, and microorganisms. For example, logging and the clearing of timber means that homes and sources of food are lost.

With the death or relocation of indigenous organisms, niches open up for those that thrive under marginal

conditions. Also, practices associated with food production can result in the creation of ideal homes for the creatures that carry pathogens (vectors). In developing countries, where ditches may be contaminated by fecal material, irrigation fields can contribute to the contamination of local water supplies.

Changes in the environment cause new interactions between agents and hosts and can potentially lead to new infectious disease threats (IOM, 2010). Human population upheavals caused by war or civil conflicts often result in the forced dislocation of large groups of people, and migration of such groups of people from rural areas to cities can be accompanied by a breakdown of public health measures. These have often been the factors in disease emergence (Fig. 15.3). Although cities have distinct advantages, such as water supplies and transportation, it was only when towns became big cities that massive die-offs became a regular part of human life. Urban life, with malnutrition, overcrowding,

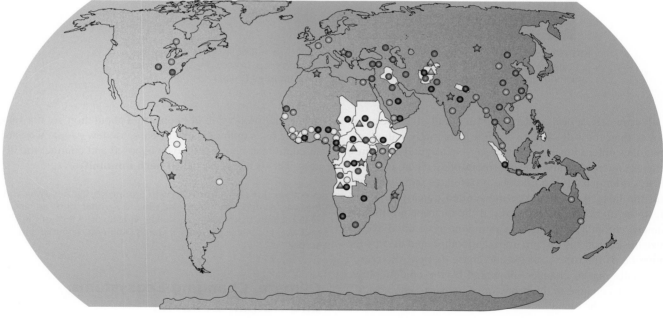

- ● Ebola, Marburg, and CCHF
- ● Influenza (H5N1)
- ○ Lassa fever
- ● Monkeypox
- ● Nipah and Hendra
- ● Rift Valley fever
- ● SARS-CoV
- ○ Yellow fever
- ● Poliovirus
- ★ Plague
- ☆ Tularemia
- △ Malaria
- △ Trypanosomiasis

Symbols: Outbreaks of emerging or reemerging infectious diseases during this period
Circles: Diseases of viral origin
Stars: Diseases of bacterial origin
Triangles: Diseases of parasitic origin
CCHF: Crimean–Congo hemorrhagic fever
SARS-CoV: Severe acute respiratory syndrome coronavirus

FIGURE 15.3 Geographic distribution of recent emerging or reemerging infectious disease outbreaks and countries affected by conflict, 1990–2006. Countries in *yellow* were affected by conflict during this period. *Symbols* represent outbreaks of emerging or reemerging infectious diseases. (From Gayer, M., Legros, D., Formenty, P., & Connolly, M. A. [2007]. *Conflict and emerging infectious diseases.* [Vol. 13, No. 11]. Geneva, Switzerland: World Health Organization.)

and poor sanitation, enhances the major pathways for transmission of infectious disease; plagues and cities have always developed together. For example, cholera outbreaks occurred four times between 1831 and 1854 in England because of the large influx of people into cities and the lack of proper sanitary services. These outbreaks resulted in a total of 10,675 deaths.

Evidence for Practice

Polio cases have decreased worldwide by over 99% since 1988, from an estimated 350,000 cases in more than 125 endemic countries to a total number of 22 wild poliovirus (WPV) cases and 96 vaccine-derived polioviruses (circulating vaccine-derived polio viruses), all types in 2017. In September 2018, the World Health Organization reported the following poliovirus update: WPV, 18 (all in endemic countries) and 36 cases of cVDPV, all types. Eight of the cVDPV cases were from endemic countries and 28 were from nonendemic countries. In 2018, the WHO reported that only three countries (Afghanistan, Nigeria, and Pakistan) remained polio-endemic countries. Nigeria had been declared polio-free in 2015; however, the detection of wild polio in Nigeria in July 2016 after 2 years was a sobering reminder that polio is a difficult disease to eradicate, especially in areas with ongoing humanitarian crises and faltering health systems. Afghanistan had the highest number of WPV cases in September 2018 at 14. The Democratic Republic of the Congo had the second highest number of cVDPV cases at 15 (WHO, 2018a, *Polio today.*)

Although the WPV is decreasing in prominence and has disappeared from all but the three endemic countries, the vaccine virus has increased its presence as a major challenge in countries that have interrupted the WPV transmission through major campaign activities but have not been able to keep up the high levels of vaccination coverage following declaration polio-free status in those countries. Until poliovirus transmission is interrupted in these countries, all countries remain at risk of importation of polio, especially vulnerable countries with weak public health and immunization services and travel or trade links to endemic countries. For an update, the global map of WPV and cVDPV cases can be found at http://polioeradication.org/polio-today/polio-now/

As a result of the global effort to eradicate the disease, more than 16 million people have been saved from paralysis. In 2016, 155 countries and territories successfully removed the polio type-2 strain from the oral polio vaccine (WHO [2016a], *Polio global eradication initiative*).

As long as a single child remains infected, children in all countries are at risk of contracting polio. Failure to eradicate polio from these last remaining strongholds could result in as many as 200,000 new cases every year, within 10 years, all over the world.

The WHO International Travel and Health recommendation is that all travelers to and from polio affected areas be fully vaccinated against polio (WHO, Poliomyelitis).

Environmental surveillance is frequently used by countries around the world, to support the detection of diseases of public health importance. Wild poliovirus type 1 (WPV1) was detected through routine environmental surveillance in 2013 in southern Israel, a nonendemic country. Israel has been free of indigenous WPV transmission since 1988. All viruses were detected in sewage only; no cases of paralytic polio have been reported. Routine immunization levels in Israel were estimated at 94% (WHO, *Poliovirus detected from environmental samples in Israel – update, 15 July 2013*.)

Evidence for Practice

The spirochete *Borrelia burgdorferi* has been identified as being responsible for most human cases of Lyme disease. In the northeastern and midwestern United States, *Borrelia burgdorferi* is transmitted by the vector *Ixodes scapularis* tick, also known as a deer tick. Global climate change can affect the distribution of vector-borne diseases. Lyme disease is one of the most commonly reported vector-borne illnesses in the United States. In 2015, 95% of confirmed Lyme disease cases were reported from 14 states, and it was the sixth most common nationally notifiable disease. However, this disease does not occur nationwide and is concentrated heavily in the Northeast and upper Midwest (CDC, Lyme disease data and *surveillance*).

Travel, Technology, and Industry

International air travel now allows people to reach any destination in the world in an average of 10 to 16 hours. Infected travelers can introduce new microbes into new environments, both while traveling to new places and returning home. An increasing number of travelers increases the chances of contact with an infectious disease. Also, adventure travelers, who venture into new environments with exotic wildlife, increase their chances of coming into contact with microbes that have never before been recognized as human pathogens.

Mass food production that processes or uses biologic products increases the chance of unknown contamination at every stage. These contaminated food products can be distributed widely, often to grocery shelves or restaurants within a day, and they may be eaten shortly thereafter. A single source of contamination has the potential to affect thousands of people in a large geographic area. A 2012 multistate outbreak of Shiga toxin–producing *Escherichia coli* O157:H7 (STEC O157:H7) linked to prepackaged organic spinach and spring mix blend grown in contaminated fields (CDC, *Shiga toxin-producing Escherichia coli O157:H7 infections linked to organic spinach and spring mix*) and the intentional contamination of Chinese milk with melamine in 2009 (food counterfeiting) are just two examples of the types of problems created by mass food production.

There have been profound changes in society within the last 100 years, perhaps few greater than the changes in healthcare technology. Infections acquired in healthcare facilities affect millions of people annually worldwide. The sickest people are at the highest risk. Microbial adaptation and change in response to the overuse of antibiotics and consequent accumulation in the environment have caused the rapid evolution of resistant pathogens. Microorganisms such as methicillin-resistant *Staphylococcus aureus* (MRSA) are now found in the community as well as in healthcare institutions. Antibiotic-resistant pathogens, one of the plagues of the 20th century, continue to be a problem in the 21st century.

✎ Practice Point

To protect travelers going to countries outside the United States, the CDC publishes its Health Information for International Travel (commonly called the *Yellow Book*) every 2 years as a reference for health professionals providing care to international travelers and is a resource for anyone interested in staying healthy abroad. It includes important travel medicine updates, including the latest information about emerging infectious disease threats such as Zika, Ebola, and Middle East respiratory syndrome (MERS), which are discussed below. It also provides vaccine recommendations for travel, updated guidance on the use of antibiotics in the treatment of travelers' diarrhea, and special considerations for unique types of travel, such as wilderness expeditions, work-related travel, and study abroad (CDC, Yellow Book, 2018).

The CDC *Yellow Book, 2018*, codifies the U.S. government's most current travel health guidelines, including pre-travel vaccine recommendations and destination-specific health advice. For example, destination-specific recommendations for popular itineraries include new sections for travelers to Cuba. In the summer of 2017, the CDC updated travel information for malaria in Cape Verde, the Dominican Republic, and Mexico. It also updated Zika travel warnings in several countries. For more information on travel vaccination recommendations, see the CDC website at https://wwwnc.cdc.gov/travel.

Source: CDC. *Yellow Book, 2018.* Retrieved on August 19, 2017, from https://wwwnc.cdc.gov/travel/page/yellowbook-home.

Lack of Political Will and Breakdown of Public Health Infrastructures

Unlike the United States, Canada, the United Kingdom, and European countries, most developing nations do not have the public health network and technologic advances required to fight against infectious diseases. Many of these countries have to choose between funding economic development initiatives and investing in a national public health infrastructure.

The 1991 outbreak of cholera in Peru is a good case study; this outbreak illustrates the complex web of causation that contributed to the onset and spread of the disease. Historically, there have been seven acknowledged cholera pandemics. The seventh pandemic of cholera commenced in 1961 in Indonesia; by 1991, it had reached Peru. Cholera is a disease transmitted through the fecal–oral route that is associated with poverty. The disease had been absent from Peru for more than 100 years. It has been suggested that human waste contaminated with *Vibrio cholerae* was discharged from a Chinese freighter offshore from infected crew members on board the ship. The microbes then found their way into plankton, which was in turn ingested by fish and shellfish. Consumption of raw shellfish is a delicacy in Peru, and one possible source of the epidemic was contaminated shellfish. Cholera infection in humans occurred because a series of complex factors existed along Peru's shores. The rapid population growth in the coastal cities exceeded the capability of the public health infrastructure to deal with fecal contamination of water supplies. The cholera outbreak in Peru cost the country U.S. $770 million due to food trade embargoes and adverse effects on tourism. The disease subsequently quickly spread to other Latin American countries (Mutreja et al., 2011; WHO, *Global epidemics and impact of cholera*).

✎ Practice Point

Infectious disease prevention requires global consciousness. Not all countries have the public health infrastructure to combat emerging infectious diseases.

RECENT EMERGING AND REEMERGING INFECTIOUS DISEASES

Severe Acute Respiratory Syndrome, 2002–2003

At least 7 of the 13 factors affecting emerging infections, identified in the 2003 IOM report, occurred during the 2002–2003 SARS outbreak. The SARS epidemic, which occurred worldwide between February and July of 2003, began in mainland China in November 2002 but was not reported to the WHO until February 2003, when the Chinese Ministry of Health reported that an outbreak of 305 cases of "atypical pneumonia," including five deaths, had occurred in Guangdong Province. By then, SARS had spread to several countries, including Hong Kong, Taiwan, Singapore, Vietnam, and Canada. Secondary cases of SARS were imported to the respective countries by a "superspreading event" that occurred through exposure to an index case of SARS from mainland China. Although the causative agent for SARS had not been identified early in the outbreak, a case definition for SARS was established, and secondary attack rates of more than 50% were observed in healthcare providers caring for clients with SARS in both Hong Kong and Vietnam (CDC, *Remembering SARS 10 years later*).

The causative agent for SARS was identified in April 2003 as a variant coronavirus (CoV), with an average incubation period of 4 to 6 days (range, 1 to 14 days) and a maximum of 10 days. Although SARS-CoV was found to be mostly transmitted by close contact with respiratory secretions and aerosols, other body fluids, such as saliva, tears, urine, and feces, also demonstrated presence of the virus. Most cases of SARS among healthcare providers occurred from contacts with clients and visitors who were not identified as having SARS and before infection control and quarantine measures were in place or, when infection control precautions were relaxed (CDC, *Remembering SARS 10 years later*).

Canada became the first SARS epicenter in the Western Hemisphere, with two clusters of SARS infection epidemiologically linked to two hospital outbreaks. Globally, the WHO received reports of SARS from 29 countries and regions; 8,096 persons with probable SARS, resulting in 774 deaths. In the United States, 8 SARS infections were documented by laboratory testing and an additional 19 probable SARS infections were reported (CDC, *Remembering SARS 10 years later*).

Isolation precautions and quarantine measures to prevent the spread of SARS-CoV were established early in the outbreak, which were effective in containing the epidemic. SARS-CoV was less transmissible than most respiratory infections; therefore, it was highly susceptible to appropriate control measures. About 30% of the early SARS cases in China were in healthcare providers, with the majority of cases occurring before the cause of SARS was identified and before correct infection control measures were in place. By the end of the epidemic, 21% of SARS cases had occurred in healthcare providers, ranging from 3% in the United States to 43% in Canada. Several secondary SARS cases also occurred in household contacts before quarantine measures were instituted.

In 2012, the National Select Agent Registry Program declared SARS-CoV a select agent. A select agent is a bacterium, virus, or toxin that has the potential to pose a severe threat to public health and safety. There have been no known cases of SARS reported anywhere in the world since 2004, when human cases of SARS-CoV infection were reported in China in an outbreak resulting from laboratory-acquired infections (CDC, 2017, *Remembering SARS 10 years later*). However, in June 2014, Chinese scientists discovered a new type of SARS-like CoV in bats in the Yunnan Province of China that could be the precursor of the SARS virus or its "relative" (Hu et al., 2013.) There is no evidence that transmission of this new SARS-like CoV to humans has occurred. Nonetheless, this discovery represents an important clue in the hunt for the source of SARS-CoV.

The main lessons learned from SARS, the first new infectious disease to emerge in the 21st century, were that (1) astute healthcare providers are likely to be the key to early detection and reporting of initial cases of new CoV infections; (2) containment of disease requires the diligent application of enhanced infection control measures at the national and local levels; and (3) control of an emerging infection necessitates swift action by healthcare providers as well as an adequate public health infrastructure.

Middle East Respiratory Syndrome Coronavirus

As of November 2018, 2,274 global laboratory-confirmed cases of Middle East respiratory syndrome (MERS) had been reported to WHO, including at least 806 deaths (case fatality rate, 35.4%). However, the majority of these cases were reported from Saudi Arabia (1896 cases, including 732 related deaths with a case–fatality rate of 38.6%) (WHO, *Middle East respiratory syndrome [MERS] situation update*, November 2018.) In May 2015, the National Health and Family Planning Commission of China notified WHO of one confirmed case of MERS-CoV. The case was a male traveler from the Republic of Korea.

The Republic of Korea reported its first laboratory-confirmed case of MERS-CoV in May 2015. By July 2015, a total of 186 MERS-CoV cases, including 36 deaths, had been reported. One of the 186 was the case that was confirmed in China and also notified by the National Focal Point of China. All transmission of these Korean MERS-CoV cases had been linked to healthcare facilities where MERS patients were treated. Several factors were identified as contributing to the spread of the infection, including lack of awareness among healthcare providers and the general public about MERS, patients' behaviors, and suboptimal infection prevention and control measures in hospitals (WHO, 2015a, *Middle East respiratory syndrome coronavirus [MERS-CoV]—Republic of Korea.*) In September 2018, the Republic of Korea notified WHO of another laboratory-confirmed case of MERS-CoV. The case was a male Korean national who visited Kuwait on business from August 16 through September 6, 2018. He returned to Korea via Dubai (WHO, 2018b, *Middle East respiratory syndrome coronavirus [MERS-CoV] infection—Republic of Korea.*)

In August 2018, the International Health Regulations National Focal Point for the United Kingdom of Great

Britain and Northern Ireland notified WHO about a laboratory-confirmed Middle East respiratory syndrome coronavirus (MERS-CoV) infection. The patient was a resident of the Kingdom of Saudi Arabia who was visiting the United Kingdom of Great Britain and Northern Ireland. This is the fifth case of MERS-CoV diagnosed in the United Kingdom of Great Britain and Northern Ireland, with the four previous cases diagnosed in 2012 and 2013 (WHO, *Middle East respiratory syndrome coronavirus [MERS-CoV]—United Kingdom of Great Britain and Northern Ireland*, 31 August 2018.

It should be noted that the recent upsurge of new cases was attributed in part due to breaches in infection prevention and control measures in healthcare settings. The WHO also has reported that MERS-CoV has been found in some camels and in some MERS patients who have had contact with camels. Therefore, in addition to a travel history, patients should be asked if they have visited farms, markets, barns, or other places where animals are present (WHO, 2014a, *MERS-CoV Summary 11 June, 2014*).

The first two imported cases of MERS-CoV infection in the United States (Indiana, Florida) were reported in May 2014. Both cases involved healthcare workers who lived and worked in Saudi Arabia and had traveled to the United States. The two cases were not linked (CDC, 2014c). A third asymptomatic Illinois patient, who had contact with the Indiana MERS case, had previously been identified through contact screening. However, further testing by the CDC found that the Illinois resident was not previously infected with MERS-CoV (CDC, *Press release*, May 28, 2014). All of the cases were transferred from the Middle East to other countries for care of the disease or returned from the Middle East and subsequently became ill. In addition, as noted above, some healthcare providers have been diagnosed with MERS-CoV infection after exposure to infected patients. Although active surveillance has identified an increase in community-acquired cases, there was no evidence of sustained spreading of MERS-CoV in community settings (CDC, Press Release [June 17, 2014]). Healthcare facilities that provide care for patients with suspected MERS-CoV infection should take appropriate measures to decrease the risk of transmission of the virus to other patients and healthcare providers by systematic implementation of infection prevention and control measures. A probable case of MERS-CoV infection is defined as a case where the patient is under investigation (PUI) with absent or inconclusive laboratory results for MERS-CoV infection who is a close contact of a laboratory-confirmed MERS-CoV case. A confirmed case is a person with laboratory confirmation of MERS-CoV infection. Confirmatory laboratory testing requires a positive PCR on at least two specific genomic targets or a single positive target with sequencing on a second (CDC, *MERS-CoV. Information for healthcare professionals*).

Based on information we have to date, the incubation period for MERS (time between when a person is exposed to MERS-CoV and when they start to have symptoms) is usually about 5 or 6 days, but can range from 2 to 14 days (*MERS-CoV. Information for healthcare professionals*). The CDC continues to work in consultation with the WHO and other partners to better understand the public health risk posed by MERS-CoV. Updated information from the WHO indicate that the period for considering evaluation for MERS-CoV infection in persons who develop severe acute lower respiratory illness days after traveling from the Middle East and other affected countries should be extended to within 14 days of travel (CDC, *MERS-CoV. Information for healthcare professionals*).

Infection Control for the Prevention of MERS-CoV Transmission

In 2015, the WHO updated the interim guidance that was published in 2013 to meet the urgent need for up-to-date information and evidence-based recommendations for the safe care of patients with probable or confirmed MERS-CoV infection. Healthcare-associated outbreaks with transmission to healthcare personnel highlight the importance of infection control procedures. It is crucial that healthcare personnel are provided with the best locally available protection for caring for MERS-CoV-infected patients and are followed up with if exposure has occurred. To prevent the transmission of *all* acute respiratory infections, respiratory hygiene/cough etiquette measures should be implemented at the first point of contact with a potentially infected person and should be incorporated into standard precautions. This includes covering the nose and mouth when coughing or sneezing, using tissues to contain respiratory secretions and disposing of them in the nearest waste receptacle after use, and hand hygiene (e.g., handwashing with nonantimicrobial soap and water, alcohol-based hand rub, or antiseptic hand wash) after having contact with respiratory secretions and contaminated objects/materials (WHO, *Infection prevention and control during healthcare for probable or confirmed cases of Middle East respiratory syndrome coronavirus (MERS-CoV) infection Interim guidance. Updated June 4, 2015*). The 2015 WHO guidelines for patients with acute respiratory infections, including suspected or confirmed MERS, called for placing the patient in a single isolation room with equal or greater than 12 air exchanges per hour (WHO, 2015). The CDC also has developed updated MERS *Interim* guidance for healthcare professionals, available at https://www.cdc.gov/coronavirus/mers/interim-guidance.html

The use of personal protective equipment (PPE) should be guided by a risk assessment concerning anticipated contact with blood, body fluids, secretions, and nonintact skin for routine patient care. When procedures include a risk of splash to the face and/or body, PPE should include the use of facial protection by either a surgical mask, and eye visor or goggles, or a face shield; *and* a gown and clean gloves. In addition to standard precautions, all individuals, including visitors and healthcare providers, in contact with patients with acute respiratory tract infection should use droplet precautions, which include wearing a surgical mask when in close contact (i.e., within approximately 3 ft) and upon entering the room of the patient; perform hand hygiene before and after contact with the patient and their surroundings, and immediately after removal of a surgical mask (CDC, MERS *Interim guidance for healthcare professionals*; Ho et al., 2017).

Additional precautions should be observed and PPE worn when performing aerosol-generating procedures, which may be associated with an increased risk of infection transmission, in particular, intubation. These include a particulate respirator (e.g., N95 respirator), eye protection (i.e., goggles or a face shield), gown, and gloves (some procedures may require sterile gloves).

These guidelines are interim ones to control transmission of the nCoV (MERS-CoV). In addition, not all suspected MERS-CoV patients would be admitted to healthcare facilities. They may prefer to stay in their homes. The CDC and WHO publications are available for MERS-CoV patient care at home and in the community. The CDC website (https://www.cdc.gov/coronavirus/mers/index.html) and the WHO website (http://apps.who.int/iris/bitstream/10665/174652/1/WHO_MERS_IPC_15.1_eng.pdf?ua=1) should be consulted for periodic updates regarding MERS-CoV recommendations and guidelines.

Clients in the United States with a history of MERS-CoV who are hospitalized with a severe febrile respiratory illness, or those who are being evaluated for MERS-CoV, should be managed using isolation precautions identical to those recommended for clients with known avian influenza. These precautions are outlined in Appendix A: "Type and duration of precautions needed for selected infections and conditions" in the CDC 2007 Guideline for isolation precautions: Preventing transmission of infectious agents in healthcare settings at https://www.cdc.gov/infectioncontrol/guidelines/isolation/appendix/type-duration-precautions.html. Clusters of severe acute respiratory illness of unknown etiology in the community also should be thoroughly investigated, and if no etiology is identified, this should prompt immediate notification of local public health officials, and testing for MERS-CoV should be conducted if indicated. In addition, any clusters of severe acute respiratory illness in healthcare personnel in the United States should be thoroughly investigated (CDC, *MERS interim guidance for healthcare professionals*).

Practice Point

Observance of infection control practices can reduce the risk of transmission of an acute respiratory illness, such as MERS-CoV infection, to healthcare providers. Community and public health nurses are educators who provide information to prevent the transmission of all respiratory infections, including MERS-CoV.

Avian Influenza

During the past century, three influenza A pandemics have occurred, and pandemic influenza will inevitably occur in the future. Although the timing and severity of the next pandemic cannot be predicted, the probability that a pandemic will occur has increased based on the recent outbreaks of influenza A (H5N1) in Asia, Europe, and Africa.

Influenza A viruses, which originate in birds, are categorized into subtypes on the basis of their surface antigens. These viruses have 16 hemagglutinin (H) surface antigen subtypes and nine neuraminidase (N) surface antigen subtypes. Only viruses of the H5 and H7 subtypes are known to cause the highly pathogenic form of type A influenza. New influenza virus variants result from frequent antigenic change (i.e., antigenic drift), which is a consequence of point mutations that occur during viral replication. These frequent changes that result from antigenic drift mean that there is a new seasonal influenza vaccine each year (CDC, *How the flu virus changes*).

Knowledge of the history of past influenza A pandemics has increased the awareness of the potential for another pandemic. Three influenza A pandemics have been reported in the past century. As noted above, the first pandemic, known as the "Spanish flu" (influenza A [H1N1]), occurred in 1918–1919 and resulted in millions of deaths worldwide, with more than 500,000 deaths in the United States. The "Spanish flu" was unique because the causative agent was very deadly, and it spread quickly across the globe within 6 months. Almost half of the people who died were young, healthy adults between 20 and 40 years of age, and many died within the first few days after infection. Others died of complications soon thereafter. The second pandemic, known as the "Asian flu" (influenza A [H2N2]), occurred in 1957–1958, and it was first identified in China in late February 1957. In less than 6 months, it spread to the United States, where it caused approximately 70,000 deaths. The highest mortality with Asian flu occurred in the elderly. The H2N2 influenza A virus that caused the pandemic of 1957 disappeared from the human population 10 years later. The third pandemic, known as "Hong Kong flu" (influenza A [H3N2]), occurred in 1968–1969. The first cases were detected in Hong Kong in early 1968. Later that year, the virus spread to the United States, where it claimed approximately 34,000 lives (Kilbourne, 2006). Influenza A (H3N2) viruses are still circulating today.

Avian Influenza A (H5N1) Outbreaks, 2003–2017

Until 1997, the risk of avian influenza was considered rare in humans. However, confirmed cases of human infection from several subtypes of avian viruses have been reported since then. Most of these human cases have resulted from contact with infected domestic poultry (e.g., chickens and ducks) or surfaces contaminated with blood and secretions/excretions from infected birds. Until 2003, the last epidemic of human infection with avian influenza A (H5N1) occurred in Hong Kong in 1997, with 18 confirmed cases and six deaths (WHO, 2011). In 2003, an outbreak of avian influenza A (H5N1), a highly pathogenic virus, spread among millions of birds (mostly chickens) across Southeast Asia. Although the H5N1 virus rarely infects humans, since 2003, a total of 860 laboratory-confirmed cases of human infection with avian influenza A(H5N1) virus, including 454 deaths, have been reported to WHO from 16 countries. The majority of cases were from Egypt, with 359 (79%) cases and 120 deaths, followed by Indonesia, with 200 cases and 168 deaths, and Vietnam, with 127 cases and 64 deaths (WHO, 2018d, *Cumulative number of A(H5N1) cases reported to WH, July 20, 2018.*) This was the largest number of documented cases since the virus first emerged in humans in 1997. Nearly all of the infections were the result of people having direct or close contact with infected poultry or contaminated surfaces (WHO, *Fact sheet: Influenza [avian and other zoonotic]*).

In 2012, Russell and colleagues reported that as few as five amino acid substitutions, or four with reassortment, might be sufficient for mammal-to-mammal transmission of A (H5N1) viruses through respiratory droplets. While the technical aspects of the study by Russell and colleagues are beyond the scope of this text, their "analyses…, using current best estimates, indicate that the remaining mutations could evolve within a single mammalian host, making the possibility of a respiratory droplet–transmissible A/H5N1 virus evolving in nature a potentially serious threat" (p. 1547).

An avian influenza virus can improve its transmissibility among humans by two mechanisms. The first is antigenic shift, a "reassortment" event, in which genetic material is exchanged between human and avian viruses during coinfection of a human or an animal such as a pig. Reassortment could result in a fully transmissible pandemic virus, which could rapidly spread throughout the world (Fig. 15.4). The second mechanism is a more gradual process of *antigenic drift*, an adaptive mutation, whereby the capability of the virus to bind to human cells increases during subsequent infections of humans. Adaptive mutation, which is expressed initially as small clusters of human cases with some evidence of human-to-human transmission, would probably give the world some time to take defensive action. If avian influenza A (H5N1) viruses gain the ability for efficient and sustained transmission among humans, an influenza **pandemic** (an epidemic occurring worldwide) could result, with potentially high rates of illness and death worldwide. Therefore, the epizootic A (H5N1) virus continues to pose an important public health threat (CDC, *Public health threat of highly pathogenic avian influenza A [H5N1] virus*).

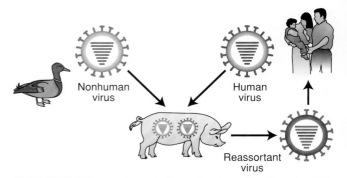

FIGURE 15.4 Reassortment: A mechanism of antigenic shift. (Adapted from National Institute of Allergy and Infectious Diseases, National Institutes of Health. Retrieved from http://www.niaid.nih.gov/topics/flu/research/basic/pages/antigenicshiftillustration.aspx.)

Infection Control for the Prevention of Avian A (H5N1) Influenza Transmission

Clients with a history of travel within 10 days to a country with avian influenza activity and who are hospitalized with a serious febrile respiratory illness, or are otherwise being evaluated for avian influenza, should be managed using isolation precautions. The isolation procedures are the same as those that were used for SARS-CoV and for suspected or confirmed MERS-CoV. In addition to standard precautions, which include careful attention to hand hygiene before and after all client contact or contact with items potentially contaminated with respiratory secretions, the CDC recommends the following enhanced isolation precautions when avian influenza is diagnosed or suspected:

- Contact precautions
- Use gloves and gown for all client contact.
- Use dedicated equipment such as stethoscopes, as well as disposable blood pressure cuffs and disposable thermometers.
- Eye protection
- Wear goggles or face shields when within 3 ft of the client.
- Airborne precautions
- Place the client in an airborne isolation room (AIR). Such rooms should have monitored negative air pressure in relation to corridor, with 6 to 12 air changes per hour (ACH), and exhaust air directly outside, or have recirculated air filtered by a high-efficiency particulate air (HEPA) filter. If an AIR is unavailable, a portable HEPA filter should be used to augment the number of ACH.
- Use a fit-tested respirator, at least as protective as a National Institute of Occupational Safety and Health (NIOSH)-approved disposable N95 filtering face piece respirator, when entering the room (CDC, *Interim guidance for infection control within healthcare settings when caring for confirmed cases,…* with novel influenza A viruses associated with severe disease).

H1N1 Influenza (Swine Flu) Pandemic, 2009–2010

In June 2009, the WHO declared a moderately severe global influenza A H1N1 pandemic, which was the first global pandemic in 40 years and the first in the 21st century. This declaration was based on the sustained worldwide spread of H1N1 from person to person, not the severity of illness caused by the virus. Although the Spanish flu was caused by an A (H1N1) virus, the 2009 virus was a similar but different type of virus. Taubenberger and colleagues (2005) proposed that the 1918 virus was not a "reassortment," virus like those that caused the smaller pandemics of 1957 and 1968. In those cases, avian flu viruses traded some genes with human-adapted flu viruses to spawn new hybrids. They posit that the 1918 virus was "an entirely avian-like virus" that somehow adapted to humans. While the 2009–2010 H1N1 virus was by no means as severe as the 1918 pandemic, it was expected that cases would continue to increase because of the onset of the influenza season in the Southern Hemisphere at that time. From April 12, 2009 to April 10, 2010, the CDC estimated that there were 60.8 million cases, 274,304 hospitalizations, and 12,469 deaths in the United States due to the A (H1N1) 2009 virus. The CDC estimated that between 151,700 and 575,400 people worldwide died from 2009 H1N1 virus infection during the first year the virus circulated. Globally, CDC estimated that 80% of (H1N1) 2009 virus–associated deaths were in people younger than 65 years of age, which differs from typical seasonal influenza epidemics during which about 70% to 90% of deaths are estimated to occur in people 65 years of age and older (CDC, *Past pandemics*).

Though this most recent influenza pandemic primarily affected children and young and middle-aged adults, the impact of the (H1N1) 2009 virus on the global population overall during the first year was less severe than that of previous pandemics.

The Department of Health and Human Services updated its pandemic influenza operational plan (DHHS, 2009) and was used during the 2009 H1N1 pandemic to describe progression of the pandemic and to help guide the response. The revised plan also incorporated the recently developed Influenza Risk Assessment Tool (IRAT). The IRAT makes an assessment of potential pandemic risk for a novel virus (i.e., new in humans) on the basis of the likelihood of emergence and the public health impact if it were to emerge, and acquire the ability to spread easily and efficiently in humans. Public health impact refers to the potential severity of human disease caused by the virus (e.g., deaths and hospitalizations), as well as the impact on society (e.g., missed workdays, strain on hospital capacity and resources, and interruption of basic public services) if a novel influenza virus were to begin spreading efficiently and sustainably among humans (CDC, *Interim guidance on use of intervals, triggers, and actions for novel influenza A* [H1N1] response [Updated 29 April 2009]). The CDC also developed a new tool for evaluating the potential effects of an emerging pandemic, the Pandemic Severity Assessment Framework (PSAF). Once a novel influenza A virus is identified by IRAT and is spreading from person-to-person in a sustained manner, public health officials use the PSAF to determine the impact of the pandemic, or how "bad" the pandemic will be. There are two main factors that can be used to determine the impact of a pandemic. The first is clinical severity, or how serious is the illness associated with infection. The second factor is transmissibility, or how easily the pandemic virus spreads from person-to-person. These two factors combined are used to guide decisions about which actions CDC recommends at a given time during the pandemic (CDC, *Pandemic Severity Assessment Framework [PSAF]*). Results of the PSAF help public health officials and healthcare professionals make timely and informed decisions, and to take appropriate actions. Using the PSAF, the 1918 pandemic can be characterized as one with very high transmissibility and very high clinical severity, while a mild or moderate pandemic, such as the 2009 H1N1 pandemic, is characterized by low to medium transmissibility and clinical severity (Fig. 15.5).

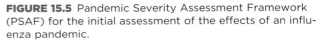

FIGURE 15.5 Pandemic Severity Assessment Framework (PSAF) for the initial assessment of the effects of an influenza pandemic.

To prevent/reduce the effects of a future pandemic, the CDC and the DHHS (2017) have recommended nonpharmaceutical mitigation strategies that can be implemented early and throughout a pandemic event (Table 15.1). The CDC also has developed checklists that identify important, specific activities that each state and local community can implement to prepare for a possible pandemic. Nurses practicing in the community should be aware of what some of these guidelines are. Many of these activities are specific to pandemic influenza, but many also pertain to any public health emergency. The CDC website at https://www.cdc.gov/flu/pandemic-resources/index.htm will have the latest guidelines to follow in the event of an influenza outbreak.

Practice Point

Stress the personal steps that everyone can take to reduce the spread of acute respiratory infection:

- Recognize symptoms of the flu and see a healthcare provider immediately if you have:
  - A temperature of greater than 100°F
  - A cough
  - A sore throat
  - An underlying condition that increases risk
- Cover your cough or sneeze

TABLE 15.1 Nonpharmaceutical Interventions (NPIs) to Prevent and Control Pandemic Influenza		
NPI Category	**Recommended NPIs**	**Timing**
Personal NPIs Personal protective measures for everyday use	Voluntary home isolation of ill persons (staying home when ill) Respiratory etiquette Hand hygiene	**Recommended at all times**
Personal protective measures reserved for pandemics	Voluntary home quarantine of exposed household members (staying home for up to 3 days when a household member is ill). If the next pandemic influenza virus transmission period is longer or shorter than 3 days, CDC will amend the recommendation. Use of face masks in community settings when ill.	**Reserved for pandemics**[a]
Community NPIs School closures and dismissals	School closures and dismissals. A school closure involves closing a school and sending all the students and staff members home. A school dismissal could involve a school staying open for staff members while the students stay home. Temporary, preemptive, coordinated dismissals of child care facilities and schools for grades K–12 (preemptive, coordinated dismissals might be implemented early during a pandemic to decrease the spread of influenza before many students and staff members become ill). Selective dismissals might be implemented by schools that serve students at high risk for complications from infection with influenza. Reactive dismissals might be implemented when many students and staff members are ill and not attending school or when many students and staff members are arriving at school ill and being sent home. Selective and reactive dismissals do not help slow disease transmission in the community.	**Reserved for pandemics**[a]
Social distancing NPI examples	Dividing classes into smaller groups and creating opportunities for distance learning (e.g., via the internet or local television or radio stations). Telecommuting and remote-meeting options in workplaces. Mass gathering modifications, postponements, or cancellations.	**Reserved for pandemics**[a]
Environmental NPIs	Routine cleaning/disinfection of frequently touched surfaces and objects in homes, child care facilities, schools, and workplaces.	**Recommended at all times**

[a]The CDC will use the Pandemic Severity Assessment Framework (PSAF) to assess pandemic severity (**low to moderate, high, very high**) to provide early and continuing guidance on use of NPIs to help slow the transmission of a novel virus.
Source: Adapted from Qualls, N., Levitt, A., Kanade, N., Wright-Jegede, N., Dopson, S., Biggerstaff, M.,…Uzicanin, A. (2017). Community mitigation guidelines to prevent pandemic influenza —United States, 2017. *Morbidity and Mortality Weekly Report, 66* (RR.1), 1–34. Retrieved on August 21, 2017, from https://www.cdc.gov/mmwr/volumes/66/rr/rr6601a1.htm.

- Wash hands often and keep hands away from your face
- Stay home and do not travel if you are ill
- Be prepared for increased illness in your schools and community

In **Case 1**, when the WHO declared that A (H1N1) influenza was pandemic in 2009, early available data suggested that the H1N1 pandemic virus was highly transmissible, and was caused by a new virus that occurred in addition to influenza viruses that circulate every year. It caused severe outcomes mostly among children, young adults, and specific groups at high risk for complications (e.g., pregnant women) rather than in adults aged ≥65 years, the group most at risk from seasonal influenza. The number of deaths among children also was more than twice as high as during a regular influenza season. Based on these data, in August 2009, the Advisory Committee on Immunization Practices recommended that children be placed higher on the priority list for receiving the new monovalent H1N1 vaccine, which became available in October 2009.

- How was the 2009 H1N1 influenza pandemic similar to the 1918 "Spanish flu?"
- How was the 2009 H1N1 influenza virus different from regular seasonal influenza virus?
- Why were children placed higher on the priority list for receiving the 2009 H1N1 vaccine?

Novel Avian Influenza A (H7N9) Virus, 2013–2017

Influenza A (H7N9) is one of a subgroup of influenza viruses that normally circulate among birds. This virus has not been previously seen in humans; however, human infections with the H7N9 virus have now been detected in China (WHO, *WHO risk assessment: Human infections with avian influenza A [H7N9] virus*). During the first wave from February to May of 2013, a total of 133 human cases and 43 deaths occurred. The second wave, which occurred from October 2013 through early June 2014, had many more cases than the first wave, with 313 cases. The total number of laboratory-confirmed cases of human infection with avian influenza A (H7N9) virus reported to WHO as of June 2014 was 450, including 165 deaths (WHO, *WHO risk assessment: Human infections with avian influenza A [H7N9] virus*). By February 2015, there were a total of 571 laboratory-confirmed cases of human infection with avian influenza A (H7N9) virus, including 212 deaths; 568 of the cases were from China (WHO, *Human infection with avian*

influenza A [H7N9] virus—China). Reports of family clusters of H7N9 have been rare, providing evidence that the virus is not easily spread from person to person. Although most cases had contact with live poultry or had visited live-animal markets before the onset of illness, the source of infection remained unclear. While the second wave of H7N9 infections had tapered off by June 2014, experts felt that cases would continue to emerge since the virus appears to be present in poultry and their environments. A fifth epidemic wave that has occurred since October 2016 has been greater than earlier waves. On August 4, 2017 the National Health and Family Planning Commission of China notified WHO of an additional laboratory-confirmed case of human infection with avian influenza A (H7N9) virus in China. This suggests that the virus continues to spread, and emphasizes that further intensive surveillance and control measures in both the human and animal health sectors remain crucial (WHO, *Influenza at the human-animal interface. Summary and assessment*, April 21, 2017 to May 16, 2017). During October 1, 2016 to August 7, 2017, the National Health and Family Planning Commission of China; CDC, Taiwan; the Hong Kong Centre for Health Protection; and the Macao CDC reported 1,557 human infections with Asian H7N9 viruses, including 605 (39%) deaths, to the WHO, making this the largest of the five epidemics of Asian H7N9 infections that have occurred since 2013 (Kile et al., 2017). As of September 2018, a total of a total of 1,567 laboratory-confirmed human cases, including at least 615 deaths, have been reported to WHO. In the latest wave (the sixth wave since October 2017), only three human cases have been detected. Also, there have been fewer A (H7N9) virus detections in poultry and environmental samples according to various reports from mainland China and the Hong Kong Special Administrative Region, China (WHO, 2018c, *Human infection with avian influenza A[H7N9] virus—China*: Updated on 5 September 2018).

Findings from this latest emerging influenza virus highlight the importance of zoonotic viruses on global health. Li and colleagues (2014) conducted an epidemiologic study of A (H7N9) influenza using the 2006 WHO case definition for human infections with A (H5N1) virus and identified through the Chinese surveillance system for pneumonia of unknown origin. A total of 139 cases with confirmed H7N9 infection had a median age of 61 years (range: 2 to 91 years), 71% were male, 73% were urban residents, and 9 were poultry workers. Except for four case clusters among family members who had provided care to case patients, most of the cases were epidemiologically unrelated. Of the data available among 131 patients, 82% had a history of exposure to live animals, including chickens. Ninety-nine percent (n = 137) were hospitalized with pneumonia or respiratory failure, with a 34% fatality rate. Analysis of 2,675 close contacts of case patients, 28 (1%) developed respiratory symptoms. However, all 28 close contacts tested negative for the H7N9 virus. Using available data and identifying the date of exposure to live poultry among 111 early cases of A

(H7N9) influenza, Gao and colleagues (2013) estimated the incubation period of A (H7N9) to be 5 days.

Early in the outbreak of novel A (H7N9) bird flu, Hu and colleagues (2013) found an emergence of antiviral resistance to oseltamivir (Tamiflu) in 3 of the 14 patients studied. While early treatment of suspected or confirmed cases of A (H7N9) with oseltamivir was advised, Wang and colleagues (2014) developed an assay to help clinicians monitor emergence of oseltamivir resistance in the A (H7N9) virus. Hu and colleagues warned: "The apparent ease with which antiviral resistance emerges in A/H7N9 viruses is concerning; it needs to be closely monitored and considered in future pandemic response plans" (p. 6).

Pure bird flu strains, such as the new H7N9 strain and the H5N1 virus, where the latter virus killed 59% of people it infected since 2003, are generally more deadly for humans. All of the reported cases of A (H7N9) up to 2016 had been from China (WHO, *WHO risk assessment: Human infections with avian influenza A* [H7N9] virus). However, ongoing surveillance can identify reassortment of zoonotic viruses that can spread human-to-human transmission, leading to a pandemic. While there may be limited person-to-person spread of the A (H7N9) virus, many people travel between China and the United States; therefore, the CDC has issued a public health alert for healthcare providers to be aware of patients who present with acute respiratory illness and a travel history to countries where the A (H7N9) virus has been confirmed (CDC, *Influenza: H7N9*). Recommendations for infection control for A (H7N9) may be found at the CDC website: https://www.cdc.gov/flu/avianflu/healthprofessionals.htm

---

Case 1: A goal of the U.S. Department of Health and Human Services (DHHS) in its Pandemic Influenza Plan 2017 Update was to sustain momentum and improve implementation of community mitigation measures. Such measures may be used from the earliest stages of an influenza pandemic, including the initial months when the most effective countermeasure, for example, a vaccine against the new pandemic virus, might not yet be broadly available.

To meet this goal, the following objective was developed: Improve public awareness and implementation of nonpharmaceutical interventions (NPIs) to slow the spread of influenza.

- Based on the data outlined in see Table 15.1, what NPIs would you consider appropriate for the 2009 A (H1N1) influenza pandemic?

West Nile Virus

Human cases of West Nile virus (WNV) infection appeared for the first time in the Western Hemisphere in New York in 1999, and by 2003, an epidemic of WNV had expanded across the United States from eastern United States to the west coast within a 3-year period. WNV has now become endemic in the United States, and its continued expansion indicates that it is permanently established in the Western Hemisphere. As of January 17, 2017, a total of 2,038 cases of WNV disease in people have been reported to CDC. Of these, 1,140 (56%) were classified as neuroinvasive disease (such as meningitis or encephalitis) and 898 (44%) were classified as non-neuroinvasive disease. In 2016, 47 states and the District of Columbia had reported WNV infections in people, birds, or mosquitoes (CDC, *West Nile virus, preliminary maps* and data for 2016). Although the incidence of WNV outside North America is low, the virus has been found in Central America, parts of South America, and the Caribbean. Recent reports have even found WNV in the Artic (ISID, 2013).

Transmission of WNV involves animals. The most common route of transmission is from the bite of an infected mosquito. Mosquitoes become infected when they feed on infected birds and then spread the disease to humans and other animals when they bite them. Symptoms typically develop between 3 and 14 days after the infected mosquito bites someone. The majority of WNV cases occur among males, with the date of onset ranging from late March to early October. However, in warmer climates, WNV infections can occur year-round.

Symptoms of WNV vary. Approximately 80% of infected people (about four out of five) do not have any symptoms. Another 20% of those who become infected have symptoms such as fever, headache, body aches, nausea, vomiting, and sometimes swollen lymph glands or a skin rash on the chest, stomach, and back. Symptoms can last for as short a period as a few days; however, some *healthy people* have become sick for several weeks. About 1 in 150 people infected with WNV develops severe illness, with severe symptoms that can include high fever, headache, neck stiffness, stupor, disorientation, coma, tremors, convulsions, muscle weakness, vision loss, numbness, and paralysis. These symptoms may last for several weeks, and neurologic effects may be permanent. People older than 50 years are more likely to develop serious symptoms of WNV if they do become sick; therefore, they should take special care to avoid mosquito bites (CDC, *West Nile virus*).

In the 2002 WNV outbreak, nonvector routes of transmission were identified, including blood transfusions, organ transplantation, and vertical transmission in utero. Nonvector WNV transmission has also been reported in laboratory workers and poultry farm workers. Because of the transfusion-related cases of WNV in 2002, the CDC has established a mechanism through state and local health departments for reporting WNV infection occurring in people who have received blood component transfusions within 4 weeks prior to onset of illness. Therefore, WNV disease should be considered in any person with a febrile or acute neurologic illness who has had recent exposure to mosquitoes, blood transfusion, or organ transplantation, especially during the summer months in areas where virus activity has been reported. Of the 2,038 reported WNV cases in 2016, 275 were presumptive viremic blood donors (PVDs). People who had no symptoms at the time of donating blood through a blood collection agency, but whose blood tested positive when screened for the presence of WNV are considered PVDs. Some PVDs develop symptoms after donation. The diagnosis of WNV should also be considered in any infant born to a mother infected with WNV during pregnancy or while breast-feeding (CDC, *West Nile virus*).

Prevention of WNV Infection

WNV is not transmitted from person to person. No isolation precautions are indicated other than standard precautions. The CDC guidelines emphasize avian, animal, mosquito, and human WNV surveillance, along with control and elimination of mosquito breeding sites such as standing water in flowerpots, buckets, and old tires.

There is no vaccine to prevent WNV infection, and although various drugs have been evaluated or empirically used for WNV disease, none have shown specific benefit to date. To prevent WNV, the CDC recommends using an insect repellant such as DEET (*N*, *N*-diethyl-m-toluamide) or picaridin when outdoors, following the directions on the package. Because mosquitoes are most active at dusk and dawn, in addition to an insect repellant, long sleeves and pants should be worn when outdoors during these hours. Screens on windows and doors will keep mosquitoes out (CDC, *West Nile virus*).

WNV disease is a nationally notifiable condition. All cases should be reported to local public health authorities. Reporting can assist local, state, and national authorities to recognize outbreaks and to implement control measures to reduce future infections. More information on WNV is available at the CDC website at http://www.cdc.gov/west-nile/index.html

Practice Point

Community and public health nurses should educate the public about how to prevent WNV infection:

- Use of Food and Drug Administration (FDA)-approved repellants for skin and/or clothing for protection from mosquito-borne diseases.
- When weather permits, wear long-sleeved shirts and long pants outdoors.
- Place mosquito netting over infant carriers when outdoors with infants.
- Consider staying indoors at dawn, dusk, and early evening, which are peak mosquito biting times.
- Install or repair window and door screens so that mosquitoes cannot come indoors.

Lyme Disease

Epidemiology of Lyme Disease

Lyme disease was first described in the late 1970s by Dr. Allen Steere. He recognized it as an important emerging infection when it appeared in a cluster of children in the Lyme, Connecticut, area, who were thought to have juvenile rheumatoid arthritis. However, it became apparent that Lyme arthritis was a late manifestation of a multisystem disease, of which some symptoms had been recognized previously in Europe and America (Steere, Coburn, & Glickstein, 2004).

Lyme disease, which is caused by a bacterium and transmitted by ticks, is the most commonly reported vector-borne disease in the United States. In 1981, Burgdorfer and colleagues discovered a previously unidentified spirochetal bacterium, subsequently named *Borrelia burgdorferi* (as noted in a previous Evidence for Practice feature). The spread of Lyme disease and its vectors have developed from the recent proliferation of deer and the process of reforestation now taking place. As a result, increasingly large numbers of people live where risk of Lyme disease is increased. The agents of these infections, which once were transmitted by an exclusively rodent-feeding vector, have now become zoonotic. The deer tick (*I. scapularis* in the northeastern and north central United States; *I. pacificus* in the western United States) is an important vector in human Lyme borreliosis along with the white-tailed deer, the preferred host of the adult deer tick. The white-tailed deer populations seem to be critical for the survival of the ticks. However, the deer is not involved in the life cycle of the spirochete (Steere et al., 2004). The life cycle of the *Ixodes* tick takes 2 years. Once a tick becomes infected with *Borrelia burgdorferi*, it remains infected for life and can transmit the organism to new hosts.

In 2015 (latest available data), the CDC reported 28,453 confirmed cases and 9,616 probable cases of Lyme disease in the United States, at an incidence rate of 8.9 per 100,000 population, and it was the sixth most common nationally notifiable disease that year. The majority (95%) of Lyme disease cases in 2015 were reported from 14 states in New England, the mid-Atlantic states, and the upper Midwest. Lyme disease does not occur nationwide and is concentrated heavily in the Northeast and upper Midwest (CDC, *Lyme disease*). Although the incidence of human Lyme disease in the northeastern United States is more than twice that in the Midwest, the prevalence of *Borrelia burgdorferi* in the tick vector is nearly identical in the two regions (Brisson, Vandermause, Meece, Reed, & Dykhuizen, 2010). Lyme disease is spreading throughout the world. Cases have been found on all continents except Antarctica. The incidence rates of Lyme disease in 2002 and 2015 were 8.2 per 100,000 and 8.9 per 100,000 population, respectively. The overall incidence rate of Lyme disease in the United States in 2015 had reached the *Healthy People 2010* targeted rate of 9.7 new cases per 100,000 population where the disease is endemic (DHHS, 2000); however, the rates were still more than five times higher in some northeastern states

(Connecticut, Maine, Pennsylvania, Rhode Island, Vermont) (CDC, *Lyme disease*).

A recent study by Hersh and colleagues (2014) found that humans in the northeastern and midwestern United States are at increasing risk of not only Lyme disease, but also coinfection with two emerging pathogens *Anaplasma phagocytophilum* and *Babesia microti*. *Borrelia burgdorferi*, *Babesia microti*, and *Anaplasma phagocytophilum* are transmitted by the same tick vector, *I. scapularis*. Although coinfection with the gram-negative bacterium *Anaplasma phagocytophilum* was found to be less common in the ticks they studied, 83% were found to be coinfected with *Borrelia burgdorferi* and *Babesia microti*. Human babesiosis, caused by *Babesia microti*, a protozoan blood parasite, has been increasing in prevalence, especially in the Northeast. Babesiosis can be asymptomatic or present with flu-like symptoms (e.g., fever, chills, body aches, weakness, and fatigue) that may not appear for weeks or months after exposure to *Babesia microti*. In addition, Krause and colleagues (2014) found that *Borrelia miyamotoi* is prevalent in southern New England. Therefore, healthcare providers should be aware that acute *Borrelia miyamotoi* infection may be misdiagnosed as Lyme disease. They also should keep in mind an increased risk of coinfection with *Borrelia burgdorferi* and *Babesia microti* when diagnosing and treating tick-borne illness. Babesiosis became a notifiable disease in 2011 (CDC, *Babesiosis*).

Symptoms and Signs of Lyme Disease

Lyme disease is diagnosed based on symptoms, physical findings (e.g., a "bull's-eye rash," which is the hallmark symptom of Lyme disease), and the possibility of exposure to infected ticks; laboratory testing is helpful if used correctly and performed with validated methods.

Exposure to Lyme disease is defined as having spent time (less than or equal to 30 days before onset of the initial skin lesion) in wooded, brushy, or grassy areas (i.e., potential tick habitats) in a county in which Lyme disease is endemic. A history of tick bite is not required. A county in which the disease is endemic is one in which at least two confirmed cases have been previously acquired or in which established populations of a known tick vector are infected with *Borrelia burgdorferi* (CDC, *Lyme disease*).

The best clinical marker of Lyme disease is the initial skin lesion (i.e., erythema migrans), which occurs in 60% to 80% of people with the disease. For purposes of surveillance, erythema migrans is defined as a skin lesion that typically begins as a red macule or papule and expands over a period of days to weeks to form a large round lesion, often with partial central clearing. Within 1 to 2 weeks of being infected with *Borrelia burgdorferi*, people may have the bull's-eye rash with fever, headache, and muscle or joint pain. Some people have Lyme disease and do not have any early symptoms. Other people have fever and other flu-like symptoms without a rash (CDC, *Lyme disease*). Figure 15.6 (CDC, *Two-tier testing for Lyme disease*).

After several days or weeks, the bacteria may spread throughout the body of an infected person. Symptoms such as rashes in other parts of the body, pain that seems to move from joint to joint, and signs of inflammation of the heart or nerves may occur. If the disease is not treated, additional symptoms, such as swelling and pain in major joints or mental changes, months after becoming infected, may occur in a few cases. People who are treated with antibiotics early in the infection generally recover quickly and completely, as do those in the later stages of the infection. Antibiotics commonly used for oral treatment include doxycycline, amoxicillin, or

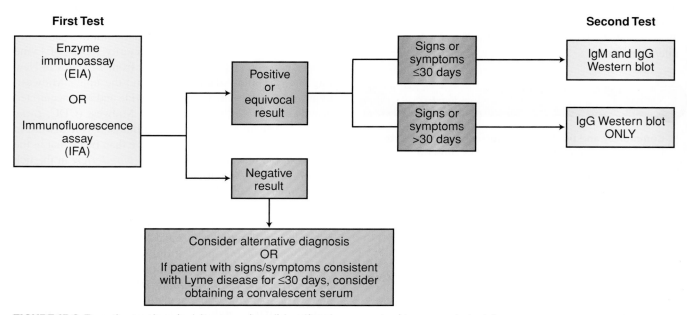

FIGURE 15.6 Two-tier testing decision tree describing the steps required to properly test for Lyme disease. *Source:* CDC. *Two-tier Testing for Lyme Disease.* Retrieved on August 15, 2017 from https://www.cdc.gov/lyme/healthcare/clinician_twotier.html.

cefuroxime axetil. Patients with certain neurologic or cardiac forms of illness may require intravenous treatment with drugs such as ceftriaxone or penicillin (CDC, *Lyme disease*). For detailed recommendations on treatment of Lyme disease, consult the 2006 guidelines for treatment of Lyme disease developed by the Infectious Diseases Society of America (IDSA, 2006) at https://doi.org/10.1086/508667

I was coming down with the flu. My mom made me go to a doctor when she saw that I had a large red sore at the site of the tick bite. The doctor found several red sores on my legs and tested me for Lyme disease. I had to be on antibiotics for 3 weeks, and then I felt fine. That experience made me very interested in infectious diseases and nursing as a career.

Student Reflection

When I was in high school, I went to an Outward Bound camp in Connecticut. It was great—we were outdoors hiking or riding almost all day, and slept outside most of the time. It was one of the most memorable times of my life. The day before we left for home, though, I found a fat tick on my thigh. We were warned about bug bites and used a spray when we remembered. I went to the camp nurse and she cleaned it out really well, so I forgot about it. After a couple of weeks, I got a nasty headache, had a fever, and felt like

Prevention of Lyme Disease

Steps to prevent Lyme disease include using insect repellant, identification and removal of deer ticks promptly, applying pesticides, and reducing tick habitat. Nymphal deer ticks are the size of poppy seeds, and adult deer ticks are the size of apple seeds (Fig. 15.7). Although interventions are inexpensive, are unlikely to be harmful, and have probably slowed the increase in Lyme disease in the United States, the epidemic continues to gain momentum.

According to the American Lyme Disease Foundation, the best precaution against Lyme disease in tick-infested

Proper tick removal

Wear protective gloves if available. Grasp the tick with a pair of tweezers as close to the skin as possible. Gently but firmly pull it straight out. If tweezers and gloves are unavailable, use a tissue or piece of cloth as a barrier to protect your hands.

Do *not* apply a lit match, petroleum jelly, nail polish remover, or other solvents.

Do *not* crush a tick with bare hands. Tick secretions may carry disease.

The tick can be killed with alcohol and disposed of in the trash or by flushing it down the toilet.

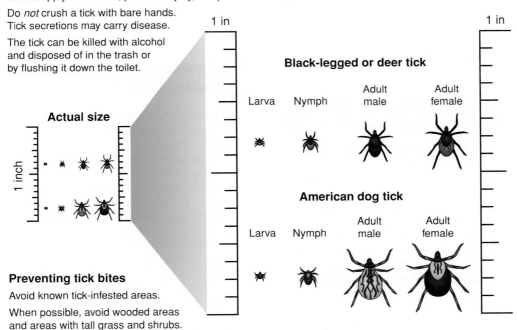

Preventing tick bites

Avoid known tick-infested areas.

When possible, avoid wooded areas and areas with tall grass and shrubs.

Wear light-colored long sleeves and long pants.

Tuck long pants into socks or boots.

Walk in the center of trails to avoid brushing against tall grass, shrubs, or brush.

Apply DEET-containing repellants primarily to clothes and sparingly to exposed skin. Follow product directions carefully and supervise children when using repellants.

Treat pets with repellants that are specifically formulated for pets.

FIGURE 15.7 Tick ID card.

15.2 Lyme Disease Combined Prevention Techniques

- Know how to identify deer ticks.
- Wear enclosed shoes and light-colored clothing with a tight weave to make it easier to spot ticks.
- Scan clothes and any exposed skin frequently for ticks while outdoors.
- Stay on cleared, well-traveled trails.
- Use insect repellant containing diethyl-meta-toluamide (DEET) on skin or insect repellant for clothes.
- Avoid sitting directly on the ground or on stone walls since they are havens for ticks and their hosts.
- Keep long hair tied back, especially when gardening.
- Do a final, full-body tick check at the end of the day for adults, children, and pets.
- Ticks tend to climb to warm, hidden areas of the head and neck if not intercepted first.
- Performed consistently, this is the most effective current prevention technique.
- Shower and shampoo on returning home; crawling ticks may be removed, but not attached ticks.
- Spin clothes in a dryer for 20 minutes to kill any unseen ticks.

Source: Adapted from American Lyme Disease Foundation. *Lyme disease.* Retrieved on August 21, 2017, from http://www.aldf.com/lyme.shtml.

areas is to avoid contact with soil, leaf litter, and vegetation as much as possible. People who garden, hike, camp, hunt, work outdoors, or otherwise spend time in brush, overgrown fields, or the woods should use the precautions listed in Box 15.2 to reduce their risk of getting Lyme disease (American Lyme Disease Foundation, *Lyme disease*).

Practice Point

Community and public health nurses must be prepared to educate the public about the signs and symptoms of Lyme disease and other tick-borne diseases, as well as the prevention of these diseases. Because the population density and percentage of infected ticks that may transmit Lyme disease and other tick-borne infections vary markedly from one region of the country to another, people should know whether infected deer ticks are active in their area or in places they may visit. There is even great variation from county to county within a state and from area to area within a county. For example, less than 5% of adult ticks south of Maryland are infected with *Borrelia burgdorferi*, whereas up to 50% are infected in areas with a high tick infection rate in the Northeast. The tick infection rate in Pacific coastal states is between 2% and 4% (American Lyme Disease Foundation). As noted above, healthcare providers should also be aware of an increased risk of coinfection with *Borrelia burgdorferi*, *Babesia microti*, and *Borrelia miyamotoi*.

Escherichia coli O157:H7

E. coli O157:H7, a Shiga toxin–producing *E. coli* (STEC), may also be referred to as verocytotoxin-producing *E. coli* (VTEC) or enterohemorrhagic *E. coli* (EHEC). This deadly toxin-producing bacterium is the one most commonly heard about in the news in association with food-borne outbreaks in the United States, and have led to national recalls of several food products (CDC, E. coli). It produces symptoms of severe abdominal cramps, bloody and nonbloody diarrhea, and vomiting, which generally resolve within 7 to 10 days.

Most people recover fully from an *E. coli* infection in 2 or 3 days; however, *E. coli* O157:H7 can cause fatal hemolytic-uremic syndrome (HUS) and renal failure in the very young and the elderly, and clients may require dialysis. HUS generally occurs up to a week after a gastrointestinal infection with *E. coli*. In these cases, HUS develops when the bacterial toxins enter the bloodstream and destroy red blood cells (CDC, *E. coli*).

Freedman and colleagues (2016) report that treating STEC infections frequently prompt consideration of antibiotic treatment, prior to or after culture results are known. However, they concluded that "such treatment may increase the risk of developing HUS. Given the lack of literature support for the value of early-in-illness antibiotics in STEC infections, and the potential for harm associated with their administration in such instances, these results can be used to promote a more unified public health recommendation against using antibiotics in individuals infected with STEC" (Freedman et al., 2016).

Practice Point

E. coli O157:H7 infections can also be caused by zoonotic transmission through contact with animals that carry the organism.

Recent cases of HUS have been associated with outbreaks of *E. coli* O157:H7 infections, which were apparently caused by contact with animals, including fairs, farm tours, and petting zoos. In July 2017, an outbreak of *E. coli* O157:H7 killed two children and sickened 10 other people in a remote community on the Utah-Arizona border. Infected farm animals followed by person-to-person contamination were the likely cause. Public health officials report that the outbreak was likely caused by animal manure containing *E. coli* O157:H7 bacteria being spread by humans (Luna et al., 2018). Experience from these and previous outbreaks underscores the necessity for adequate control measures to reduce zoonotic transmission. The CDC has developed standardized recommendations for public health officials, veterinarians, animal exhibitors, and visitors to animal exhibits; it established that handwashing is the single most important prevention step for reducing the risk for disease transmission. Other critical recommendations for venues with animals are the inclusion of transition areas between animal and nonanimal areas (e.g., where food is sold) and proper care and management of animals in public settings. In addition, as discussed in Chapter 14, the CDC recommends educating the operators and staff of animal venues, as well as visitors, about the risk of disease transmission if animal contact is possible (CDC, 2005a). More information about transmission of *E. coli* O157:H7 can be found in Chapter 14.

Tuberculosis

Epidemiology of Tuberculosis

Tuberculosis (TB) is a disease caused by *Mycobacterium tuberculosis* that is spread from person to person through the air when a person with TB disease of the lungs or throat coughs, sneezes, speaks, or sings. The TB bacteria (droplet nuclei) can stay suspended in the air for several hours, depending on the environment. Persons who breathe in the air containing these TB bacteria can become infected. The bacteria usually attack the lungs, but they can attack any part of the body such as the kidney, spine, and brain. If not treated properly, TB disease can be fatal (CDC, *Tuberculosis*). Tuberculosis remains one of the most common infectious diseases worldwide. According to the WHO, TB killed fewer people between 2000 and 2015, but was still among the top 10 causes of disease. There was an estimated 10.4 million new TB cases worldwide in 2015, and a death rate of 1.4 million among HIV-negative people, with an additional 0.4 million deaths among people living with HIV. Of the 10.4 million new TB cases in 2015, 5.9 million (56%) were among men, 3.5 million (34%) among women, and 1.0 million (10%) among children. People living with HIV accounted for 1.2 million (11%) of all new TB cases. Six countries accounted for 60% of the new cases: India, Indonesia, China, Nigeria, Pakistan, and South Africa. There also were an estimated 480, 000 new cases of multidrug-resistant TB (MDR-TB) and an additional 100,000 people with rifampicin-resistant TB (RR-TB) who were also newly eligible for MDR-TB treatment (WHO, 2016b).

Tuberculosis was once the leading cause of death in the United States. After approximately 30 years of decline, the number of reported cases of TB increased 20% between 1985 and 1992. This led to a renewed emphasis on TB control and prevention in the 1990s and actions that reversed the increase in cases.

A total of 9,557 TB cases (a rate of 3 cases per 100,000 population) were reported in the United States in 2015 and had remained at that rate for the past 3 years. However, a total of 66.4% of reported TB cases in the United States occurred among foreign-born persons in 2015. The case rate among foreign-born persons (15.1 cases/100,000 persons) was approximately 13 times higher than among U.S.-born

persons (1.2 cases/100,000 persons). The majority of these cases are among persons who have been in the United States 5 years or longer. While the rate of TB among whites in the United States was 0.6 cases per 100,000 persons in 2015, racial and ethnic minorities and foreign-born persons continue to be disproportionately affected by TB. In 2015, the highest TB rates in the United States occurred among persons who were Asian (18.2 cases/100,000), native Hawaiians and other Pacific Islanders (18.2 TB cases/100,000), black or African American (5 cases/100,000), Hispanic/Latino (4.8 cases/100,000 persons), and American Indian or Alaskan Native (6.1 cases/100,000). In addition, MDR-TB remains a threat among foreign-born people. Of the total number of reported primary MDR-TB cases overall, the percentage of MDR-TB cases decreased slightly from 1.3% (94 cases) in 2014 to 1.2% (89 cases) in 2015. Of the total number of reported MDR-TB cases, the proportion occurring among foreign-born persons increased from 31% (149 of 484) in 1993 to 85% (76 of 89 cases) in 2015 (CDC, *TB facts*). MDR-TB, defined as resistance to the two most potent "first-line" anti-TB agents, is discussed further below.

Despite successful declines in TB cases and case rates over the past 60 years, the goal of *Healthy People 2020* (DHHS, 2010) to reduce TB in the United States to 1 case per 100,000 population has not been met. As can be seen by the 2015 data above, that target has not been met yet. The improvement of TB control among racial/ethnic minorities and foreign-born persons is essential as the United States strives to prevent TB transmission and meet TB elimination goals. Vigilance for TB among homeless persons is also crucial for maintaining progress toward TB elimination among the U.S.-born population (CDC, 2015).

Practice Point

M. tuberculosis is an example of an infectious agent that can cause an infection in an individual, but not be contagious at all times.

M. tuberculosis infection occurs when a susceptible person inhales airborne droplet nuclei containing the TB bacilli, which pass through the upper respiratory tract and bronchi. When the bacilli reach the alveoli of the lungs, they are taken up by macrophages and spread throughout the body. Generally, 2 to 10 weeks after initial infection with *M. tuberculosis*, an immune response limits additional multiplication and spread of the bacilli. *M. tuberculosis* generally affects the lungs but can attack any part of the body such as the kidney, spine, and brain. If not treated properly, TB can be fatal. However, some of the TB bacilli remain dormant and viable for many years and are defined as latent TB infection. People with latent TB infection usually have a positive tuberculin skin test (TST) but no symptoms of active TB and therefore are not contagious. In many people who have latent TB infection, the *M. tuberculosis* bacteria remain inactive for a lifetime without causing active TB disease.

But in other people, especially those who have weak immune systems, the bacteria become active and cause TB disease (CDC, *Tuberculosis*). Table 15.2 for the difference between latent TB infection and active TB disease.

Symptoms and Signs of TB

Active TB infection is characterized by a chronic productive cough, low-grade fever, night sweats, and weight loss, along with a positive Mantoux tuberculin skin test (TST), which is the standard method of determining whether a person is infected with *M. tuberculosis*. People with active TB are contagious. However, certain people who are anergic (lack an immune response to an antigen) may not have a positive TST (e.g., persons with HIV) (CDC, *Tuberculin skin testing*).

Evidence for Practice

A nurse case-managed intervention, with incentives and tracking procedures to increase adherence to treatment of latent TB infection, was evaluated to determine the efficacy of the program. Twelve homeless subgroups were chosen that had characteristics previously identified in the literature as predictive

of nonadherence to treatment. These characteristics included female gender, African American ethnicity, history of military service, lifetime injection drug use, daily alcohol and drug use, poor physical health, and a history of poor mental health. Five hundred twenty homeless adults in homeless shelters in Los Angeles were followed prospectively over a period of 5 years. The intervention achieved a 91% completion rate for homeless shelter residents, and there was significantly improved latent TB infection treatment adherence in 9 of the 12 subgroups. However, daily drug users, participants with a history of injection drug use, daily alcohol users, and people who were not African American had particularly poor completion rates. It was concluded that nurse case management with incentives appears to be a good foundation for improving adherence to treatment for latent TB infection, especially for sheltered homeless populations (Nyamathi et al., 2008).

Latent TB and HIV Infections

People infected with HIV, especially those with low $CD4^+$ cell counts, develop TB disease rapidly after becoming infected with *M. tuberculosis*. Because HIV infection weakens the immune system, people with prior untreated latent TB infection and HIV infection are at very high risk of developing active TB disease (CDC, *TB and HIV coinfection*). Therefore, all people with HIV infection should be tested to find out if they have latent TB infection. If they

TABLE 15.2 Symptomatic Differences Between Latent Tuberculosis (TB) Infection and Active TB Disease

A Person With Latent TB Infection	A Person With Active TB Disease
• Has no symptoms	• Has symptoms that may include the following:
• Does not feel sick	• A bad cough that lasts 3 weeks or longer
• Cannot spread TB to others	• Pain in the chest
• Usually has a positive skin test or QuantiFERON-TB Gold In-Tube test (QFT-GIT)	• Coughing up blood or sputum
• Has a normal chest x-ray and sputum test	• Weakness or fatigue
	• Weight loss
	• No appetite
	• Chills
	• Fever
	• Sweating at night
	• May spread TB to others
	• Usually has a positive skin test or QFT-GIT
	• May have an abnormal chest x-ray or positive sputum smear or culture

Notes: QuantiFERON-TB Gold In-Tube test (QFT-GIT) is an FDA-approved indirect blood test for *M. tuberculosis* infection (including infection resulting in active disease) when used in conjunction with risk assessment, radiography, and other medical and diagnostic evaluations.
Sources: Centers for Disease Control and Prevention (CDC). *Tuberculosis fact sheets*. Retrieved from http://www.cdc.gov/tb/topics/testing.htm; Centers for Disease Control and Prevention (CDC). (2010). Updated guidelines for using interferon gamma release assays to detect *Mycobacterium tuberculosis* infection—United States, 2010. *Morbidity and Mortality Weekly Report, 59*(RR05), 1–25; Centers for Disease Control and Prevention (CDC). *Latent tuberculosis infection: A guide for primary healthcare providers*. Retrieved from https://www.cdc.gov/tb/publications/ltbi/diagnosis.htm.

have latent TB infection, they need treatment as soon as possible to prevent them from developing active TB disease. If they have active TB disease, they must take medicine to cure the disease (Lewinsohn et al., 2017; CDC, *Treatment regimens for latent TB infection*).

Prevention and Control of TB

TARGETED TUBERCULIN TESTING AND TREATMENT OF LATENT TB INFECTION

In the United States and other countries with a low incidence of TB, most new, active cases have occurred in people with latent TB infection who later developed active TB. Targeted identification and treatment of infected people at highest risk for developing disease benefits both infected people and susceptible people. Because health departments often lack access to high-risk populations and the resources necessary to undertake targeted testing programs, the participation of other healthcare providers is essential to ensure the successful implementation of community efforts to prevent TB in high-risk groups. Community sites where healthcare professionals may find people at high risk for TB and where targeted testing programs have been evaluated include neighborhood health centers, jails, homeless shelters, inner-city areas, methadone clinics, syringe/needle-exchange programs, and other community-based social service facilities (Lewinsohn et al., 2017). The WHO recommends directly observed therapy (DOT), using the most effective standardized, short-course regimens, and of fixed-dose TB drug combinations as an approach to TB control (WHO, *The five elements of DOT*).

Treating latent *M. tuberculosis* infection (LTBI) is a cornerstone of the U.S. strategy for TB elimination. Randomized controlled studies have shown that a new combination regimen of isoniazid (INH) and rifapentine administered weekly for 12 weeks as DOT is as effective for preventing TB as other regimens and is more likely to be completed than the U.S. standard regimen of 9 months of INH daily without DOT. These "first-line" treatment drugs are highly effective against nonresistant TB but much less so against MDR-TB. The new regimen is recommended as an equal alternative to the 9-month INH regimen for otherwise healthy patients aged 15 years or older who have LTBI and factors that are predictive of TB developing (e.g., recent exposure to contagious TB) (CDC, *Treatment regimens for latent TB*). Box 15.3 for people at high risk for progressing from latent TB infection to active TB disease.

TREATMENT OF ACTIVE TB

Active TB disease can be treated by taking several drugs for 6 to 9 months. There are 10 drugs currently approved by the FDA for treating TB. Of the approved drugs, the first-line anti-TB agents that form the core of treatment regimens are isoniazid (INH), rifampin (RIF), ethambutol (EMB), and pyrazinamide (PZA). Drug-susceptible TB disease treatment consists of an intensive phase of 2 months of isoniazid

---

15.3	**Factors That Influence Progression From Latent Tuberculosis (TB) Infection to Active TB Disease**

People infected with HIV

People infected with *Mycobacterium tuberculosis* within the previous 2 years

People with a history of untreated or inadequately treated TB disease, including people with chest radiograph findings consistent with previous TB

Infants and children aged <5 years who have a positive TB test result

People with any of the following clinical conditions or other immunocompromising conditions:
- Silicosis
- Diabetes mellitus
- Chronic renal failure
- Certain hematologic disorders (leukemias and lymphomas)
- Other specific malignancies (e.g., carcinoma of the head, neck, or lung)
- Body weight >10% below ideal body weight
- Prolonged corticosteroid use
- Other immunosuppressive treatments
- Organ transplant
- End-stage renal disease
- Intestinal bypass or gastrectomy

Source: Centers for Disease Control and Prevention (CDC). *Latent tuberculosis infection: A guide for primary healthcare providers.* Retrieved on August 22, 2017, from https://www.cdc.gov/tb/publications/ltbi/targeted-testing.htm#identifyingTBDisease.

(INH), rifampin (RIF), pyrazinamide (PZA), and ethambutol (EMB) followed by a continuation phase of 4 months of INH and RIF. Because of the relatively high proportion of adults with TB caused by organisms that are resistant to INH, four drugs (INH, RIF, PZA, EMB) are necessary in the intensive phase to be maximally effective. However, EMB can be discontinued as soon as the results of drug susceptibility studies demonstrate that the isolate is susceptible to INH and RIF. Pyridoxine (vitamin B6) should be given with INH to all persons at risk of neuropathy (e.g., pregnant women; breastfeeding infants; persons infected with HIV; patients with diabetes, alcoholism, malnutrition, or chronic renal failure; or those who are of advanced age (Nahid et al., 2016).

A pediatric TB expert should be involved in the treatment of TB in children and in the management of infants, young children, and immunocompromised children who have been exposed to someone with infectious TB disease. It is very important that children or anyone being treated for latent TB infection or TB disease finish the medicine and take the drugs exactly as instructed (CDC, *TB treatment for children*).

Drug susceptibility tests should be performed on initial isolates from all clients to identify what should be an effective anti-TB regimen. In addition, drug susceptibility tests should be repeated if the client continues to produce culture-positive sputum after 3 months of treatment or develops positive cultures after a period of negative cultures (Nahid et al., 2016).

Directly observed therapy (DOT) is one in which healthcare professionals observe clients to ensure that they ingest each dose of anti-TB medication to maximize the likelihood of completion of therapy. Programs using DOT as the central element in a comprehensive, client-centered approach to case management (enhanced DOT) have higher rates of treatment completion than less intensive strategies. Each client's management plan should be individualized to incorporate measures that facilitate adherence to the drug regimen. Such measures may include, for example, social service support, treatment incentives and enablers, housing assistance, referral for treatment of substance abuse, and coordination of TB services with those of other providers (Nahid et al., 2016; WHO, *The five elements of DOT*). There is no need to hospitalize a person solely because they are infectious. Outpatients should be instructed to remain at home, without visitors, until they are no longer thought to be infectious. Also, people who are particularly susceptible to developing TB disease if they become infected (small children, immunocompromised people) should not visit or live with an infected client while he or she can transmit the TB bacterium (CDC, *Treatment for TB disease;* Lewinsohn et al., 2017; Nahid et al., 2016).

DIAGNOSTIC AND PUBLIC HEALTH EVALUATION OF TB CONTACTS

By law and regulation, cases of active TB in the United States must be reported to the local health department. Reporting is essential for action by TB control programs at local, state, and national levels. TB case finding is important for understanding the magnitude and the distribution of the disease in the United States. Therefore, reporting of TB suspects promptly (prior to bacteriologic confirmation) is important. Public health services are available for epidemiologic evaluation, including the identification and examination of source cases and contacts (Lewinsohn et al., 2017).

The probability that a person who is exposed to *M. tuberculosis* will become infected depends primarily on the concentration of infectious droplet nuclei in the air and the duration of exposure to a person with infectious TB disease. The closer the proximity and the longer the duration of exposure, the higher the risk of becoming infected. Close contacts are people who share the same air space in a household or other enclosed environment for a prolonged period (days or weeks, not minutes or hours) with a person with pulmonary TB disease. A suspect TB client is a person in whom a diagnosis of TB disease is being considered, whether or not anti-TB treatment has been started. People generally should not continue to be suspected of having TB for more than 3 months (Lewinsohn et al., 2017).

Initial assessment of contacts should be accomplished within 3 days of reported exposure to a person who has active TB disease. During that initial assessment, a history of previous *M. tuberculosis* infection or disease and treatment should be taken along with any current symptoms of TB illness and medical conditions that increase the risk of TB infection. The type, duration, and intensity of exposure should be documented to provide data for high- and medium-priority contact follow-up with diagnostic tests and possible treatment. All high- and medium-priority contacts who do not have a documented previous positive TST or previous TB disease should receive a baseline Mantoux TST. The reaction to the intracutaneously injected TST is the classic example of a delayed (cellular) hypersensitivity reaction, which induces induration. Induration of 5 mm or more is considered a positive result in people who have an initial induration of 0 mm (CDC, *TB testing & diagnosis*). See Figure 15.8 for factors to consider when initiating TB contact investigation (CDC, 2005b).

Some people infected with *M. tuberculosis* may have a negative reaction to the TST if many years have passed since they became infected. They may have a positive reaction to a subsequent TST because the initial test stimulates their ability to react to the test. This is commonly referred to as the "booster phenomenon" and may incorrectly be interpreted as a skin test conversion (going from negative to positive). For this reason, the "two-step method" is recommended at the time of initial testing for individuals who may be tested periodically (e.g., healthcare workers). If the first TST result in the two-step baseline testing is positive, consider the person infected and evaluate and treat the person accordingly. If the first test result is negative, the TST should be repeated in 1 to 3 weeks. If the second test result is positive, consider the person infected and evaluate and treat the person accordingly; if both steps are negative, consider the person uninfected and classify the TST as negative at baseline testing (Fig. 15.9). Note: When Interferon–Gamma Release Assays (IGRAs) are used for serial testing, there is no need for a second test because boosting does not occur (CDC, *Latent tuberculosis infection: A guide for primary healthcare providers*).

Practice Point

Nurses in health departments and in community and public health settings may be responsible for conducting TB contact investigations. By taking a careful contact history, nurses are able to determine which contacts are at greatest risk for TB exposure. Nurses also administer a TST during evaluation of exposure. Reliable administration and reading of the TST requires standardization of procedures, training, supervision, and practice.

Questions often arise about the interpretation of TST results in people with a history of bacillus

FIGURE 15.8 Decision-making factors when initiating a tuberculosis (TB) contact investigation. AFB, acid-fast bacilli; CXR, chest radiograph; NAA, nucleic acid assay. Approved indication for NAA. (From Centers for Disease Control and Prevention [CDC]. [2005b]. Guidelines for the investigation of contacts of persons with infectious tuberculosis. *Morbidity and Mortality Weekly Report, 54*[RR15], 1–37.)

Calmette–Guérin (BCG) vaccine, HIV infection, and recent contacts with an infectious case of TB. History of BCG vaccine administration is not a contraindication for tuberculin testing. If more than 5 years have elapsed since administration of BCG vaccine, a positive tuberculin test reaction is most likely a result of *M. tuberculosis* infection (CDC, *Tuberculosis*).

TB DIAGNOSTIC TESTS

The majority of experience with diagnosing *M. tuberculosis* infection, primarily in contacts, has been with the Mantoux TST. In 2005, the CDC issued guidelines for using the FDA-approved QuantiFERON-Gold (QFT-G) test for diagnosing *M. tuberculosis* infection, including both active TB disease and latent TB infection. The 2005 guidelines indicated that QFT-G may be used in all circumstances in which a TST test was recommended, including contact investigations, evaluation of recent immigrants, and serial-testing surveillance programs for infection control (e.g., those for healthcare workers). However, the guidelines provided cautions for testing persons from selected populations, including persons

at increased risk for progression to active disease if infected (CDC, 2005b).

Two new interferon gamma (IFN-γ) release assays (IGRAs) were later approved by the Food and Drug Administration (FDA) as aids in diagnosing *M. tuberculosis infection*, both latent infection and infection manifesting as active tuberculosis. These tests are the QuantiFERON-TB Gold In-Tube test (QFT-GIT) (Cellestis Limited, Carnegie, Victoria, Australia) and the T-SPOT TB test (T-Spot) (Oxford Immunotec Limited, Abingdon, United Kingdom). The antigens, methods, and interpretation criteria for these assays differ from those for IGRAs approved previously by FDA. Control materials and antigens for QFT-GIT and T-Spot are contained in special tubes used to collect blood for the test, thus allowing more direct testing of fresh blood. Both tests are approved as indirect tests for *M. tuberculosis* infection (including infection resulting in active disease) when used in conjunction with risk assessment, radiography, and other medical and diagnostic evaluations. The FDA-approved indications for QFT-GIT and T-Spot are similar to indications for QFT-G and TST. Because of administrative and logistic difficulties associated with the TST skin test, IGRAs

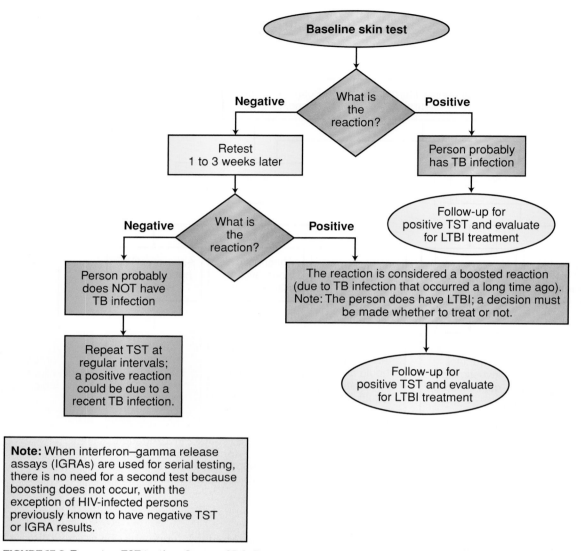

FIGURE 15.9 Two-step TST testing. *Source:* CDC. Two-step TST testing. *In Latent Tuberculosis Infection: A Guide for Primary Health Care Providers.* Retrieved from https://www.cdc.gov/tb/publications/ltbi/diagnosis.htm.

are attractive diagnostic aids for detecting *M. tuberculosis* infection. Unlike the TST, IGRA results can be available within 24 hours without the need for a second visit. As laboratory-based assays, IGRAs are not subject to the biases and errors associated with TST placement and reading. However, the cost for an IGRA is substantially greater than that for a TST. Nonetheless, this additional cost might be offset by decreasing the number of persons testing positive and the associated costs of evaluating and treating persons with positive test results. Because of these new IGRAs, the CDC updated the 2005 guidelines to include these new IGRAs in 2010, which state that TSTs and IGRAs (QFT-G, QFT-GIT, and T-Spot) should be used as aids in diagnosing infection with *M. tuberculosis*. These tests may be used for surveillance purposes or to identify persons likely to benefit from treatment, including persons who are or will be at increased risk for *M. tuberculosis* infection or for progression to active tuberculosis if infected (CDC, 2010).

In 2017, the CDC, the American Academy of Pediatrics, the American Thoracic Society, and the Infectious Disease Society of America coordinated development of updated guidelines for using IFN-γ assays for U.S. public health officials, healthcare providers, and laboratory workers to detect TB infection. They recommend performing an interferon-γ release assay (IGRA) rather than a TST in individuals 5 years or older who meet the following criteria: (1) are likely to be infected with *M. tuberculosis*, (2) have a low or intermediate risk of disease progression, (3) it has been decided that testing for LTBI is warranted, and (4) either have a history of BCG vaccination or are unlikely to return to have their TST read. However, a TST is an acceptable alternative, especially in situations where an IGRA is not available, too costly, or too burdensome. They suggest performing a TST rather than an IGRA in healthy children less than 5 years of age for whom it has been decided that diagnostic testing for LTBI is warranted. However, in situations in which an IGRA is deemed the preferred diagnostic test, some experts are willing to use IGRAs in children over 3 years of age.

While both IGRA and TST testing provide evidence for infection with *M. tuberculosis*, they cannot distinguish active from latent TB. Therefore, the diagnosis of active TB must be excluded prior to embarking on treatment for LTBI. This is typically done by determining whether or not symptoms suggestive of TB disease are present, performing a chest radiograph and, if radiographic signs of active TB (e.g., airspace opacities, pleural effusions, cavities, or changes on serial radiographs) are seen, then sampling is performed and the patient managed accordingly. They also recommend that acid-fast bacilli (AFB) smear microscopy be performed, and performing a diagnostic nucleic acid amplification test (NAAT), on the initial respiratory specimen from patients suspected of having pulmonary TB (Lewinsohn et al., 2017).

Generally, persons at high risk for developing TB disease fall into two categories:

- Persons who have been recently infected with TB bacteria
- Persons with medical conditions that weaken the immune system

Persons who have been recently infected with TB bacteria include:

- Close contacts of a person with infectious TB disease
- Persons who have emigrated from areas of the world with high rates of TB
- Children <5 years of age who have a positive TB test
- Groups with high rates of TB transmission, such as homeless persons, injection drug users, and persons with HIV infection
- Persons who work or reside with people who are at high risk for TB in facilities or institutions such as hospitals, homeless shelters, correctional facilities, nursing homes, and residential homes for those with HIV
- Persons with medical conditions that weaken the immune system (including babies and young children who often have weak immune systems).

Other people also can have weak immune systems, especially people with any of these conditions:

- HIV infection (the virus that causes AIDS)
- Substance abuse (including alcohol)
- Silicosis
- Diabetes mellitus
- Severe kidney disease
- Low body weight
- Organ transplants
- Head and neck cancer
- Medical treatments such as corticosteroids or organ transplant
- Specialized treatment for rheumatoid arthritis or Crohn disease (CDC, *TB risk factors*).

Case 2: The subsequent investigation in the Illinois TB outbreak found that all patients were homeless and had been overnight shelter guests. Excess alcohol use was common (82%), and two bars emerged as additional sites of potential transmission. Patients with outbreak-associated TB were treated successfully for TB disease.

- What screening measures would public health officials have used in this case?
- What were the risk factors in this case?

Practice Point

Best-practice nursing interventions must be tied into the role of community and public health nurses in the care and supportive aspects of TB case management. The American Thoracic Society, the CDC, and the Infectious Diseases Society of America support client-centered case management with an emphasis on evidence-based DOT options.

Multidrug-Resistant TB

Although effective drugs exist, a major reason for the failure to stem the spread of TB lies in the rise of drug-resistant strains of *M. tuberculosis*. Some strains are resistant to several drugs. MDR-TB is defined as resistance to the two most potent "first-line" anti-TB agents. MDR-TB is difficult and expensive to treat and fails to respond to the two most potent anti-TB agents (INH and RIF). In addition, extensively drug-resistant TB (XDR-TB), another emerging threat, is a rare type of MDR-TB that is resistant to the first-line TB drugs, plus resistance to any fluoroquinolone and at least one of three injectable second-line drugs (CDC, *Tuberculosis fact sheets*).

Globally in 2015, there were an estimated 480,000 new cases of MDR-TB and an additional 100,000 people with RR-TB who were also newly eligible for MDR-TB treatment. Drug resistance surveillance data show that 3.9% of new and 21% of previously treated TB cases were estimated to have had MDR/RR-TB in 2015. As in 2014, MDR-TB accounted for 3.3% of new TB cases. MDR/RR-TB caused 250,000 deaths in 2015. Most cases and deaths occurred in Asia. About 9.5% of MDR-TB cases had additional drug-resistance, XDR-TB. To date, 117 countries worldwide have reported at least one XDR-TB case (WHO [2016b], *MDR-TB 2016 update*).

In contrast to the 2011 WHO recommendations, the current WHO treatment guidelines for drug-resistant tuberculosis 2016 update did not update the policy on the use of rapid diagnostics for RR-TB, the monitoring of response to treatment, the duration of longer MDR-TB regimens, the delay in starting antiretroviral therapy in MDR-TB patients with HIV infection and models of care. For these aspects of the programmatic management of drug-resistant TB, the 2011 guidelines for the programmatic management of drug-resistant tuberculosis (WHO, 2011) continue to apply until future evidence shows a need for revision.

The main changes in the 2016 WHO recommendations are as follows:

- A shorter MDR-TB treatment regimen is recommended under specific conditions.
- Medicines used in the design of longer MDR-TB treatment regimens are now regrouped differently based upon current evidence on their effectiveness and safety. Clofazimine and linezolid are now recommended as core second-line medicines in the MDR-TB regimen while p-aminosalicylic acid is an add-on agent.
- MDR-TB treatment is recommended for all patients with RR-TB, regardless of confirmation of isoniazid resistance.
- Specific recommendations are made on the treatment of children with RR-TB or MDR-TB.
- Clarithromycin and other macrolides are no longer included among the medicines to be used for the treatment of MDR/RR-TB.
- Evidence-informed recommendations on the role of surgery are now included. Bedaquiline and delamanid have now been assigned to a specific subgroup of add-on agents. In October 2016, the WHO published its new policy on delamanid. Delamanid may now also be used alongside longer MDR-TB regimens in patients aged 6 to 17 years. Bedaquiline is still only recommended for adults (WHO, 2016b).

More information on the changes in the 2016 MDR-TB recommendations can be found at WHO treatment guidelines for drug-resistant tuberculosis: http://www.who.int/tb/areas-of-work/drug-resistant-tb/treatment/resources/en/

In **Case 2**, the average length of stay at the homeless shelter for guests was 2 weeks. During contact investigations and four mass screenings at the shelter during May 2010 to June 2011, public health officials evaluated 386 persons recently exposed to a person with an infectious outbreak case, finding six (2%) additional TB cases. As of September 2011, a total of 28 outbreak-associated cases involving shelter guests, dating back to 2007, had been recognized, indicating ongoing M. tuberculosis transmission among guests at the homeless shelter.

- To prevent future cases of TB, what treatment program should public health officials have implemented in this high-risk population?

TB Infection Control Guidelines for Healthcare Settings

The CDC updated the TB infection control guidelines for healthcare settings in 2005 (CDC, 2005c). These recommendations reflect shifts in the epidemiology of TB, advances in scientific understanding, and changes in healthcare practice that have occurred in the United States during the preceding decade. The updated TB infection control guidelines emphasize actions to maintain momentum and expertise needed to avert another TB resurgence and to eliminate the lingering threat to healthcare personnel, which is mainly from clients or others with unsuspected and undiagnosed infectious TB disease. A sample recommendation is that the term "tuberculin skin tests" (TST) be used rather than "PPD." The scope of settings in which the guidelines apply has been broadened to include laboratories and additional outpatient and nontraditional healthcare settings.

These recommendations also apply to an entire healthcare setting rather than to areas within a setting. New terms such as "airborne infection precautions" (airborne precautions) and "airborne infection isolation (AII) room" have been introduced. One of the most critical risks for healthcare-associated transmission of *M. tuberculosis* in healthcare settings is from clients with unrecognized TB disease who are not promptly handled with appropriate airborne precautions or who are moved out of an AII room too soon (e.g., clients with unrecognized TB and MDR-TB). The CDC *Guidelines for Preventing the Transmission of Mycobacterium tuberculosis in Health-Care Settings* can be found at http://www.cdc.gov/mmwr/PDF/rr/rr5417.pdf

Ebola Virus Disease

Ebola first appeared in 1976 during two simultaneous outbreaks in Nzara, Sudan, and in Yambuku, Democratic Republic of Congo. It was named from the Ebola River, which is located in Yambuku. The Ebola virus is a member of the *Filoviridae* family (filovirus), and has five distinct species:

- *Bundibugyo ebolavirus* (BDBV)
- *Reston ebolavirus* (RESTV)
- *Sudan ebolavirus* (SUDV)
- *Taï Forest ebolavirus* (TAFV)
- *Zaire ebolavirus* (EBOV) (WHO, *Ebola virus disease*)

Ebola virus disease (EVD), previously called Ebola hemorrhagic fever, is a severe, often fatal illness with a reported case fatality rate as high as 100%. The virus can be brought into human populations through close contact with blood, secretions, or other body fluids and organs of infected animals such as chimpanzees, gorillas, fruit bats, monkeys, forest antelope, and porcupines. It can be spread from person-to-person through direct contact (through broken skin or mucous membranes) with blood, secretions, excretions, or other body fluids of an infected person. Ebola virus has been found in semen up to 61 days. The virus can also be spread by indirect contact through medical equipment and the contaminated environment in contact with these fluids. Large outbreaks of EVD in Africa have been associated with BDVD, BDBV, EBOV, and SUDV since 1976, but not RESTV and TAFV. Although RESTV has been reported in China and the Philippines, it has not caused illness or death in humans to date (WHO, *Ebola virus disease*).

Large outbreaks of EVD have been reported in Africa since 1976. The last reported outbreak of EVD had occurred in the Democratic Republic of Congo in 2012. However, in the spring of 2014, an outbreak of EVD was reported in the forested areas of southeast Guinea and quickly spread to several districts. This was the first time EVD had been detected in West Africa. Confirmed cases were reported in Guinea, Liberia, and Sierra Leone. The WHO confirmed that this outbreak was caused by the Zaire ebolavirus (EBOV). The Ebola virus had been introduced into Nigeria in July 2014 by a Liberian traveler, resulting in a total of 20 cases and eight deaths. But by late October 2014, WHO had declared that Nigeria was free of Ebola virus transmission (WHO [2014b], *Nigeria ends Ebola*).

However, intense transmission of the Ebola virus continued in Guinea, Liberia, and Sierra Leone. And by the spring of 2016, the total number of reported cases of EVD in the four West African countries (Guinea, Liberia, Sierra Leone, and Nigeria) was 28,652. Of these, 15,261 were laboratory-confirmed cases; total deaths were 11,325 (case fatality rate: 39.5%), making it the worst EVD outbreak in history. Most of the later cases reported had occurred in Guinea, Liberia, and Sierra Leone, with Liberia reporting the highest death rate at 45% (CDC, *2014–2016 Ebola outbreak in West Africa*). A small number of cases of Ebola infection had been reported in the Democratic Republic of the Congo, but was not related to the ongoing outbreaks in Guinea, Liberia, and Sierra Leone (CDC, *Ebola in Democratic Republic of the Congo*).

The first imported case of Ebola infection in the United States occurred in Dallas, Texas, in September 2014 in a man who had traveled from Liberia. Two healthcare providers who had cared for that patient, who died, became ill with the Ebola virus and have since recovered. A third U.S. case of Ebola infection occurred in October 2014 in a doctor who had worked treating Ebola patients with Doctors without Borders in Guinea. He was hospitalized in New York City, and has recovered (CDC [2014b], *Cases of Ebola diagnosed in the United States*).

Although the Ebola virus posed little to no risk to the U.S. general population, in July 2014, the CDC issued a level 3 travel alert (Avoid Nonessential Travel) for Sierra Leone, Guinea, and Liberia and reminded all healthcare providers to take a good travel history to identify patients who had traveled to/from West Africa (CDC, *Travel Health Notices*, 31 July 2014).

Postarrival monitoring by state and local public health departments was an additional safeguard to exit screening of all travelers for 21 days from the date of their departure from the affected countries.

In May 2017, the WHO was notified by the Ministry of Public Health of the Democratic Republic of the Congo (DRC) of a cluster of undiagnosed illnesses and deaths with signs of EVD in the Likati Health Zone, a remote area that shares borders with the Central African Republic and two other provinces of the DRC. Cases of the disease were reported in four health districts. This was the DRC's eighth outbreak of EVD since the discovery of the virus in the country in 1976. By July 2017, WHO had declared the end of this most recent outbreak. The announcement came 42 days (two 21-day incubation cycles of the virus) after the last case of EVD. Eight cases of EVD were identified during the outbreak, with five cases laboratory-confirmed; four people died. A total of 583 contacts were closely monitored, but no known contacts developed signs or symptoms of EVD. Enhanced surveillance in the country continued, as well as strengthening of preparedness and readiness for Ebola outbreaks (WHO [2017], *Declaration of the end of Ebola virus disease outbreak in the Democratic Republic of the Congo*, 2 July 2017).

Less than a year later, in May 2018, the Ministry of Health of the DRC declared an outbreak of EVD in the Bikoro Health Zone, Equateur Province, which is 250 km from Mbandaka, the capital of Equateur Province, in an area of the country that is very hard to reach. Ebola had spread to Mabalako, a city with more than 1 million people by June 2018. This was the ninth outbreak of EVD over the last four decades in the DRC, with the eighth outbreak occurring in May 2017. The risk of more rapid spread was likely given that EVD had been found in the large urban area of Mabalako, which is right on the Congo River. With the city's location on the river along with its road and air links, the confirmation of Ebola cases there increases the risk of both local propagation and further spread within the DRC and to neighboring countries. At the time of this latest outbreak, the WHO assumed that 100 to 300 cases of EVD could occur in the DRC by July 2018 (WHO [2018e], *Strategic response plan for the Ebola virus disease outbreak, Democratic Republic of the Congo*).

By August 2018, the Ministry of Health of the DRC declared the second outbreak of EVD in the country that year in North Kivu Province, less than 2 weeks since the previous outbreak, in nearby Equateur province, was declared over (UNICEF, *The Government of the Democratic Republic of the Congo announced the end of the Ebola epidemic in the Equateur Province on 25 July 2018*). North Kivu, in the eastern part of the country, is among the most populated provinces in the country, shares borders with Uganda and Rwanda, and experiences conflict and insecurity, with over one million internally displaced people and migration of refugees to neighboring countries. By Mid-December 2018, WHO epidemiological data on EVD in the

DRC, indicated that since the beginning of the epidemic, the cumulative number of cases was 529, with 481 confirmed and 48 probable cases. In total, there have been 311 deaths (263 confirmed and 48 probable), with a case-fatality rate of 59%, and 183 patients had recovered. An increase in the case fatality rate may rise as long as the risk of the outbreak spreading to other provinces in the Democratic Republic of the Congo. This possibility remains very high as long as unrest prevents healthcare workers to identify cases and contacts (International Society for Infectious Diseases, December 15, 2018). Cumulatively, since June 2018, 19 health workers had been affected (18 confirmed and one probable), three of whom have died. All health workers' exposures occurred in health facilities outside the dedicated Ebola treatment centers (WHO, *Ebola virus disease, DRC External Report 7*). The WHO and partners continued to work with health workers and communities to increase awareness on infection prevention and control measures, as well as vaccinate those at risk of infection (WHO, *Ebola virus disease*: Democratic Republic of the Congo. 3 August 2018).

The current Ebola outbreak in the DRC demonstrates the infectious disease risks posed by globalization and rapid travel. In previous outbreaks in the DRC, the virus was confined to villages and small towns so remote that infected humans didn't travel far enough to spread the disease. Case finding had been difficult due to community resistance. Some families were concealing potential or probable Ebola cases among them. Even after some probable cases had been identified at home, their families were refusing to allow the affected family member to be quarantined and cared for in the Ebola treatment centers. Other contacts were refusing vaccination (International Society for Infectious Diseases, Ebola update (82), *ProMED Mail*, September 5, 2018).

Several weeks after the second outbreak occurred in the DRC, there were still significant threats for further spread of the disease. The Ebola outbreak in North Kivu and Ituri provinces remained active, but continued to be closely monitored, with the Ministry of Health, WHO and partners making progress in response to the outbreak. Current reports indicated that control measures were working. However, additional risks remained following the movement of several cases from Beni and Mabalako to other health zones. Continued challenges included contacts lost to follow-up, delayed recognition of EVD in health centers, poor infection control in health centers, and cases leaving health centers and refusing transfer to Ebola treatment centers (International Society for Infectious Diseases, Ebola update (93). *ProMED Mail*, September 20, 2018).

At the same time, attacks by armed rebels continued in Beni territory, following a clash between the Congolese army and the Ugandan Islamist rebels of the Allied Democratic Forces, resulting in the deaths of two Sudanese UN peacekeepers on September 3, 2018 (International Society for Infectious Diseases, Ebola update (82). *ProMED Mail*, September 5, 2018. Retrieved on September 21, 2018, from http://www.promedmail.org). Field activities were suspended in Beni in late September 2018, following clashes between rebels and the Congolese armed forces, but were to continue when calm returned to the city (International Society for Infectious Diseases, Ebola update (96). *ProMED Mail*, September 24, 2018).

Although there had been no declared travel ban to the Democratic Republic of the Congo by the WHO, and the Ebola virus posed little to no risk to the United States, the CDC reminded all healthcare providers to (1) take a good travel history to identify patients who traveled to/from affected area in the past 3 weeks, (2) know the signs and symptoms of EVD, and (3) follow infection control precautions for suspected and symptomatic cases of EVD to prevent the spread of the Ebola virus (CDC, *Travel Health Notices*).

Signs, Symptoms, and Diagnosis of EVD

EVD has an incubation period from 2 to 21 days, but the average is 8 to 10 days. Early symptoms include sudden onset of fever, muscle pain and weakness, headache, and sore throat. These symptoms are followed by vomiting, diarrhea, rash, compromised liver and kidney function, and in some cases, internal and external bleeding (CDC, *EVD* signs and symptom*s*). Before the diagnosis of EVD is made, other diseases should be ruled out, such as malaria, influenza, and typhoid fever, since these diseases may have similar signs and symptoms. Laboratory tests for a definitive diagnosis of EVD include ELISA, antigen detection tests, PCR assay, and culture isolation of the virus (CDC, *EVD diagnosis*). Studies have shown that the Ebola virus remains in semen for longer than 2 years after recovery from EVD (Fischer et al., 2017).

Prevention and Control of EVD

There is currently no vaccine against EVD; however, results of Phase I clinical trials for two vaccine candidates, developed by GlaxoSmithKline (GSK) in collaboration with the U.S. National Institute of Allergy and Infectious Diseases (NIAID), and by NewLink Genetics and Merck Vaccines USA in collaboration with the Public Health Agency of Canada, were published in 2016. Both vaccine candidates have been shown to be safe and well tolerated in humans (Agnandji et al., 2016).

Despite there being no licensed vaccine against EVD, vaccination played an integral part in the response to the 2018 Ebola outbreak in the DRC. The WHO Strategic Advisory Group of Experts on Immunization recommended in April 2017 that the Ebola vaccine be promptly deployed under the Expanded Access framework, with informed consent and in compliance with "Good Clinical Practice," if an Ebola disease outbreak occurred before the candidate vaccine was licensed. The WHO sent vaccine developed by

Merck to the DRC. Two key international actors, Doctors without Borders and the WHO, tested an Ebola vaccine during the current outbreak in DRC, in collaboration with the ministry of health. The DRC has had, as well as controlled, multiple Ebola outbreaks. The country has experienced public health teams and has had excellent collaborations with Médecins Sans Frontières (MSF) and other international organizations for many years. Fortunately, the Ministry of Health, Doctors without Borders, and the Epicenter team started preparing for such an effort before the last DRC epidemic in 2017. Because it is impossible to conduct a randomized placebo-controlled trial, Doctors Without Borders ran an open-label, single-group study to provide additional information on the vaccine's safety and effectiveness. All participants who consented to take part were included, and followed for at least 42 days (twice what is often considered to be the maximum incubation period of EVD. The plan was to start as soon as possible after the teams were on the ground in the DRC. The WHO teams started using the Ebola vaccine in the DRC in May 2018, with healthcare personnel operating in affected areas of the Ebola outbreak to be the first to be vaccinated (Haug et al., 2018).

In addition to the vaccine developed by Merck, the National Institute of Allergy and Infectious Diseases shipped 100 doses of an experimental Ebola virus treatment to the DRC, filling a request from health officials there to use the treatment in a clinical trial during the current outbreak. According to NIAID Director, Dr. Anthony Fauci, "That's not unusual in an emergency situation. If they use it in a trial or under compassionate use, informed consent would have to make it very clear that it hasn't completed a phase 1 trial" (Healio, *Infectious Disease News*, May 25, 2018).

As of mid-September 2018, 58 vaccination rings (as used in the Phase 3 study in Guinea, but randomization was discontinued), plus 24 rings of health and frontline workers had been defined. By December 15, 2018, 46,887 people had been vaccinated, including healthcare and frontline workers, and children (International Society for Infectious Diseases. Ebola update, December 15, 2018). There was one area in Ndindi where the implementation of vaccination was hampered due to community resistance (WHO, *Ebola virus disease, DRC External Report 7*).

In the absence of a licensed human vaccine and lack of effective treatment for EVD, the CDC has outlined epidemiologic risk factors, ranging from "High Risk" to "No Identifiable Risk," that should be considered when evaluating a person for EVD, classifying contacts, or considering public health actions such as monitoring and movement restrictions based on exposure. For example, use of standard contact and droplet precautions and other infection control measures in healthcare settings to prevent exposure to blood and body fluids and the potentially contaminated environment when caring for patients with suspected or confirmed EVD. It should be noted that Ebola virus can be detected in semen for months after recovery from the disease. Unprotected contact with the semen of a person who has recently recovered from Ebola may constitute a potential risk for exposure (CDC, *Epidemiologic risk factors to consider when evaluating a person for exposure to Ebola virus*).

Travelers to or are in an area affected by an Ebola outbreak, should be aware of the following:

- Practice careful hygiene. For example, wash your hands with soap and water or an alcohol-based hand sanitizer and avoid contact with blood and body fluids (such as urine, feces, saliva, sweat, urine, vomit, breast milk, semen, and vaginal fluids).
- Do not handle items that may have come in contact with an infected person's blood or body fluids (such as clothes, bedding, needles, and medical equipment).
- Avoid funeral or burial rituals that require handling the body of someone who has died from Ebola.
- Avoid contact with bats and nonhuman primates or blood, fluids and raw meat prepared from these animals (bushmeat) or meat from an unknown source.
- Avoid contact with semen from a man who had EVD until you know the virus is gone from the semen.
- Avoid facilities where Ebola patients are being treated.

These same prevention methods apply when living in or traveling to an area affected by an Ebola outbreak. After returning from an area affected by Ebola, monitor health for 21 days and seek medical care immediately if you develop symptoms of EVD (CDC, *Travel Health. Ebola in Democratic Republic of the Congo*. [Updated September 14, 2018]).

In 2015, the CDC published *Infection Prevention and Control Recommendations for Hospitalized Patients under Investigation (PUIs) for Ebola Virus Disease in U.S. Hospitals*. For historical and informational purposes, these recommendations are available at https://www.cdc.gov/vhf/ebola/healthcare-us/hospitals/infection-control.html (Last reviewed: August 30, 2018).

Zika Virus Disease

Zika is caused by the Zika virus, which is transmitted primarily through a bite from an infected vector, the Aedes species mosquito (*Aedes aegypti* and *Aedes albopictus*). Zika virus also can be transmitted through sexual contact and possible blood transfusion; however, the virus remains in semen longer than in blood. Several cases of sexually transmitted Zika infections have been reported.

The Zika virus was first discovered in 1947 and its name came from the Zika Forest in Uganda. In 1952, the first human cases of Zika were detected and since then, outbreaks of Zika have been reported in tropical Africa, Southeast Asia, and the Pacific Islands. Zika virus emerged in the

Region of the Americas on Easter Island, Chile, in 2014 and in northeast Brazil in 2015. In May 2015 in response, to the Zika outbreak, the Pan American Health Organization (PAHO), which serves as the Regional Office of the Americas for the WHO, issued recommendations to enhance surveillance for Zika virus. Subsequently, Brazilian investigators reported Guillain–Barré syndrome, which had been previously recognized among some patients with Zika virus disease, and identified an association between Zika virus infection during pregnancy and congenital microcephaly (CDC, *Zika virus*).

In February 2016, the WHO declared Zika virus–related microcephaly clusters and other neurologic disorders a Public Health Emergency of International Concern. In March 2016, PAHO developed case definitions and surveillance guidance for Zika virus disease and associated complications. Analysis of reports submitted to PAHO by countries in the region or published in national epidemiologic bulletins revealed that Zika virus transmission had extended to 48 countries and territories in the Region of the Americas by late 2016. Reported Zika virus disease cases peaked at different times in different areas during 2016. Because of ongoing transmission and the risk for recurrence of large outbreaks, response efforts, including surveillance for Zika virus disease and its complications, and vector control and other prevention activities, needs to be maintained (CDC [2017c] Zika virus transmission—Region of the Americas). In March 2016, the WHO updated its travel recommendations to advise pregnant women not to travel to areas with ongoing Zika virus outbreaks.

By the fall of 2016, 73 countries and territories had reported evidence of mosquito-borne Zika virus transmission to the WHO. Twelve countries, including the United States had reported evidence of person-to-person transmission of Zika virus, and 23 countries or territories reported microcephaly and other CNS malformations potentially associated with Zika virus infection, or suggestive of congenital infection. Most of these cases were from Brazil at 2,063 (WHO, *Situation report, Zika virus*, October 27, 2016). By March 2017, the overall global risk assessment had not changed. Zika virus continued to spread geographically to areas where competent vectors are present. Eighty-four countries, territories, or subnational areas were reporting evidence of vector-borne Zika virus transmission, with additional cases of microcephaly and other CNS malformations being reported. Although a decline in cases of Zika virus infection had been reported in some countries, or in some parts of countries, vigilance remained high (WHO, *Situation report, Zika virus*, March 10, 2017).

Although Zika was not a nationally notifiable disease in the United States in 2015, cases could be reported to ArboNET, the national surveillance system for arthropod-borne diseases. There were 61 symptomatic Zika virus disease cases reported in 2015 from travelers returning from affected areas. There were no cases acquired through presumed local mosquito-borne transmission, and no cases acquired through other routes (e.g., sexual, laboratory, or blood borne transmission). In 2015, the U.S. territories, reported nine symptomatic Zika virus disease cases, with one case in a traveler returning from an affected area, eight cases acquired through presumed local mosquito-borne transmission, and no cases acquired through other routes (CDC, *Cumulative Zika virus disease case counts in the United States, 2015–2017*). In 2016, Zika virus disease became a nationally notifiable condition. Cases are reported to CDC by state, territorial, and local health departments using standard case definitions. In February 2016, the United States reported two sexually transmitted cases of Zika virus. That year, there were 5,102 symptomatic Zika virus disease cases reported. Of these, 4,830 cases were in travelers returning from affected areas, 224 cases acquired Zika virus through presumed local mosquito-borne transmission in Florida ($n = 218$) and Texas ($n = 6$), and 48 cases were acquired through other routes, including sexual transmission ($n = 46$). Thirty-seven (80%) of these latter cases were from presumptive viremic blood donors. One case of Zika virus disease occurred through laboratory transmission, and one person-to-person case was through an unknown route. Most of the cases occurred in Florida ($n = 1,115$), New York ($n = 1,001$), and California ($n = 421$). In the U.S. territories, there were 36,079 symptomatic Zika virus disease cases reported in 2016, with 142 cases in travelers returning from affected areas, 35,937 cases acquired through presumed local mosquito-borne transmission. Almost (97%) of the cases occurred in Puerto Rico ($n = 34,963$), 322 of the cases were from presumptive viremic blood donors (CDC, *Cumulative Zika virus disease case counts in the United States*, 2015–2017).

By September 2017, the CDC reported a decline in the number of Zika virus cases in the United States at 231 symptomatic Zika virus disease cases reported, with 229 cases in travelers returning from Zika-affected areas, no cases acquired through presumed local mosquito-borne transmission, and two cases acquired through sexual transmission, and nine cases were from presumptive viremic blood donors. Most of the cases were in New York ($n = 44$), Florida ($n = 31$), California ($n = 25$), and Texas ($n = 22$). In the U.S. territories, there were 554 symptomatic Zika virus disease cases reported, 554 cases acquired through presumed local mosquito-borne transmission, and no cases in travelers returning from affected areas; however, three cases were from presumptive viremic blood donors were identified in Puerto Rico. Again, Puerto Rico reported the most cases at 474 (CDC, *Cumulative Zika virus disease case counts in the United States, 2015–2017*).

None of the 2015–2017 Zika virus disease cases reported above included congenital Zika disease cases. Pregnant women and infants who meet the following criteria are eligible for the U.S. Zika Pregnancy Registry: Pregnant women in the United States with laboratory evidence of Zika virus infection (positive or equivocal test results, regardless of whether they have symptoms) and periconceptionally, prenatally, or perinatally exposed infants born to these women. Infants with laboratory evidence of congenital Zika virus infection (positive or equivocal test results, regardless of whether they have symptoms) and their mothers are eligible for the U.S. Zika Pregnancy Registry. As of August 2017, there were 1,862 completed pregnancies with or without birth defects in the Zika Registry. Of these there were 95 live-born infants with birth defects, and eight pregnancy losses with birth defects. In the U.S. territories, there were 3,258 completed pregnancies with or without birth defects, 132 live-born infants with birth defects, and seven pregnancy losses with birth defects. The data collected through the Zika pregnancy and infant registries are used to update recommendations for clinical care, to plan for services and support for pregnant women and families affected by Zika virus, and to improve prevention of Zika virus infection during pregnancy (CDC, *Outcomes of pregnancies with laboratory evidence of possible Zika virus infection in the United States*).

Signs, Symptoms, and Diagnosis of Zika Disease

Many people infected with Zika virus won't have symptoms or will only have mild symptoms. The most common symptoms of Zika are:

- Fever
- Rash
- Headache
- Joint pain
- Red eyes
- Muscle pain

Symptoms can last for several days to a week. People usually don't get sick enough to go to the hospital, and they very rarely die of Zika. Once a person has been infected with Zika, they are likely to be protected from future infections (CDC, *Zika overview*).

Prevention and Control of Zika Disease

In July 2017, CDC issued updated interim guidance for healthcare providers caring for pregnant women with possible Zika virus exposure (CDC [2017b], Update: Interim guidance for healthcare providers caring for pregnant women with possible Zika virus exposure—United States [including U.S. territories]). However, CDC is continually updating this information. Because Zika infection during pregnancy can cause severe birth defects, pregnant women should not travel to the areas where the Zika virus is circulating. The CDC has provided areas identified as Alert Level 2 (Practice Enhanced Precautions). For a list of all Zika virus travel notices for travelers to international destinations, U.S. territories, and within the United States, see Zika travel information at https://www.cdc.gov/zika/geo/index.html

As of February 2018, the WHO Classification scheme for travelers included four categories of Zika virus transmission, which are defined as follows:

- Category 1. Area with new introduction or re-introduction with ongoing transmission
- Category 2. Area either with evidence of virus circulation before 2015 or area with ongoing transmission that is no longer in the new or re-introduction phase, but where there is no evidence of interruption
- Category 3. Area with interrupted transmission and with potential for future transmission
- Category 4. Area with established competent vector but no known documented past or current transmission. For the latest (February 2018) country category status update, see WHO. Zika virus classification at: http://apps.who.int/iris/bitstream/handle/10665/260419/zika-lassification-15Feb18-eng.pdf?sequence=1.

More than 40 Zika vaccine candidates are in the pipeline and five are entering Phase I trials, where the vaccine's safety and ability to produce an immune response will be evaluated. In the meantime, the best way to prevent diseases spread by mosquitoes is to be protected from mosquito bites:

- Use Environmental Protection Agency (EPA)-registered insect repellants.
- Wear long-sleeved shirts and long pants when outdoors.
- Sleep under a mosquito bed net if air conditioned or screened rooms are not available or if sleeping outdoors.
- Prevent sexual transmission of Zika by using condoms or not having sex (CDC, *Zika overview*).

Evidence for Practice

The diagnosis of Zika is based on a person's recent travel history, symptoms, and test results.

A blood or urine test can confirm a Zika infection. The CDC has updated the interim guidance for U.S. healthcare providers caring for pregnant women with possible Zika virus exposure. As the prevalence of Zika virus disease declines, the likelihood of false-positive test results increases. In addition, emerging epidemiologic and laboratory data indicate that Zika virus IgM antibodies can persist beyond 12 weeks after infection. Therefore, IgM test results cannot always reliably distinguish between an infection that occurred during the current pregnancy and one that occurred before the current pregnancy, particularly for women with possible Zika virus exposure before the current pregnancy. These limitations should be considered when counseling pregnant women about the risks and benefits of testing for Zika virus infection during pregnancy.

Key recommendations include the following:

1. All pregnant women in the United States and U.S. territories should be asked about possible Zika virus exposure before and during the current pregnancy, at every prenatal care visit. CDC recommends that pregnant women not travel to any area with risk for Zika virus transmission. It is also recommended that pregnant women with a sex partner who has traveled to or lives in an area with risk for Zika virus transmission use condoms or abstain from sex for the duration of the pregnancy.
2. Pregnant women with recent possible Zika virus exposure and symptoms of Zika virus disease should be tested to diagnose the cause of their symptoms. The updated recommendations include concurrent Zika virus nucleic acid test (NAT) and serologic testing as soon as possible through 12 weeks after symptom onset.
3. Asymptomatic pregnant women with ongoing possible Zika virus exposure should be offered Zika virus NAT testing three times during pregnancy: at the initiation of prenatal care, and if Zika virus RNA is not detected on clinical specimens, two additional tests should be offered during the course of the pregnancy coinciding with prenatal visits.
4. Pregnant women who have recent possible Zika virus exposure and who have a fetus with prenatal ultrasound findings consistent with congenital Zika virus syndrome should receive Zika virus testing to assist in establishing the etiology of the birth defects. Testing should include both NAT and IgM tests.
5. Asymptomatic pregnant women who have recent possible Zika virus exposure (i.e., through travel or sexual exposure) but without ongoing possible exposure are not routinely recommended to have Zika virus testing.

Sources: CDC. *Zika: Clinical Evaluation & Disease.* Retrieved on September 1, 2017, from https://www.cdc.gov/zika/hc-providers/ preparing-for-zika/clinicalevaluationdisease.html; Centers for Disease Control and Prevention. (2017b). Update: Interim guidance for healthcare providers caring for pregnant women with possible Zika virus exposure—United States (including U.S. territories), July 2017. *Morbidity and Mortality Weekly Report, 66*(29), 781–793.

REEMERGING VACCINE-PREVENTABLE DISEASES

The United States has been able to eliminate many infectious diseases because of its effective vaccination programs, which achieve high vaccine coverage in children and a strong public health system for detecting and responding to new cases and outbreaks. However, the reemergence of **vaccine-preventable disease** outbreaks continue to occur in the United States despite these vaccination programs. People who are unvaccinated for any reason, including those who refuse vaccination, risk getting infected and spreading these infectious diseases to others, including those who cannot get vaccinated because they are too young or have specific health conditions.

Measles, Mumps, and Rubella

Measles

In 2000, the United States declared that measles was eliminated from this country (the absence of endemic transmission for 12 months or more). Nonetheless, since measles cases are still common in many other countries, this disease will continue to be brought into the United States.

Measles is highly contagious, so anyone who is not protected against the disease is at risk of becoming infected. Measles is more likely to spread and cause outbreaks in U.S. communities where groups of people are unvaccinated. Several recent outbreaks of measles have been reported in the United States. The majority of people who got measles were unvaccinated.

People who are unvaccinated for any reason, including those who refuse vaccination, risk getting infected with measles and spreading it to others, including those who cannot get vaccinated because they are too young or have specific health conditions (CDC, *Measles (Rubeola) for healthcare professionals*).

Outbreaks in countries to which Americans often travel can directly contribute to an increase in measles cases in the United States. In 2011, more than 30 countries in the WHO European Region reported an increase in measles, and France was experiencing a large outbreak.

At the end of 2017, 118 cases of measles from 15 states and the District of Columbia were reported to the CDC. By mid-August 2018, a total of nine outbreaks (defined as three or more linked cases) and 124 individual cases of measles had been confirmed in 22 states and the District of Columbia. But the CDC warned at that time that there was no current multistate measles outbreak in the United States. However, while this case count was preliminary and with four more months before the end of that year, it had already exceeded the total number of measles cases for 2017 (CDC, *Measles cases and outbreaks.* [Last updated: August 22, 2018]).

Travelers with measles continue to bring the disease into the United States, and it can spread when it reaches communities where groups of people are unvaccinated. Maintaining 95% vaccine coverage is critical to public health and elimination of measles transmission. Vaccination hesitancy and movement of populations due to economic hardship are preventing this goal from being reached globally, leading to measles outbreaks. Before any international travel, infants 6 months through 11 months of age should receive one dose of MMR vaccine. Children 12 months of age and older should receive two doses of MMR vaccine separated by at least 28 days. Teenagers and adults who do not have evidence of immunity against measles should get two doses of MMR vaccine separated by at least 28 days (CDC, *Measles (Rubeola) for healthcare professionals*).

Mumps

Before there was a vaccine against mumps, the disease was a common disease in the United States and caused severe complications. Vaccination is the best way to prevent mumps. Since a vaccine became available, mumps is no longer a very common infection in the United States.

However, outbreaks still occur from year to year, with many cases occurring on college campuses. Therefore, young adults and teenager immunizations should be up to date (CDC, *Mumps for healthcare professionals*).

Rubella

Rubella was a common disease that occurred primarily among young children before the rubella vaccine was licensed in the United States in 1969. Epidemics occurred every 6 to 9 years, with the highest number of cases during the spring. Rubella was declared eliminated from the United States in 2004 (the absence of endemic transmission for 12 months or more). However, it is still commonly transmitted in many parts of the world. As a result, less than 10 cases (primarily import-related) have been reported annually in the United States since elimination was declared. Because rubella continues to circulate in other parts of the world, an estimated 100,000 infants are born with congenital rubella syndrome annually worldwide (CDC, *Rubella* [German measles, three-day measles] for healthcare professionals).

Pertussis

Pertussis (whooping cough) is a common (endemic) disease in the United States, with peaks in reported disease every 3 to 5 years and frequent outbreaks. Before the availability of pertussis vaccine in the 1940s, public health experts reported more than 200,000 cases of pertussis annually. Since widespread use of the vaccine began, incidence has decreased more than 75% compared with the pre-vaccine era. However, since the 1980s, there has been an increase in the number of reported cases of pertussis. In 2012, the last peak year, CDC reported 48,277 cases of pertussis in the United States. In the summer of 2017, an outbreak of pertussis occurred in St. Joseph County, MI, which began with one Amish family and spread throughout the community. There were 233 cases who were treated with antibiotics by the end of August. Amish religious doctrine does not prohibit vaccination; however, coverage levels for routine childhood vaccination remain low in many Amish communities. In the Michigan case, an Amish family opened their home for an immunization clinic. The Amish community also offered its community building for monthly immunizations (ISID, 2017).

The CDC believes that much of pertussis disease goes unrecognized and unreported. The best way to prevent pertussis is vaccination. There are vaccines for babies, children, preteens, teens, and adults. The childhood vaccine is called DTaP (Diphtheria, Tetanus, and Pertussis), and the pertussis booster vaccine for preteens, teens, and adults is called Tdap (Tetanus, diphtheria, and pertussis) vaccine (CDC, *Pertussis [whooping cough]*).

Immunity to pertussis wanes despite receiving vaccine as children. The Advisory Committee on Immunization Practices (ACIP, 2017a) currently recommends that adults and adolescents receive one dose of the (Tdap) booster vaccine to protect against whooping cough. A dose of Tdap is recommended for adults who expect to have close contact with an infant younger than 12 months of age. Adolescents who have already received a booster dose of Td are encouraged to receive a dose of Tdap. A 5-year interval from the last Td dose is encouraged, but an interval as short as 2 years may be used if pertussis immunity is needed. All adults should receive a booster dose of Td every 10 years. Tdap is licensed for only one lifetime dose per person. Adults who have never received a dose of Tdap should substitute it for their next booster dose. New mothers who have never received Tdap should get a dose as soon as possible after delivery. If vaccination is needed during pregnancy, Td is usually preferred over Tdap. Healthcare providers who have direct patient contact should receive a dose of Tdap. Adolescents and adults who require a tetanus-containing vaccine as part of wound management should receive a dose of Tdap instead of Td if they have not previously received Tdap. If Tdap is not available or was previously administered, Td should be administered (CDC, *Pertussis [whooping cough]*).

Eliminating Vaccine-Preventable Diseases

An objective of *Healthy People 2020* (DHHS, 2010) is to reduce, eliminate, or maintain elimination of cases of vaccine-preventable diseases. However, as discussed above, these diseases continue to cause outbreaks in the United States. Unvaccinated adults and children who travel to and from foreign countries are at risk of acquiring one of these diseases. In 2017, global vaccination coverage had stalled at 86%, with no significant changes made over the previous year. An estimated 19.5 million infants worldwide were still missing out on basic vaccines in 2017 (WHO, Immunization coverage). In October 2016, the ACIP (2017a, 2017b) approved the 2017 recommended immunization schedule for children under age 18 years or younger and for adults age 19 years or older in the United States. These ACIP recommendations were revised in February 2017, some of the recommendations included new or revised recommendations for influenza, human papillomavirus, hepatitis B, and meningococcal vaccines. The revised ACIP recommendations are available at http://www.immunize.org/acip/

Evidence for Practice

Immunization prevents illness, disability, and death from vaccine-preventable diseases. Health departments all over the United States monitor vaccination coverage to understand how well communities are protected from vaccine-preventable diseases. Vaccination coverage information is used to identify areas and groups with lower vaccination coverage so public health departments, healthcare partners, and schools can take action to help improve vaccination coverage and protect everyone from vaccine-preventable diseases. The 13th edition of *Epidemiology and Prevention of Vaccine-Preventable Diseases,* (a.k.a. the "Pink Book") offers healthcare providers the most comprehensive information on routinely used vaccines and the diseases they prevent (CDC, 2017a).

Practice Point

For better or for worse, invisible invasive organisms have been a part of life since life began. Their life cycles are so short in comparison with ours that they have multiple generations to react to obstacles in their environment, adapt to adverse conditions, and increase their strength and capacity to reproduce. Therefore, the public health system must continue to be vigilant.

ANTIBIOTIC-RESISTANT MICROORGANISMS

This chapter on emerging infectious diseases would not be complete without a discussion of emerging antibiotic-resistant pathogens. Microbial adaptation and change has led to the rapid evolution of these microorganisms, which are a result of the overuse of antibiotics and consequent accumulation in the environment. Nearly 2 million people become infected with microorganisms that are resistant to antibiotics, and at least 23,000 die each year as a direct result of these infections. Antibiotic-resistant microorganisms are now found in the community as well as in healthcare settings (CDC, *Antibiotic/antimicrobial resistance*). Antibiotics/antimicrobials are among the most commonly prescribed drugs used in healthcare and can be life-saving. However, as much as 50% of the time they are not correctly prescribed, and often are given when not necessary. Antibiotic use in food-producing animals also has contributed to the increase in antibiotic-resistance. In 2013, the CDC

outlined the top 18 antimicrobial-resistant threats in the United States. These are categorized as:

- Urgent threats
- Serious threats
- Concerning threats

Three microorganisms that pose an *urgent threat* because they have the potential to become widespread without public health attention to identify infections with these microorganisms and limit their transmission. They are:

- *Clostridium difficile* (CDIFF)
- Carbapenem-resistant Enterobacteriaceae (CRE)
- *Neisseria gonorrhoeae* (CDC, *Antibiotic/*antimicrobial resistance)

As discussed in Chapter 14, sexually transmitted diseases are a significant challenge in the United States, particularly among adolescents and young adults. Due to concerns about the development of antibiotic-resistant *N. gonorrhoeae*, the CDC recommends only one treatment regimen for gonorrhea in the United States: Dual therapy with ceftriaxone and azithromycin (CDC, *Sexually transmitted diseases*). CRE, a family of microorganisms that include Klebsiella species and *E. coli*, are untreatable and/or hard-to-treat. Healthy people usually do not get CRE infections, and they usually happen to patients in hospitals, nursing homes, and other healthcare settings. Patients whose care requires devices like ventilators, urinary catheters, or intravenous catheters, and patients who are taking long courses of certain antibiotics are most at risk for CRE infections. Some CRE bacteria have become resistant to most available antibiotics. Consequently, infections with these bacteria are very difficult to treat, and can be deadly (CDC, *Carbapenem-resistant Enterobacteriaceae*). One report cites CRE are associated with an increase in mortality (Gupta, Limbago, Patel, & Kallen, 2011).

Clostridium difficile (CDIFF) causes life-threatening diarrhea that most frequently occurs in people who have been recently under medical care and received antibiotics. Infections with CDIFF are a major cause of healthcare-associated infections worldwide. It is associated with high rates of mortality and illness, and has a case-fatality rate of up to 14% within 30 days after diagnosis. Disease recurrence further increases illness rates, reduces quality of life, and might occur in up to 27% of the incident cases. These features place a major burden on healthcare systems. The disease burden of CDIFF has been well studied in Europe and North America. Although antimicrobial drug stewardship programs have contributed to a decrease in incidence in some countries, CDIFF is still a major health burden in other countries (Ho et al., 2017). Recent reports have found that as many as 350 patients at 41 healthcare facilities in the United States and worldwide were infected or exposed to CRE from tainted endoscopes between January 2010 and October 2015 (ISID, 2016). *Serious antibiotic-resistant threats* include several microorganisms that, albeit are declining in incidence of resistance and currently have effective therapeutic agents to treat them, they may become urgent without ongoing public health monitoring and prevention activities. Tuberculosis is among the most common infectious diseases and a frequent cause of death worldwide. As describe earlier in the chapter, an important worldwide serious threat is drug-resistant TB.

Concerning threat microorganisms have a low threat of antibiotic resistance and/or have multiple therapeutic options. However, these pathogens cause severe illness and require monitoring and rapid outbreak response. The current list of all microorganism "threats" is posted on the CDC website at https://www.cdc.gov/drugresistance/biggest_threats.html

Antibiotic Stewardship

Antibiotic stewardship refers to a set of coordinated strategies to improve the use of antimicrobial medications with the goal of enhancing patient health outcomes, reducing resistance to antibiotics, and decreasing unnecessary costs.

Antimicrobial resistance has emerged as a significant healthcare quality and patient safety issue in the twenty-first century that, combined with a rapidly dwindling antimicrobial armamentarium, has resulted in a critical threat to the public health of the United States. Antimicrobial stewardship programs optimize antimicrobial use to achieve the best clinical outcomes while minimizing adverse events and limiting selective pressures that drive the emergence of resistance and may also reduce excessive costs attributable to suboptimal antimicrobial use. **Fishman et al., 2012**

In 2015, the White House hosted a Forum on antibiotic stewardship. It brought together more than 100 key leaders in healthcare and industry to develop, promote, and implement activities to ensure appropriate use and prescription of antibiotics. As early as 2012, the Society for Healthcare Epidemiology of America, the Infectious Diseases Society of America, and the Pediatric Infectious Diseases Society had issued a joint policy statement on antimicrobial stewardship. It can be accessed at http://www.shea-online.org/index.php/practice-resources/priority-topics/antimicrobial-stewardship/shea-policy-statement

CONCLUSIONS

By the middle of the 20th century, many researchers regarded the threat of infectious diseases to be significantly diminished. However, in the globally interconnected world of the 21st century, it has become clear that the threat of epidemics and pandemics remains a current and pressing possibility. Recent concerns about the potential for the influenza A (H7N9) virus to mutate so that it poses the highest potential pandemic risk has highlighted the broader problem: Conditions around the globe are set for the possible development of epidemics of zoonotic diseases that have the potential to become pandemic. Unlike other public health threats such as TB and malaria, the emergence of these zoonotic diseases represents the potential of rare events with catastrophic consequences, as seen in the 1918 influenza pandemic and the more recent HIV epidemic. To date, scientists and public health advocates have focused on surveillance as the critical tool for detecting and monitoring outbreaks of zoonotic diseases in human and animal populations, but questions remain as to how to make zoonotic disease surveillance more comprehensive and timely in human and animal populations in order to prevent or minimize the potential for outbreaks to occur in human populations. Scientists have been concerned for some time about climate change and its effect on zoonotic diseases in human and animal populations.

To address this problem, in 2010, the IOM and the National Research Council convened an expert committee. The committee's task was to provide consensus advice on the challenge of achieving sustainable global capacity for surveillance and response to emerging diseases of zoonotic origin such as avian influenza, and ways to protect the public from them. The 2-day workshop by the Committee can be summarized by the following statement: "Because it would be impossible to test every species…, the strategy must be to focus on so-called hotspots—areas with high biodiversity as well as high human population density—where zoonoses are most likely to be found." Several options are available to monitor and track emerging zoonotic diseases in humans. By conducting "smart surveillance," scientists will be able to target their resources and efforts in areas where human–animal interaction is most likely to provide conditions favorable to zoonotic diseases (IOM, 2010).

Most of the world, including the United States, lacks a skilled workforce to combat emerging diseases. There is a call to increase educational programs in applied epidemiology and infectious disease prevention and control. Nurses are the largest group of healthcare professionals; therefore, they are in a position to take leadership initiatives. Hands-on experience, such as those obtained through the CDC Epidemic Intelligence Service (EIS) 2-year postgraduate program, can equip nurses with surveillance skills.

KEY CONCEPTS

- Factors that influence the emergence or reemergence of infectious diseases are multiple, complex, and interrelated.
- Epidemics and pandemics can place sudden and intense demands on healthcare systems.
- In addition to morbidity and mortality, outbreaks of emerging and reemerging infections can disrupt economic activity and development.
- Certain zoonotic diseases can be transmitted to humans through contact with animals, birds, and insects like ticks or mosquitoes.

KEY CONCEPTS *(Continued)*

- The goal of *Healthy People 2020* (DHHS, 2010) to reduce TB in the United States to 1 case per 100,000 population has not been met.
- An objective of *Healthy People 2020* is to reduce, eliminate, or maintain elimination of cases of vaccine-preventable diseases. However, vaccine-preventable diseases are reemerging in the United States.
- The CDC's top priority for the public health response to Zika is to protect pregnant women because of the risks associated with Zika virus infection during pregnancy.
- Microbial adaptation and change has occurred in the rapid evolution of antibiotic-resistant pathogens.
- The CDC has outlined the top 18 antimicrobial-resistant threats in the United States.

- Antibiotic stewardship involves coordinated interventions designed to improve and measure the appropriate use of and prescriptions for antimicrobials.
- The Society for Healthcare Epidemiology of America, the Infectious Diseases Society of America, and the Pediatric Infectious Diseases Society have developed a joint policy statement on antibiotic stewardship.
- There is a worldwide need for a skilled public health workforce to combat emerging diseases.
- Nurses must be able to recognize new and reemerging infectious diseases, identify the conditions that foster their development, and act to protect the health of the public.

CRITICAL THINKING QUESTIONS

1. You spent last weekend hiking in the woods but forgot to bring insect repellant. Two days ago, a circular flat rash with a white center appears high on the back of your calf. It does not hurt; therefore, you decide to forget about it. Today, you develop a fever, are fatigued, and have a headache along with muscle and joint pain.
   a. Explain what may have happened.
   b. Outline your plan of action.
   c. How would you prevent similar occurrences?
2. A neighbor, who is 3 months pregnant, asks to talk to you because she has felt tired for the last 2 days, has a headache, a rash, and does not feel like eating. You take her vital signs and find that she has a low-grade fever. She has recently

traveled to an area where there is risk for Zika virus disease.
   a. To what could your neighbor have been exposed, and how could the exposure have occurred?
   b. What advice would you give your neighbor?
3. Outline the factors that have contributed to the emergence or reemergence of each of the following infectious diseases. Explain how these factors differ with each disease.
   a. Lyme disease
   b. Zika virus
   c. *E. coli* O157:H7
4. Identify at least two vaccine-preventable diseases that have not met the *Healthy People 2020* target.

REFERENCES

Advisory Committee on Immunization Practices (ACIP). (2017a). Recommended immunization schedule for adults aged 19 years or older in the United States, 2017. *Morbidity and Mortality Weekly Report, 66*(5), 136–138. doi: http://dx.doi.org/10.15585/mmwr.mm6605e2

Advisory Committee on Immunization Practices (ACIP). (2017b). *Recommended immunization schedule for children aged 18 years and younger, 2017.* Retrieved on September 6, 2017, from https://www.cdc.gov/vaccines/schedules/downloads/child/0-18yrs-child-combined-schedule.pdf

Agnandji, S. T., Huttner, A., Zinser, M. E., Njuguna, P., Dahlke, C., Fernandes, J. F.,…Siegrist, C. A. (2016). Phase 1 trials of rVSV Ebola vaccine in Africa and Europe. *New England Journal of Medicine, 374,* 1647–1660. doi: 10.1056/NEJMoa1502924.

American Lyme Disease Foundation. *Lyme disease.* Retrieved on August 21, 2017, from http://www.aldf.com/lyme.shtml

Brisson, D., Vandermause, M. F., Meece, J. K., Reed, K. D., & Dykhuizen, D. E. (2010). Evolution of northeastern and

midwestern Borrelia burgdorferi, United States. *Emerging Infectious Diseases, 16*(6), 911–917.

Centers for Disease Control and Prevention (CDC). *Measles (Rubeola) for healthcare professionals* (Last updated: May 8, 2018). Retrieved on September 23, 2018, from https://www.cdc.gov/measles/hcp/index.html

Centers for Disease Control and Prevention (CDC). *Measles cases and outbreaks.* (Last updated: August 22, 2018). Retrieved on September 23, 2018, from https://www.cdc.gov/measles/cases-outbreaks.html

Centers for Disease Control and Prevention (CDC). *Travel Health Notices.* Retrieved on June 1, 2018, from https://wwwnc.cdc.gov/travel/notices/watch/ebola-democratic-republic-of-the-congo

Centers for Disease Control and Prevention (CDC). *Travel Health. Ebola in Democratic Republic of the Congo.* [Updated September 14, 2018]. Retrieved on September 22, 2018, from https://wwwnc.cdc.gov/travel/notices/watch/ebola-democraticrepublic-of-the-congo

Centers for Disease Control and Prevention (CDC). *Zika virus.* Retrieved on September 1, 2017, from http://www.cdc.gov/zika/index.htm

Centers for Disease Control and Prevention (CDC). *Zika travel information.* Retrieved on September 2, 2017, from https://www.cdc.gov/zika/geo/index.html

Centers for Disease Control and Prevention (CDC). *Zika overview.* Retrieved on September 1, 2017, from https://www.cdc.gov/zika/about/overview.html

Centers for Disease Control and Prevention (CDC). *Yellow Book, 2018.* Retrieved on August 19, 2017, from https://wwwnc.cdc.gov/travel/page/yellowbook-home

Centers for Disease Control and Prevention (CDC). *West Nile virus, preliminary maps and data for 2016.* Retrieved on August 22, 2017, from https://www.cdc.gov/westnile/index.html

Centers for Disease Control and Prevention (CDC). *West Nile virus.* Retrieved on August 22, 2017, from http://www.cdc.gov/westnile/index.html

Centers for Disease Control and Prevention (CDC). *Two-tier testing for Lyme disease.* Retrieved on August 15, 2017, from https://www.cdc.gov/lyme/healthcare/clinician_twotier.html

Centers for Disease Control and Prevention (CDC). *Tuberculosis.* Retrieved on August 25, 2017, from https://www.cdc.gov/tb/

Centers for Disease Control and Prevention (CDC). *Tuberculin skin testing.* Retrieved on August 25, 2017, from https://www.cdc.gov/tb/publications/factsheets/testing/skintesting.htm

Centers for Disease Control and Prevention (CDC). *Treatment regimens for latent TB infection.* Retrieved on August 25, 2017, from https://www.cdc.gov/tb/topic/treatment/ltbi.htm

Centers for Disease Control and Prevention (CDC). *Treatment for TB disease.* Retrieved on August 26, 2017, from https://www.cdc.gov/tb/topic/treatment/tbdisease.htm

Centers for Disease Control and Prevention (CDC). *TB treatment for children.* Retrieved on August 26, 2017, from https://www.cdc.gov/tb/topic/populations/tbinchildren/default.htm

Centers for Disease Control and Prevention (CDC). *TB testing & diagnosis.* Retrieved on August 21, 2017, from https://www.cdc.gov/tb/topic/testing/default.htm

Centers for Disease Control and Prevention (CDC). *TB risk factors.* Retrieved on August 23, 2017, from https://www.cdc.gov/tb/topic/basics/risk.htm

Centers for Disease Control and Prevention (CDC). *Tuberculosis fact sheets.* Retrieved on August 24, 2017 from https://www.cdc.gov/tb/publications/factsheets/default.htm

Centers for Disease Control and Prevention (CDC). *Data and surveillance.* Retrieved August 15, 2017, from https://www.cdc.gov/lyme/datasurveillance/index.html

Centers for Disease Control and Prevention (CDC). *Tuberculosis fact sheets.* Retrieved on August 24, 2017 from https://www.cdc.gov/tb/publications/factsheets/default.htm

Centers for Disease Control and Prevention (CDC). *TB and HIV coinfection.* Retrieved on August 24, 2017, from https://www.cdc.gov/tb/topic/basics/tbhivcoinfection.htm

Centers for Disease Control and Prevention (CDC). *Travel Health Notices, July 31, 2014.* Retrieved on September 2, 2017, from https://www.cdc.gov/media/releases/2014/p0731-ebola.html

Centers for Disease Control and Prevention (CDC) (2015). *Strategies for elimination of tuberculosis in the United States.* Retrieved on August 25, 2017 from https://ctca2015.iescentral.com/filelibrary/file_720.pdf

Centers for Disease Control and Prevention (CDC). *Shiga toxin-producing Escherichia coli O157:H7 infections linked to organic spinach and spring mix.* Retrieved on August 14, 2017, from https://www.cdc.gov/ecoli/2012/o157h7-11-12/index.html

Centers for Disease Control and Prevention (CDC). *Sexually transmitted diseases.* Retrieved on September 3, 2017, from https://www.cdc.gov/std/default.htm

Centers for Disease Control and Prevention (CDC). *Rubella (German measles, three-day measles) for healthcare professionals.* Retrieved on September 2, 2017, from http://www.cdc.gov/rubella/hcp.html

Centers for Disease Control and Prevention (CDC). *Recommendations for infection control for A (H7N9).* Retrieved on August 6, 2017, from https://www.cdc.gov/flu/avianflu/healthprofessionals.htm

Centers for Disease Control and Prevention (CDC). *Remembering SARS 10 years later.* Retrieved on August 4, 2017, from http://www.cdc.gov/about/history/sars/timeline.htm

Centers for Disease Control and Prevention (CDC). *Public health threat of highly pathogenic avian influenza A (H5N1) virus.* Retrieved on August 20, 2017, from https://www.cdc.gov/flu/avianflu/h5n1-threat.htm

Centers for Disease Control and Prevention (CDC). *Pertussis (whooping cough).* Retrieved on September 2, 2017, from https://www.cdc.gov/pertussis/index.html

Centers for Disease Control and Prevention (CDC). *Past pandemics.* Retrieved on August 3, 2017, from https://www.cdc.gov/flu/pandemic-resources/basics/past-pandemics.html

Centers for Disease Control and Prevention (CDC). *Pandemic Severity Assessment Framework (PSAF).* Retrieved on August 22, 2017, from https://www.cdc.gov/flu/pandemic-resources/national-strategy/severity-assessment-framework.html

Centers for Disease Control and Prevention (CDC). *Pandemic influenza resources.* Retrieved on August 4, 2017, from https://www.cdc.gov/flu/pandemic-resources/index.html

Centers for Disease Control and Prevention (CDC). *Outcomes of pregnancies with laboratory evidence of possible Zika virus infection in the United States.* Retrieved on September 1, 2017, from https://www.cdc.gov/zika/reporting/pregnancy-outcomes.html

Centers for Disease Control and Prevention (CDC). *Mumps for healthcare professionals.* Retrieved on September 2, 2017, from http://www.cdc.gov/mumps/hcp.html

Centers for Disease Control and Prevention (CDC). *MERS interim guidance for healthcare professionals. Case definitions and guidance.* Retrieved on August 16, 2017, from https://www.cdc.gov/coronavirus/mers/interim-guidance.html

Centers for Disease Control and Prevention (CDC). *MERS-CoV. Information for healthcare professionals.* Retrieved on August 16, 2017, from https://www.cdc.gov/coronavirus/mers/case-def.html

Centers for Disease Control and Prevention (CDC). (Press release, June 17, 2014). *MERS-CoV.* Retrieved on August 15, 2017, from https://www.cdc.gov/media/releases/2014/p0617-mers.html

Centers for Disease Control and Prevention (CDC). (Press release, May 29, 2014). *Measles cases in the United States reach 20-year high.* Retrieved on September 2, 2017, from https://www.cdc.gov/vaccines/news/press-rel/index.html

Centers for Disease Control and Prevention (CDC). *Lyme disease data and surveillance.* Retrieved on August 15, 2017, from https://www.cdc.gov/lyme/datasurveillance/index.html

Centers for Disease Control and Prevention (CDC). *Lyme disease.* Retrieved on August 3, 2017, from http://www.cdc.gov/lyme/

Centers for Disease Control and Prevention (CDC). Latent tuberculosis infection: A guide for primary health care providers. Retrieved on August 26, 2017, from ttps://www.cdc.gov/tb/publications/ltbi/diagnosis.htm

Centers for Disease Control and Prevention (CDC). *Interim guidance on use of intervals, triggers, and actions for novel influenza A (H1N1) response* (Updated April 29, 2009). Retrieved on August 22, 2017, from http://epi.publichealth.nc.gov/cd/flu/plan/Intervals_Triggers_Actions.pdf

Centers for Disease Control and Prevention (CDC). *Interim guidance for infection control within healthcare settings when caring for confirmed cases, probable cases, and cases under investigation for infection with novel influenza A viruses associated with severe*

REFERENCES *(Continued)*

disease. Retrieved on August 3, 2017, from https://www.cdc.gov/flu/avianflu/novel-flu-infection-control.htm

Centers for Disease Control and Prevention (CDC). *Influenza: H7N9.* Retrieved on August 1, 2017, from https://www.cdc.gov/flu/avianflu/h7n9-virus.htm

Centers for Disease Control and Prevention (CDC). *Infection prevention and control recommendations for hospitalized patients under investigation (PUIs) for Ebola virus disease (EVD) in U.S. hospitals.* Retrieved on August 27, 2017, from https://www.cdc.gov/vhf/ebola/healthcare-us/hospitals/infection-control.html

Centers for Disease Control and Prevention (CDC). *How the flu virus changes.* Retrieved on August 2, 2017, from http://www.gov/about_the_flu/virus_changes/index.html

Centers for Disease Control and Prevention (CDC). *EVD signs and symptoms.* Retrieved on August 27, 2017, from http://www.cdc.gov/vhf/ebola/symptoms/index.html

Centers for Disease Control and Prevention (CDC). *EVD diagnosis.* Retrieved on August 28, 2017, from http://www.flu.gov/.http://www.cdc.gov/vhf/ebola/diagnosis/index.html

Centers for Disease Control and Prevention (CDC). *Epidemiologic risk factors to consider when evaluating a person for exposure to Ebola virus.* Retrieved on August 30, 2017, from https://www.cdc.gov/vhf/ebola/exposure/risk-factors-when-evaluating-person-for-exposure.html

Centers for Disease Control and Prevention (CDC). *E. coli.* Retrieved on August 22, 2017, from http://www.cdc.gov/ecoli/general/index.html

Centers for Disease Control and Prevention (CDC). *Colorado City, E. coli O157:H7 outbreak, farm animals, Hildale, Mohave County Department of Health, Southwest Utah Public Health Department.* Retrieved on August 22, 2017, from http://www.foodsafetynews.com/tag/farm-animals/

Centers for Disease Control and Prevention (CDC). (2014b). *Cases of Ebola diagnosed in the United States.* (Press Release September 30, 2014). Retrieved on August 24, 2017 from https://www.cdc.gov/media/releases/2014/s930-ebola-confirmed-case.html

Centers for Disease Control and Prevention (CDC). *Carbapenem-resistant Enterobacteriaceae.* Retrieved from https://www.cdc.gov/hai/organisms/cre/index.html

Centers for Disease Control and Prevention (CDC). *Babesiosis.* Retrieved on August 23, 2017, from http://www.cdc.gov/parasites/babesiosis/health_professionals/index.html

Centers for Disease Control and Prevention (CDC). *Antibiotic/antimicrobial resistance.* Retrieved on September 4, 2017, from http://www.cdc.gov/drugresistance/index.html

Centers for Disease Control and Prevention (CDC). (2010a). *2009 H1N1: Overview of a pandemic.* Retrieved on August 4, 2017, from https://www.cdc.gov/h1n1flu/yearinreview/yir3.htm

Centers for Disease Control and Prevention (CDC). (2005a). Compendium of measures to prevent disease Associated with animals in public settings, 2005. *Morbidity and Mortality Weekly Report, 54*(RR04), 1–12.

Centers for Disease Control and Prevention (CDC). (2005b). Guidelines for the investigation of contacts of persons with infectious tuberculosis. *Morbidity and Mortality Weekly Report, 54*(RR15), 1–37.

Centers for Disease Control and Prevention (CDC). (2005c). Guidelines for preventing the transmission of Mycobacterium tuberculosis in health-care settings, 2005. *Morbidity and Mortality Weekly Report, 54*(RR17), 1–141. Retrieved from http://www.cdc.gov/mmwr/PDF/rr/rr5417.pdf

Centers for Disease Control and Prevention (CDC). (2007). *Guideline for isolation precautions: Preventing transmission of infectious agents in healthcare settings.* Retrieved on August 22, 2014, from http://www.cdc.gov/coronavirus/mers/downloads/Isolation2007.pdf

Centers for Disease Control and Prevention (CDC). (2010b). Updated guidelines for using interferon gamma release assays to detect Mycobacterium tuberculosis infection—United States, 2010. *Morbidity and Mortality Weekly Report, 59*(RR05), 1–25.

Centers for Disease Control and Prevention (CDC). (2012). Tuberculosis Outbreak Associated with a Homeless Shelter—Kane County, Illinois, 2007–2011. *Morbidity and Mortality Weekly Report, 61*(11), 186–189.

Centers for Disease Control and Prevention (CDC). (2014a). *2014–2016 Ebola outbreak in West Africa.* Retrieved on August 10, 2018 from https://www.cdc.gov/vhf/ebola/history/2014-2016-outbreak/index.html

Centers for Disease Control and Prevention (CDC). (2014c). First confirmed case of Middle East respiratory syndrome coronavirus (MERS-CoV) infection in the United States, updated information. *Morbidity and Mortality Weekly Report, 63*(19), 431–436.

Centers for Disease Control and Prevention (CDC). (2017a). *Epidemiology and prevention of vaccine-preventable diseases* (3rd ed.). Retrieved on September 5, 2017, from https://www.cdc.gov/vaccines/pubs/pinkbook/index.html

Centers for Disease Control and Prevention (CDC). (2017b). Update: Interim guidance for health care providers caring for pregnant women with possible Zika virus exposure—United States (Including U.S. Territories), July 2017. *Morbidity and Mortality Weekly Report, 66*(29), 781–793.

Centers for Disease Control and Prevention (CDC). (2017c). Zika virus transmission—Region of the Americas, May 15, 2015–December 15, 2016. *Morbidity and Mortality Weekly Report, 66*(12), 329–334.

Centers for Disease Control and Prevention (CDC). *Travel Health. Ebola in Democratic Republic of the Congo.* (Updated September 14, 2018). Retrieved on September 22, 2018, from https://wwwnc.cdc.gov/travel/notices/watch/ebola-democratic-republic-of-the-congo

Department of Health and Human Services (DHHS). (2000). *Healthy People 2010.* Washington, DC: Author.

Department of Health and Human Services (DHHS). (2009). *State and local pandemic influenza planning checklist.* Washington, DC: Author.

Department of Health and Human Services (DHHS). (2010). *Healthy People 2020.* Washington, DC: Author.

Department of Health and Human Services (DHHS). (2017). *Pandemic resources.* Retrieved on August 20, 2017, from https://www.cdc.gov/flu/pandemic-resources/index.htm

Fischer, W. A., Brown, J., Wohl, D. A, Loftis, A. J., Tozay, S., Reeves, E.,…Hoover, D. (2017). Ebola virus ribonucleic acid detection in semen more than two years after resolution of acute Ebola virus infection. *Open Forum Infectious Diseases.* doi: 10.1093/ofid/ofx155. Retrieved on August 29, 2017, from https://academic.oup.com/ofid/article-lookup/doi/10.1093/ofid/ofx155

Fishman, N., Patterson, J., Saiman, L., Srinivasan, A., Trivedi, K. K., van Schooneveld, T., …Newland J. (2012). Policy Statement on Antimicrobial Stewardship by the Society for Healthcare Epidemiology of America (SHEA), the Infectious Diseases Society of America (IDSA), and the Pediatric Infectious Diseases Society (PIDS). *Infection Control & Hospital Epidemiology, 33*(4), 322–327. doi: 10.1086/665010

Freedman, S. B., Xie, J., Neufeld, M. S., Hamilton, W. L., Hartling, L., Tarr, P. I.,…Pang, X. L. (2016). Shiga toxin-producing Escherichia coli infection, antibiotics, and risk of developing hemolytic uremic syndrome: A meta-analysis. *Clinical Infectious Disease*, *62*(10), 1251–1258.

Gao, R., Cao, B., Hu, Y., Feng, Z., Wang, D., Hu, W.,...Shu, Y. (2013). Human infection with a novel avian-origin influenza A (H7N9) virus. *New England Journal of Medicine*, *368*(20), 1888–1897.

Garrett, L. (1995). *The coming plague*. New York: Penguin Group.

Gupta, N., Limbago, B. M., Patel, J. B., & Kallen, A. J. (2011). Carbapenem-resistant Enterobacteriaceae: Epidemiology and prevention. *Clinical Infectious Diseases*, *53*(1), 60–67. https://doi.org/10.1093/cid/cir202

Haug, C. J. (2018). Keeping your cool. Doing Ebola research during an emergency. *New England Journal of Medicine*. May 23, 2018. Retrieved on May 27, 2018, from https://www.nejm.org/doi/full/10.1056/NEJMp1806978

Healio. *Infectious Disease News*, May 25, 2018. Health care workers first to get Ebola vaccine in Congo outbreak. Retrieved on May 27, 2018, from https://www.healio.com/

Hersh, M. H., Ostfeld, R. S., McHenry, D. J., Tibbetts, M., Brunner, J. L, Killilea, M. E.,... Keesing, F. (2014). Co-Infection of blacklegged ticks with babesia microti and borrelia burgdorferi is higher than expected and acquired from small mammal hosts. *PLoS One*, *9*(6), e99348. doi: 10.1371/journal.pone.0099348.

Ho, J., Dai, R. Z. W., Kwong, T. N. Y., Wang, X., Zhang, L., Ip, M., ...Wong, S. H. (2017). *Disease burden of Clostridium difficile infections in adults*, Hong Kong, China, 2006–2014. Emerging Infectious Diseases. Retrieved on September 4, 2017, from https://doi.org/10.3201/eid2310.17079

Hu, Y., Lu, L. S., Song, Z., Wang, W., Hao, P., Li, J.,...Yuan, Z. (2013). Association between adverse clinical outcome in human disease caused by novel influenza A H7N9 virus and sustained viral shedding and emergence of antiviral resistance. *The Lancet*, *381*(9885), 2273–2279. doi: http://dx.doi.org/10.1016/S0140-6736(13)61125-3

Infectious Diseases Society of America (IDSA). (2006). *Guidelines for treatment of Lyme disease*. Retrieved on August 15, 2017, from http://www.idsociety.org/uploadedFiles/IDSA/Guidelines-Patient_Care/PDF_Library/Lyme%20Disease.pdf

Institute of Medicine. (1992). *Emerging Infections: Microbial Threats to Health in the United States*. Washington, DC: The National Academies Press.

Institute of Medicine (IOM). (2010). *Infectious disease movement in a borderless world: Workshop summary*. Washington, DC: The National Academies Press. Retrieved on August 15, 2017, from http://www.nap.edu/catalog.php?record_id=12758

International Society for Infectious Diseases (ISID). (2013). Climate change, disease impact: Arctic spread. *ProMED Mail*. Archive Number: 20130613.1769830. Retrieved on August 22, 2017, from http://www.promedmail.org

International Society for Infectious Diseases (ISID). (2016). Antibiotic-resistant Enterobacteriaceae – USA. *ProMED Mail*. Archive number: 2015 20160506.4205376. Retrieved on September 3, 2017, from http://www.promedmail.org

International Society for Infectious Diseases (ISID). *ProMED Mail* (September 2, 2017). Pertussis: USA. Archive Number: 20170902.5291495. Retrieved on September 3, 2017, from http://www.promedmail.org

International Society for Infectious Diseases (ISID). Ebola update (94). *ProMED Mail*, September 21, 2018. Retrieved on September 22, 2018, from http://www.promedmail.org

International Society for Infectious Diseases (ISID). Ebola update (96). *ProMED Mail*, September 24, 2018. Retrieved on September 24, 2018, from http://www.promedmail.org

International Society for Infectious Diseases (ISID). Ebola update (93). *ProMED Mail*, September 20, 2018. Retrieved on September 20, 2018, from http://www.promedmail.org

International Society for Infectious Diseases (ISID). Ebola update (82). *ProMED Mail*, September 5, 2018. Retrieved on September 5, 2018, from http://www.promedmail.org

International Society for Infectious Diseases (ISID). Ebola update (150): Democratic Republic of Congo. *ProMed Mail*, December 15, 2018. Retrieved December 15, 2018 from http://www.promedmail.org

Kilbourne, E. D. (2006). Influenza pandemics of the 20th century. *Emerging Infectious Diseases*, *12*(1), 9–14.

Kile, J. C., Ren, R., Liu, L., Greene, C. M., Roguski, K., Iuliano, A. D.,...Davis, C. T. (2017). Update: Increase in human infections with novel Asian lineage avian influenza A(H7N9) viruses during the fifth epidemic—China, October 1, 2016–August 7, 2017. *Morbidity and Mortality Weekly Report*, *66*(35), 928–932.

Krause, P. J., Narasimhan, S., Wormser, G. P., Barbour, A. G., Platonov, A. E., Brancato, J.,...Tick Borne Diseases Group. (2014). Borelia miyamotoi senso lato seroreactivity and seroprevalence in the northeastern United States. *Emerging Infectious Diseases*, *20*(7), 1183–1190.

Lewinsohn, D. M., Leonard, M. K., LoBue, P. A., Cohn, D. L, Daley, C. L., Desmond, E.,...Woods, G. L. (2017). Official American Thoracic Society/Infectious Diseases Society of America/Centers for Disease Control and Prevention Clinical Practice Guidelines: Diagnosis of Tuberculosis in Adults and Children. *Clinical Infectious Diseases*, *64*(2), 111–115. https://doi.org/10.1093/cid/ciw778

Li, Q., Zhou, L., Zhou, M., Chen, Z., Li, F., Wu, H.,...Feng, Z. (2014). Epidemiology of human infections with avian influenza A (H7N9) virus in China. *New England Journal of Medicine*, *307*(6), 520–532.

Luna, S., Krishnasamy, V., Saw, L., Smith, L.,Wagner J., Jenna Weigand, J., ... Gieraltowski, L. (2018). Outbreak of *E. coli* O157:H7 Infections Associated with Exposure to Animal Manure in a Rural Community—Arizona and Utah, June–July 2017. *Morbidity and Mortality Weekly Report (MMWR)*, *67*(23):659–662. Retrieved on December 18, 2018 from http://dx.doi.org/10.15585/mmwr.mm6723a2

Morens, D. M., Folkers, G. K., & Fauci, A. S. (2008). Emerging infections: A perpetual challenge. *Lancet Infectious Disease*, *8*(11), 710–719. doi: 10.1016/S1473-3099(08)70256-1.

Mutreja, A., Kim, D. W., Thomson, N. R., Conner, T. R., Lee, J. H., Kariuki, S.,...Dougan, G. (2011). Evidence for several waves of global transmission in the seventh cholera pandemic. *Nature*, *477*(7365), 462–465.

Nahid, P., Dorman, S. E., Alipanah, N., Barry, P. M., Brozek, J. L., & Cattamanchi, A. (2016). Executive Summary: Official American Thoracic Society/Centers for Disease Control and Prevention/Infectious Diseases Society of America Clinical Practice Guidelines: Treatment of Drug-Susceptible Tuberculosis. *Clinical Infectious Diseases*, *63*(7), 853–867. https://doi.org/10.1093/cid/ciw566

Nyamathi, A., Nahid, P., Berg, J., Burrage, J., Christiani, A., Agtash, S.,...Leake, B. (2008). Efficacy of nurse case-managed intervention for latent tuberculosis among homeless subsamples. *Nursing Research*, *57*(1), 33–39.

Smolinski, M. S., Hamburg, M. A., & Lederberg, J. (2003). *Microbial threats to health: Emergence, detection, and response*. Washington, DC: The National Academies Press.

Society for Healthcare Epidemiology of America, the Infectious Diseases Society of America, and the Pediatric Infectious Diseases Society. (2012). *Antimicrobial stewardship*. Retrieved on September 5, 2017, from http://www.shea-online.org/index.php/practice-resources/priority-topics/antimicrobial-stewardship/shea-policy-statement

Steere, A. C., Coburn, J., & Glickstein, L. (2004). The emergence of Lyme disease. *Journal of Clinical Investigation*, *113*(8), 1093–1101.

REFERENCES *(Continued)*

Taubenberger, J. K., Reid, A. H., Lourens, R. M., Wang, R., Jin, G., & Fanning, T. G. (2005). Characterization of the 1918 influenza virus polymerase genes. *(Letter) Nature*, *437*(7060), 889–893.

United Nations Children's Fund (UNICEF). *The Government of the Democratic Republic of the Congo announced the end of the Ebola virus epidemic in the Equateur Province on 25 July,* 2018. Retrieved on September 20, 2018, from https://www.unicef.org/wca/ebola-outbreak-equateur-province-democratic-republic-congo

Wang, W., Song, Z., Guan, W., Liu, Y., Zhang, X., Xu, L.,…Hu, Y. (2014). PCR for detection of oseltamivir resistance mutation in influenza A (H7N9) virus. *Emerging Infectious Diseases*, *20*(5), 847–849.

World Health Organization (WHO). Middle East respiratory syndrome (MERS) situation update November 2018. Retrieved on December 17, 2018 from http://www.emro.who.int/pandemic-epidemic-diseases/mers-cov/mers-situation-update-november-2018.html

World Health Organization (WHO). (2018d) *Cumulative number of A(H5N1) cases reported to WHO*, July 20, 2018. Retrieved on August 1, 2018, from http://www.who.int/influenza/human_animal_interface/2018_07_20_tableH5N1.pdf?ua=1

World Health Organization (WHO). *Fact sheet: Influenza (avian and other zoonotic)*, January 2018. Retrieved on March 4, 2018, from http://www.who.int/news-room/fact-sheets/detail/influenza-(avian-and-other-zoonotic)

World Health Organization (WHO). *Poliovirus detected from environmental samples in Israel—update*, July 15, 2013. Retrieved on May 10, 2017, from http://www.who.int/csr/don/2013_07_15/en/.

World Health Organization (WHO). (2018a) *Polio today*, September 18, 2018. Retrieved on September 21, 2018, from http://polioeradication.org/polio-today/polio-now/this-week/

World Health Organization (WHO). *Human infection with avian influenza A(H7N9) virus—China: Update*, September 5, 2018. Retrieved on September 21, 2018, from http://www.who.int/csr/don/05-september-2018-ah7n9-china/en/)

World Health Organization (WHO). (2015a). *Middle East respiratory syndrome coronavirus [MERS-CoV]—Republic of Korea,* 21 July 2015. Retrieved August 5, 2018, from http://www.who.int/csr/don/21-july-2015-mers-korea/en/

World Health Organization (WHO). (2018b) *Middle East respiratory syndrome coronavirus (MERS-CoV) infection—Republic of Korea,* September 12, 2018. Retrieved on September 21, 2018, from http://www.who.int/csr/don/12-september-2018-mers-republic-of-korea/en/

World Health Organization (WHO). *Middle East respiratory syndrome coronavirus* (MERS-CoV)—*United Kingdom of Great Britain and Northern Ireland,* August 31, 2018. Retrieved on September 21, 2018, from http://www.who.int/csr/don/31-august-2018-mers-united-kingdom/en/

World Health Organization (WHO). *Ebola virus disease, DRC External Report 7.* Retrieved on September 20, 2018, from https://reliefweb.int/sites/reliefweb.int/files/resources/SITREP_EVD_DRC_20180918-eng.pdf

World Health Organization (WHO). *WHO risk assessment: Human infections with avian influenza A (H7N9) virus.* Retrieved on August 15, 2017, from http://www.who.int/influenza/human_animal_interface/influenza_h7n9/Risk_Assessment/en/

World Health Organization (WHO). *Poliomyelitis.* Retrieved on August 15, 2017, from http://www.who.int/mediacentre/factsheets/fs114/en/

World Health Organization (WHO). *Middle East respiratory syndrome coronavirus (MERS-CoV)—Saudi Arabia.* Retrieved on September 9, 2017, from http://www.who.int/csr/don/6-september-2017-mers-saudi-arabia/en/

World Health Organization (WHO). (2016b). *MDR-TB 2016 update.* Retrieved on August 26, 2017, from http://www.who.int/tb/challenges/mdr/mdr_tb_factsheet.pdf?ua=1

World Health Organization (WHO). *Human infection with avian influenza A(H7N9) virus – China.* Retrieved on September 7, 2017, from http://www.who.int/csr/don/5-september-2017-ah7n9-china/en/

World Health Organization (WHO). (2018c). *Human infection with avian influenza A[H7N9] virus—China:* [Updated on September 5, 2018]. Retrieved on September 21, 2018, from http://www.who.int/csr/don/05-september-2018-ah7n9-china/en/

World Health Organization (WHO). *Immunization coverage.* Retrieved on September 3, 2017, from http://www.who.int/mediacentre/factsheets/fs378/en/

World Health Organization (WHO). (2014a). *MERS-CoV Summary 11 June, 2014.* Retrieved on September 10, 2017 from https://www.who.int/csr/disease/coronavirus_infections/MERS-CoV_summary_update_20140611.pdf?ua=1

World Health Organization (WHO). (2014b) *Nigeria ends Ebola.* Retrieved on August 21, 2017, from http://www.who.int/mediacentre/news/statements/2014/nigeria-ends-ebola/en/

World Health Organization (WHO). *Global epidemics and impact of cholera.* Retrieved on August 6, 2017, from http://www.who.int/cholera/en/

World Health Organization (WHO). *Ebola virus disease.* Retrieved on August 21, 2017, from http://www.who.int/mediacentre/factsheets/fs103/en/

World Health Organization (WHO). *The five elements of DOT.* Retrieved on August 25, 2017, from www.who.int/gtb/dots/whatisdots.htm

World Health Organization (WHO). (2018f). Zika virus classification at: http://apps.who.int/iris/bitstream/handle/10665/260419/zika-lassification-15Feb18-eng.pdf?sequence=1

World Health Organization (WHO). *Fact sheet: Influenza (Avian and other zoonotic).* Retrieved on March 4, 2018 from https://www./influenza-(avian-and-other-zoonotic)

World Health Organization (WHO). (2011). *Guidelines for the programmatic management of drug-resistant tuberculosis 2011 update.* Retrieved on August 26, 2017, from http://apps.who.int/iris/bitstream/10665/44597/1/9789241501583_eng.pdf

World Health Organization (WHO). *MERS-CoV summary,* June 11, 2014. Retrieved on August 16, 2017, from http://www.who.int/csr/disease/coronavirus_infections/MERS-CoV_summary_update_20140611.pdf?ua=1

World Health Organization (WHO). (2015b). *Infection prevention and control during health care for probable or confirmed cases of Middle East respiratory syndrome coronavirus (MERS-CoV) infection Interim guidance,* Updated June 4, 2015. Retrieved on August 23, 2017, from http://apps.who.int/iris/bitstream/10665/174652/1/WHO_MERS_IPC_15.1_eng.pdf?ua=1

World Health Organization (WHO). *Situation report, Zika virus October 27, 2016.* Retrieved on August 31, 2017, from http://apps.who.int/iris/bitstream/10665/250633/1/zikasitrep27Oct16-eng.pdf?ua=1

World Health Organization (WHO). (2016a). *Polio global eradication initiative.* Retrieved on September 20, 2018 from http://polioeradication.org/wp-content/uploads/2018/05/polio-vaccination-gpei-fact-sheet-may-2018-20180516.pdf

World Health Organization (WHO). (2016c). *Global tuberculosis report 2016.* Retrieved on August 23, 2017, from http://www.who.int/tb/publications/global_report/en/

World Health Organization (WHO). (2017). *Declaration of the end of Ebola virus disease outbreak in the Democratic Republic of the Congo,* July 2, 2017. Retrieved on May 5, 2018, from http://apps.who.int/iris/bitstream/handle/10665/255798/EbolaDRC-02072017.pdf?sequence=1

World Health Organization (WHO). *Situation report, Zika virus,* March 10, 2017. Retrieved on August 31, 2017, from http://apps. who.int/iris/bitstream/10665/254714/1/zikasitrep10Mar17-eng. pdf?ua=1

World Health Organization (WHO). *Influenza at the human-animal interface. Summary and assessment,* April 21, 2017 to May 16, 2017. Retrieved on August 21, 2017, from http://www.who.int/ influenza/human_animal_interface/Influenza_Summary_IRA_ HA_interface_05_16_2017.pdf?ua=1

World Health Organization (WHO). *Ebola situation reports: Democratic Republic of the Congo,* September 22, 2018. Retrieved on September 24, 2018, from http://www.who.int/ebola/situation-reports/drc-2018/en/)

World Health Organization (WHO). *Ebola virus disease: Democratic Republic of the Congo,* August 3, 2018. Retrieved on September 4, 2018, from http://www.who.int/csr/don/31-august-2018-ebola-drc/en/

World Health Organization (WHO). (2018e). *Strategic response plan for the ebola virus disease outbreak: Democratic Republic of the Congo.* Retrieved on June 1, 2018, from http://www.who.int/emergencies/crises/cod/DRC-ebola-disease-outbreak-response-plan-28May2018-ENfinal.pdf?ua=1&ua=1

WEB RESOURCES

Please visit thePoint® web resources for up-to-date information on this topic.

16

Violence and Abuse

Annie Lewis-O'Connor, Aitana Zermeno, and Kiara Manosalvas

> If you and I are having a single thought of violence or hatred against anyone in the world at this moment, we are contributing to the wounding of the world.
>
> **Deepak Chopra**

> Those who make peaceful revolution impossible will make violent revolution inevitable.
>
> **John F. Kennedy**

> You cannot shake hands with a clenched fist.
>
> **Golda Meir**

> From pacifist to terrorist, each person condemns violence—and then adds one cherished case in which it may be justified.
>
> **Gloria Steinem**

> Violence is immoral because it thrives on hatred rather than love. It destroys community and makes brotherhood impossible. It leaves society in monologue rather than dialogue.
>
> **Dr. Martin Luther King, Jr.**

CHAPTER HIGHLIGHTS

- Overview of violence in U.S. communities
- School violence
- Mandatory reporting of elder abuse, child maltreatment, and abuse of people with disabilities
- Intimate partner violence (IPV)
- Health consequences of exposure to IPV in children
- Model of care for victims of intentional crimes
- IPV as a major women's health problem, including impact on pregnancy
- Screening and intervention in IPV
- Risk and lethality assessment in IPV
- Role of healthcare providers: assessing for and intervening in violence and abuse

OBJECTIVES

- Identify the incidence and prevalence of intimate partner violence (IPV).
- Understand the health consequences that violence has on the health of patients and families.
- Explain the effects of IPV on adults and children.
- Summarize the models of care that have evolved in caring for victims of intentional violence.
- Describe interventional strategies (screening) and the limitations of measuring the effects of these interventions.
- Summarize the tenets of mandatory reporting laws.
- Apply nursing process in caring for and screening for IPV.

KEY TERMS

Femicide: A term used to refer to a homicide of a female person that occurs in the context of intimate partner violence (IPV).

Gender-based violence: A term used to distinguish violence which targets people, or groups of people, on the basis of their gender from other forms of violence (United Nation's Convention on the Elimination of All Forms of Discrimination against Women). It includes any act that results in, or is likely to result in, physical, sexual, or psychological harm such as rape, torture, mutilation, sexual slavery, forced impregnation, and murder.

Human rights: Basic rights and freedoms to which all humans are entitled.

Incidence: The number of cases of disease with an onset during a prescribed period of time; often expressed as a rate (e.g., the incidence of measles per 1,000 children 5 to 15 years of age during a specified year).

Intimate partner violence (IPV): A pattern of assaultive and coercive behaviors which may include inflicted physical injury, psychological abuse, sexual assault, progressive social isolation, deprivation, intimidation, and threats. These behaviors are perpetrated by someone who is, was, or wishes to be involved in an intimate or dating relationship with an adult or adolescent, and they are aimed at establishing control by one partner over the other (Family

Violence Prevention Fund, 1999).

Lethality assessment: An assessment that identifies high-risk factors for IPV.

Perpetrate: To be responsible for; commit, as in a crime.

Prevalence: Number of cases of a disease, infected persons, or people with some other attribute present during a particular interval of time; often expressed as a rate (e.g., the prevalence of diabetes per 1,000 persons during a year).

Violence: Framed in the context of "intentional" violence, or stated another way, that which is carried out by a person or persons against another person or persons when there is a conscious choice to act in a violent manner.

CASE STUDY

References to the case study are found throughout this chapter (look for the case study icon). Readers should keep the case study in mind as they read the chapter.

Kathy is a 28-year-old married woman with three children who are all younger than 6 years. The middle child has autism. Last year, Kathy had a miscarriage at 20 weeks following a fall down the stairs. She has not worked outside the home since the birth of her first child and is financially dependent on her husband. Her relationship with her husband has always been emotionally abusive, and although signs of physical abuse have been present during visits to Laura, a nurse practitioner and healthcare provider, Kathy has denied serious physical abuse except for an occasional push or shove. Sometimes, she has presented with bruises, which she has always said were accidental. After the birth of each child, Kathy has become quieter and seems sadder, and she has been noticeably depressed since her miscarriage. Recently, Kathy has admitted to Laura that she trusts her and needs her help because her husband's behavior is becoming worse and she is not sure what to do. Kathy does not wish to go to the police at this point. She denies direct harm to her children, yet she says "they must hear us arguing and fighting."

- What should Laura do to help Kathy?
- What should she consider about the safety of Kathy's children?
- What should Laura do if she becomes ambivalent about her disclosure?

Kathy has voiced her concerns related to finances, housing, and fear of retaliation by her partner—very personal information. There are several questions to consider: Does the state Kathy lives in have a mandatory reporting law for abuse against women (only six states do)? If Kathy is not ready to report the intimate partner violence to the police, what safety precautions can Laura address? If Kathy does report the violence to the police and her husband is arrested, there will be no income—how should Laura help Kathy address her economic concerns? (Also, the state budget has recently cut many services that were once available for victims of abuse.) Kathy may become homeless and unemployed, with no income for three small children and a partner who may retaliate. In addition to safety issues, there are many ethical and legal responsibilities which Laura needs to consider in developing a plan of care with the patient. It is essential that she also respects Kathy's autonomy.

OVERVIEW OF VIOLENCE

Violence in the United States is pervasive. In this chapter, **violence** is considered to be "intentional;" that is, violence is an act committed by a person or persons against another person or persons in which there is a conscious choice to act violently. When caring for the client's immediate needs, nurses should consider the cumulative exposures to violence over time and the far-reaching effects of violence on the family and the community at large. More than three decades of evidence is available to inform health practice and policy. The healthcare community is in a pivotal position to have a significant impact on the lives of clients affected by violence.

Violence has an adverse impact on society. It is estimated to cost billions of dollars per year (Dolezal, McCollum, & Callahan, 2009; Waters et al., 2004). These costs include direct medical care and rehabilitation and losses to the workforce (Corso, Mercy, Simon, Finkelstein, & Miller, 2007). The impact on families and the larger community is notable. *Healthy People 2020* has targeted injury and violence prevention as a priority. The injury prevention objectives of *Healthy People 2020* include (1) prevention and reduction of firearm-related deaths; (2) identification of improper firearm storage in homes; (3) surveillance of external causes of injury in emergency departments; (4) decreased incidents of homicide, child maltreatment, and physical assaults; (5) prevention and reduction of sexual assaults; and (6) elimination of weapon possession by adolescents on school property (*Healthy People 2020*). Such efforts require a multifaceted approach to public health that targets many settings and recognizes that social determinants of health such as exposures to violence result in poor health. Viewing violence from the many vantage points from which nurses deliver care (hospitals, home, clinics, schools, etc.) provides unique and complimentary healthcare to people experiencing violence and abuse.

Violence—look, we live in a violent world, man. This country was founded on violence. Who's kidding who? **Bruce Willis**

All forms of violent behavior can be attributed to the need for power and control. A number of factors have contributed to the prevalence of violence in the United States. Primary among those factors are the acceptability of violence in U.S. culture; racism, classism, and sexism; availability and accessibility of firearms; and lack of accountability.

Nothing is more despicable than respect based on fear.
Albert Camus

Guns

The United States is facing an escalating and unprecedented gun crisis. Each year, more than 32,000 persons die as a result of firearm-related violence, suicides, and accidents in the United States; this far surpasses the number of gun-related deaths in any other industrialized country (Richardson & Hemenway, 2011). In fact, America's gun homicide rate is more than 25 times the average of other high-income countries (Grinshteyn & Hemenway, 2016). Additionally, this violence comes at a substantial price to our nation, with a total societal cost of $174 billion in 2010 (Miller, 2015).

Firearms are the second leading cause of death due to injury after motor vehicle crashes for adults and adolescents. In 2014, there were 33,594 firearm deaths and 33,736 motor vehicle deaths, and while motor vehicle deaths in aggregate

16.1	**Gun-Related Deaths Versus Motor Vehicle Deaths, by State, 2014**

Alaska: 145 gun deaths, 87 motor vehicle deaths
Arizona: 927 gun deaths, 857 motor vehicle deaths
Colorado: 663 gun deaths, 545 motor vehicle deaths
District of Columbia: 86 gun deaths, 37 motor vehicle deaths
Illinois: 1,179 gun deaths, 1,075 motor vehicle deaths
Louisiana: 896 gun deaths, 807 motor vehicle deaths
Maryland: 546 gun deaths, 480 motor vehicle deaths
Michigan: 1,095 gun deaths, 1,014 motor vehicle deaths
Nevada: 429 gun deaths, 319 motor vehicle deaths
Oregon: 497 gun deaths, 380 motor vehicle deaths
Utah: 337 gun deaths, 261 motor vehicle deaths
Virginia: 899 gun deaths, 789 motor vehicle deaths
Washington: 702 gun deaths, 583 motor vehicle deaths

Source: Data from http://www.vpc.org/studies/gunsvscars16.pdf.

are higher than firearms deaths, firearm-related deaths outpaced motor vehicle deaths (CDC, 2016a). Box 16.1 lists several states where gun related deaths are higher than deaths from motor vehicle accidents.

The data on firearms is daunting. Nationwide, the overall gun death rate (suicides, homicides, and unintentional shootings) increased from 10.21 per 100,000 in 2009 to 11.96 per 100,000 in 2016. According to data from the CDC (2016b), on average, 96 Americans are killed every day by gun shot. Moreover, states with higher rates of gun ownership and weak gun violence prevention laws had the highest overall gun death rates in the nation (Violence Policy Center, 2017),

Dr. David Hemenway, director of the Harvard Injury Control Research Center, notes in his 2004 book *Private Guns, Public Health*, "The time Americans spend using their cars is orders of magnitude greater than the time spent using their guns. It is probable that per hour of exposure, guns are far more dangerous. Moreover, we have lots of safety regulations concerning the manufacture of motor vehicles; there are virtually no safety regulations for domestic firearms manufacturers." Nurses should be vigilant in assessing whether there is a gun present in the home and whether it is safely stored away from children (Fig. 16.1). Nurses are in key positions—in schools, clinics, offices, and hospitals—to inquire about guns in the home and provide anticipatory guidance on safety when a gun is stored in the home.

Other factors that contribute to homicides related to guns are low income, discrimination, lack of education, and lack of employment opportunities. Most often, males are the victims as well as the perpetrators of homicides. African American males are affected most frequently; in fact, African Americans are eight times more likely than white males to be murder victims (Quickstats, 2017). While African Americans constitute 14% of the population, they account for 50% of all homicide victims (Violence Policy Center, 2017). Although there has been a decline in the

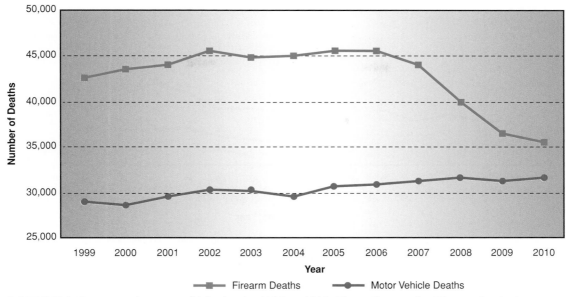

FIGURE 16.1 Firearm and motor vehicle deaths, 1999 to 2010. (From Centers for Disease Control and Prevention, National Center for Injury Prevention and Control, Division of Violence Prevention, 2008.)

homicide of intimate partners, including spouses, partners, boyfriends, and girlfriends, over the past decade, this problem remains significant and warrants conscious attention.

> Abuse a man unjustly, and you will make friends for him.
> **Douglas Horton**

School Violence

Over the past decade, the unthinkable has happened; children have been killed while at school. In December of 2012, the nation watched in horror as the news broke that Adam Lanza, 20, fatally shot 20 young elementary school children and six adult staff members in a mass murder at Sandy Hook Elementary School in Newtown, CT. Before driving to the school, Lanza had shot and killed his mother Nancy at their Newtown home. As first responders arrived, he committed suicide by shooting himself in the head. This event stimulated new debates about gun control and safety and mental health.

Five years later, the country continues to be plagued by tragic school shootings and persistent gun violence. On Wednesday, February 14, 2018, a gunman and fellow student shot and killed at least 17 students and staff at Marjory Stoneman Douglas High School in Parkland, FL. This act of senseless murder has now been marked as the deadliest school shooting since Sandy Hook. Homicide is the second leading cause of death among youths aged 5 to 18. Data from the school-associated violent death study illustrate that 1% to 2% of these deaths occur on school grounds or on the way to and from school. This underscores the importance of preventing violence in both schools and communities (Anderson et al., 2001). Firearms used in school-associated homicides and suicides came primarily from the perpetrator's home or from friends or

relatives (CDC, 2003). School shooting in the United States is a major public health concern; Kalesan and colleagues (2017) documented 154 school shootings between January 1, 2013 to December 31, 2015. However, the empirical evidence on this topic has often neglected to address two important domains—strong sentiments surrounding the Second Amendment and the culture of gun ownership in this country. Utilizing this lens, recent research has revealed that states with background check laws on firearm and ammunition purchases, higher capita mental health and K-12 education expenditures, and higher percent urban population have lower school shooting **incidence** rates (Kalesan et al., 2017).

Nurses working in educational settings must remain vigilant to the omnipresent risk factors that perpetuate violence in students. According to the data obtained from the Youth Risk Behavior Surveillance (Kann et al., 2016), 6% of students reported being threatened or injured with a weapon on school property in the preceding 12 months. Additionally, 5.6% of students reported not attending school on at least 1 day of the 30 days before the survey because they felt they would be unsafe at school or on their way to or from school. There were 20.2% of students who reported being bullied while at school in the past year, while 15.5% reported being electronically bullied via e-mail, chatrooms, instant message, websites, or texting. Finally, 15.5% of all public schools experienced one or more serious violent crimes such as rape, sexual assault, threatened or actual physical attack with a weapon, and robbery with or without a weapon. Sixty-nine percent of schools reported one or more violent incidents (Diliberti, Jackson, & Kemp, 2017). Since 1992, the Centers for Disease Control and Prevention (CDC) in partnership with the Departments of Education

FIGURE 16.2 Trends in school-associated violent deaths—1992 to 2010. (Data from Centers for Disease Control and Prevention, National Center for Injury Prevention and Control (NCIPC), http://www.cdc.gov/violenceprevention/youthviolence/schoolviolence/savd.html.)

and Justice has been conducting surveillance on school-related deaths (Fig. 16.2). Data from a number of the current national surveys are in process from collection to analysis to publication (Anderson et al., 2001; CDC, 2001, 2003; Robers, Zhang, Truman, & Snyder, 2012).

> Because in the 2 months since Newtown, more than a thousand birthdays, graduations, and anniversaries have been stolen from our lives by a bullet from a gun. **President Barack Obama**

School nurses play a pivotal role in recognizing both children who are being victimized and those who are perpetrating violence. School nurses working with teachers, school administrators, and school psychologists are in a unique position to create an environment that promotes primary prevention and intervention. By addressing and discussing with students the root causes of violence through their educational curriculum, school nurses and educators might be able to shift the paradigm to a less violent one. Schools are fertile climates for education about prevention of violence. Violence prevention should start at home and continue in school (see Chapter 22).

> Education is a vaccine for violence. **Edward James Olmos, Mexican American actor**

Practice Point

Thinking about the root causes of violence helps nurses develop primary prevention strategies (raising awareness about violence), along with secondary (identifying those at risk for being abused or perpetrating abuse) and tertiary prevention interventions (identified victim or perpetrator).

INTIMATE PARTNER VIOLENCE

Intimate Partner Violence: A Major Women's Health Problem

The phenomenon of **intimate partner violence (IPV)** differs depending on culture, discipline, theoretical framework, and philosophical perspectives. Gradually, violence against women has been recognized globally as a **human rights** violation with significant consequences for the individual, family, and community. IPV does target an individual person, but the effects on bystanders are far reaching, affecting local, state, public, and private sectors through loss of productivity, and contributing to medical and mental health costs. Although data support the belief that men are generally the perpetrators of IPV, most healthcare providers and researchers recognize that women may also, though rarely, **perpetrate** violence against their intimate partner. In the early 1990s, the international community adopted the term **gender-based violence** when referring to violence against women and girls (United Nations, 1993). This terminology appears to reflect the evolution of researchers who have sought to understand the nature of abuse that is perpetrated against females. Although there have been variations in the definition of IPV among researchers, over the past decade, these definitions have become increasingly similar. Healthcare providers see victims of IPV daily in their practice, and identification can lead to interventions that may help to decrease morbidity and mortality.

> One of the speakers asked how many women had been harassed or abused sexually in their life? There were thousands of women in the audience, and almost every one of them raised her hand. **Cheryl James (Salt), American rapper**

Investigators conducting population-based studies in the United States over the past several years have consistently reported a lifetime **prevalence** of IPV against women to be between 25% and 30%, with an annual prevalence between 2% and 12% (Black, Basile, & Breiding, 2011; Humphreys, Parker, & Campbell, 2001; Jones et al., 1999; Tjaden & Thoennes, 2000; Wilt & Olson, 1996). More recently, using a population-based national sample of women older than 18 years ($n = 1,800$) and calculating adult lifetime and prior-year prevalence of violent experiences, Moracco, Runyan, and Butts (2003) found that 60% of respondents experienced at least one form of violence since the age of 18, with 10% reporting violence in the previous year. Adult lifetime and prior-year prevalence varies by type of violence and respondents' sociodemographic characteristics. Some of the inconsistencies reported in the literature are due to variations in defining the nature of the abuse (e.g., stalking, rape, emotional abuse, or verbal abuse) and limitations in sampling. Often, purposeful and convenient sampling was used in these studies.

Extent of Intimate Partner Violence

The literature on IPV is substantial and has evolved exponentially over the past two decades. The World Health Organization's world report on violence and health (Krug, Dahlberg, Mercy, Zwi, & Lozano, 2002) found that in 48 population-based surveys from around the world, between 10% and 69% of women reported being physically assaulted by an intimate male partner at some point in their lives. This is important for nurses to recognize. Many women who have immigrated to the United States have long been exposed to violence in their country of origin, and awareness of this fact has significant implications for nursing plans of care. In addition, nurses need to know that half of all female homicide victims are murdered by their intimate partners (Petrosky et al., 2017). The majority of women killed with a gun were killed by their intimate partners (Bailey et al., 1997; Hemingway, 2004; Moracco et al., 2003). The report, which looked at 10,000 homicides between 2003 and 2014, revealed that one in 10 victims of intimate partner violence–related homicide experienced some form of violence in the month prior to being killed.

Research in the area of homicides has helped to inform nursing practice, particularly in relation to the risk to children. In a 10-city study of risk factors for intimate partner **femicide** (murder of women) or attempted femicide, Lewandowski, McFarlane, Campbell, Gary, and Barenski (2004) found that 59% of domestic violence victims had children. About 33% of the children had witnessed the incident, and 43% were the first to find the mother's body. Nurses must be aware that some 35% to 60% of children who live in homes where there is IPV are themselves physically or sexually abused (Edelson, 1999), with fathers as the most common perpetrators (McCloskey, Figueredo, & Koss, 1995).

In the context of family-centered care, it is imperative that Laura considers the safety of the children. In the hopes of preventing further abuse in Kathy's situation, Laura should know about resources in the community. If Kathy has the phone numbers of local women's shelters, food banks, mental health agencies, unemployment offices, and the Women, Infants, and Children (WIC) program, she will be able to use these resources when she is ready to do so. By providing these resources, Laura hopes to give Kathy the confidence, with the support behind her, to make the right decisions for her family. Also, and equally important, Laura gains a better understanding of the factors that affect a victim's ability to make well-informed decisions.

Dr. Jacquelyn Campbell, a pioneer nurse researcher in the area of IPV, published the earliest data on the health consequences of IPV (Campbell, 2002) and has developed and implemented a multilanguage **lethality assessment** (Campbell, 1981, 1986, 1992, 1995a, 1995b, 1995c; Campbell et al., 2003a) tool for homicide. Dr. Campbell's research indicates that factors such as access to a firearm, the abuser's use of illicit drugs, unemployment, control of daily activities, stepchildren in the home, and threats to kill the victim pose serious risks for homicide for a woman (Table 16.1; Box 16.2). In particular, the presence of a firearm in the home is a risk factor for homicide in women (Campbell et al., 2003a; Kellerman & Heron, 1999; Sorenson & Wiebe, 2004; Wiebe, 2003). These data underscore the necessity for nurses to screen clients for access to and/or presence of a gun in the home, and to provide education about safe storage.

While assessing how the abuse is affecting Kathy and her children, it is important to explore lethality risks (Box 16.3). Although the presence of lethality risk factors does not imply that Kathy is in imminent danger, the presence of these factors does warrant an in-depth assessment, such as a multilanguage danger assessment tool that is reliable and valid. Such in-depth assessments are dependent on the practice environment and the availability of social services. It is important to know what in-house and community referral resources are available.

In response to the evidence that IPV profoundly affects the health of victims and children, many professional organizations, such as the American Medical Association Council on Scientific Affairs (1992), American Nurses Association

TABLE 16.1	Risk Factors for Intimate Partner Violence
Individual risk factors	• Low self-esteem • Low income • Low academic achievement • Young age • Aggressive behavior as a child • Heavy alcohol/drug use • Depression • Anger and hostility • Antisocial personality traits • Borderline personality traits • History of being physically abused • Few friends/isolation and abused • Unemployment • Emotional dependence and insecurity • Belief in strict gender roles • Desire for power and control • Perpetrating psychological aggression in relationships • Victim of physical or psychological abuse as a child • Experiencing poor parenting • Experiencing physical discipline as a child
Relationship factors	• Economic stress • Marital conflicts (e.g., fights) • Marital instability (e.g., divorce/separation) • Dominance/control of relationship by one partner over another • Unhealthy family relationships and interactions
Community factors/societal factors	• Poverty and associated factors (e.g., overcrowding) • Low social capital—lack of institutions, relationships, and norms that shape a community's social interactions • Weak community sanctions against intimate partner violence (e.g., unwillingness of neighbors to intervene when violence is witnessed) • Traditional gender roles (e.g., women should stay at home, be submissive, not enter the workforce; men support the family and make the decisions)

(ANA) (1991), the American College of Obstetricians and Gynecologists (1993), and the Association of Women's Health, Obstetric, and Neonatal Nurses (AWHONN) established screening and routine assessment guidelines for IPV as the standard of practice. Valuable websites like Futures

16.2 Risk Factors That Indicate Significant Concern for the Safety of the Children

• Threats to kill the caretaker, children, and/or self; caretaker fears for the children's safety.
• A child was physically injured in an incident when the caretaker was the target.
• A child was coerced to participate in or witness the abuse of the caretaker.
• A weapon was used or threats were made to use a weapon, and the caretaker believed that there was intention and ability to cause harm.

Without Violence (www.futureswithoutviolence.org), Academy on Violence (www.AVA.org), and National Health Collaborative on Violence and Abuse (www.Nhcva.org) provide much information for healthcare providers.

Student Reflection

I had never been involved in screening for routine assessment guidelines until I needed some minor surgery in my sophomore year in college. In the preoperative phase of the process, a nurse asked me whether I felt safe where I lived. (My boyfriend was waiting for me in a coffee shop at the medical center where I was having my surgery.) At first, I did not expect the question, but then I understood that the nurse was asking me about IPV, and whether I was at risk. It made me really happy to see that a nurse was asking such an important assessment question. Although this situation did not apply to me, I could see how this could be an opportunity for a client to obtain help or advice. However, I also realize that this could lead to breaking emotional or financial ties with another person or dealing with the children who resulted from a relationship that has become abusive.

High rates of IPV have long been detected in emergency departments (Abbott, Johnson, Koziol-McLain, & Lowenstein, 1995; Kothari et al., 2015), prenatal clinics (Fletcher, Clements, & Bailey, 2016; Helton, McFarlane, & Anderson,

16.3 Lethality Risks

• Is there a gun in the house?
• Is the woman's partner unemployed?
• What is the worst thing the partner has ever done to the victim?
• Does the victim feel that the partner is capable of hurting her? Of carrying out his threats?
• Has the woman's partner ever been arrested?
• Is the woman's partner using drugs? Drinking excessively?

1987; Martin & Clements, 2002; McFarlane, Parker, Soeken, & Bullock, 1992); internal medicine practices, health maintenance organizations (Gin, Rucker, Frayne, & Cygan, 1992; Hamberger, Saunders, & Hovey, 1992; Jones et al., 1999), and hospitalizations when clients are admitted for behavioral health disorders, substance abuse, and suicidality (Kernic, Wolf, & Holt, 2000).

The literature has well documented the risks of IPV and pregnancy (Chang, Berg, Herndon, & Saltzman, 2005; Sarkar, 2008). Depression before, during, and after birth has been strongly correlated with IPV (Ogbonnaya, Macy, Kupper, Martin, & Bledsoe-Mansori, 2013). In a National Institutes of Health (NIH)-supported population analysis of 5 million records of California women over a 10-year period, researchers found that pregnant women who are assaulted by an intimate partner are at increased risk of giving birth to infants of reduced weight (NIH News, 2011). Although the results showed a pattern of low-weight births among women who experienced an assault, the study was not designed to establish cause and effect or explain the biologic factors for how violence against an expectant mother might cause her to deliver a low–birth-weight infant. It is now standard of practice that all pregnant women are screened for IPV during each trimester of their pregnancy, following the birth of the infant, and in cases in which there are concerns (see ACOG, http://www.acog.org/Resources_And_Publications/Committee_Opinions/Committee_on_Health_Care_for_Underserved_Women/Intimate_Partner_Violence#11a).

Women victimized by abuse are more likely to be diagnosed with serious health problems, including depression and panic attacks, as well as migraine headaches, chronic pain, arthritis, high blood pressure, gastrointestinal problems, inconsistent use of birth control, and delayed entry into prenatal care (Campbell & Lewandowski, 1997; Weiss, Lawrence, & Miller, 2002). In fact, much has been learned about how reproductive coercion—pressuring partners to get pregnant and direct interference with contraception—is a significant factor in relationships in which IPV is of concern (Miller, et al., 2010). National data show approximately 9% (or 10.3 million) women experience reproductive coercion; this number is estimated to be higher in women seeking reproductive health services (Clark, Allen, Goyal, Raker, & Gottlieb, 2014). It is essential to ask a woman about her ability to control her fertility issues and desires during reproductive healthcare visits.

In addition, women affected by IPV are more likely to engage in high-risk behaviors such as tobacco use, substance abuse, and sexual risk-taking (e.g., multiple sexual partners) (Silverman, Raj, & Clemens, 2004; Silverman, Raj, Mucci, & Hathaway, 2001). Nurses who recognize the significant impact of IPV, both acute and chronic, may be more influential in developing treatment plans with their patients that seek to intervene early, thus preventing some of the long-term mental and physical effects that are associated with IPV.

I had been, you know, held in the closet for two months and, you know, abused in all manner of ways. I was very good at doing what I was told. **Patty Hearst, kidnap ping victim**

Evidence for Practice

Validation of many of the findings from research on the long-term effects of experiencing or witnessing IPV were validated by the adverse childhood experiences (ACEs) study, one of the largest studies of its kind. This study has been a decade-long collaboration between the Division of Adult and Community Health at the CDC and Kaiser Permanente's Department of Preventive Medicine in San Diego. The researchers designed the study to examine the health and social effects of ACEs throughout the lifespan. It involved 17,337 middle-class members of the Kaiser Permanente Medical Care Program in San Diego who agreed to participate during the course of a comprehensive medical evaluation (Anda et al., 1999; Dube, Felitti, Dong, Giles, & Anda, 2003; Edwards et al., 2005; Felitti et al., 1998). It is important to note that this was a homogenous sample of middle-class Caucasians. However, the findings are significant and have important implications for practice (see www.acesconnections.com).

In this study, researchers assessed 10 categories of stressful or traumatic childhood experiences (Dong et al., 2004). They chose a broad range of ACEs that had been shown to have significant adverse health or social implications. Examples of ACEs are as follows:

- Childhood abuse (emotional, physical, and sexual)
- Neglect (emotional and physical)
- Growing up in a seriously dysfunctional household (battered mother, substance abuse, or mental illness in the home; parental separation or divorce; or a criminal household member)

In the case of participants who had a battered mother, 95% reported at least one additional ACE. The researchers also studied the relationship of childhood physical or sexual abuse, or growing up with a battered mother, to the risk of being a victim (among women) or perpetrator (among men) of IPV as an adult (Whitfield, Anda, Dube, & Felitti, 2003). Each of these three ACEs is associated with the risk of IPV; as the number of these violent childhood experiences increased, the risk of IPV also increased (CDC, 2008).

The history of Kathy's childhood or that of her husband is unknown. How an ACE score affects the ability to parent and to participate in healthy relationships is not known. The ACE score specifically considers the relationship between ACEs and health indicators, such as chronic obstructive pulmonary disease, hypertension, risky behaviors, weight, and mental health issues. It can be postulated from the ACE study that if Kathy's children remain in a home where violence is present, they would be at risk for health issues as adults.

Healthy People 2020 emphasizes a need to prevent violence and the sequelae known to result from exposure to violence, recognizing that violence leads to the following:

- Premature death
- Disability
- Poor mental health
- High medical costs
- Lost productivity

The objectives of violence prevention identified by *Healthy People 2020* are to reduce fatal and nonfatal injuries, fatal and nonfatal traumatic brain injuries, homicides, firearm injuries, and physical and sexual assaults. Preventing violence and recurrence of violence requires targeting efforts at all three levels of prevention: primary, secondary, and tertiary. There has been a great debate over the benefits of primary and secondary prevention because measuring the benefits of outcomes has intrinsic methodologic issues. However, when the United States Preventive Services Task Force (USPSTF) reviewed the literature on interventions in 2010, they found sufficient evidence to support inquiry and brief counseling for patients. The USPSTF (Moyer, 2013) recommends that clinicians screen women of childbearing age for IPV, and provide intervention services or refer women who screen positive to intervention services (http://www.uspreventiveservicestaskforce.org/uspstf12/ipvelder/ipvelderfinalrs.htm#summary).

It is well known that IPV occurs within all socioeconomic groups. Many victims and perpetrators of IPV differ in their opinions of what constitutes abuse. Opinions may be dependent on many factors: prior exposures, cultural identification, family and peer opinions, and education. Efforts to educate must be persistent, constant, multilingual, and culturally aware and must target both potential victims and potential perpetrators. Secondary prevention occurs through generalized screening and inquiry with high-risk populations.

Decades of research have indicated that some women have a higher risk of IPV (see Table 16.1). The model most widely used to understand violence is the ecologic model. This model proposes that violence is a result of factors operating at four levels: individual, relationship, community, and societal (Krug et al., 2002). Risk factors include age less than 45, low income, lack of employment, recent separation or divorce, education at the high school level or lower, and having young children (Campbell et al., 2003b). Currently under debate is how to implement policies and procedures

for the identification of perpetration of violence. Issues such as safety, what to do when a person states he or she is hurting someone, and ethical considerations require in-depth discussions with collaborative community participation.

Kathy has risk factors for IPV: a long-term emotionally abusive relationship, isolation, stressors related to having a child with autism, and financial dependence on her husband. In the context of a healthcare setting, a woman may feel that she is able to trust her provider, and thus, with proper inquiry, interventions may be offered which would assist Kathy.

Tertiary prevention (caring for victims affected by, or currently experiencing, violence) has been a major focus in the health system, and has been driven by The Joint Commission. Prior to The Joint Commission's 1998 mandate to implement policies and procedures, victims of abuse received less than optimal care within the healthcare system (The Joint Commission on Accreditation of Healthcare Organizations, 1995). Over several years, The Joint Commission required all clinical settings such as community health centers, primary care, emergency departments, and operating rooms to implement identification and interventions for victims of abuse. This was the catalyst for change within the healthcare system. Advocates working in healthcare found that this was the incentive they needed to move forward and to provide quality services for victims and their family members within the context of a healthcare environment. This movement continues to evolve today, with many hospitals and healthcare facilities employing advocates and organizing formal programs (Hathaway, Zimmer, Willis, & Silverman, 2008).

Victims of violence and abuse may often face barriers when seeking help, either immediately afterward or months or years later when the previous violence begins to affect their health. Successful programs in primary, secondary, and tertiary prevention are a critical element necessary for preventing abuse and helping victims recover while mitigating the health consequences.

Intimate Partner Violence: Health Consequences in Children Who Witness Abuse

It is alarming to consider how many children may be exposed to IPV. The most recent National Survey of Children's Exposure to Violence found that 25% of older children surveyed had witnessed a parent assault another parent (or parental partner) in their lifetime, and 5.8% had witnessed such an assault in the past year (Finkelhor, Turner, Shattuck, & Hamby, 2015). Very young children are more likely to be disproportionately represented in studies because disclosure and identification are limited due to their development and age. These young children are not always able to get out of harm's way. Adolescents often try to intervene to protect the parent being abused. Younger children, from birth to 3 years of age, have received far less attention, and thus, their responses to the IPV directed toward their mothers are less well understood (Berman, Hardesty, & Humphreys, 2004). However, author and social worker Betsy McAlister Groves succinctly addressed the impact of violence on children 8 years of age and younger in her book *Children Who See Too Much* (2002). Groves found that young children exposed to IPV during this early period have experienced physical, intellectual, emotional, and behavioral problems.

Exposure to IPV has long-lasting effects on child development, including adverse health outcomes and adjustment problems such as aggression (Bair-Merritt et al., 2015; Piotrowski, Tachie, & Cameranesi, 2017; Vu, Jouriles, McDonald, & Rosenfield, 2016). Health consequences and behavioral issues may not become prominent until long after the initial exposure to IPV, denoted as the "sleeper effect" (Vu et al., 2016). In the landmark ACEs study, a strong relationship was established between childhood trauma and adult health risk behaviors responsible for many of the leading causes of death (Felitti et al., 1998). This evidence demands that IPV be treated as a serious health risk for children.

It has been documented that IPV duration is longer when the couple has children, and children are often the reason mothers remain in, leave, or return to an abusive relationship (Nouer, Mackey, Tipton, Miller, & Connor, 2014). Children influence IPV victims' decisions to seek service providers' aid; therefore, pediatricians are encouraged to intervene in an empathetic and skillful manner (Nouer et al., 2014). The American Academy of Pediatrics (2010) has not found sufficient evidence to recommend a universal or case-by-case approach over another. However, routinely assessing for IPV leads to increased identification of victims, and disclosure is not necessary for providers to inform patients of available resources in an offensive manner. Several screening tools exist, many of which have been validated (Thackeray, Hibbard, Dowd, et al., 2010). Safely carrying out screening requires that providers be aware of issues unique to the pediatric setting: the parent is not the client and documentation in the medical record may provide information to a potential abusive partner. Moreover, the conversation should be held in private, as even small children can be affected by hearing troubling information. Creative strategies have been explored to address these issues and promising practices have been identified that include the following:

- Opening the conversation with a statement such as, "Because we know that exposure to violence is so common and has negative effects on health, I talk to all my families about safety in their homes."
- Asking mothers with a self-administered tool (written questionnaire, computer survey)

- Asking mothers directly, without the child present
- Having providers inform parents about mandatory reporting laws prior to asking questions
- Being able to screen for safety and dangerousness of the situation
- Being aware of resources and referrals (Lewis-O'Connor, 2007)

Practice Point

Some strong evidence suggests that living in a violent home has detrimental effects later in life. Knowing this and integrating this into practice help the nurse recognize and prevent long-term healthcare issues.

Screening for Intimate Partner Violence

In 2012, the USPSTF issued a recommendation in support of IPV screening and counseling (Nelson, Bougatsos, & Blazina, 2012). However, some researchers continue to have opposing views (MacMillan et al., 2009). For instance, there is no direct evidence that screening results in decreased disability or premature death.

The Affordable Care Act (ACA)—the health insurance reform legislation passed by Congress and signed into law by President Obama on March 23, 2010—helps make prevention affordable and accessible for all Americans. The ACA requires health plans to cover preventive services for women by eliminating cost sharing. Preventive services have proven evidence of improved health outcomes. Under the ACA, women's preventive healthcare screening and counseling for interpersonal and domestic violence are among eight preventive measures (http://www.hrsa.gov/womensguidelines/). The Institute of Medicine found that after reviewing the literature, there was sufficient evidence to support screening and brief counseling for IPV. When screening for IPV and assessing for risk, nurses need to make these questions a normal and routine part of healthcare assessment that fits in the context of the visit. Experts have found that wallet-size cards with information about IPV and resources can serve as a time-efficient clinical prompt from a universal education approach (Miller et al., 2010).

Screening without being prepared for a positive disclosure could be more harmful than helpful. It is important to know what resources are available and how to respond to the needs of the client before asking questions. Box 16.4 presents a sampling of questions that can be asked. Ideal screening includes questions not only about physical and sexual abuse, but also about emotional and financial abuse. Nurses should use their own language in asking these questions, need to ensure that the questions are developmentally and culturally appropriate, and use language appropriate to the client's level of comprehension.

16.4 Inquiry and Assessment for Intimate Partner Violence

Assessment for Intimate Partner Abuse

To begin the conversation about IPV, you may say "I now ask all my clients about past or current abuse in their lives because I recognize its impact on one's well-being. I ask so that I can help my clients identify help and support." Screening questions need to be culturally and developmentally framed. Such questions include the following:

- Are you currently experiencing or have you ever experienced physical or emotional harm/abuse in an intimate relationship? Has anyone ever forced you to engage in sexual activity that you did not want to participate in?
- Has your current partner ever pushed, shoved, slapped, or otherwise physically hurt you?
- Every couple has arguments and disagrees—what happens when you and your partner disagree?
- Does your partner ever make you feel afraid or scared? Tell me more.
- Are you currently being hurt by someone? Are you in a safe or unsafe situation? (When I see a client with a bruise such as this, I want to make sure he or she is safe.)

Follow-Up Questions When a Woman States That She Is Being Abused

- Can you tell me the worst thing that has ever happened? What happened? When did it happen? Where did it happen? Where were the children? Was a weapon used?
- Do you feel your partner is capable of hurting you or your children?
- What actions have you taken?
- What are your fears? What would you like me to help you with? Please help me understand what is happening. I would like to help.
- Are you in danger now? Can you tell me more about this?
- Have you ever needed emergency medical care as a result of how you were hurt? Can you tell me more about this?
- How has the abuse affected you? Do you ever think about hurting yourself, cutting, stopping eating, or purging food?
- Have you ever thought about or been granted a restraining order? What happened?
- Have you ever left? What happened? What obstacles did you face?
- What are your fears about your children? Are you worried about their safety?

Evidence for Practice

Working with victims of violence is best approached using the principles of trauma-informed care, which recognizes that patients with a history of traumatic events may feel triggered and retraumatized when accessing healthcare. Trauma survivors have reported barriers such as disjointed or chaotic care and receiving conflicting or misinformation from different providers (Lewis-O'Connor & Chadwick, 2015). To minimize distress and remove the need for the patient to retell their story, experts emphasize the need to coordinate care with warm referrals amongst multidisciplinary collaborators who are well-versed in trauma-informed care (Reeves, 2015).

People have all grown up with internalized myths, and it is imperative that healthcare providers be aware of clients' beliefs and work actively to dispel those myths so that healthcare interventions do not retraumatize clients. Victims and survivors of IPV are sensitive to nuances of words, tone of voice, and body language; so, providers must guard against making judgmental gestures, even if subtle and unintentional, because they may have an impact on the interaction between clients and providers. Healthcare professionals must take every precaution to avoid blaming victims of IPV. Victims have often lost trust in relationships, so nurses must work to build trust and not assume its existence.

Nurses can best implement the principles of trauma-sensitive care by actively listening, validating, and supporting clients as they tell their story (Box 16.5) (Elliott, Bjelajac, Fallot, Markoff, & Reed, 2005). It is imperative to keep safety issues for the victims (and children) in the forefront. Given that at the core of abusive relationships are the issues of power and control, nurses must make efforts to maximize patient autonomy. An example is explicitly asking for consent before and at each step of a sexual assault examination (Lewis-O'Connor & Chadwick, 2015). Nurses should not try to "rescue" clients; rather, they should seek to empower clients to be able to make informed decisions. It is essential to always be honest about what nurses can and cannot do, especially regarding confidentiality and mandatory reporting. Nurses should never make promises about circumstances over which they have no control, as this may cause more harm than good.

16.5 Trauma-Sensitive Care: Principles

- Demonstrate respect.
- Establish and maintain rapport.
- Share control.
- Share information.
- Respect boundaries.
- Foster a mutual learning process.
- Show compassion and avoid passing judgment.

Practice Point

The nurse's role needs to focus on sensitive communication, active listening, providing information and choices, risk assessment, medical and psychological treatment, safety planning, referral, and follow-up. Providers should be familiar with protocols that promote patient-centered assessment and interventions. When a client screens positive for IPV, it is imperative to assess for his or her safety and risk of harm. Communicating concern by validating the client's story builds trust between client and provider. Statements such as "Donna, I am so sorry that this is happening; help is available," "Thank you for sharing this with me; I would like to ask you some safety questions so that I can better understand your situation," "You are not alone and you deserve better," "This must be so difficult for you," "This is not your fault," and "I am here to help you unconditionally" are appropriate responses. We need to create systems with our patients rather than asking our patients to fit into our existing systems. While further outcomes research is warranted, centering a practice on trauma-informed principles ensures that the unique needs of this vulnerable population are met.

So many people suffer from abuse, and suffer alone. **Pamela Stephenson, Australian clinical psychologist**

Safety Assessment and Planning in Intimate Partner Violence

How an in-depth safety assessment is conducted depends on the practice environment and staff model. Whoever is conducting the safety assessment needs to seek advanced training on risk assessment, and needs to be aware of community resources. The most validated and used instrument to assess for safety is the tool developed by Campbell (1986), the lethality assessment tool. It is a 20-item tool available on the internet in English, Spanish, Portuguese, and French Creole, and recent analyses indicate it has high sensitivity (92% to 93%) and predictive value (93% to 96%) (Messing, Campbell, Sullivan Wilson, Brown, & Patchell, 2017). Campbell developed this instrument to identify women at risk of being murdered by their intimate partners. It often heightens a woman's awareness about her safety. Once the safety issues are identified, the healthcare provider can present intervention options to the client.

Safety planning involves nurse suggestions and client choices (e.g., does the client feel she is able to keep herself safe? Does she have friends or family members who could help? Does she have a supportive employer?). Components for safety planning include a crisis/disaster plan, a place to go, how to get there, and other considerations (e.g., if the abused victim stays and the abuser leaves, if victim and the abuser stay together, or if the victim decides to leave). Safety planning involves discussing measures that the client may not have considered. For example, if an argument occurs at home, the woman should stay away from (1) the kitchen because sharp instruments are there and (2) from the bathroom because the space is small and contains many hard surfaces. She should go to a room with a window or door,

carry her cell phone with 911 set to speed dial, and tell family members and neighbors. Healthcare organizations should actively partner with local shelters and court advocates, as they can assist with safety plans.

MANDATORY REPORTING OF ABUSE

When any healthcare provider suspects that abuse of an elderly person, a child, or a person with a disability has occurred, he or she is mandated to report the abuse to the appropriate agency (Box 16.6). It must be kept in mind that the data reflects the number of reported cases and not the actual number of abused people as some cases may have had multiple reports.

Elder Abuse

Starting in 2011, the Baby Boom generation (those born between 1946 and 1964) entered into the cohort of those aged 65 years and older. In 2010, there were 40.3 million people aged 65 or over. To put this in some perspective, this is 12 times the number of persons who were over the age of 65 in 1990 (https://www.census.gov/content/dam/Census/library/publications/2014/demo/p23-212.pdf).

Elder mistreatment (i.e., abuse and neglect) is defined as intentional actions that cause harm or create a serious risk of harm (whether or not harm is intended) to a vulnerable elder by a caregiver or other person who stands in a trust relationship to the elder. This includes failure by a caregiver to satisfy the elder's basic needs or to protect the elder from harm (Bonnie & Wallace, 2003). Valid incidence and prevalence rates for elder abuse and neglect are not available. The CDC website states, "While the National Center on Elder Abuse (NCEA) has collected and analyzed state adult protective services data, the number of additional data elements that might be available through healthcare, long-term care, criminal justice, fiduciary, and legal services networks has

16.6 Considerations When Making a Mandatory Report

- Talk with the adult victim about the possibility of filing a mandatory report.
- Consider the safety concerns of filing.
- Determine how the perpetrator may respond to a report being filed.
- Determine whether it will be safe to inform the children about the report.
- Identify resources available to victim (family, friends, clergy, coworkers).
- Consider filing in concert with the adult victim.
- Share concerns of safety with the child protective agency.
- Address safety planning with the nonoffending victim.
- Ask about the perpetrator's behaviors: What is the worst thing he or she has done? Does he or she own a gun? Has he or she been arrested? Does he or she use drugs? Do you think he or she is capable of hurting you or your children?

remained largely unexplored" (https://www.cdc.gov/violenceprevention/elderabuse/datasources.html).

From available data, it does appear that female elders (those aged 60 years and older) are abused at a higher rate than males and that the older one is, the more likely one is to be abused (Teaster et al., 2004). The number of aging Americans will likely continue to increase. Therefore, concern for abuse and victimization of this population will require effective proactive programs to identify elder abuse, and provide the necessary resources to prevent and treat this vulnerable population.

As a nurse, it is essential to know both the mandatory reporting laws in the state in which the nurse practices, and the policies and procedures to be followed within the workplace. Although the nurse may view the decision to report as "damaging" to the nurse–client relationship, he or she has a duty to report the abuse as mandated by the state. It is necessary to regard mandatory reports in the context of acting for the safety of the abused person, rather than reporting against the alleged perpetrator.

Child Maltreatment

Although elder abuse has been acknowledged and addressed only more recently, child maltreatment has been prevalent for centuries. The federal Child Abuse Prevention and Treatment Act (CAPTA) (42 U.S.C.A. §5106g), as amended by the Keeping Children and Families Safe Act of 2003 (U.S. Department of Health and Human Services, 2003), defines child abuse and neglect as follows:

- Any recent act, or failure to act, on the part of a parent or caretaker which results in death, serious physical or emotional harm, sexual abuse, or exploitation; or
- An act or failure to act which presents an imminent risk of serious harm

According to the most recent data available from the U.S. Department of Health and Human Services, Administration for Children and Families (2017), our rates of child maltreatment continue to be disturbing. These data report an increase, citing 676,000 cases of child maltreatment, up from 656,000 in 2012. Neglect remains the highest form for maltreatment (74.8%), with 18.2% reporting physical abuse and 8.5% reporting sexual abuse. The nationally estimated death rate for abuse and neglect stands at 2.36 per 100,000 children (https://www.acf.hhs.gov/sites/default/files/cb/cm2016.pdf). School nurses, visiting nurses, public health nurses, and pediatric nurses must be familiar with signs and symptoms for children at risk. Early identification and intervention are key to mitigating the effects on child development and well-being.

Prevention strategies that address child maltreatment offer the best hope for reducing the incidence of child abuse or neglect. Early identification may help prevent significant morbidity and mortality. Over the past decade, much attention has been given to the effects of children witnessing violence in the home. Researchers indicate that witnessing violence in the home can have significant developmental and psychological sequelae and affect health subsequently, even into adulthood (Dube et al., 2003; Groves, 2002).

> I was angry about the fact that my father would beat my mother on a daily basis, that my mother would take it in turn and beat on me. I was an abused child. I was mad about all those things, very bitter and very angry. **Rick James, American singer, songwriter, musician**

Often, the strongest protective factor in the lives of children who are exposed to domestic violence is support for the nonoffending parent. Futures Without Violence produced a document entitled *The Facts on Children and Domestic Violence* (2008). This is an excellent resource for healthcare providers. A safe, stable, and nurturing relationship with a caring adult can help a child overcome the stress associated with IPV (Middlebrooks & Audage, 2008).

As the nurse caring for Kathy, Laura needs to assess the following, using observation skills and appropriate questioning:

- Her children's current functioning
- Changes in her children's behavior
- Changes in her children's functioning as a result of the perpetrator's actions

Laura uses Boxes 16.2 and 16.6 to assess whether there is significant concern about the safety of Kathy's children. After reviewing the data and consulting with team members, Laura may decide to file a report with the child protective agency. Laura would want to share this with Kathy as a resource that could assist her.

Deciding whether a particular case may involve abuse that requires reporting is often difficult. Collaborating with others on the healthcare team ensures a well-informed decision. Nurses should remember that when they file a report for concern of child maltreatment, they are filing on behalf of the child, not against an individual person. If no report of child maltreatment is necessary, nurses should still encourage the affected mother to express her family's immediate needs, seek the support of a community domestic violence advocate, tell her about family services that meet their immediate needs, identify the family's support system, assist her in developing a safety plan, and consult with child protection experts and/or other domestic violence providers.

Abuse of Disabled People

Although overall trends in violence and abuse seem to be decreasing, Americans with disabilities seem to experience abuse disproportionately. In fact, research and the anecdotal experience of those who work with people with disabilities suggest that this population is experiencing a heightened risk of becoming victims of violence and abuse; however, research on this population is sparse.

Only limited and dated information that addresses the issues affecting this group can be found. One study found that more than 70% of women with developmental disabilities are sexually assaulted in their lifetime, which represents a 50% higher rate than the rest of the population (Sobsey & Doe, 1991; Sobsey, 1994). In another frequently cited study, Young, Nosek, Howland, Chanpong, and Rintala (1997) found that women with physical disabilities appear to be at risk of emotional, physical, and sexual abuse to the same extent as women without physical disabilities. It appears that people with cognitive disabilities, who have a desire to be accepted and "fit in," may acquiesce to behaviors they are not quite comfortable with because of fear of social isolation. Often, a person with a disability is dependent on another, and that dependency prevents him or her from recognizing abuse and seeking help. Even when a person with a disability reports a crime, the victim is often not believed, and is viewed as not credible. It was only in 1998 that Congress passed the Crime Victims with Disabilities Awareness Act. This represented the first piece of national legislation in U.S. history to address the issue of abuse of persons with disabilities. Such legislation draws attention at many levels—policy, research, advocacy, and law enforcement.

Awareness of the risks to persons in the disabled population should guide nursing practice through the tasks of assessing clients at risk, discussing prevention strategies with clients and their caregivers, and reporting concern for abuse to the local designated social service agency. Knowing the risks to this vulnerable population may help detect early signs of abuse and provide services to intervene.

Student Reflection

Long ago, I remember hearing in the news about a woman in a nursing home. Although she was in a coma, she became pregnant; a male attendant raped her. I was shocked, but thought how sensational and out of the norm this event really was. However, in thinking about vulnerability, it seems that abuse of people who are disabled, or of people who are unable to make their desires and needs known, is all too common. Becoming knowledgeable about how vulnerability can make certain groups of people more at risk for abuse helped me understand how assessment and follow-up is critical. It is as if nurses are the voice of the voiceless in many ways. Today, I asked an elderly person, who is wheelchair-bound in her private home, whether she felt safe; she thought I meant from burglars. I felt awkward in probing more about her physical, mental, and emotional safety, and I did not want to scare her. What I did do was help her develop a safety plan in the event she needed help, and helped her feel comfortable by giving her examples of how some community dwellers develop systems to protect their interests. Some useful examples might include sharing some routines with neighbors and having daily contact with a family member or friend via phone. I felt as though I had empowered her. It felt good.

INTERVENTION

Ideally, preventing exposures to violence and abuse offers the best outcomes for an individual's biopsychosocial well-being. Research on interventions has been predominately quasi-experimental and descriptive designs, as the research community is cautious about the use of randomized controlled trials (RCTs), since withholding services and/or interventions that could provide safety and well-being is contraindicated and poses ethical and moral discussions. Despite the limitations of RCTs, there is notable evidence that supports interventions for women exposed to violence.

One rigorous longitudinal RCT is the Nurse–Family Partnership program, which has been in practice for decades. The outcomes of this home visiting program for first-time mothers and babies have proven its effectiveness. Positive outcomes include improved prenatal health, fewer childhood injuries, fewer subsequent pregnancies, increased intervals between births, increased maternal employment, and improved school readiness. Most recently, a 19-year follow-up study on the program showed that it resulted in fewer girls born to high-risk mothers later entering the criminal justice system (Eckenrode et al., 2010).

Another study, the Domestic Violence Enhanced Home Visitation (DOVE) Program, which used three different designs in three different settings, showed improved outcomes with the use of perinatal home visitors (Sharps et al., 2016). In an effort to build on earlier research of evidence-based empowerment, researchers explored what facilitators and barriers exist to implementing home visiting interventions. Kilburn and colleagues (2008) developed and tested a "town and gown" partnership to assist pregnant women who were in a violent relationship based on the DOVE Program (Parker, McFarlane, Silva, Soeken, & Reel, 1999). This empowerment intervention utilized prenatal visitors (town partners) with a research-driven strategy (gown intervention). The DOVE intervention includes the following:

- A structured, tailored brochure with information regarding the cycle of violence, designed to meet each women's special needs
- Risk factors associated with increased risk of homicide
- Options available to women
- Safety planning
- IPV resources specific to their locales
- National hotline numbers

Barriers and facilitating factors to the working partnership were identified in focus groups conducted with home visitors. Barriers include the lack of knowledge and training received by healthcare professionals related to recognizing violence and warning signs, how to ask about violence, and legal options and social services. Also, issues related to the rural communities were identified, such as limited services, lack of anonymity, and the home visitor and the women knowing one another. The town/gown partnership provides home visitors with evidence-based knowledge and the hands-on experience needed to assist and empower the women they are working with. Research findings related to the effectiveness of home visiting programs with related improved health outcomes, safety, and well-being are worth replicating and implementing into practice (Eckenrode et al., 2000; Sharps et al., 2016; Olds et al., 2014; Olds, Henderson, Chamberlin, & Tatelbaum, 1986) (see more at http://www.nursefamilypartnership.org/proven-results/published-research#sthash.k55hBbXe.dpuf).

One major intervention that health providers can address with their patients is safety and risk for harm. Feder and associates (2011) conducted a cluster RCT aimed at IPV training for providers with a focus on Identification and Referral to Improve Safety (IRIS) for women experiencing domestic violence and seeking primary care. Researchers randomized 51 (61%) of 84 eligible general practices in Hackney (London) and Bristol (United Kingdom). Of these, 24 received a training and support program; 24 did not receive the program, and three dropped out before the trial began. Following the second training session, the 24 intervention practices recorded 223 referrals of patients to advocacy and the 24 control practices recorded 12 referrals (adjusted intervention rate ratio 22.1 [95% CI 11.5 to 42.4]). Intervention practices recorded 641 disclosures of domestic violence and control practices recorded 236 (adjusted intervention rate ratio 3.1 [95% CI 2.2 to 4.3]). These findings strongly support training primary care clinicians on assessment of IPV, and referral to community resources that provide services to victims of IPV.

In the clinical setting, nurses need not place pressure on themselves to take on the entire burden of safety planning for a patient, especially when it is beyond their training. The role of the healthcare provider is primarily clinical care and follow-up, discussion of the health effects of violence, referral to resources, and empathetic emotional support (Bair-Merritt et al., 2014; García-Moreno et al., 2015). This first-line support includes attentive listening that is validating, and nonjudgmental provision of referrals to trusted resources for legal protection and housing, if needed. It is up to the patient to decide her own trajectory to safety, even if it is not a linear path.

Another promising practice is the use of in-clinic IPV advocates. Using a quasi-experimental design, investigators explored the efficacy of clinic-based advocacy for IPV to increase help-seeking, reduce violence, and improve women's well-being (Coker et al., 2012). Eligible and consenting women attending one of six selected clinics in the rural Southern United States were assessed for IPV. Consenting women disclosing IPV were offered either an in-clinic advocate intervention or usual care, depending on the clinic they attended and were followed for up to 24 months. Over follow-up time, both IPV scores and depressive symptoms trended toward greater decline among women in the advocate intervention clinics relative to the usual care. In some areas of the country, such as Boston, MA, every teaching hospital employs in-house advocates.

HUMAN TRAFFICKING

Attention to human trafficking in the healthcare field has exploded in recent years due to increased awareness and research efforts. Human trafficking is defined as the recruitment, harboring, transportation, provision, or obtaining of a person for the purpose of a commercial sex act, labor, or services (UN General Assembly, 2000).

Devastatingly, human trafficking is the fastest growing industry in the world, with the United States as the second largest market for women and children trafficked into sex work (behind Germany) (Sabella, 2011). The majority of victims are women and girls, and over half of victims trafficked into the United States are children. Trafficking flourishes in situations of poverty, war, and other crises, which weaken law enforcement and increase demand for cheap labor. For minors, childhood maltreatment trauma and running away from home are the most important risk factors for domestic minor sex trafficking victimization (Choi, 2015). Contrastingly, there is minimal and conflicting evidence on demographic risk factors, so at this time they are not considered strong predictors (i.e., people of all genders, sexual orientations, races, and educational levels are at risk). In response to the rise in human trafficking, the Victims of Trafficking and Violence Protection Act, which was signed into law in October 2000 and has since undergone revision, takes steps to prevent trafficking, protect victims from revictimization and deportation, and prosecute traffickers.

Common health concerns for trafficking victims include mental health issues such as PTSD, anxiety, depression, and suicidality, as well as physical health issues such as drug abuse, STDs, urinary tract infection, infertility, unintended pregnancy, trauma to the vaginal area or other places on the body, cigarette burns, and jaw and neck disorders (Choi, 2015; Sabella, 2011). Victims often characterize the psychological damage of trafficking as more difficult to recover from than physical harm. Because exposing these health issues is risky for the trafficker, victims are usually only granted care when their condition becomes serious. Though there is no one "red flag" that will automatically point to trafficking, clinicians should be aware of the following potential indicators (Sabella 2011):

- Person doesn't speak English and accompanying person is speaking for him or her; accompanying person appears to be supervising and resists leaving him or her alone

- Person doesn't seem to know where her or she is, can't give you a home address, or his or her story about what her or she is doing in this country or his or her job doesn't make sense
- Person doesn't have ID or spending money, or someone else is holding it
- Signs of physical abuse or neglect, or signs of malnutrition, dehydration, drug use, or poor hygiene
- Signs of prolonged exposure to chemicals or airborne contaminants (in the case of labor trafficking) (Peternelj-Taylor, 2016)
- Person has a tattoo that resembles branding (e.g., "Property of __")

There are many reasons trafficking victims are unlikely to ask for help, including threats of violence to themselves or their family/friends, fear of arrest or deportation, language barrier, lack of knowledge about availability of help, shame and belief that they have put themselves in this situation, or fear that the trafficker is "testing" them by employing someone in the league to go undercover and make false offers of escape.

Despite these barriers, nurses are well positioned to identify cases of human trafficking since they are active in many health delivery settings. Forensic nurses can play an especially important role, since they are trained to perform post-trauma examinations and to testify as expert witnesses in legal cases. Internationally renowned trafficking expert Hanni Stoklosa, emphasizes that health professionals have an important role to play in identifying and caring for trafficking victims, and encourages providers to educate themselves on the topic (Chisolm-Straker & Stoklosa, 2017). In January 2018, the U.S. Department of Health and Human Services released a trafficking toolkit for healthcare providers, based on the latest research and best practices for recognizing and responding to trafficking cases (Marcias-Konstantopoulos & Owens, 2018). The screening tool is available free of charge online and consists of eight minimally invasive, close-ended questions with a focus on the core elements of trafficking: force, fraud, and coercion. The areas of inquiry concern recruitment, personal identification and travel documents, working conditions, living conditions, and violence, coercion, or threats.

Asking directly whether a person has been trafficked is usually not helpful, and it is important to talk with the person alone before asking questions that could lead to a disclosure. While the potential to uncover a human trafficking case may seem intimidating, the role of the healthcare provider is not to get a detailed account or to prove that trafficking is occurring, but rather to act on reasonable suspicion by calling a professional at a trafficking resource center for guidance.

At an organizational level, nurses can address human trafficking by staying up-to-date on trafficking research and

sharing this information by hosting a seminar, providing literature to colleagues, or displaying hotline numbers in their clinic. Efforts to respond to human trafficking are most successful when coordinated amongst an interdisciplinary team, so nurses should seek out collaborators in other relevant sectors (e.g., law enforcement, faith, and education) (Peternelj-Taylor, 2016). Nurses have already paved the way in such advances and have great potential to improve efforts to end human trafficking.

MODEL OF CARE FOR VICTIMS OF INTENTIONAL CRIMES

In the past, approaches to acute care of sexual assault victims, domestic abuse victims, and victimized children were inconsistent and suboptimal. Victims of intentional violence often found provider services degrading and received victim-blaming treatment; these experiences would often exacerbate the victim's physical and mental distress (Campbell, Wasco, Ahrens, Sefl, & Barnes, 2001). However, in the past 25 years, significant reform in providing acute forensic medical examinations has occurred, and evidence-based practice has evolved exponentially. Caring for victims of sexual assaults has evolved with the development of nationally certified Sexual Assault Nurse Examiner (SANE) programs. Model programs such as the C.A.R.E Clinic at Brigham and Women's Hospital in Boston, MA, seeks to create innovative approaches to healthcare delivery that mitigate the health consequences cause by violence, trauma, and abuse (www.brighamandwomens.org/careclinic).

> I can be changed by what happens to me but I refuse to be reduced by it. **Maya Angelou**

In response to child maltreatment and in recognizing the special needs of these children, in June 2009, the American Academy of Pediatrics developed a clinical specialty leading to board certification in child maltreatment. Most pediatric academic hospitals in the United States have child protection or children-at-risk teams made up of physicians, nurses, and social workers. Such teams evaluate cases for child maltreatment, work with state child social service agencies and law enforcement, provide education to a broad audience, and conduct research. Over the next decade, this area of specialty practice is likely to expand significantly.

 Assisting Kathy will require multiple practice disciplines coordinating and prioritizing her needs and those of her children. In Laura's institution, it is important that she be aware of policies and procedures related to IPV, child maltreatment, and abuse of the person with disabilities, as well as any resources for management of these problems. Knowing forensic nurse experts in the community will be useful for consultation.

FORENSIC NURSING

Nurses have been providing forensic-type services for centuries. From a formal educational perspective, it was not until recently that specific education in forensic nursing was offered through a traditional nursing college or university. Graduate programs in forensic nursing are likely to impact the field of forensic nursing in the future. Some nurses in the SANE program have received broader instruction; trained as forensic nurse examiners, they care for victims of all types of intentional violence. Nurses working in these areas receive advanced training that includes a didactical component and clinical practicum, which leads to eligibility for board certification.

Forensic nurses offer victims compassionate, trauma-sensitive, evidence-based care. Advanced training focuses on taking a history of the assault, collecting evidence, and providing treatment and follow-up. The field of forensic nursing is growing rapidly, with forensic nursing programs developing in all regions of the country. Forensic nurses are employed in the following areas: emergency departments, police departments, medical examiners offices, homeland security offices, correctional institutions, and mental health facilities. As the evidence grows and the field of forensic nursing evolves, options for nurses to work within a collaborative community team offer interesting opportunities for

nursing professionals. Forensic nursing focuses not only on providing client care, but its practitioners also collect evidence, counsel clients, and communicate with professionals in legal systems. Employers are asking for forensically prepared nurses who can screen and treat clients, as well as testify in court.

As with any relatively new science, it takes time to build a body of knowledge. The *Journal of Forensic Nursing* (https://journals.lww.com/forensicnursing/pages/default. aspx), a peer-reviewed journal, is now recognized as a scholarly scientific journal. The ANA and the International Association of Forensic Nurses (IAFN) released *Forensic Nursing: Scope and Standards of Practice* (2009), a comprehensive reference guide that identifies and defines the expectations for the role and practice of the forensic nurse.

A panel of nurse experts convened by the ANA and the IAFN developed the standards for forensic nurses. The guide outlines six standards for forensic nursing practice and nine standards for professional performance. Forensic nurses are among the most diverse groups of clinicians in the nursing profession with respect to client populations served, practice settings, and forensic and healthcare services provided. Forensic nurses apply a unique combination of processes rooted in nursing science, forensic science, and public health to care for clients. In addition to recommended standards of professional performance, the IAFN book's summary discussion of the scope of forensic nursing practice—including characteristics, trends, education, practice environments, and its ethical and conceptual bases—lends an informative and broad context for the reader's understanding and use of these standards.

KEY CONCEPTS

- Violence against women is a form of gender-based violence that can result in physical, sexual, or psychological harm for both the direct victims and also their dependents (children).
- Intimate partner violence is fundamentally based on the desire for control on the part of the perpetrator.
- Empowering victims of intentional violence to care for themselves and get help is assumed to be a welcomed opportunity. For many, however,

it is a difficult context that has brought them to violent, abusive relationships, and it is a difficult context which will release them from the situation.

- Although abuse and violence can be unintentional, it is the intentional violence which impels nurses to become members of a healthcare team involved in assessing and addressing policy as a way of decreasing the incidence of such acts in communities.

CRITICAL THINKING QUESTIONS

1. You live in a state that has no mandatory laws requiring professionals to report elder abuse. How would you develop support of the individual clients, families, and the community to work toward a system of mandatory reporting?
2. A mother in a pediatric setting becomes very upset when indirect questions are asked

about her children's safety at home. How would you address her feelings?
3. Discuss the positives and negatives of domestic violence shelters for women and children.
4. Compare and contrast violence in the context of heterosexual and lesbian, gay, bisexual, transsexual, and queer relationships. Are preventive solutions the same in these groups?

COMMUNITY RESOURCES

Through networking and attending local conferences on domestic violence, one can begin to build a resource directory of community partners—knowing the following resources is imperative.

- Women's shelters
- Churches/synagogues/temples
- Food banks
- Women, Infants, and Children (WIC) program

- Mental health agencies
- Unemployment offices
- Law enforcement agencies
- Advocacy centers
- Justice centers
- Support groups
- Batterer's intervention groups
- Forensic nurses

HEALTHY PEOPLE 2020 LEARNING ACTIVITY

Injury and Violence Prevention

Healthy People 2020 provides a blueprint that identifies nationwide health improvement priorities. This national consensus plan includes 42 topics, with a subset of 12 leading health indicators (LHI) and over 1,200 objectives. It offers a framework for strategic planning to promote health improvement and achieve health equity through measurable objectives and deliberate actions. The *Healthy People 2020* website is dense with important information on the development, implementation, and progress of this national plan. Learning to navigate the website to access the rich materials offered is vital to gaining a deep understanding of the national health improvement priorities, specific objectives, and initiatives seeking to achieve the national goals and objectives.

Injury and Violence Prevention is a topical area identified as a priority in *Healthy People 2020.* To learn more about this topic go to https://www.healthypeople.gov

Click on "Topics & Objectives": Topics are listed alphabetically, scroll down to "I" and click on **Injury and Violence Prevention.**

Click on the "Overview" and find the answers to the following questions:

- What is the goal for this topic?
- What are some examples of health consequences of violence?
- What factors affect the risk of unintentional injury and violence?

Click on "Objectives" and select five objectives: Analyze the data, looking specifically at any disparities, progress made, and thinking about continued barriers to achievement.

Click on "Interventions & Resources" and select three resources: Review the resources to explore how community and public health groups are working to address and improve services related to injury violence prevention across the nation.

REFERENCES

Abbott, J. T., Johnson, R., Koziol-McLain, J., & Lowenstein, S. R. (1995). Domestic violence against women: Incidence and prevalence in an emergency department population. *JAMA, 273,* 1763–1767.

American Academy of Pediatrics. (2010). Clinical report—intimate partner violence: The role of the pediatrician. Retrieved from http://pediatrics.aappublications.org/content/early/2010/04/26/peds.2010-0451..info?versioned=true

American College of Obstetricians and Gynecologists. (1993). *The obstetrician-gynecologist and primary-preventive health care.* Washington, DC: American College of Obstetricians and Gynecologists.

American Medical Association Council on Scientific Affairs. (1992). Violence against women-relevance for medical practitioners. *JAMA, 267,* 3184–3189.

American Nurses Association. (1991). *Position statement on physical violence against women.* Kansas City, MO: American Nurses Association.

Anda, R., Croft, J., Felitti, V. J., Nordenberg, D., Giles, W. H., Williamson, D. F., & Giovino G. A. (1999). Adverse childhood experiences and smoking during adolescence and adulthood. *JAMA, 82,* 1652–1658.

Anderson, M., Kaufman, J., Simon, T. R., Barrios, L., Paulozzi, L., Ryan, G., … Potter, L.; School-Associated Violent Deaths Study Group. (2001). School-associated violent deaths in the United States 1994–1999. *JAMA, 286*(21), 2695–2702.

Bailey, J., Kellerman, A., Somes, G., Banton, J., Rivara, F., & Rushforth, N. (1997). Risk factors for violent death of women in the home. *Archives of Internal Medicine, 157*(7), 777–782.

Bair-Merritt, M., Lewis-O'Connor, A., Goel, S., Amato, P., Ismailji, T., Jelley, M., … Cronholm, P. (2014). Primary care-based interventions for intimate partner violence: A systematic review. *American Journal of Preventive Medicine, 46*(2), 188–194.

Bair-Merritt, M. H., Voegtline, K., Ghazarian, S. R., Granger, D. A., Blair, C., Johnson, S. B., & Family Life Project Investigators. (2015). Maternal intimate partner violence exposure, child cortisol reactivity and child asthma. *Child Abuse & Neglect, 48,* 50–57.

Berman, H., Hardesty, J., & Humphreys, J. (2004). Children of abused women. In J. Humphreys & J. Campbell (Eds.). *Family violence and nursing practice* (pp. 150–185). Philadelphia, PA: Lippincott Williams & Wilkins.

Black, M., Basile, K., & Breiding, M. (2011). *The national intimate partner and sexual violence survey (NISVS): 2010 summary report.* Atlanta, GA: Centers for Disease Control and Prevention.

REFERENCES *(Continued)*

Bonnie, R., & Wallace, R. (Eds.) (2003). *Elder mistreatment: Abuse, neglect and exploitation in aging America.* Washington, DC: National Academies Press.

Campbell, J. C. (1981). Misogyny and homicide of women. *Advances in Nursing Science, 3,* 67–85.

Campbell, J. C. (1986). Nursing assessment for risk of homicide with battered women. *Advances in Nursing Science, 8,* 36–51.

Campbell, J. C. (1992). "If I can't have you, no one can": Power and control in homicide of female partners. In J. Radford & D. Russell (Eds.), *Femicide: The politics of woman killing.* New York: Twayne.

Campbell, J. C. (1995a). *Assessing dangerousness.* Newbury Park, CA: Sage.

Campbell, J. C. (1995b). Prediction of homicide of and by battered women. In J. Campbell (Ed.), *Assessing the risk of dangerousness: Potential for further violence of sexual offenders, batterers, and child abusers.* Newbury Park, CA: Sage.

Campbell, J. C. (1995c). Homicide of and by battered women. In J. C. Campbell (Ed.), *Assessing dangerousness: Violence by sexual offenders, batterers, and child abusers* (pp. 96–113). Thousand Oaks, CA: Sage.

Campbell, J. C. (2002). Health consequences of intimate partner violence. *Lancet, 359,* 1331–1336.

Campbell, J. C., & Lewandowski, L. A. (1997). Mental and physical effects of intimate partner violence on women and children. *Psychiatric Clinics of North America, 20,* 353–374.

Campbell, R., Wasco, S., Ahrens, C., Sefl, T., & Barnes, H. (2001). Preventing the "second rape": Rape survivors' experiences with community service providers. *Journal of Interpersonal Violence, 16,* 1239–1259.

Campbell, J. C., Webster, D., Koziol-McLain, J., Block, C., Campbell, D., Curry, M. A., … Laughon, K. (2003a). Risk factors for femicide in abusive relationships: Results from a multicity case control study. *American Journal of Public Health, 93,* 1089–1097.

Campbell, J. C., Webster, D., Koziol-McLain, J., Block, C. R., Campbell, D., Curry, M. A., … Wilt, S. A. (2003b). Assessing risk factors for intimate partner homicide. *National Institute of Justice Journal, 250,* 14–19. Retrieved from http://ncjrs.org/pdffiles1/jr000250e.pdf

Centers for Disease Control and Prevention (CDC). (2001). Temporal variations in school-associated student homicide and suicide events—United States, 1992–1999. *Morbidity and Mortality Weekly Report, 50*(31), 657–660.

Centers for Disease Control and Prevention (CDC). (2003). Source of firearms used by students in school-associated violent deaths–United States, 1992–1999. *Morbidity and Mortality Weekly Report, 52*(09), 169–172.

Centers for Disease Control and Prevention (CDC). (2008). Adverse health conditions and health risk behaviors associated with intimate partner violence—United States, 2005, *57*(5), 113–117. Retrieved from http://www.cdc.gov/mmwr/preview/mmwrhtml/mm5705a1.htm

Centers for Disease Control and Prevention (CDC). (2016a). Deaths: Final Data for 2014. National Vital Statistics Report, *65*(4). Retrieved from https://www.cdc.gov/nchs/data/nvsr/nvsr65/nvsr65_04.pdf

Centers for Disease Control and Prevention (CDC). (2016b). Fatal Injury Reports, National, Regional, and State, 1981–2016. Retrieved from https://webappa.cdc.gov/sasweb/ncipc/mortrate.html

Chang, J., Berg, C. J., Herndon, J., & Saltzman, L. (2005). Homicide: A leading cause of injury deaths among pregnant and postpartum women in the United States between 1991–1999. *American Journal of Public Health, 95,* 471–477.

Chisolm-Straker, M., & Stoklosa, H. (Eds.). (2017). *Human trafficking is a public health issue: A paradigm expansion in the United States.* New York: Springer.

Choi, K. R. (2015). Risk factors for domestic minor sex trafficking in the United States: a literature review. *Journal of Forensic Nursing, 11*(2), 66–76.

Clark, L. E., Allen, R. H., Goyal, V., Raker, C., & Gottlieb, A. S. (2014). Reproductive coercion and co-occurring intimate partner violence in obstetrics and gynecology patients. *American Journal of Obstetrics & Gynecology, 210*(1), 42-e41-48.

Coker, A., Smith, P., Whitaker, D., Le, B., Crawford, T., & Flerx, V. (2012). Effect of an in-clinic IPV advocate intervention to increase help seeking, reduce violence, and improve well-being. *Violence Against Women, 18*(1), 118–131.

Corso, P. S., Mercy, J. A., Simon, T. R., Finkelstein, E. A., & Miller, T. R. (2007). Medical costs and productivity losses due to interpersonal violence and self-directed violence. *American Journal of Preventive Medicine, 32*(6), 474–482.

Diliberti, M., Jackson, M., & Kemp, J. (2017). *Crime, violence, discipline, and safety in U.S. public schools: Findings from the school survey on crime and safety: 2015–16 (NCES 2017–122).* Washington, DC: U.S. Department of Education, National Center for Education Statistics. Retrieved from http://nces.ed.gov/pubsearch.

Dolezal, T., McCollum, D., & Callahan, M. (2009). *Hidden cost in health care: The economic impact of violence and abuse.* Eden Prairie, MN: Academy on Violence and Abuse.

Dong, M., Anda, R., Felitti, V. J., Dube, S. R., Williamson, D. F., Thompson, T. J., … Giles, W. H. (2004). The interrelatedness of multiple forms of childhood abuse, neglect, and household dysfunction. *Child Abuse and Neglect, 28,* 771–784.

Dube, S., Felitti, V. J., Dong, M., Giles, W., & Anda, R. (2003). The impact of adverse childhood experiences on health problems: Evidence from four birth cohorts dating back to 1900. *Preventive Medicine, 37,* 268–277.

Eckenrode, J., Campa, M., Luckey, D. W., Henderson, C. R., Cole, R., Kitzman, H., … & Olds, D. (2010). Long-term effects of prenatal and infancy nurse home visitation on the life course of youths: 19-year follow-up of a randomized trial. *Archives of Pediatrics & Adolescent Medicine, 164*(1), 9–15.

Eckenrode, J., Ganzel, B., Henderson, C., Smith, E., Olds, D., Powers, J., … Sidora, K. (2000). Preventing child abuse and neglect with a program of nurse home visitation the limiting effects of domestic violence. *JAMA, 284*(11), 1385–1391.

Edelson, J. (1999). Children's witnessing of adult domestic violence. *Journal of Interpersonal Violence, 14,* 839–870.

Edwards, V., Anda, R., Dube, S. R., Dong, M., Chapman, D., & Felitti, V. J. (2005). The wide-ranging health consequences of adverse childhood experiences. In K. Kendall-Tackett & S. Giacomoni (Eds.), *Child victimization: Maltreatment, bullying, and dating violence prevention and intervention.* Kingston, NJ: Civic Research Institute.

Elliott, D., Bjelajac, B., Fallot, R., Markoff, L., & Reed, R. (2005). Trauma-informed or trauma-denied: Principles and implementation of trauma-informed services for women. *Journal of Community Psychology, 33*(4), 461–477.

Family Violence Prevention Fund. (1999). *Preventing domestic violence: Clinical guidelines on routine screening.* San Francisco, CA: Family Violence Prevention Fund. Retrieved November, 2, 2009, from http://endabuse.org/userfiles/file/HealthCare/dental.pdf

Feder, G., Davies, R. A, Baird, K., Dunne, D., Eldridge, S., Griffiths, C., … Sharp, D. (2011). Identification and referral to improve safety (IRIS) of women experiencing domestic violence with a primary care training and support programme: A cluster randomized controlled trial. *Lancet, 378,* 1788–1795.

Felitti, V., Anda, R., Nordenberg, D., Williamson, D. F., Spitz, A. M., Edwards, V., … Marks, J. S. (1998). The relationship of childhood abuse and household dysfunction to many of the leading causes of death in adults. The Adverse Childhood Experiences (ACE) Study. *American Journal of Preventive Medicine, 14,* 245–258.

, Finkelhor, D., Turner, H. A., Shattuck, A., & Hamby, S. L. (2015). Prevalence of childhood exposure to violence, crime, and abuse: Results from the national survey of children's exposure to violence. *JAMA Pediatrics, 169*(8), 746–754.

Fletcher, T. R., Clements, A. D., & Bailey, B. (2016). Identifying intimate partner violence during pregnancy in prenatal care settings. *International Journal of Health Sciences Education*, 3(1), 3.

García-Moreno, C., Hegarty, K., d'Oliveira, A. F., Koziol-McLain, J., Colombini, M., & Feder, G. (2015). The health-systems response to violence against women. *The Lancet*, 385(9977), 1567–1579.

Gin, N. E., Rucker, L., Frayne, S., & Cygan, R. (1992). Prevalence of domestic violence among patients in three ambulatory care internal medicine clinics. *Journal of General Internal Medicine*, 6, 317–322.

Grinshteyn, E., & Hemenway, D. (2016). Violent death rates: The US compared with other high-income OECD countries, 2010. *The American Journal of Medicine*, 129(3), 266–273.

Groves, B. M. (2002). *Children who see too much: Lessons from the child witness to violence project.* Boston, MA: Beacon Press.

Hamberger, L. K., Saunders, D. G., & Hovey, M. (1992). Prevalence of domestic violence in community practice and rate of physician inquiry. *Family Medicine*, 24, 283–287.

Hathaway, J., Zimmer, B., Willis, G., & Silverman, J. (2008). Perceived changes in health and safety following participation in a health care-based domestic violence program. *Journal Midwifery Womens Health*, 53, 547–555.

Healthy People 2020. Understanding and Improving Health. Retrieved from http://www.health.gov/healthypeople

Helton, A., McFarlane, J., & Anderson, E. (1987). Battered and pregnant: A prevalence study. *American Journal of Public Health*, 77, 1337–1339.

Hemingway, D. (2004). *Private guns, public health.* Ann Arbor, MI: The University of Michigan Press.

Humphreys, J., Parker, B., & Campbell, J. C. (2001). Intimate partner violence against women. In D. Taylor & N. Fugate-Woods (Eds.), *Annual review of nursing research* (pp. 275–306). New York: Springer Publishing Company.

International Association of Forensic Nurses. (2009). Retrieved from www.iafn.org

Joint Commission on Accreditation of Healthcare Organizations. (1995). *Accreditation manual for hospitals.* Oakbrook Terrace, IL: JCAHO.

Jones, A. S., Gielen, A. C., Campbell, J. C., Schollengerger, J., Dienemann, J. A., Kub, J., … Wynne, E. C. (1999). Annual and lifetime prevalence of partner abuse in a sample of HMO enrollees. *Women's Health Issues*, 9, 295–305.

Kalesan, B., Lagast, K., Villarreal, M., Pino, E., Fagan, J., & Galea, S. (2017). School shootings during 2013–2015 in the USA. *Injury Prevention*, 23(5), 321–327.

Kann, L., McManus, T., Harris, W. A., Shanklin, S. L., Flint, K. H., Hawkins, J., … & Zaza, S. (2016). Youth risk behavior surveillance – United States, 2015. *Mortality and Morbidity Weekly Report: Surveillance Summaries*, 65(4), 1–180.

Kellerman, A., & Heron, S. (1999). Firearms and family violence. *Emergency Medicine Clinic North America*, 17, 699–716.

Kernic, M., Wolf, M. E., & Holt, V. (2000). Rates and relative risk of hospital admissions among women in violent intimate relationships. *American Journal of Public Health*, 90, 1416–1420.

Kilburn, E., Chang, C., Bullock, L., & Sharps, P. (2008). Facilitators and barriers for implementing home visit interventions to address intimate partner violence: Town and gown partnerships. *Nursing Clinics of North America*, 43(3), 419–435.

Kothari, C. L., Rohs, T., Davidson, S., Kothari, R. U., Klein, C., Koestner, A., … & Kutzko, K. (2015). Emergency department visits and injury hospitalizations for female and male victims and perpetrators of intimate partner violence. *Advances in Emergency Medicine*, 11 pages.

Krug, E., Dahlberg, L., Mercy, J., Zwi, A., & Lozano, R. (Eds.). (2002). *World report on violence and health.* Geneva, Switzerland: World Health Organization.

Lewandowski, L., McFarlane, J., Campbell, J. C., Gary, F., & Barenski, C. (2004). He killed my mommy: Children of murdered mothers. *Journal of Family Violence*, 19, 211–220.

Lewis-O'Connor, A. (2007). When push comes to shove: Screening mothers for intimate partner violence during a pediatric visit (Dissertation). Boston: Boston College.

Lewis-O'Connor, A., & Chadwick, M. (2015). Engaging the voice of patients affected by gender-based violence: informing practice and policy. *Journal of Forensic Nursing*, 11(4), 240–249.

MacMillan, H. L., Wathen, C. N., Jamieson, E., Boyle, M. H., Shannon, H. S., Ford-Gilboe, M.; McMaster Violence Against Women Research Group. (2009). Screening for intimate partner violence in health care settings: A randomized trial. *JAMA*, 302(5), 493–501.

Marcias-Konstantopoulos, W. & Owens, J. (2018). Adult human trafficking screening tool and guide. *U.S. Department of Health and Human Services: Administration for Children and Families Office on Trafficking in Persons.* Retrieved from https://www.acf.hhs.gov/sites/default/files/otip/adult_human_trafficking_screening_tool_and_guide.pdf

Martin, S. E., & Clements, M. L. (2002). Young children's responding to interparental conflict: Associations with marital aggression and child adjustment. *Journal of Child and Family Studies*, 11, 231–244.

McCloskey, L. A., Figuerdo, A., & Koss, M. (1995). The effects of systemic family violence on children's mental health. *Child Development*, 66, 1239–1261.

McFarlane, J., Parker, B., Soeken, K., & Bullock, L. (1992). Assessing for abuse during pregnancy: Severity and frequency of injuries and associated entry into prenatal care. *JAMA*, 26, 3176–3178.

Messing, J. T., Campbell, J., Sullivan Wilson, J., Brown, S., & Patchell, B. (2017). The lethality screen: the predictive validity of an intimate partner violence risk assessment for use by first responders. *Journal of Interpersonal Violence*, 32(2), 205–226.

Middlebrooks, J. S., & Audage, N. C. (2008). The effects of childhood stress on health across the lifespan. CDC, NCIPC. Retrieved from http://www.cdc.gov/ncipc/pub-res/pdf/Childhood_Stress.pdf

Miller, T. R. (2015). *The cost of firearm violence.* Calverton, MD: Children's Safety Network; 2012.

Miller, E., Decker, M. R., McCauley, H., Tancredi, D. J., Levenson, R. R., Waldman, J., … Silverman, J. G. (2010). Pregnancy coercion, intimate partner violence and unintended pregnancy. *Contraception*, 81, 316–322.

Miller, E., Decker, M. R., Raj, A., Reed, E., Marable, D., Silverman, J. G. (2010). Intimate partner violence and health care-seeking patterns among female users of urban adolescent clinics. *Maternal Child Health Journal*, 14(6), 910–917.

Moracco, K., Runyan, C., & Butts, J. (2003). Female intimate partner homicide: A population-based study. *Journal American Medical Women's Association*, 58, 20–25.

Moyer, V. A.; U.S. Preventive Services Task Force. (2013). Screening for intimate partner violence and abuse of elderly and vulnerable adults: U.S. Preventive Services Task Force recommendation statement. *Annals of Internal Medicine*, 158(6), 478–486.

Nelson, H. D., Bougatsos, C., & Blazina, I. (2012). Screening women for intimate partner violence: a systematic review to update the US Preventive Services Task Force recommendation. *Annals of Internal Medicine*, 156(11), 796–808.

Nouer, S. S., Mackey, S. N., Tipton, N. G., Miller, A. C., & Connor, P. D. (2014). Identifying predictors for children witnessing intimate partner violence. *Journal of Family Violence*, 29(6), 675–679.

Ogbonnaya, I. N., Macy, R., Kupper, L., Martin, S., & Bledsoe-Mansori, S. (2013). Intimate partner violence and depressive symptoms before pregnancy, during pregnancy and after infant delivery. *Journal of Interpersonal Violence*, 28, 2112–2133.

Olds, D., Henderson, C., Chamberlin, R., & Tatelbaum, R. (1986). Preventing child abuse and neglect: A randomized trial of nurse home visitation. *Pediatrics*, 78, 65–78.

Olds, D., Holmberg, J., Donelan-McCall, N., Luckey, D., Knudtson, M., & Robinson, J. (2014). Effects of home visits by paraprofessionals and by nurses on children: Follow-up of a randomized trial at ages 6 and 9 years. *JAMA Pediatrics*, 168(2), 114–121.

Parker, B., McFarlane, J., Silva, C., Soeken, K., & Reel, S. (1999). Testing an intervention to prevent further abuse to pregnant women. *Research in Nursing and Health*, 22, 59–66.

REFERENCES *(Continued)*

Peternelj-Taylor, C. (2016). Trafficking in Persons: Q&A with Dr. Donna Sabella. *Journal of Forensic Nursing 12*(1):1–4.

Petrosky, E., Blair, J. M., Betz, C. J., Fowler, K. A., Jack, S. P., & Lyons, B. H. (2017). Racial and Ethnic Differences in Homicides of Adult Women and the Role of Intimate Partner Violence—United States, 2003–2014. *MMWR. Morbidity and Mortality Weekly Report, 66*(28), 741.

Piotrowski, C. C., Tachie, R. M., & Cameranesi, M. (2017). Aggression in children exposed to intimate partner violence: a comparison of maternal, sibling, and observer perspectives. *Journal of Interpersonal Violence*, 0886260517741624.

QuickStats: Age-Adjusted Rates for Homicides, by Race/Ethnicity—United States, 1999–2015. *MMWR Morb Mortal Wkly Rep,* 2017;66:839. doi: http://dx.doi.org/10.15585/mmwr.mm6631a9

Reeves, E. (2015). A synthesis of the literature on trauma-informed care. *Issues in Mental Health Nursing, 36*(9), 698–709.

Richardson, E. G., & Hemenway, D. (2011). Homicide, suicide, and unintentional firearm fatality: comparing the United States with other high-income countries, 2003. *Journal of Trauma and Acute Care Surgery, 70*(1), 238–243.

Robers, S., Zhang, J., Truman, J., & Synder, T. D. (2012). *Indicators of school crime and safety: 2011*. Washington, DC: National Center for Education Statistics, U.S. Department of Education, and Bureau of Justice Statistics, Office of Justice Programs, U.S. Department of Justice. Retrieved from http://nces.ed.gov/pubs2012/2012002.pdf

Sabella, D. (2011). The role of the nurse in combating human trafficking. *The American Journal of Nursing, 111*(2), 28–37.

Sarkar, N. N. (2008). The impact of intimate partner violence on women's reproductive health and pregnancy outcome. *Journal of Obstetrics and Gynaecology, 28*(3), 266–271.

Sharps, P. W., Bullock, L. C., Campbell, J. C., Alhusen, J. L., Ghazarian, S. R., Bhandari, S. S., & Schminkey, D. L. (2016). Domestic Violence Enhanced Prenatal Home Visits: The DOVE Randomized Clinical Trial. *Journal of Women's Health, 25*(11), 1129–1138. PMID: 27206047.

Silverman, J. G., Raj, A., & Clements, K. (2004). Dating violence and associated sexual risk and pregnancy among adolescent girls in the United States. *Pediatrics, 114*, e220–e225.

Silverman, J., Raj, A., Mucci, L., & Hathaway, J. (2001). Dating violence against adolescent girls, associated substance use, unhealthy weight control, sexual risk behavior, pregnancy, and suicidality. *JAMA, 286*, 572–579.

Sobsey, D. (1994). *Violence and abuse in the lives of people with disabilities*. Baltimore, MD: Paul H. Brookes Publishing Co.

Sobsey, D., & Doe, T. (1991). Patterns of sexual abuse and assault. *Journal of Sexuality and Disability, 9*(3), 243–259.

Sorenson, S. B., & Wiebe, D. J. (2004). Weapons in the lives of battered women. *American Journal of Public Health, 94*, 1412–1417.

Teaster, P. B., Dugar, T., Mendiondo, M., Abner, E. L, Cecil, K. A., & Otto, J. M. (2004). *The 2004 survey of adult protective services: Abuse of adults 60 years of age and older*. Washington DC: National Center on Elder Abuse.

Thackeray, J. D., Hibbard, R., Dowd, M. D., Committee on Child Abuse and Neglect, & Committee on Injury, Violence, and Poison Prevention. (2010). Intimate partner violence: the role of the pediatrician. *Pediatrics, 125*(5), 1094–1100.

Tjaden, P., & Thoennes, N. (2000). *Extent, nature and consequences of intimate partner violence: Findings from the National Violence against Women Survey (Report publication No. NCJ-181867)*. Washington DC: U.S. Department of Justice, Office of Justice Programs.

United Nations. (1993). *Declaration on the elimination of violence against women*, Geneva: Universal Declaration of Human Rights. Retrieved November 2, 2009, from http://www.un.org/en/documents/udhr/

United Nation's General Assembly. (2000). Protocol to prevent, suppress and punish trafficking in persons, especially women and children, supplementing the United Nations convention against transnational organized crime. *GA res, 55*, 25. Retrieved from https://www.unodc.org/unodc/en/organized-crime/intro/UNTOC.html

U.S. Department of Health and Human Services, Administration for Children and Families, Children's Bureau. (2003). Child abuse and neglect. Retrieved from https://www.childwelfare.gov/can/

U.S. Department of Health and Human Services, Administration for Children and Families, Administration on Children, Youth and Families, Children's Bureau. (2017). Child maltreatment 2016. Retrieved from http://www.acf.hhs.gov/cb/research-data-technology/statistics-research/child-maltreatment. Also at https://www.acf.hhs.gov/sites/default/files/cb/cm2016.pdf

Violence Policy Center. (2017). Black Homicide Victimization in the United States: An Analysis of 2014 Homicide Data. Available at: http://www.vpc.org/studies/blackhomicide17.pdf

Vu, N. L., Jouriles, E. N., McDonald, R., & Rosenfield, D. (2016). Children's exposure to intimate partner violence: a meta-analysis of longitudinal associations with child adjustment problems. *Clinical Psychology Review, 46*, 25–33.

Waters, H., Hyder, A., Rajkotia, Y., Basu, S., Rehwinkel, J. A., & Butchart, A. The economic dimensions of interpersonal violence. Department of Injuries and Violence Prevention, World Health Organization, Geneva, 2004. Retrieved from http://apps.who.int/iris/bitstream/handle/10665/42944/9241591609.pdf?sequence=1

Weiss, H., Lawrence, B., & Miller, T. (2002). Pregnancy-associated assault hospitalizations. *Obstetrics & Gynecology, 100*, 773–780.

Whitfield, C., Anda, R., Dube, S., & Felitti, V. J. (2003). Violent childhood experiences and the risk of intimate partner violence in adults: Assessment in a large health maintenance organization. *Journal of Interpersonal Violence, 18*, 166–185.

Wiebe, D. (2003). Homicide and suicide risks associated with firearms in the home: A national case-control study. *Annals of Emergency Medicine, 41*, 771–778.

Wilt, S., & Olson, S. (1996). Prevalence of domestic violence in the United States. *Journal of the American Medical Women's Association, 51*, 77–82.

Young, M. E., Nosek, M. A., Howland, C., Chanpong, G., & Rintala, D. H. (1997). Prevalence of abuse of women with disabilities. *Archive of Physical and Medical Rehabilitation, 78*, S34–S38.

SUGGESTED READING

Bailey, J., Kellerman, A., & Somes, G. W. (1997). Risk factors for violence death of women in the home. *Annals of Internal Medicine, 157*, 777–782.

WEB RESOURCES

Please visit thePoint® for up-to-date web resources on this topic.

Chapter 17

Substance Use

Judith Shindul-Rothschild

> The basic thing nobody asks is why do people take drugs of any sort? Why do we have these accessories to normal living to live? I mean, is there something wrong with society that's making us so pressurized, that we cannot live without guarding ourselves against it?
>
> **John Lennon**
>
> Man is the only creature that refuses to be what he is.
>
> **Albert Camus**
>
> Drugs? Everyone has a choice and I choose not to do drugs.
>
> **Leonardo DiCaprio**
>
> Reality is just a crutch for people who can't cope with drugs.
>
> **Robin Williams**

CHAPTER HIGHLIGHTS

- Factors affecting prevalence rates of substance use: age, gender, race, socioeconomic level, urban or rural settings
- Population-based interventions to decrease substance use
- Evidence-based treatment protocols for substance abuse that should be incorporated by community health nurses in all practice settings
- Self-help groups: a highly effective community-based treatment with proven efficacy in sustaining recovery

OBJECTIVES

- Define substance use, substance abuse, and addiction.
- Describe the impact of substance abuse and addiction on individual people and their families, communities, and nations.
- Identify risk factors for substance misuse and abuse in individual people and populations.
- Apply evidence-based practice in the nursing care of populations most at risk for substance use disorders.
- Apply evidence-based interventions in providing nursing care in the community for clients with substance abuse.

KEY TERMS

The World Health Organization (WHO) has compiled a list of terms and definitions commonly used in population surveys and WHO research publications on substance use. The list is entitled "Lexicon of alcohol and drug terms published by the World Health Organization" and is available online. Other terms are defined by the *Diagnostic and Statistical Manual of Mental*

KEY TERMS *(continued)*

Disorders (*DSM-5*) compiled by the American Psychiatric Association (APA, 2013).

Abstinence: No use of illicit substances or alcohol in the preceding 12 months; a person is considered "abstinent."

Addiction: A term, along with habituation, which the WHO recommends be substituted with substance dependence. However, clients and practitioners commonly use addiction.

Craving: A very strong urge or desire to seek the euphoric feeling achieved by using substances (*DSM-5*).

Intoxication: A reversible syndrome that appears after ingestion of a specific substance that results in clinically significant problematic behavioral or psychological changes (e.g., belligerence, mood lability, impaired judgment, disturbances of perception,

psychomotor behavior, and interpersonal behavior [*DSM-5*]).

Remission: Early remission is defined in *DSM-5* as occurring when a person has previously met criteria for a substance use disorder but has not met the criteria for 3 to 12 months. Sustained remission occurs when a person no longer meets the criteria for substance use disorder for 12 months or more.

Substance use (in this chapter): The use of alcohol, illicit drugs, and nonmedical use of prescription medications. Illicit drugs include cannabis, cocaine, heroin, hallucinogens, inhalants, and methamphetamine. Prescription medications used nonmedically include pain relievers, tranquilizers, stimulants, and sedatives.

Substance use disorders (SUD): In *DSM-5*, SUD includes

separate criteria for alcohol, anxiolytics, caffeine, cannabis, gambling, hallucinogens, hypnotics, opioids, phencyclidine (PCP), sedatives, stimulants, and tobacco.

Tolerance: Diminished physical and/or psychological response to effects of alcohol or illicit substances. A person develops tolerance when he or she needs to use higher doses of alcohol or illicit substances to achieve the desired euphoric effect (*DSM-5*).

Withdrawal: A reduction in prolonged substance use that results in problematic behavioral, physiologic, and cognitive changes. Withdrawal causes significant impairment in social, occupational, and interpersonal functioning and is usually associated with an urge to readminister the substance to reduce the symptoms (*DSM-5*).

CASE STUDY   *References to the case study are found throughout this chapter (look for the case study icon). Readers should keep the case study in mind as they read the chapter.*

James Campbell, a 63-year-old African American man, is retired from the Boston Fire Department. His wife died 6 months ago from breast cancer, and he now lives alone next to his adult daughter. Since his wife died, Mr. Campbell has been increasingly relying on his daughter's assistance to manage his home. His daughter, who works full-time and has four children of her own, has not been able to spend as much time with her father as she would like, but she checks with him daily. Recently, she has noticed that her father's appetite seems to have decreased; he has lost so much weight that his pants are very loose around his waist. At his daughter's insistence, Mr. Campbell agrees to see a nurse practitioner at a Boston clinic for a thorough evaluation.

In the meeting with the nurse, the daughter says that she is worried about her father becoming depressed. Mr. Campbell does admit to having difficulty sleeping and says that he takes a "shot" of whiskey to help him relax. He injured his back before he retired, and sometimes, his back pain is so severe that he takes a "pain pill" that his wife was given to manage her cancer pain. Mr. Campbell's daughter believes that her mother took oxycodone (OxyContin). Mr. Campbell vehemently denies changes in mood but does admit that he gets the "jitters" during the day for no apparent reason and takes one alprazolam (Xanax), which his wife's physician prescribed for him when she was first diagnosed with cancer. His daughter says that it seems she has been filling the Xanax prescription more frequently lately.

INTERNATIONAL ASPECTS OF SUBSTANCE ABUSE

Substance use affects societies in many ways, and countries have used different models to address the impact on populations. Approaches range from strict prohibition and criminalization

to the harm reduction model, which is based on public health principles. When substances that can alter mental states are believed to lead to **addiction** and social harms or dysfunction, some governments respond by enacting laws that support strict drug prohibition. The harm reduction approach focuses on the reduction of the harmful effects of drug use and addiction without necessarily achieving **abstinence**. Most countries actually apply a model combining both harm reduction strategies and criminalization (WHO, 2014a).

Scope of Substance Use

Worldwide, mental and substance use disorders (SUD) are the leading cause of all nonfatal disease burdens, and most deaths (81%) are attributable to SUD (Whiteford et al., 2013). It is important for community health nurses to appreciate the cultural norms and differences in the use of illicit and licit substances. For example, in some cultures, such as the United States, alcohol use is viewed as normative, while in other cultures, the use of alcohol is strictly forbidden and viewed as a behavior that is one of the most stigmatized of all health conditions (WHO, 2014a). Globally, public health models that address drug and alcohol abuse focus on interventions at three points: the agent (the distributor of the substance), the host (the addicted person), and the environment (local, national, or international).

> The real problems are cultural. The problems of the people who take drugs are a cultural trap—I think there's a real problem there, the crack stuff, the hopelessness of the junkie. The urban angst. **Jerry Garcia**

Global Public Health Policies to Minimize Harms From Substance Use

Alcohol misuse is a global public health threat that poses significant social and economic costs to healthcare systems, criminal justice authorities, and social welfare systems (Fig. 17.1) (WHO, 2014a). Successful global and multinational policies

---

17.1 WHO Public Health Principles Guiding Development and Implementation of Alcohol Policies

a. Public policies and interventions to prevent and reduce alcohol-related harm should be guided and formulated by public health interests and based on clear public health goals and best available evidence.
b. Alcohol policies should be equitable and sensitive to national, religious, and cultural contexts.
c. Protection of populations at high risk for alcohol-related harm and those exposed to the harmful effects of drinking by others should be an integral part of public health policies.
d. Populations affected by the harmful use of alcohol should have access to affordable and effective prevention and care services.

Source: World Health Organization (WHO). (2014). *Global status report on alcohol and health*. Luxembourg: World Health Organization.

---

aimed at reducing social harms associated with alcohol consumption focus on availability, marketing, pricing, drinking and driving, prevention, and treatment in healthcare systems (WHO, 2014a). These aspects of a public health model are reflected in the WHO's "Guiding public health principles to reduce the harmful use of alcohol" (Box 17.1). The most common public health policies are national awareness campaigns that educate populations about the social harms associated with alcohol misuse, especially drinking and driving (WHO, 2014a).

FIGURE 17.1 Global alcohol-attributable causes of death, disease, and injury, 2012. (From WHO. [2014]. *Global status report on alcohol and health* [p. 47]. Luxembourg: World Health Organization.)

Evidence-based policy options related to health services delivery include population screening and brief intervention with referral to treatment (SBIRT), especially for high-risk populations including children, adolescents, pregnant women, and older adults (WHO, 2014a). Population-based policies designed to limit the availability of alcohol include laws regulating the minimum drinking age, licensing restrictions, marketing restrictions, and increased pricing through taxation. Other examples of policies enacted by nations or states to minimize the harm to populations from alcohol use include blood alcohol limits on driving and warning labels on alcohol beverages about the adverse effects on health (WHO, 2014a).

At the community level, strategies to reduce the harmful use of alcohol include developing policies designed for specific community events such as sporting events or festivals where subpopulations, especially youth, maybe at risk for harm from excessive substance use. Community-based policies may include restrictions on public consumption of alcohol, restrictions on the hours establishments can serve alcohol, and mandatory training for hospitality providers.

Globally, approximately 29.5 million people suffer from drug use disorders (United Nations Office on Drug and Crime [UNODC], 2017). From a public health perspective, self-administered injection of illicit substances poses the greatest risk for population health and social harms (UNODC, 2012). The United States alone accounts for almost one quarter of all opioid overdose deaths worldwide (UNODC, 2017). New synthetic derivatives of opioids such as fentanyl which vary in potency have escalated the rates of opioid-related deaths.

Hepatitis C, HIV, and tuberculosis are the leading causes of morbidity among people who inject drugs. Public health programs including opioid substitution treatment and syringe exchange programs are harm reduction strategies used in both developed and developing countries to combat the spread of hepatitis C and HIV. Opioid substitution treatment consists of administering methadone or buprenorphine in prescribed doses in programs administered by governments. There is widespread agreement among public health experts in both developed and developing countries that opioid substitution treatment programs are an effective public health strategy to reduce the social harms associated with illicit opioid use, such as prostitution, shoplifting, theft, and property crime.

The WHO recommends that public health programs for people who inject drugs be integrated into healthcare delivery systems to avoid fragmentation of services and promote implementation of evidence-based treatments. The UNODC's Global Youth Network provides information and materials to prevent drug abuse at the individual, family, school, and community level. The UNODC/WHO's Global Initiative on Primary Prevention of Substance Abuse provides information on evidence-based practices to assess substance abuse, plan prevention programs, and evaluate effectiveness of programs on preventing substance abuse. More information is available at the UNODC's websites.

In many countries, evidence-based prevention and treatment strategies have not been widely disseminated nor adequately funded by governments. Antiviral treatment for hepatitis C has been hampered by the high cost of pharmaceuticals. For marginalized populations such as the homeless, those in prison, or sex workers who maybe at greatest risk for harms associated with injection drug use, substance use treatment is often not equivalent to services available in the general population (UNODC, 2017).

National Scope of Substance Use

The United States leads the world in the portion of its citizens who abuse or are dependent on alcohol or illicit substances and is the country with the largest illicit drug market. Most Americans (65.7%) use alcohol and 17.8% report use of illicit drugs (U.S. Department of Health and Human Services [USDHHS], Office of the Surgeon General, 2016). From 2002 to 2015, deaths involving heroin increased 6.2-fold and is the leading cause of accidental deaths in the United States (National Institute on Drug Abuse [NIDA], 2017a; Presidents Commission on Combating Drug Addiction and the Opioid Crisis, 2017). Overdose deaths involving heroin or synthetic opioids increased for all demographic groups, regions, and in 30 states (Fig. 17.2) (Rudd, Seth, David, & Scholl, 2016).

If current trends continue, it is estimated that 1 in 23 women and 1 in 36 men who inject drugs will be infected with HIV in the United States (Fig. 17.3) (Centers of Disease Control and Prevention [CDC], 2016). Injection drug use, especially in rural regions of the United States, has created new public health challenges for the prevention of HIV. The CDC has embarked on a high-impact prevention strategy that includes directing federal grants, pharmaceutical treatment, and intervention programs to communities most at risk. Included in the CDC prevention strategies are culturally appropriate public service messages, syringe services, comprehensive recovery services, pre-exposure prophylaxis (PrEP), post-exposure prophylaxis (PEP), and antiretroviral therapy (ART) to treat HIV (CDC, 2016).

In the United States, rates of substance use are higher among native-born populations than immigrants. Public health researchers theorize that the "immigrant paradox" for **substance use disorders** is related to protective factors, such as community safety and family cohesion, which contribute to lower rates of substance use among immigrants upon arrival to the United States (Qureshi et al., 2014; Salas-Wright & Vaughn, 2014; Savage & Mezuk, 2014). As immigrants' length of residence in the United States increases, the rate of substance misuse also increases, suggesting that sociocultural exposures, including acculturation and discrimination, play a direct role in increasing risk among immigrants (Savage & Mezuk, 2014). Immigrant youth in particular are more susceptible to peer influence and acculturation stress and are more likely to adopt unhealthy substance use behaviors than immigrant adults (Li & Wen, 2015).

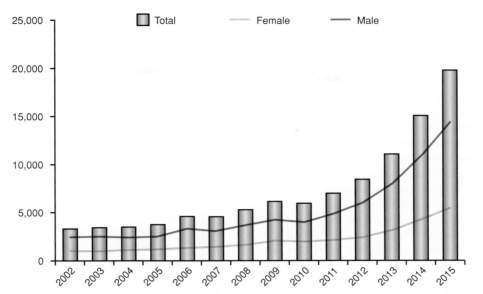

FIGURE 17.2 National overdose deaths from heroin and illicit opioids. (From National Institute on Drug Abuse (NIDA). [2017]. *National overdose deaths—2015* [p. 5]. Retrieved from https://www.drugabuse.gov/related-topics/trends-statistics/overdose-death-rates.)

Practice Point

A challenge for community health nurses caring for immigrant populations, especially youth, is to preserve protective factors to minimize the risk of substance misuse associated with longer residency in the United States.

I bought a gun and chose drugs instead. **Kurt Cobain**

Evidence for Practice

Lexicon for Behavioral Health and Primary Care Integration (Peek & The National Integration Academy Council [NIAC], 2013).

WHAT: Integrated primary and behavioral healthcare that addresses mental health and substance use, health behaviors, and life stressors for a defined population. Medical, behavioral health, and substance use treatment are core components of primary care services and are integral to improving health outcomes.

GOAL: To integrate primary and behavioral healthcare to a population so there is "no wrong door" for seeking treatment

Role of Community Health Nurses in Collaborative Care Models:

1. Screening and implementation of prevention measures
2. Promotion of health behavior change
3. Psychological support and crisis intervention
4. Chronic or complex illness case management
5. Outcome measurement of clinical, functional, and quality of life
6. Outreach to patients or families who do not follow-up and to high-risk populations

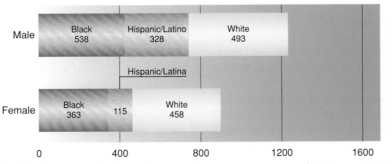

FIGURE 17.3 HIV diagnoses attributed to injection drug use by race/ethnicity and gender, 2015. (From Centers for Disease Control and Prevention [CDC]. [2016]. *HIV and injection drug use: Fast facts* [p. 1]. Retrieved on August 24, 2017, from https://www.cdc.gov/hiv/pdf/risk/cdc-hiv-idu-fact-sheet.pdf.)

Alcohol

Alcoholism is the only disease that you can get yelled at for having. **Mitch Hedberg**

The age at which Americans first use alcohol is a significant risk factor for future dependence or addiction to alcohol. Children who initially use alcohol at 14 years of age or younger are seven times more likely to become dependent on alcohol or abuse it than those who initially use alcohol when they are 21 years of age or older. Rates of alcohol use are now equivalent in adolescent males and females (13.3% and 13.3%, respectively), and the rates of alcohol dependence and abuse are now equivalent in adolescents (Substance Abuse and Mental Health Services Administration [SAMHSA], 2012a). Underage drinking is highest among those reporting two or more races as their ethnic heritage (17.5%), among Native Americans (15.2%), and among white youth (14.6) (SAMHSA, 2012a). Lower socioeconomic status and educational opportunities are two of the social factors associated with increased risk among Native Americans, but a comprehensive understanding of the root social causes is lacking (Stanley, Harness, Swaim, & Beauvais, 2014).

Drinking and driving is a serious public health concern. A positive trend is that the percentage of all Americans who reported drinking and driving continues to decline from 2002. Strict law enforcement and population-based strategies such as school-based education programs and community-based programs are credited with contributing to a decrease in the portion of Americans reporting they engaged in drinking and driving. Laws include mandatory alcohol testing for automobile drivers, sobriety checkpoints, social host laws to reduce teenage alcohol consumption by imposing liability on adults who provide alcohol to underage drinkers, lower blood alcohol levels for driving under the influence (DUI), immediate license suspension for DUI, and age-21 minimum legal drinking age restrictions. A subpopulation that continues to be at high risk for drinking and driving is young adults (18 to 25 years of age) who have almost double the rate of driving impaired than the general population (18.6%) (SAMHSA, 2012a).

Binge drinking is defined by the National Institute on Alcohol Abuse and Alcoholism (NIAAA) as five or more drinks on the same occasion for 1 day during the preceding month for men and four or more drinks on the same occasion for women. Over the past decade, there has been a steady decline in binge drinking among youth who participated in substance prevention programs (SAMHSA, 2012a). Yet, almost one fourth of all Americans over the age of 12 who drink alcohol (22.6%) still meet criteria for binge drinking (SAMHSA, 2012a).

Binge drinking peaks during young adulthood (ages of 18 and 25 years), with 39.8% of users reporting binge drinking behavior (SAMHSA, 2012a). Rates of binge alcohol use vary by race and ethnicity and are highest among American Indians (AIs) or Alaska Natives (ANs) (24.3%) (SAMHSA, 2012a). A major risk factor for problem drinking in young adults is enrollment in college. The significant difference ($p < 0.05$) in binge and heavy drinking between college students (39.1%) and their peers (35.4%) not enrolled in college has remained unchanged over the past decade and suggests campus cultural norms are a strong factor contributing to significantly higher health risks (SAMHSA, 2012a).

The nurse practitioner, Katherine, can see that Mr. Campbell has many of the risk factors for abuse of or dependence on illicit drugs but does not want to stereotype him or falsely assume that he has a drug problem. He may be depressed or in need of proper pain management. She determines that it would be appropriate to begin an evaluation of Mr. Campbell by assessing his mood, especially if he has had any suicidal ideation. In addition, he needs an evaluation for his back pain and sleep disorder.

Cannabis

Cannabis is the most frequently used illicit substance in the United States. There has been a gradual decline in cannabis use over the past 5 years in youth aged 12 to 17 years (SAMHSA, 2017a). Public health prevention strategies recognize that perceived risk can effect when, or if, an individual initiates use of an illicit substance. As states have legalized the recreational and medicinal use of cannabis, adolescents' perception that there are risks associated with smoking cannabis has decreased (NIDA, 2017b). Among adolescents who smoked cannabis in the past month, the majority (73.7%) perceived there was no physical or other risks associated with cannabis (SAMHSA, 2017a). One protective factor is that the use of cannabis is six times lower in youth who perceive parental disapproval compared to youth who perceive strong parental approval.

Tobacco

Over the past decade, the use of tobacco in the United States has continued to significantly decline (SAMHSA, 2012a). The number of Americans reporting daily cigarette smoking continues to decline across all racial/ethnic groups and ages (SAMHSA, 2017a). Over 90% of adolescents strongly disapprove of cigarette smoking by their peers (SAMHSA, 2012a). A disturbing trend is the increasing use of nonconventional tobacco products, such as e-cigarettes or hookahs among youth. Public health experts attribute the increased use of nonconventional tobacco products to a lower perceived risk of harm and confusing public health messages (Mermelstein, 2014). Past month use among teens is now higher for e-cigarettes (12.5%), than for cigarettes (10.5%) (NIDA, 2016). In educating populations, especially youth, about the risks of tobacco use, community health nurses must expand their public health interventions to include nonconventional tobacco products.

Illicit Drugs

In addition to perceived risk, public health studies have found that the availability of drugs and the ease of obtaining illicit substances are associated with initiation and use (Lipari, Williams, Copello, & Pemberton, 2016). In 2015, 27 million Americans used illicit substances or abused drugs including cocaine, opioids (i.e., heroin), hallucinogens (i.e., lysergic acid diethylamide [LSD], phencyclidine [PCP], peyote, mescaline, psilocybin mushrooms, "ecstasy" [also known as MDMA]), inhalants (i.e., nitrous oxide, amyl nitrite, cleaning fluids, gasoline, spray paint, other aerosol sprays, and glue), pain relievers (i.e., oxycodone and propoxyphene), benzodiazepines (i.e., alprazolam and lorazepam), stimulants (i.e., methamphetamine), and sedatives (i.e., phenobarbital, Seconal) (President's Commission Combating Drug Addiction and the Opioid Crisis, 2017). The rate of illicit drug use peaks in young adulthood and then declines with age (SAMHSA, 2017a). Use of any illicit substance is highest among native Hawaiians or other Pacific Islanders (OPI) and AIs or ANs (Fig. 17.4).

Beginning in the 1990s, there was a shift in the pharmacologic treatment of chronic pain by clinicians spearheaded by the designation of pain as the "fifth vital sign." This shift spurred a rapid escalation in the prescription opioids leading to three times as many prescriptions for opioids in 2015 than in 1999 and the total number of prescriptions (239 million) approximating the entire population of the United States (Brady, McCauley, & Back, 2016; Guy et al., 2017). Over half of nonmedical users of stimulants, tranquilizers,

sedatives, and pain relievers received the drug from a friend or relative for free, and four out of five stated that the drug was prescribed by one physician (SAMHSA, 2012a).

There are important public health implications for the rapid escalation and wide regional variation in opioid prescribing practices (Fig. 17.5). Prescription of opioids is significantly higher in nonmetropolitan cities and towns with higher densities of physicians, percentages of non-Hispanic whites, unemployment, and Medicaid enrollment (Guy et al., 2017). This geographic variation suggests inconsistent adherence to evidence-based treatments, including the use of nonopioid analgesics and nonpharmacologic interventions, such as exercise therapy and cognitive–behavioral therapy, to manage chronic pain. To reduce the risks associated with long-term opioid use, in 2016, CDC issued guidelines for the prescription of opioids for chronic pain not associated with palliative or end-of-life care (Dowell, Haegerich, & Chou, 2016). Many states also recently enacted public health policies mandating that prescribers participate in Prescription Drug Monitoring Programs and have imposed stricter regulations of pain clinics (Guy et al., 2017). Public health initiatives at both the national (Box 17.2) and state level are credited with recent reductions in prescription opioid–involved deaths and lowering the number of persons exposed to opioids (Dowell, Zhang, Noonan, & Hockenberry, 2016).

The most recent epidemiologic surveys on substance use in the United States help community health nurses identify populations at greatest risk for abuse and addiction. Some trends have remained stable over many years. But the latest surveys also warn of emerging trends that will pose new challenges for community health nurses. One of the greatest

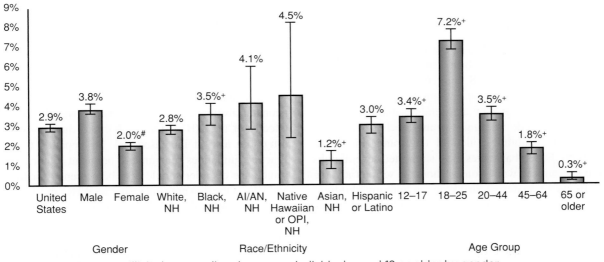

FIGURE 17.4 Past year illicit drug use disorder among individuals aged 12 or older by gender, race/ethnicity, and age group, 2015. NH, non-Hispanic. (From Substance Abuse and Mental Health Services Administration [SAMHSA]. [2017]. *Behavioral health barometer: United States, Volume 4: Indicators as measured through the 2015 National Survey on Drug Use and Health and National Survey of Substance Abuse Treatment Services* [p. 16]. HHS Pub No. SMA-17-BaroUS-16. Rockville, MD: SAMHSA.)

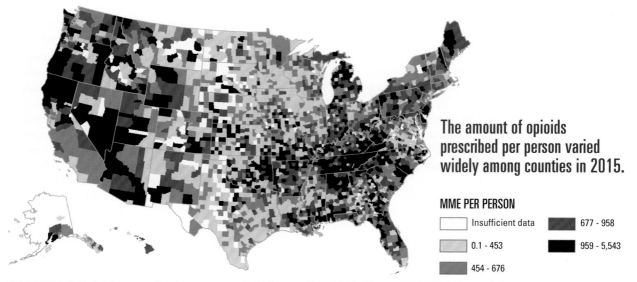

The amount of opioids prescribed per person varied widely among counties in 2015.

MME PER PERSON

☐ Insufficient data	▨ 677 - 958
☐ 0.1 - 453	■ 959 - 5,543
▩ 454 - 676	

FIGURE 17.5 Opioids prescribed per person in U.S. counties, 2015. (From CDC Vital Signs, July 2017. Retrieved from https://www.cdc.gov/vitalsigns/opioids/infographic.html#graphic-b.)

challenges will be faced by nurses in the community who provide nursing care to at-risk populations. For example, populations at greatest risk for prescription opioid overdose are white males between the ages of 35 and 44 years with a history of substance use disorder or psychiatric disorder (Brady, Giglio, Keyes, DiMaggio, & Li, 2017). How community health nurses can identify people at risk across the lifespan and intervene with evidence-based programs aimed at prevention is the focus of the next section of this chapter.

HEALTH PROFILES AND INTERVENTIONS FOR HIGH-RISK POPULATIONS

Pregnant Women

Fetal alcohol syndrome (FAS) is the leading cause of preventable developmental disability in the world (Hoyme et al., 2016). In 1981, the U.S. Surgeon General issued the first public health advisory warning about the association of alcohol use during pregnancy and fetal disabilities. An Act of Congress followed, ordering warning labels to be added to all products containing alcohol (Bertrand, Floyd, & Weber, 2005). Federal agencies have supported several public health measures to warn women about the serious adverse health effects of maternal drinking on unborn children. Alcohol use during pregnancy is a serious public health concern because of the multiple deleterious, lifelong effects of alcohol on the fetus including low IQ, hyperactivity, short attention span, distinctive facial anomalies, and structural brain defects. Given the severity of developmental disabilities associated with FAS, the WHO (2014b) issued guidelines recommending that all healthcare providers ask all pregnant women about their use of alcohol and other substances as early as possible in the pregnancy and at every

antenatal visit (Box 17.3). If pregnant women are using alcohol or drugs, the WHO (2014b) recommends brief intervention and immediate referral to detoxification services and psychosocial care.

The American College of Obstetricians and Gynecologists and the CDC also recommend screening all women of childbearing age for substance use (Reddy, Davis, Ren, & Greene, 2017). When screening women for alcohol use, community health nurses should ask women to respond to questions in the validated T-ACE questionnaire as they would before they learned that they were pregnant. Nurses should also inquire about the stage of pregnancy at which the woman reduced or eliminated her alcohol consumption. At this time there are no validated screening instruments available for illicit substance use. Urine toxic screens can supplement face-to-face interviews and provide information about the use of polysubstances, but laboratory tests must be interpreted cautiously because a negative result does not rule out past use or the intensity of past use (Reddy et al., 2017).

The rise in opioid use has resulted in a fivefold increase in neonatal abstinence syndrome (NAS) over the past decade (Reddy et al., 2017). Infants born to mothers who inject drugs are also at increased risk for hepatitis C and HIV. Practice guidelines recommend pregnant women with substance use disorder should also be screened for hepatitis C and HIV at the first prenatal visit. The WHO and the American Society of Addiction Medicine endorse medication-assisted treatment with methadone and buprenorphine over supervised opioid withdrawal for pregnant women to minimize the risk of relapse and nonadherence to prenatal care.

Opioid withdrawal symptoms in neonates may present in the first 48 hours or a week after birth with symptoms ranging from irritability to life-threatening seizures. Newborns with NAS may remain hospitalized for weeks after mothers have been discharged potentially impeding the opportunities

17.2 CDC Recommendations for Prescribing Opioids for Chronic Pain Outside Palliative and End-of-Life Care

Determining When to Initiate or Continue Opioids for Chronic Pain

1. Nonpharmacologic therapy and nonopioid pharmacologic therapy are preferred for chronic pain. Clinicians should consider opioid therapy only if expected benefits for both pain and function are anticipated to outweigh risks to the patient. If opioids are used, they should be combined with nonpharmacologic therapy and nonopioid pharmacologic therapy, as appropriate.

2. Before starting opioid therapy for chronic pain, clinicians should establish treatment goals with all patients, including realistic goals for pain and function, and should consider how opioid therapy will be discontinued if benefits do not outweigh risks. Clinicians should continue opioid therapy only if there is clinically meaningful improvement in pain and function that outweighs risks to patient safety.

3. Before starting and periodically during opioid therapy, clinicians should discuss with patients known risks and realistic benefits of opioid therapy and patient and clinician responsibilities for managing therapy.

Opioid Selection, Dosage, Duration, Follow-Up, and Discontinuation

4. When starting opioid therapy for chronic pain, clinicians should prescribe immediate-release opioids instead of extended-release/long-acting (ER/LA) opioids.

5. When opioids are started, clinicians should prescribe the lowest effective dosage. Clinicians should use caution when prescribing opioids at any dosage, should carefully reassess evidence of individual benefits and risks when considering increasing dosage to ≥50 morphine milligram equivalents (MME)/day, and should avoid increasing dosage to ≥90 MME/day or carefully justify a decision to titrate dosage to ≥90 MME/day.

6. Long-term opioid use often begins with treatment of acute pain. When opioids are used for acute pain, clinicians should prescribe the lowest effective dose of immediate-release opioids and should prescribe no greater quantity than needed for the expected duration of pain severe enough to require opioids. Three days or less will often be sufficient; more than 7 days will rarely be needed.

7. Clinicians should evaluate benefits and harms with patients within 1 to 4 weeks of starting opioid therapy for chronic pain or of dose escalation. Clinicians should evaluate benefits and harms of continued therapy with patients every 3 months or more frequently. If benefits do not outweigh harms of continued opioid therapy, clinicians should optimize other therapies and work with patients to taper opioids to lower dosages or to taper and discontinue opioids.

Assessing Risk and Addressing Harms of Opioid Use

8. Before starting and periodically during continuation of opioid therapy, clinicians should evaluate risk factors for opioid-related harms. Clinicians should incorporate into the management plan strategies to mitigate risk, including considering offering naloxone when factors that increase risk for opioid overdose, such as history of overdose, history of substance use disorder, higher opioid dosages (≥50 MME/day), or concurrent benzodiazepine use, are present.

9. Clinicians should review the patient's history of controlled substance prescriptions using state Prescription Drug Monitoring Program (PDMP) data to determine whether the patient is receiving opioid dosages or dangerous combinations that put him or her at high risk for overdose. Clinicians should review PDMP data when starting opioid therapy for chronic pain and periodically during opioid therapy for chronic pain, ranging from every prescription to every 3 months.

10. When prescribing opioids for chronic pain, clinicians should use urine drug testing before starting opioid therapy and consider urine drug testing at least annually to assess for prescribed medications as well as other controlled prescription drugs and illicit drugs.

11. Clinicians should avoid prescribing opioid pain medication and benzodiazepines concurrently whenever possible.

12. Clinicians should offer or arrange evidence-based treatment (usually medication-assisted treatment with buprenorphine or methadone in combination with behavioral therapies) for patients with opioid use disorder.

All recommendations are category A (apply to all patients outside of active cancer treatment, palliative care, and end-of-life care) except recommendation 10 (designated category B, with individual decision making required); see full guideline for evidence ratings.
Source: Dowell, D., Haegerich, T. M., & Chou, R. (2016). CDC guideline for prescribing opioids for chronic pain – United States, 2016 [p. 16]. *Morbidity and Mortality Weekly Report, 65*(1), 1–50.

for mother–infant bonding. Innovative models provide additional resources for community-based care, so newborns maybe discharged home with their mothers and if indicated, receive medication-assisted treatment for detoxification. Best practices for care of infants recovering from NAS in the home include the use of a transitional care nurse to coordinate care across healthcare settings and providers (Gregory, 2014). Families and caregivers should be provided with education to recognize the symptoms of NAS and guidance on nonpharmacologic interventions (Reddy et al., 2017). The severity of NAS symptoms can be minimized by a quiet, lowly lit, nonstimulating environment. Other infant comfort measures include swaddling, nonnutritive sucking, rocking, and gentle massage (MacMullen, Dulski, & Blobaum, 2014). Unless contraindicated, nurses should encourage women prescribed methadone or buprenorphine to breastfeed. A home safety assessment by nurses is critical to assure medication-assisted treatments are safely stored and administered.

17.3 Assessment Guideline for Identifying Fetal Alcohol Syndrome

Facial dysmorphia
   Smooth philtrum
   Thin vermillion border
   Small palpebral fissures
Growth problems
   Postnatal height, weight, or both <10th percentile
Central nervous system abnormalities
   Structural
      Head circumference <10th percentile
      Reduced size or change in shape of corpus callosum,
         cerebellum, and basal ganglia seen on MRI
   Neurologic
      Motor problems
      Seizures
   Functional
      Cognitive or intellectual deficits <3rd percentile
      Functional deficits <16th percentile in three of the following:

   1. Cognitive development
   2. Executive functioning
   3. Motor functioning delays
   4. Problems with attention or hyperactivity
   5. Problems with social skills
   6. Sensory, language, or memory problems

Source: Bertrand, J., Floyd, R. L., & Weber, M. K. (2005). Guidelines for identifying and referring persons with fetal alcohol syndrome. *Morbidity and Mortality Weekly Report Recommendations and Reports, 54*(RR11), 1–14.

One of the most widely used and scientifically proven programs to improve health outcomes for at-risk first-time mothers is the Nurse–Family Partnership (NFP) program (Dawley, Loch, & Bindrich, 2007; Donelan-McCall, Eckenrode, & Olds, 2009). The NFP pairs at-risk new mothers with community health nurses who provide hour-long visits every 2 weeks in the home for the first 2 years of an infant's life. Health education and interventions provided by the community health nurses include avoiding alcohol and drug use, nutritional counseling, smoking cessation, parenting skills, case management regarding pediatric care for their infant and primary care for the mothers, and vocational counseling to promote economic self-sufficiency (Dawley et al., 2007).

Donelan-McCall and colleagues (2009) note that the NFP has the strongest support to date of any nurse home-visiting program; scientific evidence shows that it can improve the health outcomes of children born to at-risk mothers and is cost-effective. The savings realized by the NFP programs in decreased adverse health events, emergency department visits, and the like (approximately $18,000) are twice as much as the cost per family for 2 years of nurse home visits (approximately $9,000) (Donelan-McCall et al., 2009; Lee, Aos, & Miller, 2008). Begun in 1977 by Dr. David Olds with community health nurses in Elmira, New York, today NFP is in 350 counties nationally

17.4 The Nurse–Family Partnership

Nurse–Family Partnership (NFP) is a prenatal and infancy nurse home visitation program that aims to improve the health, well-being, and self-sufficiency of low-income, first-time parents and their children. Nurses follow a detailed, visit-by-visit guide that provides information on (tracking) dietary intake; reducing cigarette, alcohol, and illegal drug use; identifying symptoms of pregnancy complications and signs of children's illnesses; communicating with healthcare professionals; promoting parent–child interactions; creating safe households; and considering educational and career options. Program objectives include decreased substance use, improved maternal economic self-sufficiency, fewer subsequent unintended pregnancies, reduced child abuse and neglect, and improved school readiness of the children. Individual programs serve a minimum of 100 to 200 families and are supported by 4 to 8 trained registered nurse home visitors (each carrying a caseload of 25 families), a nurse supervisor, and administrative support. Nurse home visits begin early in pregnancy and continue until the child's second birthday. The frequency of home visits changes with the stages of pregnancy and infancy and is adapted to the mother's needs, with a maximum of 13 visits occurring during pregnancy and 47 occurring after the child's birth.

The NFP targets women in urban, suburban, rural, and frontier areas. Races and ethnicities who have received the NFP interventions include Asian, black or African American, Hispanic or Latino, and white.

Readiness for dissemination ratings by criteria = 3.7 (0.0–4.0
   scale)
Implementation materials = 3.5
Training and support = 4.0
Quality assurance = 3.5

Source: Substance Abuse and Mental Health Services Administration (SAMHSA). (2017). Using Prevention Research to Guide Prevention Practice. *SAMHSA's Center for the Application of Prevention Technologies, 34.* Retrieved on December 17, 2018, from https://www.samhsa.gov/capt/sites/default/files/resources/preventing-youth-marijuana-use-programs-strategies-2017.pdf.

and is supported by funding from federal or state healthcare and social service grants as well as private foundations. NFP is a compelling example of how investing in preventive healthcare provided by community health nurses improves health outcomes in a cost-effective manner. SAMHSA has developed a National Registry of Evidence-based Programs and Practices, including NFP, to identify scientifically proven programs to prevent or treat mental and/or substance abuse disorders and facilitate their implementation in communities across the United States (Box 17.4). An example of a culturally tailored model using health educators indigenous to the population is Family Spirit, an organization in which trained health educators provide home-visiting intervention for AI teenage mothers (Box 17.5).

Given the marked risk for teratogenesis and obstetric complications, the American Society on Addiction Medicine recommends that pregnant women in need of substance use treatment be given the highest priority for admission and

17.5 Family Spirit

Family Spirit is a culturally tailored home-visiting intervention for American Indian teenage mothers—who generally experience high rates of substance use, school dropout, and residential instability—from pregnancy through 36 months postpartum. The intervention is designed to increase parenting competence (e.g., parenting knowledge and self-efficacy), reduce maternal psychosocial and behavioral risks that could interfere with effective parenting (e.g., drug and alcohol use, depression, externalizing problems), and promote healthy infant and toddler emotional and social adjustment (i.e., internalizing and externalizing behaviors). It also aims to prepare toddlers for early school success, promote parents' coping and life skills, and link families to appropriate community services.

Family Spirit is based on Patterson's social interaction learning model, which suggests that a parent's stressful life circumstances (e.g., unstable housing, poverty, weak family support, mental health and substance abuse issues) trigger a high level of coercive parenting associated with early childhood behavior problems that predict poor outcomes in middle and later childhood. The intervention consists of 63 structured lessons delivered one-on-one by health educators in participants' homes, starting at about 28 weeks of gestation and continuing to 36 months postpartum. The lessons, designed to correspond to the changing developmental needs of the mother and child during this period, address topics such as prenatal care, infant care, child development, family planning, and healthy living. Each home visit lasts about an hour and includes a warm-up conversation, lesson content, question-and-answer period, and review of summary handouts. Health educators, trained American Indian paraprofessionals, deliver the lessons using illustrated tabletop flipcharts. The bond formed between the health educator and mother is intended to facilitate the mother's progress toward goals. The 63 lessons can be delivered in 52 home visits, which occur weekly through 3 months postpartum and gradually become less frequent thereafter.
Family Spirit targets American Indian or Alaska native women in rural and frontier areas.

Readiness for dissemination ratings by criteria = 4.0 (0.0–4.0 scale)
Implementation materials = 4.0
Training and support = 4.0
Quality assurance = 4.0

Source: Substance Abuse and Mental Health Services Administration (SAMHSA). (2017). Using Prevention Research to Guide Prevention Practice. *SAMHSA's Center for the Application of Prevention Technologies, 18.* Retrieved on December 17, 2018, from https://www.samhsa.gov/capt/sites/default/files/resources/preventing-youth-marijuana-use-programs-strategies-2017.pdf.

treatment (Haug, Duffy, & McCaul, 2014). Six new objectives have been added to *Healthy People 2020*, including abstinence from drinking or smoking in preconception.

Evidence for Practice

A study by Jarlenski and colleagues (2017) of reproductive age women (*n* = 4498) from 2005 to 2014 found 2% reported nonmedical opioid use in the last 30 days. Among a subsample of pregnant women who reported nonmedical opioid use, 42% smoked 5 or more cigarettes a day and 51.2% ingested 5 or more alcohol drinks per day. The authors note that given these findings, public health programs need to expand polysubstance use treatment to women of reproductive age to promote recovery from substance use disorder and improve pregnancy outcomes.

Evidence for Practice

The Dartmouth-Hitchcock Medical Center Perinatal Addiction Treatment Program integrates prenatal care and postpartum care with evidence-based substance use treatment services consistent with models of integrative care endorsed by the Agency for Healthcare Research and Quality (AHRQ) and the Institute of Medicine (Goodman, 2015). Regular multidisciplinary meetings between maternity and pediatric providers in both the hospital and outpatient clinic facilitate the coordination of care for pregnant women and their infants, improve patient satisfaction, and increase attendance at prenatal visits. Maternity providers, including certified nurse midwives, nurse practitioners, and neonatal nurses, receive training in screening and brief interventions for SUD. Neonatal nurses participate in outpatient addiction recovery groups to provide education to pregnant women about the care of newborns with NAS. Colocation of midwifery services in a dedicated substance use treatment program is cost-effective and improves health outcomes for both women and newborns (Goodman, 2015).

The criminalization of health behaviors raises serious ethical questions for community health nurses who provide healthcare to people who may become targets of criminal investigations. In the case of *Ferguson v. the City of Charleston (South Carolina) (99–936)*, the Fourth Circuit Court of Appeals upheld the conviction of a pregnant woman who tested positive for cocaine and was reported to law enforcement authorities on the basis of a hospital policy adopted at the University of South Carolina Medical Center. The case was ultimately heard by the U.S. Supreme Court. Professional healthcare organizations such as the American Nurses Association (ANA), the American Public Health Association, and the American College of Obstetricians and Gynecologists submitted written testimony, termed an *amicus curiae* brief, in support of the defendant. Subsequent to the ruling of the U.S. Supreme Court, the ANA joined over 140 organizations and researchers in a public letter to the U.S. Surgeon General stating, "The ANA recognizes alcohol and other drug problems as treatable illnesses. The threat of criminal prosecution is counterproductive in that it prevents many women from seeking prenatal care and treatment for their alcohol and other drug problems" (Tillett & Osborne, 2001, p. 6).

In 2001, the U.S. Supreme Court decided in a 6-to-3 ruling that the defendant's Fourth Amendment rights had been violated, and overturned the conviction. In an analysis of the Supreme Court ruling of *Ferguson v. the City of Charleston*, the noted medical ethicist George Annas (2001) observed that the more the lines between the professional duties of physicians and nurses are blurred with those of law enforcement, the more that trust between clients and healthcare providers is eroded, and the greater the likelihood that women who are in need of prenatal care will not seek care at all.

More recently, the Child Abuse Prevention and Treatment Act was amended in 2016 (P.L. 114–198) to require states develop discharge plans for newborns born with NAS or FAS that assure adequate community resources are in place for mothers to appropriately care for their newborns in their home (USDHHS, 2016). The intent of the 2016 amendment was to assure the safety and well-being of newborns who may be at risk from alcohol or opioid exposures during pregnancy. However, Terplan and Mindoff (2017) note that the effect of the 2016 amendments to the Child Abuse Prevention and Treatment Act may be to trigger a response beyond addressing the health needs of substance-exposed newborns to removal of children and prosecution of mothers for illicit substance use. Community health nurses conduct assessments and validated screenings of pregnant women to identify populations at risk and provide evidence-based interventions to minimize harm to an unborn child. Yet the very act of professional nursing practice raises complicated ethical questions about duty to patient's confidentiality and autonomy given federal reporting mandates.

Substance Use at an Early Age

Individual, family, and community influences all contribute to the use of substances by underage children and adolescents. How much of the increased risk is due to nature (genetic vulnerabilities) or nurture (environmental influences) can partially be illuminated by studies of twins, adopted children, and genetic research. Monozygotic twin and adoption studies estimate the risk of inheritability of alcoholism at approximately 50% (Gray & Squeglia, 2018). Thus, at least half the risk of developing alcoholism may be due to factors in communities, schools, or families.

Developmental or peer influences also play a role. It is known that most adults with addiction or substance abuse disorders began using alcohol or illicit substances while in middle school. Since 2011, the percentage of adolescents initiating alcohol, marijuana, and cigarette use has declined suggesting that public health education initiatives maybe having a positive effect on delaying substance use (SAMHSA, 2017a). Despite growing rates of opioid use and deaths in adults, misuse of all prescription opioids among 12th graders in 2016 markedly declined by 45%

over the past 5 years (NIDA, 2016). Personality attributes such as poor impulse control, attention deficits, conduct disorders, and general psychological dysregulation are individual factors that have been associated with early-onset substance use. In adolescents with substance use disorder there is often a high comorbidity with the early onset of anxiety disorders, posttraumatic stress disorder, and major depression (Gray & Squeglia, 2018). However especially among youth, access to substances continues to play a central role in initiation of substance use. For example, marijuana use by adolescents is higher in states legalizing medical and recreational marijuana use compared to states where marijuana use remains illegal (NIDA, 2016). It is critical that community health nurses recognize that during middle school, risk is greatly increased if a child has any friends who have used alcohol in the past year (Strobbe, 2013). How individual vulnerabilities, social experiences, or community influences coalesce to the point where 12 to 14 year olds are initiating alcohol use is the focus of public health research.

A thorough family history for substance use and screening youth for risk factors associated with early substance use is a critical first step. The United States Preventive Services Task Force (USPSTF, 2014) recommends primary care and community-based health professionals screen youths to identify patients at risk for substance misuse. The American Academy of Pediatrics recommends the CRAFFT screening tool specifically designed for use in adolescent populations (Box 17.6). Integrative primary care and schools are ideal locations for nurses to introduce prevention and early intervention programs (Curtis, McLellan, & Gabellini, 2014).

17.6   CRAFFT Drug Screening Questionnaire for Use in Adolescents

1. Have you ever ridden in a **Car** driven by someone (including yourself) who was "high" or had been using alcohol or drugs?
2. Do you ever use alcohol or drugs to **Relax**, feel better about yourself, or fit in?
3. Do you ever use alcohol or drugs while you are by yourself, **Alone**?
4. Do you ever **Forget** things you did while using alcohol or drugs?
5. Do your family or **Friends** ever tell you that you should cut down on your drinking or drug use?
6. Have you gotten into **Trouble** while you were using alcohol or drugs?

Scoring: A "Yes" answer to two or more questions indicates the need for active intervention.

Source: Substance Abuse and Mental Health Services Administration (SAMHSA). TIP 31: *Screening and assessing adolescents for substance use disorders.* Retrieved on July 29, 2009, from http://www.ncbi.nlm.nih.gov/books/bv.fcgi?rid=hstat5.chapter.54841.

While peer influences play a role in substance use, numerous studies have found strong associations between parenting style and health risk behaviors in children. Parents who are engaged with their child, supervising and monitoring their activities, providing appropriate discipline, and sustaining positive parent–child bonds throughout adolescence can have a notable effect on adolescent substance use (Allen et al., 2016). The majority of adolescents who abuse prescription medication acquired the medication from a friend or family member (Allen et al., 2017). It is critical for community health nurses to screen for family or social experiences that are associated with the misuse of alcohol, illicit drugs, and prescription opioids in children and adolescents. Nurses can ask whether there is excessive consumption by family members and peers, if the adolescent or child has access to alcohol or prescription opioids, and if there are peers or family members who willingly provide them with access to these substances. It is the early initiation of substance misuse that is most strongly predictive of addiction in adulthood.

I mean, I inherited the disease of alcoholism, and I learned early to get help when I needed it. **Liza Minnelli**

Evidence for Practice

The SAMHSA (2017b) has developed a practical guide to provide nurses in community-based settings information to plan and deliver prevention strategies based upon SAMHSA's Strategic Prevention Framework. The Strategic Prevention Framework is a five-step process that describes evidence-based prevention strategies and tools communities can use to successfully implement prevention programs. Step One is to correctly assess the substance use, risk and protective factors, and readiness in the community to act. Step Two is to build coalitions with key stakeholders and train individuals to sustain the mission of the program. Step Three is to develop an evidence-based prevention plan that identifies outcomes for evaluating performance. Step Four is to implement culturally competent programs and policies with proven effectiveness in the community. Step Five is to evaluate program outcomes, assess the quality of the services, and identify areas for improvement. Sample materials include a pitch letter to organizations and stakeholders; sample public service announcements; sample feature articles; media kits; and detailed "how-to" plans to guide implementation of a prevention program targeting substance use among youth. To learn more about SAMHSA's *Focus on Prevention: Strategies and Programs to Prevent Substance Use,* see http://www.samhsa.gov.

The difference in substance use among Native American youth and the general adolescent population is especially pronounced among the youngest adolescents. Substance misuse is a major public health concern for Native American

youth on reservations where over half of eighth graders report alcohol and cannabis use, a pronounced increase from overall national prevalence rates for eighth graders of all ethnicities (Stanley et al., 2014). While there is no causal model to explain the higher rates of substance use among youth on reservations, social factors including greater availability from local cannabis farms, proximity to Mexico and drug gangs, lower socioeconomic status, and lower academic attainment are some of the social conditions that researchers have associated with this pronounced health disparity (Stanley et al., 2014).

Although less than 1% of adolescents report using inhalants to get high, the effects, even with first-time use, can be deadly (Lipari, 2017). The 2015 National Survey on Drug Use and Health found no differences in inhalant use by region, race, or ethnicity. Inhalant use peaks in young adolescence and diminishes with age with significantly more girls reporting inhalant use than boys (Lipari, 2017). Typical inhalants used by adolescents are common household items that contain volatile solvents such as felt-tip markers, glues, or paint thinners; computer cleaner; butane, propane, or gasoline. Fumes may be inhaled through the mouth, referred to by adolescents as "huffing," or the nose (sniffing), to achieve a short-term state of **intoxication** similar to alcohol. Adolescent inhalant users are at increased risk for delinquency, depression, suicide, and drug and alcohol use (Lipari, 2017). Given the morbidity and mortality associated with inhalant use, it is important for nurses in the community to educate adolescents, parents, teachers, and other adults interacting with youth about the serious health hazards associated with inhalant use.

Evidence for Practice

The LifeSkills Training program, an evidence-based program for prevention of drug and alcohol abuse, has been implemented in 33 rural public schools located in communities prone to methamphetamine abuse. Outcome studies of LifeSkills Training have reported statistically significant and sustained decreases in all forms of substance use, especially for higher-risk subpopulations of adolescents, including those in rural and frontier regions of the United States (Spoth, Randall, Trudeau, Shin, & Redmond, 2008, p. 66). These scientifically validated prevention efforts appear to be having an effect. In 2012, the number of Americans 12 years of age or older who used methamphetamine for the first time (133,000) was less than half the number of new users reported in 2004 (318,00). (SAMHSA, 2012a). These statistics suggest that comprehensive public health and law enforcement efforts are making a significant difference in decreasing the methamphetamine use in the United States. SAMHSA's National Registry of Evidence-Based Programs and Practices has given LifeSkills Training its highest rating for efficacy and readiness of dissemination (Box 17.7).

17.7   LifeSkills Training

LifeSkills Training (LST) is a school-based program that aims to prevent alcohol use, tobacco use, illicit substance use, and violence by targeting the major social and psychological factors that promote the initiation of substance use and other risky behaviors. LST addresses multiple risk and protective factors and teaches personal and social skills which build resilience and help youth navigate developmental tasks, including the skills necessary to understand and resist prodrug influences. LST is designed to provide information relevant to the important life transitions that adolescents and young teens face, using culturally sensitive and developmentally and age-appropriate language and content. Facilitated discussion, structured small group activities, and role-playing scenarios are used to stimulate participation and promote the acquisition of skills. Separate LST programs are offered for elementary school (grades 3–6), middle school (grades 6–9), and high school (grades 9–12).

LST targets adolescents in urban, suburban, rural, and frontier areas. Races and ethnicities who have received LST include American Indian or Alaska native, Asian, black or African American, Hispanic or Latino, and white.

Readiness for dissemination ratings by criteria = 4.0 (0.0–4.0 scale)

Implementation materials = 4.0

Training and support = 4.0

Quality assurance = 4.0

Source: Substance Abuse and Mental Health Services Administration (SAMHSA). (2017). Using Prevention Research to Guide Prevention Practice. *SAMHSA's Center for the Application of Prevention Technologies, 26.* Retrieved on December 17, 2018, from https://www.samhsa.gov/capt/sites/default/files/resources/preventing-youth-marijuana-use-programs-strategies-2017.pdf.

Population-based interventions to decrease substance use among adolescents can be conceptualized in four categories: regulatory, developmental prevention, early screening, and harm reduction (Toumbourou et al., 2007). Minimum age laws for drinking alcohol, strict enforcement of laws prohibiting drinking and driving, and enforcement of youth possession laws have proved to be effective deterrents to underage substance use (Toumbourou et al., 2007). Developmental prevention programs can be effective in deterring substance use in adolescents as well, if such prevention programs are sensitive to the significant variations in substance use in adolescence by age, ethnicity, geographic location, and gender.

Research shows that parents are the single biggest influence on children—if you are worried about your teen and drugs, talk to them. **John Walters**

In contrast to screening and education of entire populations of adolescents, a public health approach demonstrating improved efficacy with adolescents is screening with the CRAFFT tool to identify youth at risk followed by tailored brief interventions and referral to specialty treatment based upon the severity score. This approach, termed SBIRT (screening, brief intervention, referral to treatment) has been implemented in primary care, emergency rooms, school-based settings, and in shelters with homeless youth (Mitchell, Gryczynski, O'Grady, & Schwartz, 2013). In the SBIRT model, interventions are specifically targeted based on the severity of symptoms and it includes brief interventions for even mild symptoms in populations considered at-risk. The brief interventions in SBIRT consist of the chief components of motivational interviewing.

Motivational interviewing is particularly effective with adolescents because it respects the adolescents' developmental need for autonomy (Mitchell et al., 2013). The nurse partners with the adolescent to identify the harms associated with substance misuse in a nonjudgmental manner, and the nurse objectively points out inconsistencies with the adolescent's personal goals and aspirations. The nurse thoughtfully negotiates with the adolescent about the possibility of changing harmful behaviors and assists the adolescent in setting realistic goals achievable in a brief period of time. For example, a goal may be slightly decreasing the amount of alcoholic beverages consumed in a week or the weekend by a goal self-selected by the adolescent. In follow-up sessions, the nurse reinforces health promoting behaviors and the achievement of goals. Key to the successful implementation of brief interventions is that the goals be self-selected by the adolescent, that they be achievable, and that the nurse provides immediate reinforcement and encouragement for achieving the goal.

Evidence for Practice

SBIRT was implemented in two urban New York public schools during nonacademic classes (Curtis et al., 2014). All 6th- to 12th-grade students were screened with an interactive computer tool that included the CRAFFT scale. Adolescents with a CRAFFT score of zero (no use) would be given factual information and support for continuing health promoting behaviors. Those scoring 1 or 2 on the CRAFFT screen (low-risk use) would be given a motivational interview lasting between 15 and 30 minutes. Adolescents with a CRAFFT score of 3 or greater with significant levels of substance use were provided a brief intervention emphasizing the severity of substance use, telephone notification of parents, and options for referral to treatment.

In summary, community health nurses should follow the guidelines of the American Academy of Pediatrics that recommend all adolescents be screened for alcohol and drug use and that at-risk adolescents be given brief interventions and in the cases of severe misuse, referred for treatment by specialists (USPSTF, 2014). In formulating culturally appropriate evidence-based interventions, studies suggest that Hispanic youth have better outcomes when paired with

Hispanic healthcare providers, and gang youths or youth with severe substance use and complex behavioral issues benefit from family-based therapies that broadly examine social issues within the family, school, peer relationships, and the juvenile justice system (Hogue, Henderson, Ozechowski, & Robbins, 2014).

College Students and Binge Drinking

Binge drinking is defined as a consumption of alcohol that brings the blood alcohol level to 0.08% or above, which typically occurs after women consume four alcoholic beverages or men five alcoholic beverages in 2 hours (NIAAA, 2015). Although alcohol use has declined in high school students and young adults not in college, students in college deviated from similarly aged cohorts with continued high use of alcohol, especially, binge drinking (Johnston, O'Malley, Bachman, Schulenberg, & Miech, 2016). These findings suggest that the environmental influence of attending college is a significant risk factor in hazardous use of alcohol for young adults. Unlike their younger peers, who may use alcoholic beverages to cope with family dysfunction, violence, or painful emotions, college students are more likely to engage in heavy or binge drinking to enhance their mood or affective state.

Of the 60% of college students who reported consuming alcohol in the past month, approximately two out of three college students report binge drinking (NIAAA, 2015). That the majority of college students who consume alcohol engage in high-risk patterns of consumption is a major public health issue on college campuses. Binge drinking by college students is associated with a life altering health risks including physical and sexual assault, alcohol poisoning, and alcohol-related deaths. Rates of binge drinking vary by race, gender, and peer-group affiliation, suggesting that cultural and environmental influences play a strong role in the patterns of drinking behavior by college students.

That's all drugs and alcohol do, they cut off your emotions in the end. **Ringo Starr**

In 2002, the NIAAA Task Force on College Drinking received a mandate to review and disseminate evidence-based strategies to decrease alcohol use on college campuses. The NIAAA Task Force compiled their findings in a report entitled *A Call to Action: Changing the Culture of Drinking at U.S. Colleges*, which was distributed to college administrators across the United States. The NIAAA Task Force continues to systematically review the scientific evidence for programs or initiatives with demonstrated efficacy and provides periodic updates of new evidence-based programs on its website entitled "College AIM" (Alcohol Intervention Matrix) (Table 17.1).

The NIAAA (2017) created "College AIM" to provide universities and healthcare providers a matrix on individual and environmental evidence-based interventions effective for the general population of college students (see Table 17.1).

Interventions that target individual students at high risk include first year students, student athletes, members of Greek organizations, and mandated students. Consistent with recommendations from the USPSTF, one of the recommended individual-level interventions College AIM is that alcohol screening be included as a standard practice in all university student health services. To detect high-risk drinking in college students, community health nurses and physicians should specifically assess for the quantity and frequency of heavy episodic drinking. Computerized screening surveys in routine health screening may also be a useful tool for community health nurses to identify students who may be at risk. Given the wide variation among college students in their patterns of binge drinking behavior, multiple screenings are advised. An individual-level intervention relevant to nurse practitioners and physicians is the prescription of naltrexone, acamprosate, and disulfiram approved by the Food and Drug Administration (FDA) for the treatment of alcohol use disorder. College AIM also endorses the USPSTF recommendation for brief counseling sessions to reduce the frequency and intensity of alcohol use.

Evidence for Practice

Research compiled by the NIAAA has found that patterns of hazardous drinking varied by a number of demographic and environmental factors, including year in school, week in the semester, and whether the student was in residential housing on or off campus. For example, women drink more intensely in their freshman year, whereas men drink more intensely in their senior year (Kelly-Weeder, 2008). In both heavy and moderate college drinkers, drinking patterns are cyclical, with peaks 3 weeks into the semester, over holidays, and spring break (Greenbaum, Del Boca, Darkes, Wang, & Goldman, 2005). Despite the substantial patterns of alcohol abuse, studies have found that nurses and physicians screen for alcohol use in less than one third of university health services and that only 12% use standardized instruments (Foote, Wilkens, & Vavgiakis, 2004).

Practice Point

One consequence of the failure to identify high-risk students in the freshman year in college is the increased likelihood for academic failures. Wilhite, Ashenhurst, Marion, and Fromme's (2017) longitudinal study of college students found that binge drinking was a significant predictor of time to college graduation and lower odds of achieving developmental milestones in adulthood. The researchers note that these alcohol-related effects may indicate a lack of

TABLE 17.1	National Institute on Alcohol Abuse and Alcoholism (NIAAA) Evidence-Based Programs to Decrease Binge Drinking on College Campuses			
		Three-in-One Framework		
		Level of Operation		
Tier	**Strategy**	**Individuals, Including At-Risk and Dependent Drinkers**	**Student Population as Whole**	**Community**
1. Effective among college students	Combining cognitive–behavioral skills with norms clarification and motivational enhancement intervention	Yes	No	No
	Offering brief motivational enhancement interventions in student health centers and emergency rooms	Yes	No	No
	Challenging alcohol expectancies	Yes	No	No
2. Effective with general populations	Increased enforcement of minimum drinking age laws	No	Yes	Yes
	Implementation, increased publicity, and enforcement of other laws to reduce alcohol-impaired driving	No	Yes	Yes
	Restrictions on alcohol retail density	No	No	Yes
	Increased price and excise taxes on alcoholic beverages	No	No	Yes
	Responsible beverage service policies in social and commercial settings	No	Yes	Yes
	The formation of a campus/community coalition	No	Yes	Yes
3. Promising	Adopting campus-based policies to reduce high-risk use (e.g., reinstating Friday classes, eliminating keg parties, establishing alcohol-free activities, and dorms)	No	Yes	No
	Increasing enforcement at campus-based events that promote excessive drinking	No	Yes	No
	Increasing publicity about enforcement of underage drinking laws/eliminating "mixed" messages	No	Yes	Yes
	Consistently enforcing campus disciplinary actions associated with policy violations	No	Yes	No
	Conducting marketing campaigns to correct student misperceptions about alcohol use on campus	No	Yes	No
	Provision of "safe rides" programs	No	Yes	Yes
	Regulation of happy hours and sales	No	Yes	Yes
	Enhancing awareness of personal liability	Yes	Yes	Yes
	Informing new students and parents about alcohol policies and penalties	Yes	Yes	No
4. Ineffective	Informational, knowledge-based, or values clarification interventions when used alone	N/A	N/A	N/A

Source: National Institute on Alcohol Abuse and Alcoholism (NIAAA). (2007). *College drinking: Changing the culture.* Retrieved on July 24, 2009, from http://www.collegedrinkingprevention.gov/StatsSummaries/4tier.aspx.

academic engagement or the neurodegenerative effects of heavy drinking on diminishing students' cognitive functioning and development. A study by West, Graham, and Temple (2017) of binge drinking episodes over the past year by college students with learning, physical, psychiatric, sensory, or developmental disabilities, found higher rates than their nondisabled college peers. Amphetamine use was the strongest predictor of increasing the likelihood of binge drinking among students with disabilities while nursing or pre-med majors were less likely to binge drink than students in all other majors (West et al., 2017). The authors strongly recommend colleges intervene early in college orientation activities to promote safer patterns of alcohol consumption (Wilhite et al., 2017) and design programs that address the unique risks of specific populations (West et al., 2017).

Nurses in university health services are ideally positioned to identify at-risk students and use motivational interviewing to ascertain the students' readiness to change their behavior (Kelly-Weeder, 2008). Motivational interviewing begins by establishing trust, being an empathic listener, and instilling hope and positive regard—communication skills familiar to nurses, which are the foundation of the nurse–client relationship. Once the nurse establishes rapport, brief motivational interviewing consists of specific cognitive strategies such as eliciting feelings about how the drinking behavior is affecting the student's life, noting discrepancies between attitudes toward alcohol and alcohol-associated harms, emphasizing strengths, supporting life goals, and empathically supporting the student on ways to implement change, or remaining neutral when met with ambivalence (Schaus, Sole, McCoy, Mullett, & O'Brien, 2009). Outcomes studies have demonstrated that at-risk students who received brief motivational interviewing at a university health service drink less alcohol and report fewer alcohol-related harmful incidents (Ehrlich, Hague, Swisher-McClure, & Helmkamp, 2006; Schaus et al., 2009).

Decreasing underage drinking requires sustained partnerships between government agencies, schools and colleges, parents, and local communities. The role of nurses in decreasing alcohol-related events involving students of all ages may begin in school-based health services. It also includes a coordinated effort among nurses in counseling services, health clinics, primary care offices, public health agencies, and hospital emergency departments to identify students' at-risk behaviors, implement evidence-based treatments, and educate students and others. Evidence-based programs most effective in decreasing alcohol-related harms to underage populations include (1) developmental prevention programs, (2) early screening and brief intervention, (3) government laws and school policies to reduce harmful incidents, and (4) tertiary treatments for those who meet criteria for substance use disorder or other associated mental

disorders (to be reviewed later in this chapter) (Toumbourou et al., 2007). The midcourse review of *Healthy People 2020* suggests that concerted public health efforts are lowering the rates of binge drinking in the past 2 weeks by college students from 41.1% in 2007 to 35.4% in 2014, exceeding the 2020 target (National Center for Health Statistics [NCHS], 2016).

Older Adults

Katherine takes some time to ask Mr. Campbell how he thinks he is doing. She wants to begin with an open-ended question to assess how he feels about his health status. But he only responds by saying "I've got nothing to complain about" and smiles weakly. To Katherine, he appears sad and depressed. She asks him whether he has noticed that he has lost some weight, and he agrees that he has not been eating as he should. When she asks him why he thinks his appetite has changed, he says, "I really miss cooking for all the guys in the firehouse, and now that my wife is gone, I just don't have the motivation to cook for myself."

It is clear that Mr. Campbell is undergoing some major life transitions, which indicates to Katherine that she needs to screen for substance use using the Short Michigan Alcoholism Screening Test—Geriatric Version (SMAST-G). She also asks Mr. Campbell's daughter to put all the prescription medications and over-the-counter medications that her father takes at home in a brown bag and bring them to his next appointment.

Evidence for Practice

The National Guideline Clearinghouse has 68 evidence-based treatment protocols for substance abuse, including screening and treatment of older adults. The protocols recommend screening for alcohol and prescription drug use yearly for all older adults and more frequent screening if there are any major life changes or transitions, or if physical symptoms suggestive of substance abuse appear. Recommended screening instruments for older adults include the Michigan Alcoholism Screening Test—Geriatric Version (MAST-G), the CAGE questionnaire, and the Alcohol Use Disorders Identification Test (AUDIT) (Naegle, 2008). (Geriatric Nursing Resources for Care of Older Adults has more information available online.) Evidence-based practice protocols may be effective for evaluation of older adults for substance misuse or alcohol abuse (the National Guideline Clearinghouse's website has additional information). To assess prescription and nonprescription medication use among older adults, the protocols recommend the "brown bag approach"—asking the older adults to bring in all the medications they take to the practitioner in a brown bag.

Substance misuse is emerging as a major public health concern for older Americans. The "baby boom" generation, the cohort with the greatest lifetime use and dependence on both alcohol and illicit substances, is now entering older adulthood. Not only will the "baby boomers" strain healthcare services because of their sheer numbers, but unlike previous generations, epidemiologists predict the rates of substance use disorder will greatly increase given the "baby boomers'" past patterns of drug and alcohol use (Mattson, Lipari, Hays, & Van Horn, 2017). Older adults who are most at risk of being diagnosed with substance abuse disorders are those who began drinking alcohol or using illicit drugs when they were 16 years of age or younger (Han, Gfroerer, Colliver, & Penne, 2009). The number of older adults with substance abuse disorders is expected to more than double from approximately 2.8 million in 2002 to 5.7 million in 2020 (Han et al., 2009).

Evidence for Practice

A study examining trends in opioid prescriptions for noncancer pain in Medicare Part D recipients who are 65 years of age or older, found the rate of prescriptions almost doubled from 2007 to 2012 (Kuo, Raji, Chen, Hasan, & Goodwin, 2016). Prolonged prescription of opioids to Medicare Part D recipients for more than 90 days significantly increased the odds of opioid overdose requiring emergency department evaluation and hospitalization by 60%. Prescription of opioids to Medicare Part D recipients without cancer was lower in states with laws regulating pain clinics (Kuo et al., 2016). States with Prescription Drug Monitoring Programs also saw prescriptions to Medicare Part D recipients for high-potency opioids (e.g., oxycodone) decrease and the length of opioid treatment shortened (Moyo et al., 2017). The findings of these studies suggest that state regulations are having a measurable effect on decreasing the volume of opioid prescriptions to older adults for noncancer pain.

Practice Point

Chronic health conditions in older adults, such as cardiac, respiratory, kidney, and liver disorders can all be adversely affected by drug and alcohol abuse. Drug

and alcohol use also puts the older adult at greater risk for neurocognitive symptoms that can precipitate falls or other accidents that can cause skeletal injuries and hip fractures. In recognition of the unique needs and risks of substance misuse among older adults, The New Jewish Home in New York established the first in the nation nursing home–based recovery program for older adults. The program offers team-focused treatment with integrated care among medical, nursing, mental health, and addiction professionals as well as self-help groups such as Alcoholics Anonymous. Evidence-based interventions are all provided within the Jewish Home's Geriatric Substance Abuse Program for co-occurring medical, substance, and mental disorders with sensitivity to culturally diverse populations. When a resident is discharged, continuity of care to support sustaining recovery is provided by The Jewish Home's Senior Day Care and certified home care services. For more information, see https://jewishhome.org/substance-abuse/

The SAMHSA National Clearinghouse for Treatment Improvement Protocols advises that men older than 65 years drink no more than one drink a day, or two drinks in any one occasion, and that women older than 65 years drink even less (SAMHSA *Treatment Improvement Protocol for Substance Abuse Among Older Adults*, available online). However, comorbid medical conditions may substantially reduce levels of acceptable drinking in the older adult, and even much lower rates of alcohol consumption may put the older adult at risk.

Nurses should regularly screen for alcohol use using the MAST-G, which has been demonstrated to be a reliable and valid measure in older adult populations (Naegle, 2008). As of August 2016, the USPSTF is reviewing routine screening for illicit drug use across all age cohorts (USPSTF, 2016, update available online). Nurses can assess for illicit and prescription drug use by conducting a thorough health history, examining urine and blood toxicology values, as well as systematically assessing older adults for symptoms suggestive of either intoxication or **withdrawal** symptoms from illicit substances and multiple classes of prescription medications, including benzodiazepines, opioids, and sedative hypnotics. In addition, nurses should inquire whether older adults are using over-the-counter preparations with caffeine (such as diet aids), cold remedies that have anticholinergic side effects or include alcohol, and herbal remedies that can have interactive effects with either prescription or nonprescription substances.

According to SAMHSA's *Treatment Protocols for Substance Abuse Among Older Adults*, benzodiazepines should not be prescribed for longer than 4 weeks, sedative hypnotics should not be prescribed for longer than 7 to 10 days, and antihistamines should be avoided completely because of changes in mental status that can result from anticholinergic effects. Misuse or excessive use of prescription as well as nonprescription medication may be a function of diminished cognitive capacity, poor vision, language barriers, lack of understanding about drug interactions, or the propensity for schedule II medications to cause dependence and **tolerance**.

SAMHSA has characterized substance abuse among older adults as an "invisible epidemic" (Lofwall, Schuster, & Strain, 2008, p. 898). *Treatment Improvement Protocol for Substance Abuse Among Older Adults* recognizes that there are many barriers to care for the older adult which are similar to those of other age groups such as language barriers, poor access to transportation, lack of health insurance, living in rural regions, and insensitivity of healthcare practitioners to the needs of racial and ethnically diverse populations (SAMHSA, 2012b). Other barriers noted by SAMHSA (2012b) as specific to older adults are a lack of substance disorder programs targeting the unique needs of older adults, as well as a lack of public awareness about the extent of substance abuse in older populations, including among healthcare providers. In the face of these challenges, Sorrell (2017) emphasizes that nurses are ideally positioned in their roles as advocates and providers to address the gaps in substance use care for older adults especially in long-term care facilities.

Evidence for Practice

The USPSTF has found sufficient scientific evidence to recommend that positive screens for alcohol abuse be followed up with brief alcohol counseling in the primary care setting (USPSTF, 2013). It has described behavioral counseling of alcohol abuse in terms of the five As: (1) assess using standardized screening instruments; (2) advise the older adult to reduce alcohol consumption to moderate levels; (3) agree on goals for reducing alcohol use or for increasing abstinence; (4) assist clients with acquiring the motivations, self-help skills, or supports needed for behavior change; and (5) arrange follow-up counseling and treatment (USPSTF, 2013).

Practice Point

SAMHSA (2017c) has developed a toolkit entitled "Get Connected" with detailed resources for community health nurses to address the unique needs of older adults with respect to SUD. Support materials include educational curricula for healthcare providers and older adults as well as fact sheets that include tips for older adults and evidence-based treatment recommendations for clinicians.

Nurses and other health providers may mistakenly attribute the presenting signs and symptoms of substance use disorder in older adults to depression, dementia, or other medical conditions. The nursing assessment of older adults may also be complicated by the inclination of many older adults to mask their symptoms and deny that they need treatment (Han et al., 2009). Nurses in all settings must be cognizant that the symptoms of delirium in the older adult may be related to polysubstance intoxication or withdrawal. The changing profile in substance use among older adults, from alcohol to polysubstance abuse, in combination with a precipitous increase in the sheer numbers of older adults needing substance use treatment, has profound clinical and public health implications (Lofwall et al., 2008, p. 902). As health educators, community health nurses have an important role in communicating to older adult populations that the national recommendations about acceptable levels of alcohol consumption decrease as they age.

Self-help programs are widely used community-based treatments that have proven efficacy in sustaining recovery for people with substance abuse disorders. Alcoholics Anonymous (AA) and Narcotics Anonymous (NA) are the two largest self-help groups for substance dependence or abuse, and both have local peer-support groups throughout the United States. To encourage participation by older adults, AA has developed an education pamphlet that includes testimonials by older adult members entitled *AA for the Older Alcoholic—Never Too Late* (available online).

Persons Who Inject Drugs

Beginning in the 1980s, proponents of syringe exchange programs argued that by providing sterile needles to people who inject drugs, pathogens transmitted by sharing needles would be lessened, slowing the spread of HIV, hepatitis, and other blood-borne diseases. In the ensuing years, as scientific evidence accumulated demonstrating the efficacy of syringe exchange programs in decreasing the spread of HIV, the CDC, medical associations, public health agencies, and the ANA all formally endorsed syringe exchange programs as a sound public health initiative (Bluthenthal, Heinzerling, Anderson, Flynn, & Kral, 2008; Villarreal & Fogg, 2006). Syringe exchange programs are one component credited in public health prevention strategies that lowered the rate of HIV transmission in people who injected drugs in the 1980s (Paz-Bailey, 2016).

More recently with the incidence of heroin use increasing, accompanied with a rise in young people injecting drugs, there has been a resurgence of HIV and hepatitis C infection in some communities lacking public health prevention programs (Paz-Bailey, 2016). Syringe Service Programs (SSPs) have proven effectiveness in protecting people who inject drugs from blood-borne illnesses, but as of 2013 the approximately 2,000 SSPs were primarily located in metropolitan areas with few in rural or suburban communities (Paz-Bailey, 2016). To promote the expansion of SSPs in regions vulnerable to outbreaks of blood-borne diseases from injection drug use, the Consolidated Appropriations Act of 2016 provided federal funds to underwrite the costs of SSPs including staffing and treatment for medical, mental health, and substance use care. It is important to note that the federal funds

What is an **SSP?** A community-based program that provides key pathway to services to prevent drug use, HIV, and viral hepatitis

Free sterile needles and syringes

Safe disposal of needles and syringes

Referral to mental health services

Overdose treatment and education

Hepatitis A and B vaccination

Other tools to prevent HIV and hepatitis, including counseling, condoms, and PrEP (a medicine to prevent HIV)

Referral to substance use disorder treatment, including medication-assisted treatment

HIV and hepatitis testing and linkage to treatment

FIGURE 17.6 Syringe service programs: A vital part to combat opioid, HIV, and hepatitis epidemics (December 2016). (From CDC Vital Signs. Retrieved on September 5, 2017, from https://www.cdc.gov/hiv/pdf/risk/cdc-hiv-syringe-services-programs.pdf.)

may not be used for the purchase of sterile syringes for injection of illicit drugs (Fig. 17.6).

 Evidence for Practice

A quality improvement (QI) project initiated by public health nurses reflects the challenges of implementing the core components of SSPs. An audit of 46 client medical records in an opioid treatment program found the majority of records did not reflect referral of patients with positive HIV, STD, or PPD screens (Gadbois, Chin, & Dalphonse, 2016). Clinic nurses identified time constraints and difficulties with the electronic medical record limiting their ability to make referrals.

The QI project team collaborated with administrators and clinic nurses to implement new systems for referrals and shared documentation to facilitate communication between clinic nurses and the agency's STI/HIV Prevention Program. Medication reconciliation was improved by having all prescribers in the opioid treatment program enroll in the state's Prescription Monitoring Program. The opioid treatment program added new staff including primary care providers within the program to minimize referrals of clients to a local healthcare center and a nurse case manager to coordinate patient-centered care. The findings of the QI project highlight the key role of public health nurses to assure evidence-based, patient-focused care in opioid treatment facilities (Gadbois et al., 2016).

Numerous studies have demonstrated that the safest and most effective treatment for injection drug users is opioid substitution treatment with long-acting opioids such as methadone or buprenorphine (Gerra et al., 2009; Mattick, Kimber, Breen, & Davoli, 2008). Unfortunately, access to opioid substitution treatment in the United States has been limited by a lack of methadone maintenance programs or waiting lists for those that do exist. Office-based treatment with buprenorphine can also potentially expand the availability of opioid substitution treatment, but up until the passage of the Comprehensive Addiction and Recovery Act (CARA) of 2016, the number of physician participants was constrained by FDA requirements for training and accreditation. CARA temporarily expanded the eligibility to prescribe buprenorphine for SUD to nurse practitioners (NPs) and physician assistants (PAs) who complete the FDA requirements for training and are supervised by a physician who is certified to prescribe buprenorphine (Leahy, 2017). *Healthy People 2020* midcourse review (NCHS, 2016) reported admissions for injection drug use treatment increased from 255,374 in 2006 to 300,230 in 2011 and that 19.5% of the people who needed treatment for illicit drug use, received treatment exceeding the target of 17.6%.

Methamphetamine Users

Methamphetamine is a highly addictive stimulant. From 2010 to 2014, the rate of methamphetamine overdose deaths more than doubled and nearly 20% of those deaths also involved heroin (Warner, Trinidad, Bastian, Minino, & Hedegaard, 2016). Persons who inject drugs may co-inject methamphetamine, a stimulant, with heroin to counteract heroin's depressant effects. Co-injection of methamphetamine with heroin greatly increases the risk of overdose and death because methamphetamine has a shorter half-life than heroin (Meacham et al., 2016). Methamphetamines increase libido and are associated with high-risk sexual behaviors that may in turn increase the risk of HIV and STD transmission (Warner et al., 2016). Public health prevention programs for people who inject drugs described previously are an important component of treatment for methamphetamine users.

Methamphetamine maybe produced in home "laboratories" by cooking readily available ingredients (e.g., drain cleaner, fertilizer, starter fluid, and pseudoephedrine) at high heat (CDC, 2005; Denehy, 2006; McGuinness, 2006). The process is extremely hazardous and noxious odors from the toxic chemicals released in the manufacturing process can disperse and threaten the health of communities (Denehy, 2006). In contrast to other incidents involving the release of hazardous fumes or materials in communities, adverse events associated with methamphetamine "laboratories" have a much greater percentage of injured victims (31%) with most being police officers (56%) and the general public (33%) (CDC, 2005). First responders (60%) and the general public (34%) were also the most likely to require decontamination from hazardous toxins emanating from methamphetamine "laboratories" (CDC, 2005).

It is important to note that children have been found in 20% of the homes containing methamphetamine "laboratories" (CDC, 2005). Children who are chronically exposed to acetone or ammonia fumes are at grave risk for neurologic, psychological, and physical harm (Denehy, 2006; McGuinness, 2006). In addition to the signs of abuse and neglect, a distinguishing characteristic of children exposed to ammonia fumes released in methamphetamine production is a smell like the odor of cat urine (Denehy, 2006). Chemicals used in the manufacture of methamphetamine are highly explosive, and anyone in proximity to the methamphetamine "laboratory" is in danger of sustaining severe burns (Mitka, 2005). Toxic and hazardous chemicals used to manufacture methamphetamine may contaminate local neighborhoods and have necessitated the evacuation of surrounding residences (CDC, 2005).

The danger methamphetamine poses to individual people, families, and communities requires a multifaceted prevention strategy that incorporates public health and law enforcement agencies. To disrupt the availability of ingredients needed to manufacture methamphetamine, in 2000, the Methamphetamine Anti-Proliferation Act put restrictions on the amounts of pseudoephedrine that could be purchased over the counter and regulated the distribution of other key ingredients used in the manufacture of methamphetamine (Birckmayer, Fisher, Holder, & Yacoubian, 2008). Departments of Health in states with high rates of methamphetamine manufacture and addiction, launched public health education efforts using media campaigns which depict the ravaged faces of young methamphetamine addicts to graphically illustrate the morbidity associated with methamphetamine use. A pamphlet available through the National Clearinghouse for Alcohol and Drug Information entitled *Tips for Teens: The Truth About Methamphetamine*, states bluntly in bold letters, "Methamphetamine can kill you. An overdose of meth can result in heart failure. Long-term physical effects such as liver, kidney, and lung damage may also kill you."

Practice Point

Denehy (2006) urges all school nurses to be part of the solution to the methamphetamine epidemic through education of children, families, and the community about the effects of methamphetamine use, and through advocacy for prevention and treatment programs.

IMPACT ON THE COMMUNITY

The NIDA (2017c) estimates that costs to the United States from substance abuse has risen substantially over the past decade to a staggering $740 billion annually. Communities hit hardest by substance use are often ill equipped to combat the adverse effects on the quality of life in their neighborhoods, homes, and schools. The states spend $81.3 billion on substance abuse–related services, including prevention programs, family assistance, mental health, public safety, criminal justice, and healthcare (SAMHSA, 2008). The Paul Wellstone and Pete Domenici Mental Health Parity and Addiction Equity Act (MHPAEA) and the Affordable Care Act have improved private insurance coverage for substance abuse treatment (SAMHSA, 2016). Nonetheless, with the marked increase in demand for treatment, without added federal monies or private insurance reforms, the added burden on states and local government to assume the bulk of costs for substance abuse treatment may result in less access to services.

Evidence for Practice

The National Institute on Drug Abuse (2012) estimates that every dollar invested in addiction treatment programs yields a savings of between $4 and $7 in reduced drug-related crime, criminal justice costs, and theft. When savings related to healthcare are included, total savings can exceed costs by a ratio of 12 to 1.

PUBLIC HEALTH MODELS FOR POPULATIONS AT RISK

Community health nurses play a critical role in screening populations at risk for preventable disease. Population research suggests that there is a window of vulnerability for later development of addiction if initial substance use precedes age 15 (Crome & McLellan, 2013). A challenge in identifying people at risk for substance abuse is that many healthcare practitioners in primary care do not directly, or routinely, ask about alcohol or drug use across all age groups when collecting information about a person's health history. Reliable and valid screening instruments that are easy to administer are important tools to aid community health nurses in evaluating populations and individual people at risk for substance abuse. In 2004, the USPSTF issued a national recommendation that all adults in primary care should be routinely screened for alcohol use with the AUDIT-C or CAGE questionnaires (Box 17.8). The AUDIT-C, CAGE, and SMAST-G screening instruments are now available in a pocket-sized brochure to facilitate use in all primary care settings. (The SAMHSA website provides further information.)

Screening for substance use is the first step in assessing whether a person has substance use disorder. The efficacy of screening instruments is highly dependent on the candor of client responses. Putting the client at ease with a nonconfrontational request to ask a series of questions about health behaviors and beginning the conversation with less-

17.8   AUDIT-C and CAGE Screening Instruments for Alcohol Abuse

1. How often do you have a drink containing alcohol?
   0 = Never
   1 = Monthly or less
   2 = 2 to 4 times per month
   3 = 2 to 3 times per week
   4 = 4 or more per week
2. How many drinks containing alcohol do you have on a typical day?
   0 = None
   1 = 1 or 2
   2 = 3 or 4
   3 = 5 or 6
   4 = 7 or more
3. How often do you have…
   [MEN]—five or more drinks on one occasion
   [WOMEN]—four or more drinks on one occasion
   0 = Never
   1 = <Monthly
   2 = Monthly
   3 = Weekly
   4 = Daily or almost daily
4. Have you ever felt you should cut down on your drinking?
   Yes/No
5. Have people annoyed you by criticizing your drinking?
   Yes/No
6. Have you ever felt bad or guilty about your drinking?
   Yes/No
7. Have you ever had a drink first thing in the morning to steady your nerves or to get rid of a hangover?
   Yes/No

Scoring: Refer client for further evaluation if
- Three or more points on questions 1 to 3
- Six or more drinks on one occasion
- "Yes" to questions 4 to 7 and drinking in 1 to 3

Sources: AUDIT-C Overview. Retrieved on December 17, 2018 from https://www.integration.samhsa.gov/images/res/tool_auditc.pdf; CAGE-AID Overview. Retrieved on December 17, 2018 from https://www.integration.samhsa.gov/images/res/CAGEAID.pdf.

threatening questions about diet, sleep, and exercise are helpful transitions to questions pertaining to alcohol use.

The second step in assessing for SUD is to determine whether there are maladaptive behaviors that have resulted in dysfunction in health and interpersonal, social, and legal domains. In conducting a complete biopsychosocial history, two of the key indicators for risk of substance dependence are age at first use and a family history of substance use disorder. Patterns of substance abuse often occur in the context of other high-risk behaviors such as driving while intoxicated or unsafe sex practices. Legal, employment, or academic difficulties that have resulted from misuse are an important gauge of how substance use is impairing the client's ability to fulfill normal role functions.

Specific questions about misuse or abuse of substances should include a list of all substances that can result in a change in behavior or mental status. Patterns of use for caffeine, nicotine, over-the-counter medications, and herbal treatments should also be assessed. To evaluate the degree of dependence on substances, it is critical to ascertain the last time the substance was used and how much was used. In situations in which the person has experienced withdrawal symptoms in the past, nurses should ask about the typical first signs of withdrawal and what medications or treatments he or she has found helpful.

Nurses should not only gather information about the patterns of substance use, but the social contexts in which the abuse occurs. Recognition of gender, ethnic, or cultural preferences and influences are at the core of fully understanding the individualized meaning of maladaptive behaviors. It is the environmental context of the substance use behavior that can guide the nurse in evaluating what prevention strategies or interventions will be the most effective in minimizing harm. In particular, nurses should carefully note whether the client has been a victim of trauma or whether there is any physical evidence of trauma. Children or the elderly in homes where there are adults with SUD are at high risk for abuse and neglect. The ability of individual people to fulfill social role responsibilities at home, work, or school has implications not only for people with SUD but for their dependents as well.

There is high comorbidity of SUD with major mental illness. The mental status examination is a valuable tool in identifying signs and symptoms of major mental illness that co-occur with substance use. The mental status examination can alert the nurse to cognitive changes that are the result of chronic substance use and can help differentiate symptoms from other medical conditions, such as dementia or delirium. As a general rule, the more rapid the onset of symptoms is, the more likely it is that the symptoms are a product of substance use rather than a medical or psychiatric condition.

Urine and blood toxicology screens and physical assessments also aid in determining whether changes in behavior or mental status are a function of substance use or other healthcare conditions. Vital signs are crucial in assessing impending withdrawal syndromes for central nervous system depressants, or intoxication on stimulants, both of which can be fatal. The Clinical Institute Withdrawal Assessment for Alcohol tool is commonly used to assess the degree of withdrawal, and to guide nurses in the appropriate administration of benzodiazepines used for the treatment of withdrawal symptoms of central nervous system depressants (Fig. 17.7). People who are grossly intoxicated or actively withdrawing from substances have pronounced positive signs and symptoms, such as gross motor skill impairment, slurred speech, marked disorientation, confusion, or even hallucinations (Table 17.2).

In the community, nurses may encounter clients who are not seeking treatment and may deny a substance use problem, yet aspects of the history or behaviors suggest that their health status is at risk because of an underlying substance use disorder. This is particularly true for older adults whose misuse of substances can greatly exacerbate other chronic health conditions (Crome & McLellan, 2013). Fine motor tremors, shakiness, tremulous speech, sweaty palms, or restlessness may be misinterpreted as evidence of anxiety, when in fact the person is exhibiting subtle signs of withdrawal from central nervous system depressants. The condition of the person's skin is particularly illuminating about the extent and degree of substance use. Skin conditions seen with chronic substance use include dark shadows under the eyes, bruising, jaundice, burns between the fingers or inside the lips, scabs, bloody gums and nasal mucosa, decayed teeth, ascites, or needle track marks. A person's pupil size can reveal much about their current state of intoxication and the substances involved. Dilated pupils are seen with people intoxicated on stimulants, cocaine, or hallucinogens, whereas people intoxicated on opioids have constricted pupils.

A challenge for nurses in conducting a risk assessment for clients with substance use disorder is that the clients may mask symptoms or deny high-risk behaviors. More than half of clients with SUD believed that primary care providers were not able to detect their dependence or abuse (Fleming, 2005). Sometimes, clients do not allow nurses to inquire with collateral informants (such as other healthcare providers, family, friends, or school personnel) about changes in behavior or evidence of high-risk behavior that suggest the person may have a substance use disorder. It is extremely useful in conducting a health assessment of a client who may have a substance use disorder if the client gives informed consent to elicit additional information from other people who know the client well.

Nurses must always ask directly if the client has any thoughts of harming himself or herself or others. All threats of self-harm or harm to others must be taken seriously. Nurses should ask clients who appear intoxicated or express suicidal ideation whether they have access to weapons. If a client responds affirmatively, the nurse must seek a responsible adult to secure any weapons. Clients who have SUD may become less inhibited when they are intoxicated, or extremely despondent and agitated while withdrawing from substances. Any indication that the person is a danger to himself or herself or others warrants immediate referral to an emergency department for more thorough evaluation.

A person's readiness for substance use treatment varies greatly. Throughout the assessment, nurses should convey that they are a partner in helping the client access substance use services and achieve recovery. If clients disavow problems with substance use or the need for treatment, nurses can use the encounter as an opportunity to educate the clients and share concerns for their well-being. Throughout the encounter, nurses should follow the person's lead and work to problem-solve issues which they have identified are of immediate concern. An essential attribute of nurses who work with this population is the nurses' capacity to sustain

Clinical Institute Withdrawal Assessment of Alcohol Scale, Revised (CIWA-Ar)

Patient:_____ Date: _____ Time: _____ (24 hour clock, midnight = 00:00)

Pulse or heart rate, taken for one minute:_____ Blood pressure:_____

NAUSEA AND VOMITING – Ask "Do you feel sick to your stomach? Have you vomited?" Observation.
0 no nausea and no vomiting
1 mild nausea with no vomiting
2
3
4 intermittent nausea with dry heaves
5
6
7 constant nausea, frequent dry heaves and vomiting

TREMOR – Arms extended and fingers spread apart. Observation.
0 no tremor
1 not visible, but can be felt fingertip to fingertip
2
3
4 moderate, with patient's arms extended
5
6
7 severe, even with arms not extended

PAROXYSMAL SWEATS – Observation.
0 no sweat visible
1 barely perceptible sweating, palms moist
2
3
4 beads of sweat obvious on forehead
5
6
7 drenching sweats

ANXIETY – Ask "Do you feel nervous?" Observation.
0 no anxiety, at ease
1 mild anxious
2
3
4 moderately anxious, or guarded, so anxiety is inferred
5
6
7 equivalent to acute panic states as seen in severe delirium or acute schizophrenic reactions

AGITATION – Observation.
0 normal activity
1 somewhat more than normal activity
2
3
4 moderately fidgety and restless
5
6
7 paces back and forth during most of the interview, or constantly thrashes about

TACTILE DISTURBANCES – Ask "Have you any itching, pins and needles sensations, any burning, any numbness, or do you feel bugs crawling on or under your skin?" Observation.
0 none
1 very mild itching, pins and needles, burning or numbness
2 mild itching, pins and needles, burning or numbness
3 moderate itching, pins and needles, burning or numbness
4 moderately severe hallucinations
5 severe hallucinations
6 extremely severe hallucinations
7 continuous hallucinations

AUDITORY DISTURBANCES – Ask "Are you more aware of sounds around you? Are they harsh? Do they frighten you? Are you hearing anything that is disturbing to you? Are you hearing things you know are not there?" Observation.
0 not present
1 very mild harshness or ability to frighten
2 mild harshness or ability to frighten
3 moderate harshness or ability to frighten
4 moderately severe hallucinations
5 severe hallucinations
6 extremely severe hallucinations
7 continuous hallucinations

VISUAL DISTURBANCES – Ask "Does the light appear to be too bright? Is its color different? Does it hurt your eyes? Are you seeing anything that is disturbing to you? Are you seeing things you know are not there?" Observation.
0 not present
1 very mild sensitivity
2 mild sensitivity
3 moderate sensitivity
4 moderately severe hallucinations
5 severe hallucinations
6 extremely severe hallucinations
7 continuous hallucinations

HEADACHE, FULLNESS IN HEAD – Ask "Does your head feel different? Does it feel like there is a band around your head?" Do not rate for dizziness or lightheadedness. Otherwise, rate severity.
0 not present
1 very mild
2 mild
3 moderate
4 moderately severe
5 severe
6 very severe
7 extremely severe

ORIENTATION AND CLOUDING OF SENSORIUM – Ask "What day is this? Where are you? Who am I?"
0 oriented and can do serial additions
1 cannot do serial additions or is uncertain about date
2 disoriented for date by no more than 2 calendar days
3 disoriented for date by more than 2 calendar days
4 disoriented for place/or person

Total **CIWA-Ar** Score_____
Rater's Initials_____
Maximum Possible Score 67

The **CIWA-Ar** is not copyrighted and may be reproduced freely. This assessment for monitoring withdrawal symptoms requires approximately 5 minutes to administer. The maximum score is 67 (see instrument). Patients scoring less than 10 do not usually need additional medication for withdrawal.

Sullivan, J.T.; Sykora, K.; Schneiderman, J.; Naranjo, C.A.; and Sellers, E.M. Assessment of alcohol withdrawal: The revised Clinical Institute Withdrawal Assessment for Alcohol scale (**CIWA-Ar**). *British Journal of Addiction* 84:1353-1357, 1989.

FIGURE 17.7 Clinical Institute Withdrawal Assessment of Alcohol Scale, revised (CIWA-Ar). (From http://www.ireta.org/ireta_main/webinarOnDemand-files/CIWA-Ar.pdf. This scale is not copyrighted and may be used freely.)

TABLE 17.2 Nursing Assessment and Implications for Alcohol and Illicit Drug Use

Substance[a]	Dependence	Fatal in Overdose	Fatal in Withdrawal	Symptoms of Intoxication/ Overdose	Symptoms of Withdrawal	Nursing Implications in Community
Alcohol Beer Wine Spirits	Yes	Yes	Yes	Ataxia, slurred speech, disinhibition, drowsiness, hypotension, CNS depression, coma convulsions, death.	Nausea, vomiting, hypertension, tachycardia, diaphoresis, tremors, delirium tremens, coma, death. Peaks 24–35 hours.	*In overdose if awake*, induce vomiting, give activated charcoal, vital signs q15 min. *In overdose if unarousable*, maintain airway, seizure precaution, emergency transport to hospital. *In withdrawal early stage*, administer benzodiazepines. *In withdrawal late stage*, maintain airway, seizure precautions, emergency transport to hospital.
Illicit drugs Heroin	Yes	Yes	No	Constricted pupils, euphoria, slurred speech, CNS depression, coma, convulsions, death.	Yawning, rhinorrhea, cramps, bone pain, chills, fever, diaphoresis, diarrhea, irritability, panic.	*In overdose if unarousable*, administer IV naloxone stat. *In withdrawal*, administer buprenorphine, methadone. *In abrupt withdrawal*, administer clonidine.
Nonmedical Pain relievers Oxycodone Fentanyl Morphine Codeine	Yes	Yes	No	Opioid analgesics have signs and symptoms similar to heroin, including death.	Opioid analgesics have signs similar to heroin. Peak symptoms depend on half-life.	Nursing implications are the same as for heroin.
Nonmedical Tranquilizers Diazepam Alprazolam Klonopin	Yes	Rare	Yes	Benzodiazepines are CNS depressants, and effects are similar to alcohol, including death.	Benzodiazepines are CNS depressants, and effects are similar to alcohol, including death.	Nursing implications are the same as for alcohol.
Nonmedical Sedatives Meprobamate Chloral hydrate	Yes	Yes	Yes	Sedative hypnotics are CNS depressants, and effects are similar to alcohol, including death.	Sedative hypnotics are CNS depressants, and effects are similar to alcohol, including death.	Nursing implications are the same as for alcohol.

(Continued)

TABLE 17.2 Nursing Assessment and Implications for Alcohol and Illicit Drug Use *(Continued)*

Substance[a]	Dependence	Fatal in Overdose	Fatal in Withdrawal	Symptoms of Intoxication/ Overdose	Symptoms of Withdrawal	Nursing Implications in Community
Nonmedical Stimulants Amphetamine Adderall Concerta	Yes	Yes	No	Dilated pupils, insomnia, tachycardia, paranoia, hallucinations, assaultive, hyperpyrexia, coma, elevated BP, coma, stroke, death.	Craving, agitation, hypersomnia, anxiety, depression.	*In intoxication if awake,* antipsychotics, ambient cooling, seizure precautions. *In intoxication if severe,* emergency transport to hospital. *In withdrawal,* administer antidepressants, dopamine agonist.
Cocaine	Yes	Yes	No	Cocaine is a CNS stimulant, and the effects are similar to amphetamines.	Cocaine is a CNS stimulant, and the effects are similar to amphetamines.	*Nursing implications* are the same as for amphetamines.
Inhalants	Yes	Yes	Yes (chronic use)	Similar to alcohol and visual hallucinations, cardiac arrhythmias, sudden death.	In chronic use, similar to alcohol and convulsions, delirium.	*In intoxication,* rest, decrease stimulation, monitor for cardiac arrhythmias. *In overdose and withdrawal,* emergency transport to hospital.
Hallucinogens LSD MDMA Mescaline Peyote	No	Yes	No	Dilated pupils, tremor, elevated vital signs, psychosis, death.	None	*In intoxication if alert,* decrease sensory stimulation, administer benzodiazepines, or chloral hydrate.
PCP	No	Yes	No	Dilated pupils, nystagmus, hypertensive crisis, hyperthermia, death.	None	*In intoxication if alert,* can be very violent, institute safety precautions, acidify urine, administer Haldol or diazepam, decrease stimuli.
Cannabis	No	No	No	Red eyes, dry mouth, increased pulse, panic, toxic psychosis.	None	*In intoxication if psychotic,* administer antipsychotics.

[a]Nine substance use categories are defined in 2007 National Survey on Drug Use and Health (NSDUH).
BP, blood pressure; CNS, central nervous system; IV, intravenous; LSD, lysergic acid diethylamide; MDMA, 3,4-methylenedioxy-N-methylamphetamine; PCP, phencyclidine.
Source: From National Survey on Drug Use and Health (NSDUH).

unconditional positive regard as they partner with clients through an often-winding course of ambivalence, relapse, and recovery.

Practice Point

The main reason Americans who self-identify as needing treatment for alcohol or drug use and did not receive treatment stated that they had no health insurance and could not afford the cost (SAMHSA, 2013). Mandated coverage for essential services in the Patient Protection and Affordable Care Act includes substance use prevention, early intervention, treatment, and case management (Crome & McLellan, 2013). Federally qualified healthcare centers will take the lead in spearheading the integration of mental health and substance use treatment in primary care (Urada, Teruya, Gelberg, & Rawson, 2014). In response, the ANA has acknowledged that nurses must be clinically prepared to implement evidence-based screening, brief interventions, and referrals for complex substance use treatment when indicated (Savage & Finnell, 2013).

TREATMENT INTERVENTIONS FOR SUBSTANCE ABUSE

In community settings, evidence-based treatments for substance use fall into two broad modalities, pharmacologic and psychosocial. Nurses should always ask women about their pregnancy status during the assessment because some medications used in treatment may be contraindicated in pregnancy. Co-occurring substance use disorder and major mental illness affect approximately half of all people with drug abuse, and about a third of people with alcohol abuse. Ideally, the treatments for co-occurring disorders, also termed *dual diagnosis*, are fully integrated in the multidisciplinary treatment plan. The substance use treatments reviewed in this chapter will be augmented with additional psychiatric treatments in cases where a person has a dual diagnosis.

Medication-Assisted Treatments for SUD

Medication-Assisted Treatments for Alcohol-Dependent Disorders

Based on empirical evidence, APA Practice Guidelines for Substance Use Disorders (2006) recommend treatment with naltrexone, acamprosate, or disulfiram. Naltrexone and acamprosate have pharmacologic properties that diminish **craving** for alcohol, whereas disulfiram induces aversive effects if alcohol is consumed. APA Guidelines (2006) note that pharmacologic studies sponsored by the NIAAA are underway to investigate if combinations of these three med-

ications may improve outcomes for people who are dependent on alcohol.

NALTREXONE

Naltrexone (Vivitrol) mediates opiate receptors and diminishes the alcohol-induced release of dopamine thought to be involved in alcohol craving. The dosing is 50 mg a day orally or 380 mg intramuscularly (IM) every 4 weeks into alternating buttocks. Side effects associated with oral preparations of naltrexone include nausea, vomiting, and hepatotoxicity. The FDA approved a long-acting IM naltrexone in 2006 and issued a warning about adverse injection site reactions on August 12, 2008. (More information is available on the FDA's website.)

The warning reads, "Naltrexone IM should only be administered with the prepackaged 1.5-inch needle that is specifically designed for administration. Naltrexone IM should never be administered intravenously, subcutaneously, or inadvertently into fatty tissue. Nurses should not administer naltrexone IM to any client whose body habitus precludes a gluteal IM injection with the prepackaged 1.5-inch needle. Women are physiologically at higher risk for injection site reactions because of typically higher gluteal fat thickness. Nurses should advise clients to immediately report any signs of redness, pain, or swelling in the injection site."

ACAMPROSATE

Acamprosate is believed to normalize glutamate function that may contribute to craving or protracted withdrawal symptoms. Dosing is a maximum of 1,998 mg a day given in 333-mg tablets three times a day. Acamprosate is excreted through the kidneys. Creatine levels, blood urea nitrogen levels, and kidney function should be carefully monitored. Diarrhea is a common side effect.

DISULFIRAM

Disulfiram inhibits aldehyde dehydrogenase. When disulfiram is taken, and then alcohol is consumed, levels of aldehyde accumulate, which triggers flushing, nausea, and vomiting. Dosing is a maximum of 500 mg daily initially for 1 to 2 weeks followed by 250 mg daily. Clients must be carefully educated about the adverse symptoms that occur if they ingest alcohol. Nurses should alert clients that alcohol may be used in preparation of gravies, desserts, soups, ciders, mouthwash, cough syrups, and other common household items. Clients should avoid inhaling fumes from substances containing alcohol.

Medication-Assisted Treatments for Opioid Use Disorders

The APA Treatment Guidelines (2006) recommend treatment with the opioid agonists methadone and buprenorphine for both withdrawal syndromes and maintenance. Methadone or buprenorphine should be given as maintenance medications only when the client has a history of opioid dependence exceeding 1 year. Methadone and buprenorphine are dispensed only in specially licensed facilities. The number of opioid treatment programs has increased to meet demand with approximately 1,482 opioid treatment programs operating nationwide that are federally approved to dispense methadone (Alderks, 2017). Buprenorphine is available in physicians' offices, which have been licensed and approved by various states. The CARA expands the authorization to prescribe buprenorphine in office-based settings to qualifying NPs and PAs. The certification process for NPs includes additional education and authorization through the Drug Enforcement Administration (DEA). The SAMHSA Buprenorphine Information Center is available to answer any questions from nurses about buprenorphine. Nurses can assist clients in locating a provider of buprenorphine through the SAMHSA Center for Substance Abuse Treatment. SAMHSA's websites contain additional information.

METHADONE

Methadone binds to opioid receptors and blocks the euphoric and sedating effects of opiates, thus relieving the craving. The standard of once-a-day dosing of 60 to 120 mg by tablet, elixir, or diskette is followed in opioid treatment programs, which are located throughout the United States. Side effects include constipation, diaphoresis, and sexual dysfunction. Methadone prescriptions increased to 4.1 million in 2006. Levo-α-acetylmethadol (LAAM) is a form of methadone that has a longer half-life. Dosing of LAAM is 20 to 40 mg at induction, with gradual increases up to 10 days. Maintenance dose of LAAM is three times a week; each of the 3 days, the doses range from 60 to 180 mg.

Deaths associated with methadone overdose increased 262% from 2001 to 2007 to 10,361. At the request of Congress, in March 2009, the U.S. Government Accountability Office (GAO) completed a report analyzing factors associated with the steep rise in methadone deaths (GAO, 2009). It concluded that one factor associated with methadone fatalities was the increased use of methadone to treat chronic pain (GAO, 2009). To improve safety, the FDA has initiated a Risk Evaluation and Mitigation Strategy that restricts prescription authority of certain opioids to practitioners knowledgeable about the use of potent opioid medication.

Unlike when naltrexone is used in alcohol addiction, when naltrexone is used in the treatment of opioid addiction, the client should be opioid free for at least 5 days after using heroin or 7 days after using methadone; otherwise, the naltrexone will trigger withdrawal symptoms. Dosing is oral three times a week, with 100 mg on Monday and Wednesday followed by 150 mg on Friday. There is poor compliance in opioid-dependent clients for the oral route of administration. The IM route of administration has the advantage of being long acting and promoting adherence (APA, 2006).

BUPRENORPHINE

Buprenorphine (Subutex) is considered a partial opioid agonist that enables opioid-dependent people to discontinue opioids without experiencing withdrawal symptoms. Initiation of maintenance treatment should be 12 to 24 hours after last use of opioids. On the first day of treatment, clients are given a dose of 2 to 4 mg and assessed for symptoms of withdrawal over a 2-hour period. If withdrawal symptoms occur, additional doses can be given in 2-hour intervals for a maximum daily dose of 8 mg. The average daily maintenance dose is 16 mg. For use in opioid withdrawal, buprenorphine can be withdrawn over a short (3 days), moderate (10 to 14 days), or long (180 days) period. Doses may be reduced by 50% per day. Buprenorphine can be abused, and in such cases, clients can be given a combination preparation of naloxone and buprenorphine (Suboxone). Side effects include hepatic failure and central nervous system depression when taken with benzodiazepines or alcohol. Nurses should caution clients that they should avoid driving during initial induction or with any dosing changes. This information is summarized from *Buprenorphine: A Guide for Nurses* (SAMHSA, 2009). To improve treatment adherence for patients who are stabilized on buprenorphine, another option is a subdermal implant of long-acting buprenorphine (Probuphine), which delivers a constant low dose of buprenorphine over a 6-month time span.

NALOXONE

Naloxone is an opioid antagonist that blocks the opioid receptors and temporarily reverses respiratory depression associated with opioid overdose. Over 10,000 potential opioid overdoses were reversed by community-administered naloxone (CDC, 2012). Naloxone hydrochloride injection is available as a prescription treatment that can be used by family members or caregivers for the emergency treatment of an opioid overdose in a community setting. Once turned on, the handheld auto-injector provides verbal instruction to the user describing how to deliver the single dose of naloxone hydrochloride by injection to immediately reverse respiratory depression. Naloxone rescue kits include two mucosal atomization devises and two prefilled syringes with 2 mg/2 mL naloxone hydrochloride. Naloxone administered via the atomizer is given intranasally with 1 mL to each nostril (Doe-Simkins et al., 2014). Patients administered naloxone in community settings must seek emergency treatment in a medical center as the opioid antagonist effects dissipate and additional doses may be needed within 20 minutes. Currently 17 states and the District of Columbia have enacted laws permitting the distribution of naloxone rescue kits by injection or inhalation to first responders, family members, and opioid users (American Journal of Nursing [AJN], 2014). Figure 17.8.

Evidence-Based Psychosocial Treatments in Substance Use Disorders

In addition to brief motivational interviewing and social skills training (Box 17.9), additional evidence-based modalities for people with substance use disorders include cognitive–behavioral strategies that focus on relapse prevention,

FIGURE 17.8 User-friendly delivery systems for naloxone. (From Sarlin, E. [2016]. *Messages shore up support for making life-saving anti-overdose medication widely available.* NIDA Notes. Retrieved on October 10, 2017, from https://www.drugabuse.gov/news-events/nida-notes/2016/10/messages-shore-up-support-making-life-saving-anti-overdose-medication-widely-available.)

behavioral therapy that uses community reinforcement and contingency contracting, and psychodynamic and interpersonal therapies for people with dual diagnoses (APA, 2006). An example of contingency contracting is the "Prize Incentives Contingency Management for Substance Abuse" that is based upon operant conditioning principles, and use rewards to modify and change the occurrence of substance use behavior (Box 17.10).

Self-help group modalities and 12-step programs such as AA or NA are the primary source of support for people with substance use disorders. Research indicates that mutual-aid groups such as AA are also strongly associated with sustained recovery and improved health outcomes (Tusa & Burghoizer, 2013). The success of mutual self-help groups

in helping these people sustain recovery is apparent by the sheer numbers of individuals with substance use disorders who use 12-step programs as their primary mode of treatment. Yet, AA does not consider itself a treatment but rather a fellowship of people who mutually support each other to sustain sobriety one day at a time. Addressing the spiritual needs of individual people and families is an essential component of comprehensive nursing care. A philosophy of spirituality and mutual support are the guiding principles of AA and NA and make it an important resource in recovery for two million people worldwide (Galanter, 2008).

The Mental Health Parity and Addiction Equity Act compelled health insurers to provide the same level of services for mental health and substance use treatment as physical disorders. In response, treatment for substance use has been transitioning from an episodic, disease model to a chronic care model (McLellan et al., 2014). Nurses have a key role in a chronic disease model to identify populations at risk, intervene early to prevent relapse, and use case management skills to sustain recovery.

One component of the chronic care model is teaching patients self-management skills to prevent relapse and self-harm. Self-management skills to sustain recovery include health promoting behaviors to improve nutrition and physical well-being, avoiding triggers, and adopting healthy coping strategies to manage stress such as exercise or spiritual support (Bradbury-Golas, 2013; Walton-Moss, Ray, & Woodruff, 2013). Nurses apply a harm reduction approach to teach patients about sustaining sexual health to prevent HIV or other sexually transmitted diseases (Bartlett, Brown, Shattell, Wright, & Lewallen, 2013).

17.9 Project ASSERT

Project ASSERT (Alcohol and Substance Abuse Services, Education, and Referral to Treatment) is a screening, brief intervention, and referral to treatment (SBIRT) model designed for use in health clinics or emergency departments (EDs). Project ASSERT aims to reduce or eliminate unhealthy substance use through collaboration with trained nurses, peer educators, and other health professionals.

Patients with a positive screening result are engaged by interventionists with the Brief Negotiated Interview (BNI), a semiscripted, motivational interviewing counseling session that focuses on the negative consequences associated with drug use and unhealthy drinking. Using the BNI, the nurse builds rapport with the patient; asks the patient for permission to discuss drug and alcohol use; explores the pros and cons of the behavior associated with drug and alcohol use; discusses the gap between the client's real and desired quality of life; assesses the client's readiness for change in the targeted behavior; and develops an action plan, which includes direct referrals and access to substance abuse treatment.

On average, Project ASSERT is delivered in 15 minutes, although more time may be needed, depending on the severity of the patient's substance use problem and associated treatment referral needs. The face-to-face component of the intervention is completed during the course of primary care visit. After the nurse delivers the intervention, he or she follows up with each patient by telephone 10 days after the health clinic visit. This call serves as a 5- to 10-minute booster session to discuss what has transpired since the BNI and to find out whether new service referrals are needed.

Project ASSERT targets adults and adolescents in urban, suburban, rural, frontier, and tribal areas. Races and ethnicities who have received Project ASSERT interventions include Asian, black or African American, Hispanic or Latino, and white.

Readiness for dissemination ratings by criteria = 4.0 (0.0–4.0 scale)

Implementation materials = 4.0

Training and support = 4.0

Quality assurance = 4.0

Source: American Hospital Association. (2017). *Project ASSERT: To improve Alcohol & Substance Use Disorder Services, Education and Referral to Treatment.* Retrieved on December 17, 2018 https://www.aha.org/2017-10-05-improving-hospital-and-emergency-department-response-substance-use-disorders-project.

17.10 Prize Incentives Contingency Management for Substance Abuse

Prize Incentives Contingency Management for Substance Abuse is a variation of contingency management and awards prizes for abstinence and treatment compliance, such as group attendance and healthy behaviors. Over a period of 3 months, urine and breath samples are collected two or three times a week for at least the first 6 weeks and once or twice weekly thereafter. For each sample that tests negative for the target drug, clients can draw slips of paper or plastic chips from a bowl for the chance of winning a prize valued from $1 to $100. Clients may also receive draws from the prize bowl for attending counseling/group therapy sessions and completing weekly activities designed to meet goals related to health (e.g., scheduling or attending a medical or nutritionist appointment, obtaining medications, recording daily medication or food consumption, exercising at a gym), sobriety (e.g., attending 12-step meetings), employment (e.g., creating a resume), and other areas. A drug-positive sample or an unexcused absence resets the number of draws to one.

Prize Incentives targets adults with substance use disorders and has also been applied to HIV-related risk behaviors. Races and ethnicities who have received Motivational Interviewing interventions include Asian, black or African American, Hispanic or Latino, and white. The program augments existing, usual care services in community-based treatment settings for adults who primarily abuse stimulants (especially cocaine) or opioids (especially heroin) or who have multiple substance use problems.
Readiness for dissemination ratings by criteria = 4.0 (0.0–4.0 scale)
Implementation materials = 4.0
Training and support = 4.0
Quality assurance = 4.0

Source: National Institute on Drug Abuse (NIDA). (2018). *Principles of Drug Addiction Treatment: A Research Based Guide.* (3rd ed.), U.S. Department of Health and Human Services: National Institutes of Health, 45. Retrieved on December 17, 2018, from https://www.drugabuse.gov/publications/principles-drug-addiction-treatment-research-based-guide-third-edition/evidence-based-approaches-to-drug-addiction-treatment/behavioral-0.

Evidence for Practice

A systematic review of 11 trials of nurse-conducted brief intervention for alcohol use was compared to usual treatment or physician-delivered brief intervention. In community settings, 5 studies found statistically significant reductions in alcohol consumption in nurse-delivered brief intervention and 2 trials found nurses were equally effective as physicians. Policy recommendations included adoption of nurse-delivered brief interventions for substance use as an essential standard of care by the International Council of Nurses (Joseph, Basu, Dandapani, & Krishnan, 2014).

In summary, nurses in the community can implement a wide range of evidence-based programs to decrease the morbidity and mortality associated with substance use. As healthcare educators and practitioners, nurses are leaders in ensuring that evidence-based prevention programs are available in schools and other community settings. Prevention programs are the first step in decreasing the use of substances in high-risk people, and some, such as NFP and LifeSkills Training (LST), include motivational interviewing to address patterns of misuse or abuse. Motivational interviewing by nurses is an effective treatment intervention that can be delivered in a range of community settings such as primary care clinics or student health services (Kelly-Weeder, 2008) (Box 17.11). The National Registry of Evidence-based Programs and Practices lists programs that have demonstrated efficacy in treating individual people,

17.11 Motivational Interviewing Interventions in Community Settings

Motivational Interviewing (MI) is a goal-directed, client-centered counseling style for eliciting behavioral change by helping clients to explore and resolve ambivalence. The operational assumption in MI is that ambivalent attitudes or lack of resolve is the primary obstacle to behavioral change, so that the examination and resolution of ambivalence becomes its key goal. MI has been applied to a wide range of problem behaviors related to alcohol and substance abuse, as well as health promotion, medical treatment adherence, and mental health issues. Although many variations in technique exist, the MI counseling style generally includes the following elements:

- Establishing rapport with the client and listening reflectively
- Asking open-ended questions to explore the client's own motivations for change
- Affirming the client's change-related statements and efforts
- Eliciting recognition of the gap between current behavior and desired life goals
- Asking permission before providing information or advice
- Responding to resistance without direct confrontation
- Encouraging the client's self-efficacy for change
- Developing an action plan to which the client is willing to commit

MI targets adults and adolescents in urban and suburban areas. Races and ethnicities who have received MI interventions include Asian, black or African American, Hispanic or Latino, and white.
Readiness for dissemination ratings by criteria = 4.0 (0.0–4.0 scale)
Implementation materials = 4.0
Training and support = 4.0
Quality assurance = 4.0

Source: Substance Abuse and Mental Health Services Administration (SAMHSA) (2017). Using revention research to guide prevention practice. *SAMHSA's Center for the Application of Prevention Technologies, 31.* Retrieved on December 17, 2018, from https://www.samhsa.gov/capt/sites/default/files/resources/preventing-youth-marijuana-use-programs-strategies-2017.pdf.

couples, and families who are diagnosed with substance use disorder.

GOALS OF *HEALTHY PEOPLE 2020*

An estimated 23 million Americans are struggling with some form of substance use disorder in the United States—the highest proportion of any nation in the world. Community health nurses are at the forefront of strategic efforts to improve the health of Americans who abuse alcohol or illicit drugs in all segments of the population. The mid-course objectives for substance use in *Healthly People 2020* were met or exceeded for 11 objectives, however 12 were unchanged and 9 were getting worse. New objectives were added to track use of prescription medications for nonmedical purposes.

While some progress has been made in achieving targets for decreasing substance use among youth, there are also some concerning trends. The *Healthy People 2020* Midcourse Review (NCHS, 2016) found that the proportion of high school seniors who never used alcohol increased to 34%, exceeding the target, but those who reported never using drugs decreased to 50.9% away from the target, and those who used marijuana was unchanged. The *2020* targets for binge drinking behavior were exceeded for both high school seniors who engaged in binge drinking in the past 2 weeks (19.4% in 2014 down from 25.2% in 2009) and college students (34% in 2014 down from 41.1% in 2007). Decreases in high-risk alcohol use among adolescents and college students suggest public health campaigns are having a measurable positive effect. But there is notable work to be done on educating youth about the risks of marijuana and drug use.

Tragically the rates of drug and alcohol-induced deaths all increased away from the *2020* target with the exception of motor vehicle deaths associated with high blood alcohol. Consistent with the increased mortality for illicit drug use, the proportion of adults using illicit substances in the past month increased from 7.9% in 2008 to 9.4% in 2013 as did the number of adults seeking treatment for substance misuse.

> Everybody needs a way out of that pain. Many people choose drugs and alcohol. Some people obsessively exercise or develop strange dietary habits, which is what I did. At least it got me toward a path of healthier living. **Mariel Hemingway**

KEY CONCEPTS

- The United States leads the world in rates of substance use. Patterns of substance dependence vary by age, gender, race, ethnicity, and geographic location.
- Across the lifespan, the age cohorts at high risk for morbidity associated with substance use disorder include pregnant women, children younger than 14 years, college students, and older adults in the baby boom generation.
- Environmental factors, such as poverty, lack of access to health services, and the capacity of law enforcement to constrain supply, contribute to a disproportionate burden of harms associated with substance use among Native Americans, Alaskan Natives, and African Americans.
- Biopsychosocial risk factors in substance use disorder include genetic history, family history, history of trauma, early initiation, and environmental factors such as poverty or group affiliation, sexual or other abuse.
- Substance use disorders have high comorbidity with major mental illness and increase the risk for chronic health conditions such as HIV.
- Evidence-based substance use prevention programs implemented in community settings are empirically proven to be effective in decreasing substance use in targeted populations.
- Substance use treatment need not be voluntary to help people achieve recovery. The most effective treatment involves a multimodal approach with interventions such as motivational interviewing, opioid substitution programs, family therapy or couples therapy, and 12-step self-help groups.

CRITICAL THINKING QUESTIONS

1. How do you think the values of different stakeholders such as the alcohol industry, local communities, law enforcement, public health organizations, nurse researchers, nurse clinicians in alcohol treatment facilities, and college students would affect the identification of "social harms" associated with alcohol abuse or misuse?
2. In what ways are the social harms associated with substance use different across the lifespan?
3. Why are some communities disproportionately impacted by the social harms associated with illicit drug use and what are the implications for nursing practice?
4. Do you think the general public's perception of the social harms associated with alcohol, tobacco, and cannabis has changed? Why?
5. What are the essential elements needed in prevention programs to change people's perceptions of the social harms associated with substance use?
6. Contingency management incentives give prizes, cash, or vouchers for substance abstinence. What

CRITICAL THINKING QUESTIONS *(Continued)*

are your views about providing pregnant women who are actively abusing teratogenic substances monetary incentives to abstain? In framing your response, consider the ANA Code of Ethics.

7. The United States prides itself on having the premier healthcare system in the world. Yet the "immigrant" paradox suggests the longer immigrants reside in the United States, the more likely they are to adopt substance use behaviors that result in the

highest morbidity and mortality in world. How would you propose community health nurses intervene to mitigate acculturation influences on substance use?

8. How do you anticipate the legalization of cannabis in some states will impact that prevalence of cannabis use among children and adolescents? Discuss what, if any, effect there may be on development, academic attainment, and behavioral health.

COMMUNITY RESOURCES

- Local methadone treatment center
- NFP to help first-time mothers succeed
- LifeSkills training: evidence-based prevention program for schools, families, and communities

- Gatekeeper program: a proactive community training program to identify at-risk, home-dwelling older adults
- Alcoholics Anonymous
- Narcotics Anonymous

HEALTHY PEOPLE 2020 EVIDENCE-BASED RESOURCE RECOMMENDATIONS

Alcohol Misuse: Screening and Behavioral Counseling Interventions in Adults (U.S. Preventive Services Task Force, 2013)

Description of Resource: The U.S. Preventive Services Task Force (USPSTF) recommends that clinicians screen adults ages 18 or older for alcohol misuse and provide people engaged in risky or hazardous drinking with brief behavioral counseling interventions to reduce alcohol misuse. This is a B recommendation, which means the USPSTF recommends the service. There is high certainty that the net benefit is moderate or there is moderate certainty that the net benefit is moderate to substantial.

Strength of Evidence: 4 out of 4
Healthy People 2020 Topic Area(s): Substance Abuse
Healthy People 2020 Objectives: SA-9
Exercise for Students:

1. Apply evidence-based screening for alcohol misuse by comparing the use of the following screening tools for specific populations.

   a. National Institute on Alcohol Abuse and Alcoholism (NIAAA) single-item (for adults) or two-item (for adolescents) screening test, or comparable,

including the Brief Screener for Tobacco, Alcohol, and other Drugs (BSTAD) (for adolescents)

   b. Alcohol Use Disorders Identification Test (AUDIT) and its abbreviated version (AUDIT-C)

   c. CAGE questionnaire

   d. Comorbidity Alcohol Risk Evaluation Tool (CARET) (for older adults)

   e. TWEAK and T-ACE (for pregnant women)

2. What are the advantages, disadvantages, and challenges of using electronic or computer-based screening with diverse populations across the lifespan?

3. Describe how the screening process would be adapted to the unique needs of populations in these community-based settings.

   a. Primary care clinics/offices for adolescents and adults

   b. Secondary schools and universities

   c. Prenatal clinics

   d. Obstetrics/gynecology clinics

   e. Senior care centers

   f. Homes

ACKNOWLEDGE

A Special thanks to Dr. Donna White for her review and discussion of the chapter.

REFERENCES

Alderks, C. E. (2017). *Trends in the use of methadone, buprenorphine, and extended-release naltrexone at substance abuse treatment facilities: 2003–2015 (update)*. The CBHSQ Report: Center for Behavioral Health Statistics and Quality, Substance Abuse and Mental Health Services Administration. Rockville, MD. Retrieved on December 17, 2018 from https://www.samhsa.gov/data/sites/default/files/report_3192/ShortReport-3192.pdf

Allen, J. D., Casavant, M. J., Spiller, H. A., Chounthirath, T., Hodges, N. L., & Smith, G. A. (2017). Prescription opioid exposures among children and adolescents in the United States: 2000–2015. *Pediatrics*, 139(4), e20163382.

Allen, M. L., Garcia-Huidobro, D., Porta, C., Curren, D., Patel, R., Miller, J., & Borowsky, I. (2016). Effective parenting interventions to reduce youth substance use: A systematic review. *Pediatrics*, 32(2), e20154425.

American Journal of Nursing (AJN). (2014). Heroin: Life, death and politics. *American Journal of Nursing*, 114(5), 22–23.

American Psychiatric Association (APA). (2006). *Practice guidelines for the treatment of psychiatric disorders*. Arlington, VA: APA Press.

American Psychiatric Association (APA). (2013). *Diagnostic and statistical manual of mental disorders (DSM-V)* (5th ed.). Arlington, VA: APA Press.

Annas, G. J. (2001). Testing poor pregnant women for cocaine—Physicians as police investigators. *New England Journal of Medicine*, 344(22), 1729–1732.

Bartlett, R., Brown, L., Shattell, M., Wright, T., & Lewallen, L. (2013). Harm reduction: Compassionate care of persons with addictions. *MedSurg Nursing*, 22(6), 349–358.

Bertrand, J., Floyd, R. L., & Weber, M. K. (2005). Guidelines for identifying and referring persons with fetal alcohol syndrome. *Morbidity and Mortality Weekly Report*, 54(RR11), 1–17.

Birckmayer, J., Fisher, D. A., Holder, H. D., & Yacoubian, G. S. (2008). Prevention of methamphetamine abuse: Can existing evidence inform community prevention. *Journal of Drug Education*, 38(2), 147–165.

Bluthenthal, R. N., Heinzerling, K. G., Anderson, R., Flynn, N. M., & Kral, A. H. (2008). Approval of syringe exchange programs in California: Results from a local approach to HIV prevention. *American Journal of Public Health*, 98(2), 278–283.

Bradbury-Golas, K. (2013). Health promotion and prevention strategies. *Nursing Clinics of North America*, 48(3), 469–483.

Brady, J. E., Giglio, R., Keyes, K. M., DiMaggio, C., & Li, G. (2017). Risk markers for fatal and non-fatal prescription drug overdose: A meta-analysis. *Injury Epidemiology*, 4(1), 24.

Brady, K. T., McCauley, J. L., & Back, S. E. (2016). Prescription opioid misuse, abuse and treatment in the United States: An Update. *American Journal of Psychiatry*, 173(1), 18–26.

Centers for Disease Control and Prevention (CDC). (2005). Acute public health consequences of methamphetamine laboratories—16 states, January 2000–June 2004. *Morbidity and Mortality Weekly Report*, 54(14), 356–359.

Centers for Disease Control and Prevention (CDC). (2012). Community based opioid overdose prevention programs providing naloxone–United States, 2010. *Morbidity and Mortality Weekly Report*, 61(6), 101–105.

Centers for Disease Control and Prevention (CDC). (2016). *HIV and injection drug use*. Retrieved on August 24, 2017, from https://www.cdc.gov/hiv/pdf/risk/cdc-hiv-idu-fact-sheet.pdf

Crome, I. & McLellan, A.T. (2013). Editorial: A new public understanding about addiction. *Public Health Review, 35*, 1. https://doi.org/10.1007/BF03391700.

Curtis, B. L., McLellan, A. T., & Gabellini, B. N. (2014). Translating SBIRT to public school settings: An initial test of feasibility. *Journal of Substance Abuse Treatment*, 46(1), 15–21.

Dawley, K., Loch, J., & Bindrich, I. (2007). The nurse-family partnership. *American Journal of Nursing*, 107(11), 60–67.

Denehy, J. (2006). The meth epidemic: Its effect on children and communities. *Journal of School Nursing*, 22(2), 63–65.

Doe-Simkins, M., Quinn, E., Xuan, Z., Sorensen-Alawad, A., Hackman, H., Ozonoff, A., & Walley, A. Y. (2014). Overdose rescues by trained and untrained participants and change in opioid use among substance-using participants in overdose education and naloxone distribution programs: A retrospective cohort study. *BMC Public Health*, 14, 297.

Donelan-McCall, N., Eckenrode, J., & Olds, D. L. (2009). Home visiting for the prevention of child maltreatment: Lessons learned during the past 20 years. *Pediatric Clinics of North America*, 56(2), 389–403.

Dowell, D., Haegerich, T. M., & Chou, R. (2016). CDC guideline for prescribing opioids for chronic pain—United States, 2016. *Morbidity and Mortality Weekly Report*, 65(1), 1–50.

Dowell, D., Zhang, K., Noonan, R. K., & Hockenberry, J. M. (2016). Mandatory provider review and pain clinic laws reduce the amounts of opioids prescribed and overdose death rates. *Health Affairs*, 35(10), 1876–1883.

Ehrlich, P. F., Hague, A., Swisher-McClure, S., & Helmkamp, J. (2006). Screening and brief intervention for alcohol problems in a university student health clinic. *Journal of American College Health*, 54(5), 279–287.

Fleming, M. F. (2005). Screening and brief intervention in primary care settings. *Alcohol Research and Health*, 28(2), 57–62.

Foote, J., Wilkens, C., & Vavgiakis, P. (2004). A national survey of alcohol screening and referral in college health centers. *Journal of American College Health*, 52(4), 149–157.

Gadbois, C., Chin, E. D., & Dalphonse, L. (2016). Health promotion in an opioid treatment program: An evidence-based nursing quality improvement project. *Journal of Addictions Nursing*, 27(2), 127–142.

Galanter, M. (2008). Spirituality, evidence-based medicine and alcoholics anonymous. *American Journal of Psychiatry*, 165(12), 1514–1517.

Gerra, G., Maremmani, I., Capovani, B., Somaini, L., Berterame, S., Tomas-Rossello, J.,...Kleber, H. (2009). Long-acting opioid-agonists in the treatment of heroin addiction: Why should we call them "substitution"? *Substance Use & Misuse*, 44(5), 663–671.

Goodman, D. (2015). Improving access to maternity care for women with opioid use disorders: Colocation of midwifery services at an addiction treatment program. *Journal of Midwifery and Womens Health*, 60(6), 706–712.

Government Accountability Office (GAO). (2009). *Methadone associated overdose deaths: Factors contributing to increased deaths and efforts to prevent them (March. GAO-09-341)*. Washington, DC: U. S. Government Accountability Office.

Gray, K. M., & Squeglia, L. M. (2018). Research review: What have we learned about adolescent substance use? *The Journal of Child Psychology and Psychiatry*, 59(6), 618–627.

Greenbaum, P. E., Del Boca, F. K., Darkes, J., Wang, C. P., & Goldman, M. S. (2005). Variation in the drinking trajectories of freshman college students. *Journal of Consulting and Clinical Psychology*, 73(2), 229–238.

Gregory, K. E. (2014). Caring for the infant with neonatal abstinence syndrome in a community-based setting. *Journal of Perinatal & Neonatal Nursing*, 28(3), 161–163.

Guy, G. P., Zhang, K., Bohm, M. K., Losby, J., Lewis, B., Young, R.,...Dowell D. (2017). Vital signs: Changes in opioid prescribing in the United States, 2006–2015. *Morbidity and Mortality Weekly Report*, 66(26), 697–704.

Han, B., Gfroerer, J. C., Colliver, J. D., & Penne, M. A. (2009). Substance use disorder among older adults in the United States in 2020. *Addiction*, 104(1), 88–96.

Haug, N. A., Duffy, M., & McCaul, M. E. (2014). Substance abuse treatment services for pregnant women: Psychosocial and behavioral approaches. *Obstetric and Gynecology Clinics of North America*, 41, 267–296.

Hogue, A., Henderson, C. E., Ozechowski, T. J., & Robbins, M. S. (2014). Evidence base on outpatient behavioral treatments for adolescent substance use: Updates and recommendations 2007–2013. *Journal of Clinical Child & Adolescent Psychology*, 43(5), 695–720.

Hoyme, H. E., Kalberg, W. O., Elliott, A. J., Blankenship, J., Buckley, D., Marais, A. S.,...May, P. A. (2016). Updated clinical

REFERENCES *(Continued)*

guidelines for diagnosing fetal alcohol spectrum disorders. *Pediatrics, 138*(2), e20154256.

Jarlenski, M., Barry, C. L., Gollust, S., Graves, A. J., Kennedy-Hendricks, A., & Kozhimannil, K. (2017). Polysubstance use among US women of reproductive age who use opioids for nonmedical reasons. *American Journal of Public Health, 107*(8), 1308–1310.

Johnston, L. D., O'Malley, P. M., Bachman, J. G., Schulenberg, J. E., & Miech, R. A. (2016). *Monitoring the future national survey results on drug use, 1975–2015: College students and adults (Vol. 2).* Ann Arbor, MI: Institute for Social Research, The University of Michigan. Retrieved on September 4, 2017, from http://monitoringthefuture.org/pubs.html#monographs

Joseph, J., Basu, D., Dandapani, M., & Krishnan, N. (2014). Are nurse-conducted brief interventions (NCBIs) efficacious for hazardous or harmful alcohol use? A systematic review. *International Nursing Review, 61*(2), 203–210.

Kelly-Weeder, S. (2008). Binge drinking in college-aged women: Framing a gender-specific prevention strategy. *Journal of the American Academy of Nurse Practitioners, 20*(12), 577–584.

Kuo, Y. F., Raji, M. A., Chen, N. W., Hasan, H., & Goodwin, J. S. (2016). Trends in opioid prescriptions among Part D Medicare recipients from 2007 to 2012. *American Journal of Medicine, 129*(2), 221 e21–e30.

Leahy, L. G. (2017). The opioid epidemic: What does it mean for nurses? *Journal of Psychosocial Nursing, 55*(1), 18–23.

Lee, S., Aos, S., & Miller, M. (2008). *Evidence-based programs to prevent children from entering and remaining in the child welfare system: Benefits and costs for Washington (Document No. 08-07-3901).* Olympia, WA: Washington State Institute for Public Policy.

Li, K., & Wen, M. (2015). Substance use, age at migration, and length of residence among adult immigrants in the United States. *Journal of Immigrant and Minority Health,17*(1), 156–164.

Lipari, R. N. (2017). *Understanding adolescent inhalant use.* The CBHSQ Report National Survey on Drug Use and Health. June 13. Center for Behavioral Health Statistics and Quality. Rockville, MD: Substance Abuse and Mental Health Services Administration. Retrieved on August 5, 2017, from https://www.samhsa.gov/data/sites/default/files/report_3095/ShortReport-3095.pdf

Lipari, R. N., Williams, M. R., Copello, E. A. P., & Pemberton, M. R. (2016). Risk and protective factors and estimates of substance use initiation: Results from the 2015 National Survey on Drug Use and Health. *NSDUH Data Review.* Retrieved from http://www.samhsa.gov/data.

Lofwall, M. R., Schuster, A., & Strain, E. C. (2008). Changing profile of abused substances by older persons entering treatment. *The Journal of Nervous and Mental Disease, 196*(12), 898–905.

MacMullen, N. J., Dulski, L., & Blobaum, P. (2014). Evidence based intervention for neonatal abstinence syndrome. *Pediatric Nursing, 40*(4), 165–172, 203.

Mattick, R. P., Kimber, J., Breen, C., & Davoli, M. (2008). Buprenorphine maintenance versus placebo or methadone maintenance for opioid dependence. *Cochrane Database of Systematic Reviews, 16*(2), CD002207.

Mattson, M., Lipari, R. N., Hays, C., & Van Horn, S. L. (2017). *A day in the life of older adults: Substance use facts.* The CBHSQ Short Report. Center for Behavioral Health Statistics and Quality. Rockville, MD: Substance Abuse and Mental Health Services Administration.

McGuinness, T. (2006). Methamphetamine abuse. *American Journal of Nursing, 106*(12), 54–58.

McLellan, A. T., Starrels, J. L., Tai, B., Gordon, A. J., Brown, R., Ghitza, U.,...McNeely, J. (2013). Can substance use disorders be managed using the chronic care model? Review and recommendations from a NIDA consensus group. *Public Health Reviews, 35*(2). Retrieved from https://doi.org/10.1007/BF03391707

Meacham, M. C., Strathdee, S. A., Rangel, G., Armenta, R. F., Gaines, T. L., & Garfein, R. S. (2016). Prevalence and correlates of heroin-methamphetamine co-injection among persons who inject drugs in San Diego, California and Tijuana, Baja California, Mexico. *J Stud Alcohol Drugs, 77*(5), 774–781.

Mermelstein, R. J. (2014). Adapting to a changing tobacco landscape: Research implications for understanding and reducing youth tobacco use. *American Journal of Preventive Medicine, 47*(2 Suppl 1), S87–S89.

Mitchell, S. G., Gryczynski, J., O'Grady, K. E., & Schwartz, R. P. (2013). SBIRT for adolescent drug and alcohol use: Current status and future directions. *Journal of Substance Abuse Treatment, 44*(5), 463–472.

Mitka, M. (2005). Meth lab fires put heat on burn centers. *JAMA, 294*(16), 2009–1010.

Moyo, P., Simoni-Wastila, L., Griffin, B. A., Onukwugha, E., Harrington, D., Alexander, G. C., & Palumbo, F. (2017). Impact of prescription drug monitoring programs (PDMPs) on opioid utilization among Medicare beneficiaries in 10 US States. *Addiction, 112*(10), 1784–1796.

Naegle, M. A. (2008). Screening for alcohol use and misuse in older adults: using the Short Michigan Alcoholism Screening Test–Geriatric Version. *American Journal of Nursing, 108*(11), 50–58, quiz 58–59.

National Center for Health Statistics (NCHS). (2016). *Chapter 40: Substance abuse. Healthy People 2020 midcourse review.* Hyattsville, MD: U.S Government Printing Office. Retrieved on September 5, 2017, from https://www.cdc.gov/nchs/data/hpdata2020/HP2020MCR-C40-SA.pdf

National Institute on Alcohol Abuse and Alcoholism (NIAAA). (2015). *College drinking.* U.S. Department of Health and Human Services, National Institutes of Health. Retrieved on September 4, 2017, from https://www.niaaa.nih.gov/alcohol-health/special-populations-co-occurring-disorders/college-drinking

National Institute on Alcohol Abuse and Alcoholism (NIAAA). (2017). *College AIM (Alcohol Intervention Matrix).* Retrieved on September 4, 2017, from https://www.collegedrinkingprevention.gov/CollegeAIM/Introduction/default.aspx

National Institute on Drug Abuse (NIDA). (2012). *Principles of drug addiction treatment: A research-based guide* (3rd ed.). Retrieved on October 12, 2017, from https://www.drugabuse.gov/publications/principles-drug-addiction-treatment-research-based-guide-third-edition

National Institute on Drug Abuse (NIDA). (2016). *Teen substance use shows promising decline.* Washington, DC: National Institutes of Health, US Department of Health and Human Services. Retrieved from https://www.drugabuse.gov/news-events/news-releases/2016/12/teen-substance-use-shows-promising-decline

National Institute on Drug Abuse (NIDA). (2017a). *National overdose deaths – 2015.* Washington, DC: National Institutes of Health, US Department of Health and Human Services. Retrieved from https://www.drugabuse.gov/related-topics/trends-statistics/overdose-death-rates.

National Institute on Drug Abuse (NIDA). (2017b). *Marijuana.* Washington, DC: National Institutes of Health, US Department of Health and Human Services. Retrieved from https://www.drugabuse.gov/publications/research-reports/marijuana/what-scope-marijuana-use-in-united-states

National Institute on Drug Abuse (NIDA). (2017c). *Trends & statistics.* Retrieved on October 12, 2017, from https://www.drugabuse.gov/related-topics/trends-statistics

Paz-Bailey, G. (2016). *HHS Implementation Guide to Support Certain Components of Syringe Services Programs 2016.* April 27. Retrieved on September 5, 2017, from https://www.cdc.gov/hiv/

pdf/risk/cdc-hiv-syringge-Transcript_HHS_SSP_Guidance_Webinar.pdf

Peek, C. J., & The National Integration Academy Council (NIAC). (2013). *Lexicon for behavioral health and primary care integration: Concepts and definitions developed by expert consensus (AHRQ Pub. No. 13-IP001-EF)*. Rockville, MD: AHRQ. Retrieved July 22, 2014, from http://integrationacademy.ahrq.gov/sites/default/files/Lexicon.pdf

Presidents Commission on Combating Drug Addiction and the Opioid Crisis. (2017). *Interim report*. Retrieved from https://www.whitehouse.gov/sites/whitehouse.gov/files/ondcp/commission-interim-report.pdf.

Qureshi, A., Campayo, G. J., Eiroa-Orosa, F. J., Sobradiel, N., Collazos, F., Febrel Bordejé, M.,...Casas, M. (2014). Epidemiology of substance abuse among migrants compared to native born population in primary care. *American Journal on Addiction, 23*, 337–342.

Reddy, U. M., Davis, J. M., Ren, Z., & Greene, M. F. (2017). Opioid use in pregnancy, neonatal abstinence syndrome and childhood outcomes: Executive summary of a joint workshop by the Eunice Kennedy Shriver National Institute of Child Health and Human Development, American College of Obstetricians and Gynecologists, American Academy of Pediatrics, Society for Maternal-Fetal Medicine, Centers for Disease Control and Prevention, and the March of Dimes Foundation. *Obstetrics and Gynecology, 130*(1), 10–28.

Rudd, R. A., Seth, P., David, F., & Scholl, L. (2016). Increases in drug and opioid-involved overdose deaths – United States, 2010–2015. *Morbidity and Mortality Weekly Report, 65*(50-51), 1445–1452.

Salas-Wright, C. P., & Vaughn, M. G. (2014). A "refugee paradox" for substance use disorders? *Drug and Alcohol Dependence, 142*, 345–349.

Savage, C., & Finnell, D. (2013). Screening, brief intervention and referral to treatment (SBIRT). *Journal of Addictions Nursing, 24*(3), 195–198.

Savage, J. E., & Mezuk, B. (2014). Psychosocial and contextual determinants of alcohol and drug use disorders in the National Latino and Asian American study. *Drug and Alcohol Dependence, 139*, 71–78.

Schaus, J. F., Sole, M. L., McCoy, T. P., Mullett, N., & O'Brien, M. C. (2009). Alcohol screening and brief intervention in a college student health center: A randomized controlled trial. *Journal of Studies on Alcohol and Drugs*, (Suppl. 16), 131–141.

Sorrell, J. M. (2017). Substance use disorders in long-term care settings: A crisis of care for older adults. *Journal of Psychosocial Nursing, 55*(1), 24–27.

Spoth, R. L., Randall, G. K., Trudeau, L., Shin, C., & Redmond, C. (2008). Substance use outcomes 5 ½ years past baseline for partnership-based family-school preventive interventions. *Drug and Alcohol Dependence, 96*(1-2), 57–68.

Stanley, L. R., Harness, S. D., Swaim, R. C., & Beauvais, F. (2014). Rates of substance use of American Indian students in 8th, 10th and 12th grades living on or near reservations: Update, 2009–2012. *Public Health Reports, 129*, 156–163.

Strobbe, S. (2013). Addressing substance use in primary care. *The Nurse Practitioner, 38*(10), 45–53.

Substance Abuse and Mental Health Services Administration (SAMHSA), Center for Abuse Prevention. (2008). *Substance abuse prevention dollars and cents: A cost-benefit analysis. U.S. Department of Health and Human Services. (DHHS Pub. No. (SMA) 07–4298)*. Rockville, MD.

Substance Abuse and Mental Health Services Administration (SAMHSA), Center for Substance Abuse Treatment (CSAT). (2009). *Buprenorphine: A guide for nurses. Technical Assistance Publication (TAP) Series 30. (DHHS Publication No. SMA 09–4376)*. Rockville, MD: SAMHSA.

Substance Abuse and Mental Health Services Administration (SAMHSA). (2012a). *Results from the 2011 National Survey on Drug Use and Health: Summary of national findings (NSDUH Series H-44, HHS Publication No. (SMA) 12–4713)*. Rockville, MD: Substance Abuse and Mental Health Services Administration.

Substance Abuse and Mental Health Services Administration (SAMHSA), Center for Substance Abuse Treatment (CSAT). (2012b). *Substance abuse among older adults. Treatment Improvement Protocol (TIP) Series, No. 26, (HHS Publication No. (SMA) 12–3918)*. Rockville, MD: Substance Abuse and Mental Health Services Administration.

Substance Abuse and Mental Health Services Administration (SAMHSA). (2013). *Results from the 2012 National Survey on Drug Use and Health: Summary of national findings (NSDUH Series H-46, HHS Publication No. (SMA) 13–4795)*. Rockville, MD: Substance Abuse and Mental Health Services Administration. Retrieved on July 24, 2014, from http://www.samhsa.gov/data/NSDUH/2012SummNatFindDetTables/NationalFindings/NSDUHresults2012.pdf

Substance Abuse and Mental Health Services Administration (SAMHSA). (2016). *Facing Addiction in America: The Surgeon General's Report on Alcohol, Drugs, and Health*. Washington, DC: U.S. Department of Health and Human Services (HHS), Office of the Surgeon General, Retrieved august 5, 2017 from https://addiction.surgeongeneral.gov/surgeon-generals-report.pdf

Substance Abuse and Mental Health Services Administration (SAMHSA). (2017a). *Behavioral health barometer: United States, Volume 4: Indicators as measured through the 2015 National Survey on Drug Use and Health and National Survey of Substance Abuse Treatment Services*. HHS Pub No. SMA-17-BaroUS-16. Rockville, MD: SAMHSA.

Substance Abuse and Mental Health Services Administration (SAMHSA). (2017b). *Focus on prevention: Strategies and programs to prevent substance use*. HHS Pub. No. SMA10-4120. Rockville, MD: Substance Abuse and Mental Health Services Administration. Retrieved on August 5, 2017, from https://store.samhsa.gov/shin/conten// /SMA10-4120.pdf

Substance Abuse and Mental Health Services Administration (SAMHSA). (2017c). *Get connected: Linking older adults with resources on medication, alcohol and mental health*. HHS Pub. No (SMA) 03–3824. Rockville, MD: Substance Abuse and Mental Health Services Administration.

Terplan, M., & Mindoff, H. (2017). Neonatal abstinence syndrome and ethical approaches to the identification of pregnant women who use drugs. *Obstetrics and Gynecology, 129*(1), 164–167.

Tillett, J., & Osborne, K. (2001). Substance abuse by pregnant women: Legal and ethical concerns. *The Journal of Perinatal Neonatal Nursing, 14*(4), 1–11.

Toumbourou, J. W., Stockwell, T., Neighbors, C., Marlatt, G. A., Sturge, J., & Rehm, J. (2007). Interventions to reduce harm associated with adolescent substance use. *The Lancet, 369*(9570), 1391–1401.

Tusa, A. L., & Burghoizer, J. A. (2013). Came to believe: Spirituality as a mechanism of change in alcoholics anonymous. A review of the literature from 1992 to 2012. *Journal of Addictions Nursing, 24*(4), 237–246.

United Nations Office on Drug and Crime (UNODC). (2012). *World drug report*. Vienna: United Nations.

United Nations Office on Drugs and Crime (UNODC). (2017). *World drug report 2017*. Austria: United Nations publications. Retrieved from http://www.unodc.org/wdr2017/field/Booket_1_EXSUM.pdf

United States Department of Health and Human Services (USDHHS). (2016). *The Child Abuse Prevention and Treatment Act including the Justice for Victims of Trafficking Act of 2015 and the Comprehensive Addiction and Recovery Act of 2016*. Children's Bureau.

REFERENCES *(Continued)*

Retrieved from https://www.acf.hhs.gov/sites/default/files/cb/capta2016.pdf

Urada, D., Teruya, C., Gelberg, L., & Rawson, R. (2014). Integration of substance use disorder services with primary care: Health center surveys and qualitative interviews. *Substance Abuse Treatment, Prevention and Policy, 9*, 15.

U.S. Department of Health and Human Services (USDHHS), Office of the Surgeon General. (2016). *Facing addiction in America: The Surgeon General's report on alcohol, drugs and health.* Washington, DC: HHS.

U.S. Preventive Services Task Force (USPSTF). (2013). *Screening and behavioral counseling interventions in primary care to reduce alcohol misuse: Recommendation statement.* AHRQ Publication No. 12-05171-EF-3. Retrieved on July 8, 2014, from http://www.uspreventiveservicestaskforce.org/uspstf12/alcmisuse/ alcmisusefinalrs.htm

U.S. Preventive Services Task Force (USPSTF). (2014). Primary care behavioral interventions to reduce illicit drug and nonmedical pharmaceutical use in children and adolescents: Clinical summary of U.S. Preventive Services Task Force Recommendation. *Annals of Internal Medicine, 160*(9), 635–640.

U.S. Preventive Services Task Force (USPSTF). (2016). *Draft update summary: Drug use in adolescents and adults, including pregnant women: Screening.* August 2016. Retrieved on October 12, 2017, from https://www.uspreventiveservicestaskforce.org/Page/Document/UpdateSummaryDraft/drug-use-in-adolescents-and-adults-including-pregnant-women-screening

Villarreal, H., & Fogg, C. (2006). Syringe-exchange programs and HIV prevention. *American Journal of Nursing, 106*(5), 58–63.

Walton-Moss, B., Ray, E. M., & Woodruff, K. (2013). Relationship of spirituality or religion to recovery from substance abuse. *Journal of Addictions Nursing, 24*(4), 217–226.

Warner, M., Trinidad, J., Bastain, B. A., Minino, A. M., & Hedegaard, H. (2016). Drugs most frequently involved in drug overdose deaths: United States, 2010–2014. *National Vital Statistics Reports, 65*(10), 1–15.

West, S. L., Graham, C. W., & Temple, P. (2017). Rates and correlates of binge drinking among college students with disabilities, United States, 2013. *Public Health Reports, 132*(4), 496–504.

Whiteford, H. A., Degenhardt, L., Rehm, J., Baxter, A. J., Ferrari, A. J., Erskine, H.,...Vos, T. (2013). Global burden of disease attributable to mental and substance use disorders: Findings from the Global Burden of Diseases Study 2010. *Lancet, 382*(9904), 1575–1586.

Wilhite, E. R., Ashenhurst, J. R., Marion, E. N., & Fromme, K. (2017). Freshman year alcohol and marijuana use prospectively predict time to college graduation and subsequent adult roles and independence. *Journal of American College Health, 65*(6), 413–422.

World Health Organization (WHO). (2014a). *Global status report on alcohol and health.* Luxembourg: World Health Organization.

World Health Organization (WHO). (2014b). *Guidelines for the identification and management of substance use and substance use disorders in pregnancy.* Geneva: World Health Organization.

Chapter 18

Underserved Populations

Rosanna F. DeMarco

Being unwanted, unloved, uncared for, forgotten by everybody, I think that is a much greater hunger, a much greater poverty than the person who has nothing to eat.
Mother Teresa

No matter what people tell you, words and ideas can change the world.
Robin Williams

There is a lot that happens around the world we cannot control. We cannot stop earthquakes, we cannot prevent droughts, and we cannot prevent all conflict, but when we know where the hungry, the homeless and the sick exist, then we can help.
Jan Schakowsky, American Congresswoman

By trying we can easily endure adversity. Another man's, I mean.
Mark Twain

CHAPTER HIGHLIGHTS

- Vulnerable versus underserved populations
- Social determinants of health/health disparities
- Genomics and underserved populations
- Health priorities in rural areas, particularly elders
- Health priorities in gay, lesbian, bisexual, and transgender people; in people in correctional institutions; and in people who are homeless
- Access to quality care
- Chronic disease management
- Veteran's health
- Human trafficking
- Health personnel issues
- Risk, prevention, and health promotion in hard-to-reach populations

OBJECTIVES

- Identify situations that make populations underserved.
- Apply recommendations from *Healthy People 2020* initiatives to meet individual, family, and population health needs.
- Discuss creative solutions such as increased use of internet technologies to build participation and capacity in underserved populations.
- Compare and contrast population-based healthcare needs with unique needs of other population groups (urban, heterosexual, homeless dwellers).

KEY TERMS

Genomics: The study of DNA sequencing to analyze the function and structure of complete sets of DNA in a cell of an organism.

Health professional shortage area (HPSA): Geographic area, population group, or medical facility with shortages of healthcare professionals that may not allow a full complement of healthcare services.

Human trafficking: Human trafficking is the trade of humans for the purpose of forced labor, sexual slavery, or commercial sexual exploitation for the trafficker or others.

Inmate: A person who is held in a jail or prison to protect the public.

Medically underserved area (MUA): Area that is determined through calculation of a ratio of primary medical care physicians per 1,000 population, infant mortality rate, percentage of the population with incomes below the poverty level, and percentage of the population aged 65 or older.

Medically underserved population (MUP): A U.S. federal designation for those populations that face economic barriers (low-income or Medicaid-eligible populations) or cultural and/or linguistic access barriers to primary medical care services.

Trimorbidity: Three common chronic illnesses of homeless people (i.e., mental illness, chronic physical illness, and substance addiction).

Underserved population: A subgroup of the population that has a higher risk of developing health problems due to a greater exposure to health risk because of marginalization in sociocultural status, access to economic resources, age, or gender.

Veteran's health: Care or service that will promote, preserve, and restore health of those who have served in the military.

CASE STUDIES

References to the case studies are found throughout this chapter (look for the case study icon). Readers should keep the case studies in mind as they read the chapter.

CASE 1

Lydie, an 80-year-old woman, was born in France. She came to the United States in her early 20s to be a cook for a wealthy family in a metropolitan area. She became a U.S. citizen, and when she retired in her mid-50s, she settled alone in a rural community in the United States along the Canadian border—unmarried, independent, and financially secure. She bought a small farm, raised goats, made goat cheese, and swore off any primary healthcare. She basically believed that she was in charge of her health; in reality, she found primary healthcare highly inconvenient. Although she did drive, seeing a physician or a nurse practitioner required a car ride of 90 minutes, and she had too much to do on the farm to be bothered with that commute.

Lydie fell one day while milking her goats. The mail carrier, who noticed that her mail was untouched for 3 days, found her and notified the local volunteer fire department. The moment she fractured her hip in the fall was a sentinel event that spiraled into many losses, including her farm, goats, and a life of solitude, because she had no immediate family, extended family, or friends who could help her, and little access to local healthcare that would have allowed her to stay home and enter a rehabilitation phase after surgery. Lydie died in a nursing home in a metropolitan area 150 miles away from her beloved farm 4 months after her fall. She was diagnosed with hypertension, diabetes, and congestive heart failure during her time in rehabilitation and died of complications from these comorbidities.

CASE 2

Saliha, a 15-year-old girl, has been in a youth detention facility, awaiting placement to foster care. She was arrested and brought to the center for selling marijuana in the neighborhood, as well as trading sex for money. Her home situation is less than ideal. Her mother is an active intravenous drug user and the single head of the household. Saliha is the only child living at home, and her mother, who is not a positive role model, often forgets to remind her daughter to attend school. Saliha has been living at friends' homes in the neighborhood for about 18 months, saving money she earns through selling marijuana and exchanging sex for money. She gets free healthcare at the local hospital, which has a clinic for people just like her, but she rarely follows through on any of the advice she receives from the nurses and doctors.

Saliha takes a positive step toward taking care of herself that often lasts for a month and then reverts to what she is most familiar with (i.e., a disruptive life on the streets). She frequents a place where she feels the safest, where she can get food, shower, and condoms. It is a harm reduction drop-in center. She is beginning to like and trust a nurse who volunteers there on Friday afternoons.

CASE 3

Reluctantly, Jan decides to make an appointment with her gynecologist to start having an annual Pap test. Her best friend has been diagnosed with cervical cancer, and she doesn't want this to happen to her. She has stopped seeing any sort of primary care physician, more from a sense of disillusionment than anything else. Although Jan, a bisexual woman, was once married to a man, she is now in a committed relationship with a woman. The female physician assistant (PA) who sees Jan begins to ask all the routine assessment questions, including whether Jan is sexually active and uses safe sex practices. Jan says "yes." Jan senses that the PA assumes that Jan is heterosexual, because she, the PA, refers to condoms when she discusses prevention of human immunodeficiency virus/acquired immunodeficiency syndrome (HIV/AIDS). Jan wonders why the PA doesn't ask her if she is having sex with men, women, or both, as at least a way to tailor her remarks. Jan is left feeling confused by assumptions and misdirected information.

THE CONTEXT OF HEALTH RISKS

We have a responsibility as a state to protect our most vulnerable citizens: our children, seniors, people with disabilities. That is our moral obligation. But there is an economic justification too—we all pay when the basic needs of our citizens are unmet. **John Lynch, American football player**

Vulnerability

Discussions regarding the health risks of certain groups of people who have a greater disproportionate risk of poor health often identify the individual people who make up these groups as members of "vulnerable" populations. One definition of a vulnerable population comes from the seminal writing of Flaskerud and Winslow (1998)—that is, "social groups who have an increased relative risk or susceptibility to adverse health outcomes" (p. 69). Unfortunately, this definition is accurate in terms of negative outcomes complicated by struggles for the basic needs associated with a quality of life. However, vulnerability implies being a victim, with little recourse but to depend on others for help with healthcare goals and outcomes. Vulnerability seems to mean lacking sufficient ability to advance health and wellness, along with a greater need to look to others for solutions.

In reality, many people in certain groups are not served equitably by public and private healthcare infrastructures because of lack of access, racism, sexism, homophobia, and fear of what they do not understand. They constitute **underserved populations**. Here are some questions to consider about these populations.

- Why do some people have health insurance and others do not?
- Why do some have access to primary care and others end up in emergency departments for healthcare, with complex follow-up?
- How does perceived and actual discrimination contribute to decision making involved in obtaining healthcare when one is ill?

Other people who are underserved from the perspective of healthcare include many who are not discussed in this chapter. The concept of vulnerability can apply to people with specific health conditions such as depression, schizophrenia, substance abuse, posttraumatic stress disorder (PTSD), or HIV/AIDS. Even the benefits of living in a successful industrialized nation such as the United States may not include access to adequate healthcare. Unfortunately, some people continue to suffer from lack of basic assessment of their healthcare needs; from lack of assurance that the healthcare system is available and has trained professionals willing to help; and from lack of healthcare policies that specifically address the uniqueness of their needs. These people may include undocumented men, women, and children who migrate from their country to find work in rural areas; children and youth; populations with high rates of violence; frail elders who experience multiple organ failure and frequent rehospitalization; and children in foster care. In this chapter, discussion will focus on four groups of underserved people who are susceptible to adverse outcomes and, in some cases, health disparities that are generated from many social determinants of health: rural populations; prison inmates; lesbian, gay, bisexual, transgender (LGBT) people; veterans, victims of human trafficking, and the homeless.

There is a hugely underserved population out there...those who are the least capable of paying pay the highest. **James Cameron, Canadian film director**

Social Determinants of Health and Health Disparities

The World Health Organization (WHO) defines social determinants of health as "the conditions in which people are born, grow, live, work and age. These circumstances are shaped by the distribution of money, power and resources at global, national and local levels. The social determinants of health are mostly responsible for health inequities—the unfair and avoidable differences in health status seen within and between countries" (WHO, 2018a). Olshansky (2017) explains that since the nursing function is to improve patients' health, this definition is applicable to nursing practice through attention to ways to support the importance of the social determinant of health on health disparities through *Healthy People 2020* goals. Health disparities are considered the unintended effects of social determinants of health on quality, access, and outcomes of care for certain groups of individuals. The National Institutes of Health (NIH), National Library of Medicine (2018) further defines health disparities as the variation in rates of disease occurrence and disabilities between socioeconomic and/or geographically defined population groups. Because socioeconomic and/or geographically defined population groups (individuals, families, and communities) are complex and unique entities nationally and globally how to address determinants and disparities is challenging.

Olshansky (2017) provided recommendations of how nurses could increase the awareness regarding the importance of the social determinant of health factors. She recommended that the nursing education programs should provide education about the social determinants of health, integrate the concept of social determinants of health into the clinical and interprofessional practice, and partner with community organizations and agencies to advocate for policies that improve the social determinants of health.

In the end, policies are addressing social determinants of health and health disparities from a perspective of health justice.

The concept of health disparities is a form of systematic injustice and inequality in healthcare. According to *Healthy People 2020*, the term *disparities* often is interpreted to mean racial or ethnic disparities. However, many dimensions of disparity exist in the United States, particularly in health. "If a health outcome is seen in a greater or lesser extent between populations, there is disparity" (*Healthy People 2020*). Race or ethnicity, sex, sexual identity, age, disability, socioeconomic status, and geographic location all contribute to an individual's ability to achieve good health. The *Healthy People 2020* goals include a specific goal directed at eliminating health disparities and healthcare inequities. A key operational definition, which was derived from consensus building during the construction of the *Healthy People 2020* goals, defines health disparities as systematic, plausibly avoidable health differences adversely affecting socially disadvantaged groups; they may reflect social disadvantage, but causality need not be established. This definition, grounded in ethical and human rights principles, focuses on the subset of health differences reflecting social injustice, distinguishing health disparities from other health differences also warranting concerted attention, and from health differences in general (Braveman et al., 2011). In the *Healthy People 2020* federal initiatives in the United States, the following groups are identified as needing special attention and creative solutions to live a healthy life in the face of the sobering health disparities and social injustices: (1) high-risk mothers, (2) chronically ill and disabled people, (3) people living with HIV/AIDS, (4) mentally ill people, (5) substance abusers, (6) homeless people, and (7) immigrants and refugees.

> Until the great mass of the people shall be filled with the sense of responsibility for each other's welfare, social justice can never be attained. **Helen Keller**

Genomics and Underserved Populations

Genomics is defined as the study of genes and their functions, and related techniques (WHO, 2018a). The main difference between genomics and genetics is that genetics scrutinizes the functioning and composition of the single gene, whereas genomics addresses all genes and their interrelationships in order to identify their combined influence on the growth and development of the organism (WHO, 2018b). Understanding the genetic predictors of disease through genomics is a determinant of how certain individuals, families, and communities may be disproportionately affected by illness, and why public health must be part of a practical strategy that addresses discoveries in this developing science. In many communities discussed in this chapter, screening, genetic differences, access to ethical treatment, patterns of disease prevalence, and care at secondary and tertiary levels of prevention are addressed. The application of epigenetics in these communities will affect other public health interventions.

Screening will need to be reconsidered related to specific populations who may have polygenic inheritance that is linked with what we thought were common diseases (Khoury, Janssens, & Ransohoff, 2013). For example, compared to age-based criterion for breast, colorectal, and prostate cancer screening, using polygenic risk and family history may be a more efficient way to screen, with an earlier start on screening for segments of the population at higher absolute risk (Khoury et al., 2013). According to Burton and colleagues (2013), a multidisciplinary program, which used results from the Collaborative Oncological Gene-environment Study (COGS), identified genetic variants associated with breast, ovarian, and prostate cancers to model risk-stratified prevention for breast and prostate cancers. Implementing such strategies would require attention to the use and storage of genetic information, the development of risk assessment tools, new protocols for consent, and programs of professional education and public engagement as key in public health strategic plans of the future. Developing risk stratification will need to be changed to establish screening that is sensible and accessible, especially to those struggling with access from isolation or other barriers (Burton et al., 2013). We also know that different groups of people, based on gender or other key demographic characteristics, respond to preventive treatment differently because of their genetic makeup. For example, some genotypes may metabolize medications so differently that individuals, families, and communities might struggle with drug-seeking behaviors because accepted pain killers, such as codeine, may not work on common pain relief problems (Crews et al., 2012). Some populations may have specific vulnerability and may be subject to key environmental influences related to their health. Gomes and Pelosi (2013) discuss how the potential vulnerability to environmental changes can control gene expression in diseases of great interest in public health such as cancer, autoimmune diseases, and perhaps even the aging process. It is expected that in the future, epigenetics, the study of gene expression in the context of environment, will help guide lifestyle changes more precisely and modulate the development of disease, and thus will have a large role in prevention. Within this context of developing genomics, a variety of underserved populations are described in an attempt to understand the effects of a variety of factors that often yield outcomes fraught with challenges to public health. In the end, although genetics does not seem to fit with the notion of underserved populations, specialization in this area is evolving at the intersection of genomics with the specific diseases prevalent in populations currently underserved in the healthcare system. For example, there is a developing focus on highly prevalent chronic conditions (e.g., nicotine dependence, cancer, and obesity) which can help with the advances in treatment and prevention in communities of those who are underserved.

RURAL POPULATIONS

People who live in rural areas must fight social inequities and health disparities. The word "rural" can be a subjective interpretation of a geographic area, or it can be an area used to measure and compare predetermined characteristics established by the public and private sector. Definitions of rural areas can be based on administrative, land-use, or economic concepts, including variation of these three themes (Amber Waves, 2013; U.S. Department of Agriculture [USDA], 2018). Federal, state, and local public officials are interested in distinguishing rural from nonrural areas because they make decisions on resource distribution and other geopolitical needs. Therefore, creating a system that identifies the characteristics of an area with some level of fairness is imperative. For example, government agencies that use statistical criteria to identify areas as "rural" are the Office of Management and Budget (OMB), the U.S. Department of Commerce's Census Bureau, and the USDA's Economic Research Service (ERS). In many cases, these offices categorize geopolitical sectors of the country to determine areas that need support whether from the perspective of financial backing, tax credits, or personnel.

According to the USDA, metropolitan or urban areas can be defined using several criteria (USDA, 2018). Once this is done, nonmetropolitan (micropolitan statistical areas) or rural areas are defined by exclusion. Determining the criteria used has a great impact on the resulting classification of areas. The United States Census Bureau (2018) provides data to the OMB that further defines metropolitan and urban areas. Accordingly, each metropolitan statistical area must have at least one urbanized area of 50,000 or more inhabitants. Each micropolitan statistical area must have at least one urban cluster of at least 10,000 but less than 50,000 inhabitants. If specified criteria are met, a metropolitan statistical area containing a single core with a population of 2.5 million or more may be subdivided to form smaller groupings of counties referred to as "metropolitan divisions." As of 2015, there were 382 metropolitan statistical areas and 536 micropolitan statistical areas in the United States (OMB Bulletin No. 15-01, 2015).

According to the United States Census Bureau (2018), 61.7 million (25%) of the total population is rural, and according to the OMB, 55.9 million (23%) of the total population is nonmetropolitan. According to the United States Census Bureau (2018), 97.5% of the total land area is rural, and according to the OMB definition, only 84% of the total land area is nonmetropolitan. The ERS estimates that, in 1990, 43% of the rural population in the United States lived in metropolitan counties. This classification of metropolitan does not truly consider the range of population density and land types between both of these extremes in populations and land area. It can be seen that determination of whether a geopolitical area is rural may vary depending on the viewpoint. Table 18.1 for comparative data of rural and urban density between 2010 and 2000 and Box 18.1 for three primary definitions.

Rural towns aren't always idyllic. It's easy to feel trapped and be aware of social hypocrisy. **Bill Pullman, Actor**

TABLE 18.1 Urban, Urbanized Area, Urban Cluster, and Rural Population, 2010 and 2000, United States

Area	Number of 2010 Urban Areas	Population		Percentage of Total Population (%)	
		2010	2000	2010	2000
United States	3,573	308,745,538	281,421,906		
Urban		249,253,271	222,360,539	80.7	79.0
Urbanized areas	486	219,922,123	192,323,824	71.2	68.3
Urban clusters	3,087	29,331,148	30,036,715	9.5	10.7
Rural		59,492,267	59,061,367	19.3	21.0

Source: United States Census Bureau. (2018). Retrieved from http://www.census.gov/geo/reference/ua/urban-rural-2010.html.

18.1 Three Primary Definitions of Urban/Rural Areas

1. The United States Census Bureau (http://www.census.gov/population/censusdata/urdef.txt) defines an urbanized area (UA) by population density. According to this definition, each UA includes a central city and the surrounding densely settled territory that together have a population of 50,000 or more and a population density generally exceeding 1,000 people per square mile. A "county" is a political distinction and is not incorporated in the United States Census Bureau classification scheme; so one UA may cover parts of several counties. Using this definition, all persons living in UAs and in places (e.g., cities, towns, and villages) with a population of 2,500 or more outside of UAs are considered the urban population. All others are considered rural.

Classification of Urban and Rural Areas (United States Census Bureau)

Question: How is my area classified, and where are the data?

Answer: If you want to find out the number of people within a designated area (e.g., place, county, and state) or whether it is urban or rural, do the following:

Go to https://ask.census.gov/. Select American FactFinder.

Select "Data Sets" from the listing on the left-hand side of the page.

Select "SF1" (default) on the left-hand side of the page and "Detailed Tables" on the right-hand side of the page.

Select your geographic preference (e.g., county, place, and metropolitan area) and place the exact geographic names in the box below.

Select "P2 Urban and Rural" from the table selection box and add it to the box below.

View the result.

The American FactFinder also lets users see the urban/rural components of the data shown in each of the tables found in the Summary Files. Once a user accesses a table in any of the four Summary Files, it is possible to view "Geo Components" in the "Options" menu. This lets the user see the urban/rural components, in many cases with other more narrow graduations (e.g., "Urban–in central place").

2. The Office of Management and Budget (OMB) (http://www.census.gov/population/www/estimates/metrodef.html) designates areas as metropolitan on the basis of standards released in January 1980. According to this definition, each metropolitan statistical area (MSA) must include at least one city with 50,000 or more inhabitants or a UA (defined by the Bureau of the Census) with at least 50,000 inhabitants and a total MSA population of at least 100,000 (75,000 in New England). These standards provide that each MSA must include the county in which the central city is located (the central county) and additional contiguous counties (fringe counties), if they are economically and socially integrated with the central county. Any county not included in an MSA is considered nonmetropolitan. The OMB periodically reclassifies counties on the basis of census data and population estimates.

3. The Economic Resource Service (ERS) (U.S. Department of Agriculture [USDA]) (http://www.ers.usda.gov/briefing/rurality/RuralUrbCon/) uses rural–urban continuum codes to distinguish metropolitan counties by size and nonmetropolitan counties by their degree of urbanization or proximity to metro areas. USDA defines codes 0 to 3 as metropolitan and 4 to 9 as nonmetropolitan (e.g., 4 = urban population of 20,000 or more, adjacent to a metropolitan area; and 9 = completely rural or urban population of fewer than 2,500, not adjacent to a metropolitan area).

Practice Point

It is important to remember that definitions of categories, such as urban or metropolitan and nonurban or rural, change with the new perspectives and calculations based on the census. The census data collected in 2010 will no doubt shift these classifications. This is important information for community and public health nurses to know because as leaders in health promotion, initiators of disease prevention projects, or as client advocates, nurses need to know where to access data that support the rationale of needed healthcare services or personnel. The United States Census Bureau has a useful area on its website that helps health professionals know how many persons live in a certain area.

Health Personnel Issues

Whether a geographic area consists of densely or less densely populated segments, the notion of the public health core function of assurance (all people have access to healthcare) is of crucial importance in the role of the community and public health interprofessional team. Unfortunately, healthcare providers enter rural settings in small numbers, primarily because many of them enter residency or post-academic training programs in the areas where they were educated or trained, which is often not in a rural setting and fewer and fewer providers are interested in primary care (Garrison-Jakel, 2011; National Conference of State Legislatures, 2018). Policy options that may motivate healthcare personnel to engage in coming to, and staying in, rural areas of practice include scholarship programs and targeted recruitment, rural residency programs, student loan repayment, including nonphysician primary care opportunities, and international health provider or student options (National Conference of State Legislatures, 2018).

The Health Resources and Services Administration (HRSA) has developed a system for designating areas with a shortage of healthcare professionals based on certain criteria (HRSA, 2018). The HRSA then decides how to develop initiatives to train and secure health professionals to serve in these areas and to create networks of care that meet the unique needs of the populations. The use of the terms **health**

18.2 Health Professional Shortage Areas and Underserved Populations

Health professional shortage areas (HPSAs) may be designated as having a shortage of primary medical care, dental, or mental health providers. They may be urban or rural areas, population groups, or medical or other public facilities. As of September 5, 2018, there were:

- **6,863 primary care HPSAs** with 74 million residents. It would take 14,076 practitioners to meet their need for primary care providers.
- **5,710 dental HPSAs** with 56 million residents. It would take 10,275 practitioners to meet their need for dental providers.
- **5,005 mental health HPSAs** with 110 million residents. It would take 6,581 practitioners to meet their need for mental health providers.

Medically Underserved Areas/Populations

- **Medically underserved areas (MUAs)** may be an entire county or a group of contiguous counties, a group of county or civil divisions, or a group of urban census tracts in which residents have a shortage of personal health services.
- **Medically underserved populations (MUPs)** may include groups of people who face economic, cultural, or linguistic barriers to healthcare.

Source: Health Resources and Services Administration (HRSA). (2018). *Shortage areas*. Retrieved from https://data.hrsa.gov/topics/health-work-force/shortage-areas.

professional shortage areas (HPSAs), medically underserved areas (MUAs), and medically underserved populations (MUPs) is part of the system that establishes a designation that becomes the focus of federal assistance. For example, if an area is designated as an HPSA or an MUA, then the HRSA can support programs to educate personnel who are needed in these areas and provide services to these areas with the help of tax dollars. It does this by soliciting grant proposals for healthcare models to meet population needs and by fiscally supporting training of healthcare personnel to meet these needs. Box 18.2 for more information. Special attention is directed to MUPs. Underserved people may be living in the middle of a busy designated metropolitan area but are underserved for economic, cultural, or literacy reasons.

The HRSA Data Warehouse (HDW) allows users to interact with data in charts, tables/reports, maps, and tools. Visit the Data Sources and Refresh Dates page for more information about where shortage area data is available in the HDW (https://datawarehouse.hrsa.gov/topics/shortageAreas.aspx).

The chart below (Table 18.2) shows the number of currently designated HPSAs by discipline. The criteria for designation vary from one discipline to another, and there is no intrinsic relationship between them; an area may be considered to have a shortage of practitioners in any or all of the disciplines independently.

TABLE 18.2 Designated HPSAs and MUA/MUPs (2018)

Category	Item	Value
Designated HPSAs	Total designated HPSAs (by discipline)	18,084
	–> Dental health	5,866
	–> Mental health	5,042
	–> Primary care	7,176
Medically underserved areas/populations	Designated medically underserved areas/populations	4,235

 Evidence for Practice

Area Health Education Centers (AHEC, 2018) focus on strengthening the supply and distribution of primary care providers in rural and underserved areas. As noted by the Rural Health Information Hub (www.rural-healthinfo.org), AHECs "act as community liaisons with academic institutions and assist in arranging training opportunities for health professions students" (RHI-hub, 2018), prepping students for rural healthcare via:

- the recruitment and training of minority students and those from disadvantaged backgrounds
- the use of student placements in community-based clinical practices settings (with a focus on primary care)
- improvement in quality of care by promoting inter-professional education and collaboration
- facilitation of programs and continuing education resources for health professionals in rural and underserved areas
- pipeline activities that expose high school students to health careers (RHIhub, 2018)

A state directory of all AHECs is available via the National AHEC website, which lists 56 current programs (and more than 235 centers nationwide). These centers, which are funded federally via the HRSA Bureau of Health Workforce (and use other options to match their federal funding), collaborate with approximately 600 nursing and allied health schools and 120 medical schools.

Among the successful programs and activities that AHECs have created are the following (which have been tailored to the needs of the region):

- **Rural Experiences for Health Professions Students (REHPS),** based in the Yankton Rural Area Health Education Center, which placed health professions students in rural or frontier areas of South Dakota, helping to raise awareness of healthcare needs in those areas of the state

- **The Naloxone Education Empowerment Distribution Program**, organized by the San Luis Valley Area Health Education Center, operated a training and certification program (which ended in September 2016) for the administration of naloxone by healthcare workers and community members
- **Project PROMISE (Providing Rural Opportunities in Medicine through Inspiring Service and Education)** from North Carolina, which gave high school seniors the opportunity to have medical academic training, mentor relationships, and experience in working in rural medical facilities
- **The Targeted Rural Underserved Track (TRUST)** program, in locations throughout Washington, Wyoming, Alaska, Montana, and Idaho, which enabled students to return on a regular basis to learn and work in the same community
- **The Forward NM Pathways to Health Careers** program, which supported comprehensive workforce pipeline programs for middle and high school students, undergraduates, medical students, graduate students, and resident physicians
- **The MU-AHEC (University of Missouri Area Health Education Center) Summer Community Program**, which allowed second-year medical students to work under rural community-based physicians (in 4- to 8-week programs)

Source: Rural Health Information Hub (RHIhub). (2018). *Area Health Education Centers (AHEC)*. Retrieved from https://www.ruralhealthinfo.org/topics/workforce-education-and-training#ahec.

Lydie lived in a nonmetropolitan, rural area that was technically classified as an MUA. As such, she inherited many prospective problems despite the numerous benefits. By moving to a less populated area, she had more privacy, cleaner air, and less automobile traffic in a natural, country setting. However, when she became ill, shortages related to the availability of qualified, local healthcare personnel contributed significantly to primary, secondary, and tertiary prevention and her growing list of comorbid conditions and her eventual death.

- Can you determine what areas of this country are designated as MUPs, MUAs, and HPSAs?
- Does the HRSA offer scholarships for healthcare personnel to obtain their respective degrees for entry to practice?
- If the HRSA does offer support, are there contingencies? What are they?
- How would a community and public health nurse begin to address the notion of assurance for a population of interest?

Evidence for Practice

Wines (2016) describes the challenges that need to be considered to deliver an educational program in nursing (Baccalaureate Program) to those men and women who want to become nurses who live in rural areas. The author advises that rural teaching in distance programs takes motivated faculty who are willing to approach challenges using innovative techniques and exceptional communication skills. Faculty must look beyond the common hospital placements for clinical sites when in the rural environment and need to create innovative opportunities using synchronous distance learning methods and unique clinical applications. There is evidence that supports that making the effort to identify and educate motivated faculty can yield exceptional results. The challenges of creating and delivering rural programs to those who know the area and culture the best can be overcome with effort and creative approaches to the traditional profession education modalities.

Morbidity and Mortality Issues

From an epidemiologic perspective, rural population trends indicate a primarily aging population related to outward migration of youth. Despite a net loss of all levels of population leaving rural areas over the last 60 years from out-migration, more recently older retired adults and young people with families have returned to rural areas (Smith, Winkler, & Johnson, 2016). In rural areas, there is less racial diversity (residents are mostly Caucasian), although there are pockets of population diversity (Hispanics in Texas, Native Americans in Arizona and New Mexico). Other characteristics of people who live in rural areas are less college education, higher high school dropout rate, and decreased income (and thus lower socioeconomic status). On the other hand, the cost of living is lower. Families struggle with homelessness and poverty. Females head many families. Employment opportunities are few. Because of the various constraints mentioned, women and children often are the most vulnerable and suffer the most in terms of lack of adequate healthcare. Box 18.3 for more detailed information.

Bolin and colleagues (2015) describe how rural health priorities have changed little in the last decade. The health of rural America is more important than ever to the health of the United States and the world. *Rural Healthy People 2020* was to serve as a counterpart to *Healthy People 2020*, providing evidence of rural stakeholders' assessment of rural health priorities and allowing national and state rural stakeholders to reflect on and measure progress in meeting those goals. The specific aim of the *Rural Healthy People 2020* national survey was to identify rural health priorities from among the *Healthy People 2020's* (*HP2020*) national priorities (Box 18.4).

18.3 Health Factors and Effects of Living in Rural Geopolitical Areas

- Only about 10% of physicians practice in rural America despite the fact that nearly one fourth of the population lives in these areas.
- Rural residents are less likely to have employer-provided healthcare coverage or prescription drug coverage, and the rural poor are less likely to be covered by Medicaid benefits than their urban counterparts.
- Although only one third of all motor vehicle accidents occur in rural areas, two thirds of the deaths attributed to these accidents occur on rural roads.
- Rural residents are nearly twice more likely to die from unintentional injuries, other than motor vehicle accidents, than urban residents. Rural residents are also at a significantly higher risk of death by gunshot injuries than urban residents.
- Rural residents tend to be poorer. On the average, per capita income is $7,417 lower than in urban areas, and rural Americans are more likely to live below the poverty level. The disparity in incomes is even greater for minorities living in rural areas. Nearly 24% of rural children live in poverty.
- People who live in rural America rely more heavily on the federal Food Stamp Program, according to the Carsey Institute at the University of New Hampshire. The institute's analysis found that although 22% of Americans lived in rural areas in 2001, a full 31% of the nation's Food Stamp beneficiaries lived there. In all, 4.6 million rural residents received Food Stamp benefits in 2001, the analysis found.
- There are 2,157 health professional shortage areas (HPSAs) in rural and frontier areas of all states and U.S. territories compared with 910 in urban areas.
- Abuse of alcohol and use of smokeless tobacco is a significant problem among rural youth. The rate of driving under the influence (of alcohol) arrests is significantly greater in nonurban counties. Forty percent of rural 12th graders reported using alcohol while driving compared with 25% of their urban counterparts. Rural 8th graders are twice as likely to smoke cigarettes (26.1% vs. 12.7% in large metro areas.)
- Anywhere from 57% to 90% of first responders in rural areas are volunteers.
- There are 60 dentists per 100,000 population in urban areas vs. 40 per 100,000 in rural areas.
- Cerebrovascular disease was reportedly 1.45 times higher in nonmetropolitan statistical areas (non-MSAs) than in MSAs.
- Hypertension was also higher in rural than in urban areas (101.3 per 1,000 people in MSAs and 128.8 per 1,000 people in non-MSAs.)
- Twenty percent of nonmetropolitan counties lack mental health services vs. 5% of metropolitan counties. In 1999, 87% of the 1,669 mental HPSAs in the United States were in nonmetropolitan counties and home to over 30 million people.
- The suicide rate among rural males is significantly higher than in urban areas, particularly among adult men and children. The suicide rate among rural women is escalating rapidly and is approaching that of men.
- Medicare payments to rural hospitals and physicians are dramatically less than those to their urban counterparts for equivalent services. This correlates closely with the fact that more than 470 rural hospitals have closed in the past 25 years.
- Medicare clients with acute myocardial infarction (AMI) who were treated in rural hospitals were less likely than those treated in urban hospitals to receive recommended treatments and had significantly higher adjusted 30-day post-AMI death rates from all causes than those in urban hospitals.
- Rural residents have greater transportation difficulties reaching healthcare providers, often traveling great distances to reach a doctor or a hospital.
- Accidents resulting in death and serious injury account for 60% of total rural accidents vs. only 48% of urban. One reason for this increased rate of morbidity and mortality is that in rural areas, prolonged delays can occur between a crash, the call for emergency medical services (EMS), and the arrival of an EMS provider. Many of these delays are related to increased travel distances in rural areas and personnel distribution across the response area. National average response time from motor vehicle accident to EMS arrival in rural areas was 18 minutes, or 8 minutes greater than in urban areas.

Source: National Rural Health Association (NRHA). (2018). *What's different about rural health care?* Retrieved from http://www.ruralhealthweb.org/go/left/about-rural-health.

Access to healthcare continues to be the most frequently identified rural health priority. Within this priority, emergency services, primary care, and insurance generate the most concern. A total of 926 respondents in this study identified access as the most pressing priority, followed by nutrition and weight status ($n = 661$), diabetes ($n = 660$), mental health and mental disorders ($n = 651$), substance abuse ($n = 551$), heart disease and stroke ($n = 550$), physical activity and health ($n = 542$), older adults ($n = 482$), maternal infant and child health ($n = 449$), and tobacco use ($n = 429$).

Identifying challenges is a critical aspect of rural health assessment. Creative solutions to key challenges related to access to care with the input and participation of the

populations affected are critical. For example, veterans who are aging and live in rural areas are being served through a geriatric scholar program (GSP), a Department of Veterans Affairs' workforce development program directed to all disciplines working with veterans who are aging. The intent of the program is to infuse geriatric competencies in primary care using a multimodal educational program to target primary care providers and ancillary staff who work in Veteran Administration–sponsored rural clinics. GSP uses didactic presentations, webinars, audio conferences, clinical practica, and mentoring in these programs (Tumosa et al., 2012). Interprofessional teams that contain nurses are starting to make a difference in addressing the needs of people and their families in rural areas.

18.4 Ranking of Rural Health Priorities (*Healthy People 2010* and *Healthy People 2020* Goals)

1. Access to quality healthcare
2. Heart disease
3. Diabetes
4. Mental health and mental disorders
5. Oral health
6. Tobacco use
7. Substance abuse
8. Education and community-based programming
9. Maternal, infant, and child health
10. Nutrition and overweight
11. Cancer
12. Public health infrastructure
13. Immunization and infectious disease
14. Injury and violence prevention

Evidence for Practice

1. Researchers tested a computer-based electronic screening tool (eScreening) for depression and alcohol use as a way to evaluate primary care needs of rural residents (Farrell et al., 2009). eScreening uses a portable computer-based format. The study involved (1) a focus group with providers, (2) usability testing with selected rural clients using a computerized touch screen, and (3) implementation of the touch screen platform with a small sample in primary care to determine feasibility. Consumer response was extremely positive.

2. One study explored the incidence of depression in a sample of 48 people visiting a primary care clinic in rural southeastern North Carolina (Kemppainen, Taylor, Jackson, Kim-Godwin, & Kirby, 2009). Forty percent of the participants met the criteria of clinical depression according to the Center for Epidemiologic Studies Depression Scale (CES-D). Depression was highest in single, African American men who were employed, with adequate health insurance. Researchers attributed this primarily to work-related stressors in dealing with overwhelming social problems of other rural residents and their own economic problems. Critical incident interviews identified self-management strategies for depression and sources of social support.

3. A program intended to encourage relationship building, called the Rural Health Roundtable Project, has prompted change in rural communities (Pennel, Carpender, & Quiram, 2008). This project involves identifying culturally relevant, sensitive topics. In an informal, social environment where participants feel comfortable sharing, targeted questions engage participants and empower local residents. Follow-up is part of the Rural Health Roundtable Project, which has demonstrated its value as an effective tool in working with rural communities. These communities, which have fewer human and financial resources at their disposal, can use the project strategies to identify and make the most of their unique strengths when responding to public health emergencies and natural disasters. Initiated in 1999, the methodology has been refined and enhanced over the past 8 years to more effectively reach participants, promote sharing and discussions, build stakeholder networks, and encourage continued communication and collaboration. The Rural Health Roundtable Project has significant potential for replication and application to all areas of rural public health.

Elderly People

Elders, who are diverse in culture and ethnicity, face many challenges as they age in rural settings. According to Krout and Kinner (2007), most elders do not live on farms. They may be isolated in a variety of housing situations, including family homes in which they brought up their families; the children may have left the area and the parents may live as widows or widowers. They have incomes that can be up to 20% lower than that of their urban counterparts because of lower social security payments, smaller levels of assets in the bank or in property, less pension coverage, and less opportunity to make up the difference because of lack of part-time employment possibilities (Krout & Kinner, 2007). In many cases, fewer options for leisure and recreation are available to these older people.

What complicates these issues are the healthcare service components that are lacking, or are created on the basis of the primary mechanism of payment (i.e., Medicaid). Generally, there are fewer healthcare professionals—physicians, nurses, occupational therapists, and physical therapists—in rural areas, especially with expertise in gerontology, palliation, and end-of-life care. Lack of public transportation puts a burden on the elderly to find private transportation. If they are disabled or cannot drive, dependence for transportation rests on the network of friendships or connection to relatives that may or may not be in place.

It was once said that the moral test of government is how that government treats those who are in the dawn of life, the children; those who are in the twilight of life, the elderly; and those who are in the shadows of life, the sick, the needy, and the handicapped. **Hubert H. Humphrey**

 In Lydie's case, she had no relatives or friend networks available to help, primarily because she chose to live a solitary life that she thought was health promoting for her. In the end, her approach isolated her so much that she had little recourse but to deal with her healthcare issues from a preventive perspective; she prided herself on "not needing those doctors and nurses" and not seeking any primary care treatment. In her mind, toughness in not doing this was a sign of personal and spiritual strength.

When it comes to elder care in rural communities, seven factors compound disease prevention and health promotion efforts to identify and reduce modifiable risk: (1) availability, (2) accessibility, (3) affordability, (4) awareness, (5) adequacy, (6) acceptability, and (7) assessment. These are defined in Box 18.5. Community and public health nurses should discover how to deal with these issues. They should realize that they can use meeting places that seem to draw the greatest group of citizens to good effect. The nurses can work toward developing an education infrastructure to help rural citizens at least understand what modifiable risks they may be facing and how they may receive help if a coalition of requested services can be initiated. For example, in MUPs in inner cities, healthcare professionals often reach elders through churches. In rural areas, solutions may begin through education in a church, post office, or grocery store. In addition, public health nurses, in collaboration with interested citizens and other professional disciplines, can work together developing networks of volunteers to help with transportation needs or other needs that may be identified from a thorough assessment.

Student Reflection

I will never forget my experience in the rural part of a county where I volunteered one summer to help the elderly. Although I was going into my senior year in nursing school and had explained that I wanted to help the elderly with healthcare teaching, I was initially dismayed to know that I would have to go door-to-door with a team of young adults like myself and ask whether there was any need for minor home repairs. My teammates were a physical therapy student and an occupational therapy student. The idea was to help in a practical way with minor issues in the elders' homes, and while doing this work, to take the opportunity to assess health needs and provide health education. It was the best time I had as a nursing student. I really felt as though we students were preventing problems from the beginning and dealing with problems that we found from a health and safety perspective, without shaming elders into thinking they were weak or unable to care for their needs.

18.5 Factors That Compound Disease Prevention and Health Promotion

1. **A**vailability: Insufficient number and diversity of formal services and providers; lack of acceptable services and human service infrastructure
2. **A**ccessibility: Shortages of adequate, appropriate, and affordable transportation; cultural and geographic isolation
3. **A**ffordability: Poverty and inability to pay for services
4. **A**wareness: Low levels of information dissemination; literacy issues
5. **A**dequacy: Lack of service standards and evaluation; evidence-based practice compromised
6. **A**cceptability: Reluctance to ask for help
7. **A**ssessment: Lack of basic information on what is needed using research rigor and analyses

Source: Krout, J. A., & Kinner, M. (2007). Sustaining geriatric rural populations. In L. L. Morgan & P. S. Fahs (Eds.). *Conversations in the disciplines: Sustaining rural populations* (pp. 63–74). Binghamton, NY: Global Academic Publishing.

Occupational and Environmental Health Problems

Occupational health is of particular concern in rural communities, where farmers live. Although the number of people who choose farming as a lifestyle choice has been decreasing steadily over the years, people who do select it as an occupation are exposed to many dangerous conditions in an environment that puts them at risk for injury or death. Farming is a hazardous profession. The total number of agricultural fatalities has been decreasing in recent years, but according to the Bureau of Labor Statistics (2016), the only group with higher fatalities at work than those civilians working as driver/sales workers/truck drivers were farmers, ranchers, and other agricultural managers.

From a family perspective, it is often the case that parents and children help with the work on the farm so there is variability in experience and developmental knowledge. This lifestyle may contribute to injuries and a larger effect on families in general.

Finally, community and public health nurses evaluating safety must consider that farmers and their families work outdoors throughout the year in all sorts of weather and are exposed to a variety of conditions (extremes of heat and cold, snow, sleet, rain, tornados, and drought). Possible contact with chemical treatments applied to the land (e.g., pesticides, fertilizers) also adds variability to the direction of health promotion and injury prevention.

Evidence for Practice

Nilsson (2016) collected data in an international study through interviews from 20 parents of children who own and work on farms. This study examined farming parents' attitudes and experiences regarding having their children grow up on farms, focusing on four themes: (a) the most dangerous places and situations on the farm; (b) children's tasks on the farm; (c) children as a safety risk on the farm; and (d) farm risk education for children. Nilsson concluded that most farming parents were aware of the risks on the farm; however, the parents could be sometimes careless when they worked under stress or exhaustion. Some parents wanted more information, and "some wanted compulsory preventative or safety measures by manufacturers, e.g. a safety belt as standard on the extra seat in tractors. Children's friends were described as one of the greatest risks for injury due to peer pressure. Some parents mentioned that people who grow up on farms are sometimes 'blind' to the dangers. Other parents seemed to overlook the risks and had their children carrying out tasks for which they were not mentally or physically equipped. It is thus important for farming parents to be repeatedly reminded of the risks to their children and to increase their awareness of how to prevent and eliminate risks in order to avoid accidents on the farm" (Nilsson, 2016, p. 1).

Although this chapter does not explicitly address migrant or seasonal workers' conditions on farms, these circumstances have come under scrutiny in terms of sanitation, emergency healthcare, and primary care during the time of high harvest intensity. Although workers and families who are involved in farming may vary by age and education, it is consistently the case that language barriers, health literacy, and generally lower educational status compound efforts to promote health and advance prevention by those involved with rural health initiatives.

Evidence for Practice

1. In many national and international settings, a relevant and sensitive approach to helping population groups obtain healthcare assistance and guidance, involves the use of health promoters or navigators. These key people can relate to specific groups with particular healthcare needs (Pereira, Enard, Nevarez, & Jones, 2011). **There were 11 million unauthorized immigrants in the United States in 2015**, a small but statistically significant decline from the estimated 11.3 million in 2009 (Pew Research Center, 2018). The Pew Research Center's preliminary estimate of the unauthorized immigrant population in 2016 was 11.3 million, a number statistically no different from the 2009 or 2015 estimates. Unauthorized immigrants represented 3.4% of the total U.S. population in 2015 (Pew Research Center, 2018). Per Pew's research, the number of unauthorized immigrants reached a peak in 2007 at 12.2 million, with that group then representing 4% of the U.S. population.

Not all people living within the U.S. borders benefit from the healthcare system in the United States, as many Americans are without health insurance coverage despite state and federal efforts to make this not the case. For this reason, many people use emergency departments for all of their health needs. Only one in five farm workers is able to obtain health insurance through either his or her employer or the state or federal government (Pew Research Center, 2018). The lack of health insurance makes it increasingly difficult for the uninsured and undocumented populations to obtain healthcare, and more than two thirds of this population is living in poverty.

2. Another article has described a model of risk for HIV and problem drinking in Latino labor migrants in the United States (Sanchez, Silva-Suarez, Serna, & De La Rosa, 2012). Specific risks that need to be addressed for this group include stressful living and working conditions, not just drinking behaviors that may compromise safe sex practices. The broader environmental risk in this unique population of Latinos needs to be addressed with a new model for interventions.

In most rural areas, the issue of access has been addressed with managed care organizations (MCOs) since 2008 (Willging, Waitzkin, & Nicdao, 2008). MCOs build provider networks and encourage community health plans so that local providers of healthcare can control cost. Mobile clinics, school-based health programs, and telehealth systems (programs that use wireless and nonwireless electronic devices to communicate health information for educational or diagnostic purposes) are other ways by which distance between healthcare providers and family members can be addressed. At the local level, transportation volunteers and parish or church visitors can help decrease isolation and help families share health resources with adjacent rural areas. There needs to be a concentrated focus on prevention with particular emphasis on decreasing or eliminating smoking behaviors; decreasing sun exposure; reducing fat intake; and educating families about the signs and symptoms of depression, heart disease, diabetes, and cancer.

From a professional perspective, working in rural areas can have positive and negative aspects. In areas where people and communities have problems maintaining connections, it is important to create a way to interact, or network, with other professionals for professional support and diagnostic assistance. Working in a rural area offers opportunities to be creative and to "think outside the box" and not merely consider the usual care methodologies. Community and public health nurses have to use limited resources effectively.

The work of healthcare professionals in rural areas may not be as intensive as would be the case in a large medical center in an urban setting, or even in a community-based service in an urban setting. In areas where healthcare is intensive, there are also many opportunities to learn a specific discipline. What is intriguing and perhaps attractive in rural settings is the slower pace, with the opportunity to engage in relationships with communities that could be long-lasting and ultimately might prove more rewarding. Roles and disciplines are more blurred in rural areas because of lack of resources. So it may be the case that collaboration, interprofessional work, and self-care within the context of caregiving all become matters of pragmatic healthcare and intervention.

CORRECTIONAL HEALTH: UNDERSERVED POPULATIONS IN JAILS AND PRISONS

In the United States, detention centers, jails, and prisons are places that provide safety to the public by incarcerating people who have committed crimes and who are deemed a threat to society. There are a variety and levels of jails and prisons, ranging from detention centers, where **inmates** await arraignment or care decisions and where there is high turnover, to minimum- or maximum-security prisons, where there are longer lengths of stay for inmates in some cases. Generally, minimum- and maximum-security prisons are administered by the states, and penitentiaries are federally administered prisons in which inmates are incarcerated for crimes against the government. In correctional institutions, there is a disproportionate number of persons of color, regardless of youth, gender, and age (Nellis, 2016). Incarceration may be socially determined, but in the final analysis, the health of the people in this system is compromised. Many reports contain evidence that illness and injury arrive at institutions with the inmates or detainees, occur in these areas, and recycle back into neighborhoods when inmates and detainees leave.

> Maybe I won't stay out of prison. Who knows? **Jack Kevorkian**

All levels of prevention need to be addressed for all people in correctional facilities. For example, the Children's Defense Fund (CDF) has taken a leadership role in addressing the issues of children being in a "pipeline" spiraling into lives of violence and crime because of a variety of negative contributing variables leading to arrest, conviction, incarceration, and death (CDF, 2009). The CDF supports initiatives at the individual, family, community, organizational, and government levels (Box 18.6). The Cradle to Prison Pipeline is a CDF campaign designed to bring public attention to this issue.

 Where do you see community public health nurses contributing care and healing that relates to Saliha (see Box 18.5)? Give specific examples.

Most inmates are males who are African American or Latino. The average age of inmates is 37. Prisoners who are incarcerated for violent crimes have been involved in rape, murder, sodomy, kidnapping, armed robbery, and sexual offenses, and 34% are in high- or maximum-security facilities, and 40% are serving sentences of more than 10 years. However, 75% of all prisoners are nonviolent and have been incarcerated for drug possession and trafficking, bribery, and extortion. Of those who are African American, 14.5% are women and 52% are incarcerated primarily on drug possession or prostitution charges (U.S. Department of Justice, Bureau of Justice Statistics, 2018).

Many have conjectured that poverty, violence and abuse as children, lack of education, and poor self-esteem have made incarceration an area where those who are oppressed are further oppressed and exposed again to violence, mental health problems, and physical morbidities. Issues that face inmates, their families, and healthcare providers who work in prisons include security issues; despairing attitudes; overcrowding; the increased risk of communicable diseases such as tuberculosis, HIV infection, sexually transmitted infections (STIs), and hepatitis C; and fragmentation of families. Community and public health nurses may find conflicts with the will of the warden or person in charge of the area of incarceration and the standards of nursing practice. For example, state nurse practice acts are in direct conflict with participation in the highly politicized issue of capital punishment. Despite the autonomous nature of nursing practice and medicine, the decision maker in jails and prisons is often the warden or director. Thus, conflicts of interest and philosophy can and do occur (Nolan & Walsh, 2012).

After release from incarceration, inmates often face social injustices and economic problems. The ability to find appropriate shelter at a reasonable cost is becoming very difficult, as is finding social support that prevents recidivism. Trying to help families reconnect with adequate financial and rehabilitation support is extremely difficult. Literacy and job training are important family-centered approaches to maintaining a productive and financially stable life. Many men and women describe how repeating crimes that put them back in jail or prison is a way to bring them to a place where they feel protected and escape the painful realities they face on release (Nellis, 2016).

What is critical to understand about those in prison returning to their home communities is how important it is to understand the integral connection and responsibility that is mutually shared. Those in charge of prison health and those in charge of health in communities need to help each other in creating the best opportunities for all types of success for citizens. Those citizens who have health problems "upstream" will bring them "downstream" and vice versa.

> Probably the only place where a man can feel really secure is in a maximum-security prison, except for the imminent threat of release. **Germaine Greer, Australian author**

18.6   Solution Pyramid for Youth (Children's Defense Fund)

Individual People

- Mentor a child.
- Volunteer at an after-school program for youth.
- Vote in every election and advocate for children.
- Educate elected officials about the Cradle to Prison Pipeline.
- Host a house party to educate others about the Cradle to Prison Pipeline and what they can do to dismantle it.
- Volunteer with children who are homeless or in foster care.
- Organize a forum on incarcerated youth and the funding disparities between prisons and education in our nation.
- Volunteer your talents or professional services to help a single-parent, kinship care, or foster care family by babysitting, inviting them to events with their children, or providing transportation.
- Invite youth to events at the next educational level (i.e., taking a high school student to a college basketball game).

Families

- Spend quality time with your family (i.e., family game night, eating meals together).
- Join the Parents Teachers Association (PTA), a parent support group, or other school group.
- Attend school activities and/or volunteer in the classroom.
- Consistently praise your child's achievements in school and extracurricular activities.
- Establish and maintain a supportive home learning environment.
- Create daily homework routines and limit television viewing.
- Offer tutoring and homework help to your children or younger siblings.
- Offer to run errands or help around the house.
- Communicate with and listen to your child.
- Talk and actively listen to children within your extended family.
- Show affection, love, and respect to your child every day.
- Do something fun with your child or sibling.
- Adopt a foster child or become a foster parent.

Communities

- Institute a "cradle roll" within your faith-based institution or community, linking every child to a permanent, caring family member or adult mentor who can keep them on track and get them back on track if and when they stray.
- Promote learning by starting an after-school program for children.
- Ensure that at least one caring community member attends every public school student suspension meeting or court hearing.
- Encourage families to spend quality time together by hosting a movie or game night at your church.
- Start a support group for single-parent or kinship care families.
- Provide job opportunities and guidance for families and youth in need.
- Create college scholarships for children from disadvantaged, foster care, and kinship care families.
- Work with school officials to develop and adopt more child-appropriate discipline policies and procedures.

- Reach out to youth who are homeless or in foster care.
- Prepare care packages of new clothes, personal toiletries, and/or a welcome gift for children placed into foster care homes.
- Hold events to celebrate the strengths of our children and provide college scholarships and leadership opportunities to youth.
- Start a halfway house and counseling program for youth who have run away.
- Create a summer job opportunity for a youth.
- Create and distribute a community resource manual so that parents know where to turn for help for their families.

Organizations

- Invest in prevention and early intervention.
- Host a health fair to ensure that all children who are eligible for Medicaid or your state children's health insurance program are enrolled.
- Provide free tax filing assistance to low-income working families.
- Educate families about how they can apply for food stamps, Head Start, federal nutrition programs, and other similar benefits.
- Create and distribute a calendar of free family-friendly community events.
- Start a parent education program to familiarize parents about conflict resolution in the home and how to advocate for their children.
- Encourage alternatives to incarceration such as restitution, community service, electronic monitoring, drug rehabilitation treatment, or placement in a "staff secure" (but not locked) community corrections facility.
- Work to ensure that counseling, social services, education, and health and mental health services are provided to at-risk youth.
- Fund reinvestment in urban communities, such as parks, schools, and roads.
- Write annual child and gun violence reports to track the killing of children and call for effective gun control measures and nonviolent conflict resolution training.
- Host a Cradle to Prison Pipeline summit to connect and educate others about this "pipeline" and ways to dismantle it.

Government Agencies

- Bring other elected officials and leaders together to gain firsthand awareness of the status of your local children; demonstrate what is working and what is not.
- Ensure children in foster care and detention receive quality treatment to address their mental, behavioral, and emotional needs.
- Promote high-quality children's television programming and access to other quality electronic media.
- Provide high-quality early childhood development programs for all.
- Ensure all children and pregnant women access to affordable, seamless, comprehensive health coverage and services.

- Establish policies that emphasize prevention and rehabilitation to keep children out of or rescue them from the pipeline.
- Expand "second chance" programs for high school dropouts, ex-offenders, and at-risk youth to secure General Equivalency Degrees (GEDs), job training, and employment.
- Reduce repeat offender rates by focusing on treatment- and family-oriented approaches.
- Make sure that every child can read at grade level by fourth grade and graduate from high school able to succeed in post-secondary education and/or work.

- Organize state and local leadership councils or committees to create strategic plans to address the learning and developmental needs of children.
- Invest money in community-based rehabilitation centers and treatment programs to serve as an alternative to juvenile detention and prison.
- Stop the criminalization of children at increasingly younger ages.
- Create partnerships with local businesses, schools, and/or churches to create quality exit programs for those leaving the juvenile justice system as a way to start them on the "Pipeline to Success."

Source: Children's Defense Fund (CDF). *Cradle to Prison Pipeline campaign—Key immediate action steps.* Retrieved from http://www.childrensdefense.org/helping-americas-children/cradle-to-prison-pipeline-campaign/action-steps.html.

Practice Point

In the context of healthcare prevention education, one of the most important functions nurses can address when caring for people who have left correctional institutions is to discern whether the client has a health literacy challenge. Direction and encouragement of where to obtain support to advance education through a variety of extension programs and special projects can be important to preventive work at the individual, family, and community level.

Sixty percent of people entering prison today are illiterate.
Jeffrey Archer

Evidence for Practice

Out of concern that standards for pregnancy-related healthcare in jails and prisons need to be established, followed, and accredited regularly, a study specifically examined the healthcare practices of pregnant women in state prisons using a survey with 62 multiple choice questions and four open-ended questions. Wardens of 50 women's state correctional facilities were contacted to involve them in the process. Of the 50 contacted, 19 completed the survey, a 38% response rate. The findings of this study gave evidence that substandard care does exist for pregnant incarcerated women in correctional facilities. More specifically, nutritional recommendations for a healthy pregnancy are not met, adequate rest is compromised, and lower bunks are not required. Psychosocial support and education are minimal and the use of restraints, which can compromise the health and safety of the woman and her baby, continue, including during labor and delivery. A key finding was that best practices are not used generally and there is a serious need to address the unmet healthcare needs of this

marginalized population, and support legislation to limit the use of restraints with pregnant incarcerated women (Ferszt & Clarke, 2012).

Criticism abounds in terms of the quality of care offered at correctional institutions. People who end up in prison systems almost always struggle with chronic, difficult-to-change healthcare problems such as chronic mental health issues, substance addiction, proclivity to violent acts, and risky behaviors, leaving them vulnerable to STIs in general and HIV/AIDS in particular. Although part of the reason for lack of quality care relates to maintaining qualified and inspired healthcare personnel, the more formidable issue is public financing of the growing numbers of inmates' healthcare needs. Box 18.7 for commentary of a medical director in Michigan concerning prison inmates.

According to van den Bergh, Gatherer, Fraser, and Moller (2011), from a local and global perspective there are also

18.7 Summary of Study Criticizing Prison Healthcare

- The medical director for a Grand Rapids clinic serving low-income patients was the technical adviser to Michigan's prisons.
- Findings released indicate 32 changes needed to improve healthcare in the prisons.
- Infectious diseases, such as hepatitis C, need treatment.
- Inadequate care during incarceration must be addressed to face current burden in hospitals and other healthcare providers in the community on release.
- Report recommends reviving the Legislative Corrections Ombudsman, a position the legislature eliminated in 2003, and creating a permanent legislative committee to oversee prison medical care and mental healthcare.

Source: Adapted from Shellenbarger, P. (2008). Study criticizes prison health care. *The Grand Rapids [Michigan] Press.* Retrieved from http://blog.mlive.com/grpress/2008/02/study_criticizes_prison_health.html.

serious concerns related to the need for gender sensitivity directed to the care of women and their experience in prisons. Women prisoners, although a minority within all prison systems, have special health needs that are frequently neglected. The evidence in the literature includes a lack of gender sensitivity in policies and practices in prisons, violations of women's human rights, and failure to accept that imprisoned women have more and different healthcare needs compared with male prisoners. Many of these violations are related to reproductive health issues, mental health problems, drug dependencies, and histories of violence and abuse. Additional needs stem from their frequent status as a mother and usually as the primary caregiver for her children.

In Michigan, a for-profit MCO called Correctional Medical Services has been hired to address the healthcare needs of inmates in the state's correctional system. Use of this kind of organization often occurs because many healthcare professionals find it difficult to work in the conditions of correctional institutions. From a community and public health perspective, students and licensed nurses should consider the contribution they could make in these settings with regard to primary, secondary, and tertiary prevention. Whatever improvements nurses engender concerning mental health, communicable disease, and physical wellness will eventually be a positive contribution to a family, a neighborhood, and a community.

GAY, LESBIAN, BISEXUAL, TRANSGENDER, AND QUEER COMMUNITY

Not all people are attracted to people of the opposite sex all the time. Some belong to the LGBTQ community. Many people in this community have experienced actual or perceived discrimination. Part of the discrimination is not intentional but comes from a lack of thoughtful sensitivity on the part of healthcare providers in not examining the assumptions made about lifestyles based on stereotypes. Some of the problem stems from assessing and offering interventions related to health issues using the standards of heterosexual patients. Healthcare providers working with LGBTQ clients need to understand that not all of these people are openly "out of the closet" and that confidentiality is extremely important in light of active discrimination. Such discrimination may involve work, housing, health insurance, and financial support if the client is in a domestic partnership with another person.

Gay people are the sweetest, kindest, most artistic, warmest, and most thoughtful people in the world. And since the beginning of time all they've ever been is kicked. **Little Richard**

Jan is a good example of someone who is trying to approach her health in good faith, with a preventive orientation, but who may easily be persuaded to not to return to a primary care physician because of lack of consideration of her specific needs.

- How would you address the needs of healthcare professionals who wish to understand the specific needs of unique populations?
- Are there best practices that can help inform healthcare professionals related to how to assess what the specific needs may be?

Student Reflection

It was really exciting to work with my nursing professor, who is not only a clinician but also a researcher in a project about the nursing care of incarcerated women, in a detention facility for women. We worked together over a 10-week period using yoga exercise as an intervention to effect perceptions of well-being. In the first week, we measured vital signs and completed a health history, measured depression on a self-report inventory, and also asked questions about perceptions of wellness. Then we met weekly and helped the women participate in yoga. Following these meetings, we took the measurements again. Some important changes took place in perceptions of wellness, especially mental health. But what really struck me was how happy the women were to be able to do something and accomplish something while they were in prison. As I got to know them, I felt very sad that many were in jail for crimes they committed to keep themselves from becoming even poorer (sex work, selling drugs). They were poor women trying to survive, not mass murderers. Many of them talked about their children, who were in foster care or with family members. All I could think was that these women not only had to heal themselves when they left jail but also their families, or the cycle will continue.

Student Reflection

Several months ago, I was involved as a leader in an education discussion about prevention of STIs with a group of women in a drop-in center in the inner city. Boy, was I embarrassed! I assumed that everybody in the group was heterosexual. In reality, four of the women there were lesbians and had brought their significant others with them. All of the information I shared was regarding risk related to intercourse or oral sex between a man and a woman alone. After the session was over, I was really horrified when the two couples told me about the sexual orientation of people in the group. I felt as though I perpetuated assumptions about sex and did not provide helpful statistics about risk.

My instructor and I came up with a solution. We were able, with these couples' permission, to recontact some members of the group who had attended originally and asked if they would like to bring some of their friends who may be in the same type of relationship with them so we could specifically address their needs in a tailored session of prevention messages. So about a month later, we had a lesbian/bisexual safe sex session that was uniquely constructed just for these people. It was so successful that many members of the group, who vary in age from 24 to 60 years, continue to meet in a supportive capacity. It has been a bonus to see the intergenerational sharing and support.

Student Reflection

I had no idea what the "Q" meant in the LGBTQ community. I consulted my clinical faculty member and he explained that when the "Q" for QUEER is used it means an individual is questioning their identity and is uncertain of their orientation. My clinical faculty helped me understand that not everybody is sure of their identity which may make them more vulnerable in opening up and being honest with clinicians about what they are experiencing or thinking about the life's past, present, and future. Not everybody is clear about where they stand in the alphabet of LGBTQ. One of the things that I remember from this conversation is that although the word "queer" may be offensive to providers because they don't understand what it means, it is also important to let patients self-identify their orientation followed by caring acceptance on the part of the provider. Being identified as "queer" can mean different things to different people, so the best thing to do is just to say that you would like to understand more about what this means for the patient and what are the things from a health perspective that are of concern so you can address those issues directly. Finally, when it comes down to it, using or not using the word "queer" is an extremely personal choice; the important thing is to let people identify themselves, no matter what that identity might be. We all deserve the dignity to decide who we are for ourselves.

In the course of assessment, diagnosis, and treatment of LGBTQ people, community and public health nurses should be aware that partners need to be included in care decisions; be familiar with key health concerns of this population such as STIs, alcohol and substance abuse, depression, and suicide; and become comfortable with asking healthcare assessment questions that include LGBT lifestyles, so that key prevention opportunities are not missed. For example, during a physical assessment, it is essential to ask a client whether he or she has sex with men, women, or both; this information is critical in identifying further clarifying questions about high-risk behaviors and sex. No healthcare provider should assume that a client is homosexual or heterosexual based on appearance or other factors.

Evidence for Practice

1. One seminal research article has examined the literature to provide clinicians with evidence-based recommendations for care of lesbian clients (Roberts, 2006). Data organization related to specific health problems was noted frequently in the research articles. Findings and conclusions include that lesbians have previously been invisible in health services and research. Lesbians are "coming out" more and more with healthcare providers, which means that data about them can be collected. Data now show that lesbians are at risk for cancer, heart disease, depression, and alcohol abuse. Adolescent lesbians are especially at risk for smoking, as well as depression and suicide. However, screening for these conditions continues to be low in lesbians.

2. In a world where healthcare needs of the LGBTQ population is increasingly important, healthcare professionals require appropriate academic and clinical training in preparation for the increased demand for culturally competent care. Nurses are of particular interest, as they are the core direct caregivers in many healthcare settings. This research study explored the national climate around LGBTQ individuals. The conclusion is that educators need to be committed to ensure the development of knowledgeable practitioners who will be able to implement best practices in LGBTQ patient care. Attention should be paid to providing students with diverse clinical placements, access to LGBT interest groups, and clear expectations for LGBTQ-sensitive nursing care plans and course outcomes selection that promote cultural competence (Lim, Brown, & Jones, 2013).

3. One qualitative study has used ethnography to identify, describe, and classify the effect of sociostructural factors on men who have sex with men and HIV transmission risk (Natale, 2009). Included are the perceptions of HIV risk in four subgroups: HIV-positive, Latino, black, and young (18 to 24 years) men who have sex with men. Results classify participant-perceived transmission factors into sociostructural factors (e.g., social, health, economic, political, and mental health). This article also addresses significant areas of social stigma and discrimination—critical areas that need to be addressed to promote the general health of these men as well as their sexual health. It is also important to prevent and treat substance use in this population.

4. Families are of critical importance in Latino communities in the United States. Research has shown

that familism—or the cultural ideal that involves reliance on nuclear and extended family members for emotional support, connectedness, honor, loyalty, and solidarity—reduces sexual health risks among heterosexual youth, yet this relationship has not been examined among Latino bisexual teenagers. A complex construct, familism has a strong potential for providing insights into sexual health practices of bisexual Latino adolescents. One study examined how familism shapes sexual decision making regarding behavior and expressions of bisexuality in Latino adolescents living in New York City (Muñoz-Laboy et al., 2009). Twenty-five in-depth interviews and ethnographic observations in bisexual males and females (15 to 19 years of age) for 9 months were the basis for the study. Findings suggested that these bisexual Latinos value closeness to their families by maintaining family ties and seeking emotional and material support from their families. For those who wanted to keep their bisexuality private, the constant surveillance of the family network is a negative.

Bradford and Mayer (2008) have identified 10 summary points of great concern related to demographic information and the needs of LGBTQ people. These points are valid and continue to be relevant today. These points include the following:

- The four different subgroups—gay, lesbian, bisexual, and transgender people—have unique needs. There is little demographic data tailored to each of these separate groups.
- Few population-based studies have been conducted in LGBTQ groups, with the exception of HIV-related research, particularly in men who have sex with men.
- Specific questions on surveys related to sexual orientation are lacking.
- Recognition of same-sex heads of households has not always been included in survey data.
- There is confusion regarding variability of expression of one's identity, behavior, and attraction.
- Cultural contexts vary across age and developmental staging about "coming out of the closet"; some people (e.g., older gays or lesbians) may not feel comfortable with the word "queer."
- Fluidity of gender and sexual identity changes over time.
- LGBT groups tend to experience more serious physical and mental health conditions, including interpersonal violence and substance addiction.
- Particular health concerns from a prevention perspective include obesity, injury, violence, and access to healthcare facilities.
- Health professionals are poised as confidants and trusted people to make significant preventive inroads at all levels if they approach LGBTQ groups informed, with data.

One of the key goals in community and public health nursing is to begin to understand the needs of LGBTQ people through specific training that addresses the needs of each particular group. The assumption that this information is included in healthcare training programs for all healthcare disciplines is often false. Many times, students need to attend extracurricular programs that are supported by local initiatives or institutions that care for these populations because of the unique nature of the information that needs to be shared. For example, Transgender Awareness Training and Advocacy is an initiative started by Sam Lurie. He is a transgendered man, or transman, who has used his own experience as a way to help inform others of the needs of the transgender community (Transgender Awareness Training and Advocacy, 2009).

Training is meaningful only if community standards are developed so that evidenced-based practice can progress to assist people in these groups. Box 18.8 for an LGBT health access project developed and supported by the Massachusetts Department of Public Health (Massachusetts Department of Public Health, 2018).

Practice Point

When taking a sexual history, always ask whether a client is having sex with men, women, or both. This clarification is critical in offering prevention, health promotion, and risk advice. It is crucial that healthcare providers also be respectful by using the term "sexual orientation" versus "sexual preference." Although many LGBTQ people are not ashamed of their lives, many would also admit that their identity, behaviors, and attractions have caused a significant amount of personal pain related to stigma and isolation (i.e., sexual orientation may not have been their choice).

It is critical for community and public health nurses to ask questions in order to be sensitive to the LGBTQ community. This method is a healing approach that may decrease stigma and isolation.

VETERANS AND HEALTH

The brave men and women who serve their country and as a result live constantly with the war inside them exist in a world of chaos. But the turmoil they experience isn't who they are; the PTSD invades their minds and bodies. **Robert Koger**

There are 2 million reintegrated veterans in the civilian sector and 1 million veterans suffering from nonvisible or visible trauma (Conrad & Armstrong, 2016, 2017). While almost 10,000 veterans who participated in the Global War on Terror (GWOT) are receiving their healthcare in Veteran's Administration (VA) hospitals, many of them are

18.8 Community Standards of Practice for the Provision of Quality Healthcare Services to Lesbian, Gay, Bisexual, and Transgender Clients

The Gay, Lesbian, Bisexual, and Transgender Health Access Project is a collaborative, community-based program funded by the Massachusetts Department of Public Health. The project's mission is to foster the development and implementation of comprehensive, culturally appropriate, quality health promotion policies and healthcare services for lesbian, gay, bisexual, and transgendered (LGBT) people and their families. Research has indicated that fear of discrimination and stigma cause many LGBT people to postpone or decline seeking medical care. Others, once in care, sometimes withhold from their providers personal information that may be critical to their well-being.

- Working closely with consumers and clinicians across the state, the Gay, Lesbian, Bisexual, and Transgender Health Access Project works to confront the insensitivity and ignorance that many LGBT people have experienced in accessing healthcare and related services.
- In addition, the project seeks to support LGBT people in understanding and acquiring the quality care they need.
- The need for community standards emerged from several sources, including: (1) a statewide provider survey, (2) a 1997 Gay, Lesbian, Bisexual, and Transgender Health Access Project report, and (3) health concerns of the LGBT community. Among other things, these reports detailed a serious lack of LGBT awareness and understanding among healthcare providers in Massachusetts. Some believed that they had no LGBT clients or staff in their facilities; many were unsure about what their role should be in identifying and addressing LGBT issues; and a few had policies in place to guide personnel or consumers.
- To address these concerns, the Gay, Lesbian, Bisexual, and Transgender Health Access Project convened a community

working group of more than 60 consumers, providers, public, and private agency administrators and staff. The group worked to develop a framework to improve LGBT access to quality care and to assist clinicians and their facilities in creating responsive environments. This group's efforts were guided by four principles: (1) the elimination of discrimination on the basis of sexual orientation and gender identity, (2) the promotion and provision of full and equal access to services, (3) the elimination of stigmatization of LGBT people and their families, and (4) the creation of health service environments where it is safe for people to be "out" to their providers.

- The community standards of practice and quality indicators outlined in this document will guide and assist providers in achieving these goals. The standards address both agency administrative practices and service delivery components, including the following areas:
  1. Personnel
  2. Client's rights
  3. Intake and assessment
  4. Service planning and delivery
  5. Confidentiality
  6. Community outreach and health promotion
- LGBT people live in and seek healthcare and prevention services in every community in Massachusetts. Eliminating barriers to care requires both an educated and empowered consumer base and a skilled, culturally competent, sensitive, and welcoming provider community that is openly supportive of LGBT people and their families. These standards are one tool for achieving greater healthcare for all.

Source: Massachusetts Department of Health. (2013). *Gay, lesbian, bisexual and transgender health access project.* Retrieved from http://www.lgbthealth.org.

---

receiving care in a variety of settings from a variety of healthcare providers. In many cases, a veteran admitting they need care is the first hurdle to entering any healthcare system, only surpassed by the readiness of the healthcare taskforce to appropriately care for this group. Conrad and Armstrong (2016, 2017) discuss specific issues related to women veterans as an underserved and unique population but many of the points made apply to all veterans. The importance of providing cultural sensitivity in care for deployed veteran men and women is primary (Conrad & Armstrong, 2017) in addition to continual need for advocacy in care (Conrad & Armstrong, 2016).

Civilian nurses need to understand the military culture to address the health needs of the veteran men and women. Most healthcare providers do not understand the military culture that contributes to how veterans seek access to healthcare. Veterans undergo intensive training related to military values, tradition, norms, and expectations. In their training, they focus on the fundamental indoctrination of military loyalty. After discharge and reunion in the civilian

culture, few veterans forget their military experience, yet they still keep the learned value, tradition, and norms. As a result, seeking healthcare is considered weakness for some of them. Moreover, there are specific needs of women in the military. The integration of the veteran women in the civilian life after discharge from the military is significant since they will face unique obstacles and challenges, which require appropriate care for smooth transition and integration. For example, after deployment women veterans face physical, psychological, and behavioral challenges to their health that often go undiscovered. Additionally, their lower financial earning potential, lower level of education, higher family responsibility expectations, racial diversity, poverty, homelessness, and age are all issues that should be considered in care of this population. To intervene and help veteran women and men facing challenges and problems, the authors recommend screening veterans receiving care in the healthcare setting by simply asking if they served in the military or not as a standard of care and an estimate of potential health risk. Asking this simple question could help the nurses and other health providers to identify multiple health risks and healthcare needs. Increasing nurses' awareness of the needs of all veterans and providing culturally sensitive care is crucial especially in the care provided to veteran women.

Typical healthcare risks and actual challenges that have been "underserved" in healthcare systems caring for veterans include PTSD, military sexual trauma, suicide, and productive/gynecologic/urinary tract infections for women. Unfortunately, disparities in treatment received by veteran women when compared with veteran men have been observed. Examples include variation in treatment for HIV, cancer screening, and lipid-lowering therapy among others.

Evidence for Practice

Johnson and colleagues (2013) explain the unique health problems and issues that are experienced by the veterans. There is 22.5 million living military veterans. However, 75% of the veterans in the United States are receiving their healthcare needs in organizations other than VA hospitals. Therefore, it is important and significant for the non-VA nurses to understand how to provide appropriate veteran center healthcare service. Empirical data is provided to demonstrate that more and more veterans are coming into the health system across time. For example, there had been an increase in the number of veteran women between 2000 and 2010 (i.e., 1.6 to 1.8 million). This increase resulted in the need for expanding the health services provided to the veteran women including gynecology and women's clinics. The nature of military culture including the veteran identity complicated by traumatic brain injury, polytrauma, chronic pain, military sexual trauma, substance abuse, homelessness, suicidality, and hazardous exposure is a formidable list of care need areas that needs to be addressed with military cultural knowledge. Challenges faced by veterans as a unique "social determinant of their health" include perceptions of civilians lacking respect for the veteran, not fitting in the civilian life, and having high expectations of themselves compared to civilians. In addition, veterans' physical and psychological injuries caused during battle affect their transition to the civilian life. Concerns about confidentiality, embarrassment, lack of awareness about treatment and support resources, and fear of shame and stigmatization make it particularly difficult to seek out healthcare. In the end, more research is required to identify the long-term effect of military service on veteran health as well as to investigate the effectiveness of the nursing interventions.

HUMAN TRAFFICKING

In this great land of the free we call it human trafficking. And so long as we don't partake in the luxury, ignoring slavery is of no consequence. It is much easier to look away and ignore the victims. The person who ignores slavery justifies it by quickly deducing the victim is a willing participant hampered by misfortune. **D'Andre Lampkin**

Human trafficking defined as "recruitment and transportation of the people for exploitation" has severe physical and psychological impact on the survivors including, but not limited to, depression and anxiety as well as chronic physical pain (Hemmings et al., 2016). It is estimated that at least 13% of the healthcare providers had been in contact with suspected human trafficking victims without even knowing it. The healthcare system nationally and globally is lacking the detailed evidence-based guidelines that describe the assessment, planning, and application of the appropriate intervention and treatment process that are required by the victims of human trafficking. Therefore, there is an urgent need to increase the healthcare providers' readiness and awareness related to the required healthcare needs for the victims of human trafficking.

Hemmings and colleagues (2016) created a guideline for the healthcare providers to care survivors of human trafficking. The guideline was created based on a systematic review of peer-reviewed literature. Key areas that need to be addressed in caring for this group of patients include promoting disclosure, providing care, ensuring safety, supporting recovery, working in partnership, physical and psychological indicators needing to be addressed, and developing ongoing services. Healthcare needs to include detailed needs assessment, securing informed consent, and providing appropriate trauma care and culture-sensitive opportunities including an interpreter if necessary. Also noted was the need to establish collaboration and partnership relationships with agencies, such as social services and law enforcement, to create a clear treatment and referral plan for the identified trafficked cases.

Washburn (2018) points out that there are many misconceptions of victims of human trafficking including but not limited to trafficked persons are only immigrants or foreigners or the trafficked person will ask for help immediately. In fact, this vulnerable population he identifies is made up often of children, young homeless and runaway youth, refugees, immigrants, low-income people, LGBTQ, and others.

The nurse's role includes vigilance to recognize a victim of human trafficking and respond based on the approved protocol and procedures in the healthcare setting. When the nurse suspects a trafficked victim, the priority is to provide appropriate safety and care. To maintain the safety of the victim and the other healthcare personnel, the nurse should not confront the trafficking event revealed itself. In a situation where the risk is high, the nurse should notify the local law enforcement and the security. During the contact with the suspect trafficked person it is recommended that principles of a safe interview be maintained. An example of interview question that may help unravel data to create a plan of care include, "Does someone control, supervise, or monitor your work/actions?" If the screening interview resulted in suspecting an exploitation, the institution protocol should be followed. Finally, it is imperative that nurses and healthcare providers develop primary, secondary, and tertiary prevention measures to impact this evolving phenomenon. Washburn (2018) explained that the nurses could do a lot of things to develop their awareness and consequently create prevention measures. Nurses can develop anti-trafficking education program and advocate for it in different public settings. In the nursing schools, faculty could provide the student with scenarios that include human trafficking to increase the nursing students' understanding of the evolving realities of this situation.

HOMELESS POPULATIONS

Was I always going to be here? No I was not. I was going to be homeless at one time, a taxi driver, truck driver, or any kind of job that would get me a crust of bread. You never know what's going to happen. **Morgan Freeman**

Homeless people include single men, families with children led by single heads of households (women), single women (bag ladies), and children (<18 years) who lack adult supervision. In developed countries, the majority of homeless people are male and more likely to be black, veterans, unemployed, struggle with mental health challenges and/or addictions, and are victims of domestic violence (National Coalition for the Homeless, 2018). Many of these people take refuge in homeless shelters, and others live in abandoned buildings, jails, hospitals, parks, airports, and bus/train stations, as well as under bridges or in the entries to buildings.

Homelessness has many causes. Reasons for homelessness include the deinstitutionalization efforts of the 1960s to mainstream the mentally ill into society, unemployment and underemployment, domestic violence, abandonment, natural disasters and fires, disability, substance abuse and addiction, immigration, and political unrest and wars (National Coalition for the Homeless, 2018). Historically, many circumstances have led to homelessness, including freedom from slavery, westward expansion, lumber and railroad work, the Great Depression, and the aftereffects of war. In recent years, the shortage of affordable housing has been a key reason (National Coalition for the Homeless, 2018).

I lived rough, by my wits, was homeless, lived on the streets, lived on friends' floors, was happy, was miserable. **Ben Okri, Nigerian poet and novelist**

Reaching homeless people is difficult. It is not easy to provide care with trained and experienced interprofessional teams because of the inability to locate clients in the community by address or phone. Many homeless people have complications from decreased hygiene, hypothermia, and hyperthermia; suffer from lice and scabies; and have diseases or conditions such as tuberculosis, HIV infection, substance abuse and addiction, and dental problems. Even **trimorbidity** (i.e., substance addiction, mental illness, and another chronic health problem such as hypertension) is common in the homeless.

It takes much time and energy to build trust with the homeless before the many comorbidities with which they are burdened can be addressed. Some approaches to administering healthcare to the homeless have included not just offering shelter, but also offering harm reduction as a way to keep clients alive without further complicating their serious situations. For example, offering needle cleaning kits to users of intravenous drugs may decrease the use of dirty needles at the individual and population level, or providing mobile homeless units may make healthcare more accessible. Even with these efforts, homeless people may refuse assistance. To promote accessibility to healthcare for these people, community and public health nurses should approach homeless people in the following ways:

- Show respect and use a positive approach, which builds trust.
- Support primary (advocacy), secondary (tuberculosis screening), and tertiary ("detox" treatment) prevention to make it easier to cope with difficult, challenging lives.

Evidence for Practice

1. Nationally and globally, needle exchange programs and supervised injection facilities, although controversial, offer a harm reduction approach to intravenous drug users by offering clean needles for use. Operational and systematic limitations exist, including acceptable hours of operation, the location of the programs, and transportation needs. Researchers have described a novel way to measure the effectiveness of supervised injection facilities in Toronto and Ottawa, Canada. By creating a legally sanctioned place for supervised consumption of illicit drugs to decrease Hepatitis C and HIV transmission. The researchers concluded after computing direct healthcare costs and quality-adjusted life-years (QALYs over 20 years) that $50,000 is the cost-effective threshold that was maintained in three particular sites (Enns et al., 2016).

2. Researchers found that homelessness predicts attrition but not alcohol abstinence in outpatients experiencing both alcohol dependence and mental health challenges. The relationship between housing status and attrition and alcohol abstinence during treatment, were evaluated in 79 adults diagnosed with alcohol dependence and serious mental illness. Researchers found that 39% ($n = 31$) of participants reported being homeless at baseline. Individuals who were homeless were more likely to drop out of care management ($n = 10$, 62.5%) than those who

were housed ($n = 4$, 16.7%), $\chi2(1) = 8.86$, $P < 0.05$. It was concluded that individuals experiencing **homelessness** and co-occurring alcohol dependence and mental health challenges with care management had higher rates of attrition, relative to those who were housed (Leickly et al., 2017). In exploring the experience of people who are homeless, data was collected in homeless shelters and day centers including those who were actually homeless ($n = 28$), previously homeless ($n = 10$), social workers and care providers ($n = 48$), and staff ($n = 40$). Expe-

riences of end-of-life care and opinions about this approach were examined through focus groups and using qualitative analysis. Participants highlighted that conversations exploring future care preferences and palliative care with people experiencing homelessness are rare. Themes identified as challenges to such conversations included attitudes to death; the recovery-focused nature of services for people experiencing homelessness; uncertainty regarding prognosis and place of care; and fear of negative impact (Hudson et al., 2017).

KEY CONCEPTS

- In discerning community/public health practices as a nurse, one of the fundamental issues that needs to be faced are the biases and prejudices that can be barriers to understanding the needs of populations.
- Community and family assessments need to be grounded in trusting approaches that are mutually defined between health professionals and those living in situations that are less than ideal.
- Being a caregiver in a community where rural access, prison isolation, discrimination, and continuity of care are all struggles of great magnitude allows nurses to do what they do best: heal, and not necessarily fix, healthcare situations.

- A key suggestion in carrying out the core values of public health may be to check the common themes or biases that each of these groups experience "at the door" (Box 18.9).

18.9 Common Themes of Underserved Populations

- Blaming the victim, healthcare professionals, and others assuming abuse/neglect/incompetence
- Making poor choices and having the wrong priorities on the part of individuals, families, and populations
- Powerlessness and vulnerability
- Nobody cares about injury, infection, screening, preventive care

CRITICAL THINKING QUESTIONS

1. What are the ethical and moral issues that present themselves when communities/cities/states choose to address or not address the health needs of the populations covered in this chapter?
2. Are there legal obligations that you can identify in relation to rural, correctional, LGBT, or homeless health? Give specific examples and what your recourse would be to address these issues.
3. Community violence is reported as an issue in all four of the populations described in this chapter.

Identify a coalition-building approach that could unify these communities regarding this issue (refer to Chapter 16 to assist you with this answer).
4. Why is it the case that single men are prominently represented in the homeless? Is there a primary prevention program that could be a part of a public health initiative that would address this cohort specifically?

HEALTHY PEOPLE 2020 ACTIVITY

In thinking about mental health, those that are underserved or considered as "vulnerable" populations often experience many comorbid conditions that include serious mental illness (SMI). In referencing *HP2020* objective MHMD 9.1 (**Increase the proportion of adults aged 18 years and older with SMI who receive treatment**), identify how you would

evaluate the incidence and prevalence of SMI in each of the populations mentioned in this chapter and how would you go about evaluating access to mental health treatment? Consider the social determinants of health and experiences of health disparities in your answers.

COMMUNITY RESOURCES

- Rural health
  - Emergency medical services
  - Faith-based initiatives
- Correctional/prison health
  - Local jails, correctional facilities
  - Police departments
  - Detention centers for youth
  - Outreach programs directed to correctional facilities
  - Foster care agencies
- Gay, lesbian, transgender, and bisexual populations
  - Community health and neighborhood centers
- Local HIV/AIDS services
- Veterans
  - Veterans Health Administration (U.S. Department of Veterans Affairs)
- Human trafficking
  - The International Organization for Migration
  - UN Global Initiative to Fight Human Trafficking
- Homeless populations and health
  - City and state housing authorities
  - Hunger and food assistance programs
  - Health programs and clinics targeted at this group

REFERENCES

Amber Waves. (2013). *Rural America*. Retrieved on May 23, 2013, from http://www.ers.usda.gov/AmberWaves/June08/Features/RuralAmerica.htm

Area Health Education Centers (AHEC). (2018). Retrieved from https://bhw.hrsa.gov/fundingopportunities/?id=ccc4f09b-e51e-4541-988b-ddc2c7593760

Bolin, J. N., Bellamy, G. R., Ferdinand, A. O., Vuong, A. M., Kash, B. A., Schulze, A., & Helduser, J. W. (2015). Rural health people 2020: New decade, same challenges. *Journal of Rural Health, 31*(3), 326–333.

Bradford, J. B., & Mayer, K. H. (2008). Demography and the LGBT population: What we know, don't know, and how the information helps to inform clinical practice. In H. J. Makadon., K. H. Mayer., J. Potter., & H. Goldhammer (Eds.). *Fenway guide to lesbian, gay, bisexual, and transgender health* (pp. 25–44). Philadelphia, PA: American College of Physicians.

Braveman, P. A., Kumanyika, S., Fielding, J., LaVeist, T., Borrell, L. N., Manderscheid, R., & Troutman, A. (2011). Health disparities and health equity: The issue is justice. *American Journal of Public Health, 101*(Suppl. 1), S149–S155.

Bureau of Labor Statistics. (2016). *National census of fatal occupational injuries in 2016.* Retrieved from https://www.bls.gov/news.release/pdf/cfoi.pdf

Burton, H., Chowdhury, S., Dent, T., Hall, A., Pashayan, N., & Pharoah, P. (2013). Public health implications from COGS and potential for risk stratification and screening. *Nature and Genetics, 45*(4), 349–351.

Children's Defense Fund (CDF). (2009). Retrieved on June 6, 2009, from http://www.childrensdefense.org

Conard, P. L., & Armstrong, M. L. (2016). Advocating for deployed women veterans' health differences, difficulties, and disparities. *Nursing Forum, 51*(4), 225–232.

Conard, P. L., & Armstrong, M. L. (2017). Deployed women veterans: Important culturally sensitive care. *Nursing Forum, 52*(4), 225–231.

Crews, K. R., Gaedigk, A., Dunnenberger, H. M., Klein, T. E., Shen, D. D., Callaghan, J. T.,...Skaar, T. C. (2012). Clinical pharmacogenetics implementation consortium (CPIC) guidelines for codeine therapy in the context of cytochrome P450 2 D6 (CYP2D6) genotype. *Clinical Pharmacology Therapies, 91*(2), 321–326.

Enns, E. A., Zaric, G. S., Strike, C. J., Jairam, J. A., Kolla, G., & Bayoumi, A. M. (2016). Potential cost-effectiveness of supervised injection facilities in Toronto and Ottawa, Canada. *Addiction, 111*(3), 475–489.

Farrell, S. P., Zerull, L. M., Mahone, I. H., Guerlain, S., Akan, D., Hauenstein, E., & Schorling, J. (2009). Electronic screening for mental health in rural health care: Feasibility and user testing. *Computers, Informatics, Nursing, 27*(2), 93–98.

Ferszt, G. G., & Clarke, J. G. (2012). Health care of pregnant women in U.S. state prisons. *Journal of Health Care for the Poor & Underserved, 23*(2), 557–569.

Flaskerud, J., & Winslow, B. (1998). Conceptualizing vulnerable populations in health-related research. *Nursing Research, 47*(2), 69–78.

Garrison-Jakel, J. (2011). Patching the rural workforce pipeline—Why don't we do more? *Journal of Rural Health, 27*(2), 239–240.

Gomes, M. V., & Pelosi, G. G. (2013). Epigenetic vulnerability and the environmental influence on health. *Exploratory Biological Medicine (Maywood), 238*(8), 859–865.

Health Resources and Services Administration (HRSA). (2018). *Find shortage areas.* Retrieved on May 23, 2013, from http://hpsafind.hrsa.gov/

Healthy People 2020. (2018). *Disparities.* Retrieved from https://www.healthypeople.gov/2020/about/foundation-health-measures/Disparities

Hemmings, S., Jakobowitz, S., Abas, M., Bick, D., Howard, L. M., Stanley, N., &...Oram, S. (2016). Responding to the health needs of survivors of human trafficking: A systematic review. *BMC Health Services Research, 16*, 320.

Hudson, B. F., Shulman, C., Low, J., Hewett, N., Daley, J., Davis, S.,...Stone, P. (2017). Challenges to discussing palliative care with people experiencing homelessness: a qualitative study. *BMJ Open, 7*(11), E017502.

Johnson, B. S., Boudiab, L. D., Freundl, M., Anthony, M., Gmerek, G. B., & Carter, J. (2013). Enhancing veteran-centered care: A guide for nurses in non-VA settings. *AJN The American Journal of Nursing, 113*(7), 24–39.

Kemppainen, J. K., Taylor, J., Jackson, L. A., Kim-Godwin, Y. S., & Kirby, E. (2009). Incidence, sources, and self-management of depression in persons attending a rural health clinic in southeastern North Carolina. *Journal of Community Health Nursing, 26*(1), 1–13.

Khoury, M. J., Janssens, A. C., & Ransohoff, D. F. (2013). How can polygenic inheritance be used in population screening for common diseases. *Genetics and Medicine, 15*, 437–443.

Krout, J. A., & Kinner, M. (2007). Sustaining geriatric rural populations. In L. L. Morgan, & P. S. Fahs (Eds.). *Conversations in the disciplines: Sustaining rural populations* (pp. 63–74). Binghamton, NY: Global Academic Publishing.

Leickly, E., Skalisky, J., Oluwoye, O., McPherson, S. M., Srebnik, D., Roll, J. M.,...McDonell, M. G. (2017). Homelessness predicts

REFERENCES *(Continued)*

attrition but not alcohol abstinence in outpatients experiencing co-occurring alcohol dependence and serious mental illness. *Substance Abuse, 21,* 1–4.

Lim, F. A., Brown, D. V. Jr., & Jones, B. H. (2013). Lesbian, gay, bisexual, and transgender health: Fundamentals for nursing education. *Journal of Nursing Education, 52*(4), 198–203.

Massachusetts Department of Public Health. (2018). *GLBT health access project.* Retrieved from http://www.glbthealth.org

Muñoz-Laboy, M., Leau, C. J., Sriram, V., Weinstein, H. J., del Aquila, E. V., & Parker, R. (2009). Bisexual desire and familism: Latino/a bisexual young men and women in New York City. *Culture, Health & Sexuality, 1*(3), 331–344.

Natale, A. P. (2009). Denver MSM sociostructural factors: Preliminary findings of perceived HIV risk. *Journal of HIV/AIDS & Social Services, 8*(1), 35–56.

National Coalition for the Homeless. (2018). Retrieved from http://nationalhomeless.org/about-homelessness/

National Conference of State Legislatures. (2018). *Closing the gaps in the rural primary care workforce.* Retrieved from http://www.ncsl.org/research/health/closing-the-gaps-in-the-rural-primary-care-workfor.aspx

National Institutes of Health (NIH). (2018). *US National Library of Medicine, HSRIC (Health Services Research Information Central).* Retrieved from https://www.nlm.nih.gov/hsrinfo/disparities.html

National Rural Health Association (NRHA). (2018). *About rural health care.* Retrieved from https://www.ruralhealthweb.org/about-nrha/about-rural-health-care

Nellis, A. (2016). *The color of justice: Racial and ethnic disparity in state prisons.* Retrieved from https://www.sentencingproject.org/publications/color-of-justice-racial-and-ethnic-disparity-in-state-prisons/

Nilsson, K. (2016). Parents' attitudes to risk and injury to children and young people on farms. *PLoS ONE, 11*(6), e0158368.

Nolan, G., & Walsh, E. (2012). Caring in prison: The intersubjective web of professional relationships. *Journal of Forensic Nursing, 8*(4), 163–169.

Office of Management and Budget (U.S.) (OMB). (2015). *OMB bulletin no. 15-01, Revised delineations of metropolitan statistical areas, micropolitan statistical areas, and combined statistical areas, and guidance on uses of the delineations of these areas.* Retrieved from https://obamawhitehouse.archives.gov/sites/default/files/omb/bulletins/2015/15-01.pdf.

Olshansky, E. F. (2017). Social determinants of health: The role of nursing. *AJN American Journal of Nursing, 117*(12), 12.

Pennel, C. L., Carpender, S. K., & Quiram, B. J. (2008). Rural health roundtables: A strategy for collaborative engagement in and between rural communities. *Rural & Remote Health, 8*(4), 1054.

Pereira, A. N., Enard, K. R., Nevarez, L., & Jones, L. A. (2011). The role of patient navigators in eliminating health disparities. *Cancer, 117*(15 Suppl), 3543–3552.

Pew Research Center. (2018). 5 facts about illegal immigration in the U.S. Retrieved from http://www.pewresearch.org/fact-tank/2017/04/27/5-facts-about-illegal-immigration-in-the-u-s/

Roberts, S. J. (2006). Health care recommendations for lesbian women. *Journal of Obstetric, Gynecologic, and Neonatal Nursing, 35*(5), 583–591.

Rural Health Information Hub (RHIhub). (2018). *Area Health Education Centers (AHEC).* Retrieved from https://www.ruralhealthinfo.org/topics/workforce-education-and-training#ahec.

Sanchez, J., Silva-Suarez, G., Serna, C. A., & De La Rosa, M. (2012). The Latino migrant worker HIV prevention program: building a community partnership through a community health worker training program. *Family Community Health, 35*(2), 139–146.

Smith, M. N., Winkler, R. L., & Johnson, K. M. (2016). *How migration impacts rural America.* Retrieved from http://w3001.apl.wisc.edu/pdfs/b03_16.pdf

Transgender Awareness Training and Advocacy. (2009). Retrieved from http://www.tgtrain.org/

Tumosa, N., Horvath, K. J., Huh, T., Livote, E. E., Howe, J. L., Jones, L. I., & Kramer, B. J. (2012). Health care workforce development in rural America: When geriatrics expertise is 100 miles away. *Gerontology & Geriatrics Education, 33*(2), 133–151.

United States Census Bureau. (2018). *Metropolitan and micropolitan.* Retrieved from https://www.census.gov/programs-surveys/metro-micro.html

United States Department of Agriculture (USDA). (2018). *What is rural?* Retrieved from https://www.nal.usda.gov/ric/what-is-rural.

United States Department of Justice, Bureau of Justices Statistics. (2018). *Total correctional population.* Retrieved from https://www.bjs.gov/index.cfm?ty=tp&tid=11

van den Bergh, B. J., Gatherer, A., Fraser, A., & Moller, L. (2011). Imprisonment and women's health: Concerns about gender sensitivity, human rights and public health. *Bulletin of the World Health Organization, 8*(9), 689–694.

Washburn, J. (2018). What nurses need to know about human trafficking. *Journal of Christian Nursing, 35*(1), 18–25.

Willging, C. E., Waitzkin, H., & Nicdao, E. (2008). Medicaid managed care for mental health services. The survival of safety net institutions in rural settings. *Qualitative Health Research, 18*(9), 1231–1246.

Wines, M. (2016). Nursing education in rural environments. *Comprehensive Psychology, 5,* 1–8. doi: 10.1177/2165222816633322

World Health Organization (WHO). (2018a). *Social determinants of health.* Retrieved from http://www.who.int/social_determinants/sdh_definition/en/.

World Health Organization (WHO). (2018b). *Human genomics in global health.* Retrieved from http://www.who.int/genomics/geneticsVSgenomics/en/

Chapter 19

Environmental Health

*Tarah S. Somers**

TEARS OF NATURE
(A villanelle)

I think I just heard Mother Nature cry,
Or was it one more broken, falling tree?
You'd think we'd learn as time goes
speeding by.

They tell us there's a big hole in the sky,
We won't believe in something we can't see,
I think I just heard Mother Nature cry.

Coal-fired chimneys reaching up so high,
Even though the solar power's free,
You'd think we'd learn as time goes
speeding by.

We develop rocket ships that fly,
But still can't stop pollution of the sea,
I think I just heard Mother Nature cry.

Headlines: One more species set to die,
Keep it quiet...use diplomacy,
You'd think we'd learn as time goes
speeding by.

Worry on the future? Pass it by!
How can preservation start with me?
I think I just heard Mother Nature cry.
You'd think we'd learn as time goes
speeding by.

—Graeme King

CHAPTER HIGHLIGHTS

- Human health and the environment
- Assessing contaminants in the environment
- Exposure pathways
- Assessing the environment of a community
- Planning interventions to make communities healthier
- Evaluating interventions
- Environmental epidemiology
- Working toward healthy communities
- Environmental justice
- Global environmental health issues

OBJECTIVES

- Comprehend the links between human health and the environment.
- Understand how the nursing process of using assessment, intervention, and evaluation can be used to examine the impact of the environment on human health.
- Describe the concept of an exposure pathway.
- Describe several environmental conditions to consider when assessing the environment of a community.
- Understand the concept of environmental justice.
- Identify major global environmental health issues.

*The findings and conclusions in this report are those of the author and do not necessarily represent the views of the Agency for Toxic Substances and Disease Registry.

KEY TERMS

Bioavailability: The amount of a substance that is absorbed or becomes available at the site of physiologic activity.

Biomonitoring: Process of measuring contaminants in blood or urine to determine whether a person has been exposed to a contaminant and how much exposure he or she has received.

Environmental epidemiology: Field of public health science that focuses on the incidence and prevalence of disease or illness in a population from exposures in their environments.

Environmental health: A field of public health science that focuses on how the environment influences human health.

Environmental justice: The belief that no group of people should bear a disproportionate share of negative environmental health consequences (regardless of race, culture, or income).

Exposure: Contact between a contaminant and the body.

Exposure estimate: Estimated amount of contaminant that comes in direct contact with the body from inhalation, ingestion, dermal contact, or injection.

Exposure pathway: Describes how people are exposed to an environmental contaminant that originates from a specific source.

Exposure history: Process to help determine whether an individual has been exposed to environmental contaminants.

Healthy communities: Communities that optimize the physical, social, and economic environments of the community.

Risk assessment: Process to determine the likelihood or probability that adverse effects such as illness or disease will occur in a group of people because of an exposure to an environmental contaminant.

Precautionary principle: If something has the potential to cause harm to humans or the environment, then precautionary measures should be taken even if there is a lack of scientific evidence for cause and effect.

Toxicology: The study of the adverse effects of chemicals on people, animals, and the environment.

CASE STUDY *References to the case study are found throughout this chapter (look for the case study icon). Readers should keep the case study in mind as they read the chapter.*

Chris is a public health nurse in a coastal town with a long, proud history of commercial and recreational fishing. Throughout the 20th century, many industries lined the edges of the harbor, creating additional economic opportunities for the town. From 1940 to the 1970s, polychlorinated biphenyls (PCBs) were used at the transformer facility that manufactured electrical capacitors and transformers. As a result, soil and groundwater at the site, as well as at the building, are heavily contaminated with PCBs. This facility is considered the major source of historic PCB contamination of the harbor.

The facility is now fenced, and there is no public access to the contaminated soil and buildings. The community is supplied by public drinking water sources which are not connected to the site's groundwater. Commercial fishing in the harbor is banned, and all commercial fishing takes place out at sea. However, some members of the community frequently fish in the harbor, and they eat the fish they catch to supplement their diets.

The community around the harbor enjoys seasonal recreational activities along the water and sometimes boats on the water, but swimming in the harbor is difficult, since the shores are steep and rocky and there is no beach area. Access to the water can really only happen from community-owned piers.

INTRODUCTION

The environment can be considered as anything outside of ourselves whether human-made or natural. **Environmental health** is the branch of public health science that focuses on how the environment influences human health.

HUMAN HEALTH AND THE ENVIRONMENT

The environment can affect human health in many ways. Some of these effects are immediate and obvious, such as when drinking water supplies are contaminated by sewage and flood water after a hurricane. Other effects, such as contamination of a private well by arsenic, may be more difficult to discover. Where people live, work, and spend time can have direct consequences on their health. For example, living and working in highly urban environments may expose people to higher concentrations of some air pollutants, but living and working in an agricultural setting may expose them to more pesticides. **Exposure** occurs when there is contact between people and an environmental contaminant which can happen from ingesting, breathing, or touching a contaminant.

Peoples' environment can have positive or negative effects on their health. Conditions in the environment may exacerbate existing health conditions. For example, people with asthma may experience more asthmatic episodes on days when air quality is poor. The poor air quality may not cause asthma, but it may induce more frequent and severe asthma attacks in people who already have asthma.

The environment can also help improve people's health. If residents of a certain town believe that they can safely walk in their community, they may choose to walk instead of drive to the store or to schools. This can help increase their activity levels and decrease obesity or other chronic diseases. It could also lead to less pollution from cars, which, in turn, improves air quality. In some ways, the built environment can be intentionally designed to help make people healthier.

What is the use of a house if you haven't got a tolerable planet to put it on? **Henry David Thoreau**

History of Environmental Health

Historically, people often did not clearly understand the links between environment and health and did not recognize how humans influenced their environment. As nations became industrialized, the effects on the quality of air and water became more apparent. People also began to take note of the impact on ecosystems as plants, animals, or other wildlife began to disappear. Many industries were loosely, if at all, regulated, and disposal practices of hazardous materials and industrial by-products were shortsighted. Disposal of waste materials often simply involved burying or dumping the waste into lakes, rivers, or oceans in the belief that the "solution to pollution is dilution." The intent of this improper disposal of contaminants was not always malicious—people did not understand the impact that the contaminants could have on human health and ecosystems. Materials such as PCBs and asbestos were commercially available, essential to certain manufacturing processes, and were not believed to be harmful. Over time, with the development of more research and understanding, we now realize that many contaminants and hazardous materials have adverse impacts on human health.

The quality of the environment became a popular topic in the mid- to late 20th century. Books such as *Silent Spring* by Rachel Carson (1962) brought to public attention how human actions and pollution were affecting the quality of air, water, and land. In 1969, because of debris and oil in the river, the Cuyahoga River in Ohio caught on fire. The river had caught fire many times in the past, but the 1969 event caught the public's attention and helped increase awareness of how polluted some places had become. In July 1970, the White House and Congress established the Environmental Protection Agency (EPA) in response to the growing public demand for cleaner water, air, and land. The EPA had the daunting task of

---

19.1 Influential Environmental Laws

Clean Air Act
The Clean Air Act (CAA), passed in 1970, created a national program to control the damaging effects of air pollution. The Clean Air Act Amendments of 1990 went further to ensure that the air Americans breathe is safe. The CAA protects and enhances the quality of the nation's air by regulating stationary and mobile sources of air emissions. More information is available at https://www.epa.gov/clean-air-act-overview/clean-air-act-text

Clean Water Act
The Clean Water Act, passed in 1972, focuses on improving the quality of the nation's waters. It provides a comprehensive framework of standards, technical tools, and financial assistance to address the many causes of pollution and poor water quality, including municipal and industrial wastewater discharges, polluted runoff from urban and rural areas, and habitat destruction. More information is available at https://www.epa.gov/laws-regulations/summary-clean-water-act

Superfund
Superfund is the name given to the environmental program established to address abandoned hazardous waste sites. It is also the name of the fund established by the **Comprehensive Environmental Response, Compensation and Liability Act** of 1980. It allows the Environmental Protection Agency to clean up such sites and compel responsible parties to perform cleanups or reimburse the government for EPA-led cleanups. More information is available at. https://www.epa.gov/superfund/superfund-history

---

repairing the damage already done to the natural environment and to establish new criteria to making a cleaner environment a reality. For more information on the creation and current role of EPA, visit the EPA website. Several important pieces of legislation that helped highlight the importance of environmental health and protection are still used to help enforce environmental health and protection (Box 19.1).

Love Canal started it all. I visited the canal area at that time. Corroding waste disposal drums could be seen breaking up through the grounds of backyards. Trees and gardens were turning black and dying. One entire swimming pool had been popped up from its foundation, afloat now on a small sea of chemicals.... Everywhere the air had a faint, choking smell. Children returned from play with burns on their hands and faces. **Eckardt C. Beck, EPA Regional Administrator**

Today, the public has better understanding of the impact of human actions on the environment and how the environment can in turn affect human health. However, there are still many environmental health challenges that people must face, including cleaning up past, as well as ongoing contamination, deciding what to do about newly recognized issues such as climate change and energy production, and dealing with emerging scientific advances such as nanotechnology. Even though new research and developments are occurring at a historically rapid pace, there are still large gaps in peoples' knowledge about certain subjects:

- How do certain contaminants affect human health?
- How do we assess exposures to contaminants?
- How does the environment influence health?
- How do we live as a population while maintaining a healthy environment?

Loads of chemicals and hazardous wastes have been introduced into the atmosphere that didn't even exist in 1948. The environmental condition of the planet is far worse than it was 42 years ago. **Gaylord Nelson, politician and principal founder of Earth Day, 1990**

The Community Environment

The environment and its effect on human health are often considered in two ways. The first focuses on how contaminants in the environment, such as asbestos, lead, or radon, influence human health. The second focuses on how the entire environment surrounding the community, such as neighborhood safety, climate, access to grocery stores, and community design, affects health. These two ways of considering the effect of the environment on human health frequently relate to each other.

For example, lead was used in paint until the 1970s and is often found in houses built earlier. As the old paint breaks down, lead can be found in dust and old paint chips in homes (CDC, 2014). In communities with older, deteriorating housing, children can be exposed to lead. In many cases, such housing is found in poorer communities. Many low-income communities also have fewer full-service grocery stores, and all residents do not have access to necessary healthy, iron-rich foods. Sufficient blood iron can protect against some of the effects of lead exposure (EPA, 2001). Some research suggests that the combination of iron deficiency and elevated blood lead levels may work synergistically to create greater neurologic impacts in children than just iron deficiency or elevated blood lead levels. The impact of the contaminant, lead, on children's health may be greater because of characteristics of the children's community environment (CDC, 2002).

In the case of lead-based paint in the environment, it is fairly easy to determine the link between the environment and health. Sometimes, it can be challenging to determine which environmental factors have the greatest impact on health. Information about the way many contaminants affect humans is very limited. People are exposed to thousands of different things in their environment every day. One person may come into contact with a number of personal care products (e.g., shampoo, toothpaste, lotions, clothing detergent), food products (artificial colors, pesticide residue on foods, preservatives), other commercial products (e.g., inks, gasoline, dry cleaned clothing, flame retardants), and environmental contaminants (e.g., diesel particles or indoor air contaminants from cooking or burning wood) every day. In the modern world, it is nearly impossible to isolate people from all of the exposures they have every day.

The American Chemical Society, which provides the Chemical Abstracts Service (CAS) database for chemicals, had as of August 2018 in their database over "143 million unique organic and inorganic chemical substances, such as alloys, coordination compounds, minerals, mixtures, polymers and salts" (American Chemical Society, 2018, p. 1). Even if only a fraction of these chemicals eventually finds their way into the environment and humans, the burden of chemical exposure to everyone in the United States is enormous. We also have only just begun to understand how exposures to a mixture of chemicals will affect human health.

Only a small number of these chemicals have ever been tested to see how they affect human health. Many groups have called for the use of the **precautionary principle** when it comes to the use of contaminants that find their way into the environment and humans. The precautionary principle maintains that if something has the potential to cause harm to the environment or humans, then precautionary measures should be taken if there is a lack of scientific evidence concerning cause and effect (Kriebel et al., 2001). Applying the precautionary principle to new technology and chemicals may help protect the environment and human health. For example, the use of e-cigarettes is perceived by many people as "less dangerous" than smoking traditional cigarettes. Yet the safety of e-cigarettes and the chemical exposures people may get from using them is still uncertain (American Lung Association, 2016). By applying the precautionary principle, nurses can discourage the use of e-cigarettes with their patients and encourage them to consider the potential health risks. It can also be challenging to prove the existence of direct links between the environment and health status of community residents. It seems logical that if sidewalks are built, people will use them, thus improving their cardiovascular health. But is it possible to measure sidewalk use? If a community could measure sidewalk use, how could it show that using the sidewalks significantly improves cardiovascular health? Often, there is a lack of scientific data to determine how exactly the community environment impacts human health. It is also difficult to determine how genetic and behavioral factors shape the health of an individual or a population.

Practice Point

Proving causal links between exposure to environmental contaminants and health outcomes, or links between the community environment and health outcomes, is often very difficult.

Genetic and Behavioral Factors

Understanding the interaction between the environment and genetics as it relates to expression of disease is still an evolving science. The challenge for nurses is to use the best science available to assess how the environment affects human health, to formulate evidence-based or best practice interventions, and to evaluate the effectiveness of these interventions.

Hereditary factors may play an important role. Many scientists believe that there are people who are more genetically susceptible to a specific disease, but that environmental triggers play a role in determining who actually develops the disease. The interaction between genetics and the environment may help explain why some people who are exposed to specific contaminants develop certain health effects but others do not. A 2014 study showed that the certain genotype (MET rs1858830CC) and exposure to air pollution may interact to increase the risk of autism spectrum disorder (Volk et al., 2014). This type of research can help us understand how genetics and environmental exposures interact to create health outcomes.

Individual human behaviors may also interact with environmental exposures to influence human health. For example, radon, a naturally occurring radioactive compound, can be found in the basements of many homes. Exposure to this substance has been linked to lung cancer. Research has shown that people who live in a home with radon and who smoke have a greater risk of developing lung cancer than do nonsmokers who live in homes with radon. The exposure to cigarette smoke and radon seems to interact to increase the risk of lung cancer. More information about radon and health can be found on the EPA website.

Nursing and Environmental Health

Scientific understanding of how the environment affects human health has evolved since the days of Florence Nightingale, but nurses have long recognized that people's surroundings can influence their health. Even in the 19th century, nurses realized that clients who had clean food and water and fresh air had better outcomes than did those who were left in squalid conditions. Nurses can help lead the way in healthcare by understanding that clients are part of the environment and that the health of the environment has a direct impact on their health. Nurses are in a strong position to advocate for healthier environments in both the workplace and community.

Across the country, there are great examples of nurses working with communities, conducting research, and leading programs to help promote healthy people in healthy environments. Nurses are also involved in helping to ensure that the environmental impact of healthcare practices in the clinical setting and community setting are considered. For example, the group Health Care Without Harm has worldwide membership from health providers to raise awareness on issues such as safer chemicals (disinfectants, solvents in

| **19.2** | **Principles of Environmental Health for Nursing Practice** |

1. Knowledge of environmental health concepts is essential for nursing practice.
2. The Precautionary Principle guides nurses in their practice to use products and practices that do not harm human health or the environment and to take preventive action in the face of uncertainty.
3. Nurses have a right to work in an environment that is safe and healthy.
4. Healthy environments are sustained through multidisciplinary collaboration.
5. Choices of materials, products, technology, and practices in the environment that affect nursing practice are based on the best evidence available.
6. Approaches to promoting a healthy environment respect the diverse values, beliefs, cultures, and circumstances of clients and their families.
7. Nurses participate in assessing the quality of the environment in which they practice and live.
8. Nurses, other healthcare workers, clients, and communities have the right to know relevant and timely information about the potentially harmful products, chemicals, pollutants, and hazards to which they are exposed.
9. Nurses participate in research of best practices that promote a safe and healthy environment.
10. Nurses must be supported in advocating for and implementing environmental health principles in nursing practice.

Source: American Nurses Association. (2007). *Principles of environmental health for nursing practice with implementation strategies.* Silver Spring, MD: American Nurses Association.

laboratories) in healthcare, green purchasing (less toxic, minimal packaging), and medical waste management. More information about their work can be found at the Health Care Without Harm website (Health Care Without Harm, 2017).

The American Nurses Association (ANA, 2007) has created the *ANA's Principles of Environmental Health for Nursing Practice with Implementation Strategies*. These principles can help nurses incorporate principles of environmental health into nursing practice (Box 19.2). Nurses can use their core skills of assessment, intervention, and evaluation when considering the environment and its impact on individual patients or communities.

ASSESSMENT

Assessing Contaminants in the Environment

Frequently, public health professionals are asked to help assess whether a specific contaminant or contaminants in the environment are making a person or community sick.

The state public health agency asks Chris to assist with an environmental health assessment when media attention on PCBs starts drawing public concern. People start calling their local and state health departments and asking if the PCBs are making their families sick.

Chris starts by doing research on PCBs. These substances are not naturally occurring, tend to be heavy, and quickly settle out of the air to the ground or water. Being hydrophobic, once in the water, they also settle out of water into sediment. They are slow to break down, and unless they are removed, they remain in soil or sediment for a very long time. The PCBs can build up in small animals and fish. As larger fish and animals eat the smaller ones, the PCBs become increasingly concentrated in the food chain. In general, what would be good sources of information to find out more about PCBs?

If ever we had proof that our nation's pollution laws aren't working, it's reading the list of industrial chemicals in the bodies of babies who have not yet lived outside the womb.
Louise Slaughter, U.S. Congresswoman

People in communities often want to know their risk of getting sick from known or suspected exposure to a contaminant. In other words, they want a **risk assessment**—a process to determine the likelihood or probability that adverse effects such as illness or disease will occur in a group of people because of exposure to an environmental contaminant. The amount of risk can be a difficult thing to determine. There are different methods for conducting risk assessment for environmental contaminants. A simple way to understand risk is that the amount of risk equals the hazard plus exposure (risk = hazard + exposure).

The presence of a hazard alone does not determine the amount of risk the hazard poses. If a substance is hazardous, but there is no exposure to the substance, then a person is not at risk. For example, think of the sun. It is well known that exposure to too much sun can cause sunburns and put people at risk for skin cancer. However, if a person eliminates exposure by staying indoors or in the shade, he or she eliminates the risk. If a person puts on sunscreen or a hat or stays out of the sun in the middle of the day, he or she modifies the amount of risk by taking measures to reduce the exposure.

To assess exposure, one method is to think about exposure pathways. An **exposure pathway** is a process by which someone is exposed to a contaminant that originates from a specific source (Agency for Toxic Substances and Disease Registry [ATSDR], 2005). Understanding exposure pathways is important because *if the pathway is not complete or if it can be disrupted, the contaminant of concern should not affect human health*. Frequently, people incorrectly assume that if a contaminant is near their home, work, or school, they will automatically experience adverse health effects from the substance. An exposure pathway helps illustrate that proximity to a contaminant is not the deciding factor in determining its effect on humans. An exposure pathway consists of five parts: (1) source of contamination, (2) environmental media and transport, (3) point of exposure, (4) route of exposure, and (5) receptor population. Figure 19.1 shows how each of these components is related, and the following discussion describes them in more detail.

Source of Contamination

The source of contamination is used to describe what the contaminants are and from where they originate. Sometimes, a source of contamination is easy to identify (e.g., mercury coming from a former thermometer factory site). Other sources can be more difficult to identify, such as vapor intrusion into a home from contaminated groundwater. Sources of contamination can come from point or nonpoint sources. Nonpoint sources consist of many diffuse sources while a point source tends to be one specific identified source. For example, a nonpoint source of contamination could be if gasoline drips on parking lots and roads from thousands of cars and then is washed into a neighboring lake when it rains. A tanker truck carrying gasoline that crashed and spilled its contents into a pond is an example of a point source of contamination.

Knowing the type of contaminant is important to understanding its possible effect on human health. Some contaminants quickly break down in the environment, whereas others are very persistent. Contaminants that stay longer in the environment may influence health over a greater period of time. Generally, contaminants can be thought of in three categories: chemical (lead, mercury, volatile organic compounds), biologic (mold, anthrax, ricin), and radiologic (radium, radon). Table 19.1 lists some common environmental contaminants.

Environmental Media and Transport Mechanisms

Environmental media include groundwater, surface water (lakes, ponds, rivers), air, surface soil, subsurface soil, sediment, and biota (plants and animals). The environmental medium that the contaminant is in helps determine who is exposed and how they are exposed (Agency for Toxic Substances and Disease Registry, 2005).

Transport mechanisms describe how the contaminant moves from the source to the point of exposure to people. For example, if an old drum full of a contaminant is buried and leaking, knowing how that contaminant moves through the environment helps determine if only the surrounding soil is contaminated or if the contaminant is volatile and will disperse into the air or if the contaminant is likely to get into ground water (Agency for Toxic Substances and Disease Registry, 2005).

Point of Exposure

The point of exposure is the place where people come in contact with the contaminated medium, which may include

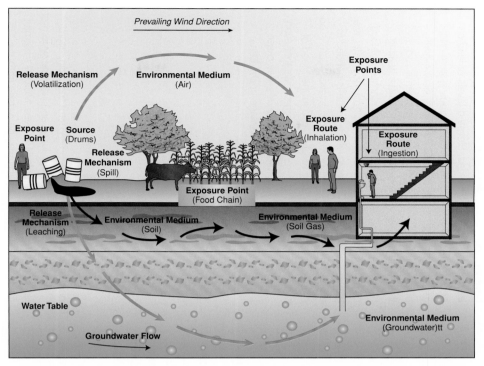

FIGURE 19.1 Exposure pathway. (Data from Agency for Toxic Substances and Disease Registry. [2005]. *Public health assessment guidance manual.* Retrieved from https://www.atsdr.cdc.gov/ HAC/phamanual/ch6.html.)

food or another item (Agency for Toxic Substances and Disease Registry, 2005). An exposure point can be a home, a playground, a lake, a business, a cloud of diesel fumes, an abandoned lot, a fish to be eaten, or a park.

Route of Exposure

The route of exposure is how the contaminant enters the body. Environmental contaminants enter the body primarily by ingestion, inhalation, or skin contact. Contaminants can come from groundwater, surface water, soil, and food (Agency for Toxic Substances and Disease Registry, 2005). Most adults do not ingest large amounts of soil. However, children may ingest soil while playing, from mouthing objects, from not washing their hands, or from pica behaviors. Contaminants can be inhaled from soil (dust), air, and aerosolized water (e.g., during showering). Dermal contact from contaminants can come from soil, water, sediment, air, or food.

Evidence for Practice

In March 2015, a family of four while on vacation in the US Virgin Islands was transported to the hospital with neurologic symptoms including weakness, severe myoclonus, fasciculations, altered sensorium, and word-finding difficulty. Three of the four family members had also vomiting and diarrhea. Three members of the family ended up intubated with mechanical ventilation. Initially, clinicians suspected ciguatera fish poisoning, however, others who had eaten the same food were not ill. An investigation revealed that an unoccupied housing unit beneath where the family was staying was fumigated with the pesticide methyl bromide two days before the family sought medical care. Methyl bromide is a pesticide first used in the 1930s but has been phased out of use. It should not be used in residential settings. In addition to the family of four, 37 other people were identified as having been potentially exposed to methyl bromide. Six of those exposed reported symptoms such as headache and fatigue which resolved on their own within a few weeks. Four of the six were emergency responders who had been to the housing complex (CDC, 2015a).

Nurses can apply this knowledge to practice by always considering the possibility of acute chemical exposure when assessing clinical symptoms and patient history. A family or group with rapid progression of the same symptoms is highly suspicious. Prompt recognition of such exposures can aid in clinical treatment, prevent further exposures, and prevent additional exposures. If a toxic exposure is suspected, those potentially exposed, such as first responders, should be alerted. Also, nurses can help community members understand how proper use of pesticides is essential to prevent exposures and health effects. Pesticides should always be used in accordance with their legal, labeled use and integrated pest management practices, which decreases the use of chemicals for controlling pests.

TABLE 19.1 Common Exposure Pathways for Selected Environmental Contaminants

Contaminant	Most Common Sources	Media and Transport	Most Common Point of Exposure	Route of Exposure	Populations of Most Concern	Health Effect
Lead	Paint before 1978. Homes built before 1978 may have lead paint on walls, windows, or other painted surfaces inside and outside the home.	As paint deteriorates, it can chip and create dust that contains lead. The chips and dust can accumulate in the house or be deposited into soil around the house.	Inside the house as chips or dust. Soil outside the house	Ingestion	Children frequently have greater exposures because they put their hands and other objects in their mouths, they may eat paint chips, and they play outside in the soil more and may ingest the soil.	Children's brains and nervous systems are sensitive to the damage done by lead. Elevated levels of lead can damage the nervous system and brain development, slow growth, create learning problems such as hyperactivity, and cause hearing problems and headaches. A blood lead level of 5 µg/dL or greater is a level at which action is needed to stop exposure. However, there is no safe level of lead in the blood of children. Research shows that even low blood lead levels may cause neurologic damage in children.
	Dust can get into air. Lead vapor if lead is heated (as if with a heat gun used to remove paint).	Inside the house	Inhalation		Children have faster respiratory rates and their breathing zone is closer to the ground, which may lead to a greater exposure.	
Mercury	Thermometers used in industry, batteries. Burning coal releases it into the air.	Intentional or accidental spills of elemental mercury	In area near a mercury spill, indoor levels can become unsafe with even small mercury spills.	Inhalation	People near the spill. Children have faster respiratory rates and their breathing zone is closer to the ground, which may lead to a greater exposure.	High levels can harm the brain, heart, kidneys, lungs, and immune system of people of all ages. Mercury's harmful effects may be passed from the mother to the fetus, causing brain damage, mental retardation, blindness, seizures, and inability to speak. Children poisoned by mercury may develop problems of their nervous and digestive systems, and kidney damage.

Contaminant	Description	Movement/Pathway	Source	Route of exposure	Who is at risk	Health effects
		Can enter the environment, settle into water, and bioaccumulate in fish	Fish	Ingestion	Pregnant women and small children	For most adults, fish eating is not a concern. Pregnant women and small children should avoid eating fish with high mercury levels such as swordfish, shark, tilefish, and king mackerel. Mercury's harmful effects may be passed from the mother to the fetus, causing brain damage, mental retardation, incoordination, blindness, seizures, and inability to speak. Children poisoned by mercury may develop problems of their nervous and digestive systems, and kidney damage.
Radon	Naturally occurring radioactive gas. Product of decaying uranium and found in soils	Moves into houses through cracks and holes in foundations	Indoor air	Inhalation	People living in homes with radon present. People who smoke	Can damage lungs. Exposure has been linked to lung cancer. Smoking combined with radon exposure is a serious health risk.
Per- and polyfluoroalkyl substances (PFAS)	Family of man-made chemicals that have been used since the 1950s. Many of the chemicals were used in firefighting foams. Some are used on consumer products for items that are "non-stick", "stain resistant" or "water proof."	In the environment the chemicals can travel long distances, move through soil, seep into groundwater, or be carried through air.	Drinking water / Consumer products	Ingestion	People who drink water contaminated with these chemicals. People can also be exposed from using consumer products that contain these chemicals.	The potential for health effects from PFAS in humans is not well understood. A few have generally been studied more extensively than other PFAS. In general, animal studies have found that animals exposed to PFAS at high levels resulted in changes in the function of the liver, thyroid, pancreas, hormone levels, and possible developmental effects. Community concerns about these chemicals have been heightened in the past several years.

(Continued)

TABLE 19.1 Common Exposure Pathways for Selected Environmental Contaminants *(Continued)*

Contaminant	Most Common Sources	Media and Transport	Most Common Point of Exposure	Route of Exposure	Populations of Most Concern	Health Effect
Polychlorinated biphenyls (PCBs)	Family of human-made organic chemicals, PCBs were domestically manufactured from 1929 until their manufacture was banned in 1979. They were used in hundreds of industrial and commercial applications, including electrical, heat transfer, and hydraulic equipment; as plasticizers in paints, plastics, and rubber products; in pigments, dyes, and carbonless copy paper; and many other industrial applications.	PCBs do not readily break down and therefore may remain for long periods of time cycling between air, water, and soil. They can be carried long distances and have been found in snow and sea water in areas far away from where they were released into the environment. As a consequence, PCBs are found all over the world. In general, the lighter the form of PCB, the further it can be transported from the source of contamination. PCBs can bioaccumulate in fish.	Fish Water Air near hazardous sites or if burning	Ingestion Inhalation	Women of childbearing age and children. People living near a contaminated site or near where PCBs may be burning	PCBs have been shown to cause a number of serious noncancer health effects in animals, including effects on the immune system, reproductive system, nervous system, endocrine system, and other health effects. PCBs have been shown to cause cancer in animals. Women who were exposed to relatively high levels of PCBs in the workplace or ate large amounts of fish contaminated with PCBs had babies who weighed slightly less than babies from women who did not have these exposures. Babies born to women who ate PCB-contaminated fish also showed abnormal responses in tests of infant behavior. Some of these behaviors, such as problems with motor skills and a decrease in short-term memory, lasted for several years. The most likely way infants will be exposed to PCBs is from breast milk.

Tetrachloroethylene (perchloroethylene [PERC])	Another name from tetrachloroethylene is PCE. Tetrachloroethylene has been found in at least 771 of the 1,430 National Priorities List sites identified by the Environmental Protection Agency (EPA). PERC is a manufactured chemical used for dry cleaning and metal degreasing.	Much of the PERC that gets into water or soil evaporates into the air, but it can contaminate groundwater and drinking water supplies.	Inhalation	Clothes from the dry cleaners, vapor intrusion—when vapors can come from contaminated groundwater or soil into a building or home.	People who live or work in a building with vapor intrusion	High concentrations of the PERC (particularly in closed, poorly ventilated areas) can cause dizziness, headache, sleepiness, confusion, nausea, difficulty in speaking and walking, unconsciousness, and death. In industry, most workers are exposed to levels lower than those causing obvious nervous system effects. The health effects of breathing in air or drinking water with low levels of PERC are not known. Tetrachloroethylene has been shown to cause liver tumors in mice and kidney tumors in male rats.
			Ingestion	Drinking water containing tetrachloroethylene	People who drink water contaminated by PERC	
Mold	Thousands of different types of molds can grow indoors and outdoors. They thrive in moist conditions.	Mold spores can travel in the air. When the spores land in favorable conditions, they will grow and produce mold.	Inhalation	Indoor and outdoor air	People who are sensitive to mold can become sick with respiratory symptoms. At high-enough levels, even people with no previous reactions to mold may experience symptoms.	Respiratory symptoms can be severe in people who are sensitive to molds. Symptoms generally will be better once exposure to mold stops. Since everyone's sensitivity to mold is different, there is no standard "safe" level of mold. When mold is seen growing in an indoor environment, it should be properly cleaned.

(Continued)

TABLE 19.1 Common Exposure Pathways for Selected Environmental Contaminants (*Continued*)

Contaminant	Most Common Sources	Media and Transport	Most Common Point of Exposure	Route of Exposure	Populations of Most Concern	Health Effect
Benzene	Benzene is a colorless liquid with a sweet odor. It evaporates into the air very quickly and dissolves slightly in water. It is highly flammable and is formed from both natural processes and human activities. Benzene is widely used in the United States; it ranks in the top 20 chemicals for production volume. Some industries use benzene to make other chemicals that are used to make plastics, resins, and nylon and other synthetic fibers. Benzene is also used to make some types of rubbers, lubricants, dyes, detergents, drugs, and pesticides.	Benzene can pass into the air from water and soil. It reacts with other chemicals in the air and breaks down within a few days. Benzene in the air can attach to rain or snow and be carried back down to the ground. It breaks down more slowly in water and soil and can pass through the soil into underground water.	Outdoor air contains low levels of benzene from tobacco smoke, automobile service stations, exhaust from motor vehicles, and industrial emissions. Air around hazardous waste sites or gas stations contains higher levels of benzene.	Inhalation	People who smoke. People who live near sites with benzene contamination.	The major effect of benzene from long-term exposure is on the blood. Benzene causes harmful effects on the bone marrow and can cause a decrease in red blood cells, leading to anemia. It can also cause excessive bleeding and can affect the immune system, increasing the chance for infection. Long-term exposure to high levels of benzene in the air can cause leukemia, particularly acute myelogenous leukemia, often referred to as AML. This is a cancer of the blood-forming organs. It is not known whether children are more susceptible to benzene poisoning than are adults. Benzene can pass from the mother's blood to a fetus. Animal studies have shown low birth weights, delayed bone formation, and bone marrow damage when pregnant animals breathed benzene.

Asbestos	Asbestos is the name given to a group of six different fibrous minerals (amosite, chrysotile, crocidolite, and the fibrous varieties of tremolite, actinolite, and anthophyllite) that occur naturally in the environment. Asbestos has been used for a wide range of manufactured goods, mostly in building materials (roofing shingles, ceiling and floor tiles, paper products, and asbestos cement products), friction products (automobile clutch, brake, and transmission parts), heat-resistant fabrics, packaging, gaskets, and coatings. Some vermiculite or talc products may contain asbestos.	Asbestos fibers can enter the air from the breakdown of natural deposits or manufactured asbestos products. Renovation of older homes or facilities containing asbestos can release it into the air.	Indoor or outdoor air	Inhalation	Workers who have worked with asbestos. Family member of people who work with asbestos. People who live or work in areas where asbestos fibers are being released into the indoor or outdoor environment.	Asbestos mainly affects the lungs and the membrane that surrounds the lungs. Breathing high levels of asbestos fibers for a long time may result in scar-like tissue in the lungs and in the pleural membrane (lining) that surrounds the lung. This disease is called asbestosis and is usually found in workers exposed to asbestos, but not in the general public. Breathing lower levels of asbestos may result in changes called plaques in the pleural membranes. Pleural plaques can occur in workers and sometimes in people living in areas with high environmental levels of asbestos. It is known that breathing asbestos can increase the risk of cancer in people. There are two types of cancer caused by exposure to asbestos: lung cancer and mesothelioma. Cigarette smoke and asbestos together significantly increase your chances of getting lung cancer.

(Continued)

TABLE 19.1 Common Exposure Pathways for Selected Environmental Contaminants (*Continued*)

Contaminant	Most Common Sources	Media and Transport	Most Common Point of Exposure	Route of Exposure	Populations of Most Concern	Health Effect
Pesticides	These chemicals are used to kill pests. There are thousands of registered pesticides in the United States. Pesticides are applied commercially and privately to protect plants and crops from pests.	Once pesticides are used on crops or to control pest infestations, they can move through the environment in a variety of ways. They may end up in water. Pesticides must be carefully used to protect human health and the environment.	Indoor or outdoor air	Inhalation Dermal contact	People who work or live close to where pesticides are applied either in an indoor or outdoor environment. People can have health effects from an exposure that occurs long after the pesticides are applied because pesticides are designed to "stick around" and rid an area of pests.	The Environmental Protection Agency regulates pesticides that are commercially available in the United States; however, there are thousands of products each with unique formulation. Without knowing the specific chemicals used in the formulation, it is impossible to predict health effects for pesticides as a group. Some pesticides have been linked to a variety of health problems. Some pesticides, such as the organophosphates and carbamates, affect the nervous system. Others may irritate the skin or eyes. Some pesticides may be carcinogens. Others may affect the hormone or endocrine system in the body.
			Drinking water Eating foods with pesticides applied or accidentally ingesting pesticides	Ingestion	People drinking water contaminated with pesticides. People who ingest pesticides when they eat foods that have had pesticides applied. Adults and more likely children who accidentally ingest pesticides.	

| Arsenic | Arsenic is a naturally occurring element widely distributed in the earth's crust. In the environment, arsenic is combined with oxygen, chlorine, and sulfur to form inorganic arsenic compounds. Inorganic arsenic compounds are mainly used to preserve wood. Copper chromate arsenate (CCA) is used to make "pressure-treated" lumber. CCA is no longer used in the United States for residential uses; it is still used in industrial applications. Organic arsenic compounds are used as pesticides, primarily on cotton fields and orchards. Arsenic was used in many industries and many former industrial sites may have arsenic contamination. Arsenic has been found in at least 1,149 of the 1,684 National Priority List sites identified by the EPA. | Arsenic occurs naturally in soil and minerals and may enter the air, water, and land from wind-blown dust and may get into water from runoff and leaching. Many common arsenic compounds can dissolve in water. Most of the arsenic in water ultimately ends up in soil or sediment. | Indoor or outdoor air Drinking water | Inhalation Ingestion | Burning of treated wood that contained CCA People whose drinking water contains high amounts of arsenic | Ingesting very high levels of arsenic can result in death. Exposure to lower levels can cause nausea and vomiting, decreased production of red and white blood cells, abnormal heart rhythm, damage to blood vessels, and a sensation of "pins and needles" in hands and feet. Ingesting or breathing low levels of inorganic arsenic for a long time can cause a darkening of the skin and the appearance of small "corns" or "warts" on the palms, soles, and torso. Skin contact with inorganic arsenic may cause redness and swelling. Almost nothing is known regarding the health effects of organic arsenic compounds in humans. Several studies have shown that ingestion of inorganic arsenic can increase the risk of skin cancer and cancer in the liver, bladder, and lungs. Inhalation of inorganic arsenic can cause increased risk of lung cancer. |

For a list of up-to-date online resources on these substances, please visit thePoint (http://thepoint.lww.com/DeMarco3e).

Receptor Population

The receptor population is the population of people who are likely to be exposed (Agency for Toxic Substances and Disease Registry, 2005). It is necessary to carefully consider and accurately identify the exposed population. For example, if a contaminant is in the groundwater, then only people with drinking wells supplied by that groundwater are likely exposed to the contaminant. People whose wells were fed by another source or people who use public water systems are not exposed.

When thinking about populations, it is also important to think about whether people are currently being exposed, whether people were exposed in the past, and whether people will continue to be exposed in the future. Thinking about when a population was or is exposed can help determine what interventions may be useful. The exposure pathway is illustrated in Figure 19.1.

Determining the Health Impact of a Completed Exposure Pathway

A completed exposure pathway does not guarantee that people will become sick. The exposure may not be great enough to cause a health effect. It is also possible we might not know enough about the toxicology of certain contaminants to understand their health effects. Given what experts know about medicine and science, it is difficult to imagine that we cannot determine with certainty whether exposure to a contaminant will lead to illness. There is often "an understandable misconception among the public that modern-day health scientists and medical professionals can precisely determine at what environmental level a particular contaminant presents a clear and predictable risk to human health future" (De Rosa, Holler, & Mehlman, 2002, p. 149). For most contaminants, toxicologic data are too limited to say for sure whether an exposure will have an effect. **Toxicology** is the study of the adverse effects of chemical, physical, or biologic agents on people, animals, and the environment (Society of Toxicology, 2017). Many of the guiding principles of toxicology will seem familiar to nurses who are familiar with pharmacology. Toxicology and pharmacology are very similar, since both require knowledge of the "dose" needed to effect a change (either positive or negative) on a human system. When people are exposed to multiple chemicals, the effects on health may be magnified; this concept should also be familiar to nurses who understand that caution must be taken with combining medications if the medications are targeting the same body systems or can damage the same organs.

To determine any possible health effects from a contaminant, an **exposure estimate** is created. An exposure estimate determines a person's level of exposure to a contaminant. Several factors are taken into account when calculating the exposure estimate, including the duration of the exposure, the concentration of the chemicals, the frequency of exposure, body size, and the bioavailability of the contaminant. **Bioavailability** is the amount of a substance that is absorbed or becomes available at the site of physiologic activity. In pharmacology, the bioavailability of a drug helps clinicians determine the necessary dose to ensure that the drug is effective. In toxicology, bioavailability helps toxicologists determine the "dose" of a certain contaminant that will cause a health effect.

Once toxicologists give an exposure estimate, health professionals compare it with standard health guidelines. If an exposure estimate is greater than the health guideline, there is a greater chance that the exposure can cause adverse health effects. Health guidelines are set to protect the whole population, including those who are most sensitive to potentially hazardous substances, such as children or the elderly. Health guidelines include safety factors designed to protect even the most sensitive members of a population; therefore, an exposure estimate above a particular health guideline

Chris considers if there is an exposure pathway that can link the contaminant to people who live in her town. She creates a table to help her determine if there are completed exposure pathways of PCBs into people. What would the exposure pathway table below look like for this site?

Source	Media and Transport	Point of Exposure	Route of Exposure	Receptor Population	Duration of Exposure

does not guarantee that an exposure will cause harm. State health agencies, as well as federal health and environmental agencies such as the ATSDR and the EPA, develop the health guidelines.

The field of toxicology is always evolving. Nurses can consult with professionals trained in the field of toxicology to help determine whether a specific exposure can lead to a health effect. State or local health departments usually have an office that deals with environmental health issues. They are a useful resource for nurses who believe they have identified an environmental health concern or who need more information about the toxicology of a specific contaminant.

Frequently, when individuals learn they have been exposed to a contaminant, they will ask their medical provider to "test" them. For some contaminants, clinical tests can determine whether someone has been exposed. For example, a blood test or urine test can determine the level of mercury in blood or urine. These levels provide information about how much mercury a person has in his or her body. These types of tests, referred to as **biomonitoring**, can be helpful for determining exposures to individual people and communities. Technology allows medical professionals to test for many chemicals in the body; however, our understanding of toxicology has not evolved as quickly as our ability to test for chemicals in a person. As health professionals we may be able to test for and find a chemical in a person, but we may not have the ability to tell the person how that level of chemical in them will affect their health. Another challenge with biomonitoring is that some chemicals may have a short half-life and do not stay in the body long enough to easily measured. If biomonitoring for a chemical exposure is being considered, medical professionals first need to be sure that the testing will provide useful clinical information for treatment of the patient.

If biomonitoring is possible, the results need to be carefully interpreted. For example, many states require at least one blood lead level be checked in young children (ages 1 to 5 years old) as part of their wellness visits for children to attend school. A single child's elevated blood lead level can alert a nurse to the lead exposure and can allow the nurse to determine whether the blood lead level is dangerously high. However, the test cannot tell exactly when or where exposure occurred or what form of lead was involved (e.g., paint chips, lead in soil, lead in drinking water, lead paint on a toy). If many children in a community have elevated blood lead levels, it alerts health professionals to a problem in that community, but again, the test alone cannot determine where exactly the children were exposed. Much information about how lead affects children is available, and medical professionals know the significance of an individual blood lead level in terms of the child's health. However, for many contaminants, even if a medical test can detect a certain level of a contaminant, data to determine whether detected levels cause an adverse health effect may be insufficient.

Evidence for Practice

Young children in Maine are routinely screened for elevated blood lead levels. As a report by the Centers for Disease Control and Prevention (CDC, 2009a) shows, between 2003 and 2007, the Maine Childhood Lead Poisoning Prevention Program (MCLPPP) identified 55 children with elevated blood lead levels. For 90% of the children, lead exposure was linked to lead hazards in the children's homes. However, for six children, there was no evidence of lead exposure inside the home. As the investigation expanded to outside of the home, researchers discovered that the six children were exposed to lead dust in their family vehicles and in child safety seats. Investigators believed that the lead dust entered the vehicles by cross contamination from family members who had high-risk lead exposure occupations (e.g., construction, painting and paint removal, metal recycling). The lead dust on the seats likely came from contamination from either clothing or articles that family members had placed in the vehicles. This was the first documented report of child lead poisoning caused by a child's exposure to lead while in a child safety seat.

Public health nurses can apply this type of information when dealing with families of children who have elevated blood lead levels. Although lead sources in the house (e.g., old chipping paint, old lead plumbing fixtures) may be the cause of the majority of lead exposure in children, nurses may need to consider other unique sources when trying to determine how children have been exposed. Asking parents about their occupations or hobbies might help a nurse discover an unexpected exposure pathway.

The CDC's Fourth National Report on Human Exposure to Environmental Chemicals (2009c) describes exposures among the US population to many environmental contaminants. This continuously updated biomonitoring report is a valuable resource for environmental health professionals. This report includes data made available from CDC's National Health and Nutrition Examination Survey (NHANES). It establishes a reference range for typical US population exposures which can be compared to individual and population measurements made in other contexts. The report also provides information about trends in US exposures over time and helps environmental health professionals learn more about the various chemicals to which Americans are exposed. In addition, it establishes a reference range that these health professionals can use for comparative purposes (i.e., is an exposure low, medium, or high), to determine whether exposures are higher in certain groups in the United States, and provides information about trends in the levels of contaminants in humans over time (CDC, 2009c). The complete report and updated tables, can be found on the CDC website (https://www.cdc.gov/exposurereport/index.html). Caution needs to be taken if a nurse wants to compare an individual's test results to data found in the CDC report to ensure laboratory analysis and collection of the samples for the individual were done with the same methodology as the CDC data.

For many contaminants, there are no medical tests to determine whether an exposure has occurred or what the health effect of the exposure might be. There are resources and professionals who work in the field of environmental and occupational health who can help a nurse decide whether medical testing is necessary or useful for an individual client or for a community. For example, the Association of Occupational and Environmental Clinics (AOEC) and the Pediatric Environmental Health Specialty Units (PEHSU) are staffed with medical providers who specialize in occupational and environmental health. These providers can provide expert advice when there is a question about a possible environmental exposure and its effects (Box 19.3.).

19.3 Association of Occupational and Environmental Clinics, Pediatric Environmental Health Specialty Units, and American College of Medical Toxicologists

Established in 1987, the Association of Occupational and Environmental Clinics (AOEC), a nonprofit organization, has grown to a network of more than 60 clinics and more than 250 individuals committed to improving the practice of occupational and environmental medicine through information sharing and collaborative research. All AOEC member clinics are multidisciplinary in staff and meet specific criteria that promote providing high-quality healthcare and patient rights. More information is available at http://www.aoec.org.

The Pediatric Environmental Health Specialty Units (PEHSU) form a respected network of experts in children's environmental health. The PEHSU were created to ensure that children and communities have access to, usually at no cost, special medical knowledge and resources for children faced with a health risk due to a natural or human-made environmental hazard. More information is available at http://www.pehsu.net/.

The American College of Medical Toxicologists (ACMT) is a professional nonprofit association that is dedicated to advancing medical toxicology. ACMT has physicians with expertise in medical toxicology and aims to advance the quality of care for patients poisoned with chemicals or other toxins. ACMT professionals can help medical providers by providing expert and timely advice on how to care for patients with poisoning or chemical exposures. More information is available at www.acmt.net.

After determining that there is at least one complete exposure pathway, the next step for Chris is to determine whether people are being exposed to high-enough levels of PCBs to make them sick. Chris meets with a member of the state environmental agency and a toxicologist from the state health department. The state has received data from fish collected in the harbor. Chris helps the toxicologist try to determine how many fish from the harbor are being eaten by local residents. With her knowledge of the local population, Chris believes that people who supplement their diets with fish from the harbor probably eat two to four fish meals a week during the warmer weather. Based on the PCB levels in the fish, Chris and the toxicologist determine that if people eat fish from the harbor two to four meals a week for 5 months a year, their exposure to PCBs is high enough to cause concern.

Some people may want to be tested to determine if they have been exposed to PCBs from the harbor. What could you do as a public health nurse to answer their questions about being tested?

Evidence for Practice

Firefighters use flame-retardant clothing for personal protection while fighting fires. Antimony oxides are often used in the production of these textiles. In 2008, the CDC received a report from a fire department chief that there was an outbreak of antimony toxicity among 30 firefighters who had elevated antimony levels detected in hair samples (CDC, 2009b). The fire department believed that exposure to the antimony in the firefighters' protective clothing caused the outbreak. The CDC administered questionnaires and collected urine antimony samples from two different groups of firefighters—one group whose clothing contained antimony and one group whose clothing did not contain antimony. The CDC found that both the groups had urine antimony levels that were not clinically significant and that wearing clothing made with antimony did not increase urine antimony levels. It should be noted that hair testing is *not* reliable or valid for measuring exposure antimony in the body (CDC, 2009b).

Public health nurses can apply this information to practice by understanding that only valid methods of testing for metals or other chemicals in the body should be used to determine whether people are being exposed to dangerous levels of a substance. Invalid tests may make people fearful that they are ill now or will be in the future. They may also lead people to seek inappropriate treatment or delay proper care. Nurses can distribute timely and accurate risk communication and health communication materials that provide useful, specific information about environmental exposure and its effects on health.

Assessing the Environment of a Community

Knowing what contaminants are in the environment and whether there are completed exposure pathways are key steps in determining how people's health is affected by the environment. However, many other environmental conditions, aside from environmental contaminants, can influence disease and injury rates. Some environmental conditions that may be important when reflecting on the potential impact of the environment on a community's health are presented in Table 19.2. This table was designed to consider many different types of communities—urban and rural, developed, developing and redeveloping—regardless of socioeconomic status.

> If a man walks in the woods for love of them half of each day, he is in danger of being regarded as a loafer. But if he spends his days as a speculator, shearing off those woods and making the earth bald before her time, he is deemed an industrious and enterprising citizen. **Henry David Thoreau**

TABLE 19.2 Community Environment and the Potential Effects on Health

Environmental Condition	Effects on Health and Examples
Access to healthy housing	Age and condition of housing can expose people to contaminants (lead, asbestos, radon, or mold), pests (cockroaches, rodents, or mosquitoes), and injuries (falls, electrocution, fire, or carbon monoxide). One major concern with housing is the quality of indoor air, which can have a direct effect on diseases such as asthma (see "Indoor air" below). Location of housing can also encourage or discourage how community members get around in their communities. For example, houses built on streets that do not connect or streets without sidewalks may encourage people to drive rather than walk even short distances—this can decrease a person's physical exercise, which increases people's risk for obesity and other health issues.
Access to potable water	Most drinking water in the United States comes from public water or private water supplies such as wells. Public drinking water supplies are tested frequently and must meet federal standards. Private water supplies are not tested regularly unless done so by the person who owns or uses the water. Both public and private water supplies can be contaminated with bacteria or chemicals; however, because public water supplies are tested regularly, contamination is likely to be identified quickly. Contaminated water can make people sick quickly or more slowly, depending on the type of contamination. In some rural communities in the United States and around the world, access to potable water is still a significant health issue. An association has also been made between lack of modern water sources and lower respiratory tract infections in young children. Droughts and floods can also impact water supplies. Floods may bring contamination into public or private water supplies and drought can limit the availability of water to communities.
Sanitation and waste removal	In most parts of the United States, sanitation services and waste removal services are taken for granted. However, there are some areas where these services are lacking. For example, in some communities that lack public sewer services, there is also a lack of septic systems because of cost or difficulty in installing a septic system. Improper disposal of human waste can create health problems from direct contact with the waste or can contaminate drinking water supplies. In some poorer countries, there are virtually no sanitation or waste removal systems. People live in and around sewage and trash. Improper disposal of trash can also encourage pests, which can carry diseases and may expose people to contaminants that leach out of the trash.
Access to green spaces	Green spaces such as parks and playgrounds can help encourage people to exercise and play. Exercise can have a positive impact on health by helping to control obesity and providing other health benefits. Exercise can also promote social development in children and provide a place for the community to gather. Green space may also help people feel better about the community they live in and have positive effects on mental health.

(Continued)

TABLE 19.2 Community Environment and the Potential Effects on Health (Continued)

Environmental Condition	Effects on Health and Examples
Ambient air	Tiny airborne particles and ground-level ozone can trigger respiratory problems, especially for people with asthma. Air pollution can aggravate health problems for the elderly and others with heart or respiratory diseases. Things to consider for ambient air include potential pollution from a variety of sources, including industry, power plants, waste sites, and vehicle traffic. Other issues to consider for ambient air include local sources of particulate matter from things such as wood burning or dust from unpaved roads or construction. Air quality is an important issue worldwide. Many poorer countries lack laws, resources, and programs to help eliminate air pollution sources, whereas more affluent countries may produce more air pollution from manufacturing, making electricity, and driving automobiles. Both situations can create air quality issues that need to be addressed on a global scale.
Indoor air	Indoor air quality can often be worse than ambient air quality. Indoor air can contain high levels of particulate matter from combustion of heating and cooking fuels, cigarette smoke, and can also contain chemical contaminants from products used in the home for cleaning and painting or even from items such as carpet or furniture. Other contaminants such as mold spores and other asthma triggers such as dust and dust mites are often also found in indoor air. Poor indoor air quality can affect both poorer and more affluent homes.
Recreational waters	Recreational waters can be an excellent resource for communities to engage in recreational activities for exercise, pleasure or even as a food source such as fishing. Unfortunately, sometimes recreational water sources can be a place where people are exposed to chemical (fuel oils, metals, etc.) or biologic contaminants (such as red tide or bacteria from sewage) that can cause harm. In pools, sometimes misuse/overuse of chemical pool cleaners can cause chemical exposures.
Abandoned buildings, vacant lots, or facilities	Abandoned properties can create physical hazards such as structurally unsound buildings and trenches where children could be hurt. These places can also increase criminal activities and may be fire risks. Abandoned cars, tires, or piles of trash create similar risks. Abandoned properties or trash can also impact resident's pride in their community and their sense of well-being. How community pride or a sense of well-being affects health can be difficult to quantify, but it does affect quality of life.
Access to healthy and safe foods	Full-service grocery stores are more likely than small convenience stores or fast food restaurants to stock healthy foods and fresh fruits and vegetables. If grocery stores are within easy access, then people may be able to include more healthy foods and fewer fast foods or processed foods into their diets. Farmers' markets and community-supported gardens may be a good source of healthy foods in a community. Food that is hunted, fished, or gathered may also be a source of healthy foods. However, all food that is purchased, grown, or gathered can be contaminated with bacteria or chemicals that can make people sick. Food safety is a challenge in all communities, and in the United States, there are programs in place to help keep consumer food products safe. Chemicals used in food production such as pesticides and herbicides can impact workers and community members where the chemicals are applied and may end up being consumed by those who eventually eat the produce. Modern food production using concentrated animal feeding operations (CAFOs) can increase the need for farmers to use chemicals and to treat and prevent animal pests and diseases that tend to spread when many animals are concentrated into small areas. Waste production from CAFOs can also pollute the environment. Worldwide, food quality and safety are critical health issues.
Access to physical activity such as biking, or other public spaces that encourage physical activity	A community that has safe sidewalks, bike paths, and/or jogging trails encourages people to exercise more, which can have positive health benefits. An absence of safe ways to walk or bike encourages dependence on automobiles, which can affect air quality and the amount of exercise that people get during the day. Also, if people are forced to walk or bike along unsafe streets or highways, there is a greater risk of pedestrian injuries.
Location of schools, public facilities, public transportation, and entertainment	Schools and other facilities such as libraries, theaters, or stores can help encourage people to walk or use public transportation rather than driving. Decreasing car dependency can improve air quality and increase the amount of exercise people engage in during the day.

Environmental Condition	Effects on Health and Examples
Safety and crime	If people feel it is unsafe in their community, they may not walk as much or allow their children to play outside. The impact of stress from living in a community that is unsafe may also affect people's physical and mental health.
Animals—strays or pests	Stray animals can discourage people from exercising in and around their communities. Other animal pests such as rodents may help spread disease.
Vectors	Vectors such as mosquitoes or ticks can transmit diseases such as those caused by the West Nile and Zika virus or Lyme bacteria. Changes in the environment can help decrease the number of vectors. For example, getting rid of standing or stagnant water can help decrease the number of mosquitoes.
Access to healthcare (primary care providers and services such as pharmacies)	If a community can easily access primary healthcare services, they may be better able to manage chronic and acute health issues. For example, if people need to drive long distances or if public transportation is difficult to use or does not exist, they may postpone receiving healthcare.
Climate	The climate may influence health in many ways. For example, very hot or very cold weather conditions may affect how often people leave their homes to exercise. Hot weather may also lead to problems with ambient air quality, which can affect people with respiratory problems. Cold climates may also affect indoor air quality if heating sources are not clean and safe. Severe storms, droughts, and flooding can also create hazards that impact people's health.
Noise	Unwanted sound can have impacts on sleep, concentration, or even conversation. Some problems related to noise include sleep disruption, high blood pressure, and loss of productivity.
Ultraviolet (UV) radiation	UV radiation comes from the sun. Exposure to UV radiation is directly linked to skin cancers. Some areas of the world have a greater UV index. Some communities also spend a greater amount of time outside, which exposes them to greater amounts of UV radiation.
Subsistence or supplemental food gathering and hunting	Some communities may subsist on or supplement their diets with locally gathered animals or plants. These food sources can help create a healthy diet if the foods are safe but may also be a source of exposure to contaminants if the foods are not safe. For example, fish is a good source of healthy protein and fats but fish caught in contaminated waters may have a negative impact on health.
Cultural practices and traditions	Some cultural practices such as using herbs or cosmetics can expose people to contaminants in those products. In some countries, manufacturing processes may not be carefully regulated to monitor for contaminants being added either intentionally or unintentionally to the products. Cultural traditions may also expose some communities to contaminants. For example, a tradition in a community might be to gather local plants or materials to create products for sale or personal use. The collection of these items may cause people to be exposed to contaminants if the plant used to make a product naturally grows in a wetland area and the wetland water is contaminated.
Natural and human-made hazards	Some communities are more vulnerable to natural hazards such as hurricanes, tornadoes, earthquakes, or other storms. These natural events can present physical hazards or chemical hazards and create community stress. Often, when power is lost, people use generators to try to heat, cool, or light their homes. Carbon monoxide poisoning after disasters, although easy to prevent with proper use of generators, and other CO generating equipment, continues to be a challenge in the United States.
Community concerns	Listening to the concerns of the community about their environment and health can provide important insight into how the environment impacts the health of the community. Listening to and addressing the concerns is vital when helping determine intervention strategies to create healthier community environments.

For a list of up-to-date online resources on these topics, please visit thePoint (http://thepoint.lww.com/DeMarco3e).

Assessing the many ways that the environment of a community can impact health is helpful to consider before interventions are developed and implemented. For example, even if community members know that exercise such as walking can help improve their health, if the town streets lack sidewalks, this discourages walking. Creating a community program to increase awareness of the benefits of exercise will not do much to increase activity levels until the issue of the sidewalks or alternative safe exercise spaces, such as parks, is addressed.

The state health department asks Chris to help it discover the steps necessary to develop interventions to disrupt the exposure pathway and keep people from being exposed to the PCBs in fish from the harbor. She determines that assessing the environment of the community may be helpful in planning successful interventions. Chris thinks about the community who eats fish caught in the harbor. For many people who fish in the harbor, fish is a major protein source in their traditional diet and a way to supplement their diets. In the harbor area, there are several small, locally owned grocery stores, which are easy to walk to without a car or public transit, and carry other traditional foods. There is also a larger national grocery store, but one needs a car to get there. English is a second language spoken by many of the people who patronize these stores.

Why is it important to understand more about the entire environment of the community and not just about the contaminated site?

Assessment of Individuals: Taking an Exposure History

Often when clients visit a clinic or health provider, the healthcare professional does not ask them about exposures to hazardous substances or contaminants. Many people also do not associate exposures at work or home with how they are feeling, and they may not think to tell a provider about an exposure. For example, a man may come to the clinic complaining about an increase in the number of times per week that he must use his rescue inhaler for asthma. Unless he is asked by the clinician about changes at home, work, or with hobbies, he may simply not think to mention that his hobby of building model planes is occupying more of his time. Without this knowledge, the practitioner may not know about the increasing exposure to glues and paints, which could irritate the client's airways, leading to more asthma symptoms.

Taking an **exposure history** can help nurses identify current or past exposures, eliminate exposures, and try to

mitigate or reduce a client's adverse health effects from exposures. The basic elements of an exposure history are found in Table 19.3.

If an exposure history reveals an exposure of concern, or if a client's illness is still possibly linked to an environmental exposure, it is important to refer that client to the appropriate resources. For example, the AOEC and the PEHSU have many useful documents and guidelines on their websites (see Box 19.3).

Local and state health departments may also have staff who can assist in finding resources for community members who have an exposure that warrants additional follow-up. In addition, a poison control center may also be able to assist with a client who has medical problems related to a suspected acute exposure, such as exposure to a pesticide.

Practice Point

Poison control centers are staffed by trained professionals who can help you evaluate a client and also help a medical professional decide on treatment options for specific exposures. The national phone number is 1-800-222-1222.

INTERVENTIONS

Planning an intervention to address environmental health issues is similar to planning any other nursing intervention. After assessing the situation, the nurse decides which intervention will best help protect and improve health. When thinking about contaminants in the environment and completed exposure pathways, the intervention is most often something designed to interrupt or break the exposure pathway. For example, if children are playing in an area with contaminated dirt or soil, placing a fence around the site to keep them away from the site is a reasonable and likely successful intervention.

From working at the local health department, Chris knows many of the clients who come to prenatal clinic and the local Women, Infants, and Children (WIC) program are members of the harbor community. Chris works with the WIC staff to determine whether women who use WIC services know about the state fishing ban in the harbor. Chris thinks about possible interventions to prevent people from eating contaminated fish from the harbor. Engineering controls such as building a fence or blocking all fishing in the harbor would be impossible to construct or enforce. The state has already banned fishing within the harbor, so new fishing bans are

TABLE 19.3 Taking an Exposure History

Subject	Types of Questions
Present work	Where do you work? At your present work, are you exposed to any types of dusts, fumes, solvents, radiation, loud noises, pesticides, or other chemicals? Do you wear personal protection equipment? Do you wear the clothing you wear at work to home? Are there any coworkers with similar symptoms?
Past work	Where are all the places you have worked in the past? What was the longest job you held? In your past jobs, were you ever exposed to any dusts, fumes, solvents, radiation, loud noises, pesticides, or other chemicals?
Home/residence	When was your home/residence built? What type of heating do you have? Have you recently done any remodeling? Where does your drinking water come from? What types of chemicals do you use at home or in the yard? Do you have mold, mildew, or water damage issues in your home?
Activities/hobbies	In what activities or hobbies do you or your family participate? Do you hunt or fish? Do you grow any of your own foods? Do you burn or melt anything? Are there any cultural practices or traditional foods?
Concerns	Do you have any concerns about current or past exposures? Do you feel like your health is being affected by past or current exposures? Have you ever felt sick after coming into contact with chemicals or other substances? Do any of your symptoms get better when you are away from home or work?

not likely to prevent fishing by members of the local community. State and federal environmental agencies are working to dredge the PCB-contaminated sediment and remove the PCBs from the harbor, but the process may take decades to complete.

What types of interventions could be used to help stop people from being exposed from this site?

When thinking about interventions to improve the environment of the entire community, it can be difficult to craft interventions to address some problems. For example, it would be nearly impossible to replace all the older deteriorating housing in a community, for reasons such as cost, even if housing quality seems to have a negative impact on health. It would also be very difficult to rebuild all roads to include sidewalks and bike lanes. However, there may be some smaller, easier-to-achieve interventions to help improve the environment of a community, such as a local

education campaign to inform people how to get rid of places were mosquitos breed to help stop the spread of mosquito borne illnesses. Interventions to make a community's environment healthier need to include the community input, be as evidence based as possible, and be feasible given the political and economic limitations. The interventions must be targeted to the community and consider language and culture.

Some interventions produce measurable results quickly, whereas other interventions might take years to produce changes. For complex or large environmental health problems, the assistance of many different community agencies and organizations, as well as local, state, tribal, or federal government support may be necessary. It is important to remember that it may take years for the community to identify a problem, develop a program to solve it (e.g., plan an intervention), and find the necessary resources, such as state or federal grants, for this program.

For example, consider a community concerned about air quality near schools. One identified source of air pollution impacting the schools is diesel exhaust from school buses. To address the problem, the community may not have the money to purchase a fleet of new less-polluting buses. Working with the local health department, the school board, and the company that is contracted to run the school buses, the community decides that it can quickly decrease diesel emissions by implementing a "no idling" policy for school buses. Now buses parked and waiting to pick up children will no longer idle. For a longer-term solution, the community decides that it would like to engage in a program such as one suggested by EPA's website for Clean School Bus USA. In this example, the community was able to create a quick, cost-effective intervention to mitigate some exposure while also working on a more permanent solution.

With Chris's help, the health department decides that an education program aimed at letting people know why harbor fish are not safe to eat while also providing alternatives to eating harbor fish could help interrupt the exposure pathway. The education program will target women of childbearing age and children because they may be most susceptible to the effects of the PCBs and because work with the WIC staff revealed that many of the clients who come to WIC were not aware of the hazards of eating fish caught in the harbor.

What information should the educational materials for this program include? What other consideration needs to be given to how the materials should be produced? Who should receive the materials and how will they receive them? How can Chris have community members participate in the development of the materials?

EVALUATION

Trying to evaluate the effectiveness of an intervention that stops exposures or makes an environment healthier can be challenging. As previously stated, some interventions may result in immediate, measurable changes, whereas others may not lead to changes for years. Here are two examples of measurable interventions:

- Suppose a city adopts a program to screen houses for lead and make the homes as lead-free as practically possible. By the end of a year, the city will be able to determine how many homes were screened and made safer.
- Suppose a town identifies contaminated private wells and decided to bring public water to supply the homes. At the end of the year, the town could count the number of people who have a safe water supply.

However, even if it is possible to measure some positive changes, it may be very difficult to measure how the

intervention positively impacted people's health. Think of the lead in housing example above and consider how a program might be viewed if, after the program was in place for a year, there was an increase in the total number of children living in the city who had elevated blood lead levels. Would the increase in numbers indicate the program was a failure? Or could the increase be caused by an increased awareness of lead as a hazard and a willingness by parents to have their children's blood lead levels tested. As more children were tested, more elevated blood lead levels were discovered. Using only the total number of children with elevated blood lead levels within the city might not be the best indicator to prove the intervention is successful.

An evaluation performed for any intervention should help decide whether the intervention has achieved its goals and whether improvements or changes need to be made. When interventions are being funded either from private or public funding sources, the entity funding the intervention often requires that some type of evaluation be performed. Sometimes, no matter how successful a program or project is, if the people running the program cannot evaluate it and communicate the results of their evaluation, the program or project may not receive the funding needed to continue.

Some types of questions to consider when evaluating an intervention include the following:

- Has the exposure pathway been interrupted?
- What does the community think about the intervention—are people satisfied?
- How has health improved?
- How many people did the intervention affect?
- Can the intervention demonstrate any cost savings?
- Is the intervention sustainable?

It is helpful to consider how an intervention will be evaluated in the process of developing the intervention. This way, it is possible to think about how to collect the necessary data either quantitatively or qualitatively to determine whether the intervention resulted in the intended outcome.

Chris tests the effectiveness of educational materials with the help of the local clinic and WIC staff. They ask clients for feedback about the materials and ask them whether they have been able to avoid eating fish from the harbor. A community member suggests that if information was available in the grocery store, more people might be able to make safer fish choices while shopping. As a result, there is outreach to owners of local grocery stores, who are asked if the educational materials can be located in the stores. The grocery store owners are receptive to posting information because fish sold in their stores is obtained from commercial fishing sources (not caught in the harbor).

Chris also works with the WIC staff to keep data on the number of clients who receive information about safe fish consumption. Why is it important to test materials before using them? Why would you want to keep data about the materials used? What other ways could be used to determine if the intervention is effective?

ENVIRONMENTAL EPIDEMIOLOGY

Epidemiology is a field of public health science that focuses on the incidence and prevalence of disease or illness in a population. This field of study is most well-known for helping to identify outbreaks of infectious diseases. Many basic principles of epidemiologic studies can be applied to the field of environmental health. **Environmental epidemiology** can help determine whether the environment is affecting people's health. One challenge in environmental epidemiology is that it is nearly impossible to create an experimental study that is generally considered the most conclusive form of epidemiologic study. In an experimental study, one group is exposed to something while another group is not exposed. It is unethical to expose a person or population to an environmental hazard or contaminant intentionally for the purposes of conducting an experimental study. For example, if we suspect that a chemical used in water treatment is harmful to health but do not know how much of an exposure would cause a health effect, it would be unethical to put various amounts of the chemical in the water supply of different communities to watch and see when people become ill. Since experimental designs cannot be used for most environmental studies, cohort studies, case-control studies, or cluster investigations are generally used for environmental epidemiology.

Case-control studies and cluster investigations are retrospective studies that first identify people who have an adverse health condition and then try to determine what exposure or exposures caused the health effect. Cohort studies are often prospective studies that go forward in time and document the characteristics or the health effects that occur (see Chapter 8). The information gained from environmental epidemiologic studies can be very helpful in trying to identify whether particular exposures have made people ill.

Major challenges to most environmental epidemiology studies include the following:

- Limited availability of data on many contaminants and their effect on health
- Limited understanding about how exposures to multiple contaminants may sicken people
- Latency between exposure and illness can be very long (e.g., even decades).
- Difficulty in generating a good exposure assessment

In addition, studies in environmental epidemiology may be

- Time-consuming to perform
- Resource-intensive in terms of personnel and money
- Inconclusive in determining whether X contaminant caused Y illness

Disease clusters occur when there seem to be an elevated number of diseases in a family, in a community, among coworkers, or among classmates. Epidemiologists who have knowledge of disease, biostatistics, and public and environmental health investigate these suspected clusters. Frequently, state or local health departments conduct these investigations. A healthcare professional should report any suspected disease cluster to the local or state health department. A variety of factors can create the appearance of a cluster where there is no increased rate of disease.

Cancer is a frequent concern for community members. For example, the local health department might receive a report that a specific neighborhood has "a lot of cancer." When the health department investigates, it finds that in the neighborhood there are many cases of cancer but that all the cancers are different types, including breast cancer, bladder cancer, prostate cancer, leukemia, and colon cancer. Unfortunately, these cancers are common, and to community members, there is a perception that their community has more cancer than other areas, but the etiology of each of these cancers is different and not linked to a common cause.

Most states have cancer registries that track all cancers diagnosed within the state. These registries can be helpful for epidemiologists to determine if a specific area has a higher-than-expected rate of cancer. However, the information from the registry needs to be considered carefully. For example, when someone is diagnosed with cancer, where they lived at time of diagnosis is put into the registry. The registry does not track whether someone just moved to that location or whether they lived their entire life at one location. Since many environmental exposures which cause cancer can take years or decades to develop, cancer registries cannot reliably show a link between cancer and exposure where people live. Other registries are also sometimes available for birth defects and diseases such as multiple sclerosis (MS) or amyotrophic lateral sclerosis (ALS). These registries, such as cancer registries, can be used by public health nurses to gather useful data. Investigating a potential cancer cluster includes (1) determining the type of cancer that is a primary cancer, (2) determining if there is a statistically significant increase in the number of expected cancers, and (3) determining if the population and geographic area which should be included in the cluster investigation (National Cancer Institute, 2014). For many suspected cancer clusters, ultimately no evidence is found to indicate that the cases of cancer represent a true cluster. A 2012 study reviewed 487 investigations for cancer clusters reported from 1990 to 2010. Only three of the investigations could link an increase in the number of cancers to a hypothesized exposure and only one investigation found a clear cause (Goodman, Naiman, Goodman, & LaKind, 2012). Because cancer is not one but many diseases, trying to find a true cancer cluster and link it to a specific environmental exposure is very challenging.

> ## Practice Point
>
> When thinking about environmental epidemiologic studies, it is important to remember how they differ from assessing an exposure pathway. An epidemiologic study often starts with people who are ill or who had a known exposure. The studies try to determine whether the illness was caused by an environmental exposure or whether people with a known exposure became sick. Assessing an exposure pathway starts with looking at specific contaminants in the environment and determining if there is a completed exposure pathway to humans.

WORKING TOWARD HEALTHY ENVIRONMENTS

Healthy Communities

Healthy communities can help mitigate exposure to harmful contaminants and also encourage good health by incorporating design principles that optimize the physical, social, and economic environment of the community. In the 20th century, builders of communities did little planning and did not consider the impact on human health and ecology from this type of development. As areas around urban centers expanded, the term "urban sprawl" or just "sprawl" described how communities edged away from urban centers. The concept of sprawl included nonexistent land use planning, dependence on automobiles, and widespread commercial development along major roads and residential areas with low population densities. While the U. S. population nearly doubled from 1950 to 2011, vehicle travel during the same time period increased sixfold (EPA, 2013). Communities developed as part of sprawl often lacked sidewalks or bike routes, and there were no routes between residential developments to allow for walking between neighborhoods.

Healthy communities help combat sprawl, and their design is gaining attention and acceptance. Terms such as *smart growth*, **healthy communities**, *green development*, *built environment*, and *healthy community design* all try to promote the concept that when health considerations are incorporated into the planning or redevelopment, the community design itself can work to make people healthier. Researchers have discovered that well-planned community growth can help lessen the environmental impacts of development.

More than 38% of carbon monoxide and nitrogen oxide emissions come from highway vehicles. Stationary sources

such as homes and businesses are also significant sources of air pollution (EPA, 2013). By working to build communities where people can decrease their transportation needs and by creating more energy-efficient buildings, communities can create healthier environments for local community members and positively impact the health of the larger national or global community. Planned, smart-growth communities can improve water quality by designing green infrastructure for storm water runoff. When rain and storm water hit impermeable structures such as paved roads, parking lots, and other surfaces, water runs off into sewer systems or directly into lakes, streams, rivers, and oceans, often taking contamination with it. Encouraging landscape design and minimizing impervious surfaces can help to keep water cleaner. Green roofs, shaded sidewalks and streets, and building with solar reflective materials can also help mitigate the "heat island" effect that makes cities and urban areas hotter than surrounding green areas.

As new communities are built or older communities are being redeveloped, nurses and public health professionals can work with planners, political leaders, developers, bankers, local boards of public health, and community groups to help ensure that the health impacts (both positive or negative) of the development are considered. Often, simple design changes can have significant health effects. For example, if a new school site is being considered, choosing a site that encourages children to safely walk to school will help increase children's activity levels and create less vehicular traffic in the community. Selection of building materials and considering the entire life cycle of materials (from where and how they are created to how they will eventually be disposed of) can also help to make communities healthier. More information on healthy communities and smart growth can be found at the ATSDR Land Reuse Program, CDC Healthy Places and EPA Smart Growth websites (https://www.atsdr.cdc.gov/sites/brownfields/overview.html; https://www.cdc.gov/healthyplaces/; https://www.epa.gov/smartgrowth).

Healthy Homes

Like the concept of healthy communities, the central premise of the healthy homes concept is that the home has a direct influence on health. Healthy Homes is a coordinated, comprehensive, and holistic approach to prevent diseases and injuries that result from housing-related hazards and deficiencies. The focus is to identify health, safety, and quality-of-life issues in the home environment and to act systematically to eliminate or mitigate problems (CDC, 2015b). The initiative seeks to provide resources, such as healthy home inspection guidelines, to educate public health professionals and to promote cross-disciplinary activities at the local, state, tribal, and federal levels to eliminate housing deficiencies and hazards.

In the past, issues such as lead (paint) and radon dominated discussions about environmental issues and housing.

These topics are still very important and deserve attention, but the more holistic healthy homes concept has continued to expand. Now, considerations about the environment and individual homes or community housing involve topics such as indoor air quality, mold and mildew mitigation and control, green building and green cleaning techniques, and integrated pest management. In addition, information is available about how older citizens can safely continue to live in their homes and communities, with new technologies and assistance that reduce hazards (such as falls and remote medical monitoring) in the home. The CDC has created a Healthy Housing Reference Manual that is available at the CDC website.

Healthy People 2020 goals include:
- 10% decrease in homes with lead paint
- 10% improvement in the number of trips made to work by walking
- 10% improvement in reducing cockroach and mouse allergens in homes
- 30% increase in homes with radon mitigation systems.

From https://www.healthypeople.gov/2020/topics-objectives/topic/environmental-health/objectives

CHILDREN'S HEALTH AND THE ENVIRONMENT

Vulnerability to the Environment

Children may be more vulnerable to environmental exposures than are adults. Several factors increase children's vulnerability, including the following:

- Children's body systems are still rapidly developing.
- Children eat, drink, and breathe more in proportion to their body size than do adults.
- Children's breathing zone is closer to the ground compared with adults.
- Children's bodies may be less able to break down and excrete contaminants.
- Children's behaviors can expose them to more contaminants. For example, young children, especially, spend time crawling and placing their hands or other objects in their mouths (EPA, 2013, 2015, 2017).
- Children spend time in places (school, day care, play spaces, gyms) outside of their homes where environmental hazards may exist. For example, children often spend more time playing outside in the dirt compared with adults.

Nurses should consider children's unique vulnerabilities to contaminants when assessing an exposure pathway. For example, lead poisoning is a problem that largely affects young children. Children living near a site with lead in the soil would likely be at greater risk from lead poisoning than the adults in the community because, as previously stated, they tend to put their hands or other objects, which may be contaminated with lead dust, into their mouths. Children who live in a community with older housing and close to a site with lead-contaminated soil may be exposed to the metal from multiple exposure pathways. Data show that children living at or below the poverty line who live in older housing are at greatest risk. There are approximately 500,000 children in the United States aged 1 to 5 with blood lead levels above 5 micrograms per deciliter (µg/dL), the reference level at which CDC recommends public health actions be initiated (CDC, 2017a). The CDC has online resources relating to lead poisoning and its prevention.

Older children and adolescents may also be at risk for exposure to environmental hazards in a way which adults are not. For example, mercury is a metal that comes from a variety of sources, including old thermometers and blood pressure cuffs. Metallic mercury is fun to play with because of the way it rolls around and forms beads. Children who find mercury frequently like to play with mercury and inadvertently track it from place to place as they share it with their friends. Most adults realize that mercury can be harmful, but most children may not realize how dangerous an object of play can be. Unfortunately, mercury has well-known health effects, and even at low levels, metallic mercury can cause health problems.

Metallic mercury exposure can cause harm before symptoms arise. The vapor from the mercury when inhaled can cause serious health problems. Even a small amount of liquid mercury can create enough mercury in the air to close a school, take buses out of circulation, or force evacuations of homes. There have been incidents where schools have been forced to stay closed for days while a mercury cleanup, which is difficult and expensive, took place. The *Don't Mess with Mercury* project, a collaboration between ATSDR and EPA, has short videos aimed at teens to help them realize the danger of mercury. The videos and other materials on mercury can be found at the website https://www.atsdr.cdc.gov/dontmesswithmercury/index.html.

When an entire community is being assessed, it is important to consider how the environment affects children, specifically. For example, a lack of safe places to play may affect children more directly than adults. Children may be at risk for more injuries if they are playing in streets or other areas that were not designed for safe play. Teens may be more likely to trespass on contaminated abandoned sites to hang out with friends or engage in activities like riding bikes. In low-income areas, the playgrounds may have more trash, rusty play equipment, and damaged surfaces, which could all contribute to an increased injury rate (CDC, 2011).

In 2015, EPA released updates to some indicators in *America's children and the environment*, 3rd edition, which has valuable information on environmental stressors' effect on children. This report provides valuable data on environmental exposures to children and trends over time. For example, as of 2009, approximately 6% of all children in the United States live within one mile of a Corrective Action or Superfund site that may not have all human health protective measures in place. This report and updates can be found at https://www.epa.gov/ace.

Student Reflection

In many respects, I don't think many of my classmates understand the impact of contaminants in the home environment. My community health practicum was in an elementary regional school in a rural setting. One little 7-year-old girl, Rebecca, who did well in school last year, was reported to have recent attention problems, and difficulty breathing, especially after recess. After talking to the family, my preceptor and I decided to make an environmental home assessment to gather more information. We found that the small two-bedroom, old farmhouse was extremely littered and crowded. All three adults in the family smoked. The only heat came from a wood stove and a small, old electric heater. There were four younger children in the house who looked frightened. While we were there, Rebecca had a coughing spell and looked very pale. Several interventions were necessary. Ultimately, Rebecca saw a physician who diagnosed asthma, and smoke was a significant trigger for her attacks. A referral to the county asthma prevention program led to a thorough assessment. Health professionals presented an educational program about asthma, its triggers, use of inhalers, and warning signs for complications to both Rebecca and her parents. By the time my practicum was finished, Rebecca was having much less trouble breathing on exertion and was doing better in the classroom.

Healthy Schools and Early Care and Education

Given how much time children spend in school and other care settings, these places should be safe from environmental exposures to the greatest extent possible. More than 55 million children (prekindergarten through grade 12) were enrolled in school in 2013 and there is an increase in expected school enrollment through 2025 (National Center for Education Statistics, 2016). Many school buildings are old and in poor condition, may contain environmental conditions that inhibit learning, and pose increased risks to the health of children and staff. Many programs and materials are available to help schools create healthy environments. These programs and materials deal with issues such as lead to green cleaning techniques, chemical management, indoor and outdoor air quality, and school site selection. The EPA has a website devoted to healthy school environments and in 2011 released the EPA Voluntary School Siting Guidelines to help communities determine the best location for schools. Healthy school information can be found at https://www. epa.gov/schools.

Environmental exposures to children attending child care and early learning facilities is also a concern for more than 8 million children (National Association of Regulatory Administrators [NARA], 2014). Such exposures can come from products used in these facilites (i.e., pesticides, cleaning products, craft materials) as well as from contamination left on site from past use or adjacent sites. In 2017, ATSDR created *Choose Safe Places for Early Care and Education* to bring awareness to the issue of where child care centers and other early education facilities are located. Information on Choose Safe Places can be found at the ATSDR website https://www.atsdr.cdc.gov/safeplaces-forece/index.html (ATSDR, 2016).

ENVIRONMENTAL JUSTICE

Environmental justice is the belief that no group of people should bear a disproportionate share of negative environmental health consequences regardless of race, culture, or income. In 1994, a White House executive order required that each federal agency makes environmental justice part of its mission. The Interagency Workgroup on Environmental Justice, established by the executive order, is charged with reducing disparities in community exposure to lead, toxic wastes, air pollution, and pesticides. It defines environmental justice as

...the fair treatment and meaningful involvement of all people regardless of race, color, national origin, or income with respect to the development, implementation, and enforcement of environmental laws, regulations, and policies. Fair treatment means that no group of people, including a racial, ethnic, or a socioeconomic group, should bear a disproportionate share of the negative environmental consequences resulting from industrial, municipal, and commercial operations or the execution of federal, state, local, and tribal programs and policies. **(CDC, 2008)**

More information about the Interagency Workgroup on Environmental Justice is available online.

Evidence for Practice

The city of Flint, Michigan, is a majority African American city where more than 40% of the population lives in poverty (Kennedy, 2016). In 2014, the city switched its water source from the Detroit Water Authority to the Flint Water system. With older water distribution pipes often containing lead, drinking water can become contaminated with lead when there is corrosion to the plumbing. With no corrosion control being used at the Flint Water System, the levels of lead in the Flint tap water increased over time.

From April 2014 to October 2015, approximately 99,000 Flint residents were affected by the changes in the water quality (CDC, 2016). Reports indicated that after the water change in April 2014, residents started to complain about their water as early as May 2014; however, a lead advisory was not issued until September 2015. In October 2015, the city switched its water systems to return to the Detroit Water Authority. A CDC report found the proportion of elevated blood lead levels in children were *significantly higher during the early period of the switch to Flint Water System compared to the previous period when residents consumed water from the Detroit Water Authority* (CDC 2016).

Living in poverty and in an area with older housing are both risk factors for children having elevated blood lead levels (CDC, 2017b). The children living in Flint at the time the water was switched were already at greater risk for having elevated blood lead levels. Nurses can apply this knowledge by recognizing how multiple environmental exposures can disproportionally affect some community members and consider how this may impact the health of individual patients or whole communities. Nurses can also help advocate for safer communities for everyone.

Many poorer or minority communities that lack political and economic power bear a disproportionate burden of environmental hazards. According to the United States Department of Agriculture (USDA, 2016), approximately 50% of 1.4 million farm workers in the United States are Hispanic. Through direct exposure to pesticides, farm workers and their families may face serious health risks. The exact number of pesticide poisonings per year is hard to determine because many cases go unreported and there is no national surveillance system for acute pesticide illness. These illnesses may make the workers and their families even more vulnerable to extreme poverty if their illness prevents them from working. Many farm workers and their families tend to live close to their work because they have few resources to travel to and from work. Living close to the field they work in often means they are exposed to pesticides while working in fields and while at home. Children may also be exposed because they live close to where the pesticides are applied. The workers may lack opportunities that would enable them to seek jobs in other industries. In addition, they may lack resources to make moving possible and if they complain, they may lose their jobs.

When we talk about environmental justice, we mean calling a halt to the poisoning and pollution of our poorest communities, from our rural areas to our inner cities. When our children's lives are no longer cut short by toxic dumps, when their minds are no longer damaged by lead paint poisoning, we will stop wasting energy and intelligence that could build a stronger, more prosperous America. **Former President Bill Clinton**

Environmental justice is an important consideration when working with tribal communities. Tribal communities often bear a disproportionate burden of impact from pollution on their tribal lands (EPA, 2014). Many tribal communities still continue to practice traditional tribal life ways, including eating traditional foods for either a majority or a portion of their diets. These traditional practices are often negatively affected by contaminated land and water. For example, if a tribal community's traditional fishing grounds are polluted, a state may issue a "no fishing" advisory, and the community may lose a large part of its traditional diet. The "no fishing" advisory may affect the tribal community more than it does the nontribal community whose diet is not as dependent on fish.

GLOBAL ENVIRONMENTAL HEALTH CHALLENGES

Climate change is happening, humans are causing it, and I think this is perhaps the most serious environmental issue facing us.
Bill Nye, American science educator and television personality

In the 21st century, there is a greater focus on world health. Modern travel and communication systems make it possible for people to go to all parts of the world. As people begin to feel more connected to their world, they may feel more vulnerable, because environmental health issues in one country can affect others. Contamination created in one country does not abide by map boundaries and may affect neighboring countries. Consumption patterns may create a situation where one country contaminates its air, water, or land while manufacturing goods for other countries. If we want to all live in a healthy environment as society moves forward, people will be forced to confront difficult issues with global consequences.

Clean Water and Sanitation

In the United States, most citizens have access to clean water and sanitation services and often take these services for granted. Worldwide, however, clean water and sanitation are not standard. According to the World Health Organization (WHO) in 2015, 844 million people still lacked basic drinking water services. Those without basic services use unprotected wells or springs, took water directly from surface water (such as rivers, lakes, ponds), or had to use more than 30 minutes to collect water. However, there has been improvement in the percent of the population with access to at least basic drinking water services by an average of 0.49% points per year between 2000 and 2015 (WHO & UNICEF, 2017). Access to basic sanitation is still a challenge in some parts of the world. The 2.3 billion people who still lacked a basic sanitation service practice open defecation, use unimproved facilities such as pit latrines or use sanitation facilities that are shared with other households (WHO & UNICEF, 2017).

There are nearly 1.7 billion cases of childhood diarrheal disease worldwide each year and it is still the second leading cause of death for children under age 5. These illnesses are preventable and treatable. Improved access to safer drinking water and basic sanitation, along with education and access to hand washing, can help decrease the burden of these illnesses. As the world's population continues to expand, access to clean water and sanitation services is likely to remain a challenge. The WHO has set goals for worldwide improvement in access to drinking water, sanitation and, hygiene. More information about these topics and the goals can be found at the WHO website (http://www.who.int/news-room/fact-sheets/detail/diarrhoeal-disease).

Air Quality

Outdoor and indoor air quality affects people in all countries. However, people in developing countries bear more than half of the burden from air pollution on human health. Exposure to particulate matter and ozone carries serious risks to health. By reducing air toxins, it is possible to reduce the morbidity and mortality of illnesses such as lung cancer, asthma, respiratory tract infections, and heart disease (WHO, 2016). As the relationship between air quality and health has become clearer, the WHO has established guidelines for countries to help decrease air pollution–related illnesses. However, reaching these guidelines is a challenge; in 2014, *92% of the world population was living in places where the WHO air quality guidelines levels were not met* (WHO, 2016).

Indoor air quality is a problem, especially in homes where biomass fuel and coal are burned for heat or cooking. Worldwide, three billion people are forced to burn fuels such as animal dung, firewood, and coal, which do not combust well and create high levels of particulate matter and carbon monoxide (WHO 2014). The burden of this exposure falls mostly on women and children, who often spend more time in the home. In 2014, the WHO set new emissions targets that will help protect health. Chronic and acute exposure to particulate matter can increase the risk of cardiovascular and respiratory diseases. Exposure to particulate matter from indoor heating and cooking sources can increase the risk of acute lower respiratory tract infections and associated deaths in young children. The 2014 WHO indoor air targets can help decrease the 4.3 million deaths per year that are believed to be linked to indoor air pollution from cooking and heating (WHO, 2014).

Weather forecast for tonight: dark. **George Carlin**

Chemical and Contaminant Exposure

Worldwide, people may be exposed to chemicals and other contaminants in ways that are very different than in the United States. Many countries lack environmental and occupational protections that we have come to appreciate. For example, mining practices in Nigeria led to an outbreak of lead poisoning in at least six villages. In this part of Nigeria, people use rudimentary tools to break apart ore to find pieces of gold. The process creates lots of lead-contaminated dust, since the ore has a high lead concentration. Much of the work is done near or in family compounds. In 2010, a multidisciplinary team surveyed two of the affected villages and collected blood from children younger than 5 years. The team found in just two villages, in the 12 months before the team arrived, 118 out of 463 (26%) children younger than 5 years had died. Parents reported that 82% of the children who died had convulsions before death, a sign of severe lead poisoning. Blood samples collected from 205 living children found that 97% had blood lead levels greater than 45 µg/dL. In the United States, children with a blood lead level of 45 µg/dL would immediately have chelation therapy started to reduce their blood lead levels. The blood lead concentrations in the children ranged from 33.3 to 445 µg/dL (CDC, 2010). The total number of deaths across all villages is not known, but according to the WHO, an estimated 2,000 children need chelation therapy. The WHO has stated of the crisis, "[S]ome children will require chelation for many months...In addition, capacities within Nigeria for the diagnosis and management of lead poisoning need further strengthening and support. A further challenge is the purchase of sufficient chelating agents: these are expensive drugs that are not available as generics" (WHO, 2011).

This story from Nigeria illustrates the potential deadly consequences when there exists a combination of limited environmental protections, lack of knowledge concerning environmental dangers by local community members, and the community members' need to earn an income. As we become a more globalized community with natural resources and materials being produced, shipped, and moved around the world faster than ever before, we need to consider the impact on the communities that produce those resources and materials and strive to protect their health as we protect ours in the United States. Just as we consider environmental justice within the United States, we must consider it on the global scale.

Climate Change

Although the extent and severity of climate change are still topics under debate, most scientists and governments agree that human activities are influencing global climate. Climate variability and change affect human health in a variety of ways. Climate change will likely cause a shift in the number and severity of natural disasters, such as heat waves, floods, and droughts. These natural disasters will have an immediate, direct impact on human health, but they will also have wider-ranging impacts on water and food supplies. Food security, already a problem for many poorer areas, will continue to be a challenge as climate change affects crop patterns.

Changes to water supplies and increased flooding may make some areas more vulnerable to diarrheal diseases. In addition, many diseases are highly sensitive to changes in climate. Experts predict that common vector-borne diseases such as malaria and dengue fever will affect larger geographic areas, as the vectors that carry the diseases find agreeable climates in expanding areas. Climate change will affect air quality and 300,000 million people with asthma and will face increased disease burden from asthma triggers such as high ozone levels and pollen. According to the WHO, between 2030 and 2050, approximately 250,000 additional deaths per year will be due to climate change. These deaths are primarily from heat exposure in elderly people, diarrhea, malaria, and childhood undernutrition (WHO, 2017).

It is necessary to realize that the effects of climate on human health will not be evenly distributed around the world. Populations in developing countries, particularly in the Small Island Developing States, arid and high mountain zones, and densely populated coastal areas, are considered to be particularly vulnerable. More than half of the world's population lives less than 40 miles from the sea making them more vulnerable to sever storms and flooding (WHO, 2017).

However, it is not only developing countries that will be affected. For example, a heat wave in Western Europe in 2003 caused approximately 70,000 more deaths that year than had been caused in previous years. Countries in Europe and the United States will feel the impact of changes to storm patterns and may also face water and food supply issues if patterns of drought or excessive rain affect agricultural areas (WHO, 2017).

Climate change has helped illustrate that humans live in a world where the health of all environments is connected. It is nearly impossible to view global environmental issues as something that happens "over there." The industrialization of countries around the world will have a direct impact on the environmental health of the entire planet. To tackle these issues, global cooperation and planning are essential. To find out more information about how climate change may impact the United States, visit the US Global Change Research Program at http://www.globalchange.gov/.

Climate adaptation is one way that public health nurses can start thinking about how to help communities deal with climate change. An example of adaptation is a community preparing to have cooling stations open for community members to seek relief during a heat wave. The community may not be able to control the extent and duration of a heat wave but they can put into place some interventions to help protect health. The CDC developed the Building Resilience Against Climate Effects (BRACE) framework to help professionals and communities start developing strategies to prepare for the health effects of climate change (CDC, 2015c). This framework and additional information can be found at the CDC website (https://www.cdc.gov/climateandhealth/BRACE.htm).

KEY CONCEPTS

- The environment has a direct impact on human health.
- The nursing process of using assessment, intervention, and evaluation can be used when thinking about how the environment affects human health and how health can be protected.
- Proximity to a contaminant or hazard is not the only factor in determining whether there is a risk to human health. For a contaminant to pose a risk, there must be a completed exposure pathway.
- When assessing a community's environment, it is helpful to think about the whole environment to

determine what components are influencing human health.
- Environmental justice is important to consider when looking at the impact of the environment on a community.
- A community environment can be built to help positively influence the health of those living in the community.
- Globally, there are still many environmental health challenges that must be faced.

CRITICAL THINKING QUESTIONS

1. You are a public health nurse and receive a call from a resident who stated "many people on Spruce Street near the old junk yard have cancer." The resident is concerned. What types of questions would you think about to begin to determine whether there could be a connection between the cancer and the site?

2. As a local public health nurse, a family is referred to you because their 3-year-old child has a blood lead level of 26 μg of lead per deciliter. Is this a high lead level? What are the likely sources of lead exposure for the child? What type of education

would you likely do for the family? Consider looking at the Center for Disease Control and Prevention's website on lead.

3. The town you live in is considering using a multi-acre abandoned site to build a mixed-use development (it will have retail facilities, residential buildings, and public space). As a public health nurse, what would you suggest the designers consider to optimize the environmental health of the development? Consider looking at the Environmental Protection Agency's website on smart growth and green building.

CRITICAL THINKING QUESTIONS *(Continued)*

4. Think of the community surrounding your school of nursing. Pick two environmental conditions and assess these conditions. Where do you think you could locate data to support your observations?

5. Why do you think it is important for the government to monitor human exposures across the United States?

6. Consider an environmental health challenge facing a developing country. What are some economically feasible interventions that could help protect community members? (Websites such as the CDC Safe Water System or the WHO Environmental Health websites might help provide some ideas.)

7. Assisting communities to adapt to climate change is a challenge we face. Pick a community near you and determine what climate change impacts they may face and what vulnerabilities they may have. Remember to consider especially vulnerable populations within those communities and identify their specific challenges. (Websites such as CDC's Climate and Health or EPA's Climate Change Adaption Resource Center might be helpful.)

REFERENCES

Agency for Toxic Substances and Disease Registry (ATSDR). (2005). *Public health assessment guidance manual*. Retrieved from https://www.atsdr.cdc.gov/hac/PHAManual/toc.html

Agency for Toxic Substances and Disease Registry (ATSDR). (2016). *Choose safe places for early care and education*. Retrieved fromhttps://www.atsdr.cdc.gov/safeplacesforece/index.html

American Chemical Society. (2018). *CAS registry—The gold standard for chemical substance information*. Retrieved from http://www.cas.org/content/chemical-substances

American Lung Association. (2016). *E-cigarettes and lung health*. Retrieved from http://www.lung.org/stop-smoking/smoking-facts/e-cigarettes-and-lung-health.html

Carson, R. (1962). *Silent spring*. New York: Houghton Mifflin Harcourt.

Centers for Disease Control and Prevention (CDC). (2002). *Managing elevated blood lead levels among young children: Recommendations from the Advisory Committee on Childhood Lead Poisoning Prevention*. Retrieved from http://www.cdc.gov/nceh/lead/CaseManagement/caseManage_main.htm

Centers for Disease Control and Prevention (CDC). (2008). *Environmental justice*. Retrieved from http://www.cdc.gov/omhd/AMH/EJ.htm

Centers for Disease Control and Prevention (CDC). (2009a). Childhood lead poisoning associated with lead dust contamination from family vehicles and child safety seats—Maine, 2008. *Morbidity and Mortality Weekly Report, 58*(32), 890–893.

Centers for Disease Control and Prevention (CDC). (2009b). Pseudo-outbreak of antimony toxicity in firefighters—Florida, 2009. *Morbidity and Mortality Weekly Report, 58*(46), 1300–1302.

Centers for Disease Control and Prevention (CDC). (2009c). *Fourth national report on human exposure to environmental chemicals*. Atlanta, GA: Department of Health and Human Services, Centers for Disease Control and Prevention. Retrieved from www.cdc.gov/exposurereport/pdf/fourthreport.pdf

Centers for Disease Control and Prevention (CDC). (2010). Notes from the field: Outbreak of acute lead poisoning among children aged <5 years—Zamfara, Nigeria, 2010. *Morbidity and Mortality Weekly Report, 59*(27), 846.

Centers for Disease Control and Prevention (CDC). (2011). School health guidelines to promote healthy eating and physical activity. *Morbidity and Mortality Weekly Report, 60*(RR05), 1–17.

Centers for Disease Control and Prevention (CDC). (2014). *Prevention tips*. Retrieved on August 16, 2017, from https://www.cdc.gov/nceh/lead/tips.htm

Centers for Disease Control and Prevention (CDC). (2015a). Severe illness from methyl bromide exposure at a Condominium Resort – U.S. Virgin Islands, March 2015. *Morbidity and Mortality Weekly Report, 64*(28), 763–766.

Centers for Disease Control and Prevention (CDC). (2015b). *Healthy Homes*. Retrieved from http://www.cdc.gov/nceh/lead/healthy-homes.htm

Centers for Disease Control and Prevention (CDC). (2015c). *CDC's Building Resilience Against Climate Effects (BRACE) Framework*. Retrieved from https://www.cdc.gov/climateandhealth/brace.htm

Centers for Disease Control and Prevention (CDC). (2016). Blood lead levels among children aged <6 – Flint, Michigan, 2013-2016. *Morbidity and Mortality Weekly Report, 65*(25), 650–654.

Centers for Disease Control and Prevention (CDC). (2017a). *Lead*. Retrieved from http://www.cdc.gov/nceh/lead/

Centers for Disease Control and Prevention (CDC). (2017b) Childhood lead poisoning indicators. Retrieved from https://ephtracking.cdc.gov/showClpIndicators

De Rosa, C. T., Holler, J. S., & Mehlman, M. A. (2002). *Impact of hazardous chemicals on public health, policy and service*. Princeton, NJ: International Toxicology Books.

Environmental Protection Agency. (2001). *Fight lead poisoning with a healthy diet*. Retrieved from https://www.epa.gov/sites/production/files/2014-02/documents/fight_lead_poisoning_with_a_healthy_diet.pdf

Environmental Protection Agency (2013). *Built and natural environments: A technical review of interactions among land use, transportation and environmental quality*. Retrieved from https://www.epa.gov/sites/production/files/2014-03/documents/our-built-and-natural-environments.pdf

Environmental Protection Agency. (2014). *EPA policy on Environmental Justice for working with federally recognized tribes and indigenous peoples*. Retrieved fromhttps://www.epa.gov/sites/production/files/2017-10/documents/ej-indigenous-policy.pdf

Environmental Protection Agency. (2015). *America's Children and the Environment*. Retrieved from https://www.epa.gov/ace

Environmental Protection Agency. (2017). *Children are not little adults!* Retrieved from https://www.epa.gov/children/children-are-not-little-adults

Goodman, M., Naiman, J. S., Goodman, D., & LaKind, J. S. (2012). Cancer clusters in the USA: What do the last twenty years of state and federal investigations tell us? *Critical Reviews in Toxicology, 42*(6), 474–490.

Health Care Without Harm. (2017). *What we do*. Retrieved from https://noharm-uscanada.org/content/us-canada/about-us

Kennedy, M. (2016). Lead-Laced Water in Flint: A step-by-step look at the makings of a crisis. *The two-way*. Retrieved from http://www.npr.org/sections/thetwo-way/2016/04/20/465545378/lead-laced-water-in-flint-a-step-by-step-look-at-the-makings-of-a-crisis.

Kriebel, D., Tickner, J., Epstein, P., Lemons, J., Levins, R., Loechler, E. L., … Stoto, M. (2001). The precautionary principle in environmental science. *Environmental Health Perspectives, 109*(9), 871–876.

National Association of Regulatory Administrators (NARA). (2014) *Research Brief #1 Trends in Child Care Licensing and Regulations Policy 2014*. Retrieved from https://childcareta.acf.hhs.gov/sites/default/files/public/center_licensing_trends_brief_2014.pdf

National Cancer Institute. (2014). *Cancer Clusters* Retrieved from https://www.cancer.gov/about-cancer/causes-prevention/risk/substances/cancer-clusters-fact-sheet#p2

National Center for Education Statistics. (2016). *Fast facts*. Retrieved from https://nces.ed.gov/fastfacts/display.asp?id=65

Society of Toxicology. (2017). What about SOT: What is toxicology. Retrieved from http://www.toxicology.org/about/

U.S. Department of Agriculture (USDA). (2016). *Farm labor, background*. Retrieved from https://www.ers.usda.gov/topics/farm-economy/farm-labor/background.aspx#Numbers

Volk, H. E., Kerin, T., Lurmann, F., Hertz-Picciotto, I., McConnell, R., & Campbell, D. B. (2014). Autism spectrum disorder: interaction of air pollution with the MET receptor tyrosine kinase gene. *Epidemiology, 25*(1), 44–47.

World Health Organization. (2011). *Nigeria: Mass lead poisoning from mining activities, Zamfara State—Update 1*. Retrieved on March 7, 2013, from http://www.who.int/csr/don/2011_11_11/en/index.html

World Health Organization. (2014). *WHO sets benchmarks to reduce health damage from indoor air pollution*. Retrieved from http://www.who.int/mediacentre/news/releases/2014/indoor-air-pollution/en/

World Health Organization. (2016). *Ambient outdoor air quality and health factsheet*. Retrieved from http://www.who.int/mediacentre/factsheets/fs313/en/

World Health Organization and the United Nations Children's Fund. (2017). *Progress on drinking water sanitation and hygiene, 2017*. Retrieved from http://apps.who.int/iris/bitstream/10665/258617/1/9789241512893-eng.pdf?ua=1

World Health Organization. (2017). *Climate change and health factsheet*. Retrieved from http://www.who.int/mediacentre/factsheets/fs266/en/

WEB RESOURCES

Please visit thePoint for up-to-date web resources on this topic.

20

Community Preparedness: Disaster and Terrorism

Merrily Evdokimoff and Joy Spellman

DOWN*
down it came
down from the autumn sky
down it came down &
every one rose &
wept in the city (my city) &
some were flying &
some were falling &
some were running &
some were burning
where were you listening

watching then?
in the shattered earth?
in the broken air?
in the oily fire?
in the tainted sea?
where were you listening
watching then when everyone rose &
lookt at the sky lookt at the
sky where they stood in my city &
wept?

—Jesse Glass

CHAPTER HIGHLIGHTS

- Public health nurses and disaster response
- Types of disasters
- Disaster management
- Public health response

- Role and responsibility of nurses in disasters
- Classification of agents
- Field response
- Skill building for field activity

OBJECTIVES

- Identify disaster types.
- Explain the disaster planning process and nursing participation.
- Understand nursing participation in a disaster.
- Promote increased competency levels through the use of Table Top Exercises (TTX), field drills, and exercises.

- Differentiate between biologic, chemical, and radiologic agents and response to exposure.
- Describe the public health response throughout the phases of an emergency response.

KEY TERMS

All-Hazards Vulnerability Study: An integrated approach to emergency preparedness that addresses a wide spectrum of emergencies.

After-action report: Retrospective analysis used to evaluate emergency response drills.

---

*Copyright 2002 by Jesse Glass. Used with permission of the author and of about.com (poetry). Available online at http://poetry.about.com/library/weekly/aa110901m.htm.

Decontamination: Process of cleaning to remove biologic, chemical, or radiologic agents.

Evacuation: Moving people from a dangerous place to safety.

Human simulation training (HST): Use of life-like/computerized models for creating increased reality during a practice scenario

Incident command system (ICS): Common organizational structure implemented to improve emergency response.

Invacuation: Moving people from one area to another within the same facility.

National Response Framework (NRF): Framework that guides how the nation conducts all-hazards incident response.

Mass casualty incident (MCI): Any incident in which emergency medical services resources, such as personnel and equipment, are overwhelmed by the number and severity of casualties.

Medical Reserve Corps (MRC) or Community Emergency Response Team (CERT): Community-based program that uses volunteers for emergency preparedness response.

National Incident Management System (NIMS): Structured, flexible framework that guides the response to disasters at all levels of government, the private sector, and nongovernmental organizations.

Personal protective equipment (PPE): Clothing and/or equipment used to protect the body from injury and illness.

Point of distribution (POD) or Emergency dispensing site (EDS): Centralized location where the public picks up emergency supplies following a disaster.

Real time: The actual time in which something occurs.

Scenario: The sequence of possible events or circumstances.

Shelter in place: The protective action of remaining in current location during an incident.

Simulation: The imitation of the features of an object or anticipated response.

Social Distancing: Action taken by Public Health officials to stop or slow down the spread of a highly contagious disease by keeping social interactions to a minimum.

Strategic National Stockpile: The supply of potentially lifesaving pharmaceuticals and medical supplies maintained by the CDC for use in a public health emergency severe enough to cause lack of local supplies.

Surveillance: A process to document and track changing information to prevent injury and illness.

Terrorism: The use of threats and/or violence to intimidate or coerce society for political purposes.

Weaponize: To convert into a weapon for use in harming others.

CASE STUDY *References to the case study are found throughout this chapter (look for the case study icon). Readers should keep the case study in mind as they read the chapter.*

Geoff, a nurse educator at the Texas Public Health Department, has played an active role in providing education and hands-on experiences involving disaster-based scenarios among community-based nurses throughout the state. Nurses require more specific knowledge about harmful agents and situations not usually seen in their practice. With state support, the public health nurses, with Geoff's leadership, decide that a certificate on biologic, chemical, and radiologic terrorism will be offered with expanded content that will build new skill sets needed in a field response.

Lessons learned from the response to the aftermath of Hurricane Harvey along the Texas coast in November 2017 are incorporated into the certificate curriculum.

Geoff will include a module on preparedness operations while working with diverse communities. The program will be delivered in the spring, followed by an emergency exercise designed to test the capability of a large city's response to a deliberate chemical attack. The community and public health nurses enrolled in the course will be key players in the planning, execution, and evaluation phases of the drill.

INTRODUCTION

The only difference between reality and fiction is that fiction has to make sense. **Tom Clancy**

Between 1900 and 2016 more than 21,000 disasters have occurred in the world (UNDRR, 2015)

Hurricanes are a major threat for the American continent and can leave behind long-lasting economic and human consequences. Constant preparedness and disaster risk reduction actions need to be taken, not only regarding direct consequences of hurricanes but also in regard to the associated disasters, such as urban flooding and dam bursting.

FIGURE 20.1 Submerged vehicle on a road outside Beaumont, Texas, in flooding from Hurricane Harvey. (*Source:* FEMA/Dominick Del Vecchio—September 2, 2017. Retrieved October 23, 2017, from https://www.fema.gov/media-library/assets/images/136115.)

Hurricanes and cyclones are extreme events that bring high destruction in terms of number of deaths and economic damages. Damage from the hurricanes of Fall, 2017 included:

Harvey: 69 deaths, 450,000 people affected and 58 billion US$ of damages.

Irma: 83 deaths, 5.7 million people affected and 50 billion US$ of damages.

Maria: 55 deaths/missing, 100,000 people affected and billions US$ of damages.

(EM-DAT, 2017)

Due to numerous natural-, weather-, and terror-related disasters, the United States has responded to in the past few years, these experiences are being used to hone emergency plans and include all levels of personnel and the public in the planning and implementation of disaster management. Recognizing the need for local government, as the first responders, to provide aid until State and Federal aid can be mobilized, there is a renewed focus on local planning. Healthcare organizations particularly have been charged with working together with local public health to be better prepared in a disaster or other **mass casualty events**. Nurses have a significant role to play in alleviating the suffering related to these disasters.

There are 2.8 million registered nurses in the United States, as well as the nursing population worldwide that provide a tremendous untapped resource that can and must be used if the nation is to adequately prepare for such events (BLS, 2016). In order for nurses to respond appropriately to mass casualty incidents (MCIs), guidelines and recommendations must be in place to ensure that they can recognize and respond to potential and occurring emergency events. Emergency preparedness for nurses begins with the recognition that effective management of a disaster event requires the integration of activities from multiple community systems including emergency response, acute and postacute care and public health (APHN, 2014).

Public health nurses (PHNs) have been responding to disasters for more than a century. Historically, nursing evolved from the actions taken by Florence Nightingale in the Crimean War. Long before the nursing process was theorized, researched, and established as part of the nursing profession, Nightingale used her skills of observation and critical thinking to improve health outcomes. Nightingale implemented principles of evidence-based nursing at that time. As she strolled through hospital wards, Nightingale was actually documenting environmental conditions and social determinants of health and their impact on the patients she was charged to keep well. Nightingale's analysis of health-related statistics, used to track outcomes, introduced epidemiology to the healthcare setting (see Chapter 6). Since that time, the PHN has continued to expand competencies by utilizing interventions that are enlightened by an evidence-based approach to improve population health. With a public health nursing workforce that understands and implements evidence-based public health practice, local health department officials and policymakers will see the benefits of evidence–based decision-making during a disaster. The *Healthy People 2020* goal for preparedness is "To strengthen and sustain communities" abilities to prevent, protect against, mitigate the effects of, respond to, and recover from incidents with negative health effects" (Healthy People, 2017).

Community and public health nursing has a broad scope of practice. For example, population-based practice may have a narrow focus (e.g., six students with diabetes in a middle school) or a broad one (e.g., a potential H7N9 pandemic). Managing a client load of six certainly seems reasonable. Doing the same within a county of 400,000 people is quite different. The role of nurses within the community is to assess the needs of the populace and ensure that service breaches are addressed. Nurses accomplish this by calling on existing agencies and institutions to find ways to serve the needs of the citizens. Collaborative effort is a significant part of response. For example, local health department nursing personnel, school nurse organizations, and volunteers from the **Medical Reserve Corps** (MRC) and Certified Emergency Response Teams (CERT) have worked in concert to provide in-school H1N1 immunization as well as engaging in **surveillance** activities. From that experience, PHNs in Texas are working at putting the knowledge and skills gained from the 2017 hurricane into evidence-based policies that may be implemented during the next event. A well-prepared cadre of community and PHNs is essential to minimize the effects of both immediate and long-range disasters.

The aftermath of the destruction of the World Trade Center in 2001 identified a lack of trained leaders and workers in all areas of public health service. The event also stimulated a growing appreciation of those who respond to large-scale events. Increased competency in disaster response became a new dimension to nursing practice. The Centers for Disease Control and Prevention (CDC) has called for the mobilization of the public health workforce to ensure the training and education of communities across the nation regarding biologic, chemical, radiologic, and explosive device attacks. It is necessary to learn how to prepare for events that are difficult to imagine, and it is even more challenging to mount a response. Multiple disasters in Texas, Florida, and Puerto Rico in a short period of time illustrate the importance of having a coordinated, multidisciplinary response to a culturally diverse population (Douglas et al., 2011).

> There cannot be a crisis next week. My schedule is already full.
> **Henry A. Kissinger**

Evidence for Practice

Lim, Lim, & Vasu (2013) surveyed physicians and nurses about their perception of their own and their institutions preparedness for a disaster. While 75% felt their institution was prepared only 36% felt they as individuals were prepared. Factors that contributed to personal preparedness included: institutional, peer, and leadership preparedness plus disaster response training. The study revealed that 80% of professionals polled were willing to act in response to such an event. Classroom study and field exercise participation among healthcare workers resulted in a significant increase in their ability and willingness to respond effectively in a disaster. This research validates the "vision" put forth by Veenema and colleagues (2016) identifying: (1) increased disaster knowledge base of nurses; (2) ability to provide direct or indirect support during a disaster; (3) promoting preparedness among individuals in the community; and (4) participating in disaster planning drills.

 What kind of data does Geoff gather in his disaster training needs assessment? How can these new findings affect the emergency planning process for healthcare facilities and the community at large? How will the needs of a diverse community be addressed in the new plan?

EMERGENCIES, DISASTERS, AND TERRORISM

Response to emergencies and disasters has been a part of the human experience since humans first walked on the earth. A nation's capacity to respond to these threats depends in part on the ability of healthcare professionals and public health officials to rapidly and effectively detect, manage, and communicate during an event resulting in mass casualties. Emergencies are considered events that require a swift, intense response on the part of existing community resources. Disasters are often unforeseen, serious, and unique events

that disrupt essential community services and cause human morbidity and mortality that cannot be alleviated unless assistance is received from others outside the community. Disasters vary by: (1) the type of onset (they often occur without warning); (2) the duration of the immediate crisis; (3) the magnitude or scope of the incident; and (4) the extent to which the event affects the community.

There are three types of disasters: natural, accidental, and terrorist attacks. Nature can wreak havoc when a tornado touches down or a hurricane obliterates a once-wide sandy beachfront. Natural disasters are widespread throughout the world. The 2017 catastrophic earthquake in Mexico is an example. The rapid occurrence in the Caribbean and United States of hurricane's Harvey, Irma, and Maria all within a month of each other emphasized the need for local disaster management organizations to mobilize quickly and deal with rapidly changing developments. Accidents include human-made disasters such as the Chernobyl meltdown in the former Soviet Union, which remains a constant reminder of the devastating effects of such a radiologic event. The near meltdown that occurred in posttsunami Japan in 2011 has been deigned to be a human-made disaster based on evidence that revealed faulty design elements in the placement of reactor cooling tanks. The shipwreck of unsafe boats filled with migrants seeking political asylum has become an increasingly frequent disaster. Active shooter attacks continue to occur throughout the world on a daily basis, and in the United States, the October 2017 attack by a "lone wolf" gunman in Nevada reminds us to be prepared for the unexpected.

Natural Disasters

Natural disasters are the result of naturally occurring events that have an impact on the environment, the economy, and the people who live in the area. Examples include earthquakes, extreme heat, floods, hurricanes, landslides, tornadoes, tsunamis, volcanic eruptions, wildfires, and winter weather. All of these conditions are threats to health.

Although many natural disasters are not predictable, it is possible to assess the circumstances that increase vulnerability to a natural disaster ahead of time and take steps to prevent complications. For example, as reports of a strengthening tropical storm in October 2017 came in to Texas state incident command center, experts tracking the storm agreed that "Harvey" would soon assume full hurricane status. With miles of ocean front coast and several counties exposed to coastal waters, a storm evacuation plan had been in place and exercised over the years. Previously identified sites to be used as shelters were activated 2 days before the hurricane made land fall. County and state health departments, the Red Cross, local and state law enforcement, and PHNs worked closely to accept the storm victims and assess their needs. On-site triaging resulted in the transfer of many storm victims for injuries and complications from existing chronic illnesses. In this instance, rapid assessment of an impending natural disaster, resource identification, and activation of an often exercised

scenario resulted in saving scores of lives. As public health practitioners gather evidence for practice, it is becoming clear that in many disaster scenarios, the displacement of people before, during, and after the event must be considered as plans are developed.

Practice Point

Many natural disasters are anticipated, such as hurricanes, rising flood waters, and temperature extremes. Include these events when planning for emergencies—a response can begin before the onset of disaster. The instillation of early warning signals can also allow for earlier warnings to take shelter or evacuate. Tornado sirens have become much more common in the Midwest. Signs of seismic activity that may indicate an impending earthquake are also being refined. Become familiar with locally designated shelter sites, evacuation routes, and early warning signals.

Accidental Disasters

Accidental incidents, broadly defined, are those that happen as a result of circumstantial factors (e.g., road conditions, human error, and physical plant deterioration) and are usually not deliberate. For example, a truck containing a toxic chemical being transported on a major highway system overturns when the driver fails to negotiate a clearly marked warning of the steep incline of the exit ramp. Evacuation of the area takes place. "Accident" implies that the incident is uncontrollable and/or unpreventable, usually with a negative outcome. But, do accidents just happen? Or can they be prevented? Over time, epidemiologists have identified ways to prevent the negative outcomes of unanticipated events by improving preparedness and awareness training and education. For instance, research findings may suggest that road signage located well before the steep incline, or consistent driver evaluation, could prevent vehicle accidents, or at least minimize their severity.

Like natural disasters, accidents may also have an impact on the environment, cost millions of dollars, and affect the lives of those involved. The 2010 collapse of the oil rig in the Gulf of Mexico and the consequent destruction of a vast, sensitive ocean environment is a good example. Preparing for accidental disaster is difficult, largely because of the possibility of human error and the setting in which it occurs. Certainly, the accidental release of nuclear materials affecting 1,000,000 people may not be seen in the same light as a medication error on the part of a nurse. In both cases, assessment of vulnerabilities with subsequent correction, followed by implementation of a preventive action, might have prevented the accident. Forgetting to complete a task can also contribute to a disastrous situation. For example, during review of an evacuation of a long-term care facility as part of a mandatory yearly exercise,

administrators find that contracts with medical transport companies were not renewed, making effective evacuation impossible. Disaster management planning is now required by Center for Medicare and Medicaid Services (CMS) for hospitals and postacute entities like clinics, home health, and dialysis sites as a requirement for receiving Medicare funding.

Evidence for Practice

Planning leaders now recognize it is essential in preparedness activities to collaborate among all levels of providers in various settings. Clear identification of roles and responsibilities as the process develops lends itself to effective response. By broadening the scope of participants in the planning process, details previously overlooked have a better chance to be included in the disaster response. Coordination within a wider community coalition assures a workable, reliable mass casualty plan.

The use of simulation supports an evidence-based approach to disaster planning by identifying methods to use empirical data in the decision-making process. This process will help emergency response planners to identify hazards and vulnerabilities through a wide variety of scenarios, learn responses to each, and develop principles or best practices that apply to a broad spectrum of disaster scenarios. Ultimately, the promotion of injury and disease prevention programs and practices will be enhanced.

Terrorism

Although there are difficulties in defining global definition of **terrorism**, the United Nations Security Council described it as "criminal acts, including against civilians, committed with the intent to cause death or serious bodily injury, or taking of hostages, with the purpose to provoke a state of terror in the general public or in a group of persons or particular persons, intimidate a population, or compel a government or an international organization to do or to abstain from doing any act" (Sanchez and Leiden, 2009. P. 67). Section 802 of the Patriot Act defines Domestic Terrorism as any unlawful act that seeks to: (1) intimidate or coerce a civilian population; (2) influence the policy of a government by intimidation or coercion; or (3) affect the conduct of a government by mass destruction, assassination, or kidnapping. (ACLU, 2017). The inclusion of intention to harm civilians for political purposes is a common thread within both definitions. The main goals of terrorism are creating fear, causing casualties, and rendering sites unusable. Fear and intimidation are potent concepts for the human psyche to process. A recent study by PEW research found that Americans are more fearful now of terrorist attacks than right after 9/11 (McGill, 2016).

Part of this new world of completely improvisational terrorism is that there were codes of war that disintegrated in the face of terrorism. **Diane Sawyer**

DISASTER PREPAREDNESS IN A CULTURALLY DIVERSE SOCIETY

It is important to integrate a community's ethnicity, race, culture, and language into emergency preparedness response and recovery plans. This requires cultural competence across all disciplines involved in the planning and implementation phases. (Addy, Browne, Blake, & Bailey, 2015). Outreach to diverse members of every community is critical to assure effective, inclusive strategies to protect all citizens. PHNs are well versed in identifying vulnerable populations within the districts in which they serve. Efforts to assure that health professionals and emergency responders become more culturally competent have gained momentum in the past few years. An increasing awareness of inequities visited upon ethnically diverse communities has emerged since Hurricane Katrina hit the Gulf Coast early in the morning of August 29, 2005. The Office of Minority Health, U.S. Department of Human Services (DHS), has developed a Cultural Competency Curriculum for Disaster Preparedness and Crisis Response that offers continuing education for those looking to enhance their skills toward the provision of competent care in disaster situations (Office of Minority Services, 2017).

Culture is the learned knowledge of values and beliefs of a particular group that are passed down through generations. These belief systems influence a person's view of the world, decisions made, and behaviors tied into those beliefs. The latest data collected in Texas have identified over 37% of population reporting a Hispanic background and an additional 3% Asian. (U.S. Census Bureau, 2016). These numbers clearly illustrate the importance of addressing multicultural influences during a disaster. A person's culture is a comforting and reassuring system at the best of times. The degree of community cohesion is seen as a determinant in survivor support. For instance, a disrupted community will not be able to provide the same level of support as one that is viewed as cohesive (McKay, 2017). Given the benefit of advanced warning as Hurricane Harvey fast approached the Texas coastline, public health leaders and emergency response teams identified designated shelters for specific county residents in an attempt to try to maintain a neighbor-to-neighbor environment. Separated family members were given the opportunity to move to a shelter where they could reunite with family and friends.

Social and economic inequality plays a large part in all areas of life; however, special attention to minority and disadvantaged neighborhoods must be given during the planning process. By most accounts, the poor and disenfranchised live in the less-desirable sections of the city, and the dwellings they occupy are not as resistant to time and natural weather extremes. They may also lack the transportation options of the more affluent during evacuation, thus depending on public transportation. PHNs recognize that many immigrant populations are not only unfamiliar with existing community resources but are reluctant to disclose their immigration status for fear of deportation.

In developing an inclusive community preparedness plan, it is important to become familiar with those community institutions that can meet the mental health needs of a diverse population. Language, and the potential barriers it may present during a disaster response, must be considered as a first step when mounting a field intervention during an event. As part of state and local planning in Texas, colleges and universities have identified volunteers who will act as interpreters for specific ethnic communities. As planning progresses, identify who the cultural brokers are within a community. By establishing solid working relationships with trusted organizations, and various cultural group leaders, PHNs can begin to educate the citizenry about plans, intended response, and community resources well before the beginning of a disastrous event. Invite leaders to participate in all phases of disaster preparedness, response, and recovery operations.

Nursing researchers established standards of practice for cultural competency to guide nurses in their practice across the world to provide "culturally congruent nursing care" (Marion, 2016). These standards are applicable to all nursing disciplines but are especially useful to PHNs whose focus is community and populations at large. Danna, Pierce, Schaubhut, Billingsley, & Bennett (2015) identified education in cultural competency and disaster management to focus on the most vulnerable populations to include: (1) older adults/seniors; (2) obstetrics/perinatal/neonatal; (3) medically needy/terminally ill; (4) children/pediatrics; (5) homeless; (6) individuals with disabilities; (7) individuals living in rural areas; (8) individuals with mental illness; and (9) individuals with limited English proficiency (LEP) (p.140). Evidence-based practice stresses the importance of implementing interventions that have proved successful among diverse populations. In terms of disaster response, although evidence is building within the scope of public health practice, nurse researchers have a fresh opportunity to test interventions used during the events surrounding Hurricane Sandy with a focus on the reduction of disparities in health outcomes among the poorest citizens.

Geoff decides to integrate evidence-based knowledge from his Hurricane Harvey experiences in 2017 into the preparedness certificate curriculum. Based on the multicultural makeup of the displaced population he cared for, he is asking each nurse participant to select two distinct cultural and ethnic groups from within the community he or she serves. What vulnerabilities, hazards, and special needs will you have identified during the community planning process? If an evacuation order is given, how will this message be conveyed to these sectors in the community? Cite specific and special needs these community members may need once transported to a shelter.

DISASTER MANAGEMENT

Disasters have a timeline, often referred to as a life cycle or phases. These include the preimpact phase (before), the impact phase (during), and the postimpact phase (after). Actions taken during these phases will affect the illness, injury, and death that occur following the incident. Although disasters vary significantly, the response to each is similar. All disaster response begins at the local level—all communities must be prepared for emergencies. The disaster management continuum illustrates the essential steps in the process (Fig. 20.2).

Just as there are distinct phases of a disaster, so too are there phases of an emergency management response. These are preparedness, mitigation, response, recovery, and evaluation. It is important to remember that during the management of any disaster, the activities carried out will frequently overlap phases. During a disaster, duties and their associated activities often cross boundaries in order to complete a task at hand.

Preparedness

Disaster preparedness plans are action plans developed in anticipation of disaster scenarios, providing a framework for response to emergency situations. They are proactive planning efforts that provide structure to a disaster response before it happens. In an all-hazards event plan, the response must be a coordinated community effort. This means engaging members of the community in ongoing preparedness activities. Working relationships can be strengthened by formalizing mutual aid agreements with regional health, police, and fire departments; volunteer organizations such as the Red Cross and other local planning groups; healthcare organizations; schools; and state response coordinators. In addition, signing memorandum of understanding (MOUs) with local providers is necessary to assure a supply of food and potable water and other supplies for disaster victims.

To ensure a successful response, steps must be taken before any incident, however minor, occurs. In this process, the risk for a given disaster is assessed, and the potential impact is evaluated. Planning for disasters involves data collection in three areas: (1) Risk Assessment (2) All Hazard Vulnerability Studies; and (3) Federal and State Response Networks. The effectiveness of the disaster plan is only as

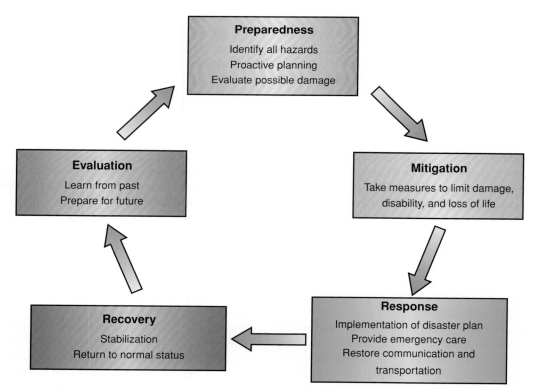

FIGURE 20.2 The disaster management continuum. (Adapted from: Veenema, T. G. [2009]. *Ready RN handbook for disaster nursing and emergency preparedness.* [pp. 3–25]. St. Louis: Mosby Elsevier.)

good as the data that underlie the planning efforts and the assumptions (Veenema, 2013). These studies identify all possible hazards, commonalities of response from the community of interest and appropriate expectations regarding Federal and State Response Networks.

The identification of all existing and potentially dangerous situations before disasters occur is the first step in planning for an effective response.

Risk Assessment

Types and combinations of hazards are unique to a community. They may involve propensity for natural disasters, chemical or radioactive spills, transportation accidents, congregation of large groups of people, and numerous other situations. Different circumstances result in different types of injuries or illness, damage, and disruption of communication and transportation. Gathering historical data about previous disasters are helpful, and proven successful nursing interventions can be noted in the growing practice of evidence-based public health. Aerial photography, satellite imagery, wireless remote sensing devices, and geographic positioning systems (GPS) are tools commonly used in hazard identification. Computer-generated pluming software is a proven means of indicating the direction in which a wind-driven chemical release may head. Once the hazards are identified, the extent of damages, interruption of services, and threats to health can be estimated. This information can be used in designing a community emergency plan.

All Hazards Vulnerability Assessment

In this process, the resources of the community that would reduce the impact of a given hazard should be identified and plans made to strengthen those resources if necessary. Disaster prevention measures may be instituted that involve the removal of identified hazards, relocation of at-risk people away from the hazard area, provision of educational materials, institution of sensors, and development of community early warning systems.

Once the potential hazards are identified, the extent of damages, interruption of services, and threats to health can be estimated. Identifying the commonalities among the potential disasters allows for a more unified approach to planning. Regardless of disaster type, the need to provide shelter for people and their pets, food, water, and healthcare are universal. The extent and type of need will vary by disaster. This information can be used in designing a community emergency plan.

Along with identifying potential unmet needs, it is important to identify those groups who are most likely to be affected in a variety of disaster events. Vulnerability varies according to the type of hazard involved, and people who are most likely to suffer injury, death, or loss of property should be identified for each hazard. In addition, the ability or capacity of the community to respond to the effects of specific disasters should be assessed. Vulnerability analysis predicts who will be affected the most and identifies community resources that are available for a response. To

keep emergency plans up-to-date, population and environment changes need to be documented with changes made to the plan accordingly.

State and Federal Response Networks

When the scope of a disaster extends beyond the capability of local and state governments to respond, the federal government is asked to provide assistance. The **National Response Framework (NRF)**, established by the U.S. Department of Homeland Security (DHS), guides the overall conduct and coordination of all-hazards incident responses. These include all disasters, whether natural, human made, or a result of terrorism, including threats to resources such as information technology and energy sources. The NRF presents a unified response that depends on the mutually supporting capabilities of federal, state, and local resources—all levels of government—working together. Federal leadership responsibilities are outlined in the NRF; however, the states have the primary responsibility for coordinating resources and capabilities and obtaining support from other states and the federal government.

National Incident Management System

The **National incident management system (NIMS)** is a structured, flexible framework that guides the response to disasters of governments at all levels, private companies, and nongovernmental organizations (NGOs). Its goal is to reduce the loss of life, property, and harm to the environment by helping departments and agencies work seamlessly to prepare for, prevent, mitigate, respond to, and recover from the effects of incidents—regardless of cause, size, location, or complexity. This process involves coordination and cooperation between public and private organizations in various emergency management and incident response activities. The NIMS is not an operational incident management or resource allocation plan. It represents a core set of doctrines, concepts, principles, terminology, and organizational processes that enable effective, efficient, and collaborative incident management. (FEMA, 2017)

In the United States, the DHS is the central organization overseeing many different agencies that focus on the safety and security of the nation. Their many responsibilities include border and transportation security; chemical, biologic, and radiologic countermeasures; informational systems and infrastructure protection; and emergency preparedness (DHS, 2017). Federal Emergency Management Administration (FEMA), as the lead agency for emergency management, has divided the states and territories into 10 regions. State, county, tribal, and municipal governments operate independently of the federal agencies in developing programs. Surrounding jurisdictions respond to a disaster as needed; thus, mutual aid agreements should be in place as the planning progresses. If the emergency is determined to be of significant magnitude that overcomes the capabilities of the state and local governments, the Secretary of Homeland Security will initiate the NRF to release federal

20.1 Disaster Preparedness and Management Competencies

- Participate in all aspects of the planning process
  - Contribute to the hazard assessment in the community
  - Conduct vulnerability and risk assessments, especially with special populations
- Identify and locate the agency's emergency response plan
  - Understand the agency's role in responding to emergencies
  - Understand your role in an emergency
  - Ensure that the plan is reviewed and updated frequently
- Describe the communication process in emergency response both within the agency, with the general public, and with personal contacts
- Recognize deviations from the norm that might indicate an emergency and describe appropriate action
- Participate in the development of data, gathering system that addresses morbidity, mortality, mental health, and infectious disease
- Apply creative problem-solving skills and flexible thinking to emergency situations, within the confines of your role
- Identify the limits of your own knowledge, skills, and authority, and referring matters that exceed these limits
- Evaluate the effectiveness of every drill and after-action response

Adapted from Gebbie, K. M., & Qureshi, K. (2002). Emergency and disaster preparedness: Core competencies for nurses. *American Journal of Nursing*, *102*(1), 46–51.

20.2 Comparison of MRC and CERT Groups

The Medical Reserve Corps (MRC) is a community-based program that organizes and utilizes local volunteers for emergency preparedness and response. MRC volunteers include medical and public health professionals such as physicians, nurses, pharmacists, dentists, veterinarians, and epidemiologists. Nonhealth professional volunteers are also included. MRCs are overseen by health departments and receive their funding through the state health departments.

Community Emergency Response Team (CERT) educates and trains professional and lay volunteers on disaster preparedness. Liability protections for CERT volunteers may be found in state and federal volunteer protection acts. Like MRC volunteers, some states have explicitly extended liability protection to CERT volunteers. CERTs are usually overseen by emergency responders such as police and fire departments and receive their funding through FEMA.

resources to local jurisdictions. Health departments and emergency management offices use the NIMS to develop a coordinated response to the disaster.

The role of state government is to supplement and facilitate local efforts before, during, and after incidents. Although the state has a crucial coordination role, local officials have the primary responsibility for community preparedness and response. Local officials are responsible for ensuring public safety and the welfare of people of that jurisdiction. The local emergency manager has the day-to-day authority and responsibility for overseeing emergency management programs and activities. Local hospitals also need to develop an emergency operations plan (EOP) that will guide the activation of resources in the event of either an internal or external disaster. The State Emergency Management Agency works closely with FEMA to assure preparation and planning have occurred on a local and state level.

Using the comprehensive data gathered from the All Hazard Vulnerability and Risk Assessments, and knowledge of Federal and State Response Networks, the probability of adverse health effects due to a specific disaster can be calculated. This is often represented as a low, medium, or high risk.

Point-of-Distribution Plans

A **point of distribution (POD) or Emergency Dispensing Site (EDS)** is a centralized location where the public picks up emergency supplies, including food, water, and medications (if necessary), following a disaster. The plan details the staffing required and procedures to be followed in the setup and deactivation of a POD/EDS.

Local departments of public health determine the need, the staffing, and the location of the POD, as well as the commodities that are to be distributed. FEMA has developed training programs to assist in planning for the execution and subsequent deactivation of PODs as a part of disaster relief efforts. This training helps states and communities coordinate with federal and nongovernmental groups as they provide much needed supplies to the public in a timely and consistent manner during and after a disaster event.

Local groups that are often instrumental in developing and running drills for EDSs or PODs are the MRC or CERT. Communities may have either or both of these groups (Box 20.2).

MRC AND CERT GROUPS

At the completion of the plan, a common way to test its relevance is through a **Table Top Exercise (TTX)** and actual drills to prepare participants for their roles and to identify gaps and elements in the plan that need revision. The TTX involves key personnel discussing simulated scenarios in an informal setting. It is used to assess plans, policies, and procedures and resolve issues before an actual disaster occurs.

Planning and practicing for a crisis is the foundation for successful communication and response. A well-trained frontline response team reduces the impact of an event. **Human simulation training** (HST) with computerized models, such as those Geoff used in the training program, are increasingly used in medical and nursing education. With this technology, trainees are assisted in applying the techniques learned in the classroom laboratory to actual situations.

During actual drills, a successful exercise using **simulation** is one in which weaknesses, mistakes, and ineffective plans are exposed. As a practice event, the opportunity to make corrections, improve certain skills, or revise disaster response plans should also be seen as a means to become a competent responder and leader. Nonclinical responders can benefit from inclusion in a simulation experience with nurses. A clearer understanding of the importance of the role of the nurse in an emergency event help the multidisciplinary team build competency and confidence. Frequent, specific-scenario–formulated training prepares the public health nurse responder to take the lead in emergency events.

Ultimately, the key starting points for emergency preparedness rest with individual people, often within households. People can contribute by reducing hazards in and around their homes, preparing emergency supply kits and household emergency plans, and monitoring emergency communications carefully. Community education regarding the contents of an emergency supply kit is an important role of the PHN. In addition to changes in public policy, educating the community regarding preparation is essential. Educating citizens on what to have in an emergency kit for themselves and their pets can help alleviate the stress of mandatory evacuations. (Box 20.3)

Geoff prepares an outline of disaster preparedness planning topics that will be included in the certification program. What topics does he choose?

In addition, he plans an emergency exercise for the end of the program. What type of geographic and demographic characteristics might have an effect on program content?

20.3 Basic Emergencies Supplies

Recommended items to include in a basic emergency supply kit:

Water, 1 gallon of water per person per day for at least 3 days, for drinking and sanitation

Food, at least a 3-day supply of nonperishable food

Battery-powered or hand crank radio and a NOAA weather radio with tone alert and extra batteries for both

Flashlight and extra batteries

First aid kit

Whistle to signal for help

Dust mask, to help filter contaminated air and plastic sheeting and duct tape to shelter-in-place

Moist towelettes, garbage bags, and plastic ties for personal sanitation

Wrench or pliers to turn off utilities

Can opener for food (if kit contains canned food)

Local map

Practice Point

An ongoing community assessment process contributes to the development and revision of an effective disaster plan.

Mitigation

Mitigation is a prevention process with two components. First, mitigation is an effort to prevent identified risks from causing a disaster. By focusing on implementation of preventive measures for reducing and eliminating identified risks before the event occurs, mitigation becomes a cost-effective primary prevention. Structural mitigation involves creation or removal of structures or alteration of the environment to remove or modify risks. The upgrading of building codes after Hurricane Andrew in Florida in 1992 resulted in decreased structural damage during Hurricane Irma in 2017. Another example is the installation of a generator to be used during a power failure. Nonstructural mitigation includes disaster training for healthcare personnel, the establishment of emergency evacuation regulations, land use planning, legislation, and insurance.

Second, mitigation involves efforts to lessen the impact of a disaster by initiating measures to limit damage, disease, disability, and loss of life among the members of a community (tertiary prevention). In this case, mitigation refers to a broad range of activities that are only accomplished satisfactorily by planning prior to the event. An example is the trimming of trees near power lines to prevent loss of power during an incident

Personal Protective Equipment

Personal protective equipment (PPE) has been used in healthcare for a century. PPE primarily refers to the use of respiratory equipment as well as gloves, gown, and/or goggles. The purpose of PPE is to prevent the transfer of the hazardous agent from the victim or the environment to healthcare practitioners. The type of agent present determines the kind of PPE required. In general, biologic, chemical, and radiologic exposures occur by breathing contaminated air, dermal contact, and/or by eating or drinking adulterated products. Nurses who have been prepared as active response team members are often issued "Go Kits" that contain various useful items, such as gloves, surgical masks, N95 masks, goggles, pencils and paper, and large trash bags. A fit-tested respirator also may be included.

The Occupational Safety and Health Administration (OSHA) has outlined four levels of personal protection and the types of equipment that should be worn in various emergency situations (Table 20.1). The agent involved and the risk of exposure are the primary determinants of the level of PPE required. If PPE is to be used, a PPE program should be implemented that addresses the hazards present; the selection, maintenance, and use of PPE; the training of employees; and monitoring of the program to ensure its

TABLE 20.1 Levels for Personal Protection in Disasters: A, B, C, and D

Level of Protection	Equipment
Level A Highest protection for respiratory tract, skin, eyes, and mucous membrane protection	SCBA, fully encapsulated water- and vapor-proof suit with a cooling system, boots, gloves, hard hat, and a two-way communication device
Level B Highest protection for respiratory tract; skin, and eye-splash resistant protection	SCBA, liquid splash-resistant clothing, hood, gloves, hard hat, boots, two-way communication device
Level C Same level of protection for skin and eyes as level B, air-purifying system for respiratory tract	Full face, air-purifying respirator rather than SCBA, liquid splash-resistant clothing, hood, gloves, hard hat, boots, two-way communication device
Level D Standard work protection from splashes, minimal skin protection, no respiratory protection	Cover suits, safety glasses, gloves, boots, and face shield

SCBA, self-contained breathing apparatus.
Occupational Safety and Health Administration Standards—29-CFR Standard number 1910.132 Personal Protective Equipment. Retrieved from http://www.osha.gov.

ongoing effectiveness. Just-in-time training (JITT) videos are available for PPE training purposes.

> ### Practice Point
>
> To ensure your safety during an emergency event, learn where PPE is located in your facility and how to use and dispose of it properly. Include your local or county HAZMAT unit at a yearly in-service on proper use of equipment.

> ### Practice Point
>
> Disasters occur locally, but their impact can extend globally.

Response

All response begins at the local level, where the disaster management plan is implemented and responders are deployed. This mobilization is multidisciplinary, and the first people on the scene will more than likely be law enforcement, fire, and ambulance crews. Reaching the victims and beginning the triaging process is essential to prevent loss of life. Response also refers to minimizing, improvising, and restoring transportation and communication systems, as well as providing food, water, and shelter to those affected. The disaster plans that are most effective are clear, easy to understand, use a structured **incident command system (ICS)**, and are frequently practiced and updated to ensure a coordinated, timely response.

Disaster response can involve fear of the unknown and the daunting prospect of serving entire communities during a very difficult time. However, by their nature, all types of disasters do not occur regularly. This is an opportunity for nurses to embrace the opportunity to test skills, practice disaster plans, and assert themselves as key members of state, regional, county, and local response organizations.

Incident Command System

When a disaster occurs, there is an immediate need for organization and management at the scene of the incident. The ICS is an on-site, flexible, all-hazards system that provides a set of personnel, policies, procedures, facilities, and equipment integrated into a common organizational structure that is designed to improve emergency response operations of all types, sizes, and complexities.

The ICS designates common titles and roles to be used in all organizations and agencies that respond to disasters. It organizes emergency response in five major functional areas: command, planning, operations, logistics, and finance and administration (Fig. 20.4). These temporary management hierarchies control funds, personnel, facilities, equipment, and communications until the requirement for management and operations no longer exists. Operations can be expanded or contracted as required. Participants are trained and approved by legitimate authorities before incidents occur so that personnel from a wide variety of agencies, jurisdictions, and backgrounds can combine rapidly into a common management structure using common terminology. The result is a unified, centrally authorized, legitimate, cost-effective emergency organization that facilitates communication and coordination of response efforts. Nurses and other healthcare professionals are encouraged to become a part of their local ICS. Basic level courses (ICS 100–200) are available online at the FEMA website.

Most countries have national agencies that oversee response in that country. Western Europe, India, Russia, the United Kingdom, Australia, and Canada refer to disaster phases as outlined above. New Zealand uses different terminology; disaster phases are known as the four Rs (reduction [mitigation], readiness [preparedness], response, and recovery).

Geoff decides that he wants to incorporate ICS into the practice sessions. How could he do this?

Practice Point

Participate in your local multidisciplinary ICS network as a part of your disaster response activities.

Field Triage

When a **mass casualty incident** occurs, rapid assessment and treatment of the victims is the utmost priority. On a disaster site, the process of field triage identifies and assesses those people who need medical care and prioritizes their needs. Triaging soldiers on the battlefield has been in practice for quite some time. In fact, field disaster response is based on evidence

FIGURE 20.3 FEMA response to Hurricane Harvey. Houston, Texas, September 6, 2017—Two volunteers pitch cardboard boxes of donated goods as they stack food, clothing, and cleaning supplies for distribution to Hurricane Harvey survivors. (*Source:* Retrieved October 23, 2017, from https://www.fema.gov/media-library/assets/images/141121. Photo by Christopher Mardorf/FEMA.)

gained by measuring successful outcomes during combat. Triage is used in mass casualty situations and in any disaster event. The victims are assessed by their presenting condition and are then color coded as to the severity of the case. A triage tag, colored tape, or ribbon is placed on each injured person after being prioritized to indicate status (Fig. 20.3; Table 20.2).

FIGURE 20.4 Incident command structure. (*Source:* Adapted from: Federal Emergency Management Agency. [2008]. National incident management system. Retrieved from http://www.fema.gov/pdf/emergency/nims/NIMS_core.pdf.)

TABLE 20.2	Color Coding for Prehospital Triage	
Red	Critical	Unstable, requiring immediate intervention
Yellow	Urgent	Stable, but may deteriorate
Green	Delayed	Injured or ill but stable and not likely to deteriorate (walking wounded)
Black	Expectant	Dead or nonsalvageable given available resources

Basic triage and rapid treatment (START) is a simple, prehospital triage system that was developed in California to assist emergency responders for use in earthquakes. Evidence based and field proven, the system separates injured people into four groups according to the severity of their injuries or illnesses (Box 20.4).

During a mass casualty incident, wherever it may occur, many different local, national, and international agencies work together in the initial rescue phase. These agencies must be able to communicate information, especially critical information about the condition of victims, effectively. With the increase of international disasters, naturally occurring and otherwise, preparedness professionals have called for a global standardized triage system with well-defined categories and instructions. This universal triage classification system includes a standardized approach to chemical, biologic, and radiologic agents as well as injuries sustained from an explosion that provides prompt information to medical providers, increasing their ability to care for victims promptly and efficiently.

Field triage is an essential topic for the nurses in the disaster management training program. What are the essential components of field triage? How does Geoff use this information in planning specific hands-on experiences?

Practice Point

Identify yourself as a nurse during an event. This helps establish your credibility as a competent responder and establishes you as part of the multidisciplinary emergency response team.

20.4 Simple Triage and Rapid Triage: The START Model

0 Those who have died
1 Injured, requiring immediate transfer
2 Injured, who can wait to be transferred
3 Injured, with minor less urgent needs

Practice Point

Become familiar with the POD/EDS plan for your facility and for your community. Make sure POD/EDS location agreements are current.

Mental Health Issues

Mental health issues during the response phase can be serious and of a permanent nature. Those especially vulnerable include the elderly and children. The Substance Abuse and Mental Health Agency (SAMSA) 2017 provides guidelines for working with victims of disasters as well as resources for those needing additional assistance. (Box 20.5)

Recovery

The recovery phase begins as the disaster ends. Many of the factors that may continue into the recovery phase and create challenges for victims include:

- Continuing death, chronic illness, and/or disability
- Population shift if recovery is prolonged
- Contamination of food and water supplies, with an increased risk of infectious diseases

20.5 Tips for Communicating With Survivors

1. Clearly identify yourself and your role.
2. Communicate calmly. Make eye contact and use an open posture (avoid crossing your arms or legs, lean forward, and stand or sit directly facing the person or group).
3. Communicate warmth. Express empathy, use a soft tone and welcoming gestures, and listen carefully.
4. Speak slowly. Repeat yourself, if necessary.
5. Do not use euphemisms. For example, state very clearly that their loved one has died or is missing.
6. Be factual and gentle and do not engage in speculation or make broad statements like "everything will be ok."
7. Acknowledge the emotions of those who are suffering. Speak to the person with respect.
8. Use concrete questions to help the person focus. Use closed-ended questions—questions the person can answer with a yes or a no, or by providing specific information—and explain why you are asking the question.
9. Listen and allow for emotional expressions or crying without interruption.
10. Do not answer questions outside of your expertise. Refer people to appropriate experts.
11. Avoid using examples from your own life, and keep the focus on those currently suffering (SAMSA, 2017).
12. Look for cues in body language, and ask if they would like to be left alone.
13. Suggest the survivor contact support resources, such as family members, medical professionals, or religious leaders.

- Collapse of local and regional healthcare access
- Increased need to provide mental health services: "psychological first aid" for disaster victims and responders

The timeline for recovery varies widely, depending upon the type and extent of the disaster. The initiation of stress debriefing and mental health services is essential in most cases. However, recovery may also involve rebuilding damaged buildings, transportation systems, and communication systems, as well as the relocation of those affected by the disaster. Communities that perform a hazard risk assessment to predict the effects of disasters on a community, and have a targeted disaster plan in place, are better prepared to address recovery issues.

Although normal operations may return, critical incident stress debriefing for staff members is important. Responders may have been exposed to traumatic situations or worked for lengths of time that left them exhausted. (Spenser & Spellman, 2013).

The impact of long term mental health issues after a disaster are just beginning to be recognized. Several studies show rates of PTSD after Hurricane Katrina as high as 62.5% among preschool children directly affected by the storm and a 50% occurrence among some groups of adults, such as female caregivers and parents of affected children. (Lamberg, 2008; Schroeder, 2017). Persons with a history of mental illness are also more likely to suffer from mental health issues after a disaster. Additional psychological health competencies have been developed due to the recognition of the long-term effects of experiencing a disaster for victims and responders (Box 20.6).

Documentation During a Disaster

During an emergency event, it is not possible or expected that normal documentation standards and protocols will be maintained. When responding to an emergency, the time, place, general assessment of the field, and the name of the Incident Commander should be noted. Events move quickly, and documentation of observations is important. However, it is not possible to document all the information that is normally required, such as victims' names. Every event is organized differently. For example, during a possible anthrax "white powder" site investigation, there were enough nurses so that one could be assigned to be the site scribe. This nurse circulated among responders and took notations as reported to her. She became the primary contact for the medical care director, an absolute necessity to obtain an accurate clinical report

 Geoff requires a plan for documentation of events during the hands-on practice sessions. What does he include and how does he plan to implement documentation in the practice sessions?

Practice Point

Time is a factor in a disaster. Note unusual incidents and appropriate essential observations and report immediately.

Evaluation

Evaluation is the foundation for evidence-based disaster response. By analyzing specific aspects of the plan and assessing the effectiveness of the plan in action, future planning efforts are enhanced. All agencies, organizations, and personnel who were involved in the disaster response should take part in the evaluation. An evaluation meeting takes place during the recovery phase immediately after the incident, eliciting observations and suggestions from participants. This provides valuable information for revisions of the Emergency Plan. Often referred to as a "hot wash" session, it is conducted while everything is fresh in one's mind, so as to not be forgotten. The more formal report, referred to as an **After Action Report** (AAR) provides a detailed list of strengths and weaknesses, successes and failures, and suggestions for improvement in future responses.

ROLES OF NURSES IN DISASTER MANAGEMENT

The ability of nurses to be calm, creative, and responsive to emergency situations is an asset, and it is imperative that roles be clearly articulated. PHNs are experts in providing health education for the various populations in a community setting. They can be proactive in providing information and developing educational materials for dissemination to an anxious public, especially for disasters that can be anticipated, such as hurricanes or tornadoes.

For most nurses, disaster preparedness planning is usually associated with the workplace. One of the first questions a nurse may ask is, "What is my role if an emergency occurs"? Nurses should be familiar with the EOP in their workplace and understand how their practice may change during an emergency or disaster. For example, a long-term care facility may become a shelter, or nurses in home healthcare agencies may be expected to be first responders. In many organizations, the nursing staff would be deployed by the operations officer. They may also take part in planning, logistics, or finance and administration. A summary of nursing competencies for disaster planning and management is outlined in Box 20.7. In addition, the Association of Community Health Nursing Educators (ACHNE) (2008) has developed competencies for entry-level nurses in response to mass casualty incidents; these competencies can be found online (See Box 20.7).

Also, some normal workplace activities will likely continue. Knowing in advance exactly what is expected of the healthcare facility during an emergency or disaster gives all staff members the opportunity to acquire the pertinent knowledge and to practice necessary skills beforehand. Today, the majority of healthcare facilities, health departments, and private industry include emergency preparedness

information as part of the orientation process for new employees. They should know the communication structure inherent in the ICS that has been established for the organization.

Public Health Nurses as First Responders

Public health nursing practice focuses on the provision of comprehensive public health services to ensure that community members have access to preventive care, immunizations, safe food and water, and assistance with services that may go beyond medical needs. An extensive knowledge of the community is the foundation for these services. Therefore, the PHN's expertise is valuable in all phases of the disaster management continuum, whether anticipating potential emergencies, developing appropriate plans, building system-wide partnerships, practicing implementation of disaster management plans and skills on a regular basis, or evaluating outcomes. By increasing clinical knowledge and skill sets associated with specific biologic, chemical, radiologic and explosive agents, PHNs are better prepared to apply their upgraded proficiencies in the field. The responsibilities of PHNs in disaster management are outlined in see Box 20.2. Even though there will be clutter, clamor, and confusion during a disaster, PHNs are not expected to function as critical care nurses in a disaster setting.

Evidence for Practice

Although public health nurses assume the lead in conducting disease surveillance activities in daily practice, their roles during a disaster response have become clearer. Working closely with members of multidisciplinary response and planning teams has secured the public health nurse's position on the disaster team. Clinical skills aside, general management skills possessed by public health nurses are a value to the team.

20.7 Responsibilities of Public Health Nurses in Disaster Management

- Assess the needs of the community as the events unfold
- Conduct surveillance for communicable disease and unmet needs
- Prevent and control the spread of disease
- Maintain communication channels to ensure accurate dissemination of information to colleagues and the public
- Organize and manage points of distribution centers and mass immunization sites as required
- Provide on-site triage as needed
- Manage behavioral responses to stress
- Ensure the health and safety of self, colleagues, and the public
- Document events and interventions

"Well-prepared PHNs bring leadership and management expertise to each phase of disaster cycle. As an integral part of the healthcare system infrastructure within their community and jurisdictions, PHNs have established linkages to community health–related networks and resources that are vital to developing disaster preparedness plans and policies at local, regional, state, and national levels. These connections between PHNs and community partners must occur in order to address complex issues such as providing mass care during the chaos of a disaster, prioritizing scarce resources, supervising spontaneous volunteers and unlicensed healthcare workers, identifying and planning for the care of populations with functional and access needs, as well as developing and maintaining effective systems of volunteers prepared to assist prior to the incident. PHNs also can use their networks

20.8 Selected Preparedness Goals from *Healthy People 2020*

PREP-1 (Developmental) Reduce the time necessary to issue official information to the public about a public health emergency

PREP-2 Reduce the time necessary to activate designated personnel in response to a public health emergency

PREP-4 Reduce the time for state public health agencies to establish after action reports and improvement plans following responses to public health emergencies and exercises

PREP-5 Increase the percentage of school districts that require schools to include specific topics in their crisis preparedness, response, and recovery plans

PREP-6 (Developmental) Increase the proportion of parents and/or guardians aware of the emergency or evacuation plan in their child(ren)'s school including the evacuation location and how to get information about the child in the event of a disaster

PREP-7 Increase the proportion of adults residing with children attending school who have an emergency plan and have household discussions of that emergency plan

PREP-8 (Developmental) Increase the proportion of adults who engage in preparedness activities for a widespread outbreak of a contagious disease after recently receiving preparedness information on outbreaks

PREP-16 Increase the percentage of Medical Reserve Corps units who participate in preparedness and public health activities

PREP-18 (Developmental) Increase the membership and diversity of HPP-funded healthcare coalitions that are engaged in collaborative emergency preparedness planning and response

PREP-20 Increase in measures to protect children during disasters

HP2020 (2017) *Preparedness Goals.* Retrieved on October 9, 2017, from https://www.healthypeople.gov/2020/topics-objectives/topic/preparedness/objectives.

across regional and state boundaries to achieve consistency in the protocols, practice standards, and operational guidelines prior to the disaster incident" (APHN, 2014, p. 11).

Outcomes and data are identified in *Healthy People 2020* related to Preparedness (Box 20.8). Several of the activities and tools identified in the disaster management continuum examined are identified, including MRCs.

20.9 What You Can Do Immediately to Be Prepared

1. Join your local MRC or CERT
2. Familiarize yourself with your community's Emergency Response Plan
3. Take the ICS Training online
4. Prepare your personal emergency kit evacuation kit (https://www.ready.gov/build-a-kit https://www.ready.gov/build-a-kit).

BIOTERRORISM

A bioterrorism event involves the intentional release of viruses, bacteria, fungi, or toxins from living organisms into the environment for the purposes of causing illness or death. Although agents may result in familiar diseases, someone intent on harming others can engineer agents to make them more deadly or to extend their life on a variety of surfaces. Biologic agents are air- or waterborne and are inhaled or ingested (Centers for Disease Control and Prevention, 2017a). For terrorists, there are some distinct advantages to using biologic versus chemical agents. The incubation periods of live agents afford the terrorist time to leave the scene of the crime before detection, whereas releases of chemicals are evident almost immediately, regardless of the circumstances. However, the use of these agents requires sophisticated expertise to weaponize resulting in long and potentially dangerous preparation times. Box 20.10 presents the advantages of biologic agents as weapons.

> How do you defeat terrorism? Don't be terrorized.
> **Salman Rushdie**

History of Bioterrorism

The world has become aware that bioterrorism is not a new tactic. History will reveal that as early as 1346, the Tartar army hurled corpses of plague victims over the walls of Caffa, a seaport on the Crimean coast, and 400 years later, Russians used the same tactic against Sweden. Using infected people as "weapons" may have contributed to the spread of plague across Europe in the 14th century. People who became victims ultimately became weapons themselves; a smallpox or plague victim approaching a village must have been a fearsome sight. Later, during the Pontiac Rebellion in 1763, the British army provided the Delaware Indians with blankets and handkerchiefs from a smallpox hospital (Barras & Greub, 2014).

20.10 Advantages of Biologics as Weapons

- Infectious via aerosol
- Organisms fairly stable in the environment
- Civilian populations are susceptible
- High morbidity and mortality rates
- Person-to-person transmission (smallpox, plague, viral hemorrhagic fever)
- Difficult to diagnose and/or treat
- Easy to obtain
- Inexpensive to produce
- Potential for dissemination over large geographic area
- Creates panic
- Can overwhelm medical services
- Perpetrators escape easily
- Previous development of organisms for biologic weapons

The word *terrorism* was first used in 1795 during the French Revolution, when the "reign of terror" was unfolding on the streets and hillsides of France. During World War I, Germany used biologic agents to infect livestock hindering troop movement. In the United States, the development of biologic warfare agents began in 1942, under President Franklin D. Roosevelt, and was not discontinued until the late 1960s. The former Soviet Union began a massive program to develop biologic weapons in the 1970s. In 1979, there was an accidental release of anthrax at a Soviet military facility, resulting in 68 deaths, and it is believed that this ultimately led to the end of the program.

Since the 1990s, worldwide there have been 19 reported bioterrorism attacks, killing approximately 1,900 and injuring over 8,500. Civilians were the most common target, followed by soldiers, prisoners of war, and government officials (Johnston, 2016). As more nations have acquired, or are seeking to acquire, biologic weapons, there are concerns that individual terrorists or terrorist groups may acquire the technologies and expertise to use these agents. **Weaponized** forms of some agents have been used against civilian populations as was the case when anthrax-contaminated mail was circulated in New Jersey, New York, and Washington, DC. Biologic agents may be used for an isolated assassination or to cause the injury or death of thousands of people. Environmental contamination could be a long-term threat.

An eye for an eye, and the whole world would be blind.
Khalil Gibran

Categories of Bioterrorism Agents

The CDC (2017a) has divided biologic agents into three categories (Box 20.12: A, B, and C). The high-priority agents in category A include organisms that pose a risk to national security. These agents: (1) can be easily disseminated or transmitted from person to person; (2) result in high mortality; (3) have the potential for major public health impact; (4) might cause public panic and social disruption; and (5) require special action for public health preparedness. "Category A" agents are discussed in the following section.

Detection of a Bioterrorism Event

Early detection of a biologic event is often difficult. The first recognition of a bioterrorism event may result from routine surveillance activities. However, a single case or a few cases of bioterrorism-related disease may not be identified. Surveillance for infectious diseases is a continual process, conducted on an everyday basis by clinicians and laboratory staff. All personnel in any healthcare-related activity should be aware of the diseases that may be associated with bioterrorism. In actuality, all people should be involved in reporting unusual events or illnesses to the local public health department. PHNs are important resources in

collecting and analyzing symptoms before a diagnosis is made. By identifying unusual spikes in disease, deliberate biologic attacks will be revealed in a timely manner. PHNs also use their system-wide relationships with their communities to track illness. Box 20.11 presents epidemiologic clues indicating that a deliberate biologic attack may have occurred.

20.11 Epidemiologic Clues of a Bioterrorism Attack

1. Single case of disease caused by an uncommon agent (e.g., glanders, smallpox, viral hemorrhagic fever, inhalational, or cutaneous anthrax) without adequate epidemiologic explanation
2. Unusual, atypical, genetically engineered, or antiquated strain of an agent (or antibiotic-resistance pattern)
3. Higher morbidity and mortality in association with a common disease or syndrome or failure of such patients to respond to usual therapy
4. Unusual disease presentation (e.g., inhalational anthrax or pneumonic plague)
5. Disease with an unusual geographic or seasonal distribution (e.g., tularemia in a nonendemic area, influenza in the summer)
6. Stable endemic disease with an unexplained increase in incidence (e.g., tularemia, plague)
7. Atypical disease transmission through aerosols, food, or water, in a mode suggesting deliberate sabotage (i.e., no other possible physical explanation)
8. No illness in persons who are not exposed to common ventilation systems (have separate closed ventilation systems) when illness is seen in persons in close proximity who have a common ventilation system
9. Several unusual or unexplained diseases coexisting in the same patient without any other explanation
10. Unusual illness that affects a large, disparate population (e.g., respiratory disease in a large population may suggest exposure to an inhalational pathogen or chemical agent)
11. Illness that is unusual (or atypical) for a given population or age group (e.g., outbreak of measles-like rash in adults)
12. Unusual pattern of death or illness among animals, (which may be unexplained or attributed to an agent of bioterrorism) that precedes or accompanies illness or death in humans
13. Unusual pattern of death or illness among humans, (which may be unexplained or attributed to an agent of bioterrorism) that precedes or accompanies illness or death in animals
14. Ill persons who seek treatment at about the same time (point source with compressed epidemic curve)
15. Similar genetic type among agents isolated from temporally or spatially distinct sources
16. Simultaneous clusters of similar illness in noncontiguous areas, domestic or foreign
17. Large numbers of cases of unexplained diseases or deaths

Source: Treadwell, T., Koo, D., Kuker, K., & Khan, A. S. (2003). Epidemiological clues to bioterrorism. *Public Health Reports, 118*(2), 92–98.

Practice Point

Report higher-than-normal cases of infectious disease, unusual occurrences, and clusters of illnesses to the local department of public health.

Bioterrorism Agents

Anthrax

Anthrax results from infection with spore-forming bacillus bacteria (*Bacillus anthracis*) that occur naturally in the soil. The resulting noncontagious acute infectious disease occurs primarily in cattle and sheep. Contact with infected animals or contaminated animal products may lead to infection in humans. In the past, anthrax, considered a wool sorter's disease, was prevalent among tanners. Cutaneous anthrax occurs from inoculation of spores under the skin, gastrointestinal and oropharyngeal anthrax occurs from ingesting contaminated meat, and inhalation anthrax occurs from spores entering the respiratory tract while breathing (Table 20.3). Without swift diagnosis and treatment, inhalational anthrax is usually fatal in approximately 90% of the cases. In 2001, weaponized anthrax spores were sent through the U.S. postal system, resulting in 22 cases and 5 deaths.

Once infection has been diagnosed, antibiotic treatment usually runs a 60-day course. Researchers have developed a protective vaccine against anthrax. Military personnel and people at high risk, such as workers in research laboratories who handle anthrax bacteria routinely or those who work with imported animal hides or furs from areas where standards are insufficient to prevent exposure, are most likely to receive the vaccine.

Postexposure prophylaxis, which combines 60 days of antibiotics plus three doses of vaccine, is effective in preventing anthrax disease from occurring after an exposure. In

20.12 Categories of Bioterrorism Agents

Category A Agents

- Pose the greatest risk to the public because they:
  Spread easily
  Result in a high mortality rate
  Cause public panic
  May affect national security
  Require special training and response and may be unfamiliar to the responding community
  Easy to obtain and "weaponize"
  Can overwhelm existing medical resources
- High-priority agents include organisms that pose a risk to national security because they:
  - Can be easily disseminated or transmitted from person to person
  - Result in high mortality rates and have the
  - potential for major public health impact
  - Might cause public panic and social disruption
  - Require special action for public health preparedness

Agents/diseases include the following:

- Anthrax (*Bacillus anthracis*)
- Botulism (*Clostridium botulinum* toxin)
- Plague (*Yersinia pestis*)
- Smallpox (variola major)
- Tularemia (*Francisella tularensis*)
- Viral hemorrhagic fevers (filoviruses [e.g., Ebola, Marburg] and arenaviruses [e.g., Lassa, Machupo]

Category B Agents

Pose less of a threat to the public. However, they are a danger because:

- They are easily available
- Can be reproduced and disseminated easily

- Surveillance and tracking will still require an intense response
- Mortality, though lower than classified "A" agents, still pose a serious public health threat

Agents/diseases include the following:

- Brucellosis (*Brucella* species)
- Epsilon toxin of *Clostridium perfringens*
- Food safety threats (e.g., *Salmonella* species, *Escherichia coli* O157:H7, *Shigella*)
- Glanders (*Burkholderia mallei*)
- Melioidosis (*Burkholderia pseudomallei*)
- Psittacosis (*Chlamydia psittaci*)
- Q fever (*Coxiella burnetii*)
- Ricin toxin from *Ricinus communis* (castor beans)
- Staphylococcal enterotoxin B
- Typhus fever (*Rickettsia prowazekii*)
- Viral encephalitis (alphaviru ses [e.g., Venezuelan equine encephalitis, Eastern equine encephalitis, Western equine encephalitis])
- Water safety threats (e.g., *Vibrio cholerae, Cryptosporidium parvum*)

Category C Agents

Include emerging pathogens and share these attributes:

- They are easily engineered for mass production and dissemination
- Their potential for high morbidity and mortality rates is significant
- Diseases include the following:

Emerging infectious diseases

- Nipah virus
- Hanta virus
- Multiple drug–resistant infectious diseases

From National Center for Environmental Health (NCEH). Retrieved from http://www.cdc.gov/nceh/; Agency for Toxic Substances and Disease Registry (ATSDR). Retrieved from http://www.atsdr.cdc.gov/; Coordinating Center for Environmental Health and Injury Prevention (CCEHIP). Retrieved from http://www.cdc.gov/about/organization/ccehip.htm.

TABLE 20.3 Bioterrorism Agents

Anthrax

Agent	*Bacillus anthracis*
	Aerobic, spore-forming bacterium
Forms of disease/systems affected	Cutaneous
	Inhalational
	Gastrointestinal
	Oropharyngeal
Transmission	Skin: direct contact with spores
	Respiratory: inhalation of aerosolized spores
	Gastrointestinal: ingestion of undercooked meat of infected animals
	No person-to-person spread
Reporting	Report suspected cases to local/state health departments
Incubation	1–7 days
Signs and symptoms	Fever, fatigue, body aches
	Inhalational: cough, chest pain, dyspnea
	Gastrointestinal: nausea, bloody diarrhea
	Cutaneous: necrotic ulcer, edema
Laboratory	Serology
	Ulcer exudate
Treatment	Ciprofloxacin or doxycycline
	Additional antimicrobials for 60 days
Postexposure prophylaxis	Ciprofloxacin or doxycycline
Mortality	High (80–90%), inhalational form

Botulism

Agent	Toxin produced by *Clostridium botulinum*
	Spore-forming bacterium found in soil and contaminated food
Forms of disease/systems affected	Neuroparalytic illness
	Foodborne ingestion of preformed toxin
	Infant ingestion of soil-producing toxin in gastrointestinal tract
	Wound infection by toxin
Transmission	Not spread from person to person
Reporting	Report suspected case to local/state health department
Incubation	12–72 hours
Signs and symptoms	Difficulty swallowing, speaking
	Double or blurred vision, dilated pupils
	Constipation (infant botulism)
	Descending flaccid paralysis
Laboratory	Stool, vomitus, suspect food samples
Treatment	Prompt diagnosis
	Antitoxin, ventilator support
Postexposure prophylaxis	None
Mortality	Low

Plague

Agent	Bacterium *Yersinia pestis*
	Found in rodents and their fleas; found throughout the world
Forms of disease/systems affected	Pneumonic (lungs)
	Bubonic (lymph glands)
	Septicemic (blood)
Transmission	Pneumonic: inhalation of aerosolized spores; spread person to person
	Bubonic: bite by an infected flea; not spread person to person
	Septicemic: multiplication of bacteria in blood; not spread person to person

Reporting	Report suspected cases to local/state health department
Incubation	1–6 days
Signs and symptoms	Pneumonic: chest pain, dyspnea, hemoptysis, sepsis, respiratory shock
	Bubonic: tender, swollen lymph glands (buboes), bacteremia, fever
	Septicemic: fever, bacteremia, sepsis
Laboratory	Blood, sputum, bubo culture
Treatment	Streptomycin, gentamicin, tetracyclines
Postexposure prophylaxis	Ciprofloxacin or doxycycline
Mortality	High (pneumonic) if untreated within 24 hours
Smallpox	
Agent	Smallpox virus
Systems affected	General viral infectious disease
Transmission	Person to person, aerosolized spread
	Contact with infected body fluids
Reporting	Declared eliminated by World Health Organization in 1980; one confirmed case constitutes an outbreak. Report case to local/state health departments
Incubation	7–12 days (12-day average)
Signs and symptoms	Influenza-like, high fever, body aches
	Early rash, raised bumps (most contagious)
	Pustular rash, raised firm bumps (contagious)
	Pustules with scab formation (contagious)
	Resolving scabs (contagious)
	Scabs resolved (noncontagious)
Laboratory	Pharyngeal or nasal swab
	Scab examination
	Serology
Treatment	Supportive intravenous therapy
	Antibiotics for secondary infections
Postexposure prophylaxis	Smallpox vaccine within 4 days of exposure
Mortality	Moderate (20–40%), unvaccinated
Tularemia	
Agent	*Francisella tularensis*
	Found in rodents, rabbits, hares (also known as rabbit fever)
	Pulmonary
Forms of disease/systems affected	Cutaneous
	Gastrointestinal
Transmission	Not spread person to person
	Cutaneous
	Gastrointestinal
	Inhalational
Reporting	Report cases to local/state health departments
Incubation	3–4 days average (up to 14)
Signs and symptoms	Fever, chills, body aches
	Dry cough
	Joint pain
	Ulcers on skin and mouth
Laboratory	Sputum, blood cultures
Treatment	Streptomycin, gentamicin
Postexposure prophylaxis	Ciprofloxacin or doxycycline
Mortality	Low, 5–15%, untreated

(Continued)

TABLE 20.3 Bioterrorism Agents *(Continued)*

Viral hemorrhagic fevers (VHFs)

Agent	Highly contagious virus; Ebola, Marburg, Lassa fever, and arenaviruses
Systems affected	General viral infectious disease
	Gastrointestinal
	Cutaneous
	Cardiovascular
Transmission	Field rodents, arthropod ticks
	Vectors not known for Ebola, Marburg
	Person-to-person spread greatest as disease progresses
Reporting	Report suspected cases to local/state health departments
Incubation	2–21 days, agent dependent
Signs and symptoms	High fever, headache, body ache
	Bloody diarrhea, mucous membrane hemorrhage
	Shock, circulatory collapse
Laboratory	Serology
Treatment	Ribavirin for Lassa fever
	Supportive therapy for other VHFs
Postexposure prophylaxis	None
Mortality	High
	80–90% Ebola-Zaire
	50–60% Ebola-Sudan
	Variable for other VHFs

an attack, PHNs may set up PODs/EDSs in their communities to administer prophylactic medications.

The **Strategic National Stockpile** enables large amounts of these medications to be made available on short notice. CDC's Strategic National Stockpile is the nation's largest supply of potentially lifesaving pharmaceuticals and medical supplies for use in a public health emergency severe enough to cause local supplies to run out. The stockpile ensures the right medicines and supplies are available when and where needed to save lives.

When state, local, tribal, and territorial responders request federal assistance to support their response efforts, the stockpile ensures that medicine and supplies get to those who need them most during an emergency. Organized for scalable response to a variety of public health threats, the repository contains enough supplies to respond to multiple large-scale emergencies, simultaneously (CDC, 2017b).

Nurses also have the responsibility to educate the public about anthrax by managing "hotlines," answering questions, providing factual information, and offering reassurance.

Botulism

Botulism is a muscle-paralyzing disease caused by the bacterium *Clostridium botulinum*, which is found in the soil worldwide. The toxin produced by the bacterium is the most potent lethal substance known to humans. The disease is relatively uncommon; in the United States, there are approximately 100 reported cases per year. Botulism is probably familiar to most consumers: beware of canned food with "popped" tops. Botulism is not spread person to person in any of its forms.

Foodborne botulism occurs when the preformed toxin is ingested and can affect people of any age. As cases are identified and confirmed, health departments have environmental inspectors, guided by epidemiologic data patterns, who work diligently to ensure that contaminated foods are removed from stores to protect against further illness.

In botulism, muscle weakness begins and descends through the body. At the point where breathing muscles are involved, ventilator assistance becomes necessary. Antitoxin must be administered because a toxin produced by *C. botulinum* is the cause of the paralysis. A supply of this antitoxin is maintained by the CDC (CDC, 2017a).

FIGURE 20.5 Triage tag.

Plague

Plague, believed to have first emerged in Egypt about 540 AD, is an infectious disease caused by the bacterium *Yersinia pestis*, found globally in rodents and their fleas. The World Health Organization (WHO) reports the occurrence of 1,000 to 3,000 cases yearly throughout the world (WHO, 2018). In the US, between 2 to 15 cases of plague are reported annually, primarily occurring in the western states (CDC, 2018). Most cases are of the bubonic form, which is the most common of the three forms of plague (see Table 20.3).

Pneumonic plague occurs when *Y. pestis* infects the lungs. Airborne transmission from person to person makes this form of plague a possible agent of choice as a bioweapon. The incubation period, 1 to 6 days, makes it possible for the bacteria to spread to others before symptoms occur. Considering this incubation period and the mobile society of the developed world, pneumonic plague can spread easily from state to state, country to country. The gap between infection and diagnosis also makes early treatment more difficult. The bacterium occurs naturally and, therefore, could be weaponized by an organization technologically savvy enough to create an aerosol.

Without early treatment, pneumonic plague has a high mortality rate. Several types of antibiotics are effective in the treatment of all forms of plague. Should there be a confirmed bioterrorism attack, prophylactic distribution of antibiotics to the public will occur from POD/EDS sites with medications supplied by the Strategic National Stockpile.

Smallpox

Smallpox is an acute, contagious, and possibly fatal disease caused by the variola virus. Humans are the only known reservoirs. The virus is contagious and spreads from person to person by contact or through inhalation of aerosols. In America, smallpox last occurred in 1949, and in the world, it last occurred in Somalia in 1977. In 1980, the WHO declared the disease eradicated. For further scientific research on the smallpox virus, the CDC has maintained stockpiles of the virus at its laboratories. Before the dissolution of the former Soviet Union, stockpiles existed at sites throughout that country. After the tragic events of September 11, 2001, officials in the United States became concerned that smallpox could become a biologic weapon.

No treatment exists for smallpox, and the only prevention available is vaccination. The vaccine is made from a virus called vaccinia, which is a "pox"-type virus related to smallpox. Unlike many other vaccines, the smallpox vaccine contains live vaccinia virus. For that reason, it is necessary to care for the vaccination site carefully to prevent the virus from spreading. In 2003, several states initiated a smallpox immunization campaign to protect citizens. For example, in New Jersey, JITT training for smallpox immunization techniques began. PHNs operated PODs throughout the state to administer vaccination to first-line healthcare workers and clinically oriented first responders. Currently, the United States has stockpiled enough smallpox vaccine to vaccinate everyone in the United States in the event of a biologic event that involves smallpox. The disease itself has been eliminated for more than three decades; therefore, the report of just one confirmed case of smallpox would be declared an outbreak. See Table 20.3 gives more information about smallpox.

Tularemia

Tularemia is a potentially serious illness caused by the bacterium *Francisella tularensis*, which occurs naturally in the Northern Hemisphere. Approximately 200 cases of tularemia are reported yearly in rural and semirural areas of the United States, mostly in the southern, central, and western states. Summer outbreaks also often occur on Martha's Vineyard in Massachusetts. The bacterium is not spread person to person, but a low infectious dose, 1 to 10 organisms, is spread by aerosol or the intradermal route. People who are infected can die if not treated quickly with the correct antibiotic. *F. tularensis* occurs naturally; thus, it could be harvested and reengineered as a bioweapon (see Table 20.3). If the organism can be aerosolized, severe respiratory illness would result.

Practice Point

Unusual, out-of-season spikes in infectious disease cases may indicate a bioterrorism attack.

Viral Hemorrhagic Fevers

Viral hemorrhagic fevers (VHFs) are a group of illnesses caused by several distinct RNA virus families. The survival of these viruses is dependent on host vectors, usually rodents, mosquitoes, and ticks. The viruses are found only in geographic areas where their host species live. However, the hosts of two VHFs, Marburg fever and Ebola fever, are unknown. Humans are infected when they accidentally come into contact with infected hosts. In some instances, humans can transmit the virus to one another.

The diseases appear to be global; however, VHFs do not occur naturally in the United States. Outbreaks are sporadic and cannot be easily predicted. In general, the term *VHF* is used to describe a severe multisystem syndrome that damages the vascular system throughout the body, and the body's ability to regulate itself is impaired. Hemorrhaging occurs, but the bleeding itself is rarely life-threatening. Although some types of hemorrhagic fever viruses can cause relatively mild illnesses, many cause severe, life-threatening conditions, and mortality is high. For example, Ebola hemorrhagic fever is a severe, often fatal viral disease in humans, and it is one of the most virulent viral diseases known to humankind. No treatment or vaccine is available, and death occurs in 50% to 90% of all cases of clinical illness.

20.13 Biosafety Levels for Infectious Agents

1. Not known to consistently cause disease in healthy adults
2. Associated with human disease
3. Hazard from percutaneous injury, ingestion, mucous membrane exposure
4. Indigenous or exotic agents with potential for aerosol transmission
5. Disease may have serious or lethal consequences
6. Dangerous/exotic agents that pose high risk of life-threatening disease, aerosol-transmitted laboratory infections; or related agents with unknown risk of transmission

From Centers for Disease Control and Prevention, Office of Health and Safety (Biosafety information page). Retrieved from http://www.cdc.gov/od/ohs/biosfty/bmbl4/bmbl4s3t.htm.

Prevention involves rodent and insect control. The 2014–2016 Ebola epidemic in West Africa required a massive international response. The arrival in a Dallas, Texas, hospital of a traveler from Liberia with Ebola and its subsequent transmission to two nurses working there led to rapid changes in domestic preparedness and response recommendations and practices in healthcare facilities nationwide. (CDC, 2016)

Ebola Precautions

The CDC classifies VHF viruses as biosafety level four (BSL-4) pathogens (Box 20.13). Once illness is confirmed, isolation is enforced along with strict infection control techniques (Fig. 20.6). The CDC, in partnership with the WHO, has developed guidelines for healthcare workers (WHO, 2017). Researchers have developed an experimental vaccine that was tested in an outbreak in Democratic Republic of the Congo in 2017 (Maxmen, 2017).

Practice Point

Maintain a library of biologic, chemical, and radiologic fact sheets from the CDC website to provide clear, accurate information to the public and fellow clinicians.

FIGURE 20.6 CDC (2017) strategic national stockpile. (Retrieved October 17, 2017, from https://www.cdc.gov/phpr/stockpile/index.htm.)

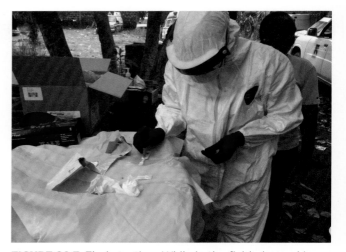

FIGURE 20.7 Ebola testing: While in the field, dressed in a full complement of personal protective equipment (PPE), this epidemiologist was implementing a rapid diagnostic test, which was used during the Ebola response to quickly test for the presence of Ebola virus. (Retrieved from: https://www.phil.cdc.gov/phil/details.asp. Public Health Service Illustration Library.)

CHEMICAL DISASTERS

The intentional or accidental spill of chemical substances can have a devastating effect both on the environment and on human health. In 1984, the release of toxic gases at Union Carbide's pesticide plant in Bhopal, India, resulted in approximately 8,000 deaths and 150,000 injuries. Severe contamination with heavy metals and toxic cancer-producing chemicals occurred at the factory site, on the surrounding land, and in the groundwater. This disaster brought the horror of industrial development to people's attention worldwide and stimulated development of environmental policy and legislation throughout the world. In response, the U.S. Congress passed the Emergency Planning and Community Right-to-Know Act (EPCRA) to address concerns about storing and handling of toxic chemicals.

Multiple chemical environmental disasters have occurred, such as the spill of 11 million gallons of crude oil into Prince William Sound by *Exxon Valdez* and the collapse of the BP oil rig that spewed huge amounts of oil from the ocean floor, to contaminate the Gulf Coast of the United States. Oil from this disaster entered the Gulf Stream and spread to the Atlantic Coast and beyond. The toxic chemical waste landfill used by Hooker Chemical in Love Canal, Niagara Falls, New York, affected hundreds of people who lived there before cleanup plans were initiated. OSHA is now responsible for developing programs to prevent chemical incidents. The Environmental Protection Agency requires all companies that use flammable and toxic substance to develop a risk management program that includes hazard assessment, a prevention program, and an emergency response program. The CDC categorization of hazardous chemicals is outlined in Table 20.4, and the characteristics of individual chemical agents can be reviewed in depth at the CDC website.

TABLE 20.4 Centers for Disease Control and Prevention Categorization of Hazardous Chemicals

Category	Action	Example
Biotoxins	Poisons that come from plants or animals	Ricin
Blister agents/vesicants	Chemicals that severely blister the eyes, respiratory tract, and skin on contact	Mustard gas
Blood agents	Poisons that affect the body by being absorbed into the blood	Cyanide
Caustics (acids)	Chemicals that burn or corrode people's skin, eyes, and mucus membranes (lining of the nose, mouth, throat, and lungs) on contact	Hydrogen fluoride
Choking/lung/pulmonary agents	Chemicals that cause severe irritation or swelling of the respiratory tract (lining of the nose and throat, lungs)	Chlorine
Incapacitating agents	Drugs that make people unable to think clearly or that cause an altered state of consciousness (possibly unconsciousness)	Fentanyl
Long-acting anticoagulants	Poisons that prevent blood from clotting properly, which can lead to uncontrolled bleeding	Super warfarin
Metals	Agents that consist of metallic poisons	Mercury
Nerve agents	Highly poisonous chemicals that work by preventing the nervous system from working properly	Sarin
Organic solvents	Agents that damage the tissues of living things by dissolving fats and oils	Benzene
Riot control agents/tear gas	Highly irritating agents normally used by law enforcement for crowd control or by individuals for protection	Mace
Toxic alcohols	Poisonous alcohols that can damage the heart, kidneys, and nervous system	Ethylene glycol
Vomiting agents	Chemicals that cause nausea and vomiting	Adamsite

From National Center for Environmental Health (NCEH)/Agency for Toxic Substances and Disease Registry (ATSDR), Coordinating Center for Environmental Health and Injury Prevention (CCEHIP).

A chemical's persistence, the length of time a chemical remains potent after its dissemination, is a factor that contributes to the classification of, and response to, a given agent. Nonpersistent chemicals lose their effectiveness in a few minutes to a few hours. For example, chlorine and other pungent gases are nonpersistent chemicals that might be used by terrorists whose goal is to take control of a site of interest. In contrast, persistent chemicals remain in the environment for weeks. For example, liquids such as blister agents and certain nerve agents are oily, and **decontamination** procedures are difficult.

Geoff works with the public health department, hospitals, and other community organizations in planning the disaster management exercise. It will be conducted in a Texas city of 100,000 residents where a deliberate release of anhydrous ammonia via a large explosive device has occurred.

Determine the characteristics of the chemical release and the type of cases that may appear for triage.

Chemicals have been used as tools of war for centuries. However, the destructive qualities of chemicals are not primarily the result of their explosive qualities. Modern chemical warfare began in World War I. At that time, available gases such as chlorine and phosgene were in use. Trench warfare was the main military formation, and soldiers were particularly vulnerable to this form of attack. In effect, attackers simply opened canisters of the gas and let prevailing winds disseminate the chemicals. During the 20th century, the development of chemical munitions, such as artillery shells, projectiles, and bombs, increased a chemical's capacity to kill and maim (Organization for Prohibition of Chemical Weapons, 2016).

Although living organisms can be biologic warfare agents, nonliving toxins produced by living organisms (e.g., botulinum and ricin) can be considered chemical agents according to the Chemical Weapons Convention. Similar to bioterrorism agents, these chemical agents can affect health through inhalation, ingestion, or skin absorption. Examples are nerve agents such as sarin and VX, gases such as the sulfur and nitrogen mustard agents, and choking agents such as phosgene (CDC, 2015). The use of the herbicide Agent Orange during the Vietnam War for defoliation became a crisis due to the genetic and cancer-causing side effects experienced by the U.S. military as well as citizens of Vietnam. (ACS, 2017) In an attempt to reduce the amount of chemical weapons, the Department of Defense began incinerating weapons at eight U.S. sites beginning in 2005. In

FIGURE 20.8 Cleanup of the crash of a small airplane. This firefighter is trying to prevent the highly volatile aviation fuel from exploding and causing a fire.

addition, industrial chemicals, poisonous chemicals found in nature, and chemicals made from compounds in everyday use can be released intentionally. Unlike biologic agents, which require an incubation period before symptoms appear, a chemical agent, when released, makes its presence known immediately through observation (explosion), self-admission (accidental), or the occurrence of rapidly emerging symptoms, such as burns, difficulty breathing, or convulsions (Spenser & Spellman, 2013) (Fig. 20.8). People may be exposed to a chemical in three ways: by breathing the chemical directly; by swallowing contaminated food, water, or medication; or by touching the chemical or coming into contact with contaminated clothing or objects.

Practice Point

You may be exposed to chemicals, even though you may not be able to see or smell anything unusual.

Fear is a defining element of chemical and biologic terrorism. In 1995, after the sarin attack in the Tokyo subway system, the "worried well" descended on the Japanese healthcare system in far greater numbers than those who were actually affected. In 2001 to 2002, the anthrax events in a New Jersey postal facility resulted in a similar response by the community. The New Jersey health department received approximately 100 calls daily, reporting "white powder" events in schools, banks, gas stations, and even doughnut shops. Recognizing that perception is reality to many people, authorities dispatched teams to investigate the reports. A nursing contingent provided telephone support for concerned citizens. No retrieved samples turned out to be anthrax, but for the 700 plus people who called in, the testing of the samples and the presence of a public health nursing team to answer questions and allay fears

was an important step toward restoring public confidence in the face of a real, or thought-to-be-real, anthrax attack. The reaction by the public, fueled by fear, would seem to be a catalyst to encourage "copycat" events. However, every report called in required a response that involved sampling, testing, and community education. To do less would not meet the standards of public health practice and disease investigation. This serves as another example of how the process itself is time-consuming and costly but essential.

The only thing we have to fear is fear itself. **Franklin D. Roosevelt**

Role of Nurses in a Chemical Disaster

In the field, the PHN's response to a chemical incident is summed up in two words: "act quickly." HAZMAT experts report to the hot zone on notification of the release of the chemical. The nurse may be asked to report to a temporary evacuation site where people exposed to the chemical are awaiting triage (Fig. 20.9). Donning PPE must be the first priority. Then assessment of the victim's ability to breathe is necessary. Maintaining adequate respiratory function tops the list for effective client management in a chemical event. Keeping the victims in a sitting position with constrictive clothing loosened or removed is necessary. If the client cannot sit, the torso should be elevated.

In the citywide disaster management drill at the end of the program on emergency preparedness that Geoff has designed, PPE is necessary. What PPE is required for exposure to anhydrous ammonia?

FIGURE 20.9 Decontamination tent. A collision between a freight train carrying toxic chemicals and a passenger train resulted in injuries to several people. Before they were transported to a local hospital, emergency medical personnel carried out on-site decontamination in this temporary facility.

Field decontamination of the victim requires removal of as many outer layers of clothing as possible and placing the victims at a good distance from unaffected population. Washing with soap—or at least water—should follow. For more thorough decontamination, field tents may be erected nearby. Victims who have been severely compromised by the chemical release will be transported to the hospital; there, they will undergo decontamination on the facility grounds before being admitted into the emergency department. The nurse leader is responsible for maintaining communication, especially updating the receiving institutions on client transfer and clinical status. The final activity is for all those working at the decontamination site to be fully decontaminated.

DECONTAMINATION TENT

During the day of the disaster management scenario, 75 "victims" plus six high-fidelity HST models are on site. Various levels of chemical injuries are represented, with the HST models representing the most seriously injured. Arrangements are made for field triage and victim transfer to four medical centers in the area. The nurse responders, the majority of whom were participants in the certificate program, don PPE and assist in the prioritizing of clients in the streets. As the triage activities begin, the nurses facilitate effective client transfer to emergency departments. There are more than 1,000 response participants, including county and local public health department personnel.

Stay or Go?

The decision to stay or go should be made quickly; as time passes, options are reduced. The decision should be made by evaluating factors specific to the event:

- The HAZMAT involved
- The population threatened
- The time span involved
- The current and predicted weather conditions
- The ability to communicate emergency information

The toxicity of the released factor influences the decision to move. Radio stations, social media and the websites of local health departments will report information about the

TABLE 20.5	Suggested Actions Following Release of a Hazardous Chemical	
Nature of Exposure	**Action**
High toxicity and short duration	Shelter in place
Low toxicity and long duration	Evacuate
High toxicity and long duration	Calculate indoor concentrations (done by HAZMAT) Evacuate, if necessary

HAZMAT, hazardous materials.

event. Generally speaking, once toxicity has been determined, actions are taken according to the level of toxicity and the duration of the event (Table 20.5).

Shelter in Place

Shelter in place is used for short-duration incidents, when moving would result in a greater hazard, or it is impractical to evacuate. People should stay inside their home, place of business, or nearest building available. It is a protective action that provides a suitable place to stay until the threat from a hazardous agent has passed. Guidelines for sheltering in place are presented in Box 20.14.

20.14 Guidelines for Sheltering in Place

- Remain inside your home or office
- Shut down heating, ventilation fan, and air conditioning systems
- Close and lock all windows and exterior doors
  - Stuff a towel tightly under each door and tape (aluminum foil or waxed paper) around the sides and top of the door
  - Cover each window and vent in the room with a single piece of plastic sheeting, seal edge with duct tape, and fill any cracks or holes with clay or similar material, such as those around pipes entering a bathroom
- Close the fireplace damper
- Go to an interior room without windows that is above ground level. Some chemicals are heavier than air and may seep into basements
- Get your disaster supplies kit
- Listen to your radio or television until you are told all is safe or you are told to evacuate

If the shelter in place order is related to an infectious disease, there may also be an order for social distancing. **Social distancing** is an action taken by Public Health officials to stop or slow down the spread of a highly contagious disease. The action may be related to a naturally occurring communicable disease event such as the H1N1 influenza pandemic of 2009 or by a bioterrorism release of a highly infectious disease. The goal is to keep social interactions to a minimum by having a minimal amount of social interactions. People are requested to stay at home and public gatherings are cancelled. In the case of the need for a POD/EDS during a social distancing event such as to provide medications or immunizations, families remain in their cars and a "drive thru" clinic is provided.

Evacuation

Evacuation occurs when there is potential for massive explosions and fire as well as for long-duration events. People must leave their homes and go to a safer area. In localized, internal events, **invacuation**, where people in a hospital or residential facility may be moved to another floor or area within the facility, may occur. Natural disasters and industrial accidents require people to evacuate, sometimes on a large scale. Based on the characteristics of the emergency, a combination of evacuation and in-place protection measures may be appropriate. People in areas downwind and in proximity to a chemical release, where concentrations are likely to be higher and less time is available for response, might be advised to shelter in place. At the same time, areas that are upwind or farther from the release might be evacuated. Evacuating upwind areas makes sense as a precautionary measure because a wind shift could rapidly place these areas in jeopardy. In fact, evacuation is most effective when it is used as a precautionary measure; thus, it is necessary to practice evacuation plans. Guidelines for evacuation are presented in Box 20.15.

Evidence for Practice

Evacuation is considered an important strategy to limit victim exposure to hazardous chemical release (HCR). However, because of the wide range of possible disaster scenarios, there is little evidence-based research to guide evacuation or sheltering decisions. A 1.5 mile area of evacuation of residents near a chemical plant in Texas after Hurricane Harvey in 2017 was taken as a preventive measure after the refrigeration system was destroyed during the hurricane and chemicals that required refrigeration were allowed to heat up, thus causing explosions and a release of gases. There was a significant lead time as temperatures were rising, thus allowing a safe, orderly evacuation.

In a study by Melnikova, Wu & Orr (2015), the most frequent public health response to chemical incidents between 1999 and 2008 was restricting access to the area (26% of incidents), public health actions (12%), evacuation (7%), decontamination (4%), and shelter-in-place (1%). Ammonia and carbon monoxide were associated with adverse health effects in the population and the most public health response actions.

Practice Point

Maintaining close contact with local HAZMAT teams guides the decision-making process for evacuation/shelter-in-place activities.

RADIOLOGIC DISASTERS

Radiation is energy that moves in the form of particles or waves, such as heat, light, radio waves, and microwaves. Ionizing radiation is a high-energy form of electromagnetic radiation. People benefit from it daily through the warmth of the sun and the use of x-ray technology. In fact, small amounts of radioactive materials are in the air, drinking water, food, and human body. It is known that excessive radiation affects the body in many ways, and often those results do not become evident for several years. The health outcome depends on: (1) the amount or dose of radiation absorbed; (2) the type of radiation; (3) the route of exposure; and (4) the length of time exposed to the dose.

When large doses are released accidentally (e.g., from a nuclear power plant) or intentionally (e.g., in a terrorist act), there is an increased risk that health effects will occur. The combined disasters of an earthquake, a tsunami, and a radiologic release in the Iwate Prefecture in Japan in 2011 is an example of a multidimensional disaster that serves as an example of a local disaster with global implications. Within days, the CDC activated their emergency operations center to respond to the health issues related to the three different disasters recorded (FDA, 2015). Very often, the terms *exposure* and *contamination* are used incorrectly or interchangeably. Internal exposure occurs when the radioactive materials enter the body by eating or drinking, whereas external exposure occurs when the radioactive source is outside the body. Contamination occurs when particles of radioactive material

20.15 Guidelines for Evacuation

- Wear long-sleeved shirts, long pants, and sturdy shoes
- Take your pets with you
- Lock your home
- Take your disaster supplies kit
- Use travel routes specified by local authorities: do not use shortcuts because certain areas may be impassable or dangerous
- Stay away from downed power lines

20.16 Radiologic Resources for Nurses

American College of Medical Toxicology Course on TICs and TIMs. American College of Medical Toxicology, http://acmt.net/Chemical_Agents_of_Opportunity.html

Centers for Disease Control and Prevention (CDC) Radiation Emergencies. Training, and Tools, http://emergency.cdc.gov/radiation/trainingguidance.asp

Nuclear Radiologic Incident Annex, https://www.fema.gov/media-library/assets/documents/25554

Radiation Decontamination Procedures, http://www.remm.nlm.gov/ext_contamination.htm/

Radiation Emergency Assistance Center/Training Site OR1SE provides expertise in the medical management of radiation incidents through the operation of the Radiation Emergency Assistance Center/Training Site (REAC/TS), a dedicated DOE facility located in Oak Ridge, Tennessee, http://orise.orau.gov/reacts

Radiation Disasters: Preparedness and Response: American College of Radiology, (2012). *Radiation Disasters: Preparedness and Response for Radiology,* http://www.acr.org/membership/legal-business-practices/disaster-preparedness

Internal Contamination Clinical Reference, CDC, http://www.emergency.cdc.gov/radiation/iccr.asp

Radiologic Terrorism: Medical Response to Mass Casualties, https://emergency.cdc.gov/radiation/masscasualties/training.asp

Radiologic Terrorism: Emergency Management Pocket Guide for Clinicians, http://www.emergency.cdc.gov/radiation/pocket.asp

REAC/TS center at the Oak Ridge National Laboratory at, http://orise.orau.gov/reacts/

Public Health Planning for Radiologic and Nuclear Terrorism, https://emergency.cdc.gov/radiation/masscasualties/publichealthplanning.asp

Virtual Community Reception Centers, CDC, http://www.emergency.cdc.gov/radiation/crc/vcrc.asp

DOE, Department of Education; ORISE, Oak Ridge Institute for Science and Education; TIC, toxic industrial chemical; TIM, toxic industrial materials.
Source: Veenema, T., & Thornton, C. (2015). Understanding nurse's role in health systems response to large-scale radiologic disasters. *Journal of Radiology Nursing, 34*(2), 64.

are deposited where they are normally not found. The Environmental Protection Agency provides additional information on radiologic risks on its website (CDC, 2017c).

"Dirty" Bombs

Deliberate release of a radioactive agent, the use of "dirty" bombs, has become an increasing concern. This is a radiologic dispersion device that uses explosives as well as radioactive materials. The act of explosion disseminates the radioactive agent. The range of a "dirty" bomb is relatively small. Exposure to a dirty bomb is via inhalation, skin, and gastrointestinal tract. This exposure may lead to health impacts, including malignancies, genetic mutations, and reproductive issues. In addition, the impact on the environment is of concern (Durakovic, 2017).

With low-level radiation, the greatest risk to the population is the blast itself. The radiation levels released are not likely to cause severe illness. For this reason, "dirty" bombs often are not considered weapons of mass destruction. Dealing with the fear that such an event would instill in the public could very well be the greatest challenge facing first responders. In addition, the economic impact of a "dirty" bomb, involving cleanup efforts and decontamination of the site, is significant.

Practice Point

In a radiologic emergency, it is necessary to decrease time spent near the source, increase distance from the source, and increase shielding from the source.

The best way to solve any problem is to remove its cause.
Martin Luther King

Role of Nurses in a Radiologic Disaster

In a radiologic event, people should leave the area quickly (distance, time); enter the nearest building (shielding); cover their noses and mouths; remove their clothes and seal them in double-thickness trash bags; shower as soon as possible (decontamination); clean and cover any open wounds; and listen to the radio, watch the television, or access the state's website. Community-based nurses are not called to the actual location. However, nurses working in a receiving station may observe dust on arrivals. It must be assumed that dust on victims is radioactive. PPE should be worn, as well as a radiation badge to measure personal exposure. People should remove their clothing and be referred for decontamination. Physical injuries are more acute than radioactive contamination. Stable victims should be moved out of the area quickly, and the people in surrounding facilities should be notified. Information should be documented; it will be used to monitor long-term health consequences. Accurate information regarding appropriate protective actions should be made available to the public.

Evidence for Practice

As noted by Veenema & Thornton (2015b), nurse involvement during a radiologic event may potentially include site response; "the establishment of community reception centers for population screening and monitoring; decontamination; shelter management; and the psychosocial support of victims, families, coworkers, and the community impacted by the event." While nurses have historically reported lack of confidence in responding to a radiologic disaster, an increased emphasis in nursing educational programs and the mandate for healthcare institutions to have emergency plans and drills with employees has begun to address this issue.

BLAST INJURIES

In the blink of an eye, an explosion and its subsequent blast can create chaos and lay waste to an area previously untouched. Explosions can occur as a result of an industrial accident, such as the fertilizer plant explosion and fire that happened in Texas, or when used as a weapon of choice by a terrorist, as witnessed during the Boston Marathon bombings in April 2013. Construction directions for makeshift devices are readily available on the internet. Such a mechanism can be inexpensive to build while producing many casualties with injuries not normally seen after naturally occurring disasters. Injuries sustained in an explosion are multisystem threatening and "war-like" in their presentation: mutilation; shrapnel wounds to bone, soft tissue, and vascular structures; and dismemberment. In the Boston attack, the limited loss of life, and saving of many critically ill victims was unprecedented. It is believed that first responders were already on the scene for the event, thus able to provide immediate first aide and transport to hospitals. In addition, the presence of numerous level I trauma units in the metropolitan also contributed to the minimal deaths among the victims. The improvisational use of tourniquets on bombing victims on-site has been documented to be an effective intervention to stop bleeding and ultimately save lives. Field stabilization of bombing victims can be incorporated into professional and volunteer responder training to sustain the survival rate of victims as seen in Boston. Also noted was the courage of fellow marathon runners and volunteers.

A concerted community effort to practice response to mass casualty events through collaborative exercises among agencies supported this coordinated response. Prior preparation in Boston included 71 MCI drills with numerous area agencies (Operation Urban Shield) to better prepare local institutions and staff to respond (City of Boston, 2014).

During a field response in an explosion-based event, there are some considerations to weigh (CDC, n.d.):

- Explosions in confined spaces are associated with higher morbidity and mortality.
- Communication with victims may be difficult due to sudden temporary deafness.
- Many injuries are not life-threatening due to blunt force trauma from flying debris.
- Open wounds have an increased chance to become infected.

- Triage and lifesaving efforts should not be delayed because of the possibility of a dirty bomb detonation.
- Detailed assessments and on-site evaluations are counterproductive to decreasing mortality.

Practice Point

The most important aspect of field response to an explosion victim in the field is stabilization and rapid transfer to a hospital.

PUBLIC HEALTH DISASTER RESPONSE

Collaboration among federal, state and local agencies include use of BioWatch. BioWatch monitors the air for biologic agents likely to be used in a bioterrorism attack. If a detection occurs, public health and other local and state officials use the information to coordinate emergency response, including prompt medical care and other actions to protect public health and safety. This combination of early warning and rapid response may potentially reduce illness and death from a bioterrorism attack. BioWatch is a cornerstone in the DHS's comprehensive strategy for countering terrorism. BioWatch jurisdictions and federal agencies work together to ensure the overall resilience of the program. Effective working relationships between federal, state, and local public health, laboratories, law enforcement, and environmental health agencies are key to BioWatch's success (DHS, 2016).

Every state department of health has established reporting requirements to ensure accurate surveillance of infectious diseases. All disasters originate as local events, and historically, local health departments respond accordingly, through stepped up surveillance activities or communication with their respective state health department. It is part of a larger emergency response effort within the region. The Health Alert Network (HAN) is a nationwide integrated information and communication system that links local and state health and safety departments. This network broadcasts and receives health alerts, offers distance learning opportunities, and provides electronic laboratory reporting and disease surveillance. In an emergency, the HAN provides essential information for an appropriate response from public health officials. People will be informed of the type of health hazard, area(s) affected, self-protection measures, evacuation routes, shelter locations, the type and location of medical facilities, and telephone numbers to call if extra help is needed.

Scope and Magnitude of Response

The scope of the disaster should become evident within the first hours of the emergency, and the magnitude of a public health response can be assessed. An act of terrorism will involve large numbers of innocent people, with a sudden increased demand for health-related services. Triage, transport, medical care, and mental health services for victims, their families, responders, and the community may be necessary. Also, recovery, transportation, and storage of human remains may be required. It is necessary to know what other agencies are involved, if an incident command post has been established and commander identified, and if state, local, or tribal operations centers have been activated. A large-scale emergency response could involve dozens of agencies at various levels of government, working together in accordance with mutual aid agreements and written emergency plans.

The public health response should be implemented in accordance with existing EOPs and procedures. As part of this joint effort, all participants should function within the incident management system adopted by the community. Once the need for the participation of the health department and PHNs has been established, key personnel should be notified. It will be necessary to coordinate with area healthcare partners and document efforts to contact participants, including unsuccessful attempts. A representative from the health department should be assigned to establish communications and act as liaison to others in the emergency operations center. The health department will take steps to ensure the safety of the response team. This may include the use of PPE and ongoing safety reports throughout the day. Throughout the event, documentation of activities should be maintained.

It is essential to constantly verify the status of the response effort. Asset and resource allocation plans will be made in response to the disaster. The mutual agreements among providers can be implemented, calling on partners to assist in the evacuation of residents, the provision of temporary shelter and food, or the transfer of the injured to hospitals outside of the affected community.

A response is always a dynamic process; therefore, an ongoing assessment of the situation should be in place. Once the health department and the regional public health system have been activated, health surveillance systems should be initiated. The needs of special populations within the jurisdiction should be addressed. The state authorities are involved at this stage, and local health authorities must confirm that the state laboratories are available so that the process of specimen collection and analysis can begin. A contact person should be identified for updates. Additional consideration should be given to the jurisdiction's policy on using volunteers during a disaster response. Often, the MRC/CERT is activated. If the incorporation of volunteers is used, the MRC/CERT contact person should be included in the communication effort.

Depending on the scope of the disaster and its nature—natural or intentional—state and, perhaps, federal representatives may be at the operations site. Specially trained response teams may be brought into the region if required. The public health authorities have the responsibility to request additional staff, supplies, and other resources as soon as the need is identified. This is carried out through the ICS. Monitoring of health resources is essential to maintain a sustained response.

As assessment and updates continue, the characteristics of the response may begin to change. The support of response personnel must be a priority. Backup shift personnel should be mobilized at the outset and deployment to the site arranged. After the acute phase of a disaster passes, specific activities related to the nature of the event should be addressed. These may include agent identification; laboratory collection and analysis; dissemination of educational materials; evacuation plans; health status assessment of responders as well as the general public affected by the event; infectious disease protocol implementation; and assessment of water supply, food safety, and vector control. The importance of veterinary services during an emergency event cannot be overlooked. Professionals in this field should be included in disaster plan development. During Hurricane Katrina, it was found people would not evacuate as they did not want to leave their pets. In response, congress passed the "Pets Evacuation and Transportation Standards (PETS) Act" and the Post-Katrina Emergency Response Act (PKEMRA) in response to public outcry about the safety and well-being of pet animals during disasters. An example of this response has been the development in Massachusetts of the State of Massachusetts Animal Response Team (SMART). The goals include:

- Minimize the threats to the health and safety of animals and humans
- Minimize the economic impact of animal emergencies
- Decrease the spread of disease to animals and humans during any emergency
- Understand the interface between human and animal health (USDA, 2017)

> The difficult we do immediately. The impossible takes a little longer. **The United States Army–Air Force**

Communication During a Disaster

Communication is one of the most important aspects of maintaining a detailed, dynamic, and broad-based response to a disaster. "Risk communication" is defined as a science-based discipline that provides an interactive exchange of information and opinions among individuals, groups, and institutions in a disaster setting. Risk communication in emergencies is used to inform the public about an event or issue to empower members of a community to protect themselves. The risk communication plan is an important component of the disaster preparedness plan; it involves identifying key decision-makers, a risk communication team, representatives for talking to media contacts, a clinical spokesperson, and a venue for conducting media updates. High-concern situations can change the rules of communication. The rapid dissemination of health messages; the adaptation of health messages for diverse audiences, locations, and circumstances; and the delivery of key risk messages at various points in time are often challenges while communicating during a disaster (Sutton, League, Sellnow, & Sellnow, 2015). Similar to emergency preparedness planning, effective risk communication occurs during all stages of the disaster cycle (Bradley, McFarland, & Clarke, 2014) (see Fig. 20.2).

The need for a strong knowledge base in emergency preparedness and the communication sciences, as well as coordination across agencies is needed to design and convey messages that meet the needs of the intended population (Marin & Witt, 2017; Miller et al., 2017)

Risk communication often involves multiple messages between multiple groups concerning the nature of risk. The perception of the risk depends on the circumstances. For example, although a voluntary evacuation may produce anxiety, it is more acceptable than one imposed on citizens. Earning trust and credibility is essential for effective risk communication. It is especially important when dealing with the fear factor associated with a deliberate attack. During this process, public health officials, nurses, and other representatives must provide clear, accurate information while minimizing the fear that may be associated with the event.

With heightened emotion, there is potential for an already bad situation to get worse. Rumors and unreliable information can create an unstable environment. Reassurance in times of crisis is essential. It is essential to listen and not interrupt. Simple statements such as "the risk is low" or "nurses are available to answer your questions at this toll-free number…" are very effective. Depending on the situation, nurses can suggest actions to decrease risk of illness or suggest that people call their primary care provider if they become ill. Trust and credibility will be compromised if these emotions are not addressed effectively. It is important to remember that feelings of fear, frustration, and anger in a crisis are to be expected, and the resulting behavior should not be taken personally.

Nurses may become the targets of this fear and frustration particularly when there is a shortage of needed materials. For example, in the initial phases of the immunization effort for H1N1 in 2009 and 2010, the demand for vaccine far outweighed the supply. Nurses often had the task of dealing with frustrated and angry people who were being told to obtain their immunizations yet could not succeed in finding available vaccine. Another example is when the shelters fill to overflowing during a MCI and people lack basic necessities. There should be backup plans in this type of situation. Sometimes, important information is not available or cannot be verified. In that case, the information should not be communicated to the public. "I don't know" is acceptable and may even increase a nurse's credibility. Under no circumstances should a nonclinical person convey or interpret clinical data. A field nurse should be identified, who will receive client reports from another clinician in the receiving facility or surge site. Medical terminology can be badly misinterpreted by someone who is unaccustomed to working in the medical professions. Erroneous messages, even if innocently transmitted, derail efforts to keep the public well informed. During a crisis, messages should be reiterated frequently. When interacting with the media, a clinician should be present to answer any questions or clarify information. Fact sheets regarding the crisis should be prepared for informing the public and shared with public information officers. The biologic, chemical, and radiologic fact sheets from the CDC should be distributed if needed.

During the disaster preparedness drill in Texas, nurses conduct triage activities and communicate with receiving hospitals to facilitate swift transfer of victims. What underlying principles are practiced when communicating with the receiving hospitals?

It takes me two weeks to prepare an impromptu speech.
Mark Twain

Geoff creates an evaluation tool to use following the disaster management exercise. What topics did Geoff include in the after-action analysis?

Results of Geoff's evaluation indicate that the use of agent-specific simulation training in the classroom enabled the nurses to increase their competency skills while raising their confidence in a nonthreatening setting. These practice sessions enable them to perform effectively in the field.

KEY CONCEPTS

- Nurses play an important role in all phases of disaster response.
- All practicing nurses should become familiar with disaster phases and their role during an event.
- Public health nurses practice principles of disaster response on a daily basis.
- Although disasters do not occur with frequency, planning with vulnerability assessment can reduce their impact on the community.

- Properly implemented triage models minimize the morbidity and mortality of people affected by the event.
- Disaster phases and the nursing process are closely aligned.
- Biologic agents have an incubation period, which delays the investigation of the use of such agents as weapons.

- Chemical agents cause illness and/or death shortly after release. Decontamination is required for most chemical exposures.
- Response during a radiologic event may potentially include site response; establishment of community reception centers and monitoring; decontamination; shelter management; and psychosocial support. Fear and intimidation are a terrorist's strongest tools in orchestrating an attack.

- During a biologic, chemical, or radiologic event, the "worried well," in addition to the injured, can overwhelm and immobilize the healthcare system.
- Policies and procedures for mass immunization clinics should be in place to adapt to an emergency POD/EDS operation.
- Public health nurses' clinical skills in agent identification, triage, and field activities may be greatly enhanced through the use of simulation technology in repeated training experiences.

CRITICAL THINKING QUESTIONS

1. Identify a disaster scenario, outline the disaster preparedness steps that should be used, and relate them to the nursing process.
2. Both your local and state health departments have confirmed reports of 16 cases of pneumonic plague among students at a large suburban college campus.
   a. Develop a just-in-time training (JITT) program on standard and droplet infection control practices for health department staff members and college residents and staff. Use the boxes, tables, and figures found in this chapter, and if necessary, consult other resources.
   b. Prepare a postexposure antibiotic prophylaxis distribution plan for your community.

3. Identify several roles that a public health nurse can function in, within the framework of a multidisciplinary planning committee. Consider how his or her assessment, implementation, and evaluation skills can be utilized in a nonclinical role.
4. Conduct a risk assessment and all hazard vulnerability studies using a community of choice, or review a disaster event taken from recent history, and identify weaknesses that contributed to the emergency. Could the event have been minimized or even prevented with accurate assessment?
5. List the emergency plans that must be in place before, during, and after a hazardous chemical release to provide essential care for clients and the community at large following the disaster.

COMMUNITY RESOURCES

- Local, county, and state public health departments
- Local Visiting Nurse Associations
- Local town hall
- Local fire department
- Local police department

- Regional Red Cross
- Regional Medical Reserve Corps (MRC) or Community Emergency Response Team (CERT)
- U.S. Homeland Security regional offices

REFERENCES

Addy, C., Browne, T., Blake, E., & Bailey, J. (2015). Enhancing interprofessional education: Integrating public health and social work perspectives. *American Journal of Public Health*, *105*(S1), S 106–109.

American Cancer Society (ACS). (2017) *Agent Orange and Cancer.* Retrieved November 2, 2017, from https://www.cancer.org/cancer/cancer-causes/agent-orange-and-cancer.html.

American Civil Liberties Union (ACLU). (2017) *How the US Patriot Act redefines "domestic terrorism.* Retrieved October 31, 2017, from https://www.aclu.org/other/how-usa-patriot-act-redefines-domestic-terrorism.

Association of Community Health Nursing Educators (ACHNE). (2008). *Disaster preparedness white paper for community/public health nursing educators.* Retrieved November 3, 2017, from http://www.achne.org/files/public/DisasterPreparedness-WhitePaper.pdf.

Association of Public Health Nurses (APHN). (2014). *The role of the public health nurse in disaster preparedness, response, and recovery.* Retrieved October 23, 2017, from http://nacchopreparedness.org/wp-content/uploads/2014/01/APHN_Role-of-PHN-in-Disaster-PRR_FINALJan14.pdf.

Barras, V.,& Greub, G. (2014) History of biological warfare and bioterrorism. *Clinical Microbiology and Medicine, 20*(6), 497–502.

Bradley D, McFarland M., & Clarke, M. (2014). The Effectiveness of disaster risk communication: A systematic review of intervention studies. *PLoS Currents.* Retrieved October 22, 2017, from http://currents.plos.org/disasters/article/the-effectiveness-of-disaster-risk-communication-a-systematic-review-of-intervention-studies/.

Bureau of Labor Statistics (BLS). (2016). *Occupational employment and wages, May 2016 29–1141 registered nurses.* Retrieved November 3, 2017, from https://www.bls.gov/oes/current/oes291141.htm#nat.

Centers for Disease Control and Prevention. (n.d.) *Blast injuries: Fact sheet for professionals.* Retrieved October 24, 2017, from http://www.calhospitalprepare.org/sites/main/files/file-attachments/blast_fact_sheet_professionals-a.pdf.

REFERENCES *(Continued)*

Centers for Disease Control and Prevention. (2012). Guidelines for field triage of Injured Patients Recommendations of the National Expert Panel on Field Triage. *Mortality and Morbidity Weekly*, *61*(11), 1–21.

Centers for Disease Control and Prevention. (2015). *Emergency preparedness and response: Sarin gas*. Retrieved November 2, 2017, from https://emergency.cdc.gov/agent/sarin/basics/facts.asp.

Centers for Disease Control and Prevention. (2016) CDC's response to the 2014–2016 Ebola epidemic—West Africa and United States. *MMWR*, *23*(16), 1–3.

Centers for Disease Control and Prevention. (2017a) *Bioterrorism agents/diseases by category*. Retrieved October 17, 2017, from https://emergency.cdc.gov/agent/agentlist-category.asp.

Centers for Disease Control and Prevention. (2017b) *Strategic national stockpile*. Retrieved October 17, 2017, from https://www.cdc.gov/phpr/stockpile/index.htm.

Centers for Disease Control and Prevention. (2017c) *Radiological Emergencies*. Retrieved November 2, 2017, from https://emergency.cdc.gov/radiation/index.asp.

Centers for Disease Control and Prevention (CDC). (2018). *Maps and Statistics: Plague in the United States*. Retrieved December 21, 2018 from https://www.cdc.gov/plague/maps/index.html.

City of Boston. (2014) *Urban shield: Boston to test region's first responders*. Retrieved October 21, 2017, from https://www.cityofboston.gov/news/default.aspx?id=8607.

Danna, D., Pierce, S., Schaubhut, R., Billingsley, L.,& Bennett, M. (2015) Educating nurses to provide culturally competent care during disasters. *Journal of Continuing Education in Nursing*, *46*(3), 135–144.

Douglas, M., Pierce, J., Rosenkoetter, M., Pacquiao, D., Callister, L., Hattar-Pollara, M., … Purnell, L. (2011). Standards of practice for culturally competent nursing care: 2011 update. *Journal of Transcultural Nursing*, *22*(4), 317–333.

Durakovic, A. (2017). Medical effects of a transuranic "dirty bomb." *Military Medicine*, *182*(3/4), e1591–e1595.

EM-DAT: International Disaster Data Base. (EM-DAT). (2017). Focus on tropical cyclones on American continent. *Cred Crunch*. Retrieved October 24, 2017, from https://reliefweb.int/sites/reliefweb.int/files/resources/CredCrunch49.pdf.

Federal Emergency Management Agency (FEMA). (2017). *National incident management agency*. Retrieved November 3, 2017, from https://www.fema.gov/national-incident-management-system.

Food and Drug Administration, US (FDA). (2015). *FDA response to the Fukushima Dai-ichi nuclear power facility incident*. Retrieved October 20, 2017, from https://www.fda.gov/newsevents/publichealthfocus/ucm247403.htm.

Healthy People. (2017). *Preparedness*. Retrieved November 2, 2017 from https://www.healthypeople.gov/2020/topics-objectives/topic/preparednesss.

Hutton, A., Veenema, T., & Gebbie, K. (2016). Review of the International Council of Nurses (ICN) Framework of Disaster Nursing Competencies. *Prehospital and Disaster Medicine*, *31*(6), 680–683.

Johnston, W. (2016). *Summary of historical attacks using chemical or biological weapons*. Retrieved October 17, 2017, from Johnston-sarchive.net/terrorism/chembioattacks.html.

Lamberg, L. (2008) Katrina's mental health impact lingers. *JAMA*, *300*(9), 1011–1013.

Lim, G. H., Lim, B. L., & Vasu, A. (2013). Survey of factors affecting health care workers' perception towards institutional and individual disaster preparedness. *Prehospital & Disaster Medicine*, *28*(4), 353–358.

Marin S., & Witt, R. (2017). Hospital nurses competencies' in disaster situations: A Qualitative study in South Brazil. *Prehospital and Disaster Medicine*, *30*(6), 548–552

Marion, L., Douglas, M., Lavin, M., Barr, N., Gazaway, S., Thomas, L., & Bickford, C. (2016). Implementing the New ANA Standard 8: Culturally congruent practice. *OJIN: The Online Journal of Issues in Nursing*, *22*(1), 9. Retrieved November 3, 2017, from http://www.nursingworld.org/MainMenuCategories/ANAMarketplace/ANAPeriodicals/OJIN/TableofContents/Vol-22-2017/No1-Jan-2017/Articles-Previous-Topics/Implementing-the-New-ANA-Standard-8.html.

Maxmen, A. (2017). *Ebola vaccine approved for use in ongoing outbreak science*. Retrieved October 17, 2017, from https://www.nature.com/news/ebola-vaccine-approved-for-use-in-ongoing-outbreak-1.22024.

McGill, A. (2016). Americans are more worried about terrorism than they were after 9/11. *The Atlantic*. Retrieved November 3, 2017, from https://www.theatlantic.com/politics/archive/2016/09/american-terrorism-fears-september-11/499004/.

McKay, J. (2017). How the shocks of disasters are impacted by the stresses of social issues. *Emergency Management*. Retrieved November 2, 2017, from http://www.govtech.com/em/disaster/How-the-shocks-of-disasters-are-impacted-by-the-stresses-of-social-issues.html.

Melnikova, N., Wu, J., & Orr, M. (2015). Public health response to acute chemical incidents—hazardous substances emergency events surveillance, nine states, 1999–2008. *MMRW*, *64*(5), 25–31.

Miller, S., Sellnow, T., Neuberger, L., Todd, A., Freihaut, R., Noyes, J., … Gamhewage, G. (2017). A systemic review of literature on effectiveness of training in emergency risk communication. *Journal of Health Communication*, *22*(7), 612–629.

Office of Minority Health, US Dept. Health and Human Services. (2017). *Cultural competency curriculum for disaster preparedness and crisis response*. Retrieved October 31, 2017, from https://cccdpcr.thinkculturalhealth.hhs.gov/.

Office of Minority Services. (2017). *Why Use Culturally and Linguistically Appropriate Services (CLAS) Throughout a Disaster?* Retrieved December 21, 2018 from https://cccdpcr.thinkculturalhealth.hhs.gov/.

Organization For The Prohibition Of Chemical Weapons. (2016) *Eliminating chemical weapons and chemical weapons production facilities Fact Sheet 6*. Retrieved November 2, 2017, from https://www.opcw.org/fileadmin/OPCW/Fact_Sheets/English/Fact_Sheet_6_-_destruction.pdf.

Sánchez, F., & Leiden, P. (2009). International legal dimensions of terrorism. *Symposium on International Humanitarian Law*. 7th edition. Boston: M. Nijhoff.

Schroeder, M. (2017). *Road map for mental wellness after a hurricane*. US News World Report. Retrieved October 23, 2017, from https://health.usnews.com/health-care/patient-advice/articles/2017-10-03/the-road-map-for-mental-wellness-after-a-hurricane.

Substance Abuse and Mental Health Agency (SAMSA). (2017). *Tips for communicating with survivors*. Retrieved September 20, 2017, from https://store.samhsa.gov/shin/content//SMA17-5036/SMA17-5036.pdf.

Sutton, J., League, C., Sellnow, T., & Sellnow. D. (2015). Terse messaging and public health in the midst of natural disasters: The Case of the Boulder flood. *Health Communication*, *30*(2), 135–143.

Spenser, L., & Spellman, J. (2013). The role and preparation of the public health nurse for disaster response. In T. Veenema (Ed.). *Disaster nursing and emergency preparedness for chemical, biological, and radiological terrorism and other hazards* (pp. 687–698). New York: Springer.

United Nations Office for Disaster Risk Reduction (UNDRR). (2015) *The human cost of natural disasters 2015L a global perspective*. Retrieved September 20, 2017, from https://reliefweb.int/report/world/human-cost-natural-disasters-2015-global-perspective.

United States Census Bureau. (2016). *Quick facts: Texas: Race and Hispanic origin*. Retrieved October 30, 2017 from https://www.census.gov/quickfacts/TX.

US Department of Agriculture (USDA). (2017). *Animal care emergency programs*. Retrieved October 21, 2017, from https://www.aphis.usda.gov/aphis/ourfocus/animalwelfare/sa_ep/ct_ep_information.

US Dep. Homeland Security (DHS). (2017). *About DHS*. Retrieved October 23, 2017, from https://www.dhs.gov/about-dhs.

US Dep. Homeland Security. (2016). *The BioWatch program*. Retrieved October 21, 2017, from https://www.dhs.gov/biowatch-program.

Veenema, T. (2013). Essentials in disaster planning. In T. Veenema (Ed.). *Disaster nursing and emergency preparedness for chemical, biological, and radiological terrorism and other hazards*. (3rd ed., pp. 1–19). New York: Springer.

Veenema, T. G., Griffin, A., Gable, A., MacIntyre, L., Simons, N., Couig, P., … Larson, E. (2016). Nurses as leaders in disaster preparedness and response—A call to action. *J of Nursing Scholarship*, 48(2), 187–200.

Veenema, T., & Thornton, C. (2015a). Disaster nursing app-for iPhone and Android developed by a recognized authority in disaster nursing, Tenor Goodwin Veenema. Free software includes: Various types of disasters, appropriate responses and planning involved. A more advanced version is available for a minimum charge.

Veenema, T., & Thornton, C. (2015b). Understanding nurse's role in health systems response to large-scale radiologic disasters. *Journal of Radiology Nursing*, 34(2), 63–72.

World Health Organization. (2017). *Haemorrhagic fevers, viral* Retrieved October 18, 2017, from http://www.who.int/topics/haemorrhagic_fevers_viral/en/.

WEB RESOURCES

For online training in Incident Command Structure: https://training.fema.gov/nims/

Medical Reserve Corps: https://mrc.hhs.gov/HomePage

Certified Emergency Response Team (CERT): https://www.ready.gov/community-emergency-response-team

Please visit thePoint for up-to-date web resources on this topic.

Part 5

Specialty Practice

Chapter 21

Community Mental Health

Judith Shindul-Rothschild

ALONE

*From childhood's hour I have not been
As others were; I have not seen
As others saw; I could not bring
My passions from a common spring.
From the same source I have not taken
My sorrow; I could not awaken
My heart to joy at the same tone;
And all I loved, I loved alone.
Then—in my childhood, in the dawn
Of a most stormy life—was drawn
From every depth of good and ill*

*The mystery which binds me still:
From the torrent, or the fountain,
From the red cliff of the mountain,
From the sun that round me rolled
In its autumn tint of gold,
From the lightning in the sky
As it passed me flying by,
From the thunder and the storm,
And the cloud that took the form
(When the rest of Heaven was blue)
Of a demon in my view.*

—Edgar Allan Poe

CHAPTER HIGHLIGHTS

- Epidemiology of mental illness from a public health perspective
- Early intervention in the treatment of schizophrenia
- Strategies to enhance treatment adherence
- Public health implications for children with behavioral disorders

- Evolution of community mental health
- Policy development and legislation for mental health services
- Role and responsibilities of the community mental health practitioner

OBJECTIVES

- Interpret the meaning of mental illness in the context of societal and cultural norms about behavior.
- Describe the scope of mental illness and the effects on morbidity and mortality worldwide.
- Describe the side effects of antipsychotic medication and its implications for nursing assessment and long-term treatment.
- Analyze emerging models of treatment that offer promise in improving the quality of life for the chronic mentally ill in communities.
- Identify the social and biologic factors associated with the incidence of mood and anxiety disorders.
- Describe public health programs to decrease the incidence of suicide, especially among youth.

- Differentiate the key signs and symptoms of attention-deficit/hyperactivity disorder and bipolar disorder in children as members of families in communities.
- Identify the motor, language, and social characteristics of infants and toddlers that are early signs of autism spectrum disorders as members of families in communities.
- Describe the policy implications in the shift in locus of care to community mental health centers for the chronic mentally ill.
- Identify the key components of psychological first aid.

KEY TERMS

Autism spectrum disorders: Also known as pervasive developmental disorders; cause severe and pervasive impairment in thinking, feeling, language, and the ability to relate to others.

"Black box" warning: Warning by the Food and Drug Administration (FDA) to advise clients and caregivers of dangers related to the use of a drug or treatment alone or in combination.

Community mental health centers: Primary care centers and neighborhood-based centers in communities with the goal of serving populations and aggregates in need of follow-up care and counseling.

Culturally competent mental health services: Mental health services by professionals who demonstrate knowledge in group values, traditions, and the cultural expression of mental illness.

Deinstitutionalization: The phenomenon of allowing patients who leave care in large, complex healthcare systems to receive care in neighborhoods and communities on an outpatient basis.

Diagnostic and Statistical Manual, 5th edition (DSM-5): The standard classification of mental disorders, published by the American Psychiatric Association and used by mental health professionals in the United States, it is intended to be applicable in a wide array of contexts and used by clinicians and researchers of many different orientations.

Early intervention programs: Specialized teams of professionals whose primary goal is to maintain the individual's current level of educational and vocational functioning through early treatment.

First-generation antipsychotics: Medications developed and used early in the science of psychiatric therapeutics.

Nonadherence: The choice to not follow directions for care; can include medications, follow-up healthcare appointments, or wellness checkups.

President's New Freedom Commission on Mental Health: Expert panel created to advise Congress and the President on how policymakers could improve mental health services for both the chronic mentally ill and children with serious mental illnesses.

Prodromal stage: Earliest stage of beginning pathology.

Psychological first aid: An evidence-informed intervention in the immediate aftermath of a disaster.

Second-generation antipsychotics: Medications developed more recently in the science of psychiatric therapeutics.

Tardive dyskinesia: Twisting movements of tongue, limbs, and torso; irreversible; often a side effect of psychotropic medication.

CASE STUDY

References to the case study are found throughout this chapter (look for the case study icon). Readers should keep the case study in mind as they read the chapter.

Carmen, a 48-year-old immigrant from Peru, is brought to the emergency department by her daughter after taking 10 mg of lorazepam (Ativan) in less than 4 hours. Her daughter describes her mother as acting "crazy" and not making any sense. Carmen lives with her mother, her husband, her two sons, her daughter, and her daughter's child. Until 2 years ago, Carmen worked cleaning houses when she sustained a back injury. She has been taking 5 mg of hydrocodone/acetaminophen (Vicodin) prn every 6 hours, but her supply ran out, and she claims that her nurse practitioner would not send in another prescription to the pharmacy. Carmen speaks some English and explains to the psychiatric nurse that she was in such pain from her back that she just wanted the pain to end. The psychiatric clinical nurse specialist contacted a primary care provider in the community, who expressed concern that Carmen was suicidal and needed additional medical evaluation for her back injury. After consulting with the primary care providers, her family, and Carmen herself, the psychiatric mental health clinical specialist admitted Carmen to a locked psychiatric unit for evaluation.

In the psychiatric unit, Carmen begins to wail loudly, slap her head with her hands, and throw her head in a backward motion against a wall. She stands rigidly against a wall and appears unresponsive to a nurse's inquiries in English about what she is experiencing. Given her daughter's concern about her mother's mental status on admission, and her current behavior and unresponsiveness to the nurses' inquiries, an order is requested for an prn dose of olanzapine (Zyprexa) 5 mg. When a student nurse asks Carmen in Spanish what is wrong, she replies that her pain is unbearable and she needs Vicodin; otherwise, she just wants to be dead.

CULTURAL CONTEXT OF MENTAL ILLNESS

Mental health and, conversely, mental illness are concepts bound by culture. Understanding of what connotes mental health is shaped by social norms that evolve from generation to generation. In Western cultures, medical science interprets any deviation from normative function of the five senses as indicative of a psychotic disorder. Hearing a voice, claiming to see an object, or having certain tactile sensations are viewed as pathologic states to be treated by psychiatric professionals. In some parts of the world, spiritual possession or healers with special powers and beliefs are culture-bound syndromes (Hwang, Myers, Abe-Kim, & Ting, 2008). Whenever health professionals are tempted to label behavior as "abnormal," it is important to always be cognizant of the values of the health professional and how these values may be in conflict with community norms. Differences in incidence by race, gender, and ethnicity are evident in many mental illnesses. It is important to determine whether these differences are a product of better surveillance and access to treatment or whether psychiatric professionals are more apt to label a behavior deviant in a certain population. Because of the stigma associated with mental disorders, many people and their families are reticent to speak publicly of their experiences and need for services. It is crucial that advocates are cognizant of the epidemiologic findings that describe the needs, trends, risk factors, and effectiveness of community mental health services. Sound epidemiologic research, both nationally and internationally, is the foundation policymakers need to formulate, plan, and implement effective community-based programs that address the needs of the mentally ill.

In Western cultures, emotional distress is most often expressed verbally, whereas in Asian or Latino cultures, somatization, specifically, physical complaints of pain, headache, or stomach aches can be a prominent symptom of depression and anxiety (Hwang et al., 2008). For Carmen, both her emotional and physical pain warrants nursing intervention and careful assessment. By alleviating her physical pain, nurses can more comprehensively assess her mental status and what, if any, symptoms of mood or psychosis would benefit from psychotropic medication.

DEFINITIONS OF MENTAL ILLNESS

Although there is no universally accepted definition of mental health, for practical purposes, widely accepted parameters of the types of behaviors that connote psychopathology must be used to measure the incidence, morbidity, and mortality of mental illness in a population. The first challenge for epidemiologists who study the prevalence of mental illness is to develop valid operational definitions and standardized measurement instruments. Since 1952, the American Psychiatric Association (APA) has been refining the diagnostic criteria that describe mental illness. This nomenclature is compiled in a text titled the *Diagnostic and Statistical Manual of Mental Disorders* (*DSM-5*) (APA, 2013). The National Comorbidity Survey (NCS) is a nationally representative survey that assesses the prevalence of major mental illnesses according to the criteria in the *DSM-5* (Kessler & Wang, 2008). Internationally, the World Mental Health initiative replicated the NCS. This allowed researchers to examine cross-cultural prevalence of major mental illnesses (Kessler & Wang, 2008).

"Normal" is just a setting on the dryer. **Barbara Johnson, author**

Practice Point

Epidemiologic studies describe the social costs of mental illness and are essential to target programs to populations in greatest need. *Healthy People 2020* identified the following key objectives in measuring progress toward improving mental health: suicide, adolescent suicide attempts, serious mental illness in homeless adults, employment of homeless adults, and the employment of people with serious mental illness and eating disorder relapses. The Centers for Disease Control and Prevention (CDC) tracks epidemiologic data to determine the extent to which target objectives for mental health and mental disorders have been reached (Fig. 21.1).

SCOPE OF MENTAL ILLNESS

Psychiatric disorders are the leading cause of disability worldwide. Every year, approximately one-third of the world's population suffers from a major mental illness, yet almost two-thirds do not receive any mental health treatment (Thornicroft, 2007). Countries that spend a larger portion of their gross domestic product on healthcare are also those countries where individuals are most likely to receive treatment for mental illness (Wang et al., 2007). Despite the prevalence of disability associated with major mental illness, these disorders are much more likely to be untreated than physical illness at every income level (Ormel et al., 2008). Those suffering from alcoholism and addictive disorders are most likely to go untreated (78%), followed by anxiety disorders (57%), depression (56%), and bipolar disorder (50%) (Thornicroft, 2007). Young African Americans and the elderly have the highest rates of unmet psychiatric care (Neighbors et al., 2007).

The mind is like an iceberg, it floats with one-seventh of its bulk above water. **Sigmund Freud**

LEGEND

✔ Target met or exceeded[2,3]	➕ Improving[4,5]	◯ Little or no detectable change[6-10]	➖ Getting worse[11,12]	Baseline only[13]	Informational[14]

Objective Description	Baseline Value (Year)	Midcourse Value (Year)	Target	Movement Toward Target[15]	Movement Away From Baseline[16]	Movement Statistically Significant[17]
Mental Health Status Improvement						
➖[11] **MHMD-1** Suicide rate (age-adjusted, per 100,000 population)	11.3 (2007)	12.6 (2013)	10.2		11.5%	Yes
➖[11] **MHMD-2** Suicide attempts by adolescents (percent grades 9–12)	1.9% (2009)	2.7% (2013)	1.7%		42.1%	Yes
➖[11] **MHMD-3** Adolescents engaging in disordered eating behaviors in an attempt to control their weight (percent, grades 9–12)	14.3% (2009)	16.7% (2013)	12.9%		16.8%	Yes
➖[11] **MHMD-4.1** Adolescents with major depressive episode in the past 12 months (percent, 12–17 years)	8.3% (2008)	10.7% (2013)	7.5%		28.9%	Yes
◯[8] **MHMD-4.2** Adults with a major depressive episode in the past 12 months (percent, 18+ years)	6.5% (2008)	6.7% (2013)	58%		3.1%	No
Treatment Expansion						
[13] **MHMD-5** Primary care facilities that provide mental health treatment on-site or by paid referral (percent)	79.0% (2006)		87.0%			
◯[6] **MHMD-6** Children with mental health problems receiving treatment (percent, 4–17 years)	68.9% (2008)	70.8% (2014)	75.8%	27.5%		No
[13] **MHMD-7** Juvenile residential facilities that screen admissions for mental health problems (percent)	58.0% (2006)		64.0%			
➖[11] **MHMD-8** Persons with serious mental illness who are employed (percent, 18+ years)	56.0% (2008)	48.5% (2013)	61.6%		13.4%	Yes
◯[6] **MHMD-9.1** Adults with serious mental illness who receive treatment (percent, 18+ years)	65.7% (2008)	68.5% (2013)	72.3%	42.4%		No
◯[8] **MHMD-9.2** Adults with major depressive episodes who receive treatment (percent, 18+ years)	69.9% (2008)	68.6% (2013)	75.9%		0.6%	No
✔[2] **MHMD-10** Persons with co-occurring substance abuse and mental disorders who receive treatment (percent, 18+ years)	3.3% (2008)	4.2% (2013)	3.6%	300.0%		No
✔[2] **MHMD-11.1** Primary care physician office visits by adults that include screening for depression (percent, 19+ years)	2.2% (2007)	2.4% (2010)	2.4%	100.0%		No

FIGURE 21.1 National Center for Health Statistics (2016). (National Center for Health Statistics. [2016]. *Chapter 28: Mental Health and Mental Disorders. Healthy People 2020 [p. 28–7]. Midcourse Review.* Hyattsville, MD: U.S. Department of Health and Human Services.)

Stigma, inequities in mental health benefits, and fragmentation in the delivery system have prevented many people, especially the elderly, those in rural areas, and ethnic minorities, from receiving appropriate mental health treatment. The failure to identify and treat young people for mental illness can have profound social consequences, including truancy, incarceration, addiction, unplanned pregnancy, poverty, and suicide.

🔎 Evidence for Practice

A panel of experts used a narrative review methodology to identify best practices to promote mental health in low and middle income countries (Petersen et al., 2016). The study concluded that *"best practice"* population level interventions include laws and regulations to control access to alcohol and lethal means of suicide. *"Good practice"* population level interventions include child protection laws, control of parasitic infections that cause neurologic disorders and public awareness campaigns. Community level intervention *"best practices"* include education programs to promote mental health for school age youth and parents of infants. Community level *"good practices"* include: training community health workers to screen for mental illness in schools or neighborhoods and assist with community-based support and recovery; integrating mental health promotion programs in the workplace; and psychoeducation for parents of youth to increase knowledge of mental disorders (Petersen et al., 2016). The authors emphasize that in low and middle income countries these population- and community-based interventions are an essential component to promoting mental health as well as early identification and referral for treatment of mental disorders (Petersen et al., 2016).

SOME MAJOR MENTAL ILLNESSES

Worldwide there has been a global shift in disease burden from communicable diseases to noncommunicable diseases, including mental and behavioral disorders (Murray et al., 2012). Major mental illness may be broadly grouped into three categories: thought disorders, mood disorders, and anxiety disorders. Often, the dysfunction that a person is experiencing in his or her thinking or mood is further complicated by substance abuse, dementia, or a medical condition. One of the top 10 causes of disability worldwide

is schizophrenia, a thought disorder characterized by psychotic thinking and profound social apathy or withdrawal.

Evidence for Practice

In 2008, the Mental Health Gap Action Programme (mhGAP) in the World Health Organization (WHO) conducted a systematic review of evidence on the treatment of major mental illness in resource-poor countries. On the basis of this scientific review, the WHO released the *"mhGAP Intervention Guide for mental, neurological, and substance use disorders in nonspecialized health settings"* (WHO, 2010). The intent of the intervention guide is to provide nonspecialist healthcare providers' evidence-based protocols to expand mental healthcare in resource-poor settings (WHO, 2010).

Schizophrenia
Epidemiology

About 1% of the world's population suffers from schizophrenia. Symptoms of schizophrenia typically first appear in late adolescence or young adulthood and persist throughout a person's life, causing significant impairment in all aspects of a person's psychosocial functioning. The exact etiology is unknown; however, genetic studies have found a high concordance of schizophrenia (40% to 50%) among monozygotic twins (Clarke, Kelleher, Clancy, & Cannon, 2012). Complications in pregnancy, delivery, viral infections, early childhood stress, head injuries, and cannabis abuse have all been

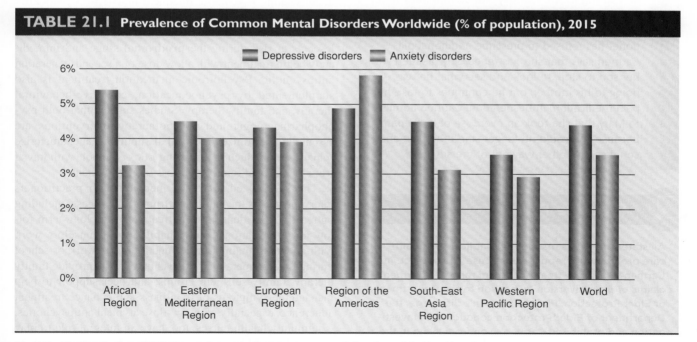

TABLE 21.1 Prevalence of Common Mental Disorders Worldwide (% of population), 2015

World Health Organization (2017). *Depression and other common mental disorders: global health estimates.* Geneva: World Health Organization. p. 12. Retrieved on September 15, 2017, from http://www.who.int/mental_health/management/depression/prevalence_global_health_estimates/en/.

implicated in increasing the risk of developing schizophrenia. Although the onset of symptoms of the disease is similar across a range of countries and cultures, there is debate among epidemiologists about cross-cultural comparisons, suggesting that the functional status of people with schizophrenia is higher in developing rather than developed countries.

Practice Point

Nurses in Western cultures need to be mindful of the fact that there are societies and cultures whose beliefs about what connotes abnormal behavior are very different from those in the United States. All social indicators are culture bound, so when epidemiologists conduct cross-cultural comparisons of mental illness and disability, they need to take these cultural differences into account.

Carmen receives a prn dose of hydrocodone/acetaminophen (Vicodin) for pain and olanzapine (Zyprexa) for agitation. Mary, a student nurse, stays with Carmen as she rested in her room, and within an hour, her restlessness, agitation, and emotional distress markedly diminished. Mary converses with Carmen in Spanish and asks her about how she manages her pain at home. Carmen explains that she believes her son, who lives with her and recently became unemployed, has been taking her Vicodin and selling it. She tearfully shares with Mary that she has been running out of Vicodin before she can refill the prescription, and her nurse practitioner has refused to prescribe additional pills. Carmen says that she has repeatedly pleaded with her son to stop, to look and see what he was doing to his mother, but he continues to take her pain medication. In desperation, Carmen admits to Mary that she took an overdose of lorazepam because she could no longer stand the pain and could see no other way out of the situation.

Practice Point

All states have laws mandating that licensed healthcare professionals report elder abuse and neglect. In Carmen's case, the treatment team reported Carmen's claims of drug diversion by her son to the Department of Elder Protection. Prior to Carmen's discharge, the Department of Elder Protection conducted an investigation and prohibited Carmen's son from living in the home with his mother.

Early Intervention Programs for First-Episode Psychosis

One of the most promising advances in the treatment of schizophrenia has been the use of **early intervention programs** for people at risk for psychosis. Early intervention programs for first-episode psychosis began in Australia in the 1980s and quickly spread to the United Kingdom, Europe, North American and Asia (McGorry, Killackey, & Yung, 2008). Detailed descriptions of the mission, goals, and services of the early intervention programs worldwide are available on the internet (Table 21.2). All these programs typically consist of specialized teams of nurses, occupational and rehabilitative therapists, and physicians, whose primary goal is to maintain the person's current level of educational and vocational functioning.

The early intervention programs are based on the theory that repeated episodes of psychosis are toxic to the brain, producing debilitating cognitive effects that may be minimized with early treatment. The hope is that if the initial treatment occurs during the first episode of psychosis, the less likely the person will be incapacitated by the disease during his or her life. The shorter the duration of untreated psychosis, termed DUP, the more likely the individual will be achieve and sustain a higher level of functioning. Researchers are also examining whether intervening even prior to the onset of psychotic behavior will improve treatment responsiveness and cognitive functioning. Early intervention programs attempt to identify at-risk people prior to the onset of hallucinations, delusions, and other symptoms of disordered thinking. Early identification is complicated by the fact that, on average, adolescents and their families delay seeking psychiatric treatment until 1 to 5 years after the onset of psychotic symptoms.

Ideally, early intervention programs identify young adolescents at risk during the **prodromal stage** and immediately begin treatment with a low dose of a second-generation antipsychotic. Psychotropic medication treatment is also supplemented by psychoeducation, cognitive-behavioral therapy, and family therapy. Studies suggest that both psychopharmacologic and psychotherapy interventions are essential to minimize the social disruptions that characterize schizophrenia, such as dropping out of school, withdrawal from friends and family, and loss of employment.

The specialized teams of mental health practitioners intervene across the entire spectrum of the illness, including outreach, early identification, treatment, and long-term follow-up. Occupational and rehabilitation counselors work with clients to maintain role functioning at work or school during the treatment phase. Psychotherapists provide family therapy, family self-help groups, and peer support to help manage the symptoms of the illness and enhance treatment adherence, especially with low-dose atypical antipsychotics. Community health nurses, too, have an integral role to play in each facet of the early intervention treatment model. In the predisease phase, primary care nurses who work in

TABLE 21.2	Early Intervention Programs for First Psychotic Episode	
Country	**Program**	**Internet Link**
Australia	Australian Early Intervention Network for Mental Health in Young People (AusEinet)	http://www.auseinet.flinders.edu.au
	Melbourne—Early Psychosis Prevention and Intervention Centre (EPPIC)	www.eppic.org.au
Canada	British Columbia—Early Psychosis Initiative (EPI)	www.mheccu.ubc.ca/projects/EPI
	Calgary—Early Psychosis Program (EPP)	www.ucalgary.ca/cdss/epp
	Vancouver—Helping Overcome Psychosis Early (HOPE)	www.hope.vancouver.bc.ca
Finland	Detection of Early Psychosis (DEEP Project)	http://www.med.utu.fi/tutkimus/ tutkimusprojektit/psykiatria3.html
France	Paris—PREPSY	http://prepsy.free.fr/
Germany	Cologne—Early Recognition and Intervention Center	http://www.kompetenznetz-schizophrenie.de/ rdkns/index.htm
Ireland	Dublin—Detection, Education and Local Team Assessment (DELTA)	http://www.deltaproject.ie/
Netherlands	Amsterdam—People with Increased Vulnerability to Psychosis (PSILON)	http://www.ypsilon.org/hulp/advies/preventi/ index.htm
New Zealand	Takapuna—Early Intervention National Training Program	http://www.werrycentre.org.nz/
Norway	Program to Reduce the Duration of Untreated Psychosis (TIPPS)	www.tips-info.com
Singapore	Early Psychosis Intervention Program (EPIP)	http://www.epip.org.sg/
Switzerland	Basil—FEPSY Project	http://www.fepsy.ch/
United Kingdom	NHS—Early Intervention in Psychosis	http://www.iris-initiative.org.uk/
United States	Albuquerque—Early Assessment and Resource Linkage for Youth (EARLY)	http://www.earlyprogram.org/
	Boston—First-Episode and Early Psychosis Program (FEPP)	www.massgeneral.org/allpsych/Schizophrenia/
	Chicago—First-Episode Psychosis Program	http://uillinoismedcenter.org/content.cfm/ psychosis
	Los Angeles—Center for the Assessment and Prevention of Prodromal States (CAPPS)	http://www.capps.ucla.edu/
	Manhattan—Center of Prevention and Evaluation (COPE)	http://cumc.columbia.edu/dept/pi/research/ clinics/pc.html
	New Haven—Prevention Through Risk Identification and Prevention (PRIME)	www.ynhh.org/ynhph/ynhph.html
	Pittsburgh—Services for the Treatment of Early Psychosis (STEP)	http://www.upmc.com/services/behavioral-health/pages/early-psychoses.aspx
	Portland, Maine—Prevent Mental Illness With Early Detection	http://www.preventmentalillness.org/pier_home. html
	Salem, Oregon—Prevent Mental Illness With Early Detection	http://www.preventmentalillness.org/pier_home. html

Schizophrenia.com. Retrieved on June 3, 2013, from http://www.schizophrenia.com/earlypsychosis.htm#ill; National Alliance for the Mentally Ill. Retrieved on May 28, 2013, from http://www.nami.org/FirstEpisode/clinics_ psychosis.jpg.

schools or pediatrician's offices are well positioned to identify youth who may be at risk. During the acute phase, nurses assess the therapeutic efficacy of antipsychotic treatment and educate clients and their families about how antipsychotic medication can help alleviate symptoms of the illness and the importance of treatment adherence. During the maintenance phase, nurses play a critical role in helping families and clients adhere to treatment recommendations and manage some of the residual symptoms of the disease.

The prodromal signs and symptoms suggesting that a young adolescent is at risk for developing psychosis are not unlike those behaviors exhibited during normal adolescent development. Screening tools to identify adolescents at risk for developing schizophrenia have been developed by practitioners in Germany, Australia, the United Kingdom, and the United States. The Structured Interview for Prodromal Symptoms and the Scale of Prodromal Symptoms are two widely used scales in the United States developed by researchers at Yale University (Miller et al., 2002). Specific prodromal signs and symptoms manifested in adolescence include sleep disturbance, anxiety, irritability, deterioration in role function, depressed mood, social withdrawal, poor concentration, suspiciousness, loss of motivation, and perceptual disturbances (Yung et al., 2007). Early identification of psychosis and administration of low-dose antipsychotic medication may help mitigate the chronic, debilitating course of schizophrenia and significantly improve long-term outcomes.

Evidence for Practice

A systematic review of early intervention programs in schizophrenia found that the screening criteria for identifying prodromal symptoms were nonspecific and mental health professionals were hesitant to identify patients at high-risk (Cheng & Schepp, 2016). Cheng & Schepp (2016) emphasize that community mental health nurses need training and screening tools to appropriately identify at-risk individuals who can benefit from early intervention for psychosis.

Primary Prevention Programs

One of the challenges for researchers is to better understand the relationship between substance abuse, the onset of psychotic symptoms, and relapse. Originally, it had been presumed that adolescents who are susceptible to mental illness abuse cannabis or other illicit substances as a means of self-medication. There is empirical evidence that cannabis use is a component cause of schizophrenia and increases the risk two- to fourfold (Clarke, Kelleher, Clancy, & Cannon, 2012). Each episode of psychosis is an assault to the neural mechanisms in the brain. Extensive studies have shown that cannabis use may increase risk of developing psychosis in at-risk individuals.

The possibility that the amount, duration, and strength of cannabis may be a precursor to the development of schizophrenia has significant implications for both drug education programs and early intervention programs for psychosis. Public health education campaigns should continue to educate adolescents about the potential adverse effects of cannabis use, especially on mental health. Encouraging even modest declines in an individual's dose and duration of cannabis use may delay conversion to psychosis or attenuate psychotic symptoms. The more conversion to psychosis can be delayed or avoided, the greater the likelihood that neurocognitive function maybe preserved.

> Legislating marijuana into legitimacy does not make it safe.
> **Chittaranjan Andrade (2016, e742)**

There has been a significant downward trend in the use of cannabis by middle-school age youth attributed to the success of drug educational programs (National Institute on Drug Abuse, 2016). Nationally, cannabis use among high school seniors has remained stable except in states where cannabis is legal for medical or recreational use. Significantly more high school seniors in states where cannabis is legal consume cannabis edibles or smoke cannabis than in states where cannabis is not legal (National Institute on Drug Abuse, 2016). A future area for epidemiologic research will be to examine whether the rise in the use of cannabis and synthetic cannabinoid substances is correlated with an increase in the prevalence and morbidity of schizophrenia in the United States.

Enhancing Treatment Adherence in Schizophrenia

Nonadherence with medication is the most common factor associated with relapse and recurrence of psychotic symptoms. One of the largest studies of treatment efficacy for patients diagnosed with schizophrenia, the Clinical Antipsychotic Trials of Intervention of Effectiveness (CATIE) study, found that 74% of the patients discontinued their medication before 18 months (Levine, Rabinowitz, Faries, Lawson, & Ascher-Svanum, 2012). The longer and more frequently patients diagnosed with schizophrenia experience psychotic symptoms, the greater the gray matter atrophy in the prefrontal cortex and greater the impairment of executive cognitive function (Morton & Zubek, 2013). A common feature of all early intervention programs is to educate the client and the family about how nonadherence to the medication regime can lead to relapse. To be maximally effective, both the client and the family must be educated about the morbidity associated with untreated psychotic symptoms, especially in light of growing evidence that the more frequent the psychotic episodes, the greater and more lasting the negative effects on cognitive function.

Nursing interventions to enhance medication adherence applicable to those with chronic mental illness may include oral and written reminders, self-monitoring tools, cues, and positive reinforcements by both the nurse and the family. Psychoeducation by community health nurses should teach clients and families about the signs of impending relapse, how medication can help remit the more debilitating negative symptoms of the disease, and the importance of lifestyle changes, especially avoiding use of illicit substances. Psychosocial interventions for clients with chronic mental illness also include employment or vocational training, social skills development, and coaching, with an emphasis on problem solving and motivational interviewing. Family support groups, training in cognitive-behavioral approaches, and basic communication strategies are particularly helpful for families who are trying to manage medication administration in the home.

In addition to psychosocial interventions, which can be prohibitively expensive and difficult to implement in resource-poor countries, long-acting injectable antipsychotic (LAI) medications are another strategy to promote recovery from psychosis. A long-acting injectable form of antipsychotic should not be administered until it is clear how the client responds to oral forms of the medication. The first-generation antipsychotics haloperidol decanoate and fluphenazine decanoate, and the second-generation antipsychotics risperidone microsphere, olanzapine pamoate, paliperidone palmitate, aripiprazole monohydrate, or lauroxil, are antipsychotics available as long-acting preparations. LAI vary in duration from 1 to 4 months (Stevens, Dawson, & Zummo, 2016).

Evidence for Practice

A comparison of treatment adherence with LAI versus oral antipsychotic medication for individuals with schizophrenia found that over a 1-year period, individuals on LAI antipsychotics were 20% less likely to discontinue their medication (Greene, Yan, Chang, Hartry, Touya, & Broder, 2017). A systematic review also concluded there is sufficient empiric evidence supporting a correlation between LAIs and treatment adherence for first-episode psychosis or recent-onset schizophrenia (Kim, Lee, Yang, Park, & Chung, 2012). Yet there are wide cross-cultural variations in prescribing LAIs with over half of the mental health prescribers in the United Kingdom likely to prescribe LAIs in first-episode psychosis compared to less than half of the prescribers in the United States (Kim et al., 2012).

Student Reflection

In the following conversation, two nursing students discuss the use of antipsychotic medication.

Student 1: Obviously, all patients have the right to refuse treatment, especially injections of antipsychotic medication, unless they pose an immediate danger to themselves or others. But it seems inhumane not to offer chronic mentally ill patients the option of taking their antipsychotic medication by injection, especially those who become so impaired they can't take care of themselves and put themselves at risk.

Student 2: I heard that some community outreach programs in England provide financial incentives for patients to receive their injections (Claassen, 2007).

Student 1: Don't you think that is unethical, to bribe a patient to take the medication by offering money or gifts?

Student 2: Well, what is the alternative, the community has rights, too, and what if a chronic mentally ill person is so psychotic that he or she is wandering the streets intimidating people? If I worked in a mental health center and I was directed to give a gift to entice a patient to take medication, I wouldn't have any problem with doing that—the patient can refuse both if he or she wants to.

Student 1: I think it would be better to go to court and seek a court order on the basis of the medical evidence and the patient's mental health history rather than to offer the patient a bribe, especially since most of the patients receiving the injectable medication are disproportionately incarcerated, uninsured, or poor people, who may belong to ethnic minorities (Glazer, 2007).

Medication adherence is also complicated in clients with schizophrenia because all antipsychotic medications have side effects that can interfere with normal daily functioning. Some side effects, especially with **first-generation antipsychotics** (e.g., haloperidol and fluphenazine), can be life-threatening and physically debilitating. Of particular concern with the first-generation antipsychotics is the risk of developing **tardive dyskinesia** (TD). This condition, which is irreversible, is characterized by twisting movements of tongue, limbs, and torso. The longer the clients are on the first-generation antipsychotics, the greater the risk of acquiring TD. Because TD is permanently disfiguring, nurses in the community should routinely screen patients for subtle symptoms of TD using the Abnormal Involuntary Movement Scale (Guy, 1976). Some of the other debilitating side effects of the first-generation antipsychotics include akathisia (extreme restlessness in the limbs), dystonia (severe stiffness in muscles, most prominently the neck), blurred vision, urinary retention, and neuroleptic malignant syndrome.

The **second-generation antipsychotics** have fewer extrapyramidal symptoms and are much less likely to cause TD but have greater risks of metabolic syndrome. Metabolic syndrome is an adverse effect of treatment with second-generation antipsychotics (such as clozapine, olanzapine, quetiapine, risperidone, and ziprasidone) that develops as a result of pronounced weight gain, dyslipidemia, and hyperglycemia. Clients may experience weight gain on all of the antipsychotics; however, almost half of all patients on the second-generation antipsychotics experience a 20% increase in weight. Evidence is mounting that the second-generation antipsychotics, in particular clozapine and olanzapine, may increase the risk of developing new-onset type 2 diabetes.

At this time, regulations mandating regular monitoring of the client's weight and other symptoms associated with type 2 diabetes have not been promulgated by the FDA. In 2004, the APA and the American Diabetes Association (ADA) developed consensus guidelines to screen clients on second-generation antipsychotics for the development of cardiovascular diseases and type 2 diabetes (Table 21.3). The ADA and the APA emphasize that given the significant risk for developing hyperglycemia, the consensus guidelines should be considered a basic standard of care for all schizophrenic patients prescribed the second-generation antipsychotics.

Studies have shown that neither class of antipsychotics is superior in treating the positive and negative symptoms of schizophrenia and both have risks of adverse effects. One exception is clozapine, which has been shown to be superior in treating both the positive and negative symptoms of schizophrenia. It is important to note that clozapine has been associated with life-threatening agranulocytosis. The FDA has established a national clozapine registry and mandates white blood cell (WBC) counts within 24 hours of the initial dose, weekly for 6 months, and then every 2 weeks. Pharmacists may only dispense enough clozapine until the next WBC count test and must receive notification of the laboratory results prior to dispensing any additional medication. Like the other second-generation antipsychotics, clozapine causes weight gain, which is one of the most common side effects of the drug that contributes to nonadherence. The World Psychiatric Association has recommended that government funding agencies provide coverage for a broad array of medication treatment options to allow individualized treatment based on safety, tolerability, and efficacy of first- and second-generation antipsychotics (Tandon et al., 2008).

> ### Practice Point
>
> All antipsychotics have untoward effects that can compromise treatment adherence and physical health. Community health nurses must carefully monitor clients especially for TD, agranulocytosis, and metabolic syndrome, which can be a precursor to type 2 diabetes. Patients with schizophrenia have a two- to threefold increased risk of death mostly from metabolic syndrome and it is a major public health concern for this population (Ventriglio, Gentile, Stella, & Bellomi, 2015).

High-Risk Populations

The unemployed, the poor, and the homeless all report higher levels of depression, anxiety, schizophrenia, and substance abuse than the general population (WHO, 2008). Whether these social conditions trigger the symptoms of depression, anxiety, and psychosis or the debilitating effects of these illnesses lead to loss of employment, housing, and subsequent poverty is a source of debate within the field of epidemiology. The rising number of mentally ill clients who are homeless has steadily increased in the United States as state governments embarked on a systematic plan to "deinstitutionalize" the mentally ill. The goal of **deinstitutionalization** is to replace state hospitals with smaller group homes, half-way houses, or other supported living arrangements that integrate, rather than separate, the chronic mentally ill in the community. Tragically, the services available in the community seldom have kept pace with the demand for services. The gap in community-based services persists in all developed countries because of fiscal and political constraints.

In the United States, local officials resist proposals to site-supported living arrangements in their community. At the state level, mental health appropriations for community-based care are rarely fully funded. At the federal level, both Congress and the White House have continued to tighten

TABLE 21.3 Recommendations for Monitoring Patients Taking Second-Generation Antipsychotics							
	Baseline	**4 Weeks**	**8 Weeks**	**12 Weeks**	**Quarterly**	**Annually**	**5 Years**
Personal and family history	X					X	
Body mass index (weight)	X	X	X	X	X	X	X
Waist circumference	X					X	
Blood pressure	X			X		X	
Fasting blood glucose	X			X		X	X
Fasting lipid profile	X			X			

American Diabetes Association; American Psychiatric Association; American Association of Clinical Endocrinologists; North American Association for the Study of Obesity. (2004). North American Association for the study of obesity. Consensus development conference on antipsychotic drugs and obesity and diabetes. *Journal of Clinical Psychiatry, 65,* 267–272.

eligibility criteria for social security disability—the primary financial resource for the chronic mentally ill who cannot work. Other federal programs in the Departments of Health and Human Services, Labor, Education, and Veterans Affairs that target homeless people have been "level funded." Therefore, funding has not kept pace with inflation. As government resources for the poor and disabled erode, shelters have been transformed from temporary to permanent housing. On the streets of any urban area, the failure to integrate the chronic mentally ill is glaringly apparent.

Practice Point

Individuals who have chronic mental illness are eligible to receive supplemental security income (SSI). However Martone (2014) notes that no where in the United States can the chronic mentally-ill receiving SSI find affordable housing. Without additional federal or state funding to support community-based housing for the chronic mentally ill, homelessness will continue to be a significant public health issue.

Role of Community Mental Health Teams in the Treatment of Schizophrenia

Prior to the community mental health movement and the deinstitutionalization of the mentally ill, people with chronic mental illness would be "warehoused," or confined to state hospitals for prolonged periods, many for life. Deinstitutionalization began as a humane initiative to end this "warehousing." But tragically, insufficient housing and the lack of other social supports in the community often results in homelessness for people with chronic mental illness. The burden of providing supportive care for the severe and persistently mentally ill has increasingly fallen to community agencies and families.

As a person with schizophrenia becomes less capable of managing social role responsibilities, families are faced with the burden of assuming the locus of care and support. Respite services, day-treatment facilities, and sheltered workshops are a few of the outpatient services that help alleviate the daily burden of care for families. Within families, caregiver burden is disproportionately shouldered by women, often the mother of the person with chronic mental illness. Women at greatest risk for burnout from the burden of care are Caucasian mothers caring for young adults with bipolar disorder in the home (Zauszniewski, Bekhet, & Suresky, 2008).

Families of people with chronic mental illness assume many of the economic costs associated with custodial care, but significant costs are also incurred by federal and local governments. People with schizophrenia are one of the largest beneficiaries of the federal and state welfare system. Federal, state, and local funds support care for people with chronic mental illness in homeless shelters, jails, long-term care facilities, and state mental hospitals. Too often, clients with chronic mental illness slip into no-care zones, adrift

between the social welfare and healthcare sectors. The fragmentation of care among a myriad of institutions and professionals makes collaboration and continuity of care a major challenge for providers.

To address these shortcomings in the delivery of care, the WHO (2013) Mental Health Gap Action Program recommends training community health workers in underresourced countries to provide evidence-based interventions for common mental health needs. Community health workers may be referred to as promotorales, paraprofessionals, or lay counselors (Barnett, Gonzalez, Miranda, Chavira, & Lau, 2017). Unlike standard treatment approaches, community health workers provide supportive mental healthcare in the client's home, school, or places of worship instead of medical setting. Ideally, community mental health teams are composed of a variety of mental health professionals including, nurses, physicians, social workers, and occupational and rehabilitation therapists, who can care for the more complex mental health needs of families and individuals. However in underresourced countries or regions, there is compelling evidence that community health workers improve the mental health outcomes for individuals and families (Barnett et al., 2017).

Internationally, several studies are evaluating the effectiveness of community mental health teams and early intervention programs, including the EDIE study in the United Kingdom, the LifeSPAN study in Australia, the OPUS study in Denmark, the PRIME study in the United States, and the TIPS study in Norway (Marshall & Lockwood, 2005). ACT is an evidence-based treatment for the chronically mentally ill that includes interdisciplinary teams, with a focus on medication management, housing, and rehabilitation. Findings thus far indicate that the most effective aspects of ACT are those that target psychosocial functioning, including vocational skills and supported employment, activities of daily living, and social relationships (Mueser, Deavers, Penn, & Cassisi, 2013).

Clients with schizophrenia often have a myriad of comorbid chronic health conditions. Obesity, hypertension, and severe cardiac and metabolic complications all are prevalent to much higher degrees in people with schizophrenia due to higher rates of smoking, poor nutrition, and lack of exercise. The social apathy associated with the disease, limited access to healthcare services, and social stigma make it difficult for clients with schizophrenia to advocate for their healthcare needs. As client advocates, an important role of the community health nurse is to ensure that the primary healthcare needs of the chronic mentally ill are met in a variety of community-based agencies.

Practice Point

A promising research initiative from the National Institute of Mental Health (NIMH), Recovery After an Initial Schizophrenia Episode (RAISE), is a network approach to integrate early intervention models with

ACT (Narayan, Mohwinckel, Pisano, Yang, & Manji, 2013). The goal of RAISE is to integrate community-based biopsychosocial treatment in the early stages of schizophrenia to minimize relapse, morbidity, and disability associated with chronic mental illness.

Mood and Anxiety Disorders

Epidemiology

SOCIAL FACTORS

Unlike schizophrenia, for which the incidence is stable across cultures worldwide, there is substantial variation in the incidence of mood disorders and suicide. Noted sociologist Emile Durkheim wrote in 1925, "Man is the more vulnerable to self-destruction the more he is detached from any collectivity. The extent that familial society is more or less cohesive, tightly-knit and strong—man is more or less strongly attached to life" (Durkheim, 1972), p. 13). By the end of the century, epidemiologic studies empirically validated Durkheim's theories that social factors do play a prominent role in the incidence of mood and anxiety disorders.

Globally, suicide ranks as one of the top causes of preventable deaths. Public health organizations in the United States and worldwide have targeted populations at-risk for harm reduction initiatives and prevention programs. A population approach holds the greatest promise for lowering the rate of suicide because predicting who will commit suicide is challenging. Past self-harm behavior is the strongest predictor of risk for suicide but 60% of individuals who commit suicide did not have a previous attempt (Christensen, Cuijpers, & Reynolds, 2016).

Populations at Risk for Suicide

One of the most pressing public health concerns for community mental health nurses is to address the precipitous increase in the rate of suicide, especially among young adults (Box 21.1). Worldwide, suicide among adolescents is the second leading cause of death (Centers for Disease Control and Prevention, 2013a; World Health Organization, 2012). Youth suicide is highest in developed countries and in South East Asia (Abraham & Sher, 2017). Suicide rates vary by gender with males having higher rates in developed countries and females having higher rates in rural

---

21.1 Evidence-Based Intervention to Promote Mental Health in Children

Cultural Adaptation of Cognitive Behavioral Therapy (CBT) for Puerto Rican Youth

Cultural Adaptation of Cognitive Behavioral Therapy (CBT) for Puerto Rican Youth is a short-term intervention for Puerto Rican adolescents aged 13–17 years who are primarily Spanish-speaking and have severe symptoms of depression. The intervention was informed in consideration of culturally sensitive criteria (i.e., language, developmental, and socioeconomic factors). Puerto Rican adolescents identified as having symptoms of depression received the intervention after being referred by local schools, clinics, and mental health professionals.

Areas of interest	Mental health treatment
Outcomes	**Review date: December 2010** Symptoms of depression Internalizing symptoms Externalizing symptoms Self-concept
Outcome categories	Mental health Social functioning
Ages	13–17 (Adolescent)
Genders	Male Female
Races/ethnicities	Hispanic or Latino
Settings	Outpatient Other community settings
Geographic locations	Urban
Implementation history	This intervention was first implemented in 1992 at the University of Puerto Rico, Río Piedras Campus. Since then, 198 Puerto Rican adolescents have received this intervention.
NIH funding/ CER studies	Partially/fully funded by National Institutes of Health: Yes Evaluated in comparative effectiveness research studies: Yes

Source: SAMHSA's National Registry of Evidence-Based Programs and Practices. Retrieved May 28, 2013, from http://www.nrepp.samhsa.gov/ViewIntervention.aspx?id=219.

communities in China and India (Abraham & Sher, 2017). In addition to a history of trauma, mood or substance disorder, a significant social risk factor is social isolation especially among immigrant or indigenous populations, homeless youth, or those in foster care (Abraham & Sher, 2017). In areas of the world where there is civil violence, terrorism, war or natural disasters, the impact of trauma to a community on the risk for suicide in youth is less certain (Abraham & Sher, 2017). Societal protective factors include family and social cohesion with strong adherence to cultural or religious beliefs that actively discourage suicide (Abraham & Sher, 2017).

The WHO recommends three evidenced-based population strategies to reduce suicide, including:

1. Restrict access to means of self-harm/suicide
2. Develop policies to reduce harmful use of alcohol as a component of suicide prevention
3. Encourage the media to provide information about where to seek help and avoid sensationalizing suicide (World Health Organization, 2012)

The most common lethal means of suicide varies by country and access. Globally, pesticide poisonings are a major cause of fatalities in non-Western countries whereas in the United States, firearms, opioids, and over the counter medications such as aspirin and acetaminophen are often used in suicide (Abraham & Sher, 2017). Government prohibition of toxic pesticides was an effective harm reduction intervention in both South Korea and Sri Lanka (Global Burden of Disease Collaboration, 2016). In Sri Lanka, bans on toxic pesticides cut the suicide rate in half (Patel et al., 2016).

In the United States, suicide now surpasses motor vehicle accidents as a leading cause of death (Centers for Disease Control and Prevention, 2013b). In addition to age, gender differences are significant, with rates of completed suicides more than twice as high for men than for women, and retired, divorced, white men at highest risk (Fig. 21.2). In 2014 the suicide rate for females aged 10 to 14 had the largest percent increase (200%) over the past decade than all other age groups (Curtin, Warner, Hedegaard, 2016). Self-harm behaviors, such as cutting or burning of the skin, has also increased significantly among adolescent girls (Mojtabai, Olfson, & Han, 2016). Adolescents in lower socioeconomic groups and American Indian/Alaskan Native youth have the highest rates of mortality from suicide (Shain, 2016). Almost half of adolescents who committed suicide used a firearm (Shain, 2016) (Figs. 21.3 and 21.4).

In October of 2004, the U.S. FDA mandated the following warning to be added to the drug information insert included in all antidepressant packaging:

- Antidepressants increase the risk of suicidal thinking and behavior (suicidality) in children and adolescents with major depressive disorder and other psychiatric disorders.
- Anyone considering the use of an antidepressant in a child or adolescent for any clinical use must balance the risk of increased suicidality with the clinical need.
- Patients who are started on therapy should be observed closely for clinical worsening, suicidality, or unusual changes in behavior.
- Families and caregivers should be advised to closely observe the patient and to communicate with the prescriber.

Up until the issuance of what is termed by the FDA as a **"Black box" warning**, there had been a steady rise in the

FIGURE 21.2 *Healthy People 2020* target to decrease suicide by gender. (National Vital Statistics System—Mortality [NVSS-M], CDC/NCHS. Retrieved May 29, 2013, from http://www.healthypeople.gov/2020/topicsobjectives2020/nationalsnapshot.aspx?topicId=28.)

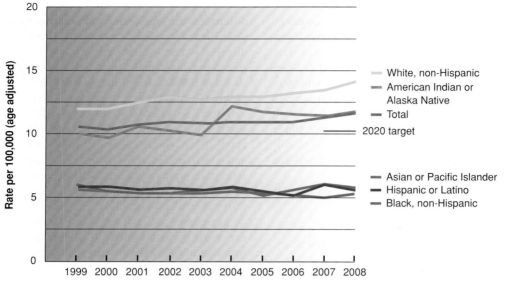

FIGURE 21.3 *Healthy People 2020* target to decrease suicide by ethnicity. (National Vital Statistics System—Mortality [NVSS-M], CDC/NCHS. Retrieved May 29, 2013, from http://www.healthy-people.gov/2020/topicsobjectives2020/nationalsnapshot.aspx?topicId=28.)

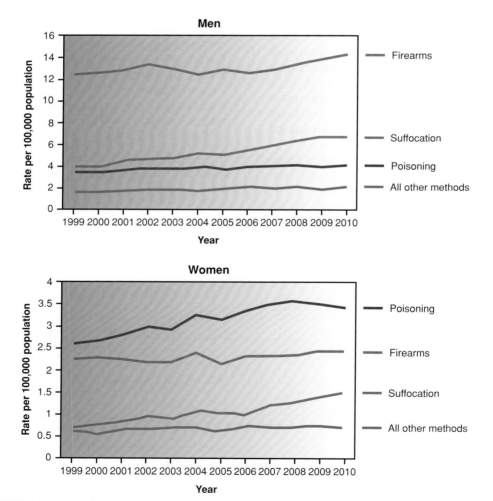

FIGURE 21.4 Trends in suicide rates by gender and means 1999 to 2010. (Centers for Disease Control and Prevention. [2013]. Suicide among adults aged 35–64. Years—United States, 1999–2010. *Morbidity and Mortality Weekly Report*, *62*[17], 325.)

use of SSRIs by pediatric practitioners. In the wake of the FDA warning, there are recent indications that the number of adolescents being prescribed antidepressants is beginning to decline. Now the concern expressed by pediatric practitioners is how to best weigh the risks and benefits of treatment with antidepressants so that the gains achieved over the past decade in lowering the rates of suicide among youth are not reversed.

The National Strategy for Suicide Prevention (NSSP) is a public health initiative launched by the federal government to prevent suicide through public health education and community-wide interventions that restore cohesiveness among community members (National Strategy for Suicide Prevention, 2012). A key feature of the NSSP is to disseminate public health programs about suicide prevention widely, among a wide range of institutions in society, especially schools. Community health nurses, who may practice in nontraditional settings (i.e., parish nurses, senior or recreational centers, and people's workplaces), are ideally positioned to implement many of the proposed program initiatives.

A man who has not passed through the inferno of his passions has never overcome them. **Carl Jung**

One of the objectives of NSSP is to limit access to lethal means of attempting suicide. Firearm access is a risk factor for suicide in the United States (U.S. Department of Health and Human Services, 2012). Often, suicide is an impulsive act that may be prevented if the means of completing the suicide was removed. The rate of completed suicides has been significantly reduced in many countries by a public health strategy termed *means restriction* (U.S. Department of Health and Human Services, 2012). A higher number of firearm laws in a state are associated with a lower rate of suicides from firearms fatalities (Fleegler, Lee, Monuteaux, Hemenway, & Mannix, 2013). Unfortunately, in American society, the power of the National Rifle Association, the availability of firearms, and the cultural value of personal freedom have thwarted enacting any meaningful restrictions on firearms.

Community health nurses can promote "means restriction," especially in families where there is a member at risk for suicide. Families who own firearms should be encouraged to secure firearms using trigger locks and locking bullets in a separate location from the firearm. If a client informs the nurse that he or she is having thoughts of taking an overdose, then prescription or over-the-counter medications that may be fatal in overdose should be removed or secured in a safe location. Although families might presume that removing the instrumental means of harm is an ineffective gesture, the community health nurse must reassure the family that their actions are sending a strong, unambiguous message to the potential victim that people care about them and will take any necessary steps to ensure their safety.

Practice Point

One of the factors that may explain the marked increase in suicide among preteen girls is the rise in cyberbullying. Middle school girls in particular report the highest rates of being victimized by cyberbullying and victims are twice as likely to have attempted suicide (Messias, Kindrick & Castro, 2014). The U.S. Department of Health and Human Services has created a public health media campaign at: www.stopbullying.gov. The website describes prevention strategies for parents and schools as well specific guidance to report cyberbullying to online service providers, police, and schools.

Nursing Interventions for Mood and Anxiety Disorders

The symptoms of major depression or anxiety commonly seen in community settings are fatigue, headache, backache, gastrointestinal complaints, anhedonia, and sleep and appetite disturbance. Clients who are exhibiting these somatic signs as well as mood symptoms should be asked directly if they have had any thoughts of harming themselves. If a client responds in the affirmative, the nurse needs to ascertain if the client has a specific plan and the means to carry out the plan.

Nonsuicidal self-injury is a growing public health problem especially among young adults. Epidemiologic reports indicate those young adults at highest risk are the unemployed, women, those with only a high school education, and those with a history of mood, anxiety, or personality disorders (Olfson et al., 2017). Nonsuicidal self-injury should always be interpreted as a cry for help. Community mental health nurses can play an important role in implementing community-based initiatives to prevent suicide and suicide attempts, especially among youth.

Evidence for Practice

A study of homeless youth in Texas found that homeless youth had higher rates of depression than the general population and were significantly more likely to abuse synthetic marijuana and alcohol (Narendorf, Cross, Maria, Swank & Bordnick, 2017). The authors conclude that homeless youth with untreated depression are misusing alcohol or synthetic marijuana to "self-medicate" their mood symptoms instead of seeking mental health treatment from healthcare professionals due to stigma and barriers to accessing mental health services. The Runaway and Homeless Youth Program funded by the U.S. Department of Health and Human Services provides grants to community agencies to provide mental and physical health services as well as individual and family counseling. For more information on how to apply for grants to address the unmet needs of homeless youth see: https://www.acf.hhs.gov/fysb/resource/rhy-fact-sheet.

Nursing Interventions for Hoarding Disorder

In the revision to the DSM-5 a new category of mental disorder was added under the category of obsessive-compulsive disorder to address the serious personal and public health implications of hoarding behavior. To be diagnosed with hoarding disorder, a person must accumulate, and not discard, items to such a degree that it significantly impairs their ability to perform basic skills of daily living. A residence may become so cluttered with waste that it is a health, fire, and safety hazard. Left unchecked, hoarding behavior has severe public health and sanitation implications for families, neighbors, and the community at large. The more longstanding the hoarding behavior, the poorer the prognosis and more difficult it becomes to change hoarding behavior (Burton, Arnold & Soreni, 2015).

Multimodal treatment for hoarding is similar to that of obsessive-compulsive disorder with the use of antidepressants and cognitive behavioral therapy. An essential component to treatment includes family support and involvement in treatment. The burden of hoarding behaviors on families is equivalent to, or greater than, living with an individual who has dementia (Drury, Ajmi, de la Cruz, Nordsletten, & Mataix-Cols, 2014). In most cases, the hoarding behavior first appeared in childhood or adolescence. About 25% of children diagnosed with autism spectrum disorder exhibit hoarding symptoms (Storch et al., 2016). The more parents accommodate to the child's hoarding behavior to avoid outbursts, the greater the likelihood treatment will be ineffective. Parents should be encouraged to restrict the space for desired items and if the space is full, then direct the child to discard items before others are added (Morris, Jaffee, Goodwin, & Franklin, 2016).

Community health nurses play an important role in identifying adults suffering from hoarding disorder because most do not seek treatment or acknowledge problematic hoarding behaviors (Brakoulias & Milicevic, 2015). A home assessment to determine the extent of hazards and if additional resources are necessary to clean and declutter the home, is the first stage of intervention by community health nurses (Murphy, 2014). Often the hoarder has limited insight about the adverse consequences of their behavior and contests the need to declutter. To overcome such an impasse, Murphy (2014) advises inviting a group of concerned family members to describe, in a nonjudgmental way, the adverse effects of the person's hoarding behavior. If the person expresses a willingness to declutter, the community health nurse can assist the person develop a timeline for achieving reasonable goals. Any behavior change is difficult and for a person with hoarding disorder, strong emotional attachments to inanimate objects or animals can make relinquishing these belongings all the more challenging. If the community health nurse identifies immediate health, fire, or safety hazards then it is appropriate to also enlist the assistance of the local fire department, board of health, and building inspection services (Murphy, 2014). Hoarding is a chronic condition and periodic check-ins by the community health nurse are essential components to sustaining a clean, safe, and de-cluttered home (Raeburn, Hungerford, Escott, & Cleary, 2015).

Attention-Deficit/Hyperactivity Disorders and Disruptive Behavior Disorders in Children

Approximately 1 in 10 youths have severe emotional disturbance with substantial functional impairment (Williams, Scott & Aarons, 2017). Disruptive behavior disorders, such as oppositional defiant disorder and conduct disorder, are often diagnosed as co-occurring with attention deficit hyperactivity disorder. Disruptive behavior disorders in childhood and adolescence account for the majority of psychiatric hospitalizations for children and half of all outpatient psychiatric treatment (Oruche et al., 2015).

The overlap in symptoms among ADHD, bipolar disorder, and disruptive behavior disorders makes it difficult for the school nurse to correctly identify students at risk and make referrals for appropriate treatment. Hyperactivity and impulsivity, hallmarks of ADHD, may also be displayed by children with bipolar disorder. Because the pharmacologic treatment for both conditions is vastly different—in ADHD, children are prescribed stimulants and in bipolar disorder, children are prescribed second-generation antipsychotics and mood stabilizers—it is important that clinicians recognize the subtle features that distinguish the two disorders.

The main characteristics that help healthcare practitioners, including school nurses, differentiate ADHD from bipolar disorder are the pervasiveness of the symptoms and the predominant symptoms. In children with ADHD, hyperactivity and impulsivity are evident in all spheres of the child's life. There is a constancy and pervasiveness of the hyperactivity in school, at home, and in activities. Distractibility and unrelenting motor behavior (e.g., always being in motion, begin unable to sit still and attend to a task) are the symptoms that cause the most distress for parents and teachers. Unlike bipolar disorder, mood and anxiety symptoms are not predominant in ADHD; generally, teachers and parents do not characterize the child with ADHD as angry, irritable, and moody.

Children diagnosed with bipolar disorder have a predominance of mood symptoms such as irritability, sleep disturbances, and anxiety (Kowatch, 2016). For a child with bipolar disorder, the slightest frustration can set off a flood of crying, screaming, or anxiety symptoms. Unlike toddlers who have temper tantrums that are time limited, children with bipolar disorder can have rage episodes that can last from 2 to 3 hours. In general, children who are angry and frustrated can be comforted by adults. However, children with bipolar disorder appear inconsolable. Angry or aggressive outbursts are unpredictable and episodic, varying from day to day and moment to moment. Because these violent outbursts overlap with symptoms seen in disruptive behavior disorders, oppositional defiant disorder is often diagnosed with bipolar disorder in children.

Family history may also alert the clinician to the possibility a child has bipolar disorder rather than ADHD. Most children with bipolar disorder had a family history of mood disorder. If parents or siblings report that they have experienced performance difficulties in school or work, it is important for the diagnostician to determine whether the poor performance was due to mood symptoms (such as depression) or motor behavior (such as impulsivity). If the social role functioning of a family member was disrupted primarily by mood symptoms, this may suggest that the child is more at risk for bipolar disorder than for ADHD.

Finally, clinicians, as well as school nurses, should carefully observe for improvement in target symptoms with medication treatment. With ADHD, there should be some improvement in symptoms after an adequate trial of psychostimulants. Similarly, with bipolar disorder, there should be an improvement in symptoms after treatment with second-generation antipsychotics. The danger in failing to make a proper diagnosis is that if children with bipolar disorder are prescribed antidepressant or stimulant drugs, there can be an exacerbation of suicidality, hostility, and agitation. Current estimates are that 20% to 40% of children initially diagnosed with depression will develop bipolar disorder. It is crucial for school nurses to carefully monitor any child on antidepressants for a worsening of symptoms, especially any indications of disinhibition.

Multidisciplinary collaboration among teachers, therapists, and primary care providers is a central feature of comprehensive treatment for the child with any behavioral disorder. Psychotherapies, specifically cognitive-behavioral therapy and family therapy, have been demonstrated to be effective in the management of depression but not as effective as antidepressants alone. Self-help groups for families are of enormous benefit in helping families cope with the child's disruptive behaviors that can quickly lead to caregiver burnout.

The role of the school nurse is integral to helping the child or adolescent understand the nature of the disorder; the purpose and side effects of medication; and the importance of maintaining a healthy lifestyle, including good sleep hygiene, avoidance of caffeine, relaxation techniques, and abstinence from illicit drugs. It may sound like a tall order for the school nurse, but there is compelling evidence that young adults and children respond positively to primary interventions, education, and support from caring adults. Often, a depressed child will come to the health office with somatic complaints such as headache, gastrointestinal upset, or fatigue. The school nurse's office can be an oasis of calm and comfort in the midst of the daily demands of school life. Empathy, active listening, and unconditional positive regard are the cornerstones to developing a therapeutic alliance—an alliance that can make a significant positive impact on the quality of a child's experience in school.

Practice Point

A study of 15 primary caretakers of adolescents' with disruptive behavior disorders identified major challenges in managing the adolescents' aggressive and defiant behavior and the resulting inactions with police, school, and mental health professionals (Oruche et al, 2015). Based on their findings, the authors advise that in addition to assessing specific behaviors that are challenging for caregivers, community health nurses should also inquire about interactions with the school, police, and other child welfare agencies that also significantly contribute to caregiver burden.

The Precipitous Rise in Autism—A Public Health Crisis

Throughout the world, there has been an increase in the prevalence rate of autism that is not explained by improved screening or changes in diagnostic criteria. Epidemiologic surveys of autism in America, Western Pacific, and Europe do not statistically differ with a global mean prevalence of 1 child out of 160 having a pervasive developmental disorder (Elsabbagh et al., 2012). Based on parent self-report, in 2013 the CDC estimates that 1 in 50 children in the United States has autism, which represents a 2% increase in all age groups in 5 years (Blumberg et al., 2013). Given the public health implications of the growing numbers of children worldwide diagnosed with autism, the foundation, "Autism Speaks" has partnered with the WHO and the CDC to enhance collaboration among researchers investigating the causes of pervasive developmental disorders and improve healthcare services, especially in developing countries (Elsabbagh et al., 2012).

Etiologic factors under investigation include genetic, biologic, developmental, and environmental agents. The heritability of autism is high, with an increased recurrence risk of 12% to 20% in siblings of a child diagnosed with autism (Chase & Leboyer, 2012). A genetic test for autism in a population of central European decent has been developed with a level of diagnostic accuracy and offers promising insights in genetic testing research for other ethnic populations (Skafidas et al., 2012). While specific alleles contribute to risk, there is growing research evidence that environmental factors and the interaction between the environment and genes also play an important role in the etiology of autism. For example, epidemiologic studies of unaffected siblings find fewer prenatal and perinatal exposures and complications than with the affected sibling (Chase & Leboyer, 2012).

Given the upsurge in autism cases, epidemiologists are investigating potential exposures that effect entire populations. The list of causative environmental agents includes exposures in utero, to the mother, and in infancy. Exposures during pregnancy associated with increased risk of developing autism include medications such as antibiotics, valproic acid, SSRIs, and misoprostol as well as substances such as ethanol, thalidomide, and the insecticide chlorpyrifos (Atladóttir, Henriksen, Schendel, & Parner, 2012; Chase, &

Leboyer, 2012; Croen, Grether, Yoshida, Odouli, & Hendrick, 2011; Duchan & Patel, 2012).

Given the profound public health implications for the rising rate of autism among U.S. children, in 2006 Congress created a federal advisory committee, the Interagency Autism Coordinating Committee (IACC) to accelerate progress in autism research and services. In 2011, Congress reauthorized the IACC, which is assisted by the Office of Autism Research Coordination (OARC), to communicate directly to Congress, other government agencies, and the public the latest information about federally supported autism research. The 2012 IACC Strategic Plan documents the magnitude of groundbreaking research and advances in treatment with the explicit goal of improving the quality of life for autistic children and their families (Interagency Autism Coordinating Committee, 2012).

Most research investigating the genetic and environmental risk factors for autism has been conducted with populations in developed countries. Yet unlocking the clues about the role of parental age, complications in pregnancy or medications taken in pregnancy can best be elucidated with cross-cultural comparisons for these and other associated risk factors. Even in the United States, prevalence rates of autism are higher in more affluent communities (Durkin et al., 2010). The Global Autism Public Health Initiative has partnerships in 42 nations to expand epidemiologic research globally in an effort to identify how genes and the environment may interact to increase the risk for autism. Epidemiology research on environmental factors associated with autism, both in the United States and abroad, is critical in providing public health nurses specific targets for education and prevention with at-risk populations.

PUBLIC HEALTH INITIATIVES IN AUTISM

Public health organizations have an important role in promoting screening programs and providing information about treatment resources. In the past, diagnosis of autism was often delayed until preschool because clinicians would look for evidence of language impairments before making a definitive diagnosis. More recently, the emphasis is on screening for prodromal symptoms in infancy with the hope that some of the more debilitating features of the disorder might be mitigated with early intervention and treatment. A goal of *Healthy People 2020* is to increase the proportion of young children with an **autism spectrum disorder** (ASD) and other developmental delays who are screened, evaluated, and enrolled in early intervention programs. The CDC's "Learn the Signs—Act Early" is a health education campaign targeting parents, educators, and healthcare providers promoting awareness of child development and information about early intervention programs. In the United States, Hispanic and African American children have been diagnosed later and enter treatment for autism later than Caucasian children. The CDC's "Learn the Signs—Act Early" education effort includes parent-friendly materials that are customizable for populations with health disparities to improve case finding and referral. The foundation "Autism Speaks" has partnered with the Ad Council to create Spanish language educational ads for the media, church groups, and other community organizations to also enhance outreach to Latino and black communities.

✏️ Practice Point

In 2013, the diagnostic criteria for autistic disorder in *DSM-5* eliminated the diagnosis of Asperger syndrome, and the category of pervasive developmental disorders was replaced with ASD (APA, 2013). Public health and school nurses should be aware of parents' heightened concerns that the more precise diagnostic criteria will be used to deny their child special education services (Halfon & Kuo, 2013). When educating parents of newborns about normal developmental milestones, it is important for community health nurses to encourage parents to report any concerns they may have about their child's social or language development.

EVOLUTION OF COMMUNITY MENTAL HEALTH

In the United States, community-based treatment of the mentally ill gained momentum as World War II veterans returned home exhibiting the symptoms of posttraumatic stress disorder (PTSD). There was a recognition that witnessing or experiencing a horrific traumatic event could have debilitating effects on the mind. The stigma associated with mental illness also began to subside in the wake of the tragic 1942 Cocoanut Grove fire in Boston, in which hundreds of trapped victims died and scores of survivors and their families sought mental health services. Through his pioneering work with people traumatized by the Cocoanut Grove fire, Dr. Erich Lindemann developed the concept of crisis intervention and promoted the notion that those suffering from mental illness can be best healed with their own communities among family and social institutions who cared and supported them.

By the early 1960s, a scathing report by the Joint Commission on Mental Health and Illness about conditions in state-supported psychiatric hospitals prompted the adoption of the Community Mental Health Center (CMHC) Act and federal initiatives to revamp mental healthcare delivery (Dixon & Goldman, 2004). Initially, the populations to be served by CMHCs were those suffering from acute, not chronic, mental illnesses (Dixon & Goldman, 2004). In the coming decades, more than 700 CMHCs funded by the federal government were created, and through outreach services, many younger and less-debilitated individuals received mental health services than ever before (Feldman, 2004). One of the distinctive features of these mental health centers was that treatment was to be population based. Each **community mental health center** was responsible for providing a range of mental health services to people who lived in a specific geographic area that was not to exceed 200,000 people. The services mandated by the CMHC Act included inpatient, outpatient, day treatment, and emergency treatment, as well as consultation and education to the community (Feldman, 2004). It was a sweeping agenda, with profound implications for the continued viability of state-run psychiatric hospitals.

Aided by advances in the development of pharmacologic treatment of the mentally ill, the numbers of patients treated in state mental hospitals precipitously declined. Coupled with changes in involuntary commitment regulations that made the confinement of patients against their will unlawful except in extreme instances of a clear danger to themselves or others, more and more mentally ill found themselves homeless. CMHCs had paved the way for mental health services to be provided for those who were acutely ill. However, few resources were in place at these centers to provide the range of supportive care needed by the overwhelming numbers of mentally ill who were rapidly being discharged from state hospitals.

The deinstitutionalization trend began as a humane effort to reduce the stigma associated with mental illness and reintegrate those suffering from mental illness into community-based settings. Indeed, some of the patients with chronic mental illness who qualified for income support through Social Security Disability were transferred to long-term care facilities, half-way houses, and supportive housing. However, in all too many cases, vast numbers of those discharged from state hospitals fell into a no-care zone—homeless, living on the streets or in shelters.

In hindsight, as originally conceived, the CMHCs were ill prepared, financially or organizationally, to meet the housing, income, employment, and rehabilitation needs of people with chronic mental illness. By the 1980s, the President's Commission for Mental Health offered a new agenda to the CMHCs that shifted the funding to rehabilitation, affordable housing, and vocational training (Geller, 2000). The shift to a more pragmatic treatment model recognized that clients with severe mental illness would likely have a lifelong dependency on services aimed at sustaining their independence and social functioning.

On the state level, community health nurses responsible for case management must negotiate with separate agencies for mental health services, criminal justice, substance abuse, and housing services. Coupled with the split at the federal level between the Social Security Administration, Medicare, and Medicaid, it is easy to see how a family or provider would have difficulty accessing or coordinating care. By reallocating federal expenditures to the state level, it is hoped that the states will be able to provide a comprehensive model of care that encompasses the entire spectrum of services for the chronic mentally ill within one entity.

Since deinstitutionalization began, there has been an outcry of frustration from nurses in the community about the lack of supportive services to meet the needs of people with chronic mental illness. Community mental health nurses have been forceful advocates at the state, national, and local level to ensure that policies and programs are in place to provide a safe haven for those no longer confined to state-run psychiatric hospitals. These state hospitals remain the provider of last resort for clients with intractable symptoms.

Over a decade ago, Geller (2000) warned that by solely focusing on the locus of care or where the care is given, without regard to the humane character, appropriateness, or quality of care, there is a risk that the very conditions deinstitutionalization sought to ameliorate will be recreated. One of the future goals for community health nurses will be to find innovative ways to partner with families in designing and implementing mental health programs that reflect the values, traditions, and beliefs of their community.

Carmen's treatment team begins planning for the psychiatric care she will need in the community from the day she is admitted. The case manager contacts day programs near Carmen's home and negotiates with Medicare disability reviewers to approve outpatient treatment for 2 weeks. At discharge, Carmen's mood is much improved, and she is reassured that a referral to a pain specialist is pending. Although the day-treatment program is near her residence, she has to rely on family members for rides. She is hesitant to ask her family for them, and at home, unexpected financial expenses mean that she does not fill her prescriptions for both pain management and depression. Carmen is readmitted to the hospital less than a month after her original discharge. She returns in severe pain, saying that she is "too much of a burden" to her family and "what is the point of living." During the second hospitalization, the case manager is able to arrange for transportation to and from day treatment and enroll Carmen in a low-cost medication administration program offered by a pharmaceutical company to improve her adherence with the treatment plan.

LEGISLATION FOR PARITY IN MENTAL HEALTH INSURANCE BENEFITS

The United States maintains the unique distinction of having a private health insurance system that allocates benefits based on where a person is employed. Because health insurance is a substantial cost to employers, myriad strategies have been used to contain healthcare costs. One of these strategies is that traditionally, in private health insurance, there have been different benefits, copays, and insurance limits for mental health versus medical health conditions.

Beginning in 1993, Congress debated the merits of legislating equal benefits for all healthcare conditions. Proponents of parity cite research evidence that many mental disorders are more responsive to treatment than common medical conditions and that with early treatment, the more chronic, residual effects of mental disorders maybe lessened. More than 365 organizations representing a wide array of public interest groups, local governments, and healthcare providers, including the American Psychiatric Nurses Association and the American Nurses Association, support mental health parity.

After 3 years of debate, the Mental Health Parity Act (MHPA) was enacted, requiring that lifetime and annual ceilings on expenditures for mental healthcare not be lower than those for physical illness. In an important concession, MHPA only applied to employer-based insurance that served 50 or more employees, exempting small businesses or people who were self-insured, and it excluded certain psychiatric conditions. As can be found with all public policies, ingenious strategies were devised to thwart the spirit of the 1996 parity law. For example, some private insurance plans set limits on inpatient days for psychiatric treatment or increased the copays and deductible charges for mental healthcare.

In the original legislation, it was stipulated that the provisions of the MHPA would expire, or "sunset," in 6 years. After a 12-year battle on Capitol Hill and in the White House, in October of 2008, the Paul Wellstone and Pete Domenici Mental Health Parity and Addiction Equity Act (MHPAEA) of 2008 was passed by Congress and signed by President Bush. The MHPAEA of 2008 expands the MHPA of 1996 and mandates that by January 1, 2010, health insurance plans covering 50 or more employees provide equal benefits for medical, surgical, mental health, and substance use treatment. All health insurance coverages, including deductibles, co-payments, coinsurance, and out-of-pocket expenses, and all treatment limitations, including frequency of treatment, number of visits, days of coverage, or other similar limits, will be the same regardless of health need or diagnosis. Those opposed to the MHPA argued that health insurance costs to employers and individuals would increase significantly if benefits for mental and medical conditions were equal. To date, mental health parity has not led to increased health insurance costs (Mark, Vandivort-Warren, & Miller, 2012).

The passage of the Patient Protection and Affordable Care Act (PPACA) in 2010 assured that behavioral health would be an essential benefit for all insurance plans. Starting in 2014, the PPACA requires all individual and small group plans to comply with the provisions of the MHPAEA. The goal of the PPACA coupled with the MHPAEA was to extend behavioral health insurance benefits to more than 60 million Americans. Yet 2 years later, a quarter of insurance plans were not adhering to these requirements. Instead these insurers instituted multiple barriers to mental healthcare including prior authorization requirements, denials of claims, insufficient numbers of approved behavioral health providers, and limits on coverage for psychiatric medications (Medford-Davis & Beall, 2017).

A promising provision in the PPACA is incentives to integrate mental and medical healthcare service through patient-centered medical homes. The model medical home provides person-centered care through a team of providers that coordinate all primary healthcare including mental healthcare. The aim of patient-centered medical homes is to improve outcomes of care, especially for the chronic mentally ill, the majority of whom also have comorbid medical conditions.

Evidence for Practice

A cluster randomized trial investigated if the Depression CAREPATH intervention would decrease hospital readmissions for Medicare recipients with co-occurring depression and medical conditions (Bruce, Lohman, Greenberg, Bao and Raue, 2016). The CAREPATH intervention used by home health nurses included assessment of mood symptoms with the PHQ-9, case management with specialist providers, patient education to promote medication adherence, application of practice protocols for depression symptom management and routine evaluation of behavioral health outcomes. Bruce and colleagues (2016) reported that patients who were referred to CAREPATH prior to hospital discharge had a 55% lower rate of readmission than those who received routine home healthcare. The findings suggest that a patient-centered medical home model that integrates management of depression with home health nursing care can significantly lower the rates of readmission for depressed older adults.

ROLES AND RESPONSIBILITIES OF THE COMMUNITY MENTAL HEALTH PRACTITIONER

Throughout this chapter, the roles of the community health nurse as teacher, clinician, and advocate have been described. Mental health is a leading health indicator in the U.S. *Healthy People 2020* program (see Fig. 21.1), and mental health promotion and disease prevention are an integral part of nursing practice. Box 21.2 outlines selected primary, secondary, and tertiary levels of prevention that help reduce risk, identify and limit disabilities, and reduce complications of mental health problems.

Providing population-based care that addresses the cultural diversity of a community remains one of the most pressing challenges facing all health providers. The WHO and the PPACA have cited the application of culturally sensitive care for people suffering from mental illness as one of the most pressing goals in the new millennium. There is not a single path to achieve this objective, although there is unanimity on the importance of providing mental health services that are sensitive to the cultural needs and expectations of clients and their families.

21.2 Levels of Prevention in Community Mental Health

Primary

- Educate families and community groups about mental health issues, symptoms of stress, and barriers to seeking help
- Foster availability of support services for community groups, such as prenatal and parent education sessions, bereavement sessions, and caregiver support

Secondary

- Screen for mental health disorders
- Refer high-risk people for diagnostic services
- Provide mental health services following stressful community events

Tertiary

- Promote support groups for people with mental health disorders
- Initiate health promotion activities as a part of rehabilitation services.

Developing a therapeutic alliance is the cornerstone to culturally sensitive nursing care. The Substance Abuse and Mental Health Services Administration (SAMHSA) has developed cultural competence standards for mental healthcare services (see link https://www.samhsa.gov/section-223/cultural-competency). For example, one of the implementation guidelines is that bilingual mental health staff be certified in language proficiency and cultural competence. The outcome benchmark recommended by SAMHSA is that 90% of racial/ethnic consumers of mental health services be satisfied with the communication styles of mental health specialists. In addition, culturally competent nursing care plans must identify and involve a range of community resources, including native societies, healers, spiritual leaders, and community organizations. Culturally competent community health nurses must demonstrate knowledge in group values, traditions, and the cultural expression of mental illness. In turn, therapeutic interventions described in the treatment plan should reflect the client's cultural values. Education and outreach programs must be designed to include specific information that addresses the unique cultural needs of a community.

Almost a decade ago, the Surgeon General's Report on Mental Health (U.S. Department of Health and Human Services, 1999) urged researchers to investigate differences in access to care and treatment response by culture, race, or ethnicity. More recently, the PPACA also highlighted the importance of expanding access to culturally competent mental health services (Nardi, Waite, & Killian, 2012). It is important to acknowledge that health insurance reform alone will not be sufficient to erase racial and ethnic healthcare disparities. Disparities in access and response to mental health treatment exist by age, gender, race, ethnic background, socioeconomic status, and geographic location (Dougherty, 2004). Clinic hours, transportation, stigma, and the availability of culturally competent mental health providers are some of the roadblocks marginalized populations face when attempting to access mental health services (Alegria et al., 2012). Community health nurses can play a critical role in advancing nursing knowledge and understanding of how models of nursing care can be developed that account for cultural differences in access to care, treatment responsiveness, and adherence. Mental health parity will never be fully realized until systems of culturally sensitive care meet the needs for treatment in every community (McCarty, 2013).

Practice Point

Community health nurses should seek certification in cultural competence and incorporate the standards of cultural competence developed by SAMHSA into treatment plans and programs that provide mental health services.

PSYCHOLOGICAL FIRST AID

Populations Traumatized by Disasters

Since 1970, the incidence of natural disasters throughout the world has been rising and irrespective of the socioeconomic status of the country, lifetime exposure to natural disasters is high, ranging from 4.4% to 7.5% (Kessler, McLaughlin, Koenen, Petukhova, Hill, & The WHO World Mental Health Consortium, 2012). Globally, there were 168 natural disasters and 150 human-made disasters, resulting in 20 million fatalities, 50 million casualties, and 2000 million homeless in 2012 (Sigma, 2013). Population's hardest hit were in Asia where over 1,900 people died or were missing from Typhoon Bopha and Africa where three million people were displaced from floods. The same year, more than 45,000 people, the majority of whom were civilians and children, were victims of terrorist attacks with 64% of all attacks occurring in Afghanistan, Iraq, and Pakistan (U.S. Department of State, 2012).

In the United States, the incidence of natural disasters has been increasing since 1998 (FEMA, 2013). Back to back hurricanes causing historic flooding and record property damage in Texas, Florida Puerto Rico and the Virgin Islands have tested the federal and volunteer disaster relief efforts as never before. "Rampage shootings," characterized by a male engaging in a shooting spree within institutions familiar to him, but toward victims that may be unknown, have also been increasing in the United States since the 1990s (Harris & Harris, 2012, p. 1054). Four terrorist attacks, including the First World Trade Center bombing in 1993, the Oklahoma City bombing in 1995, the 9/11 attacks in 2001, and the Boston

Marathon bombing in 2013, resulted in over 3,000 deaths and 2,000 injuries to U.S. civilians (National Consortium for the Study of Terrorism and Responses to Terrorism, 2012).

Populations at Risk for Psychological Trauma

Natural and human-made disasters inflict psychological impacts on populations that are 4 to 50 times greater than the number of physical injuries (McCabe, Barnett, Taylor, & Links, 2010).

Studies of the psychological effects of disasters find considerable variation in prevalence rates among populations, ranging from 14% to 76% for prolonged grief reactions, to 5% to 68% for PTSD, and to 10% to 45% for major depression (Kristensen, Weisaeth, & Heir, 2012). Population risk factors for developing disaster-associated PTSD include female gender; older adult age; Hispanic ethnicity; lower education level; personal injury; witnessing in injury or death, especially among family or friends; and prior history of psychiatric illness, especially PTSD, major depression, or panic disorder (North, Oliver, & Pandya, 2012). Psychological harms are also greater when a community is victimized by a terrorist attack or a rampage shooting rather than a natural disaster. The challenge for public health nurses is how best to intervene to minimize psychological harms when an entire community or a population has been traumatized.

In the 1950s, the federal government requested that the APA develop guidelines for providing psychological support to communities affected by disasters. Building on the principles of crisis intervention originated by Eric Lindeman, a brief therapeutic intervention was developed termed *psychological first aid* (Forbes, 2011). Psychological first aid is designed to be delivered by disaster relief workers, including nurses who are often on the front lines of a disaster in a variety of community-based settings.

The core features of psychological first aid are to protect, connect, and direct (Fig. 21.5). Nurses can protect victims of a disaster by, first and foremost, providing food, clothing, and shelter. **Psychological first aid** is the fundamental principles of therapeutic communication such as active listening, allowing silence, allowing the expression of emotions, and paraphrasing these reactions to convey understanding and compassion. Similar to the nursing process, the first steps of psychological first aid include assessment of physical and psychological well-being, coping skills, and social supports. Victims should be assessed for severe psychological reactions especially suicidal or homicidal ideation and directed to mental health disaster specialists.

The second stage of psychological first aid mirrors the intervention phase of the nursing process. The most immediate concern for many survivors is their desire to be reunited with friends, family, and social and spiritual supports. Connection with family and loved ones can be challenging in the aftermath of a disaster. Relief workers have developed innovative strategies to reunite families and friends as

Psychological First Aid for First Responders

When you work with people during and after a disaster, you are working with people who may be having reactions of confusion, fear, hopelessness, sleeplessness, anxiety, grief, shock, guilt, shame, and loss of confidence in themselves and others. Your early contacts with them can help alleviate their painful emotions and promote hope and healing.

Your goal in providing this psychological first aid is to promote an environment of safety, calm, connectedness, self-efficacy, empowerment, and hope.

DO:

Promote Safety:

- Help people meet basic needs for food and shelter, and obtain emergency medical attention.
- Provide repeated, simple, and accurate information on how to get these basic needs.

Promote Calm:

- Listen to people who wish to share their stories and emotions, and remember that there is no right or wrong way to feel.
- Be friendly and compassionate even if people are being difficult.
- Offer accurate information about the disaster or trauma, and the relief efforts underway to help victims understand the situation.

Promote Connectedness:

- Help people contact friends and loved ones.
- Keep families together. Keep children with parents or other close relatives whenever possible.

Promote Self-Efficacy:

- Give practical suggestions that steer people toward helping themselves.
- Engage people in meeting their own needs.

Promote Help:

- Find out the types and locations of government and nongovernment services and direct people to those services that are available.
- When they express fear or worry, remind people (if you know) that more help and services are on the way.

DO NOT:

- Force people to share their stories with you, especially very personal details.
- Give simple reassurances like "everything will be OK" or "at least you survived."
- Tell people what you think they should be feeling, thinking, or how they should have acted earlier.
- Tell people why you think they have suffered by alluding to personal behaviors or beliefs of victims.
- Make promises that may not be kept.
- Criticize existing services or relief activities in front of people in need of these services. [1]

Information Clearinghouses

National Mental Health Information Center (NMHIC)
P.O. Box 42557, Washington, DC 20015
(800) 789-2647 (English and Español)
(866) 889-2647 (TDD)
www.mentalhealth.samhsa.gov

National Clearinghouse for Alcohol and Drug Information (NCADI)
P.O. Box 2345, Rockville, MD 20847-2345
(800) 729-6686 (English and Español)
(800) 487-4889 (TDD)
www.ncadi.samhsa.gov

Treatment Locators

Mental Health Services Locator
(800) 789-2647 (English and Español)
(866) 889-2647 (TDD)
www.mentalhealth.samhsa.gov/databases

Substance Abuse Treatment Facility Locator
(800) 662-HELP (4357) (Toll-Free,
24-Hour English and Español
Treatment Referral Service)
(800) 487-4889 (TDD)
www.findtreatment.samhsa.gov

Hotlines

National Suicide Prevention Lifeline
(800) 273-TALK (8255)
(800) 799-4889 (TDD)

SAMHSA National Helpline
(800) 662-HELP (4357) (English and Español)
(800) 487-4889 (TDD)

Workplace Helpline
(800) WORKPLACE (967-5752)
www.workplace.samhsa.gov/helpline/
helpline.htm

FIGURE 21.5 SAMHSA psychological first aid for first responders. (*SAMHSA psychological first aid for first responders: Tips for emergency and disaster workers.* U.S. Department of Health and Human Services. NMH05-0210. Washington, DC: U.S. Government Printing Office. Retrieved May 29, 2013, from http://store.samhsa.gov/shin/content/NMH05-0210/NMH05-0210.pdf.)

TABLE 21.4 Evidence-Based Psychological Interventions for Mass Casualties

Phase	Preincident	Impact (0–48 hours)	Rescue (0–1 week)	Recovery (1–4 weeks)	Return to Life (2 weeks–2 years)
Goals	Preparation, improve coping	Survival, communication	Adjustment	Appraisal/planning	Reintegration
Behavior	Preparation vs. denial	Fight/flight, freeze, surrender, etc.	Resilience vs. exhaustion	Grief, reappraisal, intrusive memories, narrative formation	Adjustment vs. phobias, posttraumatic stress disorder, avoidance, depression, etc.
Role of all helpers	Prepare, train, gain knowledge	Rescue, protect	Orient, provide for needs	Respond with sensitivity	Continue assistance
Role of mental health professionals	**Prepare** Train. Gain Knowledge. Collaborate. Inform and influence policy. Set structures for rapid response.	**Basic needs** Establish safety/security/survival Ensure food and shelter Provide orientation. Facilitate communication with family, friends, and community Assess the environment for ongoing threat/toxin **Psychological first aid** Support and "presence" for those who are most distressed Keep families together and facilitate reunion with loved ones Provide information and education (i.e., services), foster communication Protect survivors from further harm Reduce physiological arousal **Monitoring the impact on environment** Observe and listen to those most affected Monitor the environment for stressors **Technical assistance, consultation, and training** Improve capacity of organizations and caregivers to provide what is needed to reestablish community structure, foster family recovery/resilience, and safeguard the community. Provide to: • relevant organizations • other caregivers and responders • leaders	**Needs assessment** Assess current status, how well needs are being addressed Recovery environment What additional interventions are needed for Group Population Individual Triage Clinical assessment Refer when indicated Identify vulnerable, high-risk individuals and groups Emergency hospitalization or outpatient treatment **Outreach and information dissemination** Make contact with and identify people who have not requested services (i.e., "therapy by walking around") **Outreach and information dissemination** Inform people about different services, coping, recovery process, etc. (e.g., by using established community structures, fliers, web sites) **Fostering resilience and recovery** Social interactions Coping skills training Education about stress response, traumatic reminders, coping, normal vs. abnormal functioning, risk factors, services Group and family support Foster natural social support Look after the bereaved Repair organizational fabric Operational debriefings, when this is standing procedure in responder organizations Spiritual support	**Monitor the recovery environment** Observe and listen to those most affected Monitor the environment for toxins Monitor past and ongoing threats Monitor services that are being provided	**Treatment** Reduce or ameliorate symptoms or improve functioning via • Individual, family, and group psychotherapy • Pharmacotherapy • Short-term or long-term hospitalization

quickly as possible. Disaster mental health nurses may meet with families to gather information for the identification process in the event of death. Nurses can minimize retraumatization by limiting the number of individuals, victims and survivors, interact with to "tell their story" and the number of individuals who witness the horror of aftermath.

In the third stage of psychological first aid, nurses act as advocates and direct survivors to relief agencies. Nurses actively partner with survivors in practical problem-solving to address specific, immediate concerns. It is critical that nurses not make promises or conjecture about the availability of resources. Information to survivors must be credible, culturally and linguistically appropriate, timely, and specific as to where and when resources may arrive, such as transportation, assistance for dependents, medical care, or housing. During this stage, nurses provide psychoeducation on bereavement for individuals, families, and communities who are coping with multiple losses.

Families, survivors, and first responders benefit from education about expected behavioral responses to avoid pathologizing normal grief reactions. Expected psychological reactions may include guilt or shame, anger, frequent crying or blunting of emotions, difficulty concentrating, uncharacteristic social isolation, and inability to forget sensory images of trauma. Expected physical reactions may include headaches, fatigue, gastrointestinal disturbance, pain, disrupted sleep, and disrupted eating (too much or too little). Deep breathing, yoga, prayer, and spiritual reflection can help diminish anxiety for those exhibiting expected psychological responses. As much as possible, encourage individuals to engage in group activities to facilitate social cohesion, hope, and resilience.

Survivors or first responders experiencing moderate to severe psychological reactions, including suicidal or homicidal ideation, should be directed to disaster mental health specialists. Moderate psychological reactions include nightmares, intrusive daytime images, bodily sensations related to traumatic experience, excessive physical startle reflex, extreme anxiety alternating with numbing, and difficulty modulating anger. Cognitive behavioral therapies are evidence-based interventions that can help individuals cope with the moderate symptoms of emotional distress (Everly, Barnett, & Links, 2012). Symptoms of major mental illness such as dissociation, panic attacks, agoraphobia, depression or substance abuse, in addition to the inability to perform basic self-care, or threats of violence against others or self would warrant immediate emergency treatment.

In disasters, ordinary people emerge as innovative problem solvers who are responsive to the needs of others around them. This prosocial response has been documented by researchers over several decades in countless disasters and highlights the resilience of communities even in the face of horrific traumatic events (McCabe et al., 2012). Resilience is built on the self and community perception of having the ability to cope and respond flexibly to the unexpected. Faith-based organizations, social clubs, and local schools are a few of the indigenous community supports that provide extraordinary services in disasters and are vital to long-term psychological recovery (McCabe et al., 2011) (Table 21.4).

Evidence for Practice

In 2009, a scientific review by the Advisory Council to the American Red Cross determined that psychological first aid was an evidenced-informed intervention that can be used effectively by trained volunteers to address the basic needs of individuals in the immediate aftermath of a disaster (Fox et al., 2012). The same year, the WHO Mental Health Guidelines Development Group concluded that psychological first aid, and not psychological debriefing, should be provided to populations affected by disaster (WHO, 2011) (Box 21.3). The U.S. Medical Reserve Corps training manual on psychological first aid (Brymer et al., 2006) and the WHO state there is insufficient evidence on the efficacy of debriefing and caution there is a risk that the systematic ventilation of feelings maybe triggering and hinder, rather than support, the recovery of survivors and first responders.

21.3 WHO Psychological First Aid in Different Cultures

Consider the Following Questions as You Prepare to Offer PFA in Different Cultures:

Dress	Do I need to dress a certain way to be respectful? Will affected people be in need of certain clothing items to keep their dignity and customs?
Language	What is the customary way of greeting people in this culture? What language do they speak?
Gender, Age and Power	Should affected women only be approached by women helpers? Who may I approach? (In other words, the head of the family or community?)
Touching and Behavior	What are the usual customs around touching people? Is it all right to hold someone's hand or touch their shoulder? Are there special things to consider in terms of behavior around the elderly, children, women, or others?
Beliefs and Religion	Who are the different ethnic and religious groups among the affected people? What beliefs of practices are important to the people affected? How might they understand of explain what has happened?

World Health Organization. (2011). (*Psychological first aid: Guide for field workers*. Geneva: WHO, War Trauma Foundation and World Vision International. Retrieved May 28, 2013, from http://whqlibdoc.who.int/publications/2011/9789241548205_eng.pdf.)

KEY CONCEPTS

- Genetic, biologic, and environmental risk factors all influence the incidence of mental illness.
- Early intervention can minimize the morbidity associated with mental illness.
- Adherence to psychopharmacology and psychotherapy enhances recovery from mental illness.
- The continuum of care for the chronic mentally ill includes community services, such as supportive housing and employment.
- Public health initiatives to educate communities about mental health can be effective in lowering the incidence of high-risk behaviors such as suicide.
- Psychological first aid is recommended to help support survivors and first responders to natural and intentional disasters.

CRITICAL THINKING QUESTIONS

You are a school nurse in a middle school when Jamal comes to the nurse's office requesting medication for a headache. You notice that his eyes are red, and it appears as if he has been crying. You ask if he is hurt, but he denies it. The phone rings in the office, and a teacher tells you that a female student has approached her concerned about Jamal. The teacher tells you that Jamal sent her a text message saying that he flunked his biology examination and wished he was dead.

1. What is the most immediate nursing assessment that should be evaluated?
2. If Jamal is hesitant to share his thoughts with you, what could you say or do to develop a therapeutic alliance?
3. What other collateral sources of information would you contact to evaluate the risk of suicide associated with the text message? Would you leave Jamal alone to discuss the situation with other colleagues?
4. If Jamal shared with you a suicide plan that includes harming himself with a weapon, what would be your first nursing intervention?
5. If you determined Jamal was at risk for self-harm, to whom would you refer Jamal?
6. How would you continue to assess Jamal's mental health while he was a student in the middle school?
7. How might health insurance, transportation, and family circumstances influence Jamal's ability to access mental health services?
8. What educational program would you develop for the middle school to educate students about ways to cope with stress and how to respond if a friend needs support?

HEALTHY PEOPLE 2020 EVIDENCE-BASED RESOURCE RECOMMENDATIONS

Mental Health and Mental Illness: Collaborative Care for the Management of Depressive Disorders (The Community Guide, 2016)

Developed by: Community Preventive Services Task Force. Collaborative care for the management of depressive disorders is an interdisciplinary model of person-centered medical home that uses nurse case managers to link primary care providers, patients, and mental health specialists.

***Healthy People 2020* topic area(s):** Access to health services; mental health and mental disorders

***Healthy People 2020* objectives:** MHMD-11, MHMD-4, AHS-5

Strength of recommendation: 4 out of 4

Exercise for Students

Apply the core components of collaborative care in caring for a client in a community-based setting by:

1. Demonstrating evidence-based screening for depressive disorders by using the PHQ-9 for adults or the HEADSSS for children and adolescents
2. Provide patient and family education to promote treatment adherence
3. Apply evidence-based protocols for the proactive management of diagnosed depressive disorders
4. Mobilize clinical and community support for active patient engagement in treatment goal setting and self-management (Fig. 21.6)

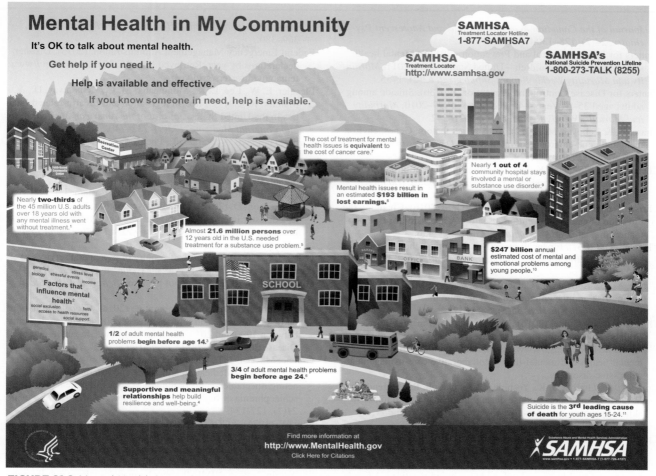

FIGURE 21.6 Mental Health in My Community: Information Graphic. (SAMHSA. [2013]. Retrieved on August 5, 2017, from https://store.samhsa.gov/product/Mental-Health-in-My-Community-Information-Graphic/SMA13-4725. References available at: https://store.samhsa.gov/shin/content/SMA13-4725/SMA13-4725_Reference.pdf.)

REFERENCES

Abraham, Z. K., & Sher, L. (2017). Adolescent suicide as a global public health issues. *International Journal of Adolescent Medicine and Health*. [Epub ahead of print]. doi: 10.1515/ijamh-2017-0036.

Alegria, M., Lin, J., Chen, C. N., Duan, N., Cook, B., & Meng, X. L. (2012). The impact of insurance coverage in diminishing racial and ethnic disparities in behavioral health services. *Health Services Research*, *47*(3, Pt. 2), 1322–1344.

American Psychiatric Association. (2013). *Diagnostic and statistical manual of mental disorders* (5th ed.). Arlington, VA: American Psychiatric Publishing.

Andrade, C. (2016). Cannabis and neuropsychiatry, 2: The longitudinal risk of psychosis as an adverse outcome. *Clinical and Practical Psychopharmacology*, *77*(6), e739–e742.

Atladóttir, H. O., Henriksen, T. B., Schendel, D. E., & Parner, E. T. (2012). Autism after infection, febrile episodes, and antibiotic use during pregnancy: An exploratory study. *Pediatrics*, *130*(6), e1447–e1454.

Barnett, M. L., Gonzalez, A., Miranda, J., Chavira, D. A., & Lau, A. S. (2017). Mobilizing community health workers to address mental health disparities for underserved populations: A systematic review. *Adm Policy and Mental Health*, *45*(2), 195–211.

Blumberg, S. J., Bramlett, M. D., Kogan, M. D., Schieve, L. A., Jones, J. R., & Lu, M. C. (2013). *Changes in prevalence of parent-reported autism spectrum disorder in school-aged U.S. children: 2007 to 2011–2012. National Health Statistics Reports, 65*. Hyattsville, MD: National Center for Health Statistics.

Brakoulias, V., & Milicevic, D. (2015). Assessment and treatment of hoarding disorder. *Australasian Psychiatry*, *23*(4), 358–360.

Bruce, M. L., Lohman, M. C., Greenberg, R. L., Bao, Y., & Raue, P. J. (2016). Integrating depression care management into Medicare home health reduces risk of 30 and 60-day hospitalizations: The depression care for patients at home cluster-randomized trial. *Journal of the American Geriatric Society*, *64*(11),2196–2203.

Brymer, M., Jacobs, A., Layne, C., Pynoos, R., Ruzek, J., Steinberg, A., & Watson, P. (2006). *Psychological first aid: Medical reserve corps field operations guide*. Washington, DC: National Child Traumatic Stress and Network National Center for PTSD. Retrieved November 18, 2014, from http://www.naccho.org/topics/emergency/MRC/resources/upload/MRC-PFA-Field-Operations-Guide.pdf

Burton, C. L., Arnold, P. D. & Soreni, N. (2015). Three reasons why studying hoarding in children and adolescents is important.

REFERENCES *(Continued)*

Journal of the Canadian Academy of Child and Adolescent Psychiatry, 24(2), 128–130.

Centers for Disease Control and Prevention. (2013a). Mental health surveillance among children—United States, 2005–2011. *Morbidity and Mortality Weekly Report, Supplement, 62*(2), 1–35.

Centers for Disease Control and Prevention. (2013b). Suicide among adults aged 35–64 Years—United States, 1999–2010. *Morbidity and Mortality Weekly Report, 62*(17), 321–342.

Chase, P., & Leboyer, M. (2012). Autism risk factors: Genes, environment and gene-environment interactions. *Dialogues in Clinical Neuroscience, 14*(3), 281–292.

Cheng, S. C., & Schepp, K. G. (2016). Early intervention in schizophrenia: A literature review. *Archives of Psychiatric Nursing, 30*(6), 774–781.

Christensen, H., Cuijpers, P., & Reynolds, C. F. (2016). Changing the direction of suicide prevention research: A necessity for true population impact. *JAMA Psychiatry, 73*(5), 435–436.

Claassen, D. (2007). Financial incentives for antipsychotic depot medication: Ethical issues. *Journal of Medical Ethics, 33*(4), 189–193.

Clarke, M. C., Kelleher, I., Clancy, M., & Cannon, M. (2012). Predicting risk and the emergence of schizophrenia. *The Psychiatric Clinics of North America, 35*(3), 585–612.

The Community Guide. (2016). Mental health and mental illness: Collaborative care for the management of depressive disorders. Available from https://www.thecommunityguide.org/findings/mental-health-and-mental-illness-collaborative-care-management-depressive-disorders.

Croen, L. A., Grether, J. K., Yoshida, C. K., Odouli, R., & Hendrick, V. (2011). Antidepressant use during pregnancy and childhood autism spectrum disorders. *Archives of General Psychiatry, 68*(11), 1104–1112.

Curtin, S. C., Warne, M., & Hedegaard, H. (2016). Increase in suicide in the United States, 1999–2014. *NCHC Data Brief*, (241), 1–8.

Dixon, L., & Goldman, H. (2004). Forty years of progress in community mental health: The role of evidence-based practices. *Administration and Policy in Mental Health and Mental Health Services Research, 31*(5), 381–392.

Doughtery, R. H. (2004). Reducing disparity in behavioral health services: A report from the American College of Mental Health Administration. *Administration and Policy in Mental Health, 31*(3), 253–263.

Drury, H., Ajmi, S., Fernández de la Cruz, L., Nordsletten, A. E., & Mataix-Cols, D. (2014). Caregiver burden, family accommodation, health and well-being in relative of individuals with hoarding disorder. *Journal of Affective Disorders, 159*, 7–14.

Duchan, E., & Patel, D. R. (2012). Epidemiology of autism spectrum disorders. *Pediatric Clinics North America, 59*(1), 27–43.

Durkheim, E. (1972). *Selected writings [Introduction by A. Giddens]*. New York: Cambridge University Press.

Durkin, M. S., Maenner, M. J., Meaney, F. J., Levy, S. E., DiGuiseppi, C., Nicholas, J. S.... Schieve, L. A. (2010). Socioeconomic inequality in the prevalence of autism spectrum disorder: Evidence from a U.S. cross-sectional study. *PLOS ONE, 5*(7), e11551.

Elsabbagh, M., Divan, G., Koh, Y., Kim, Y. S., Kauchali, S., Marcin, C.,...Fombonne, E. (2012). Global prevalence of autism and other pervasive developmental disorders. *Autism Research, 5*(3), 160–179.

Everly, G. A., Barnett, D. J., & Links, J. M. (2012). The Johns Hopkins model of psychological first aid (RAPID-PFA): Curriculum development and content validation. *International Journal of Emergency Mental Health, 14*(2), 95–103.

Feldman, S. (2004). Reflections on the 40th anniversary of the Community Mental Health Centers Act. *Administration and Policy in Mental Health and Mental Health Services Research, 31*(5), 369–380.

Federal Emergency Management Administration. (2013). Disaster declarations by year. Retrieved May 25, 2013, from http://www.fema.gov/disasters/grid/year.

Fleegler, E. W., Lee, L. K., Monuteaux, M. C., Hemenway, D., & Mannix, R. (2013). Firearm legislation and firearm-related fatalities in the United States. *Journal of the American Medical Association Internal Medicine, 173*(9), 732–740.

Forbes, D., Lewis, V., Varker, T., Phelps, A., O'Donnell, M., Wade D. J.,...Creamer, M. (2011). Psychological first aid following trauma: Implementation and evaluation framework for high-risk organizations. *Psychiatry, 74*(3), 224–239.

Fox, J. H., Burkle, F. M., Bass, J., Pia, F. A., Epstein, J. L., & Markenson, D. (2012). The effectiveness of psychological first aid as a disaster intervention tool: Research analysis of peer reviewed literature from 1990–2010. *Disaster Med Public Health Preparedness, 6*(3), 247–252.

Geller, J. L. (2000). The last half-century of psychiatric services as reflected in Psychiatric Services. *Psychiatric Services, 51*(1), 41–67.

Glazer, W. M. (2007). The depot paradox. *Behavioral Healthcare, 27*(5), 44–46.

Global Burden of Disease Collaborative (2016). Global and national burden of diseases and injuries among children and adolescents between 1990 and 2013: Findings from the Global Burden of Disease 2013 Study. *JAMA Pediatrics, 170*(3), 267–287.

Greene, M., Yan, J. T., Chang, E., Hartry, A., Touya, M., & Broder, M. S. (2017). Medication adherence and discontinuation of long-acting injectable versus oral antipsychotics in patients with schizophrenia or bipolar disorder. *Journal of Medical Economics, 21*(2), 127–134.

Guy, W. (1976). *ECDEU assessment manual for psychopharmacology: Revised (DHEW publication number ADM 76-338)*. Rockville, MD: U.S. Department of Health, Education and Welfare, Public Health Service, Alcohol, Drug Abuse and Mental Health Administration, NIMH Psychopharmacology Research Branch, Division of Extramural Research Programs.

Halfon, N., & Kuo, A. A. (2013). What DSM-5 could mean to children with autism and their families. *Journal of the American Medical Association Pediatrics, 167*(7), 608–613.

Harris, J. M., & Harris, R. B. (2012). Rampage violence requires a new type of research. *American Journal of Public Health, 102*(6), 1054–1057.

Hwang, W. C., Myers, H. F., Abe-Kim, J., & Ting, J. Y. (2008). A conceptual paradigm for understanding culture's impact on mental health: The cultural influences on mental health (CIMH) model. *Clinical Psychology Review, 28*(2), 211–227.

Interagency Autism Coordinating Committee. (2012). *IACC strategic plan for autism spectrum disorder (ASD) research—2012 update*. Washington, DC: U.S. Department of Health and Human Services. Retrieved May 27, 2013, from http://iacc.hhs.gov/strategic-plan/2012/index.shtml.

Jackman, K., Honig, J., & Bockting, W. (2016). Nonsuicidal self-injury among lesbian, gay, bisexual and transgender populations: An integrative review. *Journal of Clinical Nursing, 25*(23–24), 3438–3543.

Kellett, S., Matuozzo, H., & Kotecha, C. (2015). Effectiveness of cognitive-behaviour therapy for hoarding disorder in people with mild intellectual disabilities. *Research in Developmental Disabilities, 47*, 385–392.

Kessler, R. C., McLaughlin, K. A., Koenen, K. C., Petukhova, M., Hill, E. D., & WHO World Mental Health Survey Consortium. (2012). The importance of secondary trauma exposure for post-disaster mental disorder. *Epidemiology and Psychiatric Sciences, 21*(1), 35–45.

Kessler, R. C., & Wang, P. S. (2008). The descriptive epidemiology of commonly occurring mental disorders in the United States. *Annual Review of Public Health, 29*, 115–129.

Kim, B., Lee, S. H., Yang, Y. K., Park, J. I., & Chung, Y. C. (2012). Long-acting injectable antipsychotics for first-episode schizophrenia: The pros and cons. *Schizophrenia Research and Treatment, 2012*, 560836. doi:10.1155/2012/560836. Advance online publication.

Kowatch, R. A. (2016). Diagnosis, phenomenology, differential diagnosis and comorbidity of pediatric bipolar disorder. *Journal of Clinical Psychiatry, 77*(Suppl E1), e01.

Kristensen, P., Weisaeth, L., & Heir, T. (2012). Bereavement and mental health after sudden and violent losses: A review. *Psychiatry, 75*(1), 76–97.

Levine, S. Z., Rabinowitz, J., Faries, D., Lawson, A. H., & Ascher-Svanum, H. (2012). Treatment response trajectories and antipsychotic medications: Examination of up to 18 months of treatment in the CATIE chronic schizophrenia trial. *Schizophrenia Research, 137*(1–3), 141–146. Retrieved from http://dx.doi.org.proxy.bc.edu/10.1016/j.schres.2012.01.014.

Mark, T. L., Vandivort-Warren, R., & Miller, K. (2012). Mental health spending by private insurance: Implications for the mental health parity and addiction equity act. *Psychiatric Services, 63*(4), 313–318.

Marshall, M., & Lockwood, A. (2005). Early intervention for psychosis. In: *The Cochrane Collaboration*. New York: John Wiley.

Martone, K. (2014). The impact of failed housing policy on the public behavioral health system. *Psychiatric Services, 65*(3), 313–314.

Mataix-Cols, D. (2014). Hoarding disorder. *NEJM, 370*, 2023–2030.

McCabe, O. L., Marum, F., Mosley, A., Gwon, H. S., Langlieb, A., Everly, G. S.,...Links, J. M. (2012). Community capacity building in disaster mental health resilience: A pilot study of an academic/faith partnership model. *International Journal of Emergency Mental Health, 14*(2), 112–122.

McCabe, O. L., Perry, C., Azur, M., Taylor, H. G., Bailey, M., & Links, J. M. (2011). Psychological first-aid training for paraprofessionals: A systems-based model for enhancing capacity of rural emergency responses. *Prehospital and Disaster Medicine, 26*(4), 251–258.

McCabe, O. L., Barnett, D. J., Taylor, H. G., & Links, J. M. (2010). Ready, willing, and able: A framework for improving the public health emergency preparedness system. *Disaster Medicine and Public Health Preparedness, 4*(2), 161–168.

McCarty, D. (2013). Parity: An ongoing challenge and research opportunity. *American Journal of Psychiatry, 170*(2), 140–142.

McGorry, P. D., Killackey, E., & Yung, A. (2008). Early intervention in psychosis: Concepts, evidence and future directions. *World Psychiatry, 7*(3), 148–156.

Medford-Davis, L. N., & Beall, R. C. (2017). The changing health policy environment and behavioral health services delivery. *Psychiatric Clinics of North America, 40*(3), 533–540.

Messias, E., Kindrick, K. & Castro, J. (2014). School bullying, cyberbullying or both: Correlates of teen suicidality in the 2011 CDC Youth Risk Behavior Survey. *Comprehensive Psychiatry, 55*(5), 1063–1068.

Miller, T. J., McGlashan, T. H., Rosen, J. L., Somjee, L., Markovich, P. J., Stein, K., & Woods, S. W. (2002). Prospective diagnosis of the initial prodrome for schizophrenia based on the structured interview for prodromal syndromes: Preliminary evidence of interrater reliability and predictive validity. *American Journal of Psychiatry, 159*(5), 863–865.

Mojtabai, R., Olfson, M., & Han, B. (2016). National trends in the prevalence and treatment of depression in adolescents and young adults. *Pediatrics, 138*(6), e2011878.

Morris, S. H., Jaffee, S. R., Goodwin, G. P., & Franklin, M. E. (2016). Hoarding in children and adolescents: A review. *Child Psychiatry and Human Development, 47*(5),740–750.

Morton, N. K., & Zubek, D. (2013). Adherence challenges and long-acting injectable antipsychotic treatment in patients with schizophrenia. *Journal of Psychosocial Nursing, 51*(3), 13–18.

Mueser, K. T., Deavers, F., Penn, D. L., & Cassisi, J. E. (2013). Psychosocial treatments for schizophrenia. *Annual Review of Clinical Psychology, 9*, 465–497.

Murphy, K. (2014). The high cost of hoarding disorder. *Nursing Management, 45*(6), 20–26.

Murray, C. J. L., Vos, T., Lozano, R., Naghavi, M., Flaxman, A. D., Michaud, C.,...Memish, Z. A. (2012). Disability-adjusted life years (DALYs) for 291 diseases and injuries in 21 regions, 1990–2010: A systematic analysis for the Global Burden of Disease Study 2010. *Lancet, 380*(9859), 2197–2223.

Narayan, V. A., Mohwinckel, M., Pisano, G., Yang, M., & Manji, H. K. (2013). Beyond magic bullets: True innovation in health care. *Nature Reviews. Drug Discovery, 12*, 85–86.

Nardi, D., Waite, R., & Killian, P. (2012). Establishing standards for culturally competent mental health care. *Journal of Psychosocial Nursing and Mental Health Services, 50*(7), 3–5.

Narendorf, S. C., Cross, M. B., Maria, D. S., Swank, P. R., & Bordnick, P. S. (2017). Relations between mental health diagnoses, mental health treatment and substance use in homeless youth. *Drug and Alcohol dependence, 175*, 1–8.

National Center for Health Statistics. (2016). *Chapter 28: Mental Health and Mental Disorders. Healthy People 2020. Midcourse Review*. Hyattsville, MD: HHS.

National Consortium for the Study of Terrorism and Responses to Terrorism. (2012). Global terrorism database 1993–2012. Retrieved May 25, 2013, from http://www.start.umd.edu/gtd.

National Institute on Drug Abuse. (2016). *Teen substance use shows promising decline*. Retrieved on Sept 4, 2017, from https://d14rmgtrwzf5a.cloudfront.net/sites/default/files/2016_mtf_press_release_final_cleared_12.12.16.pdf.

National Strategy for Suicide Prevention—Revised. (2012). Retrieved on September 17, 2017, from https://www.surgeongeneral.gov/library/reports/national-strategy-suicide-prevention/overview.pdf.

Neighbors, H. W., Caldwell, C., Williams, D. R., Nesse, R., Taylor, R. J., Bullard, K. M.,...Jackson, J. S. (2007). Race, ethnicity and the use of services for mental disorders: Results from the National Survey of American Life. *Archives of General Psychiatry, 64*(4), 485–494.

North, C. S., Oliver, J., & Pandya, A. (2012). Examining a comprehensive model of disaster-related posttraumatic stress disorder in systematically studied survivors of 10 disasters. *American Journal of Public Health, 102*(10), e40–e48.

Olfson, M., Blanco, C., Wall, M., Liu, S. M., Saha, T. D., Rickering, R. P., & Grant, B. F. (2017). National trends in suicide attempts among adults in the United States. *JAMA Psychiatry, 74*(11), 1095–1103.

Ormel, J., Petukhova, M., Chatterji, S., Aguilar-Gaxiola, S., Alonso, J., Angermeyer, M. C.,...Kessler, R. C. (2008). Disability and treatment of specific mental and physical disorders across the world. *British Journal of Psychiatry, 192*(5), 368–375.

Oruche, U. M., Draucker, C. B., Al-Khattab, H., Cravens, H. A., Lowry, B., & Lindsey, L. M. (2015). The challenges for primary caregivers of adolescents with disruptive behavior disorders. *Journal of Family Nursing, 21*(1), 149–167.

Patel, V., Chisholm, D., Parikh, R., Charlson, F. J,. Degenhardt, L., Dua, T.,...Whiteford, H.(2016). Addressing the burden of mental, neurological and substance use disorders: Key messages from Disease Control Priorities. *Lancet, 387*(10028), 1672–1685.

Petersen, I., Evans-Lacko, S., Semau, M., Barry, M. M., Chisholm, D., Gronholm, P.,...Thornicroft, G. (2016). Promotion, prevention and protection: Interventions at the population and community levels for mental, neurological and substance use disorders in low and middle income countries. *International Journal of Mental Health Systems, 10*(30), 1–13.

REFERENCES *(Continued)*

President's New Freedom Commission on Mental Health. (2003). *Achieving the promise: Transforming mental health care in America (Final Report. No. SMA-03-3832)*. Rockville, MD: Department of Health and Human Services. Retrieved on November 18, 2014, from http://govinfo.library.unt.edu/mentalhealthcommission/reports/FinalReport/downloads/FinalReport.pdf.

Raeburn, T., Hungerford, C., Escott, P. & Cleary, M. (2015). Supporting recovery from hoarding and squalor: Insights from a community case study. *Journal of Psychiatric and Mental Health Nursing, 22*(8), 634–639.

Shain, B. (2016). Suicide and suicide attempts in adolescents. *American Academy of Pediatrics, 138*(1), e20161420.

Sigma. (2013). *Natural catastrophes and manmade disasters in 2012: A year of extreme weather events in the US (No. 2)*. Zurich, Switzerland: Swiss Re Ltd. Retrieved from http://media.swissre.com/documents/sigma2_2013_EN.pdf.

Skafidas, E., Testa, R., Zantomio, D., Chana, G., Everall, I. P., & Pantelis, C. (2012). Predicting the diagnosis of autism spectrum disorder using gene pathway analysis. *Molecular Psychiatry, 19*(4), 504–510.

Smith, G. L. & McGuinness, T. M. (2017). Adolescent psychosocial assessment: The HEEADSS. *Journal of Psychosocial Nursing and Mental Health Services, 55*(5), 24–27.

Stevens, G. L., Dawson, G., & Zummo, J. (2016). Clinical benefits and impact of early use of long-acting injectable antipsychotics for schizophrenia. *Early Intervention in Psychiatry, 10*(5), 365–377.

Storch, E. A., Nadeau, J. M., Johnco, C., Timpano, K., McBride, N., Mutch, P.J.,...Murphy, T. A. (2016). Hoarding in youth with autism spectrum disorders and anxiety: incidence, clinical correlates and behavioral treatment response. *Journal of Autism and Developmental Disorders, 46*, 1602–1612.

Substance Abuse and Mental Health Services Administration. (2013). Mental Health in My Community: Information Graphic. Retrieved on August 5, 2017, from https://store.samhsa.gov/product/Mental-Health-in-My-Community-Information-Graphic/SMA13-4725. References available from https://store.samhsa.gov/shin/content/SMA13-4725/SMA13-4725_Reference.pdf.

Tandon, R., Belmaker, R. H., Gattaz, W. F., Lopez-Ibor, J. J., Jr., Okasha, A., Singh, B.,...Section of Pharmacopsychiatry, World Psychiatric Association. (2008). World Psychiatric Association Pharmacopsychiatry Section statement on comparative effectiveness of antipsychotics in the treatment of schizophrenia. *Schizophrenia Research, 100*(1–3), 20–38.

Thornicroft, G. (2007). Most people with mental illness are not treated. *The Lancet, 370*(9590), 807–808.

Tolin, D. F., Frost, R. O., & Steketee, G. (2013). *Buried in treasures: Help for compulsive acquiring, saving and hoarding* (2nd ed.). New York: Oxford University Press.

U.S. Department of Health and Human Services. (1999). *Mental health: A report of the surgeon general*. U.S. Department of Health and Human Services, Substance Abuse and Mental Health Services Administration, Center for Mental Health Services, National Institutes of Health, National Institute of Mental Health.

U.S. Department of Health and Human Services. (2012). *Office of the Surgeon General and National Action Alliance for Suicide Prevention. 2012 National strategy for suicide prevention: Goals and objectives for action*. Washington, DC: U.S. Department of Health and Human Services.

U.S. Department of State. (2012). *National Counterterrorism Center: Annex of statistical information. Office of the Coordinator for Counterterrorism. Country reports on terrorism, 2011*. Retrieved May 25, 2013, from http://www.state.gov/j/ct/rls/crt/2011/195555.htm.

Ventriglio, A., Gentile, A., Stella, E. & Bellomo, A. (2015). Metabolic issues in patients affected by schizophrenia clinical characteristics and medical management. *Frontiers in Neuroscience, 9*, 297.

Wang, P. S., Aguilar-Gaxiola, S., Alonso, J., Angermeyer, M. C., Borges, G., Bromet, E. J.,...Wells, J. E. (2007). Use of mental health services for anxiety, mood, and substance disorders in 17 countries in the WHO world mental health surveys. *Lancet, 370*(9590), 841–850.

Williams, N. J., Scott, L. & Aarons, G. A. (2017). Prevalence of serious emotional disturbance among U.S. children: A meta-analysis. *Psychiatric Services in Advance, 69*(1):32–40.

World Health Organization. (2017). *Depression and other common mental disorders: Global health estimates*. Geneva: World Health Organization.

World Health Organization. (2013). *Mental Health Action Plan 2013-2020*. Geneva: World Health Organization.

World Health Organization. (2012). *Public health action for the prevention of suicide*. Geneva: World Health Organization.

World Health Organization. (2011). *Psychological first aid: Guide for field workers*. Geneva: WHO, War Trauma Foundation, and World Vision International.

World Health Organization. (2010). *mhGAP intervention guide for mental, neurological and substance use disorders in non-specialized health settings: Mental Health Gap Action Programme (mhGAP)*. Geneva: Author.

World Health Organization. (2008). *Mental Health Gap Action Programme: Scaling up care for mental, neurological, and substance use disorders*. Geneva: Author.

Yung, A. R., McGorry, P. D., Francey, S. M., Nelson, B., Baker, K., Phillips, L. J.,...Amminger, G. P. (2007). PACE: A specialised service for young people at risk of psychotic disorders. *Medical Journal of Australia, 187*(Suppl. 7), S43–S46.

Zauszniewski, J. A., Bekhet, A. K., & Suresky, M. K. (2008). Factors associated with perceived burden, resourcefulness and quality of life in female family members of adults with serious mental illness. *Journal of the American Psychiatric Nurses Association, 14*(2), 125–135.

Chapter 22

School Health

Pamela Pershing DiNapoli

> Computers are useless. They can only give you answers.
> **Pablo Picasso**

> Education is what remains after one has forgotten what one has learned in school.
> **Albert Einstein**

> Home computers are being called upon to perform many new functions, including the consumption of homework formerly eaten by the dog.
> **Doug Larson**

CHAPTER HIGHLIGHTS

- Historical perspectives of school health
- Components and organization of school health programs
- School health scope of services
- Health assessment and screening of school-aged children
- Development, implementation, and evaluation of preventive health programs
- Common health concerns in schools

OBJECTIVES

- Trace the history of school health practice.
- Explain the scope of the school nurse's role in the provision of healthcare.
- Identify useful sources for tracking epidemiology of common health concerns.
- Use best practice guidelines to address common preventable health concerns of the student population.

KEY TERMS

Americans with Disabilities Act (ADA): Wide-ranging federal legislation enacted in 1990 that is intended to make American society more accessible to people with disabilities.

Coordinated school health: A systematic approach to school health recommended by the CDC as a strategy for improving students' health and learning in the nation's schools.

Council on School Health: Coalition of a wide range of community stakeholders, including family and student representatives, who contribute to the development of action plans designed to improve the health and safety of the students.

Early Periodic Screening, Diagnosis, and Treatment (EPSDT): Program mandated by a federal law passed in 1969 that required that children and adolescents younger than 21 have access to periodic screenings.

Electronic bullying: Any kind of repeated aggression perpetrated through information technology, such

KEY TERMS *(continued)*

as the internet, to intentionally harm or harass another individual.

Every Student Succeeds Act (ESSA): Replaced and updated the No Child Left Behind Act (NCLB) and supersedes Individuals with Disabilities Education Act (IDEA) the federal law enacted in 1990 and reauthorized in 1997 designed to protect the rights of students with disabilities by ensuring that every individual receives a free appropriate public education, regardless of ability. ESSA promotes equitable general education for all students, as well as protects the supports and services necessary for individuals with disabilities.

Food Allergy and Anaphylaxis Management Act (FAAMA): Requires the U.S. Secretary of Health and Human Services to develop and make available to schools a voluntary policy to manage the risk of food allergy and anaphylaxis in schools and provide for school-based food allergy management incentive grants to support implementation of food allergy management guidelines in public schools.

Individual education plan (IEP): A plan developed by a multidisciplinary team to provide education and services to any student that has an identified disability to correspond with individual needs in the least restrictive environment.

Individuals with Disabilities Education Act (IDEA): Federal law designated in 1990, reauthorized in 1997 and redesignated in 2015. As the Every Student Succeeds Act (ESSA) was designed to protect the rights of students with disabilities by ensuring that everyone receives a free appropriate public education, regardless of ability.

School Health Index: An online self-assessment and planning tool that schools can use to improve their health and safety policies and programs.

School health nursing: Specialized practice of nursing that protects and promotes student health, facilitates optimal development, and advances academic success. School nurses, grounded in ethical and evidence-based practice, are the leaders who bridge healthcare and education, provide care coordination, advocate for quality student-centered care, and collaborate to design systems that allow individuals and communities to develop their full potential.

Whole School, Whole Community, Whole Child (WSCC): Combines and builds on the coordinated school health model and the Association for Supervision and Curriculum Development's (ASCD) Whole Child approach to education to promote improved health and educational outcomes for children in schools.

Youth Risk Behavior Surveillance Survey (YRBSS): Biannual report of the common risk behaviors that influence the health of youth in the United States.

CASE STUDY

References to the case study are found throughout this chapter (look for the case study icon). Readers should keep the case study in mind as they read the chapter.

Susan is the school nurse in a rural elementary school for children in kindergarten through grade 5. The school has approximately 300 students, who present Susan with many challenges. One child with special health needs is in a wheelchair, is catheterized twice a day while at school, and receives a tube feeding at lunch. Two children who have type 1 diabetes—one requires blood sugar monitoring and insulin injections at a minimum of once daily, while the other has a continuous insulin pump. Several children have allergies ranging from severe peanut allergies to bee stings. In addition, Susan administers daily medications to 18 students at various times; these medications include methylphenidate (Ritalin), gabapentin (Neurontin), carbamazepine (Carbatrol), and Lactaid.

Susan uses a computerized database to track the visits of the children to her office, which average 30 per day. Reasons for visits include playground injuries and acute illnesses with symptoms such as vomiting, fever, or headache.

INTRODUCTION

Many people outside of the school environment have little understanding of the scope of the roles and responsibilities of the school nurse. Currently there are more than 55 million children enrolled in nearly 125,000 U.S. schools. The association recommendation is a ratio of one nurse for every 750 students. However, it is estimated that only 41% of schools have full-time RNs, with school nurses frequently serving several schools. Findings from the National Association of School Nurses (NASN) 2016 School Nurses Survey indicate that school nurses cover, on average, three buildings and serve an average of 924 to 1,072 students (Mangena & Maughan, 2015). As such, schools represent one of the greatest opportunities to communicate important health messages to America's children and youth (AAP, 2016).

The role of the school nurse, first introduced in the early 1900s, has changed dramatically over the years. These changes closely parallel the increasing number of complex health issues being seen within the school system. Although the school nurse is often seen merely as someone who applies adhesive bandages or who serves as a parent substitute for children having difficulty adjusting to the school setting, the role of the school nurse has evolved to where it is now recognized as a specialty area in nursing. The scope of the role in promoting wellness includes administrative, educational, clerical, and supportive responsibilities, along with encouragement of school wellness policies, such as physical activity in daily practice (Avery, Johnson, Cousins, & Hamilton, 2013). This chapter describes **school health nursing** and illustrates how the school nurse has become a cornerstone in providing healthcare and health promotion to school-aged children and their families.

In 2017, the NASN revised their definition of school nursing to being, "a specialized practice of nursing, protects and promotes student health, facilitates optimal development, and advances academic success. School nurses, grounded in ethical and evidence-based practice, are the leaders who bridge healthcare and education, provide care coordination, advocate for quality student-centered care, and collaborate to design systems that allow individuals and communities to develop their full potential" (NASN, 2017).

Therefore, school nurses:

- Help encourage positive responses to normal development.
- Help promote health and safety.
- Help solve actual and potential problems.
- Help promote academic success.
- Provide case management services.
- Work with others to develop student and family capacity for adaptation, self-management, and continued growth.

HISTORICAL PERSPECTIVES

The history of school nursing can be traced back to 1902, when Lillian Wald, working in a New York City public school, saw that school nursing services were a way to decrease excessive absenteeism. At that time, the role of nurses in schools was limited to the treatment of minor contagious diseases, the conduct of health education programs, and the use of home visits to demonstrate recommended treatments to family. Historically, the scope of school health services was often the function of public health nurses contracted through municipal health departments. However, soon the first city-wide school nursing program in the world was established. Lina Rogers (Struthers) became the first school nurse in New York City and is credited with providing evidence-based nursing care across the city (Rollins, 2011; Vessey & McGowan, 2006).

During the following decades, there was a dramatic increase in the number of school nurses in the United States. The last Health Resources and Services Administration

(HRSA) health workforce survey done in 2008 estimated that 1.9% of licensed registered nurses worked in the school environment in the United States (HRSA, 2010). As the number of school nurses increased, the role of the school nurse became more focused on screening and referral. The **Early Periodic Screening, Diagnosis, and Treatment (EPSDT)** program provided for by Section 1905(a) in Title XIX of the Social Security Act, which was passed in 1965, was an influential factor promoting this key school nursing role in screening and referral. EPSDT recognized that schools can be a focal point from which to identify children with problems, to increase students' access to both preventive and curative health services, and to ensure appropriate use of healthcare resources for children and adolescents who received Medicaid and were younger than 21 (http://www.cms.gov/Regulations-and-Guidance).

However, the strongest influence on school nursing practice came with the passage of the Education for All Handicapped Children Act of 1975 (Public Law 94-142). Children who had previously been unable to attend school because of chronic or complex medical issues were now entitled to a public education, and they began attending public schools. School nurses were now providing more complex care for conditions such as seizure disorders, asthma, cardiac conditions, cystic fibrosis, quadriplegia, and life-threatening allergies (Robert Wood Johnson Foundation, 2010). For example, peanut allergy, the most common cause of anaphylaxis, is a medical emergency that requires immediate treatment with an epinephrine (adrenaline) injector (EpiPen, Twinject) and a trip to the emergency department.

Today, given the wide range of health needs in the student population, it is not uncommon for school nurses to record up to 100 visits in a single day. With the increase in these complex conditions came the need to perform high-tech skills, such as tube feedings, catheterizations, and suctioning. The inclusion of children with special needs led to a change in the EPSDT program. The School Health-Related Services Plan Section 1905(r)(5) of the Social Security Act (the Act) requires that any medically necessary healthcare service listed in Section 1905(a) of the Act be provided to an EPSDT recipient even if the service is not available under that state's Medicaid plan. An amendment required identification of children who have a learning problem due to a medical problem that requires special services. Once the child is identified, an **Individual Education Plan (IEP)** or 504 plan, which lists services needed by the child, is completed by the school. The schools employ people with special training to assist children with special needs. The IEP is reviewed annually and eligibility is reviewed every three years. The school nurse is an integral member of the IEP and should advocate for his or her role during all special education meetings. Box 22.1 lists the direct medical services reimbursable by Medicaid when performed by a school as part of the IEP and when consistent with state Medicaid regulations.

The **Individuals with Disabilities Education Act (IDEA)**, originally the Education for all Handicapped

22.1 Direct Medical Services Reimbursable by Medicaid

1. Providing health/mental health services contained in an IEP.
2. Medical/health assessment and evaluation as part of the development of an IEP.
3. Conducting medical/health assessments/evaluations and diagnostic testing and preparing related reports.
4. Providing personal aide services.
5. Providing speech, occupational, physical and other therapies.
6. Administering first aid, or prescribed injection or medication.
7. Providing direct clinical/treatment services.
8. Performing developmental assessments.
9. Providing counseling services to treat health, mental health, or substance abuse conditions.
10. Developing a treatment plan (medical plan of care) for a student if provided as a medical service.
11. Targeted case management (if provided or covered as a medical service under Medicaid).
12. Transportation (if covered as a medical service under Medicaid).
13. Activities that are services, or components of services, listed in the state's Medicaid plan.

Source: https://www.cms.gov.

Children Act, has undergone several legislative amendments in recent years. Lawmakers made these changes to accommodate the changing climate for disabled people in the United States and to promote the belief that "improving educational results for children with disabilities is an essential element of our national policy of ensuring equality of opportunity, full participation, independent living, and economic self-sufficiency for individuals with disabilities" (Individuals with Disabilities Education Improvement Act of 2004). The IDEA requires students be evaluated based on academic achievement, functional performance, cognitive functioning, communication status, health, hearing and vision, motor abilities, and social-emotional status (Department of Education, https://sites.ed.gov/idea/, n.d.). The most recent change came when the IDEA was amended in December of 2015 through Public Law 114-95, the **Every Student Succeeds Act (ESSA)**, which attempts to ensure success by focusing on the best teaching and learning strategies for all students, including gifted and talented students, and not just authorized for children with disabilities. States are accountable for protecting the general education, as well as the supports and services necessary for individuals with disabilities to succeed as provided under the IDEA (Department of Education, https://sites.ed.gov/idea/, n.d.).

You have got to keep autistic children engaged with the world. You cannot let them tune out. **Temple Grandin**

Danielle is a student with special health needs who attends the school where Susan works as a nurse. Susan must catheterize her twice daily while at school, and while Danielle's aide can assist with her tube feedings, Susan has primary responsibility for programming and attaching the pump to Danielle's "MIC-KEY button."

ROLE OF THE SCHOOL NURSE

The school nurse provides a critical link between the child, the family, and the education and healthcare systems. Each of the 50 states has a state nurse practice act that regulate the profession of nursing, including school nursing. *The Scope and Standards of Professional School Nursing Practice* (American Nurses Association & National Association of School Nurses, 2017) defines the practice of school health nurses.

Building on the evidence-based principles of the school nursing standards for competent quality care, the NASN developed a Framework for 21st Century School Nursing Practice (the Framework), which provides structure and focus for student-centered nursing care that occurs within the context of the students' family and school community. Surrounding the students, family, and school community are the nonhierarchical, overlapping key principles of care coordination, leadership, quality improvement, and community/public health (NASN, http://www.nasn.org/nasn/nasn-resources/professional-topics/framework). It should be acknowledged that many school health programs suffer as a result of inconsistency and ambiguity in the practice of school nursing. In an effort to prioritize the learning and health needs of students, the **Whole School, Whole Community, Whole Child model (WSCC)** was developed by the Association for Supervision and Curriculum Development (ASCD) and the Centers for Disease Control and Prevention (CDC). The WSCC model outlines the 10 recommended components of a comprehensive school health program, as summarized in Table 22.1.

Provision of health services by the school nurse is the anchor of the school health program. To address the diverse needs of students, the school nurse must adopt the central management position for all children and adolescents in the school. The role that emerges within the context of this management position requires that the nurse have skills in health assessment, including skills in the identification of common problems that impact a child's learning, such as vision impairment, attention-deficit/hyperactivity disorder (ADHD), and scoliosis. Screening is also a valuable tool in identifying and treating problems that may result in a child being excluded from school, such as infestation with lice, or other communicable diseases. Health promotion, health education, and child health advocacy are key components of the school nurse's role. Many nurses take on the

TABLE 22.1 Comprehensive School Health Programs

Recommended Components	Description
Health education	Curricula and instruction for students in pre-K through grade 12 that address a variety of topics such as alcohol and other drug use and abuse, healthy eating/nutrition, mental and emotional health, personal health and wellness, physical activity, safety and injury prevention, sexual health, tobacco use, and violence prevention
Nutrition and environment services	Provides students with opportunities to learn about and practice healthy eating through available foods and beverages, nutrition education, and messages about food in the cafeteria and throughout the school campus
Employee wellness	A coordinated set of programs, policies, benefits, and environmental supports designed to address multiple risk factors (e.g., lack of physical activity, tobacco use) and health conditions (e.g., diabetes, depression) to meet the health and safety needs of all employees
Social and emotional school climate	A climate that promotes health, growth, and development by providing a safe and supportive learning environment
Physical environment	A physical environment that protect occupants from physical threats (e.g., crime, violence, traffic, and injuries) and biologic and chemical agents in the air, water, or soil
Health services	Intervene with actual and potential health problems, in addition to wellness promotion, preventive services and staff, student and parent education; complement the provision of care coordination services
Counseling, psychological and social services	Services include psychological, psychoeducational, and psychosocial assessments; direct and indirect interventions to address psychological, academic, and social barriers to learning
Community involvement	Community groups, organizations, and local businesses create partnerships with schools, share resources, and volunteer to support student learning, development, and health-related activities
Family engagement	Families and school staff work together to support and improve the learning, development, and health of students
Physical education and physical activity	Provides the opportunity for students to learn key concepts and practice critical skills needed to establish and maintain physically active lifestyles throughout childhood, adolescence and into adulthood

Source: Centers for Disease Control and Prevention. Components of the Whole School, Whole Community, Whole Child (WSCC). Retrieved from https://www.cdc.gov/healthyschools/wscc/components.htm.

expanded role of certified health educator and function increasingly as valuable classroom teachers. The nurse needs to collaborate with other members of the school health services team to integrate comprehensive wellness policies and practices into school action plans, as a provision of participating in federal programs such as WSCC, ESSA, and Child Nutrition Programs (CDC, https://www.cdc.gov/healthyschools).

> Hugs can do great amounts of good—especially for children.
> **Diana, Princess of Wales**

Practice Point

School nursing requires autonomous practice and independent decision-making.

Health Assessment

Typically, there are three types of school health service visits that require the nurse to use assessment skills. The first type of visit is for acute illness (e.g., vomiting, fever, or headache) and playground injury. The nurse can easily use physical assessment skills and knowledge of first aid to address these issues. For example, peanut allergy, the most common cause of anaphylaxis, is a medical emergency that requires immediate treatment with an epinephrine (adrenaline) injector (EpiPen, Twinject) and a trip to the emergency department.

The second type is for typical screenings, often begun when the child enters school (immunization status) and may be continued as the child grows and is at risk for problems that may impact learning, such as vision impairment. Routine screening may require referral and follow-up. The third type of visit is for counseling. Students may seek out the school nurse for advice and support regarding daily stressors encountered in the social framework of the school, such as being picked on or bullied by others. These visits require that the nurse assess the child individually. In addition, there are visits that are part of population-based screening programs that may include periodic vision and hearing tests, height and weight measurements (e.g., to calculate body mass index [BMI]), or immunization checks; these may result in health teaching activities.

Individual Health Assessment

The individual assessment of the child is specific to the need for the visit and may not occur in the health office. In any case, health assessment should be the responsibility of a licensed healthcare professional in the school setting. Within the school, a variety of data sources are available to the nurse to use in completing a thorough assessment of the child's chief complaint. The nurse should begin by collecting subjective data gathered from the child, teacher, or parent, or any other witness to the complaint. Data should include location, frequency, duration and severity, quality, quantity, setting, associated symptoms, and precipitating factors that make the symptom better or worse. Objective data provide information that makes the nurse's job of understanding the complaint easier. These data should include any information or signs pertinent to the illness, such as fever.

Practice Point

The child's chief complaint may only be the tip of the iceberg. Use all data sources available to assess the problem.

Collectively, this information guides the actions taken by the nurse. These actions might include treatment, referral to a healthcare provider, and notification of a parent and/or sending the child home. Individual school policy dictates the extent to which the nurse is able to treat the presenting symptoms.

Danielle also receives occupational and physical therapy services while at school. Susan must incorporate data gathered from the treatment notes, as well as from the special medical services treatment providers who monitor Danielle's medical care within her home. It is important that Susan maintains frequent communication with this team to ensure close monitoring of Danielle's healthcare needs.

Population-Based Assessment

There are no federal laws requiring that periodic screening be provided by the schools, although as a public health concern consistent with EPSDT, these screenings are often a major part of the school health program. The screenings may be essential to the early detection of, and intervention in, problems that may affect academic success.

In addition, people often ask a school nurse why he or she performs periodic screening and how schools use this information. Screening programs typically begin when the child enters school and may continue in different forms throughout the child's education. Before implementing a screening program, schools should address these questions. For example, it is helpful if the health education curriculum addresses the conditions being assessed in the screening process. That way everyone, including the school staff, students, and families, is fully informed. It is necessary to develop clear procedures that evaluate the results of screening tests and stipulate how the results will be reported. In addition, it is essential to establish what the desired screening outcomes are and to emphasize those that fall outside of the targeted benchmarks.

The school nurse should play a major role in planning these screenings and will need to spend the required time to develop a successful program. For example, in response to the obesity epidemic, many schools are implementing walking programs or similar exercise programs to encourage the recommended 60 minutes a day of physical activity. Box 22.2 lists the school health screenings that school nurses frequently coordinate.

Practice Point

The Screening, Brief Intervention, and Referral to Treatment (SBIRT) tool focuses on early detection, risk assessment, brief counseling and referral intervention that can be utilized in the school setting to reinforce healthy behaviors and address safety issues (https://www.samhsa.gov/sbirt).

Health Promotion and Assessment of School Health Needs

Healthy People 2020 has acknowledged the need for targeted data collection and health promotion efforts regarding the common health concerns of children and adolescents (USDHHS, *Healthy People 2020*, 2018). One tool, the **Youth Risk Behavior Surveillance Survey (YRBSS)**, is a voluntary, biannual survey of the common risk behaviors

22.2 Typical School Health Screenings

- Immunization Screening
- Vision Screening
- Hearing Screening
- Postural Screening
- Body Mass Index Screening

influencing the health of the nation's youth. These risk behaviors are identified because of their potential impact on the long-term health and well-being of youth. Box 22.3 illustrates the six behavior categories for which statistics are typically reported. The CDC's YRBSS website (https://www.cdc.gov/healthyyouth/data/yrbs/index.htm) is a source of additional information about this data collection tool.

A second data collection tool is the **School Health Index**, which focuses on how schools can promote physical activity, healthy eating, and adoption of a tobacco-free lifestyle, and a wide range of safety-related behaviors in an attempt to counter common risk behaviors (CDC, 2014). There are two versions of the index, one for elementary schools and the other for middle schools and high schools. These can be obtained in print form or can be used online. The importance of the School Health Index is its ability to help schools identify the strengths and weaknesses of a particular school's policies and programs for promoting health and safety. On the basis of this assessment, school personnel can develop an action plan, which is then incorporated into a school's overall improvement plan to promote the health and safety of the students. The CDC developed the School Health Index Self-Assessment and Planning Guide for the following purposes (CDC, n.d.):

- Enabling schools to identify the strengths and weaknesses of health and safety policies and programs
- Enabling schools to develop an action plan for improving student health, which can be incorporated into the school improvement plan

22.3 Youth Risk Behavior Surveillance Survey Risk Behavior Categories

- Behaviors that contribute to unintentional injuries and violence
- Sexual behaviors related to unintended pregnancy and sexually transmitted diseases, including HIV infection
- Alcohol and other drug use
- Tobacco use
- Unhealthy dietary behaviors
- Inadequate physical activity

- Engaging teachers, parents, students, and the community in promoting health-enhancing behaviors and better health

Evidence for Practice

- Along with the School Health Index, the CDC has several standardized adolescent and school health tools that assist in assessment, planning, implementing, and evaluating school health programs.
- The CDC's Division of Adolescent and School Health and School Health Services websites provide more information (https://www.cdc.gov/healthyyouth/; https://www.cdc.gov/healthyschools/). Tools are available to the school nurse and other health professionals responsible for the provision of the continuum of healthcare services.
- Health Education Curriculum Analysis Tool (HECAT), which helps schools, school districts, and other school personnel responsible for curricular redesign and continuous quality improvement to analyze health education programs on the basis of alignment with national health education standards and characteristics of effective health education curricula.
- Physical Education Curriculum Analysis Tool (PECAT), which enables users to analyze written physical education curricula based on alignment with national standards, guidelines, and best practices for quality physical education programs.
- Healthy Students, Promising Futures which helps Local Education Agencies (LEA) link to state and local agencies to improve school-based health. Opportunities include helping families and students to enroll in health insurance and expanding services to at-risk students (https://www2.ed.gov/admins/lead/safety/healthy-students/toolkit.pdf).

School health advisory councils consisting of a wide range of community stakeholders hold the greatest potential for addressing the health needs of students to support their physical, cognitive, and emotional development. Based on past CDC recommendations, approximately one-third of the nation's schools had school health councils. Many states mandate by law that schools have councils that develop and evaluate school health action plans. The development of these councils has significantly improved the odds that schools have comprehensive policies and programs that address common health concerns. The WSCC advocates for the integration and alignment between health and education acknowledging the interrelatedness between learning and health (Lewallen et al., 2015).

The establishment of school-based health centers (SBHCs) and services complement the work of the school nurse as a model of primary healthcare in the schools. SBHCs are specifically designed to fill gaps in health services, including those to prevent teen pregnancy. The appearance of SBHCs began in the early 1980s. Today, more than 2,000 SBHCs exist in 49 of 50 states. The SBHCs do not take the place of existing nursing services, but they enhance health services by decreasing barriers to needed healthcare. The National Association of Pediatric Nurse Practitioners advocates SBHCs as a necessary component of comprehensive healthcare for children. The SBHCs are located where the children are and can effectively treat problems affecting children's health.

The Affordable Care Act appropriated $200 million from 2010 through 2013 for the centers, to build new facilities, purchase equipment, and expand services (Wall Street Journal, 2012). This infusion of money enabled those SBHCs receiving funding to increase capacity by over 50%. Subsequently, the Department of Child, Adolescent and Family Health SBHCs have established key performance measures to ensure continued quality, growth and sustainability of SBHCs (School-Based Health Alliance, https://www.sbh4all.org/resources/quality-counts/five-performance-measures/).

> ### ✎ Practice Point
>
> Collaboration across the community, school, and health sectors to meet the needs and support the full potential of each child is the most important step that schools can take to improve their comprehensive school health program.

Susan is the chair of the School District Wellness Committee. The Wellness Committee was formed primarily to oversee the nutrition and physical activity needs of the school community as part of an overall commitment to wellness. The committee has recently implemented a before-school walking program to encourage children to engage in at least 60 minutes of physical activity per day.

The School Nurse as Health Educator

Schools, where children and adolescents spend one-third of their day, present an ideal setting for providing health education. A health education curriculum is an important part of a comprehensive kindergarten to grade 12 school health program. Consistent with the WSCC program, evidence-based health education programs may vary in their approach but should be age-appropriate and should focus on developing and enhancing social and emotional strengths (ASCD & CDC, 2014).

Programs that serve to increase self-esteem, develop social skills, and increase understanding of issues such as peer influence and decision-making should be considered. Some professionals have recommended that the school nurse's role in health education should be that of a resource person or consultant and not necessarily that of a teacher. This opinion is contrary to that of the NASN, which considers health education an important intervention to be implemented as a primary responsibility of the school nurse.

Whether or not the school nurse is in the classroom, health education is a priority. The school nurse must seek to accomplish health teaching in encounters with students and families, in the classroom, in individual counseling sessions (e.g., teaching a child how and when to use his or her EpiPen), and in group meetings. Despite the existence of National Health Education Standards, the Society for Public Health Education reports that health education in schools is a low priority (SOPHE, 2018). By adopting the eight National Health Education Standards, schools increase the likelihood that children will adopt lifelong health-promoting behaviors. It is recommended that the focus of health education be skill-based and address the health promotion concerns identified in the National Health Objectives of *Healthy People 2020*. This includes focusing on protective factors that support health-enhancing behaviors related to nutrition, physical activity, and safe use of social media, and that promote the avoidance of drug, alcohol and tobacco use, and the prevention of bullying and other forms of violence.

Emergency Preparedness

An essential role of the school nurse is to be prepared for emergencies, yet as few as 75% have any specialized training in emergency care beyond basic life support. Emergency preparedness does not address a specific hazard but addresses the planning, response, and recovery needs within a local community, such as a school. An example of a training program offered to provide nurses with knowledge and skills to respond to a mass casualty is the School Emergency Triage Training (SETT) program offered by the NASN. It is the position of NASN that the school nurse has the skills to provide leadership in all phases of emergency preparedness and response. Doyle (2013) has identified four roles that by virtue of the school nurses' specialized education can be performed in an emergency situation: prevention, preparedness, response, and recovery.

COMMON HEALTH CONCERNS

It is easier to build strong children than to repair broken men.
Frederick Douglass

Substance Use: Drugs and Alcohol

Epidemiology

The National Survey on Drug Use and Health (NSDUH) is sponsored by the Center for Behavioral Health Statistics and Quality, a division of the Substance Abuse and Mental Health Services Administration (SAMHSA). SAMHSA is the primary source of data on drug and alcohol use in the civilian population. NSDUH tracks indicators of substance use and mental health among people aged 12 years or older, and further aggregates data by age group, including youths ages 12 to 17 and young adults ages 18 to 25. The most current estimate of illicit drug use among youths ages 12 to 17 years is 8.8%, whereas among young adults ages 18 to 25, the estimate is 23.2%. The most commonly reported illicit drug used in these age groups is marijuana. From 2002 to 2015, the prevalence of marijuana use has declined in youths ages 12 to 17 (8.2% to 7.0%), but has increased steadily in young adults. In 2015, about one in five young adults ages 18 to 25 (19.8%) were current users of marijuana. A recent addition to the survey was related to prescription drug (psychotherapeutics) misuse, defined as use in any way not directed by a prescriber of any drug in the following categories: pain relievers, tranquilizers, stimulants, and sedatives. About 2% of adolescents (one in 50) and 5.1% of young adults were current misusers of psychotherapeutic drugs. Pain relievers were the substance most often misused.

NSDUH also collects data on current alcohol use, including binge drinking and heavy use. Although the estimated alcohol use among adolescents decreased between 2002 and 2015, about one in 10 adolescents aged 12 to 17 years were current alcohol users in 2015. About 5.8% of these current drinkers were binge drinkers, defined as having five or more drinks on the same occasion on at least one day in the past 30 days, and about one in 100 were heavy drinkers, defined as having five or more drinks on the same occasion on five or more days in the past 30 days (SAMHSA, 2017).

Best Practices: Drug and Alcohol Prevention

Based on the trends in drug and alcohol use, the school nurse should consider introducing prevention during the three periods when the interventions are most likely to produce results: (1) the primary prevention or inoculation phase, which is designed to introduce knowledge; (2) the secondary prevention or early relevance phase, when information is likely to have meaning and applicability to students; and (3) the tertiary prevention or later relevance phase, when young people are actually being exposed to new situations involving experimentation. Programs and booster sessions should be implemented throughout these periods (National Registry of Evidence-Based Programs and Practices [NREPP], n.d.). There is an extensive body of research related to the effectiveness of school-based substance abuse programs. The SAMHSA has collated a series of evidence-based programs with the potential to produce sustained behavior change (NREPP). The NREPP website (www.nrepp.samhsa.gov) is a searchable database of interventions that have been evaluated in comparative effectiveness research. It is important to assess the needs and interests of the group carefully prior to the selection of any program. Providing school drug education programs that are meaningful and motivating to the participants should also be considered. Integrating the goals of the child's grade in school with developmentally appropriate prevention programs is essential. For example, is the goal of the program nonuse, delayed use, or harm minimization? In addition, the school nurse should design programs that are behavior-focused and use teaching and learning principles and interactive techniques that give students an opportunity to practice new skills, rather than relying on knowledge-based programs.

> ### Practice Point
>
> Classroom-based drug education should be made routinely available in schools as a cost-effective method for the prevention of drug abuse.

It is clear that a substantial number of adolescents will experiment with substances and that given the limited funding available in many schools for prevention programming evidence-based prevention strategies must be initiated as early as elementary school to prevent initiation (Singh, Jimerson, & Renshaw, 2011).

Substance Use: Smoking

Epidemiology

Tobacco use, including smokeless tobacco products continue to be the leading cause of preventable disease in the United States. Among adolescents who reported current tobacco use, 30.3% used tobacco products other than cigarettes, but did not smoke cigarettes. During the late 1990s, the overall downward trend in current cigarette smoking among high school students began to slow, as observed by the National Youth Tobacco Survey (NYTS) and other national surveys. However, some of this decline may reflect the use of electronic vaporizing devices for delivering nicotine, such as e-cigarettes. For example, data from the most recent NYTS indicates that more than a quarter-million middle school and high school students in 2013 (263,000) never smoked a conventional cigarette, but used e-cigarettes (Bunnell et al., 2015). A recent surgeon general's report on this trend indicates there has been a 900% increase since 2011 (U.S. Department of Health and Human Services, Office of the Surgeon General, 2016). Findings from 2015 indicated that 2.4 million high school students and 620,000 middle school students reported having used an e-cigarette at least one time in the past

30 days. E-cigarettes are tobacco products that deliver nicotine and are associated with the initiation of the use of other tobacco products. Serious unintended consequence of this trend is the increase in accidental poisoning due to exposure to liquid nicotine and passive exposure to nicotine.

The *Healthy People 2020* objectives also specifically target adolescent tobacco use. Specific objectives include reducing the reported use of tobacco products in the previous 12 months from 7.7% to 5.7%. Also included are objectives to decrease the initiation of smokeless tobacco and cigars among children and adolescents, aged 12 to 17 years. *Healthy People 2020* suggests that effective prevention approaches for improving health behaviors in adolescents must include school-based prevention programs, as well as community-wide strategies that address the overall social context of health risk behaviors.

Best Practices: Prevention of Tobacco Use

In the early 1990s and to the extent that tobacco use was linked to increases in smoking-related illnesses, the tobacco industry made a legal agreement, following a lawsuit co-sponsored by the states of Texas, Florida, Mississippi and Minnesota, to put an end to all marketing efforts that primarily target cigarette use by minors. In 1998, the Attorneys General of the 46 remaining states signed the Multistate Settlement Agreement (MSA) with the four largest tobacco companies in the United States to settle state suits that were initiated to recover costs associated with treating smoking-related illnesses. Conditions of the agreement included restrictions on tobacco advertising and marketing. As youth spend up to 25% of their waking hours in school and are thus a captive audience for tobacco prevention programming, programming should start with tobacco prevention education before students begin to smoke. The CDC supports school-based tobacco prevention and control programs that include targeted, evidence-based interventions combined with comprehensive policies and practice. CDC guidelines for school-based tobacco prevention can be found in Box 22.4.

- Prohibit tobacco use at all school facilities and events at all times.
- Encourage and help students and staff to quit using tobacco.
- Provide developmentally appropriate instruction in grades K–12 that addresses the social and psychological causes of tobacco use.
- Are part of a **coordinated school health** program through which teachers, students, families, administrators, and community leaders deliver consistent messages about tobacco use.
- Are implemented within the context of and reinforced by communitywide efforts to prevent tobacco use and addiction.

There is sufficient evidence that school-based tobacco prevention can produce at least short-term effects and reduce the prevalence of tobacco use among school-aged youth.

22.4 Recommendations for School-Based Tobacco Prevention Programs

1. Develop and enforce a school policy on tobacco use.
2. Provide instruction about the short- and long-term negative physiologic and social consequences of tobacco use, social influences on tobacco use, peer norms regarding tobacco use, and refusal skills.
3. Provide tobacco-use prevention education in kindergarten through 12th grade; this instruction should be especially intensive in junior high or middle school and should be reinforced in high school.
4. Provide program-specific training for teachers.
5. Involve parents or families in support of school-based programs to prevent tobacco use.
6. Support cessation efforts among students and all school staff who use tobacco.
7. Assess the tobacco-use prevention program at regular intervals.

Source: From Centers for Disease Control and Prevention. *Tobacco use prevention in schools: Guidelines and strategies.* Retrieved on September 9, 2017, from https://www.cdc.gov/healthyschools/tobacco/strategies.htm.

Practice Point

Strategies to prevent tobacco use, including e-cigarettes, in schools should begin with specific training of both the school personnel, who interact with the adolescents on a daily basis, and the student peer leaders involved with the program.

Sexual Behavior and Teenage Pregnancy

On average, 70% of adolescents have a preventive health visit only every four years. Despite recommendations for annual screening, particularly for adolescents engaging in high-risk behavior, such as sexual activity, there are many barriers to this type of preventive healthcare in primary care. These barriers include limited evidence that behavior counseling is effective, limited confidence in primary care providers to provide counseling, and perceived lack of interest by adolescents to receive counseling (Ham & Allen, 2012). This clearly represents missed opportunities for important dialogues that may prevent detrimental outcomes of sexual behavior, including unintended pregnancy and sexually transmitted infections. Students attending school should have the opportunity to receive knowledgeable and accessible sexual behavior education and counseling. Evidence supports the effectiveness of high-intensity school-based education and counseling in group settings as a way to reduce rates of consequences of high-risk sexual behavior (Manlove, Fish, & Moore, 2015; SIECUS, n.d.).

Epidemiology

Childbearing among teenagers has continued to decrease since 1991. Most recent birth rates have been reported as 22.3 births for every 1,000 adolescent females ages 15 to 19. Most adolescents who give birth are aged 18 to 19 years. Although also declining in number, birth rates continue to be higher among Hispanic and black adolescents (CDC, 2016a). While reasons for the declines are not clear, teens seem to be delaying onset of sexual activity, and more of those who are sexually active seem to be using birth control than in previous years. Long-acting reversible birth control can be a good option for a teenaged woman. Implants and intrauterine devices (IUDs) are two types. These do not require her to do anything on a regular basis, such as take a pill each day. For the past 10 years, the prevalence of adolescent pregnancy has been declining, but the ramifications for those teenagers who do become mothers are long-lasting, keeping adolescent pregnancy on the list of major public health problems. There is a strong association between teenage pregnancy and child well-being. Morbidity associated with children of teenage pregnancy includes higher rates of preterm birth and low birth weight (CDC, 2012).

Best Practices: Pregnancy Prevention

Evidence-based teen pregnancy prevention programs are those that have demonstrated, in at least one program evaluation, a positive effect on preventing teen pregnancies, sexually transmitted infections, or sexual risk behaviors. The Adolescent Family Life (AFL) program, created in 1981 (Title XX of the Public Health Service Act), was the first federal program to focus on adolescents. From 1998 to 2009, the program relied heavily on abstinence-only education. In 2010, a new Teen Pregnancy Prevention program was funded to provide "medically accurate and age-appropriate programs that reduce pregnancy." The Patient Protection and Affordable Care Act (ACA) enables states to operate a new Personal Responsibility Education Program (PREP), which is a comprehensive approach to teen pregnancy prevention that educates adolescents on both abstinence and contraception to prevent pregnancy and STDs. Finally, the Title V Abstinence Education Block Grant is available to states specifically for abstinence-only education. State Abstinence Education Grant Programs continue to provide funds for programs offering mentoring, counseling, or adult supervision programs to promote abstinence.

Since 2009, the U.S. Department of Health and Human Services (USDHHS) has sponsored an independent systematic review of the teen pregnancy prevention literature to identify programs with evidence of effectiveness in reducing teen pregnancy, sexually transmitted infections, and associated sexual risk behaviors. The American Academy of Pediatricians, the American Academy of Family Physicians, and the American Medical Association all endorse sex and contraceptive counseling performed by healthcare professionals as the model to be used to promote responsible sexual behavior and reduce teen pregnancy. The most recent YRBSS reports that the prevalence of sexual intercourse among high school students nationwide is 41.2% of students; 30.1% of students are currently sexually active. The prevalence of having ever had sexual intercourse was higher among males (43.2%) than females (39.2%); of these, 3.9% had had sexual intercourse for the first time before age 13. The prevalence of not having used any method of birth control to prevent pregnancy ranged from 7.2% to 20.0% (USDHHS, 2016). In previous surveys, the reasons that female students gave for not using contraceptives consistently included the belief that pregnancy will not affect them, the desire to become pregnant, "cultural" beliefs, and fear.

Despite evidence that supports SBHC and the school nurse as a pivotal access point to contraceptive counseling, barriers continue to exist. The ACA of 2010 that provided significant funding for SBHCs, particularly those that serve Medicaid-eligible populations, expired in 2013. Funding for SBHCs remains an issue. Most available on-site services include abstinence counseling (84%), pregnancy testing (81%), and counseling for birth control (70%); however, about 60% are prohibited from dispensing contraception, thus limiting access (Ethier et al., 2011).

Practice Point

A multidisciplinary team consisting of nurse practitioners, educators, school nurses, social service workers, and other professionals should collaborate to meet the needs of children and adolescents.

Student Reflection

My community health clinical experience was in a city high school in Massachusetts. During my time there, I became acutely aware of the student issues regarding STIs, teen pregnancy, and the lack of sexual health information. The statistics of STI rates are frightening: one in four of American girls have had an STI, and in one year in Massachusetts, syphilis increased by 20%, gonorrhea by 12%, and chlamydia infections by 8.3%. An annual questionnaire given in high schools around the state found that in 2015, 64% of teens have had intercourse by the time they graduate from high school, and many more engage in a range of other sexual activities. Only 50% of the students said that their parents had talked to them about sex!

There also were a high number of teenage pregnancies in the high school. Along with my teacher, I became involved in presenting seminars for students who were currently pregnant or had recently had a child. The groups were small to create an intimate nonjudgmental or nonthreatening atmosphere. The teen mothers-to-be learned what to expect in pregnancy and the changes that their bodies would be going through. They learned how to stay healthy—about the right things to eat, things to avoid eating, when to see a doctor, how to know when to go to the hospital, and seeking father and family support. We also discussed the labor process and postpartum issues, in particular postpartum depression and shaken baby syndrome. Then the group learned about lifestyle changes when the baby arrives. This included feeding and sleeping patterns, along with crying issues. We demonstrated changing a diaper and washing the baby and practiced using dolls. At all times, the students had the opportunity to ask questions and clear up any misconceptions or concerns. We also supplied information about STIs, contraception, and safe sex. Pamphlets, magazines, posters, fact sheets, contact information, and other resources were available.

I believe that a nurse has a responsibility to be proactive by encouraging clients to make healthy decisions and live a healthy lifestyle without pressuring them. By providing students with information, we empowered students and gave them the opportunity to make their own informed decisions. In the evaluations completed by the students, they found the interventions "catchy, current, and something that they could relate to."

Sexually Transmitted Infections

Epidemiology

Sexually transmitted infections are among the most common infectious diseases nationwide. Young people (aged 13 to 24) account for half of the 20 million new sexually transmitted infections in the United States. Among young people (aged 13 to 24) diagnosed with HIV in 2015, 81% were gay and bisexual males (USDHHS/CDC, 2016). Accurate measures of STIs in this population are difficult to obtain because many affected people have few, if any, identifiable symptoms and others delay seeking treatment. Provisions in the Affordable Care Act of 2010 extended the coverage for dependent children, allowing dependent children to remain on their parents' insurance plans until the child reached 26 years of age (CDC, 2017a). Additional provisions in the Act promote clinical preventative services by requiring that insurance plans cover key preventative services, which include some screening and testing services for STDs, without charging a deductible or co-pay (Fox & Shaw, 2015). One aim of these provisions was to assure access to preventative and treatment STD services for adolescents and young adults, however the CDC (2017a) reported that 22.6% of survey respondents aged 15 to 17 and 8.2% aged 20 to 22 who were on their parents' private insurance would not access these services due to questions about confidentiality and the possibility of their parents finding out about their sexual health. Additional information can be found in Chapter 3.

Practice Point

Making HIV testing a routine part of healthcare for adolescents and adults 13 to 64 years of age is one of the most important strategies recommended by the CDC for reducing the spread of HIV (CDC, 2017b).

School Relevance

The school nurse's role as a case finder is extremely important because the nurse is in a good position to provide the necessary counseling and referral for STI treatment. However, school health personnel should know that symptomatic adolescents who are suspected of having an STI cannot be excluded from school. In addition, health personnel should also be aware that federal law stipulates that adolescents can go directly to a health department–operated STI clinic for diagnosis and treatment of their disease without parental consent. In some cases where communication with parents does not occur, the student may choose not to seek treatment for what could ultimately result in long-term consequences of the infection. If this is the case, school health personnel should preserve the student's privacy while assisting the student with contacting the health department and arranging for necessary diagnosis and treatment. Finally, health professionals should assist in the identification of all sexual contacts involved so they can be warned and treated. In many cases, it may be easier to locate and speak with these students at school (Borawski, Tufts, Trapl, Hayman, Yoder, & Lovegreen, 2015).

Practice Point

It is rare for a person to contract an STI without some form of sexual contact. Although as many as 50% of teens are sexually active by the end of high school, not all are engaging in heterosexual contact. Students should be aware that sexual contact may involve mouth-to-genital contact, either homosexual or heterosexual.

Nutrition

Epidemiology

Obesity in children and adolescents is a serious health concern. From 1999 to 2015, there was a significant increase in the prevalence of obesity (with rates ranging from 10.6% to 13.9%). Trends indicate that an estimated one in five children and adolescents aged 2 to 19 are obese (Ogden et al., 2016). Children and adolescents (2 to 19 years) are considered overweight with a BMI) between ≥85th and <95th percentile, and obese with a BMI ≥95th percentile. This is largely a result of overeating and insufficient exercise, which lead to an energy imbalance. Obese children and adolescents are at risk for many of the health problems currently seen in adults. They are more likely to have conditions such as high blood pressure, high cholesterol, and type 2 diabetes that are risk factors for cardiovascular disease (CDC, 2016b). In addition, children and adolescents who are obese are more likely to remain obese as adults. Although in recent years the obesity epidemic in children and adolescents appears to be stabilizing, it remains at an unacceptably high level.

Continued obesity in children may result in an epidemic of cardiovascular disease and type 2 diabetes in the adolescent population. Cardiovascular disease is already the fifth leading cause of preventable death among adolescents, and there has been a marked increase in insulin resistance and type 2 diabetes. The National Health Objectives of *Healthy People 2020* address cardiovascular disease prevention in adolescents by focusing on physical inactivity and obesity. The 2015 YRBSS report indicates that 48.6% of children in the United States engage in exercise that results in sweating or hard breathing for the recommended 60 minutes per day, five or more days per week and 27.1% on all seven days (CDC, 2016b). Exercise can be linked to both physical and emotional well-being by decreasing cardiovascular risk factors, reducing feelings of depression and anxiety, and stimulating an overall improvement in psychological health and academic functioning.

> This might be the first generation where kids are dying at a younger age than their parents and it's related primarily to the obesity problem. **Judy Davis, Australian actress**

Adolescents, both in school and out, have wide access to foods with low nutritional value and high levels of fat and calories through vending machines, à la carte lunches, and snack bars. Although the USDA school-based nutrition programs have played a key role in contributing to improvement in overall health indicators in adolescents, there is no legislation banning foods sold outside of the cafeteria. The food environment in schools often serves to reinforce poor eating habits. Schools are the primary setting for engaging children in the establishment of lifelong positive behaviors. However, the matter of food choices should also be addressed using broad-based environmental and public health policy approaches.

Best Practices: Nutrition

In the Child Nutrition and WIC Reauthorization Act of 2004, the U.S. Congress established a requirement that all school districts with a federally funded school meals program develop and implement wellness policies that address nutrition and physical activity by the start of the 2006 to 2007 school year (Section 204). The CDC has established a self-assessment and planning tool (School Health Index) and guidelines that can be used in school health programs in an effort to improve the food environments of school-aged children and adolescents. These current CDC guidelines

focus on changing the social norms and environments of adolescents. In addition to school-based prevention, the guidelines recommend policy and regulatory strategies, community participation, establishment of public and private partnerships, strategic use of media, development of local programs, coordination of statewide and local activities, linkage of school-based activities to community activities, and use of data collection and evaluation techniques, such as the School Health Index (described previously) to monitor program impact.

Practice Point

An extension of the CDC website gives access to the School Health Index at no cost to the school. Based on the results of the assessment, a school can strengthen existing school health programs. For example, a school may choose to implement *CDC Guidelines to Promote Lifelong Healthy Eating*, which identify strategies most likely to be effective in promoting lifelong healthy eating among young people. Alternatively, it may choose to implement *CDC Guidelines to Promote Lifelong Physical Activity*, which identify strategies most likely to be effective in helping young people adopt and maintain a physically active lifestyle.

Joe, who is 10 years old, is in the fifth grade in the school where Susan works. When he was 8, he was diagnosed with ADHD. Joe also has a severe peanut allergy and must avoid any contact with peanuts and peanut-containing products. Using yearly height and weight screenings, Susan has found that Joe's body mass index is in the 99th percentile, which indicates obesity. Using the nine CDC guidelines, synthesized research, and best practices related to promoting healthy eating and physical activity in schools, identify Joe's needs and plan interventions to address each of these nutritional issues (https://www.cdc.gov/healthyschools/npao/pdf/mmwr-school-health-guidelines.pdf.).

Student Reflection

During my clinical rotation in community health, I encountered several high school students struggling with eating disorders, a common problem in this age group. One particular case that I found interesting involved a senior boy on the wrestling team who came to the health office because he was not feeling well. He complained of being tired and feeling worn out; he said that he just felt like he needed to go home and rest. After calling his mother, he transferred the call to the nurse. The nurse explained to his mother that her son was not feeling well and asked whether he could be dismissed. The mother stated, "I know what is wrong with him. The wrestling coach told him to only drink water for the past two days because of the match tomorrow. That's why he is not feeling well." The mother said that she was very concerned about this practice. However, she did not want to make a big deal out of the situation because she did not want the coach to bully her son, who loves wrestling. She agreed to let her son come home. However, I couldn't help but think of this boy, who was putting wrestling ahead of eating; he was at risk for an eating disorder.

This is a disturbing situation. However, no matter how much education is provided to students, I do not think the situation will change unless the teachers and coaches are involved and see the necessity of promoting healthy eating.

Violence

I have a theory because I was being beaten up a lot by people outside of school; it was almost like if I could make myself sick enough they'd take sympathy on me. **Daniel Johns, Australian musician**

Violence was declared a public health emergency in 1985, and since then, violence prevention has been a national health promotion objective. However, the incidence of youth violence remains higher in the United States than in most developed countries. The YRBSS (USDHHS/CDC, 2016) measures a number of behaviors that contribute to violence including carrying a weapon (e.g., gun, knife, or club) (16.2%), carrying a gun (5.3%), physical fighting (22.6.8%), and carrying a weapon on school property (4.1%). YRBSS also measures intimate partner violence including dating violence. Of students who reported dating, 10.6% had been forced to do unwanted sexual things. Another type of violence among children and adolescents is bullying; 20.1% of students had been bullied on school property, and 15.5% reported experiencing **electronic bullying**, defined as bullying through e-mail, chat rooms, instant messaging, websites, or texting. These numbers have remained relatively stable over time. Although the news media has recently devoted much attention to the potential dangers of technology, face-to-face verbal and physical aggression is more common than electronic bullying. The most dramatic result of bullying is suicide; 8.6% of adolescents have attempted suicide.

The tongue like a sharp knife...kills without drawing blood. **Buddha**

In response to an increased awareness to bullying—specifically defined as unwanted, aggressive behavior

---

| **22.5** | **Bullying Prevention** |

Assess bullying.
Engage parents and youth.
Set policies and rules.
Build a safe environment.
Educate about bullying.

Source: https://www.stopbullying.gov/prevention/at-school/index.html.

among school-aged children that involves a real or perceived power imbalance—numerous prevention and intervention programs have been implemented that have now made children and adolescents safer in school than anywhere else. The school nurse should be aware that students who are bullied at school are likely to feel disconnected or dislike school. They have lower academic success and school attendance records. Box 22.5 lists elements of successful bullying prevention efforts.

The many new technologies available have positively impacted students' education; however, concerns have been raised by educators and parents about the potential dangers that also exist through inappropriate use of the technologies. In an attempt to prevent unsafe and inappropriate use of these technologies, an increasing number of school systems are developing policies that address these concerns, specifically limiting the use of cell phones by students while in school, and controlling access to websites on school computers (Hertz & David-Ferdon, 2008). The CDC has published a brief for educators and caregivers to address the issue of electronic media and youth violence. Suggestions for educators, policymakers, caregivers, and parents to address electronic bullying are summarized in Boxes 22.6 and 22.7.

Evidence for Practice

A recent study by Foshee and colleagues (2013), examined the negative consequences of dating violence among adolescents. The study measured the consequences of both physical (including hitting, slapping or being hit) and psychological victimization (hurting feelings, saying insulting things, controlling behaviors). The researchers found that the consequences varied by type of violence and by gender. Victims of physical violence were more likely to smoke cigarettes, girls were more likely to use marijuana, and boys were more likely to have close friends. Victims of psychological violence increase the probability of alcohol use and internalizing the symptoms of this violence. The results of the study confirm that dating violence has detrimental consequences and that identification of both physical and psychological violence is important to implement evidence-based prevention strategies.

22.6 Electronic Media and Youth Violence

- **Explore current bullying prevention policies and work collaboratively to develop new policies.** States, school districts, and boards of education must work in conjunction with attorneys to develop policies that protect the rights of all students and also meet the needs of the state or district and those it serves. In addition, it is also helpful to involve representatives from the student body, students, families, and community members in the development of the policy. The policy should also be based upon evidence from research and on best practices.
- **Explore current programs to prevent bullying and youth violence.** Many of the programs developed to prevent face-to-face aggression address topics such as school climate and peer influences that are likely to be important for prevention of electronic aggression.
- **Offer training on electronic aggression for educators and administrators.** The training should include the definition of electronic aggression, characteristics of victims and perpetrators, related school or district policies, information about recent incidents of electronic violence in the district, and resources available to educators and caregivers if they have concerns.
- **Talk to adolescents.** Providing young people opportunities to discuss their concerns through, for example, creative writing assignments is an excellent way to begin a classroom dialogue about using electronic media safely and about the impact and consequences of inappropriate use. Technology safety could easily be integrated into the standard health education curricula. Educators and researchers should explore with adolescents how electronic media can be used as tools to prevent electronic aggression and other adolescent health problems.
- **Work with information technology (IT) personnel and support staff.** Administrators must create the infrastructure and support necessary for classroom teachers to work with IT staff to keep abreast of issues affecting young people and develop strategies to minimize risk.
- **Create a positive school atmosphere.** Research indicates that students who feel connected to their school, who think their teachers care about them and are fair, and who think the school rules are clear and fair are less likely to perpetrate any type of violence or aggression, including electronic aggression.
- **Have an action plan in place to address incidents.** Be proactive in developing a thoughtful plan to address problems and concerns. Having a plan in place may make young people more likely to come forward with concerns and may support the appropriate handling of a situation when it arises. Create an atmosphere that encourages a dialogue between educators and young people and between families and young people about their electronic experiences.

Source: Hertz, M. F., & David-Ferdon, C. (2008). *Electronic media and youth violence: A CDC issue brief for educators and caregivers.* Atlanta, GA: Centers for Disease Control and Prevention.

22.7 Cyberbullying: Suggestions for Parents and Caregivers

1. **Talk to your child.** Just as you would ask children where they are going and whom they are going to be with whenever they leave the house, ask where they are going and whom they are with when they are on the internet. Talk with teens to come up with a solution to prevent or address victimization that does not punish the teen.
2. **Develop rules.** Together with your child, develop rules about acceptable and safe behavior for all the electronic media they use and what they should do if they become a victim of electronic aggression or they witness or know about another teen being victimized.
3. **Explore the internet.** Visit the websites your child frequents. Remember that young people can learn new information on the internet, interact with and learn about people from diverse backgrounds, and express themselves to others who may have similar thoughts and experiences. Technology is not going away, so forbidding young people to access electronic media may not be a good long-term solution. Together, parents and youth can come up with ways to maximize the benefits of technology and decrease its risks.
4. **Talk with other parents and/or caregivers.** Discuss strategies that are effective as well as those that do not work.
5. **Encourage your school or school district to conduct a class for caregivers about electronic aggression.** Review school or district policies on the topic, recent incidents in the community, and resources available to caregivers who have concerns.
6. **Keep current.** Keep current on what new devices and features your child is using. You need to know "where they are going" and explore these websites yourself. Ask your teenager to educate you. This may help strengthen parent–child communication and bonding, which is important for other adolescent health issues as well.

Source: Hertz, M. F., & David-Ferdon, C. (2008). *Electronic media and youth violence: A CDC issue brief for educators and caregivers.* Atlanta, GA: Centers for Disease Control and Prevention.

Practice Point

Ineffective programs are characterized by assumptions about the cause-and-effect relationships that result in violence in schools. For example, there is an assumption that exposure to media violence causes violence. In fact, the problem of youth violence extends beyond the exposure to media into the social context of youth. School health programs must work instead to construct a culture of nonviolence.

 Susan has become aware that some of the children have been making fun of Joe because of his daily visits to the nurse's office. Joe confides in her that children sometimes pick on him because he takes medicine and cannot eat peanuts. Today, a student pushed a peanut butter sandwich into his face and laughed when he got upset. Identify specific interventions that should be taken to stop this bullying.

Student Reflection

During my clinical rotation in community health, I assisted a school nurse at an elementary school. I worked with many emotionally distressed students in need of emotional support. Often, they were homesick, frustrated with an assignment, or just needed time away from the stress of the classroom. I listened to the children's worries, offered advice on how to cope with their sadness, and called their parents if necessary. However, everything I had been taught and all the experience I had could not have prepared me for a visit I received.

A teacher entered the nurse's office, looking rather disturbed, and asked to speak to myself and my teacher (the school nurse) in a separate room. The teacher said that a student, very upset, had told the teacher that her father hits her and that she is too scared to go home because he might hit her again. The teacher calmed the student down, telling her that she would be protected. The nurse called the social worker, and everyone met to decide the best action to take to protect this child.

First, the nurse called the Department of Children and Families (DCF) so it could file a report. The DCF said that because its staff believed that the current situation could be one where it was unsafe for the student to return home, a representative was going to come to the school. The DCF requested that the nurse call the student to the office and that the child was to be inspected for any signs of physical abuse.

It was very difficult for the teacher/nurse to have to ask the child, who trusts the nurse and had developed a relationship with the nurse, to take off her clothes so that we could observe for signs of abuse. During the examination, the student was tearful; however, it appeared that she trusted us and she provided more information about the potential abuse. She said "he hits me but I hate when I see the blood coming from there (her bottom)." This made me very concerned, since it was unclear whether she was talking about blood from where she got hit on the bottom, or if there was some kind of sexual abuse involved. We did not see any signs of physical abuse.

The DCF wanted information about both her and her brother, including their friends, their demeanor in the nurse's office, medical record information, and the nurses' interactions with the parents of the children. I was not able to be very helpful, since I had not had a lot of interactions with the children, but my teacher had a wealth of information. She was able to look back at her electronic log and see that the boy had visited the nurse's office on five occasions, tearfully seeking emotional support. The nurse also said that the father was "difficult to deal with," and on one occasion left a message threatening to call the nurse's boss because the nurse was requesting records that the children had received a physical examination.

During the next 10-day period, the DCF investigators visited the children's home, talked with both the children and parents, and decided not to open the case. I had a lot of different feelings and mixed emotions during this time, and this case helped shape my philosophy and value system regarding community and public health nursing. First, I was horrified. I wanted the father to be locked up immediately and the children to be protected. However, soon I realized there were DCF procedures and nursing procedures that had to be followed. Having to check the child for hit marks really upset me. I thought that it was unfair that the nurse had to break this child's trust, which might affect the student's willingness to come to the nurse's office in the future. However, we worked hard to make the examination as painless as possible.

THE SCHOOL NURSE AS A CHILD ADVOCATE

Advocacy plays a central role in school health personnel's responsibility for the overall physical and emotional well-being of the children and adolescents they serve. Advocacy involves both teaching children and empowering others who care for the children to ensure quality care. Key components of the advocacy role include collaboration and policy-making. School nurses often spend more time with specific students than any other adult during the school day (Alexandropoulou, 2013). The advocacy role emerges from this caregiving process.

As an advocate, the school nurse needs to find a balance between empowering parents and others external to the school to pursue healthcare for the child. The child with a chronic health condition presents a unique challenge for nurses as advocates. The nurse must often mediate between educators, parents, and physicians to ensure children with chronic health conditions can function to their maximum potential. As many as 10% to 15% of children in schools are affected with chronic conditions, such as asthma, diabetes, and seizure disorders, that require daily treatment (USDHHS, National Heart, Lung, and Blood Institute, 2013). The nurse as advocate has two important roles: spreading knowledge and networking. Spreading knowledge does not ensure health, but a person's sense of being able to control his or her own healthcare does promote healthy behaviors. This sense of control comes from the provision of adequate resources. Networking is also important. Working together, the school nurse, parents, teachers, and healthcare providers can ensure that the child with special healthcare needs has access to all educational resources and opportunities. Knowledge of federal laws, including the **Americans with Disabilities Act (ADA)**, IDEA, Section 504, Family Educational Rights and Privacy Act of 1974 (FERPA), and **Food Allergy and Anaphylaxis Management Act (FAAMA)** is essential (see definitions at the beginning of the chapter). The school nurse who has identified a pupil in the school who has special healthcare needs, working within the constructs of the Framework for 21st Century School Nursing Practice (NASN, 2016), plays an important role by coordinating the interests of families, education, healthcare systems, public health, insurance, and community agencies. A meeting arranged to provide health accommodations—a 504 plan, IEP, or other school plan—has the potential to improve the long-term outcomes for the child. Children may represent themselves in these meetings if appropriate, but at a minimum should have representation by the family, school health staff, special education coordinator, and any person trained to assist the student or who has primary responsibility for the student. As an advocate, the school health staff should (USDHHS, National Heart, Lung, and Blood Institute, 2013) do the following:

- Provide education and communication necessary to ensure that the student's health and educational needs are met.
- Implement strategies to reduce disruptions in the student's school activities.
- Communicate with families and healthcare providers as authorized.
- Ensure the student receives prescribed medications and treatments and that staff who interact with the student on a regular basis are knowledgeable about these needs.
- Provide a safe and healthy school environment to promote learning.

Today, in addition to her routine activities, Susan is participating in a transition planning meeting about Joe. He will be going to middle school next year, and his parents have asked for a transition planning meeting. For his ADHD, he currently takes 20 mg of Ritalin in the morning before school and 10 mg at lunch time. His severe peanut allergy requires that an EpiPen be kept in the nurse's office. His 504 plan, which was developed when he was diagnosed, allows Joe to take his medication midday, provides for a peanut-free lunch environment, and suggests that Joe's desk be positioned in such a way that distractions are limited.

- Who should be included in the planning meeting?

- What topics should be discussed? Prepare an anaphylaxis algorithm for Joe.
- What are Susan's responsibilities regarding this transition meeting?

Joe's parents are hoping that he can stop taking his medication. Lately, Susan has had to send a messenger to remind him to take it. She knows that Joe's transition into middle school will be important in the development of his self-esteem. A strong sense of self-esteem will be a protective factor against engaging in health risk behaviors in middle school. What recommendations can Susan make that would help resolve this situation?

Practice Point

With the attention and scrutiny given to personal health information in all settings, and as a result of federal legislation, it is imperative for school nurses to revisit policies and procedures for protecting the privacy of student and family health information.

THE FUTURE OF SCHOOL HEALTH: WHOLE SCHOOL, WHOLE COMMUNITY, WHOLE CHILD (WSCC) MODEL

For each of the common health problems discussed in this chapter, it should be made clear that a single focused approach to prevention based only on education, that is, one that is approached only by teaching, has a minimal effect. The National Association of School Nurses has endorsed the provision of comprehensive school health services, called the Whole School, Whole Community, Whole Child model, as one possible solution (https://www.cdc.gov/healthyyouth/wscc/index.htm). This model serves as a blueprint for policy and practice for the 21st century school nurse. The collaborative design uses the resources of a community (including health educators, counseling, psychological services, nutrition, the environment, and the family) to provide support services and to promote changes throughout the school environment to improve the health and well-being of students. Nurses have long been aware of the importance of practicing within context to implement and sustain change. As a result of the groundbreaking findings from the National Longitudinal Study of Adolescent Health, school connectedness has become a key focus point in the provision of primary healthcare (CDC, 2009). Research has identified the importance of the link between schools and community within a prevention framework. Community-driven programs that encourage key stakeholders, including students, to set the agenda and create solutions are more likely to create a supportive environment for engaging in health-promoting behaviors.

In the political sphere of the provision of quality public education, schools have been challenged to rethink and redesign efforts to educate children. These reforms will undoubtedly continue to challenge the school nurse. The success of any education program must be linked to the social environment. School nurses have the expertise in assessment, education, and advocacy necessary to play a major role in meeting the needs of children and adolescents to ensure academic success.

KEY CONCEPTS

- Since the passage of PL 94-142 in 1975, school nurses provide more complex care for conditions such as seizure disorders, asthma, cardiac conditions, cystic fibrosis, quadriplegia, and life-threatening allergies while facing new and emerging trends in the management of behavioral health issues.
- The role that emerges within the context of this management position requires the nurse to have skills in health assessment, health promotion, skills as a health educator, and the ability to work as a child health advocate.
- Data from the Youth Risk Behavior Surveillance Survey (YRBSS), a biannual report of the common risk behaviors influencing the health of our nation's youth, can be used by the school nurse as a tool for monitoring trends both locally and nationally.
- There are online clearinghouses of school-based, evidence-based programs for the prevention of common health risk behaviors.
- School nurses play a key advocacy role that includes collaboration and policy-making, often participating in school district wellness committees.
- The future of school nursing is providing a prevention framework that links the community and the school.

CRITICAL THINKING QUESTIONS

The school nurse has a unique role in the provision of school health services for children with special health needs, including children with chronic illnesses and disabilities with various degrees of severity. This case describes the role of the school nurse caring for a child with type 1 diabetes.

Susan has two students with type 1 diabetes in her school, one requires blood glucose monitoring and daily insulin injections, while the other has a continuous insulin infusion pump. The incidence of type 1 diabetes presents a complex challenge to school healthcare providers. Type 1 diabetes ranks as the second most common chronic illness in childhood, second only to asthma. The American Diabetes Association (ADA, 2015) reports that about 193,000 Americans under age 20 live with diabetes and 17,900 are diagnosed with type 1 diabetes annually, and another 5,300 with type 2 diabetes. Children with diabetes are considered disabled and as such are protected under federal laws that prohibit discrimination against children with disabilities. Studies show that the majority of school personnel have an inadequate understanding of effective diabetes management. It is best for the student to monitor blood glucose and respond to the results as quickly as possible to avoid possible complications.

- What are the essential elements of a diabetes medical management plan for each student with diabetes in the school?
- When the school nurse is unavailable, who is legally responsible for providing care to a child with diabetes?
- What expectations should the school nurse have of the students in diabetes care?

COMMUNITY RESOURCES

- Local and county public health departments
- State and local police departments
- Local community centers
- Town parks and recreation departments
- Primary care physicians
- Advanced nurse practitioners
- YMCA and YWCA programs
- Local amusement centers

REFERENCES

Alexandropoulou, M. (2013). The health promoting school and the school nurse: A content analysis of school staff's views. *British Journal of School Nursing, 8*(3), 134–141.

American Academy of Pediatrics Council on School Health. (2016). Role of the school nurse in providing school health services. *Pediatrics, 137*(6), 1–7 e20160852.

American Diabetes Association. (2015). Retrieved from http://www.diabetes.org/

American Nurses Association & National Association of School Nurses. (2017). *School nursing: Scope and standards of practice* (3rd ed.). Silver Spring, MD: Nursesbooks.org.

ASCD & CDC. (2014). *Whole school, whole community, whole child*. Retrieved from http://www.ascd.org/ASCD/pdf/siteASCD/publications/wholechild/wscc-a-collaborative-approach.pdf

Avery, G., Johnson, T., Cousins, M., & Hamilton, B. (2013). The school wellness nurse: A model for bridging gaps in school wellness programs. *Pediatric Nursing, 39*(1), 13–17.

Borawski, E. A., Tufts, K. A., Trapl, E. S., Hayman, L. L., Yoder, L. D., & Lovegreen, L. D. (2015). Effectiveness of health education teachers and school nurses teaching sexually transmitted infections/human immunodeficiency virus prevention knowledge and skills in high school. *The Journal of School Health, 85*(3), 189–196. Retrieved from http://doi.org/10.1111/josh.12234

Bunnell, R. E., Agaku, I. T., Arrazola, R. A., Apelberg, B. J., Caraballo, R. S., Corey, C. G., … King, B. A. (2015). Intentions to smoke cigarettes among never-smoking US middle and high school electronic cigarette users: National Youth Tobacco Survey, 2011–2013. *Nicotine & Tobacco Research, 17*(2), 228–235.

Centers for Disease Control and Prevention. (2009). *School connectedness: Strategies for increasing protective factors among youth*. Atlanta, GA: U.S. Department of Health and Human Services.

Centers for Disease Control and Prevention. (2012). Births: Final data for 2010. *National Vital Statistics Report, 61*(1). Retrieved from http://www.cdc.gov/nchs/data/nvsr/nvsr61/nvsr61_01.pdf

Centers for Disease Control and Prevention. (2016a). *Continued declines in teen births in the United States, 2015*. Retrieved from https://www.cdc.gov/nchs/products/databriefs/db259.htm

Centers for Disease Control and Prevention. (2016b). *Childhood overweight and obesity*. Retrieved from https://www.cdc.gov/obesity/childhood/

Centers for Disease Control and Prevention. (2017a). Confidentiality issues and use of STD services among sexually experienced persons aged 15–25 years. *Morbidity and Mortality Weekly Report, 66*(9), 237–241.

Centers for Disease Control and Prevention. (2017b). *HIV/AIDS*. Retrieved from https://www.cdc.gov/hiv/basics/prevention.html

Centers for Disease Control and Prevention. (n.d.). *The school health index (SHI): Self-assessment & planning guide 2014*. Retrieved from http://www.cdc.gov/healthyyouth/shi/

Doyle, J. (2013). Emergency management, crisis response, and the school nurse's role. In J. Selekman (ed.). *School nursing: A comprehensive text* (2nd ed, pp.1216–1244). Philadelphia, PA: F.A. Davis Company.

Ethier, K. A., Dittus, P. J., DeRoas, C. J., Chung, E. Q., Martinez, E., & Kerndt, P. R. (2011). School-based health center access, reproductive health care, and contraceptive use among sexually experienced high school students. *Journal of Adolescent Health, 48*(6), 562–565.

Foshee, V. A., Reyes, H. L., Gottfredson, N. C., Chang, L. Y., Ennett, S. T. (2013). A longitudinal examination of psychological, behavioral, academic, and relationship consequences of dating abuse victimization among a primarily rural sample of adolescents. *Journal of Adolescent Health, 53*(6):723–729.

Fox, J. B., & Shaw, F. E. (2015). Clinical preventative coverage and the affordable care act. *American Journal of Public Health, 105*(1), e7–e10.

Ham, P. & Allen, C. (2012). Adolescent health screening and counseling. *American Family Physician, 86*(12), 109–116.

Health Resources and Services Administration. (2010). *The registered nurse population*. Retrieved from http://bhpr.hrsa.gov/healthworkforce/rnsurveys/rnsurveyinitial2008.pdf

Hertz, M. F., & David-Ferdon, C. (2008). *Electronic media and youth violence: A CDC issue brief for educators and caregivers*. Atlanta, GA: Centers for Disease Control and Prevention. Retrieved from http://www.cdc.gov/ViolencePrevention/youthviolence/electronic-aggression/index.html

Lewallen, T. C., Hunt, H., Potts-Datema, W., Zaza, S., & Giles, W. (2015), The whole school, whole community, whole child model: A new approach for improving educational attainment and healthy development for students. *The Journal of School Health, 85*(11), 729–739.

Mangena, A. S., & Maughan, E. (2015). The 2015 NASN School Nurse Survey: developing and providing leadership to advance school nursing practice. *NASN School Nurse, 30*(6), 328–335.

Manlove, J., Fish, H., & Moore, K. A. (2015). Programs to improve adolescent sexual and reproductive health in the US: A review of evidence. *Adolescent Health, Medicine and Therapeutics, 6*, 47–79.

National Association of School Nurses (NASN). (2016). Framework for 21st Century Nursing Practice. *NASN School Nurse*, 45–53. doi: 10.1177/1942602X15618644

NASN. (2017). *Definition of school nursing*. Retrieved from https://www.nasn.org/nasn/about-nasn/about

NREPP. (n.d.). *NREPP implementation strategies*. Retrieved from https://nrepp.samhsa.gov

Ogden, C. L., Carroll, M. D., Lawman, H. G., Fryar, C. D., Kruszon-Moran, D., Kit, B. K., & Flegal, K. M. (2016). Trends in Obesity Prevalence Among Children and Adolescents in the United States, 1988–1994 Through 2013–2014. *JAMA, 315*(21), 2292–2299.

Robert Wood Johnson Foundation. (2010). *Unlocking the potential of school nursing: Keeping children healthy, in school, and ready to learn*. Retrieved from http://www.rwjf.org/files/research/cnf 14.pdf

Rollins, J A. (2011). Every child deserves a school nurse. *Pediatric Nursing, 37*(5), 225–226.

SIECUS (Sexuality Information and Education Council of the United States). (n.d.). *Evidence-based and more comprehensive approaches to pregnancy-HIV/STD-prevention and sexuality education*. Retrieved from http://www.siecus.org/indexcfm?fuseaction=page.viewPage&pageID=1342&nodeID=1

Singh, R., Jimerson, S., & Renshaw, T. (2011). A summary and synthesis of contemporary empirical evidence regarding the effects of the Drug Abuse Resistance Education Program (D.A.R.E.). *Contemporary School Psychology, 15*, 93–102.

SOPHE (Society for Public Health Education). (2018) *School health*. Retrieved from https://www.sophe.org/focus-areas/school-health/

Substance Abuse and Mental Health Services Administration (SAMHSA). (2017). *Key substance use and mental health indicators in the United States: Results from the 2016 National Survey on Drug Use and Health (HHS Publication No. SMA 17–5044, NSDUH Series H-52)*. Rockville, MD: Center for Behavioral Health Statistics and Quality, Substance Abuse and Mental Health Services Administration. Retrieved from https://www.samhsa.gov/data/

REFERENCES *(Continued)*

U.S. Department of Education. (n.d.). IDEA: Individuals with Disabilities Education Act. Retrieved from https://sites.ed.gov/idea/

U.S. Department of Health and Human Services. *Healthy People 2020*. (2018) Retrieved from http://healthypeople.gov/2020/topicsobjectives2020/objectiveslist.aspx?topicId=11

U.S. Department of Health and Human Services, National Heart, Lung, and Blood Institute. (2013). *Health information for the public*. Retrieved from http://www.nhlbi.nih.gov/health

U.S. Department of Health and Human Services, Office of the Surgeon General. (2016) *E-cigarette use among youth and young adults: A report of the Surgeon General*. Retrieved from

https://e-cigarettes.surgeongeneral.gov/documents/2016_sgr_full_report_non-508.pdf

U.S. Department of Health and Human Services/Centers for Disease Control and Prevention (USDHHS/CDC). (2016). Youth risk behavior surveillance—United States, 2015. *Morbidity and Mortality Weekly Report, 65*(6), 1–174.

Vessey, J. A., & McGowan, K. A. (2006). A successful public health experiment: School nursing. *Pediatric Nursing, 32*(3), 255–257.

Wall Street Journal. (2012). *School nurses' new role in children's health*. Retrieved from http://online.wsj.com/article/SB10000872396390444358804578016221407143166.html

WEB RESOURCES

Please visit thePoint® for up-to-date web resources on this topic.

Chapter 23

Faith-Oriented Communities and Health Ministries in Faith Communities

Susan K. Chase

Faith is taking the first step even when you don't see the whole staircase.
Martin Luther King Jr.

Fear knocked at the door. Faith answered. No one was there.
Author unknown

CIRCLES

We are circles, in circles

Brushing and touching

Reaching and breaching

Our narrow confines

Giving and needing

Following, leading

Calling and heeding

Reciting our lines

—Anonymous

CHAPTER HIGHLIGHTS

- Faith communities as centers for community health
- Cultural and developmental features of faith community work
- Integration of body, mind, and spirit in whole-person health
- Health promotion in faith communities

OBJECTIVES

- Differentiate faith community nursing from community health nursing.
- Describe various models of faith community nursing practice.
- Explain scope and standards of faith community nursing practice.
- Give examples of community assessments and interventions used by faith community nurses.

KEY TERMS

Congregation: An organized group of people who share religious beliefs, customs, or practices. The congregation has an internal governance structure and may be independent or affiliated to local or national denominations. It is a community within the larger community.

Congregation-based model: A faith community nurse serving a particular faith community by virtue of a contract or job description; supports the concept of a faith community nurse who can be paid or serve as a volunteer.

Faith community nursing: A specialty practice of nursing having registered nurses contribute to the health and wholeness of people in the context of a faith community. The faith community nurse is part of the ministry staff of the congregation and serves the illness needs of individual people, families, and the entire faith community. This

KEY TERMS *(continued)*

broader term is the preferred term, and is used in settings in which the word "parish" may have no meaning or association, but many original documents used "parish nursing" as the title for the role.

Institution-based model: The faith community nurse serves a health system with assignment to particular congregational settings. In this model, the parish or faith community nurse serves as liaison and helps plan and coordinate care, particularly at times of transition.

Parish nursing: Equivalent to faith community nursing; it was the original term describing the practice.

Spiritual care: Care of the human spirit that may include dealing with the meaning of health, illness or loss, relationships with God and others, and which has the goal of peace.

CASE STUDY

References to the case study are found throughout this chapter (look for the case study icon). Readers should keep the case study in mind as they read the chapter.

Mary is the faith community nurse in a medium-sized suburban congregation. She conducted a monthly blood pressure screening session between the two services on Sunday morning. Matilda Swenson, a 76-year-old Swedish immigrant, who is active in the church despite the fact that she does not drive, has Mary check her blood pressure every month. The readings and notes for the past several months are shown below:

Medications: Advil for arthritis; no known drug allergies

Primary MD: Dexter Smith

June: 154/92 mm Hg; instructed patient to call her physician and notify him of the reading; gave pt a copy of her readings

July: 148/88 mm Hg; asked whether pt had called her physician and she had not. Repeated importance of contacting MD. Pt reported that she only went to rheumatologist for arthritis and they never checked her BP. Instructed pt to reconnect with primary care MD and report BP readings

September 2 (Labor Day weekend): 184/98 mm Hg; asked whether Mary could contact MD with pt present. Pt agreed. Drove pt home and called on-call service for advice. Learned that primary care physician had left the service but that the covering MD was available. Discussed with MD whether to go to the ER, but MD tells Mary to have pt call first thing Tuesday AM for an appointment. Called a friend of pt who was a member of the congregation who agreed to drive pt to MD Tuesday AM. Reported plan to clergy to support follow-up

September 4: Called to follow up on appointment. Learned that MD had switched pt from Advil to Tylenol for her arthritis pain and started her on atenolol for BP management. Planned to call in 3 days to check on pain level and medication compliance

October: 134/78 mm Hg. Reviewed mild exercise and low-salt diet; reinforced following medication plan. Pain control acceptable

Mrs. Swenson had been most bothered by her arthritis pain and had not found a new primary care physician when her previous physician left the practice. Her hypertension was causing her no symptoms, and arranging appointments was difficult. By assisting her in activating appropriate care, Mary helped Mrs. Swenson control her hypertension. Medications (nonsteroidal antiinflammatory drugs), smoking, or alcohol consumption sometimes exacerbates elevated blood pressure. At least in part, because of Mary's efforts, Mrs. Swenson has felt better cared for by her new healthcare team, and her new treatment plan helps to increase her comfort and function and to reduce her health risks.

Mary records the number of home and hospital visits that she makes and keeps track of services used for referrals. She also keeps track of how many seniors in the congregation are able to maintain independent living with her support. She compiles an annual report showing who had access to health ministry in the year, including the numbers of people who belong, and who do not belong, to the congregation. Some health-related programs are open to the community, which is seen as an outreach for the congregation. Documenting participation by both members and nonmembers of the congregation is important in sustaining support for faith community nursing programs.

NURSING IN FAITH COMMUNITIES

Faith community nursing is a specialty practice of nursing that sees the faith community as a source of health, healing, and wholeness, and that sees the entire community as the recipient of care. Faith community or parish nurses have specialized education in spiritual care and health promotion in working in the faith community setting. They see the faith community as the focus and context of care, and their work has a goal of providing health promotion, health screening, and health teaching as well as caring for individuals, families, and groups associated with the congregation. The faith community nurse does not replace activities that a community health or visiting nurse service would provide. There are no direct care activities such as dressing changes or injections regularly performed. The faith community nurse considers the needs of congregation members and makes referrals and advocates for quality care for congregation members. Additionally, the faith community provides a context that promotes the values, beliefs, and cultural practices of a community to support and enhance the experience of health as well as faith. In addition to providing health promotion activities, the faith community nurse provides guidance to members of the faith community as they act out their faith and provide care to other members of the community. In this way, the faith community nurse supports the ministry of the faith community itself. Nursing in faith communities combines the worlds of ministry and community nursing. The faith community nurse meets the needs of a particular community—the faith community. This chapter will focus on the activities of faith community nurses as providers and supporters of health in the particular community organized around a faith stance.

> Faith consists in believing when it is beyond the power of reason to believe. **Voltaire**

For community nurses, health is not the mere absence of disease. The faith community nurse "focuses on the intentional care of the spirit, as well as on the promotion of holistic health, and prevention or minimization of illness within the context of a faith community" (American Nurses Association [ANA], 2012, p. 5). Faith community nurses also establish programs that support health promotion for individual people and groups in the congregation.

> ### Practice Point
>
> When a faith community member is diagnosed with a new chronic illness such as diabetes, consider the mental and spiritual issues that might be raised as the entire family deals with the new diagnosis. Assess the family for signs of stress and help them work through what the diagnosis means to them spiritually.

HISTORY OF FAITH COMMUNITY NURSING

Faith community nursing is a fairly recent concept; however, in ancient times, families and religious communities served as a primary source of health and illness care. Religious groups and monasteries established the first hospitals that were designed to provide "hospitality." Religious orders of both men and women delivered healthcare to the poor as they acted out their faith. For the individual person, the faith tradition provides the basis for many health beliefs and practices. Understanding a person's religious and spiritual background is important in establishing healthcare priorities. Linking to the history of the congregation provides access to resources such as denominational materials.

> Diseases of the soul are more dangerous and more numerous than those of the body. **Cicero**

Granger Westberg, a Lutheran minister and hospital chaplain, began "parish nursing" in the 1980s. He had been involved in grant-funded holistic health programming, hospital chaplaincy, and community outreach by the healthcare system. Pastor Westberg consistently used the term "wholistic" to emphasize the wholeness of person which faith community nursing exemplifies. He made the observation that all churches had a number of nurses as members and that these nurses formed an informal network of advice and support because congregation members looked to them as sources of advice and information.

The Lutheran General Hospital established an interfaith outreach program where nurses from several Chicago area congregations were paid in part by their congregations and in part by a grant to provide services in their congregations and to come together for regular training and support. This holistic care model was linked to the hospital through the chaplaincy program. The hospital saw the **parish nursing** program as a kind of outreach to the community. The role was new, so no organized curriculum existed. As part of a grant-funded program, the nurses met regularly and asked for help on issues that arose during their care, such as health counseling, grief and loss, health promotion, **spiritual care**, and leading prayer. The parish nurses were already competent nurses, but they needed additional training in community health concepts and principles. In addition, they needed more knowledge and skill in spiritual care because this was part of their role. Over the years, the congregations assumed more responsibility for the financial support of the nurses, who eventually received full support from the congregation.

MODELS OF FAITH COMMUNITY PRACTICE

Currently, faith community nurses work either on a volunteer basis or in paid positions. Some work in an individual congregation, and others are based in a healthcare system which has links to several congregations. In any case, the principles of parish or faith community nursing apply. Table 23.1 shows the variety of faith community nurse models (Solari-Twadell & McDermott, 1999).

In a paid **congregation-based model**, the nurse is hired by the faith community to provide faith community nursing services. There is a job description, a clear list of resources or advisors, and a plan for evaluation. The advantage of this model is that the congregation clearly commits to supporting the program, and the nurse is a named member of the

TABLE 23.1	Models of Faith Community Nursing Practice	
	Paid	**Unpaid**
Based in congregation	Paid and based in congregation	Volunteer and based in congregation
Based in health system	Paid and affiliated with health system	Volunteer and affiliated with health system

congregational staff. Potential problems can exist if the congregation staff members do not understand the role of the nurse. The role of the faith community nurse is different from that of (1) a chaplain who conducts hospital and home visits, in that the faith community nurse can help interpret and advocate for healthcare services, or (2) a visiting nurse service, in that the faith community nurse knows the members of the congregation over time and sees them in states of illness and health and in that the faith community nurse is not employed to do specific technical skills requiring medical orders that congregation members might need. Overall, the strength of this model is that the faith community nurse is committed for a set number of hours to develop the faith-based nursing program for the entire faith community.

The parish pays Mary to work 20 hours a week for the parish, and she has an office on the church property. She can conduct individual assessments and teaching in this space or use larger meeting rooms for educational programs.

In an unpaid congregation-based model, a faith community nurse volunteers his or her services in a congregational setting. Even though unpaid, this faith community nurse provides the same standard of care in the services as those provided by a paid nurse. Just as with the paid model, the congregation should have an advisory committee, with a job description and an evaluation method, so that the program can develop. The faith community nurse might need to ask for these things or develop them for the congregation. Even unpaid faith community nurses require a budget for supplies, resources, and continuing education. One disadvantage to having an unpaid faith community nurse is that this person may not be recognized as a member of the ministry team, and will probably have fewer hours to offer in service. One advantage is that the faith community nurse can limit how much time he or she offers, and can maintain other employment. This allows nurses who work in clinical or educational settings to offer their services to the congregation as both a professional volunteer activity and as a lay ministry. It also allows a congregation that cannot financially

support a faith community nursing program to receive some of its benefits.

Often, new programs are started using an unpaid, congregation-based model. After the benefit of the program is demonstrated, a paid model can be supported. Both paid and unpaid congregation-based models share a disadvantage. The nurse usually operates independently, with little assistance from other nurses, and there is little support for developing new approaches to care. Faith community nurses often form informal networks to offer such encouragement to independent faith community nurses and attend regional and national conferences for faith community nurses to learn and share ideas.

Practice Point

In an unpaid congregation-based model, the faith community nurse must be creative in securing resources to support the program. Obtaining small-grant funding can help, and making a case for an item in the parish budget can help obtain blood pressure equipment, including large-sized cuffs, health reference books, and teaching handouts for specific conditions.

In a paid **institution-based model**, a faith community nurse is employed by a health system, hospital, or community agency. The benefit to the agency is that the faith community nurse can serve as an ambassador and referral agent for the institution. For example, a religiously affiliated hospital can support the services of faith community nurses in key feeder congregations, so that clients discharged from the hospital have coordinated transition to the home congregation setting. Discharge coordination or "transitional care" can result in smoother transitions for patients and can reduce costs for the hospital system. The faith community nurse does not provide direct nursing care services, but supports the patient and family members in assuming self-care and in engaging the healthcare system appropriately. One advantage of this model is that the faith community nurse is connected to other healthcare providers for clinical and personal support. Reports and accountability for practice lie with the healthcare system. The faith community nurse who works within this model may not be considered by members of the congregation to be "one of their own" as much as with the congregation-based community model.

In an unpaid institution-based model, which is the least often used, some hospitals or care systems may support their nursing staff by allowing time off, sometimes with pay, as these nurses volunteer their time in congregation settings. This can be an advantage for the nurse who wants to have time to offer services to his or her own congregation, but also wants to maintain primary identification with a healthcare institution. This can be an advantage for the institution, since community nursing activities are consistent with its mission and it receives referrals, and patients discharged from the institution benefit from coordinated transitional care. Evidence indicates that there is need for follow-up care for older persons with diabetes. Transition care provided by a faith community nurse might have reduced the hospital readmission rates. Further research is needed to test such models.

Evidence for Practice

A research study followed 96 patients who were over the age of 65 after discharge from at least a 48-hour stay in a community hospital and who were diabetic but for whom diabetes was not the reason for the admission. Patients were in good glucose control when entering the hospital. Phone calls were made at 1 week and 1 month following discharge to assess transitional care issues. Both quantitative and qualitative data were collected. Multimorbidity was found in 75% of patients, most commonly from coronary artery disease, diabetic neuropathy, and chronic kidney disease. Diabetes-related complications were evident in 46% of respondents. Unplanned care events occurred for 41% of participants, most requiring unplanned provider visit and 21% requiring hospital readmission. "Results of this study suggest that home recovery transition of an older person with diabetes is dynamic, and transition outcomes are influenced by multiple persona and community transition conditions" (LaManna, Bushy, Norris, & Chase, 2016, p. 81).

Whatever the practice setting or the organizational structure of the faith community nurse, having a theoretic model for driving practice can help to organize both activities and reports. A model is useful when explaining a new practice to audiences such as congregation councils and members themselves. One model was developed by conducting a grounded theory analysis of case reports of faith community nurse network in a southern U.S. state. The analysis revealed a multistep model of practice: "(1) entering the private world, (2) connecting to faith, (3) mutually transforming experience, and (4) sustaining health" (Dyess & Chase, 2012, p. 224). Nurses reported that, at times, a task such as taking a blood pressure established a relationship of caring, and doing this simple task opened the door to deeper conversations. The encounter almost always had a faith component which included reflection or prayer. The experience transformed both patient and nurse in sharing their human experience in a faith context, and finally, health was supported through comfort as well as active intervention.

THE UNIQUENESS OF FAITH COMMUNITIES

Regardless of the model chosen, the prospective faith community nurse must consider certain factors when setting up a faith community nursing program. A **congregation** is a group of people with its own structure, and the faith community nurse must work within this structure. Where the program will fit into the congregation in organizational terms is one of the first things to consider. Even if the faith community nurse is in a paid model, most of the congregation members that the nurse will be working with are volunteers. Assumptions about communication or accountability that work in healthcare agencies will not necessarily apply in this setting. The faith community nurse must discover whether there is already a committee or commission which focuses on health concerns. Perhaps there is a social ministry group or an outreach group in the congregation. Understanding the structure of the congregation as a whole is important to support coordination with ongoing ministry activities in the congregation. Otherwise, long-time volunteers or leaders might be offended. This is part of the assessment process that will be discussed in more detail later in this chapter.

The pastor, rabbi, or other congregational leader can be a great source of information about structure. If no suitable group exists, the faith community nurse needs to assemble an advisory board (King, 2011). The advisory board offers leadership, establishes policy, and helps develop guidelines. Having the support of an advisory board is essential for solving problems and avoiding pitfalls. Membership of the board can vary but might include the pastor, a spiritual director, designated health professionals, and interested lay people. The advisory board can help develop support for a budget for the program. When new members join the advisory board, they will need orientation about the faith community nursing program. By providing new members of the board with articles about faith community nursing, past annual reports of the congregation, and written job descriptions and evaluation forms, the faith community nurse assists the new member in becoming an active participant in the program. Meetings can take place as often as once a month. Meeting less than six times a year means that members will not have as much participation as they might like, and support for the faith community nurse might be diminished.

Relationship With the Clergy

Supportive relationships with the spiritual head of the congregation are important for the success of a faith community nursing program. Unless the pastor has worked with a faith community nurse before, repeated explanations will most likely be necessary. One common misconception is that the faith community nurse is a private visiting nurse for the congregation. Faith community nurses do not provide direct hands-on nursing care. Rather, they provide confidential professional nursing that includes assessment, teaching, referral, and counseling. An important resource on activities that faith community nurses offer can be found in the ANA's *Faith Community Nursing: Scope and Standards of Practice* (2012) which can be shared with clergy or others for guidance. If a member of the congregation is in need of visiting nurse services, the faith community nurse provides an appropriate referral.

Evidence for Practice

One interview study explored the experiences of chronically ill seniors who were members of an established faith community nurse's practice in a large suburban congregation. Despite the fact that individuals had from two to nine different diseases and were taking two to 19 different medications, the seniors reported that their lives were connected to others, and that they felt they were living well. They were connected to the goodness of God in their lives, and most were caregivers for others, which gave their lives meaning (Dyess & Chase, 2010).

In another study, researchers developed a survey that explored clergy members' commitment to health-related programming, and their experience with "congregational health ministers," a term used to include faith community nurses and other health professionals such as social workers, therapists, or pharmacists who were working in the congregational setting. Nearly 350 pastors from 80 different denominations returned the survey. The pastors fell into five main categories: mainline Protestant, conservative Protestant, African American Protestant, Roman Catholic, and other (Catanzaro, Meador, Koenig, Kuchibhatla, & Clipp, 2006). The groups with the most experience with congregational health ministers were mainline Protestant and Catholic, and congregations that were large, suburban, and financially well off. Pastors with congregational health ministries in place in their settings reported more frequent health promotion programming in their setting. The most common reported reason for starting a health program in the church was that a nurse who was a member proposed it (Catanzaro et al., 2006). This study shows that individual nurses can influence health programming in their own faith communities.

members of the community. This is consistent with most models of community healthcare. To assess the health of the faith community, principles of epidemiology, which were discussed earlier in this book, can be applied. The faith community group may be smaller than some other aggregate groups, but the same principles are appropriate. Although epidemiology began with tracing the patterns of infectious disease in the community at large, within the faith community, goals such as reducing disease risk factors, reducing the burden of chronic illness, and promoting health become more prominent than infectious disease. Nevertheless, principles of epidemiology can be used as a method to determine patterns of illness for the faith community, and risk factor assessment helps the nurse decide what programs to provide.

One of the major tools of epidemiology is statistics. Florence Nightingale was an early user of statistics to gather support for the changes she wanted to make in the British healthcare system. Similarly, faith community nurses can use statistics in two ways. First, the nurse should gather general demographic data about the faith community, including age, family structure, and proximity of residence to a healthcare facility and other health resources. These data can be summarized with descriptive statistics that can be used to generate reports and to assist planning. Second, the nurse should use data about various diseases from comparison groups, such as public health prevalence data. Is swine flu (H1N1) or methicillin-resistant *Staphylococcus aureus* infection becoming more prevalent in the area? County health departments publish data on certain reportable diseases which can be useful in planning screening or educational programs. It helps to compare the rate of cardiac events or strokes in a faith community which has wellness programs with rates for the same conditions in the region or nation. Using these data, the faith community nurse can demonstrate both the need for programming and the effectiveness of the programs conducted. See Community Resources for further information.

In the case study, the morning that Mary detects the highest blood pressure reading, she communicates her concern about Mrs. Swenson's health issue to the pastor, Mr. Dryden. She wants him to be fully informed about his parishioner. Being new in her position, Mary wants him to develop trust in how the program is operating. This way, if Mrs. Swenson needed to be admitted to hospital, he would not be surprised. He would also be able to set up a clergy visit.

Faith Community as Community

Faith community nursing is focused on the entire community of faith, not just on individual people who happen to be

Evidence for Practice

A research review of faith community health promotion for African Americans pointed out that using practice sites away from traditional healthcare systems can increase access to effective diabetes health education programs. Fourteen studies were reviewed. Overall, these studies showed the effectiveness of using culturally appropriate messages with the faith community as the recruitment source and the place for delivering the material. The studies used a collaborative approach in designing and carrying out their activities. Patient outcomes included increased vegetable usage, weight loss, and lowered HbA1c levels (Newlin, Dyess, Allard, Chase, & Melkus, 2011).

Practice Point

Developing a needs-and-skills inventory is a good way to determine what kinds of programs a congregation might value. Do people want information regarding specific high-impact conditions such as diabetes or heart disease risk, or do they care more about learning how to support the functioning of their aging parents? Sometimes, people are reluctant to admit to having weaknesses, but they want to help the health ministry. For example, a homebound person could have the "job" of writing cards to people who are in the hospital or who are having birthdays.

Another way to consider a congregation's social patterns is to explore the various ways members relate to one another, both individually and in groups. Faith communities often develop around ethnic groups. Roman Catholic parishes might be predominantly Irish, Italian, Polish, or Hispanic. Lutheran congregations might be German, Swedish, Finnish, or Norwegian. Congregations in areas with high immigration rates will likely be oriented around specific groups. Jewish congregations share ethnic as well as religious commonalities. Are gatherings planned around major life events such as weddings, funerals, baptisms, or other entry rituals? (Are regular feast or holy days important to the group?) Understanding ethnic roots can help the parish nurse understand preferences and traditions that might affect health issues (Breisch, Hurley, & Moore, 2013). In all cases, the faith community nurse needs to be careful to avoid stereotyping, and to assess each individual person's perspective. However, celebrating ethnic background is a wonderful way to build community and make all people feel welcome.

The secret of health for both mind and body is not to mourn for the past, nor to worry about the future, but to live the present moment wisely and earnestly. **Buddha**

Faith community nurses engage in primary, secondary, and tertiary prevention activities in their congregations. Primary prevention activities include programs on walking or other forms of exercise to maintain health, smoking cessation programs, and heart-healthy eating programs. Secondary prevention includes screening for hypertension or hyperglycemia, and setting up screenings such as mammogram vans or other tests to diagnose problems early. Tertiary prevention is another important focus where faith community nurses work to minimize the effect of health problems and maximize function for people with conditions such as diabetes, stroke, or injury.

Faith communities are also part of a larger geographic or public community. Federal support for faith initiatives has increased in recent years. The congregation can be a site for health-related programming for entire communities. For some people in these communities, this may be the only health resource. One such program in central Texas organized a coalition that included state health departments, healthcare organizations, faith communities, county and city health departments, and local colleges and universities (Patillo, Chesley, Castles, & Sutter, 2002). Working together over 3 years, the coalition offered workshops to more than 1,000 nurses and prepared 54 nurses with the full parish nurse educational programs. The work of this coalition allowed the number of active congregational programs to increase from five to 53, established web links to state health department resources, and offered services to Hispanic migrant families without health insurance. Students from local colleges and universities gained experience in conducting events such as health fairs.

ROLES OF THE FAITH COMMUNITY NURSE

Faith community nurses perform several roles which are similar to nurses' roles in many settings, but which often have a different emphasis. For example, as many community health nurses do, faith community nurses maintain lists of community and healthcare referrals. On the other hand, the faith community nurse's role as patient advocate may be unique because the faith community nurse has an ongoing relationship with the congregation member, may know family members, and can directly follow up on recommendations and additional referrals. Faith community nurses do health teaching in a variety of settings. These may include group settings for topical areas such as general health promotion, end-of-life planning, or healthy lifestyle activities. Faith community nurses may also do individual teaching for congregation members with specific health conditions. The ministry to the congregation as a whole often leads the faith community nurse to organize and support volunteer groups, such as home visitors, drivers to appointments, or volunteers to provide meals to families who have members just home from the hospital. Faith community nurses can also lead or convene groups with specialty leaders such as bereavement or family caregiver groups. Perhaps more importantly, faith community nurses provide spiritual care based in the belief structures of the congregation. This may include assisting the congregation member to discern God's presence in a difficult time or to use spiritual resources as a support. The roles and activities of faith community nurses are varied. One of the functions of the health cabinet or other congregational group is to assist the faith community nurse in planning and evaluating activities.

Mary has several roles as a faith community nurse. Her primary responsibility is to empower Mrs. Swenson to make healthcare choices that promote better long-term health. Describe four roles that Mary assumes as a faith community nurse.

Evidence for Practice

One study reported on the activities and roles of parish nurses. A statewide survey was completed by 72 parish nurses, most of whom were volunteers who worked less than 10 hours a week. The largest denominations represented were Catholic (25) and Methodist (23) (King & Tessaro, 2009). Activities reported by the parish nurses were blood pressure screening (70%), physical health counseling (45%), health education relating to exercise (31%), and nutrition (29%). The nurses also provided counseling on spiritual health (28%) and bereavement (21%), and they offered support to clients engaged in weight control (25%) and stress reduction (25%). The range of services and support provided by parish nurses in this study reflects a balance of body, mind, and spiritual concerns. In the parish setting, nurses can truly provide holistic care.

An additional survey of nurses in a large Catholic healthcare system (McGinnis & Zoske, 2008, p. 179) revealed that parish nurses, in addition to health promotion, "provide chronic disease management that is often lacking in our current healthcare systems." These activities included case management, advocacy, collaborating with other health professionals, and assisting clients in adapting to functional limitations.

HEALTHY PEOPLE 2020 PRIORITIES

Where do faith community nurses obtain guidance for planning, programming, and prioritizing their activities? Some of the best sources are national guidelines to support health such as *Healthy People 2020* (U.S. Department of Health and Human Services, n.d.). *Healthy People 2020* is the program sponsored by the federal government to help set health goals for the United States as a whole. The *Healthy People 2020* framework can guide faith community nurse programming. Introducing the model to the congregation starting with the health cabinet or advisory group can support program development. Leading health indicators are listed in Box 23.1.

Most of these health indicators are issues that can be addressed in congregation-wide health promotion programs. The midcourse report indicates that outcomes are actually worsening for mental and oral health, with little or no improvement in diabetes outcomes. Physical activity for all age groups in the congregation can be supported through hiking clubs, senior exercise programs, or by sponsoring an aerobics group in one of the church rooms. Denominationally related weight management programs are available which a church could sponsor. Smoking cessation materials can be prominently displayed. Alcohol and substance abuse problems can be

23.1 *Healthy People 2020* Leading Health Indicators

- Physical activity
- Overweight and obesity
- Tobacco use
- Substance abuse
- Responsible sexual behavior
- Mental health
- Injury and violence
- Environmental quality
- Immunization
- Access to healthcare

Source: Office of Disease Prevention and Health Promotion, United States Department of Health and Human Services. Retrieved from http://www.healthypeople.gov.

addressed individually, or by having the church be the site of a 12-step program. Parental groups can develop and support the teaching of healthy sexuality. In any congregation, the parish nurse must be alert to signs of domestic violence which can include child abuse or neglect, elder abuse or neglect, or partner violence. Individual referrals and support can be important. Mental health is often a hidden health problem. Knowledge of risk, and insight into high-risk situations, can assist the faith community nurse in appropriate assessment and response, specifically for referrals. To ensure that each member of the congregation obtains appropriate care, the nurse can counsel members individually about access to care, or offer resources in a reading area or library at the faith community.

Practice Point

Periodically review the *Healthy People 2020* or other such initiatives and reflect on what health programming suggested by these groups would benefit the congregation. Would adding a senior exercise group both help maintain socialization and improve function? Would a youth group focused on safety reduce the risk of traumatic injury or death for the younger members of the congregation?

Student Reflection

In community health, we try to think of ways of reaching people with health programs before they get sick and need acute care. When I was placed with a faith community for my experience, I realized that this is real community care. This is where people come together regularly, and there is always a chance for a health program, either with new mothers or with senior citizens. At my site, we sponsored a new mothers group, and used the church nursery for child care for the toddlers, so that the mothers could focus on the classes on nutrition. They shared a lot of wisdom with each other, too.

SCOPE AND STANDARDS OF PRACTICE

Faith community nurses function by virtue of their license to practice nursing. The vast majority of nurses in the United States are employees of hospitals, long-term care facilities, or home care agencies. In contrast, the faith community nurse functions more independently. The resources of the nursing profession as a whole, including the ANA's *Faith Community Nursing: Scope and Standards of Practice* (2012) are important guides to the faith community nurse. In terms of well-developed policies or procedures, the faith community nurse may not have the same level of structure as the nurse who works in a complex healthcare system. The ANA Standards of Care for Faith Community Nursing Practice are organized around the steps of the nursing process (Table 23.2).

How do faith community nurses actually spend their time? Using focus groups, researchers have conducted studies of parish nurses themselves. This method brings together people who have shared an experience to discuss and share

TABLE 23.2 Standards of Care for Parish Nursing Practice

Standard	Sample Criteria
Assessment	Collects comprehensive, appropriate data
	Collaborates with others in selecting and collecting data
	Data may include the following:
	Demographics, including living arrangements
	Health and illness incidence
	Functional status
	Spiritual issues
	Psychological issues
	Social issues in the community
	Community services and resources
	Assessment is an ongoing process
	Assessment data are used to form diagnoses
Diagnosis	Identifies actual and high-risk diagnoses and potential areas for growth, with attention to strengths
	Makes holistic diagnoses that include body–mind–spirit issues
	Uses accepted standardized nomenclature in documentation
	Diagnoses are recorded and communicated to support health and healing
Outcome identification	Expected outcomes are determined for each diagnosis, preferably with the client's participation
	Outcomes are measurable
	Outcomes are adapted to the particularities of the client, including cultural aspects and are achievable
Planning	Plans for health promotion are developed at every opportunity
	Plans specify activities and who should perform them
	Plans include evidence-based approaches
	Particular strengths and weaknesses of each client/family/group are considered
	Plans include a consideration of the client's values/beliefs/customs
	Plans include follow-up activities
Implementation	Interventions are mutually developed with the people involved
	Interventions are within the legal, professional, and contractual scope of practice
	Activities include the use of appropriate technology
	Interventions are recorded in standardized language to provide for continuity of care
Evaluation	Evaluation includes care of individuals, families, and groups using outcome criteria
	Evaluation of the major programs of the parish nurse is ongoing
	Revisions of plans and programs are based on evaluation data

Source: Adapted from American Nurses Association. (2012). *Faith community nursing: Scope and standards of practice* (2nd ed.). Silver Spring, MD: American Nurses Association.

their impressions of that experience with a researcher. The researcher then analyzes the discussion and presents the findings. One study involved 17 faith community nurses from a hospital-sponsored program of volunteer nurses. These nurses discussed the attributes of the care that they delivered in their parish settings. Investigators used a focus group and telephone interviews (Chase-Ziolek & Iris, 2002). The faith community nurses reported that their most important contributions to their congregation were health promotion and prevention of disease, advocacy, health education, health counseling, psychosocial support, and spiritual care. They stated that the congregational setting provided a personal relationship which extended over time, and which integrated faith and health in a way that was rewarding to them and their patients. The nurses also reported that having the time to meet such a wide range of needs, and contend with differences in beliefs, even in the congregational setting, presented a challenge.

To determine the perceptions of members of the congregation about parish nursing, researchers conducted an ethnographic study of faith community nursing in two congregations, one predominantly African American and one predominantly white (Tuck & Wallace, 2000; Wallace, Tuck, Boland, & Witucki, 2002). Ethnographic studies consider the language and culture of a particular group of people. This study showed that congregants were grateful for the easy access to health information that the faith community nurse provided. They also reported that the parish nurse was able to combine health and spirituality issues, and helped people more actively promote their own health. Specifically, many congregants described a successful, faith community approach to weight loss.

THE NURSING PROCESS IN FAITH COMMUNITY NURSING

In all interactions, the faith community nurse should keep in mind that the nursing process is the basis of the caring relationship (ANA, 2012). Individual assessments may include blood pressure, gait stability, home assessment for safety, assessing for distress related to grieving for the recently widowed, and assessment of knowledge regarding self-management of medical diagnoses and chronic illness. Family assessments might include stress assessment for the family with a new baby, support of the wife who is transporting her husband for chemotherapy, or strategizing with parents of teenagers whose behavior has been troubling. Community assessments can include assessing whether healthcare is accessible to members of the congregation, and determining whether a recent industry closing will create personal or financial stress for members of the congregation.

Assessment and Diagnosis

Epidemiologic principles are useful in planning faith community nurse programming. When assessing the health of a faith community, the community as a whole is the target of concern. Several key questions need to be addressed:

- What are the common health problems experienced by members of this community? The faith community nurse visits members in the hospital, and in counseling individual members, he or she begins to see patterns that affect the congregation as a whole.
- What are the chief demographic groups in the congregation? A large number of elderly people means that health programs need to be planned with an understanding of major health problems of the elderly, and should include support for maximizing functional status. A large number of young families means that programs need to include parenting support. Young mothers groups can provide socialization and encouragement to an important segment of the congregation. An active youth group means that health programs can be woven into activities in which the youth group participates.
- What are the health assets of the faith community? Churches and synagogues have a rich group of volunteers who can assist their communities by providing meals after hospitalization, transportation to physician visits or treatments, hospital visits by specially trained visitors, and support groups for a variety of conditions. Assessing for strength is the key focus of community health assessment.
- What environmental health concerns exist in the congregation? The congregation is rooted in a local community. Members include people who have lived in the community for generations, as well as newcomers. By being active in the particular community, members become active in environmental health concerns. For example, the first meeting to address an observation of a cluster of cases of childhood leukemia was in a church in the community. A successful book and movie, *A Civil Action* (Harr, 1995), tells how a toxic waste dump endangered the health of a Massachusetts community. The book shows how members of the community came together in a faith community setting to begin to address their concerns about the safety of their local environment.

The purpose of an assessment is to provide baseline data and support reporting and planning. A health assessment can be thought of as a needs assessment for developing congregational programming. Faith community nursing is often misunderstood because concepts of community health are frequently not understood by the general public, who see healthcare as physician-dominated and disease-focused. Fortunately, the importance of self-care and active participation in maintaining a person's own health has become widely accepted today. Faith community assessment can lead to important health programming in a rich community setting. North American Nursing Diagnosis Association-International (NANDA-I) regularly updates the list and organization of nursing diagnoses (NANDA-I, 2017). Many of these are applicable to the community as a whole. Domains of nursing

TABLE 23.3 Nursing Diagnoses Appropriate to the Faith Community Setting

Individual	Family	Community
Ineffective health maintenance	Impaired home maintenance	Lack of health-seeking behaviors
Impaired swallowing	Risk for imbalanced nutrition: more than body requirements	Imbalanced nutrition: more than body requirements
Impaired physical mobility	Risk for activity intolerance	Deficient diversional activity
Impaired memory	Deficient knowledge: asthma management	Deficient knowledge: resources for Alzheimer's caregivers
Chronic low self-esteem	Caregiver role strain	Powerlessness
Death anxiety	Chronic sorrow	Diminished readiness for enhanced community coping
Risk-prone health behavior	Compromised family coping	Ineffective protection
Risk for loneliness	Decisional conflict	Risk of other-directed violence

Source: Adapted from North American Nursing Diagnosis Association-International. (2012). *Nursing diagnoses: Definitions and classification 2012–2014* (H. Herdman, ed.). Philadelphia, PA: Author.

diagnoses include health promotion, nutrition, activity/rest, role-relationships, coping/stress tolerance, and life principles. Diagnoses under the domain of life principles include decisional conflict, readiness for enhanced spiritual well-being, and spiritual distress. These domains are clearly aligned with the practice of faith community nurses.

such as the NANDA (Herdman & Kamitsuru, 2017), the Omaha System (Martin, 2005), or some other recognizable nomenclature system. Diagnoses can be made for individual people, families, or the entire faith community. Table 23.3 lists diagnoses that would be appropriate for each of these three levels.

Mary maintains records of blood pressure trends and current medications for all church members who come for blood pressure screening. This assists her in detecting patterns of concern. What other assessment data would Mary gather that would be helpful, particularly for the senior citizens in the congregation? A monthly senior luncheon held at the church hall allows for socializing among the senior members of the congregation as well as those in the surrounding community. A program is associated with the luncheon, and every year Mary presents a talk about a health-related topic related to her activities. Suggest three possible topics for Mary to consider for her presentation.

Mary identifies that Mrs. Swenson has several diagnoses that need intervention. Based on what you know about Mrs. Swenson from this case study, name three of these nursing diagnoses.

Interventions and Outcomes

Outcomes may seem to be the end point in the nursing process, but before choosing interventions, it is necessary to determine which outcomes are desirable and achievable (Bulechek, Butcher, & Dochterman, 2008). This choice must include preferences of the client, family, and community and must include consideration of people's values and beliefs and resources as well as best available evidence for what actions are likely to have positive benefits for the patient. Nurses should individualize outcomes for diagnoses based on these factors. For example, for the diagnosis of ineffective therapeutic regimen management, the outcome for one person might involve independent management of diabetic testing and medication management. The outcome for another person might involve following the advice of a visiting nurse and taking medications as prescribed. Outcomes for the community as a whole might include acceptance of health status, caregiver emotional health, pain level control, decision-making, or self-care (Moorhead, Johnson, Maas, & Swanson, 2008). When nurses have determined

Practice Point

Ask a faith community nurse to share his or her best practices. Find out what documentation system the local health department uses. Does this nurse use a similar type? Perhaps if all nurses used a common format, they could combine reports and better evaluate the health of the community.

Diagnoses for faith community nurses should include nursing diagnoses as identified by organizations outcomes, they can select interventions that support attainment of those specific outcomes.

Planning in the context of the faith community includes care of individual people, as well as care of the entire faith community. For example, the faith community nurse might assess the health risk factors of members of the community as high risk for cardiovascular illness and plan programs for heart health, including (1) nutrition programs using the church kitchen to plan and prepare healthy, tasty food; (2) hypertension screening; and (3) an exercise program in the church basement.

Faith and prayer are the vitamins of the soul; man cannot live in health without them. **Mahalia Jackson**

Evidence for Practice

Ann Solari-Twadell, one of the key leaders in parish nursing, has conducted research on the interventions that active faith community nurses most often use. This study used a detailed survey based on the current version of the Nursing Intervention Classification (NIC) (Solari-Twadell, 2002; Solari-Twadell & Hackbarth, 2010), including interventions from the behavioral domain such as coping assistance, patient education, communication enhancement, and cognitive therapy. Physiologic interventions reported by nurses included activity management and nutrition education. One intervention not included in the NIC which faith community nurses reported as essential was "prayer." Prayer was listed as an activity in the NIC under the intervention labeled *spiritual growth facilitation*. One intervention listed under community was program development. This groundbreaking research is the most extensive report to date of the specific interventions that faith community nurses actually use, and it can be the basis for documentation systems, as well as for faith community nurse educational program development.

Weis, Schank, Coenen, and Matheus (2002) conducted a research study to examine the most frequent diagnoses and interventions reported by faith community nurses when working with groups of parishioners. They collected data from 22 faith communities over a 5-month period. The groups represented a variety of ages and included both men and women. In addition to quantitative data recorded by the faith community nurses, 10 participated in a focus group interview about what it is like working with groups of congregation members and whether documentation labels fit. The majority of group activities (56%) were for disease prevention, such as smoking cessation. Of group sessions, 18% were for illness management concerns, such as asthma or arthritis.

Although this study did not use as extensive a data collection instrument as the Solari-Twadell study, it showed that the nursing diagnoses selected for the group activities include health-seeking behavior, potential for spiritual well-being, knowledge deficit, anxiety, social isolation, and altered family processes. The interventions selected included active listening, health screening, support system enhancement, and presence. Other interventions for the groups included spiritual and emotional support. The nurses in the focus groups validated that these labels were a good description of their activities with congregation groups (Weis et al., 2002).

Community-Level Interventions

Of particular concern in community health is the disparity that some groups experience in gaining access to appropriate care. Faith community settings can be a unique and powerful approach to filling gaps in care. Recent immigrants and people without English language skill are particularly vulnerable to health risks. One faith community nursing intervention project focused on 100 Mexican American women with gestational diabetes (Mendelson, McNeese-Smith, Koniak-Griffin, Nyamathi, & Lu, 2008). Participants in the study completed the Health Promoting Lifestyle Profile (HPLP-II), which was used to measure the effect of a randomized trial of a parish nurse intervention program. This program consisted of a 9-hour educational program regarding nutrition, with a spiritual message related to health and wholeness consistent with the belief system of the participant. Participants not selected for the intervention received the usual care. Outcomes were scores of the HPLP-II 3 weeks after the session, maternal glucose (hemoglobin A1C [Hgb A1C]) on admission for delivery, and birth weight of the infant to detect macrosomia, a common result of gestational diabetes. The study showed that scores on the HPLP-II for the parish nurse intervention group were significantly higher in stress management, health responsibility, physical activity, and spirituality. The study did not show differences in Hgb A1C or macrosomia. The sample size may have been too low to show an effect, and the intervention may need to be designed for more of a nurse "dose," that is, more engagement to show lasting effect.

Implementation requires carrying out interventions in ways that are well supported by nursing textbooks, clinical evidence, or national guidelines. Interventions classified by the NIC (Bulechek et al., 2008) or the Omaha System (Topaz, Golfenshtein, & Bowles, 2014) can target individual people, families, and communities. The internet provides access to guidelines for screening and managing many health concerns.

 ## Student Reflection

At first, when I began assisting a faith community nurse, I was uncomfortable talking with patients about faith issues because I did not feel prepared by my college courses in how to do this. Once I realized that I did not have to have all the answers about religious issues, I relaxed about listening to how people's faith gave their lives meaning. I finally got up the courage to ask whether the patient wanted to share a prayer at the end of a visit, and I found she was praying for me, too. That was a beautiful moment, and it did not matter what denomination we belonged to, which was different. I now feel comfortable including spiritual care in my interventions with patients.

Community-Level Outcomes and Documentation of Practice

Nurses need to evaluate outcomes for individual people, families, and communities. Did individuals, families, and groups meet the outcomes that were set for them? Did they maximize their rehabilitation following surgery? Did families successfully bond with their new babies? Did the shut-ins in the congregation feel the warmth of the holiday season through visits, calls, or cards? Documentation systems which report health status of clients or communities before and after faith community nursing interventions are able to show the difference nursing makes in this setting.

Faith community nurses have begun to document the outcomes of their practice, including its effect on costs of care (Brown, 2006; Miller & Carson, 2010; Rydholm, 2006; Rydholm et al., 2008). Rydholm reports on the work of faith community nurses in supporting community resources, and as informal caregivers who provide many of the services needed by elders and those with chronic illnesses. By gathering the stories of parish nurses, this researcher has documented "an interruption of downward-spiraling illnesses through rapid access to care" (Rydholm, 2006, p. 10). Some of the issues addressed were unsteadiness in movement, syncope, medication confusion, hypertensive crises, and shortness of breath. By coordinating care at an early stage, faith community nurses reduced more expensive hospitalizations. Brown (2006) reviewed parish nurse documentation and showed that healthcare costs were reduced by parish nurses who reduced emergency department visits through advocacy and referral.

Rydholm and colleagues (2008) reported a study of 1,061 notes by 75 faith community nurses who worked in Minnesota which were made during the care of 713 older adults. Researchers uncovered the needs of elders which were met by the faith community nurses, including end-of-life care, access and referral, guidance, providing adaptive equipment, and offering calm and motivating support. These elements are consistent with the case study at the beginning of the chapter. Without access to a faith community nurse, elders and people with chronic illness may develop serious complications, lose their ability to live independently, or enter the healthcare system through the emergency department, which is unnecessarily expensive.

Evidence for Practice

In addition to health promotion, parish nurses provide for the sick and dying. O'Brien (2006) conducted a qualitative research study of parish nursing for elders near the end of life. Using a theory of spiritual well-being in illness that she had developed, she observed a parish nurse care for 15 elders at the end of life. The nurse used the Spiritual Well-Being Interview Guide and continued to visit the elders, two to four times over 8 months. The elders exhibited five identifiable nursing diagnoses: spiritual alienation, spiritual anxiety, spiritual anger, spiritual loss, and spiritual peace. Interventions offered included sharing prayer and scripture, spiritual presence, and pastoral counseling. By dealing with the meaning of their health and illness, the parish nurse was able to assist some of the elders who were in distress in achieving some peace in their lives.

It is important to document faith community nursing, which allows people to see how this new specialty is actually practiced. One study (Burkhart & Androwich, 2004) reported that an existing documentation system, the NIC, was used to code free-form charts from 170 health records from 13 parish nurses at seven sites, including urban, suburban, and rural settings. The investigators conducted this research to determine whether the system could capture the actions of parish nurses in 1,607 separate interactions. Experts coded notes separately and checked their accuracy by comparing their coding choices. Overall, 93% of interactions fit existing categories, with 117 different interventions identified. The study made several recommendations for new or modified interventions to fit the community practice of parish nursing.

In the Burkhart and Androwich (2004) study, the most frequently used interventions were surveillance, spiritual support, admission care, medication management, emotional support, referral, and vital sign monitoring. The interventions in NIC are organized into domains. The most frequently used domains were safety, behavioral, and health system activities. The NIC labels describing spiritual care worked well in this setting. The new interventions that were proposed included scheduling appointments, communication with patient, case closure, community transport, supply management (community), and dying care (community). Faith community nursing extends such care to the community, so recommendations were made to adjust the interventions as published by the research group which developed the NIC classification. This research showed that one published and accessible system was able to capture most of the faith community nurse activities recorded in parish nurse notes.

In a state of the science paper, Dyess, Chase, and Newlin (2010) reported that four main areas of evidence exist related to faith community nursing

(1) the development of new faith community nursing practices, (2) actions and roles that were reported by faith community nurses, (3) the evaluation and documentation of faith community nursing practices, and (4) perceptions of faith community nursing by congregation members. The authors point out that further research is needed in the area of demonstrating the outcomes of faith community practices.

ETHICAL CONSIDERATIONS

All the ethical principles that guide nursing practice in general apply to nursing in faith communities. On the surface, it might seem that ethics would not be a problem where practice is independent, and where the community might be expected to share common values because of a common faith. In most cases, this is true. The parish nurse works to empower members of the congregation to take charge of their health. This can enhance their autonomy. The faith community nurse is also guided by beneficence, the act of doing good. This is an even more stringent requirement than nonmaleficence: the need to do no harm.

However, ethics do play a role in faith community nursing. One area where parish nurses can commit an ethical breach comes up often in the family context of a congregation. This area is the need to protect confidentiality. One member of the congregation might ask how another member, who is in the hospital, is doing. Because of the professional code requiring confidentiality, the parish nurse has more restrictions that the average person might have on what can be shared in everyday conversations in the congregation. The parish nurse is bound by professional confidentiality not to reveal information about the health of patients, even if they are known to members of the congregation. Refusing to share information in a way that does not seem cold is a delicate art. One way to avoid this conflict is to explain to congregants early in the program, and often thereafter, that confidentiality for each member will be maintained. Often, the nurse can simply say, "I am sure that she would appreciate a call or a card;" this relieves pressure to share much information. In annual reviews, and in meetings with the advisory committee, issues of confidentiality or other general ethical issues can be discussed, and annual reports use group or aggregate data only, so they are unlikely to betray a confidence.

Whoever seeks to set one religion against another seeks to destroy all religion. **Franklin D. Roosevelt**

EDUCATION FOR FAITH COMMUNITY NURSING

Continuing education programs are often used to educate faith community nurses for their role. The Westberg Institute, formerly the International Parish Nurse Resource Center and renamed to honor the founder of faith community nurse, Lutheran Pastor Granger Westberg, has developed a curriculum which can be delivered in a continuing education format, or through a more formal academic program for college credit. The curriculum for all participants is developed at the baccalaureate nurse level, even though many faith community nurses have diploma or associate degree preparation. Others may have master's degrees in community health, theology, or in advanced practice roles, such as nurse practitioner or clinical nurse specialist. The second edition of *Faith Community Nursing: Scope and Standards of Practice* (ANA, 2012) includes guides for advanced practice nurses as well as registered nurses. The scope of practice and breadth of faith community programs is in part determined by the educational preparation of the faith community nurse. A study designed to compare activities of faith community nurses who had, and had not, completed the endorsed education program from the Westberg Institute (Mosack, Medvene, & Wescott, 2006) found that for 265 nurses in a statewide network, those who had completed a particular educational program (53%) worked more hours per month and were more likely to provide health screening, health education, and referrals, especially referrals to those services which were nonmedical sources, such as social services and mental health services. The Westberg Institute is now a part of the Church Health Center based in Memphis, TN (https://westberginstitute.org/give//). Among the roles of the Church Health Center are developing the curriculum for the preparation of faith community nurses, and identifying the seven specific functions that parish nurses perform in faith community work. These functions are derived from activities that all nurses may engage in, but some of these activities differ in faith community nursing (Table 23.4). Additionally, the Health Ministries Association offers a membership organization for nurses and others in health ministry, as well as training programs for prospective faith community nurses (https://hmassoc.org/).

Certification for Faith Community Nursing is now available through the America Nurses Credentialing Association (ANCC). It uses a portfolio process which is well-described on the AACN Website (http://www.nursecredentialing.org/FaithCommunityNursing).

In response to the need for community health experiences and in conjunction with faith community and other community initiatives, student nurses in academic programs can have clinical practice experiences in faith community settings (King, 2011). Students are not actually asked to function fully as faith community nurses. The role of the parish nurse includes spiritual care consistent with the faith and values of the congregation, which may be beyond appropriate expectations for the student, but many of the health screening and promotion activities can be performed by students with supervision.

TABLE 23.4 Functions of the Faith Community Nurse

Function	Examples
Integrator of faith and health	Spiritual care Spiritual assessment Sharing scripture Therapeutic listening
Personal health counselor	Therapeutic communication Assessing for emotional distress Assessing for suicide risk
Health educator	Individual health teaching Group health teaching Provider of health resources
Health advocate	Empowerment of members of the congregation Empowerment of the congregation to improve the health of the community
Referral agent	Maintaining lists of local providers/agencies Communicating with referrals
Coordinator of volunteers	Assessing for needs for volunteer services Recruiting and training volunteers Scheduling and supporting volunteers Commissioning and recognizing volunteers
Accessing and developing support groups	Referring congregation members to existing support groups Developing support groups for congregation members

KEY CONCEPTS

- Faith community nursing provides health promotion, health screening, and health teaching as well as care for individual people and groups associated with the congregation.
- A variety of faith community nursing models exist. In the congregation-based model, the nurse is hired by the faith community to provide faith community nursing services.

- The steps of the nursing process are applied to the faith community.
- Values, cultural practices, and faith are a part of health.
- The body, mind, and spirit of community members are the primary focus of nursing in faith communities.

CRITICAL THINKING QUESTIONS

1. The congregation is happy to hear that a nurse wishes to establish a faith community nursing ministry in their setting. They are concerned about liability and require that the nurse not "write anything down" because they believe that any written documentation would provide the basis for legal suits. How should the parish nurse respond?
2. What sources of information are best for planning educational programs for parishioners? How does the parish nurse select materials?
3. An 86-year-old male parishioner is on hospice care at home, and his daughter, a nurse, has been trying to meet all his physical needs around the clock. The pastor, who had made a home visit, calls the faith community nurse to express his concern that the daughter is becoming "burned out." How can the faith community nurse engage the faith community as a whole to provide volunteer support to this family?
4. The faith community nurse decides to increase health awareness by holding a health fair. What types of exhibitors would be good to include? Would the health fair be any different when held in the congregational setting than in another community setting? In what ways?

COMMUNITY RESOURCES

- Start with the Westberg Institute (https://westberginstitute.org/), formerly the International Parish Nurse Resource Center. They have directories of active programs.
- In your area, contact church offices to determine whether the individual congregations have health-related programs.
- Visit the website for the Health Ministry Association (https://hmassoc.org/). They have general health information and access to a membership organization. If your college has a chaplain or ministry center, ask the staff there whether they know of programs in your area.
- Hospitals, particularly those with religious affiliations, may have an active faith community link.
- Check out Community Commons (https://www.communitycommons.org/). It offers maps and surveys that can be searched by zip codes to determine health concerns and resources available in specific communities. Individual accounts can be opened and searches and reports saved for future use.

REFERENCES

American Nurses Association. (2012). *Faith community nursing: Scope and standards of practice* (2nd ed.). Silver Spring, MD: Author.

Breisch, A. J., Hurley, P. S., & Moore, L. (2013). Faith community nursing: Innovative practice in faith-based settings. *Tar Heel Nurse*, *75*(3), 12, 16.

Brown, A. (2006). Documenting the value of faith community nursing: 2. Faith nursing online. *Creative Nursing*, *12*(2), 13.

Bulechek, G. A., Butcher, H., & Dochterman, J. M. (Eds.). (2008). *Nursing interventions classification (NIC)* (5th ed.). St. Louis, MO: Elsevier.

Burkhart, L., & Androwich, I. (2004). Measuring the domain completeness of the nursing interventions classification in parish nurse documentation. *Computers, Informatics, Nursing*, *22*(2), 72–82.

Catanzaro, A. M., Meador, K. G., Koenig, H. G., Kurchibhatla, M., & Clipp, E. C. (2006). Congregational health ministries: A national study of pastors' views. *Public Health Nursing*, *24*(1), 6–17.

Chase-Ziolek, M., & Iris, M. (2002). Nurses' perspectives on the distinctive aspects of providing nursing care in a congregational setting. *Journal of Community Health Nursing*, *19*(3), 173–186.

Dyess, S. M., & Chase, S. K. (2010). Caring for adults living with a chronic illness through communities of faith. *International Journal for Human Caring*, *14*(4), 38–44.

Dyess, S. M., & Chase, S. K. (2012). Sustaining health in faith community nursing practice: Emerging processes that support the development of a middle-range theory. *Holistic Nursing Practice*, *26*(4), 221–227.

Dyess, S. M., Chase, S. K., & Newlin, K. (2010). State of research for faith community nursing 2009. *Journal of Religion and Health*, *49*(2), 188–199.

Harr, J. (1995). *A civil action*. New York: Random House.

Herdman, T. H., & Kamitsuru, S. (Eds.). (2017). *NANDA International, Inc. Nursing Diagnoses: Definitions and Classification 2018–2020, Eleventh Edition* © 2017 NANDA International, ISBN 978-1-62623-929-6. Oxford, Wiley Blackwell.

King, M. A. (2011). Parish nursing: Holistic care in faith communities. *Holistic Nursing Practice*, *25*(6), 309–315.

King, M. A., & Tessaro, I. (2009). Parish nursing: Promoting healthy lifestyles in the church. *Journal of Christian Nursing*, *26*(1), 22–24.

LaManna, J. B., Bushy, A., Norris, A. E., Chase, S. K. (2016). Early and intermediate hospital-to-home transition outcomes of older adults diagnosed with diabetes. *The Diabetes Educator*, *42*(1), 72–86.

Martin, K. (2005). The Omaha System: *A Key to Practice, Documentation, and Information Management* (Reprinted 2nd ed). Omaha, NE: Health Connections Press. ISBN no. 978-0-9825727-1-9.

McGinnis, S. L., & Zoske, F. M. (2008). The emerging role of faith community nurses in prevention and management of chronic disease. *Policy, Politics & Nursing*, *9*(3), 173–180.

Mendelson, S. G., McNeese-Smith, D., Koniak-Griffin, D., Nyamathi, A., & Lu, M. C. (2008). A community-based parish nurse intervention program for Mexican American women with gestational diabetes. *Journal of Obstetric, Gynecologic and Neonatal Nursing*, *37*, 415–425.

Miller, S., & Carson, S. (2010). A documentation approach for faith community nursing. *Creative Nursing*, *16*(3), 122–131.

Moorhead, S., Johnson, M., Maas, M. L., & Swanson, E. (Eds.). (2008). *Nursing outcomes classification (NOC)* (4th ed.). St. Louis, MO: Elsevier.

Mosack, V., Medvene, L. J., & Wescott, J. (2006). Differences between parish nurses and parish nurse associates: Results of a statewide survey of an ecumenical network. *Public Health Nursing*, *23*(4), 347–353.

Newlin, K., Dyess, S. M., Allard, E., Chase, S., & Melkus, G. (2011). A methodological review of faith-based health promotion literature: Advancing the science to expand delivery of diabetes education to Black Americans. *Journal of Religion and Health*, *51*(4), 1075–1097.

O'Brien, M. E. (2006). Parish nursing: Meeting spiritual needs of elders near the end of life. *Journal of Christian Nursing*, *23*(1), 28–33.

Patillo, M. M., Chesley, D., Castles, P., & Sutter, R. (2002). Faith community nursing: Parish nursing/health ministry collaboration model in central Texas. *Family & Community Health*, *25*(3), 41–51.

Rydholm, L. (2006). Documenting the value of faith community nursing: 1. Saving hundreds, making cents: A study of current realities. *Creative Nursing*, *12*(2), 10–12.

Rydholm, L., Moone, R., Thornquist, L., Alexander, W., Gustafson, V., & Speece B. (2008). Care of community-dwelling older adults by Faith Community Nurses. *Journal of Gerontological Nursing*, *34*(4), 18–29.

Solari-Twadell, P. A. (2002). The differentiation of the ministry of parish nursing practice within congregations (Unpublished dissertation). Loyola University of Chicago.

Solari-Twadell, P. A., & Hackbarth, D. P. (2010). Evidence for a new paradigm of the ministry of parish nursing practice using the nursing intervention classification system. *Nursing Outlook*, *58*, 69–75.

Solari-Twadell, P. A., & McDermott, M. (Eds). (1999). *Parish nursing: Promoting whole person health within faith communities.* Thousand Oaks, CA: Sage Publishing.

Topaz, M., Golfenshtein, N., & Bowles, K.H. (2014). The Omaha system: A systematic review of the recent literature. *Journal of the American Informatics Association, 21*(1), 163–170.

Tuck, I., & Wallace, D. C. (2000). Exploring parish nursing from an ethnographic perspective. *Journal of Transcultural Nursing, 11*(4), 290–299.

U. S. Department of Health and Human Services. (n.d.). Healthy People *2020*. Retrieved April 28, 2009, from http://www.healthypeople.gov/

Wallace, D. C., Tuck, I., Boland, C. S., & Witucki, J. M. (2002). Client perceptions of parish nursing. *Public Health Nursing, 19*(2), 128–135.

Weis, D. M., Schank, M. J., Coenen, A., & Matheus, R. (2002). Parish nurse practice with client aggregates. *Journal of Community Health Nursing, 19*(2), 105–113.

24

Palliative and End-of-Life Care

Patricia Tabloski

DYING

The sun kept setting, setting still;
No hue of afternoon
Upon the village I perceived,—
From house to house 't was noon.
The dusk kept dropping, dropping still;
No dew upon the grass,
But only on my forehead stopped,
And wandered in my face.

My feet kept drowsing, drowsing still
My fingers were awake;
Yet why so little sound myself
Unto my seeming make?
How well I knew the light before!
I could not see it now.
'T is dying, I am doing; but
I'm not afraid to know.

—Emily Dickinson

CHAPTER HIGHLIGHTS

- Social trends in aging and dying
- Palliative and hospice care for persons across the lifespan
- Caring for a person at the end of life
- Strategies for managing pain and common symptoms

OBJECTIVES

- Describe the role of the community health nurse in providing quality end-of-life care for seriously ill persons and their families.
- Recognize changes in demographics, economics, and service delivery that require improved nursing interventions at the end of life.
- Identify the diverse settings for end-of-life care and the role of the nurse in each setting.
- Describe how pain and presence of troublesome symptoms affect the dying person.
- Explore pharmacologic and alternative methods of treating pain.
- Identify the signs of approaching death.
- Describe appropriate nursing interventions when caring for the dying.
- Describe postmortem care.
- Discuss family support during the grief and bereavement period.

KEY TERMS

Adjuvant drugs: Medications used along with analgesics to increase the effectiveness of the drugs to treat pain and associated symptoms.

Advance directives: Documents signed by a person indicating his or her choice or wishes for medical treatment or naming of another to make choices if the person is unable to do so.

Bereavement: A period of time or state of mind where feelings of loss, grief, or mourning are experienced by the survivor after the death of a loved one.

Breakthrough pain: Pain that is experienced despite the fact that a person is receiving scheduled pain relief medication.

Comfort measures only (CMO): A plan of care that specifies nursing interventions designed not to treat disease but to improve pain, function, or quality of life.

Grief: Feelings of despair, sadness, and remorse in response to the loss of a loved one.

Healthcare proxy: A person designated to make healthcare decisions for another in the event that he or she is unable to make such decisions because of illness or disability.

Hospice care: Care of persons and families who have 6 months or less to live in what they consider their home.

Mourning: The outward social expressions of loss

often dictated by cultural norms, customs, rituals, and tradition.

Palliative care: Interdisciplinary team-based care for persons and family members experiencing life-threatening illness or injury that addresses their physical, emotional, social, and spiritual needs.

Postmortem care: Care provided by nurses to the body after death.

CASE STUDY *References to the case study are found throughout this chapter (look for the case study icon). Readers should keep the case study in mind as they read the chapter.*

Louise Clark is an 86-year-old woman who has just been discharged from a long-term care facility to her home. She spent 3 weeks at the facility after a 6-day acute care hospitalization for pneumonia and weight loss. Mrs. Clark, whose husband died 10 years ago, now lives alone with the help of her daughter, Mary, who lives nearby. Mary helps with cooking, shopping, and cleaning but is feeling overwhelmed; she is concerned that her mother may need more day-to-day assistance but does not want to consider permanent nursing home placement at this time.

Mrs. Clark has been diagnosed with several chronic conditions common to older persons, including macular degeneration, heart failure, and atrial fibrillation. The drugs and all the care related to these conditions were prescribed by primary care and emergency department physicians from whom she has received care over the last several years.

It is apparent to Mrs. Clark's family that she is failing and seems to be on a downhill trajectory, but her physician continues to state that "she is doing just fine for a woman her age." Mrs. Clark has named her daughter Mary as her healthcare proxy but has never given her specific information about the kind of care she would like as she gets older, other than to say she does not want to suffer needless pain and medical intervention

near the end of her life as her husband did the year before he died.

Mrs. Clark received home care visits to assess and monitor her cardiovascular status. Her functional status has varied and at times she has been unable to leave her home without much effort. A home care nurse came to visit her for 2 months and then referred her to the local elder care services to acquire homemaker and home health aide assistance with bathing, meals, and light housekeeping. Mrs. Clark has had two emergency department visits and three admissions to the acute care hospital in the last year. These visits were related to falls, exacerbation of heart failure, and pneumonia. After each hospitalization, Mrs. Clark improved but never returned to her prehospitalization function.

Mary is concerned that it is now less safe for her mom to live at home alone despite the help of her family and professional services and feels that more services are required to ensure her mom's safety. She was told that in order to qualify for more services she would need to become Medicaid eligible by "spending down" to $2,000 in order to receive the additional care she needed. Mrs. Clark is hesitant to spend down as she wanted to leave a small inheritance to her daughter.

NURSING AND PERSONS WITH CHRONIC DISEASE

Something began me
And it had no beginning
Something will end me
And it has no end.
Carl Sandburg

The number of adults of all ages in the United States with chronic progressive illness is growing dramatically. Approximately one half of adults (about 117 million people) have one or more chronic health conditions. Additionally, one in four adults have two or more chronic conditions, many of which are considered disabling (Ward, Schiller, & Goodman, 2014). Greater numbers of vulnerable adults and children with multiple chronic conditions are residing in the community, resulting in such problems as strained caregiver systems, shortages of homecare workers and supportive services, increasing numbers of frail older adults with limited decision-making capacity, and dwindling financial resources (Ringer, Hazzan, Agarwal, Mutsaers, & Papaioannou, 2017). Community- and home-based end-of-life palliative care and hospice services are necessary because of an increase in the aging population, an increase in the number of people who wish to receive advanced care and die in their own homes, and a decrease in the number of family caregivers available for care (Ringer, et al., 2017). Strained family caregivers are documented to be at increased risk of depression, financial strain, and diminished quality of life.

In its publication *Dying in America: Improving Quality and Honoring Individual Preferences Near the End of Life* (2015), the Institute of Medicine (IOM) summarized key issues facing seriously ill and dying persons receiving care at the end of life. The report warned of the dangers associated with current end-of-life care including increasing medicalization of natural death, depersonalization of the dying, and rising costs and patient burden resulting from overly aggressive and/or futile care. Many medical centers currently provide palliative care services to their seriously ill patients but community-based palliative care programs are often not part of the integrated health system and a gap in care exists for many persons after discharge to the community. This is especially true if the person does not meet hospice admission criteria. To qualify for hospice care, the person must be expected to live for 6 months or less and agree to forgo aggressive disease treatment. However, palliative care is applicable early in the course of illness and can be delivered in conjunction with other therapies that are intended to prolong life, such as chemotherapy or radiation therapy, and includes testing needed to better understand and manage distressing clinical complications (World Health Organization [WHO], 2017). Key concepts of both hospice and palliative care include compassionate care delivered by a highly functional expert interprofessional team, holistic focus, emphasis on pain management and symptom control, and focus on improvement of quality of life.

In 2015, 94% of hospice patients were 65 years of age or older and more than 47% were 85 years of age or older. The median length of care in hospice was 23 days. Pediatric patients (younger than 24 years of age) and younger adults (25 to 64 years of age) accounted for approximately 5% of hospice admissions (National Hospice and Palliative Care Organization [NHPCO], 2016). Cancer was the most common principle diagnosis accounting for more than 27% of the persons receiving care. It is thought that younger adults and children with life-threatening or life-limiting conditions are often not referred for hospice care for a variety of reasons, including patient, family, and caregiver's fear of acknowledging the seriousness of the underlying condition, lack of knowledge regarding the services and benefits offered by a pediatric hospice, scarcity of hospices offering

pediatric services, and lack of reimbursement by many insurance companies (Center to Advance Palliative Care [CAPC], 2017). However, with the passage of the Patient Protection and Affordable Care Act of 2010, hospice care for children was expanded and children who are enrolled in the Medicaid or Children's Health Insurance Program (CHIP) hospice benefit may continue to receive care for their terminal condition. This change in pediatric hospice eligibility signaled a potential increase in demand for pediatric hospice services, however currently only 28% of hospices provide community-based services to children and the average number of pediatric patients cared for ranged from 0 to 10 patients per year (NHPCO, 2015). See Table 24.1 for core components of pediatric palliative and hospice care.

Because of nursing's holistic focus, nurses in all settings, including community health nurses, are uniquely qualified to provide comprehensive, effective, compassionate, and cost-effective care to persons at the end of life. The Hospice and Palliative Nurses Association (HPNA, 2015) has issued a position statement declaring that professional nursing care is critical to achieving goals of care at the end of life, and that support of hospice and palliative care research and education is necessary to ensure delivery of such care.

Among the members of the healthcare team, nurses spend the most time and have the most frequent and continuous contact with patients and families at the end of life (American Nurses Association [ANA], 2016; HPNA, 2015). Patients of all ages and their families look to their nurse to educate, support, and guide them throughout serious illness and, if need be, the dying process. This intimate position allows the nurse to advocate for improved quality of life for the person with serious illness. According to HPNA (2015), "when faced with serious illness, people turn to professional nurses for education, support, and guidance" (p. 2). Informed understanding of the person's values, wishes, and goals allows the nurse to attend to each person's physical, emotional, psychosocial, and spiritual needs.

TABLE 24.1 Core Components of Pediatric Palliative and Hospice Care
• Patient- and family-centered care
• Respecting and partnering with patients and families
• Pursuing care that is high quality, readily accessible, and equitable
• Providing care across the age span and life span, integrated into the continuum of care
• Ensuring that all clinicians can provide basic palliative care and consult specialists in a timely manner
• Improving care through research and quality improvement efforts

Source: American Academy of Pediatrics, 2013.

Evidence for Practice

A systematic literature review surveying the unmet needs of persons receiving palliative care and their caregivers who received home-based palliative care services was conducted to identify ways care can be improved. The most frequently reported unmet need was effective communication with and between healthcare professionals. The researchers found that lack of communication negatively impacted the psychosocial care received by seriously ill persons and their caregivers. Physical care needs were met, indicating that the palliative home care services were delivering satisfactory care in this domain, but could improve communication to prevent or reduce suffering in areas such as psychosocial domains (Ventura, Burney, Brooker, Fletcher, & Ricciardelli, 2013). Quality of life issues that are crucial to address include self-esteem, adaptation to illness, social functioning, relationships, and spirituality.

Failure to acknowledge the presence and nature of distress experienced by seriously ill persons and their families may result in fragmentation of care, anxiety, and discomfort. Aggressive treatment of one condition may exacerbate the optimal functioning of other health problems. Through specialized end-of-life education with emphasis on therapeutic communication and pain and symptom management, the community health nurse can foster comfort and dignity for seriously ill persons, as well as for those with life-threatening illness; clarify goals of care; decrease unnecessary hospitalization; and prevent the administration of futile, aggressive end-of-life care.

Seriously ill persons and their families look to nurses to educate, support, and guide them throughout the illness trajectory. This intimate position allows nurses to advocate for improved quality of life for people with serious illness. According to HPNA (2015), "achieving quality of life, especially at the end of life, is contingent upon competent, 'state of the art' professional nursing care." Informed understanding of the individual's values, wishes, and goals allows nurses to attend to the physical, emotional, psychosocial, and spiritual needs of each person.

> Let us live so that when we come to die even the undertaker will be sorry. **Mark Twain**

Student Reflection

I was assigned to visit Mrs. Clark during my community health rotation with my preceptor, Julie, an experienced home care nurse. At first I was frightened.

I thought such a frail older person should be in the hospital, where she could be safe and nurses could look after her 24 hours a day. Julie explained to me that caring for older persons at the end of their lives is complicated; nurses can provide physical care and manage pain and symptoms in the home while attending to the psychological, social, and spiritual needs of the older adult and the family. Hospice and palliative care services can offer a number of benefits to frail persons living at home, including access to a multidisciplinary team skilled in the management of pain and symptoms that often accompany advanced disease. After Julie discussed the possibility of a hospice referral with Mrs. Clark and her daughter, everyone (including me) felt a lot better.

Hospice and palliative care nurses acknowledge and accept death as a natural process and realize that they can be instrumental in helping people achieve the kind of death they desire. Obtaining the services needed to promote safety can help alleviate the fears of professional and lay caregivers, and persons residing in their homes in need of skilled nursing services will benefit from appropriate referrals and visiting nurse services. In addition, chronically ill persons may benefit from friendly visitor programs, home-delivered meals, community-based van or transportation services, and homemaker services. A person receiving hospice care has access to additional services. Typically, hospice provides for home health aide five times a week for people with Medicare or who have private insurance with a hospice benefit in place. In 1982, the Medicare Hospice Benefit was enacted and authorized care in the person's home, and in 2015 Medicare spending per person receiving benefits was $11,510 (NHPCO, 2016). In 2015, close to 25% of Medicare hospice spending was for persons with the principle diagnosis of dementia. Close to 45% of deaths of persons in hospice care occurred in the home, 32% in nursing facilities, 15% in inpatient hospices, and 8% in acute care hospitals. The Centers for Medicare & Medicaid Services' definition of hospice is presented in Box 24.1. Seriously ill persons can access Medicare hospice benefits if they meet *all* of the conditions listed in Box 24.2.

Generally, hospice care includes services that are reasonable and necessary for the comfort and management of a terminal illness. According to the NHPCO (2017), the 10 components of quality in hospice care include the following:

- **Patient- and-Family-Centered Care**
  Providing care and services that are responsive to the needs and exceed the expectations of those served.
- **Ethical Behavior and Consumer Rights**
  Upholding high standards of ethical conduct and advocating for the rights of patients and their family caregivers.

24.1 Definition of Hospice

- Hospice provides comfort and support services to people who are terminally ill. It helps them live out the time they have remaining to the fullest extent possible.
- Hospice care is provided by a specially trained team that cares for the "whole person," including his or her physical, emotional, social, and spiritual needs.
- Hospice provides support to family members caring for a terminally ill person.
- Hospice is generally given in the home.
- Hospice services may include drugs, physical care, counseling, equipment, and supplies for the terminal and related condition(s).
- Hospice is not only for people with cancer.
- Hospice does not shorten or prolong life.
- Hospice focuses on comfort, not on curing an illness.

Source: National Hospice and Palliative Care Organization. (2013). *NHPCO facts and figures: Hospice care in America.* Alexandria, VA: NHCPO.

- **Clinical Excellence and Safety**
  Ensuring clinical excellence and promoting safety through standards of practice.
- **Inclusion and Access**
  Promoting inclusiveness in the community by ensuring that all people—regardless of race, ethnicity, color, religion, gender, disability, sexual orientation, age, or other characteristics—have access to programs and services.
- **Organizational Excellence**
  Building a culture of quality and accountability within our organization that values collaboration and communication and ensures ethical business practices.
- **Workforce Excellence**
  Fostering a collaborative, interdisciplinary environment that promotes inclusion, individual accountability, and

24.2 Conditions That Must Be Met to Obtain Medicare Hospice Benefits

- The patient is eligible for Medicare Part A (Hospital Insurance).
- A physician and the hospice medical director certify that the patient is terminally ill and has 6 months or less to live if the illness runs its normal course.
- The patient signs a statement choosing hospice care instead of other Medicare-covered benefits to treat the terminal illness. Medicare will still pay for covered benefits and treatment of any other health problems not related to the terminal illness.
- The patient receives care from a Medicare-approved hospice program.

Source: Center for Medicare and Medicaid Services (2018). *Medicare Hospice Benefits.* Retrieved from https://www.medicare.gov/Pubs/pdf/02154-Medicare-Hospice-Benefits.pdf.

workforce excellence through professional development, training, and support to all staff and volunteers.
- **Standards**
  Adopting the NHPCO Standards of Practice for Hospice Programs and/or the National Consensus Project's Clinical Practice Guidelines for Quality Palliative Care as the foundation for an organization.
- **Compliance With Laws and Regulations**
  Ensuring compliance with all applicable laws, regulations, and professional standards of practice, and implementing systems and processes that prevent fraud and abuse.
- **Stewardship and Accountability**
  Developing a qualified and diverse governance structure and senior leadership who share the responsibilities of fiscal and managerial oversight.
- **Performance Measurement**
  Collecting, analyzing, and actively using performance measurement data to foster quality assessment and performance improvement in all areas of care and services (NHPCO, 2017).

> Hospice does not speed up or slow down the dying process. It does not prolong life and it does not hasten death.
> **National Hospice Foundation**

Healthcare reform and benefits covered by Medicare are currently under debate in the U.S. Congress; therefore, it is wise to visit the Medicare website (http://www.medicare.gov) and/or consult with a knowledgeable social worker to obtain the most current and accurate information regarding services covered. The healthcare reform act has expanded services covered under the hospice benefit in an effort to improve care of the person nearing the end of life. At present, a person can get Medicare hospice benefits when they meet all of the following conditions:

- They are eligible for Medicare Part A (Hospital Insurance).
- The physician or nurse practitioner and the hospice medical director certify that the person is terminally ill and has 6 months or less to live if the illness runs its normal course.
- The person accepts comfort care rather than curative care.
- The person signs a statement choosing hospice care instead of other Medicare-covered treatments for terminal illness or other related conditions.

Medicare covers the following hospice services when they are needed to care for the person with terminal illness and related condition(s):

- Doctor services
- Nursing care
- Medical equipment (such as wheelchairs or walkers)
- Medical supplies (such as bandages and catheters)
- Drugs for symptom control or pain relief (may require a small co-payment)

- Hospice aide and homemaker services
- Physical and occupational therapy
- Speech–language pathology services
- Social worker services
- Dietary counseling
- Grief and loss counseling for the ill person and family
- Short-term inpatient care (for pain and symptom management)
- Short-term respite care (may require a small co-payment)
- Any other Medicare-covered services needed to manage pain and other symptoms related to the terminal illness, as recommended by the hospice team (Medicare.gov, 2017)

Palliative care for children can reduce a child's pain, help manage other distressing symptoms, and provide important emotional support to the child and family throughout the course of an illness. Research has shown that pediatric palliative care services may also increase overall satisfaction with care for patients and their families. Yet, many healthcare providers continue to hesitate to recommend palliative care for the youngest patients, and parents and caregivers are often unaware of its benefits (National Institutes of Health, 2014). See Box 24.3 for Pediatric Palliative Care Referral Criteria.

Viewing death as a natural process, not a medical failure, is of utmost importance. Some caregivers consider that death is not normal and when it occurs, someone is at fault. Of course, nurses know that this is not true; in many serious progressive illnesses, death is an expected outcome. Nurses who help patients die comfortably and with dignity provide the following principles of quality person-centered care (National Consensus Project [NCP] for Quality Palliative Care, 2013):

- Providing care and services that are responsive to the needs and exceed the expectations of those we serve.

24.3 Pediatric Palliative Care Referral Criteria

- Perinatal/neonatal: Life-threatening diagnoses made months to hours before birth of the neonate in the few days, weeks, or months of life
- Neurologic conditions: Hypoxic injury, birth trauma, structural malformation of the CNS, metabolic diseases, genetic or congenital syndromes
- Congenital heart defects: Ventricle malformation, pulmonary vein stenosis, cardiomyopathy, pulmonary hypertension, coarctation of the aorta, posttransplant care
- Other diagnoses: Cystic fibrosis, solid organ transplant, oncology, primary immunodeficiency disorders, acquired immunodeficiency disorder, acute leukemia

Source: Adapted from Stroupe, L. M. (2013). Process improvement for pediatric supportive care. *Journal of Hospice and Palliative Nursing*, *15*(8), 479–484.

- The ill person and family compose the unit of care.
- The hospice interdisciplinary team, in collaboration with the patient, family, and caregiver, develops and maintains a person-, family-, and caregiver-directed, individualized, safe, and coordinated plan of palliative care.
- Addressing loss, grief, and bereavement needs begins with the initial assessment at the time of admission to the hospice and continues throughout the course of care.
- Anticipatory mourning services are provided to help patients, families, and caregivers cope with the multitude of losses that occur during the illness and eventual death of the patient. Bereavement services are provided after death and are based on a number of factors, including a bereavement risk assessment which assesses intensity of grief, coping and adapting abilities of the survivors and their individual needs, and the benefits and burdens of treatment.

To supply this care, nurses must be well educated, have appropriate supports in the clinical setting, and develop a close collaborative partnership with palliative care service providers and hospice programs.

Student Reflection

I was amazed at how quickly my home health nurse preceptor mobilized community-based resources. After making several phone calls to her professional colleagues (all of whom she knew by their first names!), she was quickly able to get the needed services in place. It really illustrated the importance of communication and teamwork.

Nurses must be confident in their clinical skills when caring for the dying—awareness of the ethical, spiritual, and legal issues they may confront while providing end-of-life care is essential. Many nurses believe that the first step in the process is confronting their own personal fears about death and dying. By addressing their own fears, nurses are better able to help seriously ill persons and families when they are confronted with impending death. The nurse may then more objectively recognize and respect the person's and family's values and choices which guide their decisions at the end of life. Table 24.2 identifies common problems that interfere with quality end-of-life nursing care.

DEATH IN THE UNITED STATES
Stages in the Dying Process

Elisabeth Kübler-Ross, a psychiatrist at the University of Chicago, was also a pioneer for end-of-life care; the early hospice movement was supported by her research. Kübler-Ross (1969) interviewed hundreds of dying persons and published her findings in *On Death and Dying: What the Dying*

TABLE 24.2 Problems That Interfere With Quality End-of-Life Community-Based Nursing Care

Problem	Potential Outcomes
The community health nurse may hesitate to discuss a hospice referral.	Hospice services are not initiated in a timely manner; may come too late to initiate advanced care planning and to support end-of-life choices.
The patient has not discussed his or her end-of-life preferences for care.	Professional caregivers and families may not have the appropriate information to institute a plan of care that meets the patient's expectations, including provision of appropriate interventions.
Financial matters and insurance approvals have not been obtained.	Needed services may be denied or delayed by a lengthy appeal process.
Funeral wishes, organ donation, and establishment of a will have not been specified.	Same-sex partners may be excluded from involvement, valuable organs are not available to others in need, and families may argue over inheritance and disposition of property.

Have to Teach Doctors, Nurses, Clergy, and Their Own Families. It was through her efforts that healthcare providers began to understand the needs of dying persons. Her work also emphasized the need for pain relief in terminally ill persons. The outcome of this research was the development of the "stages of dying." These stages include denial, anger, bargaining, and acceptance. It must be remembered that a dying person may not exhibit all of these stages, or may move quickly through a stage, only to return to it at a later time.

Evidence for Practice

Although Kübler-Ross' framework stimulated research and changed practice in the field of end-of-life care, the concept may not be as simple as described. Today, not all researchers agree with Kübler-Ross, and some claim that her research cannot be replicated (Konigsberg, 2011). Today, there are over 25 instruments widely used to measure grief, and each one differs from the other. It is difficult to categorize and synthesize all of the current research, most of which tends to describe complex and unique emotional responses to grief. Nurses will often find they need to think beyond the basic five stages.

Specialized Care at the End of Life

During the mid-1900s, technologic advances dictated that sick people should go to hospitals where they could safely receive "high-tech" care. Surgery, antibiotics, and advanced testing techniques became the focus of healthcare, shifting away from the provision of care to the pursuit of cure. Table 24.3 illustrates the changing demographic and social trends surrounding the cause of death in the years 1900 and 2015. In 2014, the 10 leading causes of death, accounting for 80% of all death in the United States, include heart disease, malignant neoplasms, chronic lower respiratory disease, accidents, stroke, Alzheimer disease, diabetes mellitus, influenza and pneumonia, renal disease, and suicide

TABLE 24.3 Cause of Death and Demographic/Social Trends

	1900	2015
Focus of care	Comfort	Cure
Primary cause of death	Infectious diseases—e.g., pneumonia, influenza	Chronic illnesses—e.g., heart disease, cancer
Average life expectancy	50 years	78.8 years
Number of older persons (>65)	3.1 million	467.8 million
Place of death	Home	Institutions
Caregivers	Family	Professional healthcare providers
Disease trajectory	Short, downward trend	Prolonged, variable, peaks and valleys
Functional decline at the end of life	Short-term—expected and surprise	Lingering expected—frailty

Source: Centers for Disease Control and Prevention. (2017). *FastStats: Death and mortality*. Retrieved from http://www.cdc.gov/nchs/fastats.death.htm.

(Centers for Disease Control and Prevention [CDC], 2017a). Often, the exact cause of death is difficult to determine in seriously ill adults. The person with Alzheimer disease may fall, fracture a hip, and die shortly after the injury. However, the actual cause of the fall may have been a myocardial infarction that was not detected. The death certificate may indicate a fall or Alzheimer disease as the cause of death, whereas the true cause was the myocardial infarction. Some people think that these difficult-to-categorize deaths may be deemed "natural deaths" or deaths that occur because of numerous unspecified causes, including advanced age, organ failure, and impact of comorbidities.

In children in 2014, the main causes of death for those aged 1 to 4 years were accidents, congenital malformations, and assault due to homicide, and for those aged 5 to 14 years causes of death included accidents, cancer, and suicide (CDC, 2017b). Infant mortality rates have declined from 2005 to 2014 by 15%. The poisoning death rate among teens aged 15 to 19 years nearly doubled, from 1.7 to 4.2 per 100,000, in part because of an increase in prescription drug overdoses (e.g., opioid pain relievers). Childhood motor vehicle traffic-related death rates declined 41%; however, these deaths remain the leading cause of death by unintentional injury. Malignant neoplasms, heart disease, congenital anomalies, sudden infant death syndrome, homicide, and suicide remain significant threats to the health of children and adolescents. It is thought that 25% of all childhood deaths are preventable (NHPCO, 2015).

In the past century, social changes and technologic advancements had shifted the goals of modern healthcare from care to cure. Over the decades, the experience of serious illness, death, and dying in the United States has evolved. What was once a short, rapid decline, which often occurred in the relative comfort of one's own home, now encompasses a trajectory of chronic illness with steady decline, periodic crises, the need for ongoing aggressive treatment, and finally death. Adults with chronic and progressive illnesses often lack coordinated care, with multiple episodic and unplanned emergency department visits which focus on single systems, quick diagnosis, and cure. As a result, seriously ill adults are at risk for polypharmacy, falls, functional decline, and institutionalization (NHPCO, 2017).

Mrs. Clark has stated that she feels as if she is on a merry-go-round because she is in and out of the hospital so often. She says "I never want to go back to the cold, noisy hospital again. Please help me stay here in my home with my TV, my cats, and my memories."

NURSING CARE WHEN DEATH IS IMMINENT

Hospice care can be provided in many settings, including the person's home, hospital, nursing home, assisted-living facility, and inpatient hospice facility. When surveyed, most Americans express a preference to die in their own homes; however, many still die in institutional settings (NHPCO, 2017). However, the past 20 years have seen a shift in the trends in place of death, with increasing numbers of people dying in their homes and long-term care settings, and decreasing numbers of people dying in the hospital.

Not only are fewer people dying in the hospital, older adults are spending less time in the hospital at the end of life. A recent report of the Dartmouth Atlas Project revealed that the average number of days older adults spend in the hospital before death, as well as the percentage of deaths associated with an intensive care stay, has declined in recent years (The Dartmouth Institute for Health Policy and Clinical Practice, 2013). The report also demonstrated that increasing numbers of older adults are choosing hospice care at the end of life.

Data from numerous studies demonstrate high degrees of symptom distress in persons in hospitals and nursing homes; high use of burdensome technologies in seriously ill persons; caregiver burden on families; and communication problems among ill persons, families, and caregivers about the goals of care and medical decisions that should follow (Last Acts, 2002; NHPCO, 2017; Quill, 2000; SUPPORT Principal Investigators, 1995). Seriously ill persons who die at home avoid some of these problems. However, the reality of dying at home is often more complicated. Family caregivers are often stressed or may not be ever present; the home environment may be small, chaotic, or even unsafe; symptom control may be more difficult; and the provision of basic nursing care such as bathing and grooming may be difficult for ill persons and caregivers. Additionally, some caregivers and seriously ill persons may prefer more supportive inpatient care at the end of life (Lysaght & Ersek, 2013).

It requires more courage to suffer than to die.
Napoleon Bonaparte

Evidence for Practice

Research at the Dartmouth Atlas for Healthcare has provided evidence that populations living in regions with lower intensity of care in the last 6 months of life did not have higher mortality rates than those living in regions with higher care intensity. More than 80% of ill persons say that they wish to avoid hospitalization and intensive care during the terminal phase of illness, but those wishes are often overridden by other factors. If more intense intervention does not improve life expectancy, and if most ill persons prefer less care when more intensive care is likely to be futile, the fundamental question is whether the quality of care in regions with fewer resources and more conservative practice styles is more appropriate than in regions where more aggressive treatment is the norm (The Dartmouth Institute for Health Policy and Clinical Practice, 2013). All healthcare providers, including nurses, must work together and advocate for improvement in the quality of care provided at the end of life.

Decisions About Level of Care

Wherever seriously ill persons spend their last days, these persons and their families face difficult decisions about end-of-life care. Uncertain prognoses may affect decision making on the part of these persons, their families, and their healthcare providers, which perhaps leads to unnecessary interventions and treatments. Older people, especially, are at risk for overly aggressive care because they have high comorbidity rates and an increased likelihood of dementia (Ward et al., 2014). For some older persons, medical treatments offer little or no benefit, and at the same time may be painful or increase the burden of living; such care may be futile. Nurses, physicians, social workers, clergy, and others are responsible for counseling ill persons and families about making decisions regarding the type and level of care the person wishes to receive for the remainder of his/her life. After the decision has been reached, it is usually noted in the person's chart by the nurse or any other member of the healthcare team, so that the entire healthcare team is aware of the person's wishes. Of course, the ill person is always able to reverse these decisions.

Comfort Measures Only

A dying person may decide to receive **comfort measures only (CMO)**—that is, allow death to occur naturally while maximizing comfort. CMO is the preferred choice when the person confronts his or her mortality and considers less aggressive treatment. A nurse should review the use of life-sustaining technologies with the seriously ill person. Those persons who wish to have CMO may receive traditional hospice care, with healthcare professionals focused on quality of life rather than on the length of life.

The physician or advanced practice nurse usually orders CMO when the ill person, family, and staff are in agreement that the best care for the person is not to prolong the dying process, but to keep the dying person comfortable. Comfort becomes the focus of care when cure is no longer an attainable goal, expected quality of life is unacceptable, and comfort is a priority for the dying person and family (Moneymaker, 2005). This does not mean that nursing care or treatments stop. Assessment and management of any physical conditions, activities of daily living, and behaviors, as well as pain, continue on a daily basis. Provision of excellent nursing care at the end of life can be a challenge, especially when the family has been told by the physician that "nothing more can be done." The designation of a person as CMO does not signal the end of care, but rather shifts the focus of care from aggressive treatment of the disease to active nursing interventions to improve function, comfort, and quality of life.

Advance Directives

Many Americans are fearful of death and hesitate to discuss end-of-life preferences with their families and significant others. This can be problematic when the person becomes very ill or incapacitated, and the healthcare professionals consult for assistance in medical decision making. People of all ages should begin to discuss these issues with others who may be called on to make decisions in the case of serious illness or injury. This should occur in a noncrisis situation when the person has time to discuss the issue in depth, ask questions, and think about the risks and benefits of various interventions. Personal values, past experiences, cultural beliefs, religious preferences, medical knowledge, family orientation, and life experiences all help determine the end-of-life preferences. Each person and his or her family should provide input into treatment decisions which are then based on goals of care, assessment of risk and benefit, best evidence, and personal preferences.

Advance directives are legal documents that allow people to convey their wishes for end-of-life care and include living wills, durable powers of attorney for healthcare, and healthcare proxies. Legal requirements for advance directives vary from state to state; some state laws mandate the use of living wills, and others require designation of a healthcare proxy or durable power of attorney for healthcare. All of these documents go into effect when the person is no longer able to communicate his or her wishes. Living wills are documents in which persons describe their wishes regarding treatment intended to sustain life. This may include acceptance or limitation of life-sustaining treatment in the face of a life-threatening illness. It is necessary to copy a living will and share it with others; the physician, nurse, family members, and significant others should have copies and should indicate their willingness to comply with the terms stated therein. Many people place the living will in a safety deposit box so that others, who may not wish to honor it, cannot gain access to it. A **healthcare proxy** or durable power of attorney for healthcare is a person (and an alternate if the primary proxy is not available) designated to make decisions for the person if he or she is unable to do so. The person should then discuss his or her wishes with the proxy to ensure appropriate end-of-life care. The healthcare proxy is responsible for medical decisions only if the ill person is unable to do this, and does not have legitimate input into any other areas of the person's affairs (e.g., financial). It is necessary to make multiple copies of the proxy form, and healthcare providers and family members (including proxies) should keep them readily accessible.

Decision making around the time of death raises many legal and ethical questions. Public debate and scrutiny help shape the ethical outcome of medical dilemmas. Healthcare professionals must work within the limits of the law and their professional standards of practice. Established ethical principles and moral norms play a vital role in determining healthcare issues.

In 1976, the Karen Ann Quinlan case brought life-sustaining medical treatment to the forefront of the U.S. legal system. A medical intervention, procedure, or administration of medicine to prevent the moment of death is seen as life sustaining. This includes cardiopulmonary resuscitation (CPR), renal dialysis, use of ventilators, insertion of feeding tubes, total parenteral nutrition, chemotherapies, and other life-prolonging interventions. When questions regarding the initiation, ongoing use, and removal of life-sustaining technologies arise, and there are no advance directives in place, ethical and emotional issues arise. Many healthcare institutions have formed ethics committees to address these issues and to provide guidance and advice to the clinician, ill person, and family. If the ill person lacks a responsible family member, the courts may appoint a legal guardian. This is a cumbersome and difficult process, and naming a healthcare proxy or completing a living will prevents this process.

In 1990, the U.S. Supreme Court declared that all Americans have a right to make healthcare decisions. Even if a person is deemed currently incompetent or unable to make his or her own decisions, the person's previous wishes become the determining factor concerning care. The Patient Self-Determination Act became a federal law in 1991. This act states that the person must understand that he or she may refuse medical treatment, care, procedures, medicines, and other similar procedures. It also states that all persons must receive information about their right to prepare advance directives.

Most healthcare institutions have developed policies concerning self-determination which comply with specific state laws. In order to provide proper care as determined by the state statutes, it is necessary for the interdisciplinary team to form a collaborative relationship with the ill person and family. When the ill person is unable to make decisions, the healthcare team must consider the person's diagnosis, the benefit or burden of treatment, the effect on the prognosis, and expressed verbal patient preference. Family members, other concerned people, or surrogates may take part in the decision-making process. Reevaluation must be ongoing because the person's situation changes throughout the course of illness and treatment. Although a person's decision-making capacity may be fluctuating or limited, the individual may sometimes be able to understand some aspects of the medical situation, and even express preferences through nonverbal communication.

ARTIFICIAL NUTRITION AND HYDRATION

The decision to institute artificial nutrition and hydration should take into account possible benefits and risks. It has traditionally been assumed that artificial nutrition and hydration meet several therapeutic goals: prolonging life, preventing aspiration pneumonia and "starvation," maintaining independence and physical function, improving nutritional status, assisting in healing of pressure ulcers, and decreasing suffering and discomfort at the end of life (ANA, 2017; HPNA, 2015). However, the literature does not support this. Studies have shown that nursing home residents living with feeding tubes have similar survival rates to those living without these tubes, and that aspiration rates are higher in persons with feeding tubes (Lacey, 2005). Furthermore, artificial nutrition and nutritional supplements do not enhance the strength and physical function of frail elderly people and can also cause harm due to decreased caloric needs at the end of life (ANA, 2017; HPNA, 2011). Also, contrary to expectations, most actively dying persons do not experience hunger, even if they have inadequate caloric intake. In fact, risks such as increased infection, sensory deprivation, and restraint use have led researchers and palliative care experts to discourage the use of feeding tubes in dying persons and those with advanced dementia. To explore alternatives to artificial nutrition techniques, collaboration with other healthcare professionals (nutritionists and speech therapists) is indicated.

Dying persons, who feel strongly that they do not want feeding tubes inserted, should inform their healthcare proxies, and specify this in their living wills. Administration of artificial nutrition and hydration is a medical treatment, and thus a person can accept or reject it. This right reflects respect for patient autonomy.

CARDIOPULMONARY RESUSCITATION

CPR is the process of restarting the heart and/or lungs after one or both have stopped working. Traditionally, CPR is for people who are experiencing cardiac or respiratory arrest; simply put, CPR is most successful when it occurs in the hospital, specifically in the intensive care unit. However, when the seriously ill adult is frail, has multiple chronic conditions, and is nearing the end of life, CPR is significantly less effective. Current federal law mandates that long-term care facilities must ask residents (or their surrogates) whether they wish to receive CPR in the event of a cardiac or respiratory arrest. Research on CPR performed on elderly nursing home residents consistently shows very poor outcomes. Survival following CPR is less than 5% in this population, with most studies showing 0% survival. In such persons, the poor outcome of CPR in nursing home residents and those nearing the end of life is more likely a result of the irreversibility of the underlying diseases that end in cardiopulmonary arrest (American Medical Directors Association, 2013). Deciding to put a do-not-resuscitate (DNR) order in place usually involves the ill person, his or her family, the nurse, physician, and others on the healthcare team. In most healthcare facilities, the physician or primary healthcare provider must write the DNR order in the chart for it to be legal using a standardized form such as POLST (provider order for life-sustaining treatment); if no order is written, CPR is administered by default if the need arises. It can be very upsetting for the nurse to provide CPR to a dying person, and the person may suffer injury from anoxia, broken ribs, and aspiration.

When the nurse approaches the seriously ill person and the family for clarification of the person's "code" status, it is best to discuss the issue as fully and objectively as possible. It is necessary to present the facts with empathy, and express the idea that clinicians will support whatever reasonable decision is made. This conversation should be part of an ongoing discussion of the person's wishes and goals for end-of-life care. According to the ANA, "the efficacy and desirability of CPR attempts, a balancing of benefits and burdens to the ill person, and therapeutic goals should be considered" (ANA, 2012, p. 2). The nurse should emphasize that the decision not to resuscitate is *not* condemning that person to death. Rather, the nurse is helping the person decide whether medical intervention *might* reverse the death process and even prohibit a peaceful death. The process of letting go may be painful for both the dying person and the family.

Euthanasia and Physician-Assisted Suicide

> Death is not the greatest of evils; it is worse to want to die, and not be able to. **Sophocles**

Active euthanasia, or mercy killing, is the practice of ending the life of a terminally ill person, at the request of the person, for the purpose of limiting suffering. Active euthanasia is illegal throughout most of the United States, but legislators continue to sponsor bills in support of this action, and much public debate is ongoing concerning this issue. Rarely, a medication given for pain relief may have the unintended consequence of shortening the dying person's life; however, because the intent of the medication is relief of pain and not the hastening of death, this is not considered euthanasia.

In 1994, Oregon voters approved physician-assisted suicide, which refers to a physician acting to aid a person in ending his or her life. Terminally ill residents of Oregon may receive prescriptions for lethal medications from their physician for self-administration. Currently (2018), it is legal in the states of Washington, Vermont, Oregon, California, Colorado, Washington, DC, Montana, and Hawaii (ProCon, 2018). The ANA (2013) does not endorse the concept of participation of nurses in the process of euthanasia, mercy killing, or assisted suicide.

Cultural and Religious Issues

People of many cultural backgrounds reside in the United States. Culture encompasses dimensions such as race, ethnicity, gender, age, abilities/disabilities, sexual orientation, religion and spirituality, and socioeconomic status (Cain, Surbone, Elk, and Kagawa-Singer, 2018). An ever-changing system, culture is shaped over time as beliefs, values, and lifestyle patterns are passed from generation to generation. Sensitivity and empathy are essential when caring for a dying person from a different culture. Each person is a unique individual with cultural preferences that influence the specialized needs of the person, the family, and their caregivers.

Evidence for Practice

Despite efforts to improve access to palliative care to all seriously ill persons, improvements are not reaching minority populations (Spruill, Mayer, & Hamilton, 2013). In a classic study, the SUPPORT Principal Investigators (1995) reported that the healthcare system expended fewer resources on African Americans than on others with similar disease processes. Despite a higher incidence rate of cancer, shorter survival time after diagnosis, and higher cancer death rates, African Americans made up only 8.2% of the population who used hospice in 2015, and they were less likely to use hospice services compared with other racial groups (Spruill et al., 2013). In general, some minority persons often have an underlying mistrust of the healthcare system, and the literature has frequently described cases in which African Americans desire aggressive life-sustaining interventions in the face of terminal disease. These persons may choose feeding tubes and CPR because of fears of being denied healthcare similar in scope to that of Caucasians.

Religion and spirituality play an important role in the forming of beliefs and practices which are paramount when death is imminent. Feelings of guilt, remorse, comfort, or peacefulness may all relate to religious beliefs. Religious customs are extremely important to many dying persons, and as death nears, concerns or fears may intensify. It is helpful to know a person's religious preference; the nurse should remember that each person's spiritual reactions are highly individualized. Requests by family or ill persons to seek spiritual counseling should be met with respect. Many healthcare facilities have chaplains, clergy, social workers, and others to assist staff. The nurse should ensure that spiritual care is made available to a person at the end of life.

At times, a religious belief may help the person determine the type of end-of-life care to request. The nurse must be aware of concerns the ill person may have, and respond therapeutically. The age-old question of why this is happening may take on religious tones or thoughts. The ill person may discuss or allude to punishment, atonement, God's will, or hope for a miracle. The nurse should follow the person's lead in determining spiritual needs and beliefs. Serious illnesses frequently initiate a search for life's meaning, and questions may arise regarding the person's purpose in life. Religious or spiritual beliefs may even influence the emotional response to pain.

When discussing religion or spirituality with the ill person, it is important to assist the person in seeking meaning. Nurses who believe they are unable to assist ill persons in discussions of spirituality should make referrals to others on the team who have skills and knowledge in this area.

Specific rituals and practices are found in different faiths and religions. It is common for a person of the Roman Catholic faith to wish to receive the sacrament of the anointing of the sick to give spiritual strength and prepare for death. A religious item such as a rosary or medal may bring comfort. A person who is Jewish may want to see a rabbi and participate in prayers. Burial takes place as soon as possible after death and before the Sabbath. A person who is Muslim may prefer that a family member be notified as soon as death occurs. It is best to wait for this person, since special washing and shrouding procedures should take place after death. Placement in a position that faces Mecca is sometimes preferred. If there is no family member to prepare the body, the staff may do so provided that they wear gloves. The burial of the body should occur as soon as possible, and cremation is not acceptable. Table 24.4 summarizes some religious beliefs and rituals practiced at the end of life.

PALLIATIVE CARE

Palliative care is interdisciplinary team-based care that is focused on the relief of suffering for persons with serious illness. It attempts to achieve the best possible quality of life, not only for seriously ill persons but also for their families (NHPCO, 2016). Nursing interventions which help enhance the quality of persons' lives, reduce pain and suffering, optimize functionality, and promote appropriate goal setting and decision making are integral to the provision of excellent palliative care (HPNA, 2011).

Regardless of the stage of the disease or the need for curative therapies, palliative care is appropriate for persons with life-limiting, serious illness. It may be concurrent with life-prolonging care, or may be the main focus of care (NHPCO, 2016). Although ill persons may be of any age, even children, palliative care is especially appropriate when provided to older people who have the following:

- Acute, serious, life-threatening illness (e.g., stroke, trauma, major myocardial infarction, and cancer, where

TABLE 24.4 Religion and End-of-Life Care

Religion	Belief	Ritual
Christian	Christians believe in an afterlife and the resurrection of Jesus Christ.	Catholic • Anointing the sick by a priest • Reconciliation and communion • Funeral held 2–3 days after death Protestant • No last rites • Anointing of the sick by some Others • Mormons will administer a sacrament • Jehovah's Witnesses will not receive blood transfusions • Some sects have hands-on healing techniques
Judaism	Death confers meaning to life.	Euthanasia is prohibited. Burial usually takes place within 24 hours. The funeral or shiva is held after the burial. Autopsy, organ donation, and cremation are not allowed. A rabbi is usually called when death is near.
Muslim	Muslims believe in an afterlife. The purpose of worldly life is to prepare for eternal life.	As death approaches, the patient is positioned supine facing Mecca. The room is perfumed, and anyone who is unclean leaves the room. Prayer occurs five times a day. Discussion of death and grief counseling are discouraged. Euthanasia is not allowed by law. Organ donation is allowed. Autopsy is discouraged.
Buddhist	Belief in the afterlife through the pursuit of perfection in worldly life.	End-of-life decisions are made with much family consultation. Families often do not want the patient to know the diagnosis to hide bad news. The elderly do not talk about funeral arrangements and often defer to physicians to make treatment decisions for them.

Source: Data from Cheng, B. (1997). Cultural clash between providers of majority culture and patients of Chinese culture. *Journal of Long-Term Health Care, 16,* 39–43.; Kirkwood, N. (1993). *A hospital handbook on multiculturalism and religion.* Sydney, Australia: Millennium Books.; Ross, H. (2000). Islamic tradition at the end of life. Unpublished manuscript.

cure or reversibility may or may not be a realistic goal, but the burden of treatment is high)
- Progressive chronic illness (e.g., end-stage dementia, congestive heart failure, renal or liver failure, and frailty)

Palliative care may occur in all settings, including hospitals, outpatient clinics, long-term care facilities, or the home. The person and family are supported during the dying and **bereavement**, when they may experience feelings of loss after the death of a loved one. The care provided emphasizes quality of life and living as fully as possible up until the moment of death.

The future and growth of palliative care will be largely determined by its acceptance within the medical model, and by reimbursement for palliative care services. The focus of palliative care includes the following:

- Controlling symptoms
- Coordinating care
- Reducing unnecessary tests and futile interventions
- Ongoing conversations with the ill person and family (NHPCO, 2017)

I am not afraid of death, I just don't want to be there when it happens. **Woody Allen**

HOSPICE CARE

Through expert medical care, pain and symptom management, and emotional and spiritual support, **hospice care** provides support for people in the last phase of life-limiting illness, so that they may live as fully and comfortably as possible (NHPCO, 2017). In 2014, an estimated 1.651 million persons received services from hospice. This estimate includes the following:

- 83.3% of persons died while in hospice care
- 6.3% revoked hospice care (changed their minds and opted to return to aggressive care)
- 6.9% were discharged and deemed no longer terminally ill (known as "live" discharges) (NHPCO, 2017)

The work of nurse leaders such as Florence Wald, Dame Cicely Saunders (also a physician), and Jeanne Quint Benoliel highlighted the need for "competent, expert, evidence-based care provided in a way that embodies compassion, respect for dignity, and an appreciation for the whole person and the family" (NHPCO, 2017). Another nurse leader, Harriet Goetz, published an approach to care for the dying in 1962, emphasizing therapeutic communication and symptom management techniques to provide comfort. Current standards of comprehensive and compassionate hospice and palliative nursing care are built upon the foundation of the work of these nurse leaders.

When two physicians determine that a seriously ill person has 6 months or less to live, and the dying person and family agree to provide care and comfort as opposed to aggressive medical intervention, loved ones often seek hospice. Hospice care focuses on the whole person by caring for the body, mind, and spirit. The goal is for the person to live his or her last days as fully and comfortably as possible. To achieve this goal, a multidisciplinary team of physicians, nurses, therapists, home health aides, pharmacists, pastoral counselors, social workers, and trained lay volunteers assist the family and caregivers in providing care (Fig. 24.1). The hospice nurse assumes the role of specialist in the management of pain and control of symptoms, and assesses the ill person's and family's coping mechanisms, available resources for the provision of care, the ill person's wishes, and the support systems in place.

Hospice personnel may work with caregivers and ill persons in the home, nursing homes, other long-term care settings, and hospitals. Hospitals may have affiliated hospices, and some home health agencies promote their own home care hospices. Freestanding hospices that provide a homelike atmosphere in which care is provided by trained staff at the facility are also available, and these hospices may be a good option for persons who prefer a home death but do not have the necessary resources and support to safely remain in their homes. All hospices encourage family involvement and promote death with dignity. Because the experience of the dying and death of a loved one deeply affects the family, supportive care is provided to family and caregivers throughout the illness trajectory and for a period after the death has occurred.

CARING FOR PERSONS AT THE END OF LIFE

The nurse providing quality end-of-life care to a seriously ill person and his or her family assumes the role of expert clinician. As an expert clinician, the community health nurse acts autonomously and completes physical, psychological, social, and spiritual assessments, and this nurse designs and implements plans of care (in collaboration with the ill person, family, and interdisciplinary team) to meet the ill person's needs. Many validated instruments are available for use for healthcare professionals, including instruments for the assessment of pain and symptoms, mental health and mood, meaning in life and spirituality, functional assessment, quality of life, and caregiver strain. See the Toolkit of Instruments to Measure End-of-Life Care website (http://www.chcr.brown.edu/pcoc/resourceguide/resourceguide.pdf) for online copies and instructions for use of these various instruments.

Nurses who regularly assist seriously ill persons and families to understand changes in their health status and the implications of these changes can alleviate many commonly held fears. Common fears and concerns of the dying include the following:

- Death itself
- Thoughts of a long or painful death

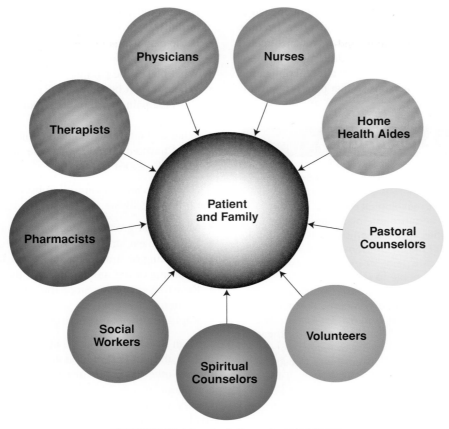

FIGURE 24.1 Interdisciplinary hospice team.

- Facing death alone
- Dying in a nursing home, hospital, or rest home
- Loss of body control, such as bowel or bladder incontinence
- Not being able to make decisions concerning care
- Loss of consciousness
- Financial costs and becoming a burden on others
- Dying before having a chance to put personal affairs in order

The community health nurse can assist the ill person to address some of these fears by ensuring comfort and support. Often, the nurse is present for the patient and family and can communicate compassion through caring acts. For instance, the small act of adjusting the ill person's position so he or she can see the television a little better can be greatly appreciated by the patient and family. When a person is diagnosed with a serious illness, life continues for an indefinite period; many persons live much longer than their prognosis predicts. The timing of a natural death is unpredictable, and it is difficult to predict exactly when death will occur. It is essential that each person have the opportunity to live life fully each day until the moment of death rather than engaging in a long, tedious dying trajectory. Therefore, accurate and timely deliverance of nursing care and addressing potential problem areas are of prime importance. The

nurse's assessment guides the interdisciplinary team in providing individualized care with respect for the person's wishes. The goal of the nurse is to help the seriously ill person achieve the best possible quality of life through relief of suffering, control of symptoms, and restoration of functional capacity while remaining sensitive to personal values, cultural practices, and religious beliefs (NHPCO, 2017).

Pain Management

Merciful relief of pain is essential for quality end-of-life care in dying persons, and nurses, including community health nurses, have a primary role in the assessment and management of pain at the end of life (ANA, 2016). According to the ANA, nurses are responsible for assessing pain and administering medications and providing other measures of comfort to alleviate troublesome symptoms. Many patients and families fear pain during the dying process. However, through ongoing assessment of levels of pain, administration of pain medication, and evaluation of the effectiveness of the pain management plan, nurses may help alleviate the distress associated with untreated pain in dying persons.

Pain is associated with many negative outcomes in dying persons. It has the potential to hasten death and is associated with needless suffering at the end of life. People in pain do not eat or drink well, do not move around, cannot engage in meaningful conversations with others, and often become isolated to save energy and cope with the pain. Untreated pain is related to sleeplessness, psychological distress, fatigue, and restlessness, and nurses have a moral obligation to advocate on behalf of ill persons so that pain is appropriately managed (ANA, 2016).

Evidence for Practice

Although efforts are under way to improve pain treatment at the end of life, there is growing evidence that improvements are not reaching all persons. Groups at particular risk for undertreatment of pain include older adults, minorities, and women (IOM, 2015). Inadequate pain relief may stem from the person's inability to communicate pain; for example, some older persons may be unable to report their pain because of delirium, dementia, aphasia, motor weakness, language barriers, and other factors. Furthermore, minority persons are at high risk for inadequate pain relief at the end of life. Possible barriers for these persons include disparities in access to many treatment options at the end of life, insensitivity to cultural differences in attitudes toward death and end-of-life care, and mistrust of the healthcare system (Spruill et al., 2013). The provision of culturally sensitive care is a necessary component of effective and comprehensive end-of-life care. Cultural preferences dictate how nurses assess and treat pain, provide for privacy, interact with the family, and deliver postmortem care after death.

Practice Point

At the end of life, assessing and managing pain, as well as relieving symptoms, is a primary responsibility of the hospice nurse. Untreated pain near the end of life is a nursing emergency and requires aggressive nursing intervention to ensure a comfortable and dignified death.

Pain Assessment

Pain assessment, including a thorough history, guides the development of a comprehensive pain management plan. Pain is a subjective experience, with self-report being the gold standard by which pain is measured. Accurate pain assessment is the basis of pain treatment, and physicians or nurses should perform it in a systematic and ongoing manner. Helpful questions may include the following:

- How bad is the pain? (It may help to use the facility pain indicator such as smiley face or rate the pain on a scale of 1 to 10.)
- How would you describe the pain (e.g., sharp, shooting, or dull)?
- Is the pain accompanied by other troublesome symptoms such as nausea or diarrhea?
- What makes the pain go away?
- Where does it hurt the most?
- Does the pain interfere with your ability to eat and sleep?
- What do you think is causing your pain?
- What have you done to alleviate the pain in the past? (ELNEC, 2006)

The nurse should carefully observe the dying person for the following signs:

- Moaning or groaning at rest or with movement
- Failure to eat, drink, or respond to the presence of others
- Grimacing or strained facial expression
- Guarding or not moving parts of the body
- Resisting care or noncooperation with therapeutic interventions
- Rapid heartbeat, diaphoresis, or change in vital signs

If an ill person has a potential reason for pain at the end of life, the nurse should assume that pain is present until proven otherwise. For instance, even in the absence of a complaint, if a bed-bound person has excoriated skin secondary to urinary incontinence, the nurse should aggressively treat the area with a moisture barrier and a soothing cream to alleviate pain and discomfort even though the patient has not complained of pain.

After conducting a complete pain assessment, the nurse shares the information with other members of the healthcare team, including the physician, advanced practice nurse, pharmacist, and others. This collaboration is essential to achieve adequate pain control.

Types of Pain in Dying Persons

Pain at the end of life is complex and multifactorial, and prevalence varies according to diagnosis and other factors. Pain in the terminally ill may be both nociceptive and neuropathic (Markman & Narasimhan, 2016). It is important to differentiate between these types of pain for the pain to be appropriately managed. Nociceptive pain is the signal the brain imparts when there is tissue inflammation or damage. Cardiac ischemia and arthritis are examples of nociceptive pain. Nociceptive pain can be divided into two categories: somatic pain, which is characterized by aching, throbbing, or stabbing due to skin, muscle, or bone injury, and visceral pain, which is characterized by gnawing, cramping, or aching due to injury of the internal organs. Nociceptive pain usually resolves when the injury heals, and initial treatment involves nonopioid pain relievers. Acetaminophen is usually the first choice, followed by nonsteroidal anti-inflammatory drugs (NSAIDs); if no relief, then physicians and advanced practice nurses may choose opioids. Neuropathic pain, which occurs when nerves have been damaged, commonly affects older adults and takes the form of diabetic neuropathy, postherpetic neuralgia, or poststroke syndrome. The pain associated with these conditions is often described as burning, electrical, or tingling. Difficult to relieve with routine pain medications, neuropathic pain may be deep and severe. At times, anticonvulsants, antidepressants, and opioids are used for pain relief.

> Mrs. Clark continues to become weaker and frailer at home, and she has developed severe pain in her left hip. You consult with the hospice physician, who recommends morphine. Mary fears that giving her mother morphine will hasten her death. What is your response?

Many healthcare providers, patients, and families believe that pain management with opioids shortens life; conversely, significant evidence exists to the contrary (ANA, 2016). Inadequate pain relief hastens death by increasing physiologic stress, potentially diminishing immunocompetency, decreasing mobility, worsening risk of pneumonia and thromboembolism, and increasing the work of breathing and myocardial oxygen requirements (Fine & MacLow, 2006). Unrelieved pain at the end of life can cause psychological distress and spiritual death and is often associated with negative outcomes, such as decreased quality of life (Markman & Narasimhan, 2016). Nurses can play a key role by teaching dying persons and families that aggressive pain control and relief of pain is an indicator of quality nursing care.

Pain Relief During the Dying Process

Various nonpharmacologic and pharmacologic methods of pain control may be implemented to control pain in the dying person. Some nonpharmacologic approaches to reducing pain may include providing a glass of warm milk to promote sleep, a back rub, a change of position, a favorite peaceful musical selection, spending time listening to the person, and/or visits from a priest, minister, or rabbi to meet spiritual needs. Nonpharmacologic methods can be used with pharmacologic therapy, and often augment the therapeutic effects of the drugs, resulting in the use of smaller doses.

Pharmacologic methods require close collaboration between the nurse, the physician, and the pharmacist to ensure the use of the correct medication, dosing regimen, and route of administration. These experts still use the model of pain relief developed by the WHO (1990) as the basis for the pharmacologic approach to pain management. It advocates a stepwise approach for pain treatment on the basis of the presence of mild, moderate, and severe or unrelenting pain. If the person has neuropathic pain, mild pain (1–3 on the 0–10 scale) requires the use of **adjuvant drugs** (nonopioid medications such as antidepressants and muscle

relaxants). Moderate pain (4–6 on the pain scale) necessitates the use of low doses of opioids; the use of nonopioids and adjuvants may continue. Severe pain (7–10 on the pain scale) requires the use of higher opioid doses. Persons presenting with severe pain should receive higher doses initially, rather than risking prolonged periods of uncontrolled pain while medications are titrated up from lower doses. It is necessary to titrate medications on the basis of the person's goals, requirements for supplemental analgesics, pain intensity, severity of undesirable or adverse drug effects, measures of functionality, sleep, emotional state, and person's or caregiver's report of the impact of pain on quality of life (ANA, 2016).

Whatever drugs are chosen, it is important to administer them routinely, and not on an as-needed (prn) basis, to prevent the unpleasant experience of the person perceiving pain and then waiting for pain relief. Long-acting drugs (sustained-release formulations) are ideal because they provide consistent pain relief. Short-acting or immediate-release agents are excellent prn medications, and their only use should be for control of **breakthrough pain**. Breakthrough pain is defined as "intermittent episodes of moderate to severe pain that occur in spite of control of baseline continuous pain" (Markman & Narasimhan, 2016). Common in persons with advanced disease, breakthrough pain may occur with specific activities (physical therapy, activities of daily living) and end-of-dose failure (pain that occurs near the end of the usual dosing interval of regularly scheduled medications), and it may also be spontaneous. Breakthrough pain requires prompt treatment to avoid the fear or memory of pain and to prevent decreased functional ability. Dying persons who consistently experience breakthrough pain should have their healthcare provider increase the dosage of their regularly scheduled, long-acting pain medications.

Types of Drugs Used to Control Pain
NONOPIOID ANALGESICS

Common types of drugs in this category include acetaminophen and NSAIDs, which may be used alone or in combination with adjuvant drugs to enhance their effect. These drugs are very effective for the treatment of mild to moderate pain. Persons with normal liver function should take 4 g or less daily to avoid liver damage. It is essential to use these drugs with caution in individuals with liver disease or who have a history of significant alcohol use and a dose of less than 3 g daily is recommended for these persons. NSAIDs can cause gastric irritation by inhibiting prostaglandin formation. Decreased prostaglandin synthesis results in thinning of the mucous lining that protects the stomach; this may result in gastrointestinal bleeding, especially in older adults. Other common side effects of NSAIDS are renal dysfunction and impaired platelet aggregation.

A newer class of NSAIDs selectively blocks the cyclooxygenase-2 (COX-2) enzyme, and there appears to be less risk of gastrointestinal bleeding with these drugs. However, studies have suggested that this benefit may not extend beyond 6 to 12 months (Reuben et al., 2017). Furthermore, these drugs have been linked to increased risk of heart attack and stroke when used for prolonged periods. The U.S. Food and Drug Administration (FDA) has withdrawn several of these drugs, but others continue to be used cautiously.

OPIOIDS

Many experts consider opioids to be the most useful agents for pain management in persons with advanced illness (IOM, 2015). These medications block receptors in the central nervous system and prevent the release of chemicals involved in pain transmission. Examples are codeine, morphine, hydromorphone, fentanyl, methadone, and oxycodone. The WHO considers morphine to be the gold standard for the relief of cancer pain. Adverse effects are rare, and the only absolute contraindication for use is a history of a hypersensitivity reaction (rash, wheeze, or edema). Respiratory depression may occur with titration of opioid analgesics; however, this rarely occurs at the end of life (Reuben et al., 2017). Most often, the respiratory rate becomes slower as the result of the dying process, not opioids. Constipation and sedation are two troublesome symptoms that are often associated with opioid use. Meperidine and propoxyphene are not recommended for use in older people because of their ineffectiveness in treating pain and their association with serious side effects. As disease progresses and organ function deteriorates, the potential for accumulation of the toxic metabolites of these drugs can lead to seizures, delirium, and tremors.

Some people with pain need higher levels of opioids than others and may fear reporting their pain is a sign of weakness. Others may fear addiction to opioid medications and refuse medication, resulting in needless suffering. When used as prescribed in seriously ill or dying persons, opioid medications improve activity levels and quality of life and ease suffering. Patients should be urged to use these medications without fear of addiction or feelings of guilt by interpreting their use as a sign of weakness.

Opioids often involve side effects such as nausea and feeling of lethargy that usually gradually resolve within 1 to 3 days. Other side effects, such as constipation, do not resolve without treatment. Over time, persons in pain will become opioid tolerant, meaning their bodies have adjusted to the medication and higher doses will be needed to relieve their pain. This is to be anticipated by the nurse, and the ill person should be reassured that this does not mean they are addicted but rather their body has become adjusted to the medication and the same dose does not work as well as it once did.

ADJUVANT ANALGESICS

A wide array of nonopioid medications from several pharmacologic classes has been shown to improve pain relief when used concomitantly with pain medications. Such adjuvant medications include muscle relaxants, corticosteroids, anticonvulsants, antidepressants, and topical medications. Their use may enhance the effectiveness of other types of drugs, allowing improved treatment of pain at lower doses with decreased risk of side effects. Clinicians may prescribe them at any step of the "analgesic ladder" developed by the WHO (1990).

Routes of Administration

Usually, physicians prefer the oral route of administration because it is the easiest and most comfortable for the ill person. However, many routes of administration are available at the end of life when the person can no longer swallow. Pain medication may be administered by the following routes.

ORAL

Tablets, liquids, and capsules are administered orally to control pain. Long-acting or sustained-release tablets can control pain for up to 24 hours. Persons who are able to swallow can use this method until very close to the time of death. It is possible to mix liquid medications in juice and to open capsules and mix the contents in applesauce. For an oral medication, a higher dose of medication is usually necessary because of the first-pass effect (deactivation that occurs when medication passes through the liver).

ORAL MUCOSA

Even when the person can no longer swallow, it is possible to deliver medication to the oral or buccal mucosa, from which it is absorbed. Placement of highly concentrated liquids such as morphine onto the mucosa involves using a dropper. Liquid morphine has a short half-life and duration of action; thus, more frequent administration may be necessary.

RECTAL

Some medications are available in suppository form, and the rectal route may be useful when the person can no longer swallow or has problems with nausea and vomiting. The rectal route is invasive, and it may be difficult for family members to deliver medication using this route. In addition, if the ill person cannot move easily, the positioning required for suppository insertion may be problematic.

TRANSDERMAL

Medications such as the fentanyl patch require placement on the skin of the upper body every 72 hours for relief of pain. However, because of changes in blood flow, metabolism, and fat distribution, some persons do not achieve or maintain stable drug levels and adequate pain relief. Peak onset may be delayed up to 24 hours, necessitating coverage with short-acting agents during the initial day of treatment.

TOPICAL

Topical capsaicin and local anesthetics (EMLA) can be useful for pain associated with postherpetic neuralgia and arthritis, and prior to invasive procedures such as insertion of IV lines or injections. When applied in small amounts to confined areas, as is recommended, topical medications usually result in little systemic absorption.

PARENTERAL

The IV and subcutaneous routes are useful when the person is unable to swallow (intramuscular administration is inappropriate in the palliative care setting) (Paice & Fine, 2006). Pain may be associated with these methods of delivery. The IV route provides rapid drug delivery and pain relief, although risks of infection increase because of the need for vascular access. If the IV route is used, it is important to use the appropriate fluid delivery system and the smallest amount of fluid possible. This minimizes the risk of volume overload, which may lead to excess secretions and difficulty breathing. Subcutaneous administration is slower to take effect, with infusion of 2 to 3 mL/h the easiest to absorb.

INTRASPINAL

The administration of drugs into or around the spinal cord via the epidural or intrathecal route is reserved for those persons who cannot achieve pain control in any other manner. The complexity of equipment used to deliver medications in this way leads to increased costs, and caregiver burden is a potential risk. Furthermore, risk of infection is a significant concern.

Tolerance

Persons who are managed with opioid analgesics over a period of time invariably develop tolerance or a "state of adaptation in which exposure to a drug induces changes that result in a diminution of one or more of the drug's effects over time" (Paice & Fine, 2006, p. 135). Medication dosages that were once therapeutic are no longer effective, especially as disease worsens. According to the ANA (2016), when pain and other distressing symptoms are present, the person should have appropriate and sufficient medication by appropriate routes to control symptoms, in whatever dosage, and by whatever route is needed to relieve pain and increase comfort. It is imperative not to undertreat pain. As pain increases, it is essential to explore underlying causes, medicate the person promptly, monitor the response to medication, and inform other team members about the effectiveness of the pain relief plan. The goal is to eliminate pain and help dying persons to improve the quality of their life through relief of suffering. Dying persons may need more pain medication than the normal range for the prescribed drug. Organic changes are occurring rapidly and systems are closing down; thus, absorption levels of drugs are also diminishing.

Preventing and Managing Adverse Effects

CONSTIPATION

Most opioid analgesics slow the movement of material in the intestinal tract and result in poor bowel elimination.

Constipation may contribute to increased pain in dying persons, and it is extremely important that the nurse monitor the bowels carefully. It is necessary to initiate a prophylactic bowel regimen when using opioid analgesics. This includes the use of stool softeners (e.g., docusate sodium) and bowel stimulants (e.g., senna). Senna tea and fruits may also be helpful, and nurses should encourage patients to increase their fluid intake, if possible. Ill persons should avoid using bulking agents (e.g., psyllium) to prevent fecal impaction.

SEDATION

Many persons experience sedation when opioid analgesics are initiated; however, this effect should subside within 24 to 48 hours. If this condition continues after 24 to 48 hours, and clinicians have checked and managed other correctable causes the opioid dose should be reduced and the person observed for improvement in level of consciousness. Although sedation is commonly cited as a reason for avoiding opioids in older adults, evidence to support this claim is lacking (Bishop & Morrison, 2007).

RESPIRATORY DEPRESSION

As previously discussed, respiratory depression is often a concern for healthcare providers when using opioids for pain management; however, it is rarely a clinically significant problem for opioid-tolerant persons (Reuben et al., 2017). Most people develop a tolerance to respiratory depression within 5 to 7 days. If respiratory depression (respiratory rate <8 breaths/min or O_2 saturation <90%) occurs, it usually has a multifactorial etiology.

NAUSEA AND VOMITING

Nausea and vomiting are common with the use of opioids in opioid-naive persons (those who have never used an opioid drug before) due to the activation of the chemoreceptor trigger zone in the medulla, vestibular sensitivity, and delayed gastric emptying (McPherson & Uritsky, 2011). Antiemetics that the person has used successfully in the past may be scheduled for 2 to 3 days with a gradual tapering of the dose. Symptoms should subside within a few days if the underlying cause is the opioid analgesic (McPherson & Uritsky, 2011).

MYOCLONUS

Myoclonic jerking movements may be associated with high-dose opioid therapy (especially morphine). If this occurs, an alternate opioid should be used.

PRURITUS

Pruritus is most commonly associated with the use of morphine and is related in part to a release of histamine caused by the drug. Treatment with antihistamines (e.g., diphenhydramine) is effective but is very likely to cause sedation in older adults.

Management of Distressing Symptoms at the End of Life

Secretions

At the end of life, it may not be easy to manage secretions. Painful xerostomia (dry mouth) can contribute to difficulty swallowing and impede clear speech; this is often exacerbated by the use of supplemental oxygen and reliance on open-mouthed breathing. Frequent mouth care at this time is crucial for making the person comfortable. It is necessary to provide oral care using soft swabs several times a day, and whenever the mouth has a foul odor or appears to be causing problems for the ill person. The nurse may instruct family members about the use of oral swabs or moistened cloths, allowing them to participate actively in their loved one's care. Alcohol-based products or those that contain perfume, lemon, or glycerin can be irritating and drying, and their use is discouraged. A salt–soda solution (1 teaspoon salt, 1 teaspoon baking soda, 1 quart tepid water) or artificial saliva used every 30 minutes may minimize dry mouth and the associated sensation of thirst (Emanuel, Ferris, von Gunten, Hauser, & Von Roenn, 2009). It is acceptable to offer ice chips to relieve the feeling of dryness as long as the swallowing reflex is present. To prevent aspiration, the nurse should remind caregivers not to give oral fluids when the person can no longer swallow. Soothing ointments or petroleum jelly may be applied to the lips to prevent painful cracking or drying. With increasing debility, oral thrush may appear, and clinicians should prescribe oral antifungal medications (e.g., nystatin swish and swallow).

As death approaches and the person becomes increasingly sedated, the blink reflex decreases, resulting in dry eyes. Opened or half-opened eyelids become dry and irritated. When this occurs, the nurse or other caregiver provides frequent eye care to promote comfort. Artificial tears or ophthalmic saline solutions may be used to prevent drying of the eyes. The appearance of a loved one with half-open eyes, redness, or puffiness may be disturbing to family members and should be avoided if possible.

Anorexia and Dehydration

Most dying persons stop eating and drinking, and anorexia and dehydration are common and normal at the end of life. If the ill person chooses to refuse food and drink, the nurse should consider this a rational decision and offer emotional and psychological support. Most experts believe that dehydration at the end of life does not cause distress and may actually initiate release of endorphins, resulting in a sense of well-being (ANA, 2016). Another benefit of dehydration is the decreased risk of lung congestion due to pulmonary edema, which leads to noisy, labored respirations, a sensation of breathlessness, and cough. By eliminating noisy respirations, the dying person seems more comfortable, and quiet breath sounds decrease anxiety for family members. Oliguria (production of less than 15 cc of urine per hour) is another favorable outcome because the person does not need to be positioned to use the bedpan or urinal frequently. When the dying person stops eating, the nurse can reassure the family that anorexia may result in ketosis, leading to a peaceful state of mind and decreased pain. Furthermore, research has shown that initiation of parenteral or enteral nutrition at this time neither improves symptom control nor lengthens life (Emanuel et al., 2009).

Mrs. Clark has stopped eating, and her daughter is concerned that she is hungry. Mary asks you if a feeding tube would help her mother get stronger and live longer. How would you answer her?

Skin Integrity

It is necessary to monitor skin integrity carefully at the end of life because increased fatigue may result in decreased movement, resulting in pressure over bony prominences. Edema, bruising, dryness, and venous pooling may occur. Repositioning of the dying person is essential, using lift or draw sheets, being careful to avoid shearing forces. Pressure-reducing surfaces, such as air mattresses or air beds, may help in alleviating pressure without needing to reposition the dying person frequently. To promote comfort and reduce the risk of skin breakdown, the nurse or caregivers may provide gentle massage. Family members may feel comfortable applying lotion to the back or hands of the dying person, again allowing participation in the care of their loved one. The nurse should tell them not to massage areas of nonblanching erythema and actual breakdown; this exacerbates ongoing tissue damage.

Incontinence

Bowel and bladder incontinence are frequent occurrences at the end of life. Seepage from body orifices may become uncontrolled, and it becomes necessary to have protective pads or briefs. It is extremely important to prevent decubitus ulcers from forming at this time because further breakdown is common due to contact with urine and feces. Barrier creams and change of position may also help maintain skin integrity. The nurse should discourage the use of indwelling urinary catheters if at all possible because they are often associated with distressing and painful urinary tract infections.

> ### ✎ Practice Point
>
> Confusion, restlessness, and agitation are common but distressing symptoms of terminal delirium.

> ### ✎ Practice Point
>
> Pleasant conversation or music at the bedside of the comatose person may be therapeutic and reassuring to the dying person.

Terminal Delirium

Terminal delirium can be a distressing phenomenon for families and caregivers. Typically, terminal delirium presents as "the abrupt onset of fluctuating confusion, inattention, and reduced awareness of the environment…and may include hallucinations and disturbances in sleep-wake cycles" (Hosker & Bennett, 2016, p. 1). Visual, auditory, and olfactory hallucinations may occur. It is important for the nurse to understand that this condition is often irreversible and that the dying person's experience of the delirium may be very different from what is witnessed by caregivers (Hosker & Bennett, 2016). In older adults, delirium is often a presenting aspect of acute illness or exacerbation of chronic illness. Further complicating the issue, delirium may exist concomitantly with dementia in older adults (Koll et al., 2016).

Management of delirium includes identification and treatment of underlying causes (infection, electrolyte imbalances), reduction of environmental stimuli, provision of a safe environment, and reduction of anxiety. It is necessary to discontinue all nonessential medications (those not needed for comfort) when goals of care so dictate, and to continue pain medications and other agents used for comfort, such as benzodiazepines (lorazepam) and neuroleptics (haloperidol).

Eventually, neurologic changes occur in dying persons, and they slip from a lethargic state into an unconscious state (which may include periods of lucidness), then coma, and finally death. Family members frequently ask how much longer their loved one will live. The anxiety and distress of family and friends at this time may be great. Waiting for death is not an easy task, and time may pass slowly. This may be frustrating to those who are at the bedside. Extra support and encouragement at the crucial hours before death occurs are often necessary.

It is impossible to know exactly what unconscious persons at the end of life can hear; however, data from operating rooms and "near-death" experiences suggest that persons near the end of life may be more aware of their environment than they are able to show (Emanuel et al., 2009). Although obtunded and comatose persons may not be able to communicate, it is believed that their sense of hearing is intact. People present at the bedside must not say or discuss anything they would not want the dying person to hear. Nursing interventions at this time include encouraging family members to "let go" and give the terminal patient permission to die. Family members can assure their loved one that he or she will be "okay" and thank the person for loving them. The nurse should allow display of appropriate gestures of affection and provide privacy. Table 24.5 outlines suggested strategies for the management of common symptoms in dying persons.

NURSING CARE OF PERSONS WHO ARE CLOSE TO DEATH

Preparing for Death

The knowledge or presumption that death is imminent may cause anxiety for the staff, family, and the dying person. Watching the body shut down life processes can bring feelings of helplessness and anxiety. Questions of an afterlife, unresolved emotional or social issues, concerns centered around family members and their acceptance of death, and financial matters are common issues generated at the end of life. It is part of the nursing role to attempt to allay the fears of ill persons and families at this time. Nurses must also remember to support themselves through this difficult period, recognizing and accepting an array of personal feelings. They may need individual support, as well as team support from outside the healthcare facility, to express and accept their true feelings. By doing this, it may be possible to prevent burnout.

In the context of terminal illness, hope is an ever-changing phenomenon. Healthcare professionals should never deny hope for the dying person and family. Hope for a cure is not unusual for both the ill person and family throughout the illness trajectory. As the disease progresses, the seriously ill person may hope for small things to make the present situation more tolerable, such as a favorite meal or a visit from a family member. Hope for a dying person may focus on living to see a grandchild graduate from college or the birth of a great-grandchild. Near the end of life, hopes may include such things as a comfortable death or death in the home. It is not unusual for dying persons to hope to speak with loved ones before they die.

Nurses should realize that the will to live is extremely strong in many persons confronting death, especially when there is a sense of unfinished business. Dying persons sometimes need reassurance from their families and caregivers that all is well and it is "OK" to let go.

> Mary is able to obtain Visiting Nurse Association (VNA) care and grant her mother's wish to remain in her own home until the end of her life. As Mrs. Clark approaches the final moments of her life, Mary sits quietly at her mother's bedside. Mary notices that her mother is becoming dusky in color and that she seems to be having trouble breathing. Mary turns to you for advice and reassurance that her mother is not suffering. How would you respond?

TABLE 24.5 Suggested Strategies for the Management of Common Symptoms in Dying Patients

Problem	Suggested Nursing Intervention
Constipation	Stimulants such as prune juice, senna, or lactulose. Avoid bulking agents (psyllium) in patients with inadequate fluid intake to avoid impaction. Monitor bowel function. Do not allow the patient to go longer than 3 days without a bowel movement. A mineral oil enema may be necessary to prevent impaction.
Delirium	Treat underlying cause if possible (fever, urinary tract infection, pain). Avoid use of physical restraints, sleep disruption, excessive medications. Urge family to remain with the patient, and have staff frequently visit and speak to and touch the patient. Use alternative interventions such as massage and music.
Dyspnea	Treat underlying cause if known (bronchospasm, hypoxia). Administer opioids to slow respiratory rate. Maintain the patient in a sitting position if possible. Minimize exertion by spreading out interventions and treatments. Provide humidified oxygen for comfort. Use alternative interventions such as massage and music.
Decubitus ulcers	Use appropriate positioning techniques, changing position every 2 hours. Keep the patient's skin clean and dry. Use special mattress pads to relieve pressure.
Cough	Assess and treat underlying cause such as postnasal drip or obstruction. Use chest physical therapy, cool humidified air, elevate head of the bed, and suction secretions as necessary. Cough suppressants may be used for comfort.
Anorexia and cachexia	The etiology of cachexia is rarely reversible in advanced disease, and aggressive nutritional treatment does not improve survival or quality of life and may create discomfort for the dying patient whose body is shutting down. Provide excellent mouth care. Treat oral problems such as candidiasis (thrush). Treat constipation, nausea, and vomiting, if present, as underlying causes. Assess the room for problem odors and try to minimize as much as possible. Generally, parenteral or enteral nutrition is useful only for patients with an appetite who cannot swallow. Offer the patient's favorite food and fluids as tolerated.
Nausea and vomiting	This occurs in up to 70% of patients at the end of life. Causes include metabolic disturbances, visceral disturbances, vestibular problems, medication side effects, emotional upset, and radiation. Assess cause and treat if possible (i.e., remove offending medication). Treatment medications include anticholinergics, steroids, benzodiazepines, and antiemetics (ondansetron and granisetron). Anticipate this and administer medications, if needed, before symptoms occur. Position the patient to prevent aspiration. Use complementary therapies such as music, relaxation, hypnosis, and acupuncture.
Fatigue	Fatigue is a subjective sense of tiredness or lack of energy that interferes with usual functioning. It may be disease related, treatment related, or psychological. If tolerated, exercise can improve function and sleep. Frequent rest periods and transfusions for very anemic patients may improve quality of life.
Anxiety	Anxiety may be a side effect of many medications such as stimulants and corticosteroids, or a paradoxical reaction to analgesics. Antidepressants and benzodiazepines may be beneficial.

Source: Data from Emanuel, L. L., Ferris, F. D., von Gunten, C. F., Hauser, J. M., & Von Roenn, J. H. (2009). *The last hours of living: Practical advice for clinicians.* Retrieved from www.medscape.com; End-of-Life Nursing Education Consortium. (2006). *Promoting advanced practice nursing in palliative care.* Duarte, CA: City of Hope National Medical Center and Washington, DC: American Association of Colleges of Nursing.

The Dying Process

> Under the wide and starry sky,
> Dig the grave and let me lie. (from *Requiem*)
> **Robert Louis Stevenson, while dying from tuberculosis**

Before death, the nurse must explain many physiologic processes to patients (if possible) and their families and caregivers. An expected set of physiologic changes typically occurs when death is imminent and is related to gradual hypoxia, respiratory acidosis, and renal failure. The nurse plays an integral role in assisting the family members who witness these changes to plan for the actual death. Expected changes include the following:

- Buildup of saliva and oropharyngeal secretions due to loss of the ability to swallow may lead to gurgling, crackling, or rattling sounds with breathing. This is sometimes referred to as the "death rattle," although this terminology should be avoided because it is often distressing to family members.
- Changes in respiratory patterns (shallow breaths with periods of apnea) may indicate significant neurologic declines, with Cheyne–Stokes respirations often heralding the impending death.

- Skin may appear dusky or gray and feel cold or clammy. Mottling of the lower extremities may take place days or hours before the actual death.
- Eyes may appear discolored, deeper set, or bruised.

Observing these body changes can be disturbing to family members. Although it is extremely difficult to assure the dying person or family that death will happen within a certain time frame, the nurse's approach and explanations of the death process are reassuring to those present. Some family members may want to be present when death occurs, and others may want to be nearby but not physically present; it is important that the nurse support whatever decision is comfortable for the family and ill person. Furthermore, patients may wish to be alone and die quietly with no one present because it may be difficult for the dying person to have loved ones near. Others find comfort in having family or professional caregivers in attendance. The dying process is as individual as living.

When respirations cease and a stethoscope does not detect breath sounds or heart sounds, the nurse should check the person's carotid pulses with the stethoscope or fingers. Next, the nurse should check the eyes for pupillary light reflex. If the pupils are fixed and dilated and the heart has stopped beating, the clinician can pronounce that the person is dead. Other signs of death include pale and waxen skin; lower body temperature; and relaxed muscles and sphincters, with released urine and stool (Emanuel et al., 2009). The nurse should note the time death occurred and put it on the person's chart, notify the attending physician of the death, and make careful notes in the person's chart to document the time the physician has been notified, and any directions received regarding postmortem care. There are certain settings where a nurse may make the death pronouncement, including long-term care. It is necessary to notify members of the interdisciplinary healthcare team of the death and express your condolences to the family. Even if the family is expecting the death, the actual occurrence of death comes as a shock and requires gentleness and empathy. If family members are present, the nurse should give them sufficient time to spend with the deceased before the body is removed.

Student Reflection

Today, Mrs. Clark died quietly in her home. Even though her daughter, Mary, was there with her through every step of the process, she seemed shocked and sad when her mother took her last breath. She cried for a few minutes and then took my hand and smiled saying, "Thank you for helping me through this. I never could have done this for Mom without you." I cried a little bit also—tears of sadness, because I would miss Mrs. Clark, as well as tears of joy, because I knew I had helped her achieve the kind of death she wanted. I felt I had been a "good nurse."

Nursing Care After Death

One of the most difficult but essential parts of nursing is providing **postmortem care**. It is essential that the nurse does this promptly, quietly, efficiently, and with dignity, thereby communicating to the family that the deceased person was valued and respected. To promote comfort and ease anxiety at a time of stress, the nurse should honor the family's wishes about performing any religious or cultural rituals and practices. The nurse may also invite the family members to talk about their loved one and encourage the family members to touch and hold the person's body as they feel comfortable. If possible, before death occurs, the nurse should straighten the limbs and place the head on a pillow. If the death is suspicious or occurs outside of a healthcare facility, the coroner may request that the body be left undisturbed until an autopsy can be performed. However, the coroner does not investigate most deaths of seriously ill persons who die in their own homes.

After the pronouncement, the nurse should glove, remove all tubes, replace soiled dressings, pad the anal area in case of drainage, and gently wash the body to remove any discharges. The body should lie on its back, with head and shoulders elevated on a pillow. The nurse should grasp the eyelashes and gently pull the lids down. Insertion of dentures is necessary. It is important not to tie or secure any body parts because this may cause skin indentations. The nurse should place a clean gown on the body and pull a clean sheet up to the shoulders. When the body is moved or the extremities repositioned, the body may produce respiratory-type sounds or the chest may appear to rise and fall. Although this can be alarming, it is only the sound of air leaving the lungs. The nurse may want to check for respiration sounds again to be certain that the person is dead. The nurse should prepare necessary paperwork for the removal of the body from the facility; call the funeral home, morgue, or other personnel for the removal of the body; and note the time in the chart, as well as who was called, and again chart when the body was released and to whom. It is advisable to also note whether eyeglasses, dentures, or any personal artifacts were released with the body and to whom they were given. If the facility requires that the body be identified with a tag, it is necessary to secure it properly.

Grief

The bitterest tears shed over graves are for words left unsaid and deeds left undone. **Harriet Beecher Stowe**

Although the death may be expected, it may be met with shock by people who are left behind. Rationalizations (e.g., he lived a long life) may help ease the initial numbness of the actual death. Statements of relief, such as "he or she is no longer in pain," may help the bereaved cope with the immediate loss. The grieving process is considered difficult work that may last for years, and it is hard to endure at times. Past death experiences, emotional health, religious beliefs, and support of friends and family all are factors which may help ease the grief process. Bereavement is the process one undergoes after a loss. **Grief** is the emotion felt after the loss. The period of **mourning** is the recovery from the loss.

Several studies have shown that the accumulation of losses compounds the effects of grief and bereavement associated with death in older adults (Konigsberg, 2011). The widow or widower may experience grief for many years. Phases of grief may include some of the following:

Numb shock: The widow or widower cannot believe the spouse's death occurred. This phase is marked by shock, emotional dullness, and restless behavior that may include stupor and withdrawal. It may include physical characteristics such as nausea or insomnia. One wants to protect oneself from the feeling of loss.

Emotional turmoil or depression: Alarm or panic-type reactions occur. Emotional expression may include crying, low mood, sleep disturbance, and anorexia. Anger, guilt, or longing for the deceased may take place. The widow or widower may also become preoccupied with the meaning of the loss.

Reorganization or resolution: Reorganization eventually takes place, and coping strategies and positive outlooks emerge. A final resolution phase leads to acceptance of the loss. The widow or widower may return to prior levels of functioning.

When the full effects of death and its associated consequences set in, so do regret, self-doubt, and at times, despair. Life's purpose becomes confusing, and mood swings are prevalent. Being alone in the house may be a major problem. Research has shown that an active listener for reminiscence is helpful to the older adult during grief work. The nurse may also encourage the surviving spouse to focus on activities such as volunteer work. While actively participating in such activities, older adults often find the affection and companionship they need at this time.

Caring for the Caregiver

Most community health nurses not only care for the seriously ill person but also support and guide family caregivers. To prevent feelings of stress and burnout, those people who care for the dying need support and an opportunity to express emotional responses and grief. A periodic assessment might be beneficial for the caregivers who provide end-of-life care. Some questions may include the following:

- What have you done to meet your own needs today?
- Have you laughed today?
- Did you eat properly, rest enough, exercise, and play today?
- What have you felt today?
- Do you have something to look forward to?

Caregivers need to care for themselves to prevent anger, frustration, and anxiety. This makes it possible for the caregivers to continue to be sensitive to the needs of the dying person.

> I didn't attend the funeral, but I sent a nice letter saying I approved of it. **Mark Twain**

COMPLEMENTARY AND ALTERNATIVE THERAPIES

Seriously ill persons and families may request complementary and alternative medicine (CAM) concomitantly with hospice and palliative care. Use of CAM has great potential when integrated with traditional medical practices in end-of-life care. Traditional medicine may share the spotlight with such therapies as acupuncture, massage therapy, Reiki therapy, chiropractic care, and herbal medicine. In 1998, the National Institutes of Health initiated the National Center for Complementary and Alternative Medicine (NCCAM) now renamed National Center for Complementary and Integrative Health (NCCIH). NCCIH is dedicated to exploring complementary and alternative healing practices in the context of rigorous science, training researchers, and disseminating authoritative information to the public and professionals. Although for many complementary therapies rigorous evidence of effectiveness is lacking, many persons who have used integrative health therapies at the end of life have reported that these therapies have physical, psychosocial, and spiritual benefits.

The CDC reports that in 2007, 41.8% of hospice care providers offered CAM services, had a CAM provider on staff or under contract, or both. Among hospice care providers offering CAM, over one half offered massage (71.7%), supportive group therapy (69.0%), music therapy (62.2%), pet therapy (58.6%), or guided imagery or relaxation (52.7%) (Berkovitz, Sengupta, Jones, & Harris-Kojetin, 2011). Massage and mind–body interventions are cited as successful strategies for easing anxiety, emotional distress, nausea, and pain while improving overall comfort levels (HPNA, 2015).

Within the context of quality end-of-life care, the nurse must respect the unique needs of each seriously ill person and his or her family. Several factors may cause people with serious illness to seek complementary therapies: they may hope that these alternative methods will succeed where traditional medicine has failed, they may be attempting to regain control over life-threatening disease, or they may hope to achieve relief of suffering and improved quality of life. HPNA (2015) has developed a position statement regarding the use of complementary therapies in end-of-life care. According to this position statement, nurses working in end-of-life care need to learn about the many types of complementary therapies because the goals of CAM to reduce suffering and enhance comfort are consistent with the goals of palliative care and hospice nurses. Nurses should also be aware of the increasing use of complementary therapies, recognize the role of CAM in symptom relief, and support the appropriate practice of complementary therapies to promote holistic end-of-life care (HPNA, 2015).

KEY CONCEPTS

- Studies have documented that the American healthcare system has substantial shortcomings in the care of seriously ill persons and their families.
- Many persons die in pain or suffering from adverse symptoms.
- Aggressive care that carries a high burden of treatment is often delivered inappropriately to seriously ill persons because of communication barriers and lack of planning.
- The community health nurse can play a key role on the interdisciplinary team and serve as advocate, educator, care provider, and planner of quality end-of-life care.
- Pain and symptom control are crucial to the delivery of quality end-of-life care.
- Cultural and ethnic variations are key factors to be considered when providing end-of-life care.
- Palliative care and hospice programs can assist the nurse in the delivery of quality end-of-life care to seriously ill persons and their families.
- Families often rely on the nurse for support and assistance during the dying process and afterward in the mourning and grieving period.

CRITICAL THINKING QUESTIONS

1. Speak to nurses and nursing assistants who work in one of your clinical rotations about the assessment of pain in the dying person. What factors do they identify as important?
2. Explain possible reasons why caring for dying persons at the end of life may be difficult. Tell a story in a small group of fellow students and observe their reactions.
3. Keep a clinical journal of your feelings and experiences as you begin to become proficient in providing end-of-life care to seriously ill persons and their families.
4. Identify a few key people in your life who can help you as you struggle to become proficient in the provision of end-of-life care.
5. Identify key people in your life who helped you to come to terms with and understand death.
6. Establish your own advance directive and name a healthcare proxy.

COMMUNITY RESOURCES

- Local hospitals that have hospital-based palliative care or hospice home care programs
- Local palliative care specialists
- Visiting nurse associations
- Volunteer church groups and friendly visitors
- Elder affairs
- Local and state health departments
- State and Federal offices of Medicare and Medicaid
- Specialty disease organizations such as the American Cancer Society, The Alzheimer's Association, The American Heart Association, and others as needed

REFERENCES

American Academy of Pediatrics. (2013). Pediatric palliative care and hospice care commitments, guidelines, and recommendations. *Pediatrics, 132*, 966–972.

American Medical Directors Association. (2013). *White paper on surrogate decision-making and advance care planning in long-term care.* Retrieved from http://www.amda.com/governance/whitepapers/surrogate/clinical.cfm?printPage=1&;

American Nurses Association. (2012). *Position statement on nursing care and do-not-resuscitate (DNR) and allow natural death (AND) decisions.* Retrieved from http://www.nursingworld.org/dnrposition

American Nurses Association. (2013). *Position statements: Euthanasia, assisted suicide, and aid in dying.* Retrieved from https://www.nursingworld.org/~4af287/globalassets/docs/ana/ethics/euthanasia-assisted-suicideaid-in-dying_ps042513.pdf

American Nurses Association. (2016). *Position statement on nurses' roles and responsibilities in providing care and support at the end of life.* Retrieved from https://www.nursingworld.org/~4af078/globalassets/docs/ana/ethics/endoflife-positionstatement.pdf

American Nurses Association. (2017). *Position Statement: Nutrition and hydration at the end of life.* Retrieved from https://www.nursingworld.org/~4af0ed/globalassets/docs/ana/ethics/ps_nutrition-and-hydration-at-the-end-of-life_2017june7.pdf

Berkovitz, A., Sengupta, M., Jones, A., & Harris-Kojetin, L. D.; Centers for Disease Control and Prevention. (2011). *Complementary and alternative therapies in hospice: The national home and hospice care survey–United States, 2007. National Health Statistics Reports.* Retrieved from http://www.cdc.gov/nchs/data/nhsr/nhsr033.pdf

Bishop, T. F., & Morrison, R. S. (2007). Geriatric palliative care—part I: Pain and symptom management. *Clinical Geriatrics, 15*(1), 25–32.

Cain, C. L., Surbone, A., Elk, R., & Kagawa-Singer, M. (2018). Culture and palliative care: Preferences, communication, meaning, and mutual decision making. *Journal of Pain and Symptom Management, 55*(5), 1408–1419.

Center to Advance Palliative Care (CAPC). (2017). *Pediatric palliative care.* Retrieved from https://www.capc.org/topics/pediatric-palliative-care/

REFERENCES *(Continued)*

Centers for Disease Control and Prevention (CDC). (2017a). *Health, United States, 2015.* Retrieved from https://www.cdc.gov/nchs/data/hus/hus15.pdf#019

Centers for Disease Control and Prevention (CDC). (2017b). *Drug overdose deaths among adolescents aged 15–19 in the United States: 1999–2015.* Retrieved from https://www.cdc.gov/nchs/products/databriefs/db282.htm

The Dartmouth Institute for Health Policy and Clinical Practice. (2013). *End of life care.* Retrieved from http://www.dartmouthatlas.org/data/topic/topic.aspx?cat=18

Emanuel, L. L., Ferris, F. D., von Gunten, C. F., Hauser, J. M., & Von Roenn, J. H. (2009). *The last hours of living: Practical advice for clinicians.* Retrieved from https://www.medscape.com/viewarticle/716463_3

End-of-life Nursing Education Consortium [ELNEC]. (2006). *Promoting advance practice nursing in palliative care.* Duarte City, CA: City of Hope National Medical Center and American Association of Colleges of Nursing.

Fine, P. G., & MacLow, C., (2006). *Principles of pain management at the end of life.* Retrieved from http://www.medscape.com.

Hosker, C. M., & Bennett, M. I. (2016). Delirium and agitation at the end of life. *British Medical Journal, 353,* i3085. Retrieved from http://eprints.whiterose.ac.uk/101456/1/16.157.pdf

Hospice and Palliative Nurses Association. (2011). *HPNA position statement: Artificial nutrition and hydration in advanced illness.* Retrieved from http://www.hpna.org

Hospice and Palliative Nurses Association. (2015). *HPNA position statement: Value of the professional nurse in palliative care.* Retrieved from https://advancingexpertcare.org/HPNA/Leadership/Position_Statements/HPNA/Leadership_Advocacy/Position_Statements.aspx?hkey=a794c17f-c88f-42d9-a09f-caf413e42aa3

Institute of Medicine (IOM). (2015). *Dying in America: Improving quality and honoring individual preferences near the end of life.* Washington, DC: The National Academies Press.

Koll, T., Pergolotti, M., Holmes, H. M., Pieters, H. C., van Londen, G. J., Marcum, Z. A.,...& Steer, C. B. (2016). Supportive care in older adults with cancer: across the continuum. *Current Oncology Reports, 18*(8), 51–61.

Konigsberg, R. D. (2011). *The truth about grief.* New York: Simon and Schuster.

Kübler-Ross, E. (1969). *On death and dying: What the dying have to teach doctors, nurses, clergy, and their own families.* New York: MacMillan.

Lacey, D. (2005). Tube feeding, antibiotics, and hospitalization of nursing home residents with end-stage dementia: Perceptions of key medical decision-makers. *American Journal of Alzheimer's Disease and Other Dementias, 20*(4), 211–219.

Last Acts. (2002). *Means to a better end: A report on dying in America today.* Retrieved on August 27, 2007, from www.lastacts.org

Lysaght, S., & Ersek, M. (2013). Settings of care within hospice: New options and questions about dying "At Home." *Journal of Hospice and Palliative Nursing, 15*(3), 171–176.

Markman, J., & Narasimhan, S. (2016). Overview of pain. *Merck Manual.* Retrieved from http://www.merckmanuals.com/professional/neurologic-disorders/pain/overview-of-pain.

McPherson, M. L., & Uritsky, T. J. (2011). Pharmacotherapy of pain in older adults: Opioid and adjuvant. In F. M. Gloth, III (Ed.). *Handbook of pain relief in older adults: An evidence-based approach* (pp. 83–95). New York: Springer.

Medicare.gov. (2017). *Medicare part A coverage: Hospice.* Retrieved from https://www.medicare.gov/what-medicare-covers/part-a/part-a-coverage-hospice.html

Moneymaker, K. (2005). Comfort measures only. *Journal of Palliative Medicine, 8*(3), 688.

National Consensus Project (NCP) for Quality Palliative Care. (2013). *Clinical practice guidelines for quality palliative care.* Retrieved from www.nationalconsensusproject.org

National Hospice and Palliative Care Organization (NHPCO). (2015). *Facts and figures: Pediatric palliative and hospice care in America.* Retrieved from https://www.nhpco.org/sites/default/files/public/quality/Pediatric_Facts-Figures.pdf

National Hospice and Palliative Care Organization (NHPCO). (2016). *Facts and figures: Hospice care in America.* Retrieved from https://www.nhpco.org/sites/default/files/public/Statistics_Research/2016_Facts_Figures.pdf

National Hospice and Palliative Care Organization. (2017). *Ten components of quality care.* Alexandria, VA: NHPCO. Retrieved from https://www.nhpco.org/quality/10-components-quality-care

National Institutes of Health. (2014). *NIH makes palliative care more attainable for pediatric patients and their families.* Retrieved from http://www.nih.gov/news/health/jan2014/ninr-08.htm

Paice, J. A., & Fine, P. G. (2006). Pain at the end of life. In B. R. Ferrell & N. Coyle (Eds.). *Textbook of palliative nursing* (pp. 131–153). Oxford: Oxford University Press.

ProCon. (2018). *State-by-state guide to physician-assisted suicide. Understand the issues.* Understand each other. Retrieved from https://euthanasia.procon.org/view.resource.php?resourceID=000132

Quill, T. (2000). Perspectives on care at the close of life. Initiating end-of-life discussion with seriously ill patients: Addressing the "elephant in the room." *Journal of the American Medical Association, 284*(19), 2501–2507.

Reuben, D., Herr, K., Pacala, J., Pollock, B., Potter, J., & Semla, T. (2017). *Geriatrics at your fingertips* (19th ed.). New York: American Geriatrics Society.

Ringer, T., Hazzan, A. A., Agarwal, A., Mutsaers, A., & Papaioannou, A. (2017). Relationship between family caregiver burden and physical frailty in older adults without dementia: a systematic review. *Systematic Reviews, BioMed Central, 6*(1), 55. Retrieved from https://systematicreviewsjournal.biomedcentral.com/articles/10.1186/s13643-017-0447-1

Spruill, A., Mayer, D., & Hamilton, J. (2013). Barriers in hospice use among African Americans with cancer. *Journal of Hospice and Palliative Nursing, 15*(3), 136–144.

SUPPORT Principal Investigators. (1995). A controlled trial to improve care for seriously ill hospitalized patients. The study to understand prognoses and preferences for outcomes and risks of treatment. *Journal of the American Medical Association, 274*(20), 1591–1598.

Ventura, A. D., Burney, S., Brooker, J., Fletcher, J., & Ricciardelli, L. (2013). Home-based palliative care: A systematic literature review of self-reported unmet needs of patients and carers. *Palliative Medicine, 28*(5), 391–402.

Ward, B. W., Schiller, J. S., & Goodman, R. A. (2014). Multiple chronic conditions among US adults: a 2012 update. *Prevention of Chronic Disease, 11,* E62.

World Health Organization. (1990). *Cancer pain relief and palliative care Technical Report Series, 804.* Geneva, Switzerland: Author.

World Health Organization (WHO). (2017). *WHO definition of palliative care.* Retrieved from http://www.who.int/cancer/palliative/definition/en/

Chapter 25

Occupational Health Nursing

Christine Pontus and
Patricia Goyette

Everything that is really great and inspiring is created by the individual who can labor in freedom.
Albert Einstein

If you cannot work with love but only with distaste, it is better that you should leave your work.
Khalil Gibran

Oh, you hate your job? Why didn't you say so? There's a support group for that. It's called everybody, and they meet at the bar.
Drew Carey

CHAPTER HIGHLIGHTS

- Characteristics of the worker and workplace
- Roles and responsibilities of occupational health nurses
- Models for occupational health practice
- Worker and workplace assessment
- Health promotion in workplace settings
- Use of epidemiologic techniques in occupational health
- Emergency preparedness and disaster management
- Emerging issues in occupational health nursing practice

OBJECTIVES

- Explain the role of nursing in occupational health.
- State current trends in the U.S. workforce.
- Describe the four types of exposures and hazards in the workplace.
- Provide examples of common work-related injuries and illnesses.
- Explain the interaction of agent, host, and environment as applied to the workplace.
- Outline the steps involved in both worker and workplace assessment.
- Describe potential benefits to both workers and businesses in offering health promotion programs.
- Explain how principles of epidemiology are applied to occupational health.
- Assess specific components within an emergency preparedness plan that will vary from industry to industry based on risk.
- Describe how emerging technology, such as nanotechnology may impact occupational health practice.

KEY TERMS

American Association of Occupational Health Nurses (AAOHN): Professional association for nurses working in a business setting, dedicated to the health and safety of workers, worker populations, and community groups.

Biologic hazards: Hazards resulting from living organisms that cause adverse effects on people.

KEY TERMS *(continued)*

Chemical hazards: Generated from liquids, solids, dusts, fumes, vapors, and gases.

Ergonomics: Study of the relationship between people and their working environments.

Nanotechnology: Manipulation of matter on a near-atomic scale to produce new structures, materials, and devices; generally defined as engineered structures, devices, and systems.

Nanomaterials: Things that have a length scale between 1 and 100 nm.

National Institute of Occupational Safety and Health (NIOSH): The federal agency established to help ensure safe and healthy working conditions by conducting scientific research, gathering information, and providing education and training in occupational safety and health.

Occupational health history: An assessment of the characteristics of the workers' present jobs, a chronologic record of all past work and potential exposures, an occupational exposure inventory, and a list of other exposures in the home or community.

Occupational Safety and Health Administration (OSHA): The federal agency that sets exposure standards and is responsible for enforcement of safety and health legislation.

Physical hazards: Hazards that result from the transfer of physical energy to workers.

Psychosocial hazards: All organizational factors and interpersonal relationships in the workplace that may affect the health of the workers.

Root cause analysis: A process for understanding and solving a problem, with the goal of determining what happened, why it happened, and what can be done to prevent its reoccurrence.

Workplace walk-through: A complete survey of the workplace, inside and outside, compiling information as to the presence of hazards, the location of entries and exits, the availability of emergency equipment, and potential trouble spots.

CASE STUDIES

References to the case studies are found throughout this chapter (look for the case study icon). Readers should keep the case studies in mind as they read the chapter.

CASE 1

A 32-year-old female bank employee suddenly stops breathing while at work. A coworker calls rescue (911), and emergency medical technicians rush her to the hospital. Later, physicians determine that she suffered respiratory arrest related to an anaphylactic reaction. An occupational health nurse (OHN) investigates both the hospitalization and the workers' compensation claim because the incident occurred at the place of employment. This investigation clarifies the incident and identifies its underlying cause, so that measures can be taken to prevent it from happening to other workers.

On receiving the case briefing from both the loss prevention and the claims management departments, the OHN reviews the file and speaks to the worker and her supervisor. The worker said that she had an anaphylactic reaction and that her supervisor told her not to return to work until physicians discovered and medically confirmed the cause of her reaction. She has an appointment with an allergist about a possible allergy.

CASE 2

At the opening of business on a Friday morning, four people enter the occupational health clinic at a factory. The employees complain of nausea, vomiting, diarrhea, fatigue, and headache. The OHN, concerned that a common exposure caused these workers to become ill, discovers that all four attended the company picnic the day before. A phone call to human resources reveals that more employees who attended the picnic have called in sick with complaints of nausea, vomiting, and diarrhea. At the picnic, the food included hamburgers; sausage and pepper sandwiches; potato, chicken, and tossed salad; and beverages such as chocolate milk, soda, and water. The OHN talks to the kitchen manager. Apparently, there have been recent problems with heat regulators, a refrigeration unit, newly hired help, and the training of cafeteria workers. The nurse immediately calls the Department of Public Health.

INTRODUCTION

Occupational health nurses (OHNs) can be found in as many diverse settings as there are types of employment for workers. They observe and care for the community, group, business, or organization as a whole. This chapter presents an overview of the discipline, work, regulations, and conditions associated with the healthcare of the workforce, both nationally and internationally. It is hoped that this information will heighten an awareness of the kinds of care provided in the community workplace environment.

THE WORKER AND THE WORKPLACE

Work is an integral part of life for most people, providing challenging and worthwhile experiences that evolve and change over time. On average, employed adults spend about one third of their time at work. Health risks are inherent in every industry, and as the workplace changes, the risk that workers will experience adverse health effects related to employment also changes. Although the potential for serious adverse health effects from exposure to dangerous substances or less-than-optimal conditions is associated with every occupation, the majority of workers do not experience hazards in the workplace. The common workplace exposures and hazards listed in Table 25.1 indicate that there are a wide variety of potential threats to health. The specialty of occupational health focuses on the identification and control of risks to health which occur as a result of physical, chemical, and other workplace hazards. The goal is to establish and maintain a safe and healthy environment for workers. Occupational health is closely allied to the specialty of environmental health, a field of public health science that focuses on how the environment influences human health (see Chapter 19). **Ergonomics**, the study of the relationship between people and their working environment, emerged during the 20th century. Also called biotechnology and human engineering, ergonomics is the applied science of equipment design, intended to maximize productivity by reducing operator fatigue and discomfort.

Designing your product for monetization first and people second will probably leave you with neither. **Tara Hunt, marketing consultant**

In July 2017, there were approximately 160 million people in the workforce in the United States, an increase from 2015 workforce of 157 million (U.S. Department of Labor, Bureau of Labor Statistics [BLS], 2017). The U.S. Bureau of Labor Statistics also indicates that 3.3 of 100 workers in all industries, including state and local governments, have a reportable injury or illness. In contrast, in 2015, when state and local governments, which are responsible for protection of the public, were removed from the calculations, there were 3.0 cases per 100 workers in private industry. The trends illustrated in Figure 25.1 show that small companies have a lower rate of injury and illness over time, and companies with between 50 and 249 employees have consistently had the highest rates. The trends shown in Figure 25.2 indicate the private industries that had at least 50,000 nonfatal occupational injuries and illnesses in 2015, and showed that general medical and surgical hospitals were at the top of the list.

Table 25.2 shows the incidence rates of occupational injuries and illnesses by industry and case types in 2015. The case rate reflects the total number of reportable events that occurred, the majority of which are mild, such as strains and sprains. The case rate for days away from work indicates that a more serious injury or illness occurred that required time away from work. The resulting costs amount to billions of dollars each year. The injuries and illnesses occur at places of business; therefore, this spreads the costs to consumers in the form of higher prices, to workers in the form of lower wages, and to taxpayers.

Injuries were the most common result of workplace hazards. The majority of the 2.9 million nonfatal workplace injuries and illnesses reported in 2015 were injuries. Seventy-five percent of these injuries occurred in

TABLE 25.1 Common Workplace Hazards and Exposures

Biologic Hazards	Chemical Exposures	Physical Hazards	Psychosocial Factors
Infectious agents	Hazardous drug and toxin exposures	Electric and magnetic fields	Sexual harassment
Contaminated body fluids	Diesel exhaust	Ultraviolet radiation	Psychological stress
Poisonous plants	Aerosols	Cold stress	Interpersonal problems
Insects, scorpions, spiders	Respirable particulate matter and fumes	Heat stress	Assaults and violent acts
Venomous snakes	Take-home toxins (reached workers' home and families)	Noise Vibration Lighting	Bodily reaction and exertion
	Substances in cleaning solutions, for example, floor strippers, disinfection, and sterilization products	Falls Fires and vibration Particulate inhalation Unsafe machinery and equipment Abrasive blasting Inadequate workstations Transportation accidents	

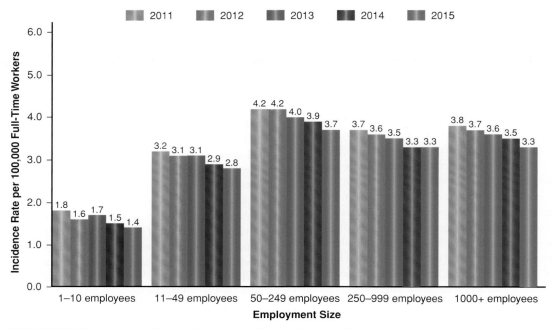

FIGURE 25.1 Total recordable nonfatal occupational injury and illness incidence rates by employment size class, private industry, 2011 to 2015. (From Bureau of Labor Statistics, U.S. Department of Labor. [2017]. *Workplace Injuries and Illnesses—2016*. Retrieved from http://www.bls.gov/news.release/pdf/osh.pdf.)

service-providing industries such as healthcare, professional, and technical businesses (U.S. Department of Labor, BLS, 2016a). Table 25.3 indicates that the highest incidence rate of injuries resulting in days away from work occurred from sprains, strains, and tears, followed by cuts and bruises. Workplace illnesses, most of which are associated with repetitive strain (i.e., carpal tunnel), accounted for only 0.5% of the total injury and illness cases in 2015 contributing to the most days away from work (U.S. Department of Labor, BLS, 2016b).

Unfortunately, deaths do occur in the workplace. In 2015, a total of 4,836 workers in the United States died as a result of injuries sustained at work. Figure 25.3 shows the number and rate of fatal occupational injuries by industry sector in 2015. Note that Figure 25.3 depicts that the number of fatal injuries related to transportation is the highest. Figure 25.4 shows the manner in which these occupational fatalities occurred. More work-related fatalities resulted from transportation incidents than from any other event. In 2015, 3.4% of all workers had an injury or illness related to the

FIGURE 25.2 Industries with at least 50,000 nonfatal occupational injuries and illnesses, private industry, 2015. (From U.S. Bureau of Labor Statistics, U.S. Department of Labor. [2016]. *Number of nonfatal occupational injuries and illnesses by industry and case type 2015*. Retrieved from https://www.bls.gov/news.release/pdf/osh.pdf.)

Industry	Case Rate (%)	Case Rate for Days away from Work (%)
Natural resources and mining	3.7	2.2
Construction	3.5	2.0
Manufacturing	3.8	2.2
Service providing	2.9	1.5
Trade, transportation, and utilities	3.6	2.2
Information	1.3	0.8
Financial activities	1.1	0.6
Professional and business services	1.4	0.7
Education and health services	4.0	1.9
Leisure and hospitality	3.5	1.5
Other services	2.3	1.2
Public administration	4.0	2.0
Total for all industries, including state and local government	3.3	1.0

TABLE 25.2 Incidence Rates of Nonfatal Occupational Injuries and Illnesses by Industry and Case Types, 2015

Source: U.S. Bureau of Labor Statistics, U.S. Department of Labor Statistics. (2016). *Incidence rates of nonfatal occupational injuries and illnesses by industry and case types, 2015*. Retrieved from http://www.bls.gov/news.release/osh.htm.

Characteristics	Incidence Rate Per 10,000 Full-Time Workers	Median Days Away From Work
Sprains, strains, tears	38.0	10
Cuts, lacerations, punctures	8.1	4
Bruises, contusions	9.1	3
Fractures	8.9	31
Multiple traumatic injuries	2.8	10
Heat (thermal) burns	1.6	5
Carpal tunnel syndrome	0.5	28
Amputations	0.5	22
Chemical burns	0.3	3
Tendonitis	0.2	14

TABLE 25.3 Statistics on Occupational Injuries and Illnesses, Involving Days Away From Work in Private Industry, State Government, and Local Government, 2015

Source: U.S. Bureau of Labor Statistics, *Survey of Occupational Injuries and Illnesses, in cooperation with participating state agencies.* https://www.bls.gov/news.release/osh2.htm.

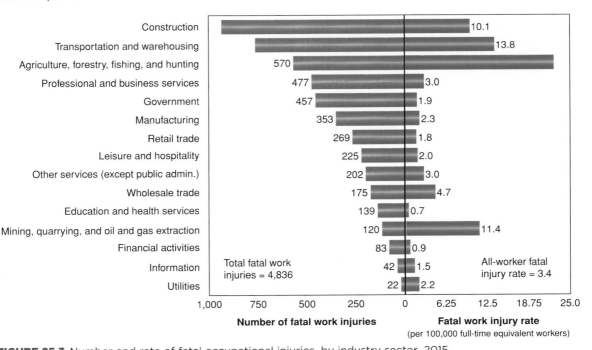

FIGURE 25.3 Number and rate of fatal occupational injuries, by industry sector, 2015. *Note:* Fatal injury rates exclude workers under the age of 16 years, volunteers, and resident military. The number of fatal work injuries represents total published fatal injuries before the exclusions. For additional information on the fatal work injury rate methodology, please see https://www.bls.gov/news.release/archives/cfoi_12162016.pdf. (*Source:* U.S. Bureau of Labor Statistics, Current Population Survey, Census of Fatal Occupational Injuries, 2016.)

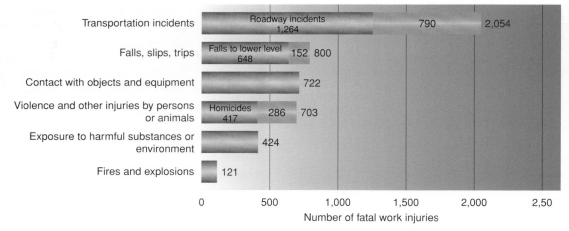

FIGURE 25.4 Fatal occupational injuries in 2015 (National Census Preliminary Report). (Bureau of Labor Statistics, U.S. Department of Labor. [2017]. *National census of fatal occupational injuries in 2015.* Retrieved from https://www.bls.gov/iif/oshwc/cfoi/cfch0014.pdf.)

workplace; these statistics reflect a slight decrease from 2011 (U.S. Department of Labor, BLS, 2016c).

Occupational health is a responsibility assumed by nurses worldwide. The World Health Organization (WHO) (2001) published a document describing the role of the OHN in workplace health management. This document reflects WHO's global plan to protect and promote workers' health in the workplace, enabling people to increase control over their health and avoid workplace hazards to their health.

OCCUPATIONAL HEALTH NURSING

Occupational health nursing and environmental health nursing are intertwined (see Chapter 19). The **American Association of Occupational Health Nurses (AAOHN)** represents both specialties. Occupational/environmental health nursing is defined as a specialty practice which provides for and delivers health and safety programs and services to workers, worker populations, and community groups. Practice focuses on promotion and restoration of health, prevention of injury and illness, and protection from occupational and environmental hazards. Practitioners combine their knowledge of public health and business with their healthcare expertise to provide a safe and healthy work and community environment. The clients may be individual workers, the work community, or the organization as a whole. This nursing specialty is multidisciplinary, practiced through the integration of knowledge from a variety of disciplines, including nursing, medicine, social and behavioral sciences, management, public health, and occupational health specialties such as toxicology, industrial hygiene, and ergonomics.

History

The earliest record of occupational health nursing, originally called industrial nursing, began a few years after

Florence Nightingale opened the "Nightingale Training School for Nurses" in 1860. In 1867, J. & J. Colman, a mustard company, hired Phillipa Flowerday in Norwich, Great Britain. Many consider her employment at this company the earliest recorded evidence of a company specifically hiring an industrial nurse to work in the dispensary and provide home care services to workers and their families.

In 1885, the Vermont Marble Company hired Ada Mayo Stewart to care for employees and their families, and she may have been one of the first "industrial nurses." Often arriving by bicycle, Ada conducted home visits providing care for ill workers and focused on teaching healthy living habits to families. In 1888, a group of coal mining companies hired Betty Moulder, a graduate of what is now Philadelphia General Hospital, to provide nursing care for injured and ill workers and their families. Unfortunately, not much information is available about her duties, background, or accomplishments.

Industrial nursing grew rapidly along with the growth of industry in the early 20th century. People recognized that the provision of health services in the workplace led to more worker productivity. Factories employed nurses to combat the spread of infectious diseases such as tuberculosis, and to address health-related problems resulting from labor shortages during World War I. There were several thousand industrial nurses by World War II, and the establishment of educational programs along with professional organizations followed. The AAOHN formed in 1942, with 16 states represented by 300 nurses, and some member nurses created the American Association of Industrial Nurses (AAIN). The intent of AAOHN was to improve occupational health program services while enhancing career opportunities for occupational and environmental health nurses (AAOHN, n.d.a).

In the United States, Congress passed several laws in the 1960s and 1970s to protect the safety and health of workers, leading to an increased need for OHNs. The 1968 Mine Safety and Health Act required the first prevention programs for workers. In 1970 came the Occupational Safety and Health Act, which established two government agencies, the **Occupational Safety and Health Administration (OSHA)**, and the **National Institute of Occupational Safety and Health (NIOSH)**. The mission of OSHA is to prevent work-related injuries, illnesses, and fatalities by setting federal standards regulating workers' exposures to potentially toxic substances. Regulations, data, and information regarding compliance assistance, training programs, and consultation are available at the OSHA website. The purpose of NIOSH is to help ensure safe and healthy working conditions by conducting scientific research, gathering information, and providing education and training in occupational safety and health. The organization provides leadership worldwide by fostering the translation of new knowledge into products and services. The NIOSH website contains more information about its activities.

Standards of Practice

OHNs can be found in almost every industry, from manufacturing and construction to public administration and leisure and hospitality businesses. They collaborate with employees, employers, members of the occupational health and safety team, and other professionals to (1) identify health and safety needs, (2) prioritize interventions, (3) develop and implement interventions and programs, and (4) evaluate care and service delivery (AAOHN, 2012a). Their scope of practice encompasses a broad range of activities that are discussed later in this chapter.

As the professional association for occupational and environmental health nurses, the AAOHN establishes and promulgates standards to define and advance the practice within a framework for evaluation. These statements describe the accountability of the practitioner and reflect the values and priorities of the profession. AAOHN has identified 11 professional practice standards that describe a competent level of performance with regard to the nursing process and professional roles of the occupational and environmental health nurse. Criteria developed for each standard are key indicators of competent practice and permit occupational and environmental health nurses to evaluate their practice relative to the standards (AAOHN, 2012b). These standards can be accessed online.

The AAOHN identifies nine categories of competency in occupational and environmental health nursing. OHN competencies are associated with specific guidelines as they relate to all OHNs who function in various workplace settings. Different settings require different levels of competency and specific skill sets. Benner (1984) identified five stages of competency in clinical nursing practice: novice, advanced beginner, competent, proficient, and expert. Within each stage are levels of achievement that are expressed in measurable behavioral objectives. AAOHN has cross-referenced and

stated behavioral objectives for the OHN in three of these stages: competent, proficient, and expert. This establishes criteria for individual nurses and those in management positions to use in their own professional development. AAOHN (2007) competency levels in occupational and environmental health nursing are listed in Box 25.1.

> The nicest thing about standards is that there are so many of them to choose from. **Ken Olsen, founder, Digital Equipment Corporation**

Environmental issues, conditions, and activities unique to OHN practice are addressed in the AAOHN Delivery of Occupational and Environmental Health Services position statement (AAOHN, 2012a). AAOHN makes the assertion that based on training, education, and experience, the licensed OHNs are in the best position to deliver comprehensive occupational and environmental health services and

25.1 AAOHN Competency Levels in Occupational and Environmental Health Nursing

Competent—A nurse who is confident and a master with an ability to cope with specific situations. There is less of a need to rely on the judgment of peers and other professionals (Benner, 1984). Example: A competent occupational and environmental health nurse recognizes a range of practice issues and functions comfortably in roles as clinician, coordinator, and case manager following company procedures, utilizing assessment checklists and clinical protocols to provide treatment.

Proficient—A nurse with the ability to perceive client situations based on past experiences, with focus on relevant aspects of the situation. The nurse is able to predict expected events in certain situations and recognize that protocols must be altered at times to meet the needs of the client (Benner, 1984). Example: A proficient occupational and environmental health nurse quickly obtains the information needed for accurate assessment and moves quickly to the critical aspects of a problem, within priority setting and structural goals, in response to a client's situation. The nurse usually possesses sophisticated clinical or managerial skills in the work and/or community environment.

Expert—A nurse having extensive experience with a broad knowledge base that enables one to grasp a situation quickly and initiate action. The nurse has a sense of salience grounded in practice guiding actions and priorities (Benner, 1984). Example: An expert occupational and environmental health nurse provides leadership in developing occupational safety and health policy within the organization, functions in upper executive or management roles, serves as a consultant to business and government, and designs and conducts significant research.

Source: Used with permission from American Association of Occupational Health Nurses. (2007). Competencies in occupational and environmental health nursing. *American Association of Occupational Health Nurses,* 55(11), 442–447.

workplace programs. Today, the scope of practice is broad, including disease management, environmental health, emergency preparedness, and disaster planning in response to natural, technologic, and human hazards in the work and community environment (AAOHN, n.d.a).

The OHN must also adhere to a code of ethics that is based on the belief that the goal of occupational and environmental health nurses is to promote workers' health and safety. The purpose of the AAOHN Code of Ethics is to serve as a guide for registered professional nurses to maintain and pursue professionally recognized ethical behavior when providing occupational health services (AAOHN, 2012a).

Founded in 1972, the American Board of Occupational Health Nurses (ABOHN) is an independent nursing specialty certification board. ABOHN is the sole certifying body for OHNs in the United States. Standards of nursing practice are used to validate an individual registered nurse's qualifications, knowledge, and practice in specific areas of occupational health nursing (ABOHN, 2012a). ABOHN awards four credentials: Certified Occupational Health Nurse (COHN), Certified Occupational Health Nurse–Specialist (COHN–S), Case Management (CM), and Safety Management (SM). More information can be obtained from the ABOHN website (ABOHN, 2012b).

CONCEPTUAL FRAMEWORKS

The Epidemiologic Triad

The epidemiologic triad, discussed in detail in Chapter 6, is very helpful in occupational health nursing practice as a means to understand the complex relationships among the workers, hazards in the workplace, and hazards in the environment (Fig. 25.5).

Practice Point

Applying the epidemiologic triad model to the specific workplace helps OHNs understand the interaction between hazards, workers, and the environment.

FIGURE 25.5 The epidemiologic triad for the workplace.

Host

In the epidemiologic triad, each worker is a host within the work population. Each person (host) has his or her own innate, nonmodifiable characteristics, some of which put him or her at risk for workplace injury or illness. For example, age, gender, and ethnicity are nonmodifiable characteristics, whereas lifestyle, work practice, and to some degree, health status are modifiable characteristics. New workers with less than one year of experience are the most susceptible to injury. In contrast, older workers, who may have chronic illness, hearing loss, vision difficulties, or delayed reaction times, may adversely react to workplace hazards more frequently. Some workers are hypersusceptible, developing reactions, even though their exposure levels are below those determined to be safe.

Agent

The agents in the epidemiologic triad are workplace hazards classified as **biologic**, **chemical**, **physical**, or **psychosocial hazards** (see Table 25.1).

BIOLOGIC AGENTS

Biologic agents include hazards from living organisms that have adverse effects. Although human illness often occurs from exposure to microorganisms, toxins released from microorganisms, insects, or animals are also biologic agents. Healthcare settings are particularly vulnerable to biologic hazards, and transmission of resistant infectious organisms is a major concern (see Chapter 14). Healthcare personnel are cognizant of potential exposures, but many workers such as maintenance workers, security personnel, and cleaners may be inadvertently exposed by trash, soiled linens, and contaminated equipment, which may result in illness.

CHEMICAL AGENTS

As industry grows, there is increasing general chemical contamination at work, at home, and in the community. Less than one percent of the two million chemicals used in industry have been studied for their effects on humans. Through ingestion, respiration, and injury, these environmental chemicals enter the body, and although exposure may be less than the maximal exposure standards (if they exist), the chemicals often accumulate, leading to a potentially chronic or life-threatening condition. There are many examples of illnesses resulting from chemical exposures. It has been known for decades that miners exposed to coal dust can suffer from pneumoconiosis, or black lung disease. Inhalation of asbestos may cause mesothelioma, a rare form of cancer found in the lining of the heart, lungs, abdomen, or the internal reproductive organs. Radiation exposure during pregnancy can result in congenital malformations, as can exposure to heavy metals and antineoplastic drugs. Interaction between the various chemicals entering the body also occurs, making it very difficult to predict the effects on health.

PHYSICAL AGENTS

Physical agents are sources of energy that may lead to injury or illness. Vibration produced through use of power tools may contribute to Raynaud phenomenon, which is vasoconstriction of the small arteries in fingers or toes, triggered by cold or emotional upset. Vibrations associated with some power tools and trucks may adversely affect internal organs. Other common physical agents are radiation, temperature extremes, noise, lighting, falls, and unsafe equipment. Monitoring exposure to such agents and use of personal protective equipment such as preventive clothes, eye guards, and hearing protection are common practice in industry.

Evidence for Practice

Initial recognition of latex allergy occurred in the late 1970s. Healthcare workers are at risk through exposure to latex gloves or medical products containing latex. It is estimated that 8% to 12% of healthcare workers are latex-sensitive (OSHA, n.d.f). Hundreds of everyday products contain latex. Repeated exposure to the protein in natural latex can make a person more likely to develop a latex allergy. It usually begins within minutes of exposure but can sometimes occur hours later. It produces varied symptoms, which commonly include runny nose, sneezing, itchy eyes, scratchy throat, hives, and itchy burning sensations. However, it can involve more severe symptoms including asthma marked by difficult breathing, coughing spells, and wheezing; cardiovascular and gastrointestinal ailments; and in rare cases, anaphylaxis and death (CDC, 2013). Healthcare workers with suspected latex allergy may use nonlatex nitrile, synthetic rubber, or vinyl gloves.

PSYCHOSOCIAL AGENTS

Psychosocial agents include all organizational factors and interpersonal relationships in the workplace that may affect the health of the workers. Psychosocial hazards are as real as physical hazards, and if not recognized and controlled, they potentially can have a very negative impact. Studies have found that workers who have a high expectation for productivity, yet little or no control over their workplace and little reward for their efforts, are at risk for psychosocial distress. Stress, anger, and frustration can result in aggressive behavior, harassment, sabotage of the work or the work of others, poor physical and mental health, and disregard of safety measures. These feelings are enhanced if there is a perception of employer unfairness. Multiple studies have indicated that nurses have a wide range of occupational factors linked to stress such as work overload, time pressure, exposure to infectious diseases, needlestick injuries, and understaffing (NIOSH, 2008). Linked to psychosocial hazards are issues such as workplace violence. There are several risk factors

25.2 Workplace Violence Risk Factors in Health Care

Patient, Client, and Setting-Related Risk Factors

Working directly with people who have a history of violence, abuse drugs or alcohol, gang members, and relatives of patients or clients

Transporting patients and clients

Working alone in a facility or in patients' homes

Poor environmental design of the workplace that may block employees' vision or interfere with their escape from a violent incident

Poorly lit corridors, rooms, parking lots, and other areas

Lack of means of emergency communication

Prevalence of firearms, knives and other weapons among patients and their families and friends

Working in neighborhoods with high crime rates

Organizational Risk Factors

Lack of facility policies and staff training for recognizing and managing escalating hostile and assaultive behaviors from patients, clients, visitors, or staff

Working when understaffed—especially during mealtimes and visiting hours

High worker turnover

Inadequate security and mental health personnel on site

Long waits for patients or clients and overcrowded, uncomfortable waiting rooms

Unrestricted movement of the public in clinics and hospitals

Perception that violence is tolerated and victims will not be able to report the incident to police and/or press charges

Source: U.S. Department of Labor Occupational Safety and Health Administration. (2016). *Guidelines for Preventing Workplace Violence for Healthcare and Social Service Workers.* Retrieved on September 13, 2017, from https://www.osha.gov/Publications/osha3148.pdf.

related to workplace violence in healthcare (Box 25.2). Employers have increasingly developed strategies to manage the risks associated with psychosocial hazards. Examples include identifying the psychosocial hazards at the workplace, assessing ways to decentralize control, addressing workers' concerns about the workplace, and implementing systems to enable workers to report unacceptable behavior.

Of all man's miseries the bitterest is this, to know so much and to have control over nothing. **Herodotus**

Evidence for Practice

The National Institute of Occupational Safety and Health (2008) defines occupational stress as "the harmful physical and emotional responses that occur when the requirements of the job do not match the capabilities, resources, or needs of the worker." Strategies recommended by NIOSH to reduce workers' stress include distribution of workloads that are matched with workers' capabilities and resources, clearly defined workers' roles and responsibilities, as well as methods to improve communication within the organization. NIOSH also suggests that workers be offered opportunities to participate in decisions and actions affecting their jobs. This process reduces uncertainty about career development and future employment prospects. OHNs should be cognizant of stress in the workplace and incorporate the strategies recommended by NIOSH in planning interventions.

Environment

The workplace exists within an external environment with specific geologic and atmospheric characteristics, air and water quality, and presence or absence of environmental pollution. Sometimes unanticipated results come from a difficult mix of agent, host, and environment characteristics. For example, patients in the intensive care unit of a major Chicago hospital were negatively affected by automobile exhaust from a highway a few hundred feet away. Replacing the air conditioning system solved the problem. Economic and political decisions can affect the public health infrastructure and, therefore, the health of a society. Factors such as adequate housing, literacy, crowding, culture, customs, and availability and accessibility of healthcare services are issues to be addressed. Social problems occurring from alcohol and substance abuse, infectious diseases, and poverty can have an impact on workforce productivity.

Practice Point

There is a level of acceptable risk in any work setting. The primary goal is to lower the accepted level of risk of injury and illness associated with employment.

Practice Models

Figure 25.6 illustrates the Hanasaari model. This framework takes into account all the factors affecting people at work, a total environment concept. A group of OHNs developed this model at a workshop in Hanasaari, Finland, in 1989. Endorsed by the Federation of Occupational Health Nurses within the European Union (FOHNEU), it is now the basis for practice, education, and research throughout the European Union. The model presents an outer circle that represents the total global concept, covering all aspects of health and safety affecting the worker population in the general environment. Extending out from the center (occupational health nursing) are the social, political, ecologic, organizational, and economic factors that influence the global environment. The man-work-health triangle indicates that the total environment can have a significant effect on workplace

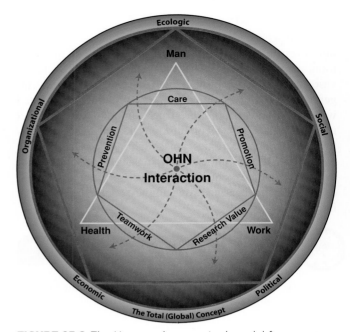

FIGURE 25.6 The Hanasaari conceptual model for occupational health nursing (OHN). OHN is presented in the center of the model. The *curving circle of arrows* represents flexibility, influence, and eventual improvement in the health of people at work and in the total community environment. (From Alston, R. M., et al. [1989]. Workshop for Occupational Health Nurses, Hanasaari, Finland [Unpublished manuscript]. Retrieved from http://www.fohneu.org/hanasaari_conceptual_model_for_o.htm.)

health. Political and social policies, for example, either expand or contract the development of occupational health.

A more recent model proposed by Thomason and Lagowski (2008) is one of collaboration and reciprocation while using the nursing process. Earlier models have not focused on the key concept of engaging clients in reciprocal relationships. This approach suggests that the OHN should use leadership and interpersonal relationship skills which foster communication and respect through continuous feedback from workers and community. The model provides a means of engaging and collaborating with clients in restoring and maintaining health, well-being, and workplace safety. Figure 25.7 illustrates the five steps of collaboration between the nurse and the client.

One of the tests of leadership is the ability to recognize a problem before it becomes an emergency. **Arnold Glasgow, psychologist**

The OHN must deal with individual, family, and community issues that often involve medical, legal, and regulatory factors. Forces may contradict and hinder health and safety priorities unless the OHN can communicate and act to resolve the issues. For example, a system's approach can be very effective within a single department or division. However, the same system may fail when interfacing with other activities of the workplace within a community. It is

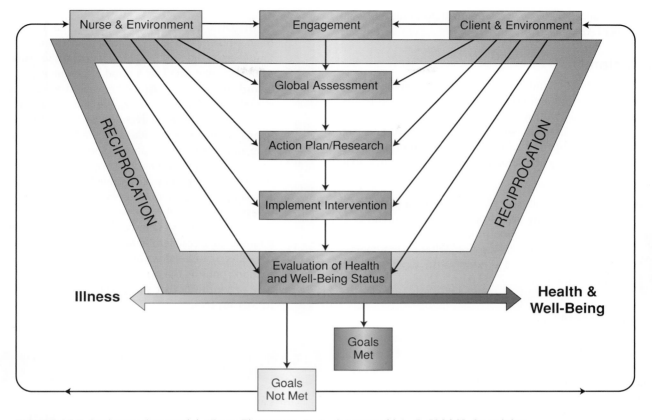

FIGURE 25.7 Reciprocation model. (From Thomason, D. A., & Lagowski, L. R. [2008]. Sustaining a healthy work force in the 21st century—A model for collaborating through reciprocation. *Journal of American Association of Occupational Health Nursing, 56*[12], 503–513.)

often the workers who take the responsibility to correct an unplanned problem, and they may choose to put themselves at risk. Without recognition, support, and ongoing communication with workers, the risk may not be apparent. It is through reciprocation during these crucial moments of a worker's life that an OHN can help sustain and maintain worker and community health.

A large number of OHNs find employment in the field as individual, privately contracted professionals. It is common for many occupational and environmental health nurses to work in more than one designated role concurrently while employed by the same company (Zichello & Sheridan, 2008). One particular practice model includes corporate OHNs who often have a master's degree. They can be responsible for managing the implementation of occupational health goals and objectives for other nurses in various facilities.

The ABOHN (2012b) conducted a 2011 Occupational Health Nursing Practice Analysis. Respondents revealed the majority of nurses are female (95.1%; male, 4.9%), and most do not have global responsibility. Nurses spend the greatest amount of time in two practice areas: health and wellness activities, and case management (ABOHN, 2012b). Midsize to larger companies may have more than one occupational and/or environmental health nurse on site. In large

companies, there can be nurses and physicians, including advanced practice nurses, in nurse practitioner roles.

There are various ways nurses enter and function in OHN positions. Most employers conduct a job search for an OHN, OHN manager, or a nurse practitioner and are specific about the education and experience required. Many employers look for a board-certified (ABOHN) nurse who has at least a bachelor of science in nursing, with three to five years' nursing experience. Some employers search for an advanced practice nurse or nurse practitioner who is prepared at the master's level. In recent years, licensed practical nurses (LPNs) and licensed vocational nurses (LVNs) are found to work in specific roles and function as team members with other OHNs who may delegate and manage activity as necessary (AAOHN, 2012a).

OCCUPATIONAL HEALTH NURSING: PRACTICE

Following their job analysis study, the ABOHN determined and designated functional roles and responsibilities for the occupational and environmental health nurse. Occupational health nursing practice requires a wide variety of roles and functions, and specific responsibilities vary. Roles include clinician, case manager, counselor, health promotion specialist, manager/administrator, educator, and researcher (ABOHN, 2012a).

Clinician

The OHN acts as a clinician whose primary responsibilities are to prevent work and non–work-related health problems, and to restore as well as maintain the health of workers. Assessments of hazards, surveillance of the workers and workplace, investigation of illness, and monitoring events that lead to an injury are fundamental to achieving this goal.

As in the case of an outbreak of illness following the company picnic, frequent communication from employees brings a problem to a nurse's attention. What assessments should be performed as soon as the workers arrive at the clinic?

Worker Assessment

Along with the traditional history and physical assessment, an **occupational health history** of every worker is an essential component of OHN practice. Components include characteristics of the worker's present jobs, a chronologic record of all past work and potential exposures, an occupational exposure inventory, and a list of other exposures in the home or community. Particular emphasis should include any individual characteristics that may predispose the worker to increased risk in a particular job. This information provides an understanding of a worker's current health status and the potential impact of exposures on health and future job performance.

Nurses have an opportunity to teach about workplace hazards and prevention measures when performing worker assessments. Assessments may take place before the worker begins the job, on a periodic basis, when the worker is being transferred to a different job with different exposures, and when an exposure, illness, or injury occurs. The goal of assessments is to identify the agent, host, and environmental characteristics which could place the worker at risk, and to take preventive steps to eliminate or reduce adverse exposures.

Following a work-related illness or injury, an initial physical assessment, including documentation and medical case record initiation, is required. Direct care and treatment of injuries is provided, often using established medical protocols. Referrals are then made for further evaluation as required. However, illnesses and injuries are often symptoms of problems in the workplace. The concept of root cause analysis (RCA), discussed shortly, can be applied when performing an accident investigation after an injury.

In Case 2, the OHN conducts a telephone interview with the employee who had an anaphylactic reaction. What type of information should the OHN obtain?

The OHN discovers that the employee had been a nurse who left hospital employment four years earlier and began working in the bank. At the hospital, she had a good attendance record. She left the hospital because she was having difficulty doing her work; she had a rash on her hands and a general low energy level. Her hands would begin to heal and she felt better on long weekends and vacations. She was not asthmatic, had never experienced any respiratory problems, and had never received a diagnosis of an allergy. However, on further questioning and investigation, the OHN learns that the woman's mother was a nurse who could not work in a hospital setting because of a latex allergy. (She was also allergic to bananas and avocados.) This information confirms the possibility of an inherited type of sensitivity that a physician would need to further explore.

✎ Practice Point

OHNs are more likely to notice the influence of work–health interactions if the worker assessment data are complete. The assessment involves continuous monitoring and surveillance of workers and their environment.

Workplace Assessment

A **workplace walk-through** is a technique for an assessment of the workplace. This process leads to an understanding of the work process, the requirements for the various jobs, the materials involved, the presence of actual or potential hazards, and the work practices of the employees (Peek-Asa et al., 2009). It is a complete survey of the workplace, inside and outside, compiling information as to the presence of hazards, the location of entries and exits, the availability of emergency equipment, and potential trouble spots (Box 25.3). If the organization employs a health and safety officer or risk manager, the workplace walk-through analysis will be a shared responsibility.

It is helpful to use a team approach during this process, soliciting the help of employees in gathering the information. OSHA strongly encourages maximum employee participation in the walk-through. Better-informed and more alert employees can assist in identifying and correcting potential injury and illness hazards in one's workplace. Talking with employees during the walk-through helps identify the nature and extent of specific hazards. The assessment should be comprehensive, thorough, and take place frequently because conditions may change daily. A system for corrective action should be in place when improvement is needed.

25.3 Workplace Walk-Through—Evaluation of Workplace Hazards

Alarms and detection devices
Occupancy, building diagrams
Exits
Fire prevention plans
Procedures for processing, receiving, shipping, and storage
Condition of buildings and grounds
Housekeeping program for fall prevention
Heating, ventilation, air-conditioning systems
Electricity
Lighting
Presence of guards for machine use
Worker training procedures
Hand and power tools
Hazardous materials
Maintenance and servicing of machines and equipment
(control of hazardous energy)
Personal protective equipment use
Emergency action plans

In Case 1, the OHN also finds that renovation and construction was occurring on the floors above the employee's office and in adjacent offices when the worker became ill. Fellow employees state that they noticed an odor on the day their coworker was rushed to the hospital. Five employees detected the odor, and two of them experienced headaches, with symptoms such as light-headedness and itchy, watering eyes. They became alarmed when their coworker started to have serious difficulty breathing.

The construction supervisor states that walls in the adjacent office space were being painted, carpets installed, seams glued, and general cleaning done in nearby areas the day of the incident. Immediately, the nurse asks the supervisor what type of paint was used the day of the incident. The OHN also wants to know what material the carpet was made of, and the types of glue and cleaning products used. A combination of environmental factors such as chemicals, fumes, vapor, dust, heat, or moisture may create an adverse condition for some people.

Case Manager

Case manager responsibilities include coordination and management of services for ill or injured workers, including various aspects related to group health, workers' compensation, and regulations pertaining to the Family Medical Leave Act (FMLA) (AAOHN, n.d.a). Case managers are as concerned with prevention as they are with healthcare after an accident. The overall goal is to do everything that can be done to prevent accidents and minimize illness.

The case manager tracks each incident that relates to employees' health and safety, beginning immediately after the onset of an illness or injury, and continuing through rehabilitation and return to work. Following the initial event, case managers gather case characteristics that provide detailed information about the circumstances of workplace injuries and illness that required one or more days away from work. There are four basic case characteristics: nature of the workplace incident, the part of the body involved, the source of the illness or injury and the circumstances that resulted in the exposure or event. After case managers record this information for ongoing monitoring of the workplace, they perform an RCA.

Root Cause Analysis

Root cause analysis (RCA) is a process for understanding and solving a problem with the goal of determining what happened, why it happened, and what can be done to prevent its recurrence. Sometimes, determination of the problem is easy; however, the process can be more complicated.

There are usually three basic types of causes: (1) tangible physical causes in which materials or machines have failed; (2) human causes when people did something wrong, either by commission or omission; or (3) organizational causes in which the policies or procedures used to make decisions were faulty. RCA incorporates all three types of causes, and it is possible to apply this method in almost any situation. It involves investigating the patterns of negative effects, finding hidden flaws in the system, and discovering specific actions that contributed to the problem. This often means that RCA reveals more than one root cause. By tracing actions back to their origins, the person using RCA can determine where the problem started and how it contributed to the illness or injury that occurred. RCA is the application of the scientific method to a specific workplace problem when applied to occupational health settings. The steps of RCA are outlined in Box 25.4.

In Case 2, explain the steps that the OHN would take in initiating an RCA of the outbreak of illness following the company picnic. (Refer to Chapter 14 to review the steps in investigating an outbreak.)

Counselor/Consultant

The OHN acts as an advisor in selecting, developing, implementing, and evaluating occupational health and safety services within both organizations and communities. As a clinician and nurse consultant, it is the role of the OHN to investigate all possible material and chemical exposures that could lead to an adverse reaction in workers. By law, workers and their advocates have a right to know the substances to which they may be exposed, and therefore, they may request the requisite information. A material safety data

25.4 Root Cause Analysis Process in Occupational Health

Define the Problem
- Define the characteristics of the case.
- Determine the circumstances under which it occurred.

Collect Data
- Determine whether similar illnesses or injuries occurred in the past.
- Compare similarities and differences.
- Create a timeline related to the problem.
- Determine the impact of the problem.

Identify Possible Causal Factors
- Convene people involved in the situation to discuss cause.
- Determine the sequence of events that led to the illness or injury.
- Identify the conditions that allowed the problem to occur.
- Identify other problems that could be related to the problem.
- Create a chart of possible causal factors.
- Identify causal factors and possible interrelationships.

Identify the Root Cause(s)
- Identify the true causes of the illness or injury.
- Determine why the causal factor(s) exist.
- Determine the real reason the problem occurred.

Recommend and Implement Solutions
- Identify ways to prevent the problem from happening again.
- Plan for implementation of solutions.
- Identify who will be responsible.
- Determine the risks of implementing the solution.

Evaluate the Outcome
- Develop and implement an evaluation plan.

sheet (MSDS) provides information to employers from the manufacturer or producer of substances.

In addition to counseling people about work-related illnesses and injuries, OHNs also counsel groups regarding issues such as substance abuse, psychosocial needs, wellness/health promotion concerns, and work-related issues. The OHN may also assume primary responsibility for managing a variety of employee assistance programs. Often, an off-site provider or group is contracted to offer workers and their families counseling and other crisis intervention services. The nurse may also handle referrals to community resources while coordinating follow-up care for workers (AAOHN, n.d.a).

When we turn to one another for counsel we reduce the number of our enemies. **Khalil Gibran**

In Case 1, after learning about the renovation, the OHN asks for a list of materials and the MSDSs for the substances used that day. The construction supervisor supplies

names of the materials, a phone number to obtain a list of materials, as well as the MSDSs that addressed all the elements of the substances used during the renovation project.

Review of the MSDSs reveals that latex paint was used the day of the episode, along with cleaners and glues containing volatile organic compounds (VOCs). VOCs consist of a variety of chemicals that may have short- and long-term adverse health effects. Thousands of products emit VOCs, including paints, lacquers, paint strippers, adhesives, glues, cleaning supplies, pesticides, building materials, and furnishings. Concentrations of VOCs are consistently greater indoors than outdoors (U.S. Environmental Protection Agency [EPA], 2012a).

Health Promotion Specialist

As a health promotion specialist, the OHN participates in the development and management of a multidimensional, broad-range health promotion program that supports the business objectives of the organization. Health promotion and illness and injury prevention is a function that the OHN performs along a continuum for the worker population. The objective is to create an environment for the worker that provides a sense of balance among work, family, personal, health, and psychosocial concerns (AAOHN, n.d.a). *Healthy People 2020* Occupational Health and Safety Objectives for the United States are presented in Box 25.5.

25.5 *Healthy People 2020* Occupational Health and Safety Objectives

OSH-1 Reduce deaths from work-related injuries.
OSH-2 Reduce nonfatal work-related injuries.
OSH-3 Reduce the rate of injury and illness cases involving days away from work due to overexertion or repetitive motion.
OSH-4 Reduce pneumoconiosis deaths.
OSH-5 Reduce deaths from work-related homicides.
OSH-6 Reduce deaths from work-related assaults.
OSH-7 Reduce the proportion of persons who have elevated blood lead concentrations from work exposures.
OSH-8 Reduce occupational skin diseases or disorders among full-time workers.
OSH-9 (Developmental) Increase the proportion of employees who have access to programs that prevent or reduce employee stress.
OSH-10 Reduce new cases of work-related, noise-induced hearing loss.

Source: From Healthypeople.gov. (2013). *Healthy People 2020: Occupational safety and health.* Retrieved from http://www.healthypeople.gov/2020/topicsobjectives2020/objectiveslist.aspx?topicId=30.

Educating all employees and administrative staff regarding the exposures and hazards associated with the workplace is the foundation of health promotion efforts. Corporate nurse educators often design programs that are used to educate workers in multiple settings, with state, regional, national, or international audiences (Dirksen, 2006). Programs are conducted through webcasts, satellite broadcasts, webinars, or established websites.

The health promotion frameworks discussed in Chapter 5 have a particular application in occupational health and safety. For example, the OHN has a unique opportunity to contribute to the current *Healthy People* prevention agenda. He or she can use leading health indicators and national occupational health and safety objectives to assess the status of the workplace. This information is useful for identifying prevention objectives for the workplace, and implementation of specific interventions and action plans. The actual prevention activities performed at any given time are a result of many changing variables in the organization, and a balance among primary, secondary, and tertiary prevention efforts is essential. For example, the nurse who is concentrating on developing strategies to prevent work site injuries and disease (primary prevention) may have little time or resources for testing individual employees for risk factors that increase the potential for illness or injury (secondary prevention).

Historically, the OHN has been involved with workers in a supportive role to maintain health at the work site. In the 1989 work by Michael O'Donnell, the seminal definition of health promotion gave OHNs interested in the pursuit of wellness a relevant rationale to pursue this approach. According to O'Donnell (Fig. 25.8), optimal health includes a balance of physical, emotional, social, spiritual, and intellectual health. The nurse can contribute toward this end by creating an environment that develops awareness and encourages behavior change (O'Donnell, 2009).

A common health and safety promotion program in occupational settings involves preservation of sight and hearing. Within a company eye protection program, the OHN often works collaboratively with the safety director and/or human resources personnel in the oversight of these programs. The OHN has a role in coordinating administration of eye examinations for those employees who need prescription safety eyeglasses. There are several approaches that a company can take when establishing and maintaining a hearing protection program. The OHN may become a certified hearing

FIGURE 25.8 O'Donnell health promotion model. (O'Donnell, M. P. [2009] Definition of health promotion 2.0: Embracing passion, enhancing motivation, recognizing dynamic balance, and creating opportunities. *American Journal of Health Promotion, 24*[1], iv–iv.)

conservationist and carry out the required monitoring of noise levels within specific facilities, work areas, and departments. He or she may oversee or manage the distribution of hearing protection to workers, conduct education as needed, administer audiometric testing at the work site, manage the feedback of hearing tests results to employees, and ensure follow-up with a physician when needed.

Manager/Administrator

The responsibilities of the OHN frequently include participation in the development, management, and evaluation of the entire health and safety program of the organization in conjunction with both the medical and safety directors. Written policies and procedures consistent with organizational goals and objectives are required to ensure compliance with legal, regulatory, and ethical standards. Often, a company may ask the OHN to prepare a business plan that justifies the cost for establishing health promotion programs. This plan, by necessity, justifies how the program will be implemented within the organizational culture by using key approaches such as working with teams and choosing relevant and sensitive interventions.

Constant surveillance, monitoring, and auditing of the safety conditions of the workplace is essential. This includes monitoring individual employees in their immediate work environment. A health record can be kept on employees separate from their other employment records. This process often starts with an initial physical examination appropriate to the type of work that is going to be done. The physical examination helps ensure fitness for the job and provides a baseline for future comparison. Often, an employee's health and safety orientation and training follows, with issuance of proper personal safety protection. The OHN schedules routine safety meetings stressing health-related issues, such as safety gear and proper lifting techniques, on a proactive basis and conducts them thereafter on a need-to-know basis. An example of this is the introduction of a hazardous substance into the work area requiring more detailed information to ensure job safety. When injured employees do not return to work, the OHN may initiate or oversee a workers' compensation claim on behalf of the employee to ensure that the worker receives workers' compensation benefits.

OSHA Compliance

The need to comply with OSHA standards is often the starting point for initiation of safety measures. The U.S. Department of Labor collects data from employers about occupational injuries and illness across the country. The OSHA designs and distributes record-keeping forms called the *OSHA log*. The OHN is usually responsible for filling out the OSHA log. This injury log is a record of accidents and illness that occur within a given year at every workplace facility employing 10 or more people. It is used to report total injuries and illness annually to OSHA and must be posted at the work site.

Other Legal Responsibilities

In addition, the OHN works with employers on compliance with regulations and laws affecting workers and the workplace. These regulations and laws include state and federal regulations dictated by FMLA and the Health Insurance Portability and Accountability Act (HIPAA) (AAOHN, n.d.a). The OHN may be responsible for record-keeping and tracking employees who need to utilize FMLA, including securing the privacy of these records. According to FMLA, an employee is eligible to exercise his or her right after working a minimum of 12 months and at least 1,250 hours. In the case of serious illness affecting themselves or family members, when all conditions are met under this act, employees can leave work for up to 12 weeks and return to work without penalty. The OHN involved with managing FMLA for an organization sends out communication to all employees who apply. The nurse helps ensure that the worker(s) or physician(s) is in compliance with the regulation by submitting the proper paperwork to the employer.

The OHN is also responsible for the privacy and record-keeping of occupational health and safety information as it relates to individuals at the workplace. The HIPAA mandates that all medical information be held in confidence. One way to ensure privacy is to keep all health-related information in a separate, secured file and storage area other than the business or human resource files.

Researcher

As researchers, OHNs contribute to the future of the profession by identifying, analyzing, monitoring, measuring, and evaluating the effects of workplace exposures and hazards for workers and members of the community. They gather and use health and hazard data to select and implement preventive and control measures in a continual process. Examples include analysis of the effects of toxic chemical exposure, development of plans to prevent work-related accidents, and an analysis of groups, not just individual people, to detect patterns, trends, changes, and commonalities, as in pandemic situations (AAOHN, n.d.a; Dirksen, 2006).

The National Occupational Research Agenda (NORA) is a partnership program to stimulate innovative research and improved practices for safer, healthier workplaces. The program is directed toward the study of disease and injury, the work environment and the workforce, and the various research methods which are used to study occupational health. Released in 1996, NORA has become a research framework for NIOSH and the nation. Diverse parties collaborate to identify the most critical issues in workplace safety and health. NORA is composed of councils which focus on specific sectors of industry, such as construction, agriculture, or healthcare. The councils develop goals and strategies for the nation, and encourage partnerships to address the goals and promote improved workplace practices, all using open processes. The partners then work together to develop goals and objectives addressing these needs. All interested people have an opportunity to participate in this process through the CDC website.

Practice Point

The recognition of conditions that may harm the individual worker or members of the community is a crucial responsibility of the OHN.

IMPLEMENTING HEALTH PROMOTION IN THE WORKPLACE

It is imperative that management be involved in all stages of the health promotion effort. The company may give the OHN complete responsibility to create the initial vision and implement the plan, but constant communication with management is necessary to ensure that the plan is meeting the organization's expectations.

Balance theory is a systems approach that can be used by OHNs to help them organize a prevention model. The balance theory states that one element in the system influences other elements, having the potential to be positive or negative depending on the effect one part plays on another (Brunette, 2006). When using the balance theory, each workplace system is examined and categorized into five areas:

1. Organization
2. Tasks
3. Tools and technologies
4. Physical environment
5. People

The scenario in Case 2 illustrates the dynamic of the balance theory. The systems breakdown in this case involves operational and SM policy and procedure, machinery, and training of personnel. Identify several check-and-balance procedures that need to be in place to ensure a decreased health and safety risk for worker populations.

Developing a Team Approach

In creating a wellness team, it is essential to include key people, such as health professionals and interested parties in the workplace, who can help to identify company or organizational needs. Team members can contribute to the development of a plan of action based on national and local trends. They can also help with the distribution of surveys and answer questions.

Collecting data for presentation to management, such as projected healthcare costs based on current utilization trends, is one way to initiate a program. Insurance companies can provide reports of medical usage (utilization reviews) on the basis of diagnosis and/or categories of visits made to providers. The OHN may have the team review health insurance data; research national leading health indicators; or conduct interviews, workplace assessments, or on-site surveys to help determine the findings and outcome of the data.

Choosing Interventions

Interventions that are appropriate for a company or work site(s) through assessment of health promotion programs depend on the findings of an employee-needs assessment which is conducted by and for the organization. It is important that the team members who are involved know the purpose of the needs assessment prior to the actual method chosen, and the need for follow-up and future planning.

A good start for a small to midsize company is to conduct a needs assessment with a general health promotion questionnaire. The questionnaire or survey can ask employees basic lifestyle questions, such as number of hours worked each week. Consumption of alcohol, diet, and smoking, exercise activity level, hours of sleep, and existing medical coverage is an excellent place to begin collecting data. The OHN should also watch for workers who take a second job to earn extra money, which may lead to fatigue and injury on and off the job.

It is important for a team to know what percentage of the working population has access to medical care because health promotion efforts depend on available resources. Some employees have medical coverage provided by a spouse or significant other working at another company. Others simply cannot afford medical insurance, and they are often referred to as the working poor (Luhby, 2012; Shipler, 2004).

The passing of the Massachusetts healthcare reform act made the Commonwealth the first state in the United States to address the problem of inadequate health insurance for all citizens. It is mandated by law that healthcare coverage be offered by all employers to workers. The state requires submission of proof of purchase or coverage for health insurance for both employer and employees to avoid a fine. Employers need to show they offered healthcare insurance, and if an employee declines, the employer must have the worker submit proof of healthcare insurance to be ready to present to the state if necessary. Workers must be ready to pay a fine on their state income tax return if they do not show proof of healthcare insurance (MassResources, 2013).

Practice Point

A proactive prevention approach in occupational health incorporates the belief that there are no accidents but only events that were not noticed or managed correctly with proper intervention.

IMPLEMENTING A PROGRAM: EXAMPLE, SMOKING CESSATION

Step I

The OHN makes a presentation to management to support offering a smoking cessation program. It is important to state the method that will be used to obtain the data (e.g., using a survey, questionnaire, or by direct interview). The OHN and/or the team could present the number of employees (by percentage) who smoke and the number of employees who say they would participate in a smoking cessation program if offered.

Step II

To initiate the program, the OHN sends out a memo calling appointed team members to attend a meeting. The team conducts an information-gathering meeting to point out why a smoking cessation program is needed, based on current smoking behaviors in the company. This includes statistics shared about smoking behaviors and risk at the local, state, and national levels. It is best if the OHN is prepared with a meeting agenda and educational information to hand out to attendees for review.

Step III

The OHN and/or the team presents the following information to justify the cost involved with conducting a smoking cessation program. Statement of fact: It is documented that workplace smoking, and especially the secondhand smoke associated with it, causes death and long-term illness. Direct medical costs for employers and schools include the following:

- Increased absenteeism
- Higher cleaning costs
- Decreased productivity
- Higher insurance premiums (health, fire)
- Increased property damage resulting from tobacco use by smokers

Step IV

The OHN and/or the team should provide take-home information, such as a copy of U.S. Morbidity and Mortality Figures Related to Tobacco Use from the CDC Fact Sheet. It is also necessary to review handout material with the group for discussion.

Step V

The OHN and/or the team should review the economics of smoking. For example, each year, the United States spends nearly $170 billion on medical care to treat smoking-related disease in adults, according to the CDC (CDC, 2017). Together with absenteeism and regular smoke breaks, the annual cost is estimated to be $3,077 per worker. The OHN can present the number of smokers currently working in the company and multiply that number by the projected cost of $3,077 per worker a year. An estimated dollar figure would show that the cost to initiate a smoking cessation program justifies the investment.

The following is an example of the initiation of a smoking cessation program and how it might progress once it is approved by management. A realistic goal would be to reach and help 4% of the smoking population become nonsmokers by the end of year 1 of the program. With more education and incentives for employees, the program could similarly affect an additional 1% after 2 more years.

Items such as cost of a program and incentives may be part of the program for those who need more support to quit smoking. The program is best offered when most workers are interested and can attend it. Time of day is important. Ideally, program times are set up during lunch time or directly after work, with experts who know how to work with people who may wish to discontinue smoking.

The OHN and/or team may send follow-up letters to participants periodically to offer continued support and information, and to provide tips about diet and activities that support the employee's new nonsmoking behavior. Invitations to join activities, such as baseball, rowing, or bowling leagues to help people replace old behaviors may help. Finally, program planners should anticipate that there will be those who relapse, and they should provide reassurance for continuing with the program. It is necessary to establish a plan of action to support these workers who want to begin the process again.

Much of what the OHN does in health promotion is to support employees in their choice of behaviors that are more life-enhancing. In 2012, Truth Initiative (formerly Legacy) and AAOHN developed a partnership with two primary goals. First, Truth Initiative and AAOHN would develop a survey together that would assess such topics as the smoking behavior of its members, the availability of tobacco cessation resources to offer workers, and tobacco cessation training, among other smoking related topics. Second, Truth Initiative would offer BecomeAnEX.org, a free quit smoking program that helps adult smokers relearn life without cigarettes, to AAOHN members as a resource for themselves and for their workers (AAOHN, n.d.b). Creating an opportunity to affect people and the quality of their lives at the work site is a logical place to begin.

Student Reflection

After working several years in the hospital, I realized that many patients were there because of needless accidents and diseases that could be prevented. Knowing how devastating the consequences of acute and chronic diseases can be, I decided to focus on health promotion and prevention of disabilities in the community when I returned to the university. I really enjoyed my experience in a health promotion program in the workplace. It allowed me to apply both my nursing and previously acquired knowledge while learning something new.

The project required tracking, quantifying, and systematically measuring the outcome of a simple nursing intervention, monitoring the employees' blood pressure (BP). The key to the success of this program had to do with consistent follow-up, continued monitoring, and referral for medical treatment as needed.

The first step was to conduct a facility-wide volunteer BP screening. All employees who were being screened received a questionnaire that contained general history questions such as the following:

Have you had high BP in the past?
Are you currently under a doctor's care?
Are you being treated for high BP?
Are you taking medication?
Are you overweight?
Do you exercise?

Advertisements for the program appeared in the company newsletter. Employees who participated for 5 consecutive weeks of BP monitoring received stipends for use in the company cafeteria. Individuals who were interested signed up and had their BP taken systematically, department by department, in the building where they worked. Workers with extremely elevated BP received an immediate referral to a healthcare provider for follow-up care. Nurses asked workers with no known history of elevated BP, but who showed two out of three moderately elevated readings at week 3, to return periodically to continue their screenings. With the workers' consent, nurses also gathered weight information and further investigated diet and medical history. At this point, the nurses recommended that workers who continued to show consistent moderate elevations see their physician.

The process continued with workers who showed slight elevations while working on goals involving exercise and diet. This experience showed me that most workers respond well when given the education and the support associated with the BP screening and monitoring program. Throughout this project, I was able to track progress and demonstrate the potential to increase quality of life, reduce medical costs, and prevent further disease such as stroke, heart attack, and kidney disease. The workplace does indeed have a captive audience; when approached in the right manner, these workers are very interested in maintaining and pursuing their health.

EPIDEMIOLOGY AND OCCUPATIONAL HEALTH

The use of epidemiology as a tool for assessing the hazards of workers has a long and productive history. Ancient Egyptian documents told about the difficult life of workers, and other early historical publications addressed the hazards of working with heavy metals and mining. In the 17th century, the Italian physician Ramazzini outlined the health hazards of chemicals, dust, metals, repetitive or violent motions, odd postures, and other disease-causative agents encountered by workers in 52 occupations. The first physician to clearly recognize the relationship between healthy workers and economic productivity, Ramazzini is now considered the father of occupational medicine.

Occupational epidemiology today deals specifically with the study of distribution and determinants of states of health related to hazardous exposures and conditions found in the workplace. In other words, epidemiologic methods are applied to populations of workers. The nurse needs to explain trends and potential or real hazards, based on epidemiologic reports, to workers, managers, and community representatives (Lukes, 2007). The epidemiologic data, plus the documented need in the workplace, are the rationale for recommending health promotion programs.

Epidemiologic Surveillance

Health surveillance is an essential concept in occupational health. The need to carefully monitor both the employee and the work environment to detect any health risk and thereby be able to initiate health protective behaviors is critical. "A strong health surveillance program, implemented by the OHN or nurse manager, is an essential component of an employer's effort to promote workers' optimal health and safety, thus preserving the company's valuable human and financial resources" (AAOHN, 2015). Workplace health surveillance includes physical examinations and the tracking of injuries, illness, hazards, and exposures both in individual people and for groups of workers. Every industry should have monitoring procedures in place that are specific to the setting. For example, biomonitoring assesses the total body burden of a hazardous chemical in a worker through laboratory tests of body fluid specimens. The best practice is to use noninvasive procedures as much as possible.

Evidence for Practice

According to the CDC (2015a), occupational exposure to bloodborne pathogens from needlesticks and other sharps injuries is a serious problem, resulting in approximately 385,000 needlesticks and other sharps-related injuries to hospital-based healthcare personnel each year. Similar injuries occur in other healthcare settings, such as nursing homes, clinics, emergency care services, and private homes. Sharps injuries are primarily associated with occupational transmission of hepatitis B virus (HBV), hepatitis C virus (HCV), and human immunodeficiency virus (HIV), but they have also been implicated in the transmission of more than 20 other pathogens. In 2011, the CDC released surveillance data from 1981 to 2010 documenting 24 cases of acquired HIV among nurses. Table 25.4 shows 2015 Hepatitis C outbreaks in the United States, by setting.

The National Institute for Occupational Safety and Health (NIOSH) released two new modules that allow for the tracking of sharps incidents and blood and body fluid exposures among healthcare workers

TABLE 25.4 Hepatitis C Outbreaks by Setting—United States, 2015		
Setting	**State**	**Outbreak-Associated Infections**
Outpatient		
Prolotherapy clinic	California	5
Insulin infusion clinic	California	9
Pain management clinic	Michigan	2
Cardiology clinic	West Virginia	5
Hospital		
Hospital	Utah	>7
Hemodialysis		
Outpatient hemodialysis facility		
Outpatient hemodialysis facility	New Jersey	2
Outpatient hemodialysis facility	New Jersey	2
Outpatient hemodialysis facility	New Jersey	2
Outpatient hemodialysis facility	Pennsylvania	3
Outpatient hemodialysis facility	Pennsylvania	3
Outpatient hemodialysis facility	Pennsylvania	2
Outpatient hemodialysis facility	California	3

Source: Center for Disease Control (CDC). (2017). Viral hepatitis. Retrieved on September 16, 2017, from https://www.cdc.gov/hepatitis/statistics/2015surveillance/Table1.1.htm.

using a system uniquely available for U.S. healthcare facilities on a free, voluntary basis. The system, Occupational Health Safety Network (OHSN), collects existing injury data (e.g., date of injury or illness, location of incident, description of illness, days away from work, and other data collected in OSHA logs) among healthcare personnel to (1) help identify job titles at highest risk for injury in their own facility, (2) develop interventions for the safety and health of hospital staff, and (3) objectively measure impact over time (NIOSH, 2017).

Incidence

Workers often come to an OHN with symptoms. If there happens to be more than one worker from the same department with consistent symptoms and objective findings, the OHN may immediately begin to suspect that a cluster or cohort is forming. Clusters are aggregations of disease diagnoses collected from a specific population within a distinct period of time or space. Documenting the number of cases of an injury or disease is an important responsibility of the OHN (Eisen, Wegman, & O'Neill, 2006).

The calculation of incidence rates is a helpful tool in understanding the severity of a workplace problem. For example, the nurse can tally the number of workers whose scores on a hearing test change when compared with the previous year's results. The yearly occurrence rate of hearing loss among workers is determined by dividing the number of workers who have changes in their recorded hearing test(s) by the number of workers at risk during that year. If 56 of 1,000 employees have more difficulty hearing at certain frequencies this year than last, then the yearly incidence rate for hearing loss is 56 divided by 1,000, or 0.056%. It is 5.6% for the current year (see Chapter 7).

The OHN should calculate specific rates for population subgroups, often by age, sex, or exposure. For example, it may be beneficial to calculate an injury rate during several different activities. The OHN might find it helpful to calculate a rate for hearing loss among workers who perform a work-related activity such as operating loud machines in a specific department at the workplace (Lukes, 2007).

Prevalence

Prevalence reflects the total burden of the injury or illness that exists in the population—in this case, the workplace. It includes both new cases and existing cases. Using the example of hearing loss, the prevalence rate indicates the extent of hearing loss in the workplace. When hearing loss has occurred, it is imperative that people be protected through a hearing conservation program. In most cases, once the damage begins, the person without protective equipment or a transfer to a quieter environment is at greater risk for more hearing loss at an increasing rate. Prevalence rises over time if working conditions are not corrected (Lukes, 2007).

Ratios

Ratios can compare and involve groups of workers in settings. Hearing tests may be given to workers from different departments within the same facility, or to workers who do the same type of work in another facility or building in another state or country. This approach adds clarity when comparing the number of affected workers in an organization that employs workers located in various geographic locations. The ratio of workers who incurred the greatest hearing loss from the previous year may be compared by facility, department, or task. This can provide information about different groups and how noise, injury, or disease affects them over a specific period of time (Lukes, 2007).

Epidemiologic Studies

Two types of epidemiologic studies are common in investigating occupational health issues in the workplace: cohort and case-control studies. First, prospective, cohort epidemiologic studies investigate workers who have been exposed to a variety of chemical, biologic, or physical agents (see Table 25.1). The purpose of these follow-up studies is to determine whether the risk of adverse health outcomes is increased after the event. Second, epidemiologic studies may involve the evaluation of workers who have already experienced a common adverse health outcome. In this case, the outcome has already occurred, so the purpose of these case-control studies is to investigate, retrospectively, what agent or set of agents may explain their condition. Chapter 8 discusses these methods in more detail.

Ecologic studies are types of epidemiologic studies that compare the rates of exposures and diseases in different populations. Aggregate data on exposure and disease are gathered, rather than data pertaining to individuals. This could be data from a group of workers within an organization, facility, community, state, or nation. Average exposures and disease rates are compared between two groups in different locations during the same time (Eisen et al., 2006). Ecologic studies are the fastest and easiest of epidemiologic studies related to the OHN practice. These approaches study the relationships between variables when research or funds are limited.

Case 2 demonstrates that actions lead to an outcome and that actions further unfold in a sequence of related events. The OHN learns that at the time of the outbreak, one of the refrigerator units was about to be replaced because of higher-than-normal holding temperatures. Also, there had been a turnover of kitchen staff in the last few weeks. Apparently, the department was short on kitchen help on the day of the picnic, and there was no record of the daily temperatures required that morning.

Holding food at correct temperatures is essential to avoid food-borne illness. "Cooked food is safe only after it's been heated to a high enough temperature to kill harmful bacteria. Color and texture alone won't tell you whether your food is done" (U.S. Department of Health & Human Services [HHS], n.d.a). For hot food, this temperature must be 140°F (60°C). For cold food, this temperature must be 40°F (4°C) or colder. Keeping food within the recommended temperatures is necessary to prevent microbial growth (U.S. Department of Agriculture, 2013).

By calculating attack (incidence) rates associated with the various foods, the OHN determines that the sausage was contaminated. Most of the people who ate the sausage manifested symptoms of food poisoning, establishing the relationship between ingestion and sickness (Aschengrau & Seage, 2003; Lukes, 2007).

EMERGENCY PREPAREDNESS PLANNING AND DISASTER MANAGEMENT

As a member of the emergency planning committee in the workplace, the OHN contributes to the design and implementation of the emergency preparedness plan. The plan ensures a line of communication with emergency management teams. Having an emergency planning committee composed of representatives from all departments is the best way to establish emergency planning in business environments. Committee members meet on a regular basis and have access to all relevant health and safety information, so that they can make responsible, informed decisions. The committees annually review documentation and update the existing emergency plans. This includes all state and federal laws that apply to the facility and type of business operation (OSHA, 2010).

Components of an Emergency Preparedness Plan

The goals of an emergency plan are to anticipate emergencies and to establish clear reporting instructions for employees. The plan names key personnel who will assume necessary tasks. It establishes emergency escape routes, and procedures to identify workers and visitors with and without disabilities. The plan ensures that predesignated areas have been arranged and employees have participated in actual drills (OSHA, n.d.b).

The committee is responsible for conducting a vulnerability analysis best utilizing an all-hazards approach. Committee members review the types of emergencies that are likely to occur at the facility and what resources will be needed to respond. Major natural emergencies are fires, floods, hurricanes, tornadoes, earthquakes, and winter storms. Human-made or technologic events include fires, violence, bomb threats, transportation accidents, industrial accidents, civil disturbance, radiation, and unintentional or intentional release of chemicals or infectious organisms (bioterrorism) (Federal Emergency Management Agency [FEMA], 2013).

Next, the committee reviews existing internal resources such as personnel, security systems, sprinkler and alarm systems, transportation and heavy equipment, shelters (for providing shelter in place), and firefighting apparatus (OSHA, n.d.d, n.d.e). If a facility is located near a river or body of water, it is necessary to have a plan to deal with flooding, one of the most common hazards in the United States (FEMA 2014).

Key components of the emergency plan involve alarms, reporting, communication, evacuation, a system for counting the occupants, procedures for staff who do not immediately evacuate, and rescue and medical services. (A list of key personnel, training for all staff, drills, with an approach to conduct an assessment following an emergency evacuation plan, must identify escape routes that are clearly marked and meet the criteria within the key components.) It is essential that the plan discuss how workers and visitors with and without disabilities will be assisted through the evacuation routes and where they will reassemble for verification of safe evacuation (OSHA, n.d.c, n.d.d).

Critical Functions of the Plan

The OHN helps ensure that procedures are established for people who attend to critical functions in the facility and who do not leave the building immediately. Floor captains are responsible for making sure everyone gets out of the building. This includes people who administer first aid and those trained to use fire extinguishers (OSHA, n.d.c).

Internal rescue and medical services depend highly on the location of the facility and its proximity to police, fire, and external rescue services. According to the hazard communication standard (OSHA, n.d.a), employers must have personal protective equipment available for those who work with and around hazardous material and chemicals (Fig. 25.9). They also must have procedures to decontaminate workers who work with and around hazardous material

FIGURE 25.9 Personal protective equipment: personal fit testing for emergency preparedness.

and chemicals. Another important aspect of every plan is *shelter in place*. A shelter-in-place policy and procedure must be established for emergencies such as hurricanes, tornadoes, high winds, or chemical releases in buildings such as healthcare and correctional facilities. Having drills on a regular basis helps ensure that workers know what they are to do in an emergency. When alarms go off, evacuation needs to occur quickly and in an orderly manner. The intent of the drill is to reduce confusion and panic (OSHA, n.d.b, n.d.c). Chapter 20 discusses emergency preparedness in further detail.

A plan for resuming operations following an emergency is necessary. The OHN may conduct a needs assessment that identifies the immediate and ongoing needs of the staff and the organization following an emergency. It is essential that counseling services are available for employees who may suffer from symptoms of posttraumatic stress. The committee periodically evaluates and modifies the plan to update key personnel lists, emergency contacts, and telephone numbers. Floor plans, changes of department location, and ongoing work in the building should be kept current (OSHA, 2010, n.d.b).

NANOTECHNOLOGY AND OCCUPATIONAL SAFETY AND HEALTH

Nanotechnology is among the emerging technologies impacting healthcare today. The National Institute for Occupational Safety and Health (NIOSH) defines **nanotechnology** as the manipulation of matter on a near-atomic scale to produce new structures, materials, and devices, and is generally defined as engineered structures, devices, and systems. **Nanomaterials** (Fig. 25.10) are defined as those things that have a length scale between 1 and 100 nm. At this size, materials begin to exhibit unique properties that affect physical, chemical, and biologic behavior (NIOSH, n.d.)

Nanotechnology offers the promise of vast improvements in many sectors such as consumer products, energy, materials, manufacturing, and medicine. Figure 25.10 shows a novel nanomaterial, a bamboo-like structure of nitrogen-doped carbon nanotubes, that can be utilized in diagnosing and treating previously inaccessible tumors. Despite the promising offers, there are also concerns about potential health hazards to workers, the environment, and consumers. For example, "nano-sized particles may be more likely to reach the bloodstream and pass through the blood-brain barrier than larger particles of the same composition and thus may represent a unique health hazard" (Centers for Diseases Control and Prevention [CDC], 2015b). Furthermore, products containing nanoparticles such as antibacterial products utilizing nanoparticles of titanium dioxide (TiO_2) or silver, for example, are already being used and possibly affecting individuals handling them. "Some toxicological studies show that animals exposed to titanium dioxide (TiO_2) and carbon nanotubes (CNTs) have displayed pulmonary

FIGURE 25.10 Diagnosing and treating previously inaccessible tumors with novel hybrid nanomaterials. This image shows the bamboo-like structure of nitrogen-doped carbon nanotubes, 50 nm in diameter and 500 to 1000 nm in length, to which 10-nm spherical gold particles have been linked. This novel material can be traced in the body by using x-ray and heat from exposure to laser energy. This combination may allow surgeons to identify and treat tumors that are inaccessible to current surgical techniques. (*Source:* National Cancer Institute [2016]. Creator: Julia Chifman, PhD., and Ravi Nandan Singh, PhD. https://visualsonline.cancer.gov/details.cfm?imageid=10865.)

inflammation, and perhaps the most troubling finding is that CNTs can cause asbestos-like pathology in mice" (NIOSH, 2013). Workers within nanotechnology-related industries have the potential to be exposed to uniquely engineered materials with novel sizes, shapes, and physical and chemical properties. Occupational health risks associated with manufacturing and using nanomaterials are not yet clearly understood.

NIOSH is the federal agency that conducts research and makes recommendations to prevent work-related injuries, illnesses, and deaths. It is conducting an extensive and multi-faceted research program with partners to better understand the occupational health and safety implications of nanotechnology. NIOSH has issued recommendations for controlling worker exposures to engineered nanomaterials during the manufacture and industrial use of those materials. These recommendations are based on technologies now applied in the various industries that use nanomaterials, and on control methods that have been shown to be effective in reducing occupational exposures in other industries.

Healthy People 2020 addresses the benefits and potential environmental and health impact of nanotechnology. Although improvements in occupational safety and health surveillance are ongoing, there are several emerging areas in which national data systems are not yet available or merit further research. For example, there are recognized data gaps in understanding the safety and health effects of exposure to nanoparticles—the ultrafine, manipulated particles used in many industries (U.S. Department of Health & Human Services [HHS], n.d.b).

With over 1,000 nanomaterial-containing products ranging from cosmetics to medical products already on the market, it is essential that occupational safety and health implications are explored to ensure a safe and healthy work environment. OHNs may find themselves at the forefront of managing workers' exposures and illness related to nanomaterials. "Occupational health nurses should maintain a heightened sense of awareness regarding the presence of nanomaterials in the workplace, current safety strategies being used, as well as developments of nanoscience, about emerging safety issues and methods in order to properly advocate for safe working environments" (Goyette & Journaey, 2014).

KEY CONCEPTS

- The primary responsibility of the OHN is that of injury prevention and health promotion, including recognition of conditions that may harm the individual worker or the community.
- The occupational health nursing process begins with assessment of both the worker and the workplace.
- Disciplines that guide the occupational nurse in understanding the agent, host, and environment relationship are epidemiology, toxicology, industrial hygiene, and safety principles.
- Advocating for patients, clients, or groups is a continual process in occupational health nursing.
- The knowledge base generated through epidemiologic studies is used to identify and prevent injury and disease.
- The recognition of adverse conditions, and the initiation of proven practice interventions, supports individuals and groups in both their work and community environments.
- With good occupational health surveillance programs in place, it is possible to proactively identify employees at risk by tracking incidence and prevalence of injuries and illness and their causes.
- The nurse must have the autonomy and skills to take action and reduce possible exposure or harm to workers.
- An understanding of regulatory, legal, and economic functions and their relationship to business production, workers, and the community environment is an essential component of occupational health nursing practice.
- Occupational health nurses must be abreast of emerging technologies with the potential to impact nursing practice.

CRITICAL THINKING QUESTIONS

1. When the population's rate is unknown, the OHN may want to use a national or state rate to compare information that is being obtained at the work site. For example, if 10% of those who participate in a company's health screening indicate they are smokers, what generalizations, if any, can be made by the OHN about the smoking rate of the company's population if a smoking assessment has not been done? Does 10% represent the true percentage of smokers? Does the company have the same or higher smoking rate as the rest of the state (e.g., approximately 25%). What percentages of workers who smoke avoid health screening?

2. Choose an occupational setting and describe the process of risk assessment you would initiate in that setting.

3. Review Figures 25.1 to 25.3, as well as Table 25.3. What are some of the factors that contributed to the decline in rates of injury and illness at the workplace? What confounding factors might be present?

4. In Case 1, the OHN deduced possible substances (agents) to which workers could be exposed. The next steps are to determine how the substances are delivered to the workers (host) and to investigate the characteristics of the workplace which lead to transmission of the substances (environment). The OHN inquires about the heating, ventilation, and air conditioning (HVAC) system at the bank. One of the questions asked concerned the position of the air vents which deliver air into the office space, and its relationship with the renovation work. The OHN learns that neither an extra exhaust system was provided for the project nor was any provision made to deal with particulates of construction materials which may have been in the air. Use this information to develop an epidemiologic triangle that identifies the interactions between the harmful substances (agent), the workers (host), and the workplace (environment).

HEALTHY PEOPLE 2020 LEARNING ACTIVITY

Occupational Safety and Health

Healthy People 2020 provides a blueprint to identify nationwide health improvement priorities. This national consensus plan includes 42 topics, with a subset of 12 leading health indicators (LHIs) and over 1,200 objectives. It offers a framework for strategic planning to promote health improvement and achieve health equity through measurable objectives and deliberate actions. The *Healthy People 2020* website is dense with important information on the development, implementation, and progress of this national plan. Learning to navigate the website, to access the rich materials offered is vital to gain a deep understanding of the national health improvement priorities, specific objectives, and initiatives seeking to achieve the national goals and objectives.

Occupational Safety and Health is a topical area identified as a priority in *Healthy People 2020*. To learn more about this topic go to https://www.healthypeople.gov. Topics are listed alphabetically;

scroll down to "O" and click on Occupational Safety and Health to read about the topic. Then, click on the link for "Overview" to find the answers to the following questions:

1. What is the goal for this topic?
2. What are the 10 sectors focused by National Occupational Research Agenda (NORA)?
3. What are emerging issues in occupational safety and health?

Once you've answered those questions, click on the link for "Objectives" and then select one of the objectives. Analyze the data, looking specifically at any disparities, progress made, and thinking about continued barriers to achievement. Then, click on the link for "Resources and Interventions" and select *Occupational Safety and Health Resources*. Review the resources and interventions to explore evidence-based resources and consumer information related to occupational safety and health to address and prevent occupational injuries and/or illnesses.

REFERENCES

American Association of Occupational Health Nurses (AAOHN). (2007). Competencies in occupational and environmental health nursing. *American Association of Occupational Health Nurses*, 55(11), 442–447.

American Association of Occupational Health Nurses (AAOHN). (2012a). *Code of ethics*. Retrieved on August 29, 2017, from

http://www.aaohn.org/component/content/article/12-practice/10-code-of-ethics.html

American Association of Occupational Health Nurses (AAOHN). (2012b). *Delivery of occupational and environmental health services*. Retrieved on September 10, 2017 from http://aaohn.org/p/do/sd/topic=28&sid=1157

American Association of Occupational Health Nurses (AAOHN). (2015). *Occupational health surveillance.* Retrieved on September 3, 2017 from http://aaohn.org/d/do/40

American Association of Occupational Health Nurses (AAOHN). (n.d.a). *Careers: Profession of occupational and environmental health nursing.* Retrieved from on August 30, 2017, from http://www.aaohn.org/careers/profession-of-occupation-environmental-health-nursing

American Association of Occupational Health Nurses (AAOHN). (n.d.b). *Clinical practice.* Retrieved on September 2, 2017, from http://aaohn.org/page/clinical-practice

American Board of Occupational Health Nurses, Inc. (2012a). *Eligibility.* Retrieved on August 30, 2017, from http://www.abohn.org/eligibility.cfm

American Board of Occupational Health Nurses, Inc. (2012b). *Occupational health nursing 2011 practice analysis.* Retrieved on August 30, 2017, from https://www.abohn.org/sites/default/files/ABOHN%202011%20Practice%20Analysis%20Report.pdf

Aschengrau, A., & Seage, G. R., III. (2003). *Essentials of epidemiology in public health.* Sudbury, MA: Jones and Bartlett.

Benner, P. (1984). From novice to expert: Excellence and power in clinical nursing practice. Menlo Park, CA: Addison-Wesley.

Brunette, M. J. (2006). Safety. In B. S. Levy, D. H. Wegman, S. L. Baron, & R. K. Sokas (Eds.), *Occupational and environmental health: Recognizing and preventing disease and injury* (pp. 218–237). Philadelphia, PA: Lippincott Williams & Wilkins.

Centers for Disease Control and Prevention (CDC). (2013). *Infection control.* Retrieved on August 28, 2017, from https://www.cdc.gov/oralhealth/infectioncontrol/faq/latex.htm

Centers for Disease Control and Prevention (CDC). (2015a). *Sharps safety for healthcare settings.* Retrieved on September 19, 2017, from https://www.cdc.gov/sharpssafety/index.html

Center for Disease Control and Prevention (CDC). (2015b). *Feasibility of industry-wide studies of workers exposed to nano-tubes.* Retrieved on August 29, 2017, from https://www.cdc.gov/niosh/programs/manuf/noragoals/projects/927zeyg.html

Centers for Disease Control and Prevention (CDC). (2017). *Smoking and tobacco use.* Retrieved on September 3, 2017, from https://www.cdc.gov/tobacco/data_statistics/index.htm, https://www.cdc.gov/hepatitis/statistics/2015surveillance/Table1.1.htm

Dirksen, M. E. (2006). Occupational and environmental health nursing: An overview. In M. K. Salazar (Ed.). *Core curriculum for occupational & environmental health nursing* (3rd ed., pp. 3–34). St. Louis, MO: Saunders.

Eisen, E. A., Wegman, D. H., & O'Neill, M. S. (2006). Epidemiology. In B. S. Levy, D. H. Wegman, S. L. Baron, & R. K. Sokas (Eds.). *Occupational and environmental health: Recognizing and preventing disease and injury* (pp. 172–179). Philadelphia, PA: Lippincott Williams & Wilkins.

Federal Emergency Management Agency. (2013). *Incident command system.* Retrieved on August 27, 2017, from https://training.fema.gov/emiweb/downloads/is111_unit%204.pdf

Federal Emergency Management Agency. (2014). *How to prepare for a flood.* Retrieved August 27, 2017, from https://www.fema.gov/media-library-data/1409002852888-3c5d1f64f12d-f02aa801901cc7c311ca/how_to_prepare_flood_033014_508.pdf

Goyette, P., & Journeay, W. S. (2014). Nanotechnology and Occupational Health. *OOHNA Journal, 33*(1), 40–45.

Luhby, T. (2012). America's near poor: 30 million and struggling. *CNN Money.* Retrieved on August 30, 2017, from http://money.cnn.com/2012/10/24/news/economy/americans-poverty/index.html

Lukes, E. (2007). Epidemiology basics for occupational health nurses. *American Association of Occupational Health Nurses, 55*(1), 26–31.

MassResources. (2013). *Massachusetts health insurance requirements—Health Care Reform Act.* Retrieved on August 30, 2017, from http://www.massresources.org/health-reform

National Cancer Institute (2016). Diagnosing and Treating Previously Inaccessible Tumors with Novel Hybrid Nanomaterials. *Visuals Online.* Retrieved on August 17, 2017, https://visualsonline.cancer.gov/details.cfm?imageid=10865

National Institute for Occupational Safety and Health (NIOSH). (2008). NIOSH publication and products: Publication exposure to stress: Occupational hazards in hospitals. (NIOSH Publication Number 2008–136). Accessed August 29, 2017. Retrieved from http://www.cdc.gov/niosh/docs/2008-136

National Institute for Occupational Safety and Health (NIOSH). (n.d.). *Nanotechnology.* August 16, 2017, from https://www.cdc.gov/niosh/topics/nanotech/default.html

National Institute for Occupational Safety and Health (NIOSH). (2013). *Current strategies for engineering controls in nanomaterial production and downstream handling processes.* Cincinnati, OH: U.S. Department of Health and Human Services, Centers for Disease Control and Prevention, Publication No. 2014–102.

National Institute for Occupational Safety and Health (NIOSH). (2017). *Occupational Safety and Health Network Now Tracks Sharps Injuries and Blood and Body Fluid Exposures.* Retrieved on September 20, 2017 from https://www.cdc.gov/niosh/updates/upd-03-27-17.html

Occupational Safety and Health Administration (OSHA). (2010). Getting started–General preparedness and response. Retrieved on August 16, 2017, from http://www.osha.gov/SLTC/emergencypreparedness/gettingstarted.html

Occupational Safety and Health Administration (OSHA). (n.d.a). *Evacuation plans and procedures: Employee alarm systems.* Retrieved on August 16, 2017, from http://www.osha.gov/SLTC/etools/evacuation/alarms.html

Occupational Safety and Health Administration (OSHA). (n.d.b). *Hazard communication standard final rule.* Retrieved on August 16, 2017, from http://www.osha.gov/dsg/hazcom/HCSFactsheet.html

Occupational Safety and Health Administration (OSHA). (n.d.c). *Evacuation plans and procedures: Develop and implement an emergency action plan.* Retrieved on August 16, 2017, from http://www.osha.gov/SLTC/etools/evacuation/implementation.html

Occupational Safety and Health Administration (OSHA). (n.d.d). *Evacuation plans and procedures: Fire, rescue and medical services.* Retrieved on August 16, 2017, from http://www.osha.gov/SLTC/etools/evacuation/fire_med_service.html

Occupational Safety and Health Administration (OSHA). (n.d.e). *Evacuation plans and procedures: Maintenance, safeguards, and operational features for exit routes.* Retrieved on August 16, 2017, from http://www.osha.gov/SLTC/etools/evacuation/egress.html

Occupational Safety and Health Administration (OSHA). (n.d.f). *Guidance on preparing workplaces for an influenza pandemic.* Retrieved on August 16, 2017, from http://www.osha.gov/Publications/OSHA3327pandemic.pdf

Occupational Safety and Health Administration (OSHA). (2016). *Guidelines for preventing workplace violence for healthcare and social service workers.* Retrieved on September 13, 2017, from https://www.osha.gov/Publications/osha3148.pdf

O'Donnell, M. (2009). Definition of health promotion 2.0: Embracing passion, enhancing motivation, recognizing dynamic balance, and creating opportunities. *American Journal of Health Promotion, 24*(1), iv–iv. doi: http://dx.doi.org/10.4278/ajhp.24.1.iv

Peek-Asa, C., Casteel, C., Allareddy, V., Nocera, M., Goldmacher, S., OHagan, E., … Harrison, R. (2009). Workplace violence prevention programs in psychiatric units and facilities. *Archives of Psychiatric Nursing, 23*(2), 166–176.

Shipler, D. (2004). *The working poor: Invisible in America.* New York, NY: Alfred A. Knopf.

Thomason, D. A., & Lagowski, L. R. (2008). Sustaining a healthy work force in the 21st century; a model for collaborating through reciprocation. *Journal of American Association of Occupational Health Nursing, 56*(12), 503–513.

REFERENCES *(Continued)*

U.S. Department of Agriculture. (2013). *Food safety and inspection services: Regulations and policies.* Retrieved on August 18, 2017, from http://www.fsis.usda.gov/Regulations_&_Policies/index.asp

U.S. Department of Health & Human Services. FoodSafety.gov. (n.d.a). *Cook to the right temperature.* Retrieve on September, 3, 2017 from https://www.foodsafety.gov/keep/basics/cook/index.html

U.S. Department of Health and Human Services. Office of Disease Prevention and Health Promotion. (n.d.b). *Healthy People 2020.* Washington, DC. Retrieved on August 12, 2017, from https://www.healthypeople.gov/2020/topics-objectives/topic/occupational-safety-and-health

U.S. Department of Labor, Bureau of Labor Statistics. (2016a). *Incidence rates of non-fatal occupational injuries and illnesses by industry and case types, 2015.* Retrieved on August 18, 2017, from https://www.bls.gov/opub/ted/2015/75-percent-of-occupational-injuries-in-2014-occurred-in-service-providing-industries.htm

U.S. Department of Labor, Bureau of Labor Statistics. (2016b). *Economic news release: Occupational injuries and illnesses news release.* Retrieved on August 18, 2017, from http://www.bls.gov/news.release/osh.htm

U.S. Department of Labor, Bureau of Labor Statistics. *National census of fatal occupational injuries in 2015.* (2016c). Retrieved on August 18, 2017, from https://www.bls.gov/news.release/archives/cfoi_12162016.pdf

U.S. Department of Labor, Bureau of Labor Statistics. (2017). *Economic news release: Occupational injuries and illnesses news release.* Retrieved on September 4, 2017, from https://www.bls.gov/news.release/pdf/empsit.pdf

U.S. Environmental Protection Agency. (2012a). *An introduction to indoor air quality.* Retrieved on August 18, 2017, from http://www.epa.gov/iaq/voc.html

World Health Organization. (2001). *The role of the occupational health nurse in workplace health management.* Retrieved on August 28, 2017, from http://www.who.int/occupational_health/regions/en/oeheurnursing.pdf

Zichello, C., & Sheridan, J. (2008). Occupational health nurses and workers' compensation insurance programs. *Journal of the American Association of Occupational Health Nurses, 56*(11), 455–458.

WEB RESOURCES

Please visit thePoint® for up-to-date web resources on this topic.

Index

Note: Page numbers followed by b, f, or t indicate text in boxes, figures, or tables, respectively.